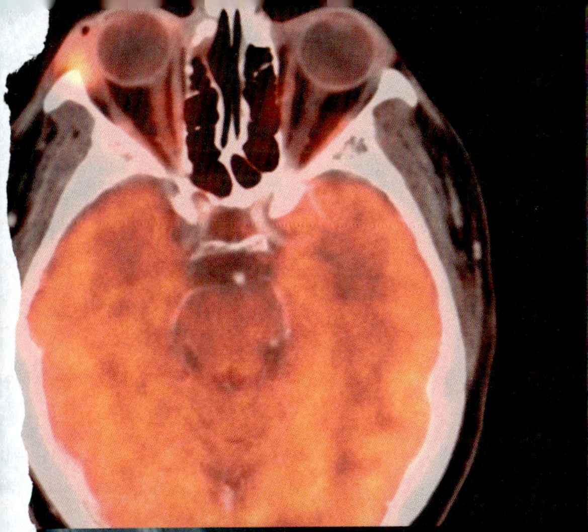
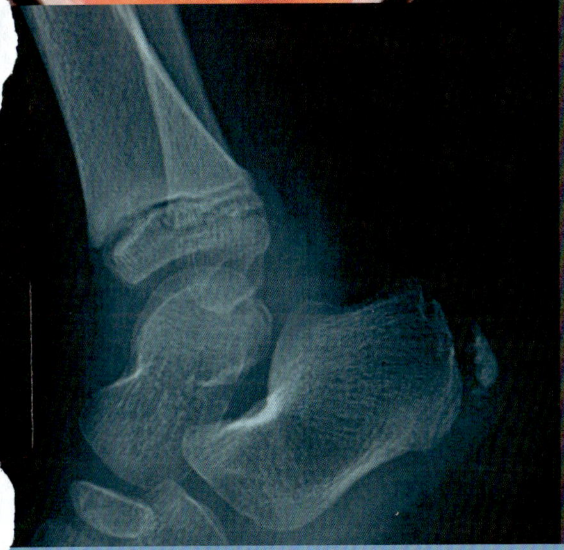
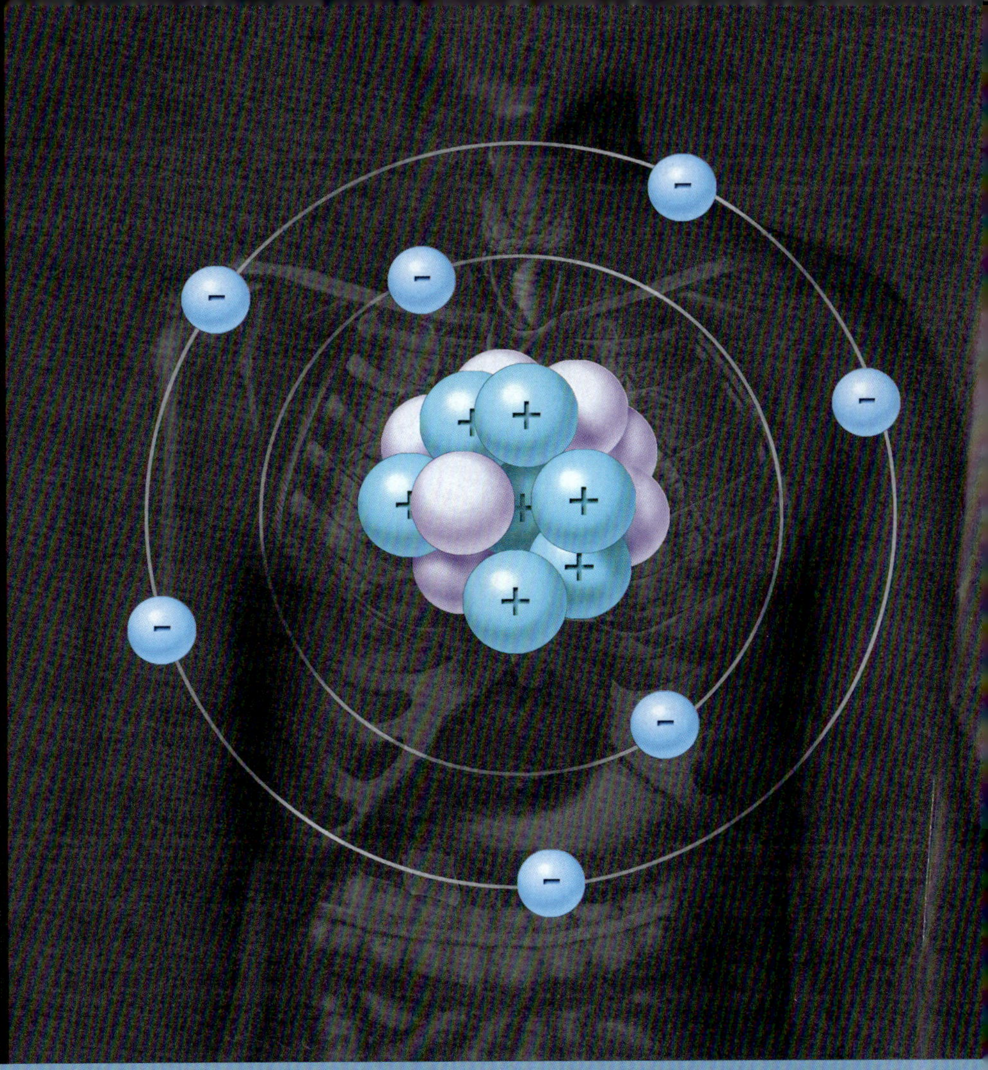

Diagnostic Imaging

Nuclear Medicine

SECOND EDITION

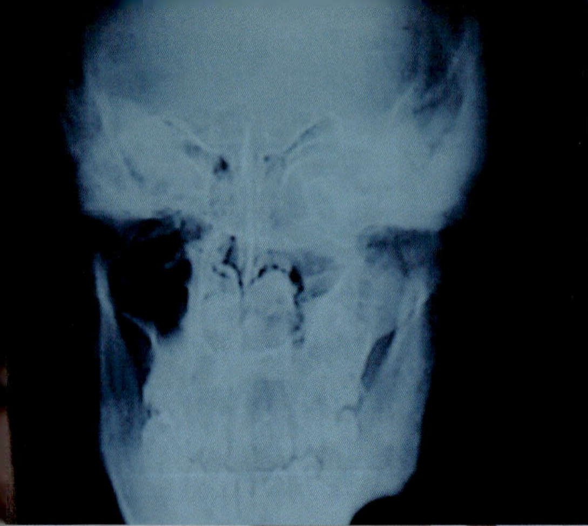

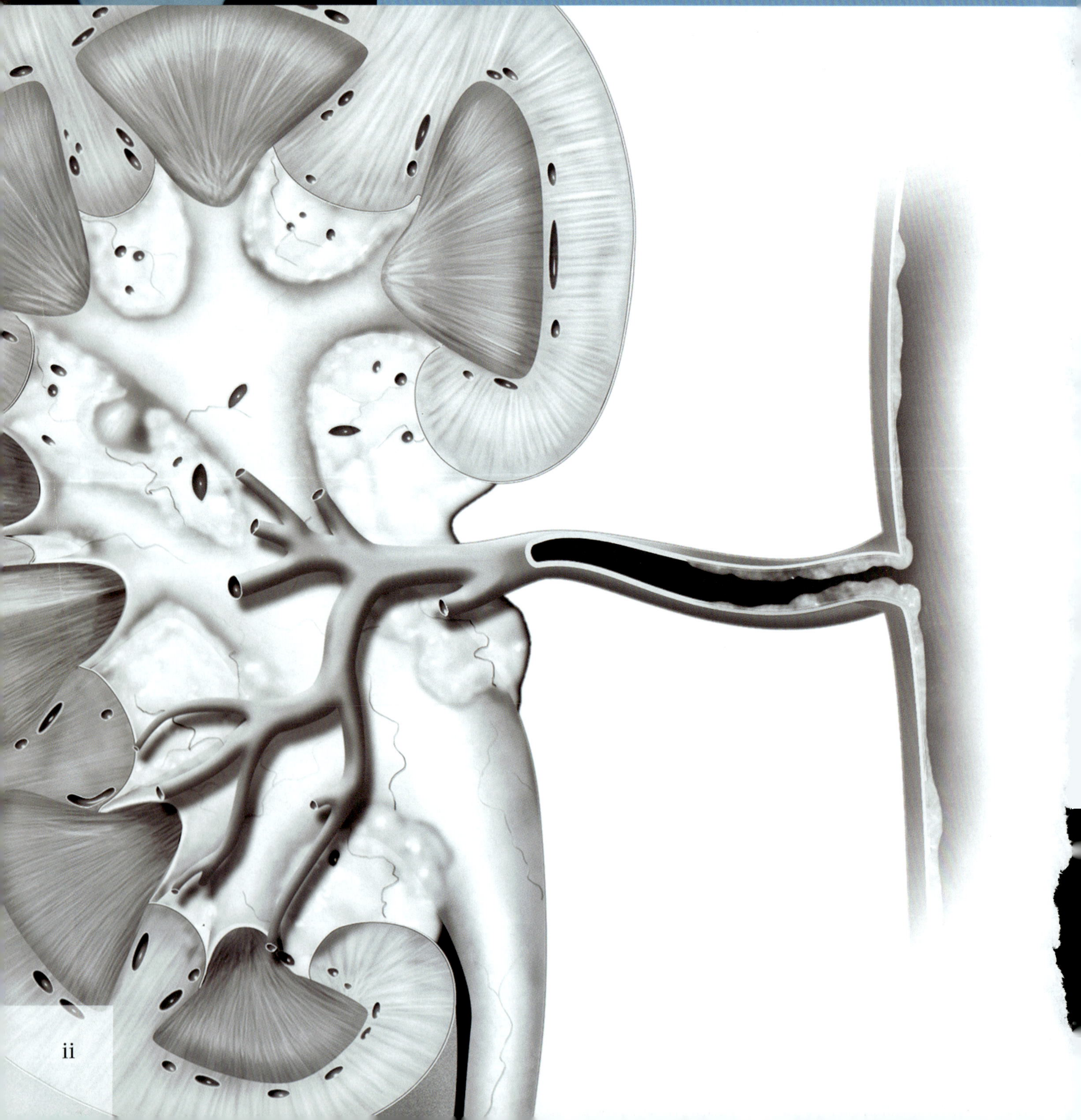

Diagnostic Imaging

Nuclear Medicine

SECOND EDITION

Paige Bennett, MD

Associate Professor
Nuclear Medicine and Molecular Imaging
Department of Radiology
Wake Forest School of Medicine
Winston-Salem, North Carolina

Umesh D. Oza, MD

Diagnostic Radiology Residency Program Director
Baylor University Medical Center at Dallas
Clinical Associate Professor
Texas A&M Health Science Center College of Medicine
College Station, Texas

Andrew T. Trout, MD

Assistant Professor of Radiology and Pediatrics
Department of Radiology
Cincinnati Children's Hospital Medical Center
Cincinnati, Ohio

Akiva Mintz, MD, PhD, MHA, CFA

Vice Chair of Finance, Department of Radiology
Section Head, Nuclear Medicine and Molecular Imaging
Department of Radiology and Neurosurgery
Leader, Translational Imaging Program
Assistant Director, Wake Forest Clinical & Translational Science Institute (CTSI)
Wake Forest School of Medicine
Winston-Salem, North Carolina

ELSEVIER

1600 John F. Kennedy Blvd.
Ste 1800
Philadelphia, PA 19103-2899

DIAGNOSTIC IMAGING: NUCLEAR MEDICINE, SECOND EDITION ISBN: 978-0-323-37753-9

Publisher Cataloging-in-Publication Data

Diagnostic imaging. Nuclear medicine / [edited by] Paige Bennett and Umesh D. Oza.
2nd edition.
pages ; cm
Nuclear medicine
Includes bibliographical references and index.
ISBN 978-0-323-37753-9 (hardback)
1. Diagnostic imaging--Handbooks, manuals, etc. 2. Nuclear medicine--Handbooks, manuals, etc.
I. Bennett, Paige. II. Oza, Umesh D. III. Title: Nuclear medicine.
[DNLM: 1. Diagnostic Imaging--methods--Atlases. 2. Nuclear Medicine--methods--Atlases.
3. Radiopharmaceuticals--Atlases. WN 39]
RC78.7.D53 D5282 2015
616.07/57--dc23

International Standard Book Number: 978-0-323-37753-9

Cover Designer: Tom M. Olson, BA
Cover Art: Richard Coombs, MS

Printed in Canada by Friesens, Altona, Manitoba, Canada

Last digit is the print number: 9 8 7 6 5 4 3 2 1

Dedications

This book is dedicated to my family.
To Diane and Ted Bennett, who love me the most.
To Betsy, Sidney, and Lee Andrew Clark, the loves of my life.
To my extended family of friends, Dr. Kathryn Morton, Cecilia Vargas Ortega.
Nothing matters without all of you.
Thank you to everyone who works with Amirsys: Your professionalism, leadership, and vision created the Diagnostic Imaging series, of which we are all proud to be a part.
Arthur Gelsinger and Dr. Umesh Oza: You made this endeavor fun. Double thanks.

PB

While we have laboriously poured heart, soul, and spirit into this textbook to impart the leading edge of nuclear medical knowledge to the next generation, there has been an equally and painstaking devotion paid to us by loved ones and mentors that have dedicated time, wisdom, guidance, and advice that cannot, and should not, go unrecognized. To my beautiful wife, Komel, thank you for your strength, guidance, and unwavering resolve. To my children, Quaid and Willa, you are my driving force. I want for you what you have given me — courage to strive for better, enjoy life to the absolute fullest, and run with wild abandon. To my loving parents, Dhruv and Surekha, thank you for your lifelong sacrifice, instilling discipline and confidence and single-minded focus raising three successful children. To Rishi and Veena, thank you for your unconditional love and steadfast support. A project of this magnitude reflects the hard efforts of many underrecognized people. I extend my deepest gratitude to all of you — thank you!

UDO

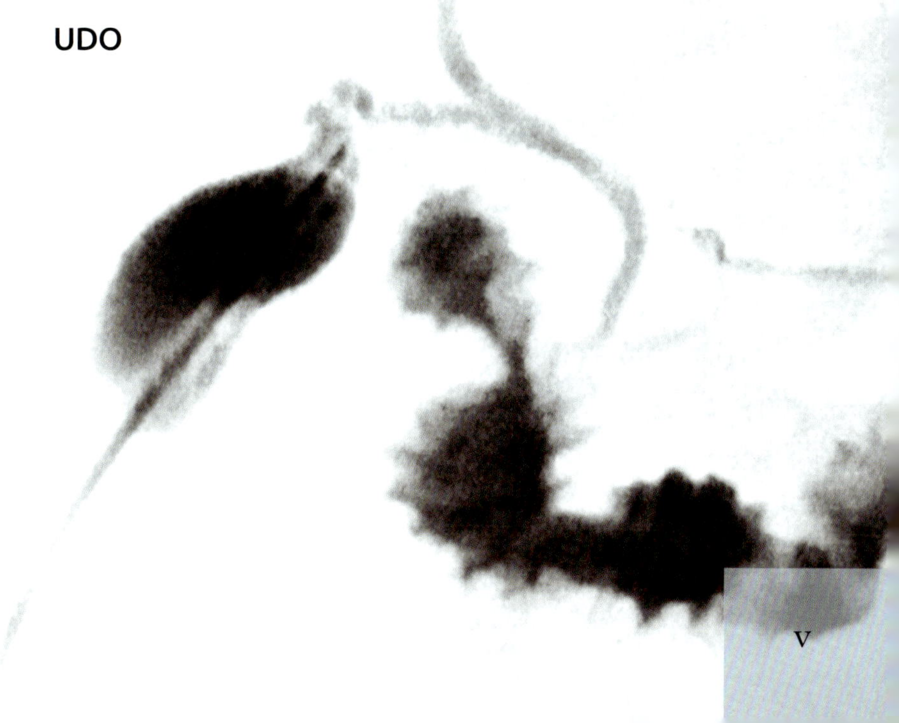

Contributing Authors

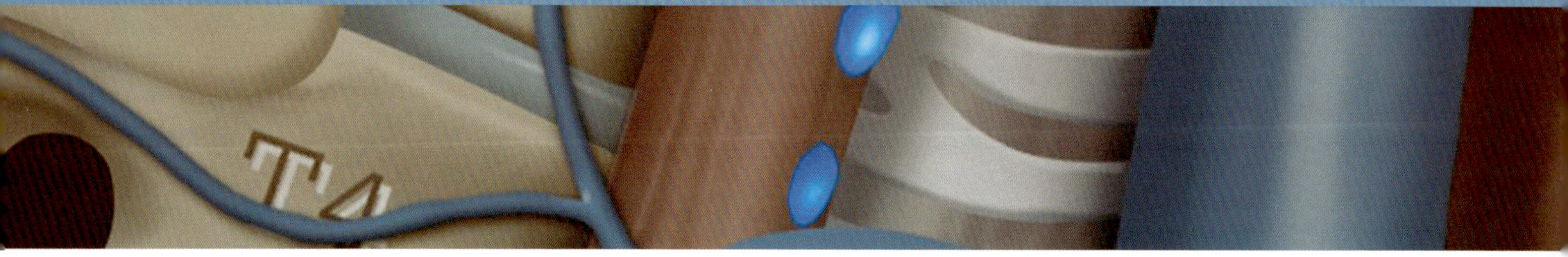

Angela P. Bruner, PhD, DABR
Director, Radiation Safety Officer, Medical Physicist
Radiation Safety & Medical Physics
Baylor Scott & White Health - North Texas
Dallas, Texas

Hollins Clark, MD
Associate Professor
Department of Radiology
Wake Forest School of Medicine
Winston-Salem, North Carolina

Pushpender Gupta, MBBS
Assistant Professor
Department of Radiology
Wake Forest School of Medicine
Winston-Salem, North Carolina

John M. Holbert, MD, FACR
Professor of Diagnostic Radiology
Department of Radiology
Wake Forest School of Medicine
Winston-Salem, North Carolina

Brian Kouri, MD
Associate Professor
Department of Radiology
Wake Forest School of Medicine
Winston-Salem, North Carolina

Shane C. Masters, MD, PhD
Assistant Professor
Department of Radiology
Wake Forest School of Medicine
Winston-Salem, North Carolina

Anita Thomas, MD
Associate Professor
Department of Radiology
Wake Forest School of Medicine
Winston-Salem, North Carolina

Christopher T. Whitlow, MD, PhD, MHA
Section Head, Neuroradiology
Associate Professor
Department of Radiology
Wake Forest School of Medicine
Winston-Salem, North Carolina

Matthew Bennett, MD
Department of Radiology
Wake Forest Baptist Medical Center
Winston-Salem, North Carolina

Todd Michael Danziger, MD
Department of Radiology
Wake Forest Baptist Medical Center
Winston-Salem, North Carolina

James Patrick Davidson, MD
Department of Radiology
Wake Forest Baptist Medical Center
Winston-Salem, North Carolina

Trevor Downing, MD
Department of Radiology
Wake Forest Baptist Medical Center
Winston-Salem, North Carolina

Christopher R. McAdams, MD
Department of Radiology
Wake Forest Baptist Medical Center
Winston-Salem, North Carolina

Amie M. McPherson, MD
Department of Radiology
Wake Forest Baptist Medical Center
Winston-Salem, North Carolina

Virginia Barnes Planz, MD
Department of Radiology
Wake Forest Baptist Medical Center
Winston-Salem, North Carolina

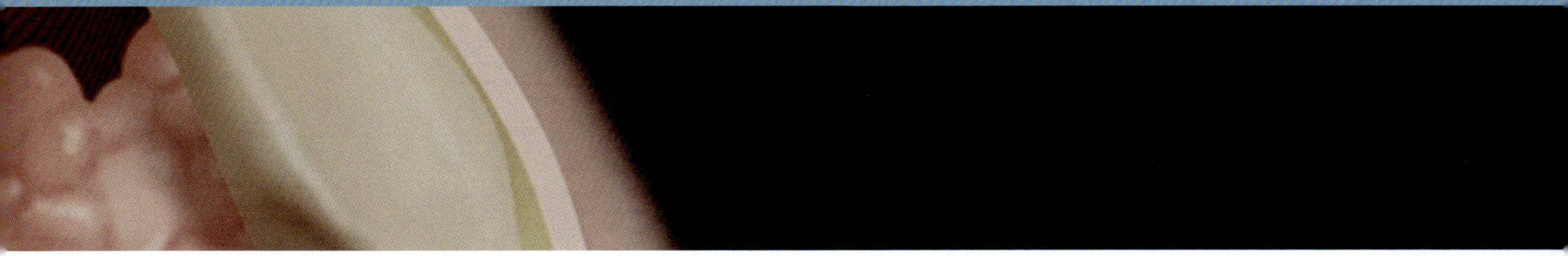

Colin Segovis, MD, PhD
Department of Radiology
Wake Forest Baptist Medical Center
Winston-Salem, North Carolina

Valerie E. Stine, MD
Department of Radiology
Wake Forest Baptist Medical Center
Winston-Salem, North Carolina

Pavani Thotakura, MD
Department of Radiology
Wake Forest Baptist Medical Center
Winston-Salem, North Carolina

Paula Vergara-Wentland, MD
Department of Radiology
Wake Forest Baptist Medical Center
Winston-Salem, North Carolina

Bimal Vyas, MD, MS
Department of Radiology
Wake Forest Baptist Medical Center
Winston-Salem, North Carolina

Amanda Jo Lott Marcellino, MD
Department of Otolaryngology
Wake Forest Baptist Medical Center
Winston-Salem, North Carolina

Ashley C. Mays, MD
Department of Otolaryngology
Wake Forest Baptist Medical Center
Winston-Salem, North Carolina

T. Alex McKnight, MD
Department of Otolaryngology
Wake Forest Baptist Medical Center
Winston-Salem, North Carolina

Kelli Y. Ha, MD
Department of Radiology, Breast Imaging
Baylor University Medical Center
Dallas, Texas

Tejaswini Vasamsetty, MD
Research Assistant
Department of Radiology
Wake Forest School of Medicine
Winston-Salem, North Carolina

John Bailey, MD
Wake Forest School of Medicine
Winston-Salem, North Carolina

Aidan Burke, MD
Wake Forest School of Medicine
Winston-Salem, North Carolina

Daniel G. Hampton, MD
Wake Forest School of Medicine
Winston-Salem, North Carolina

Katarina Kesty, MD, MBA
Wake Forest School of Medicine
Winston-Salem, North Carolina

Zachary Allen Lindsey, MD
Wake Forest School of Medicine
Winston-Salem, North Carolina

Charlotte Myers, MD
Wake Forest School of Medicine
Winston-Salem, North Carolina

Bryan J. Neth, BS
Wake Forest School of Medicine
Winston-Salem, North Carolina

Brad Perry, MD
Wake Forest School of Medicine
Winston-Salem, North Carolina

G. Lance White, MD
Wake Forest School of Medicine
Winston-Salem, North Carolina

Preface

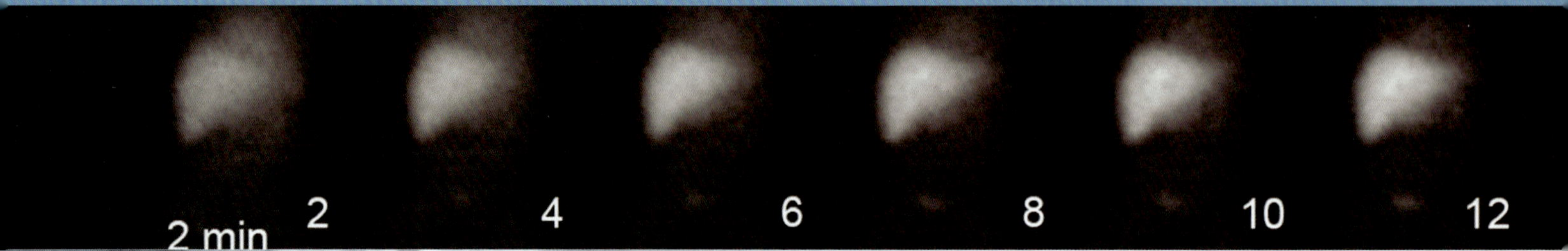

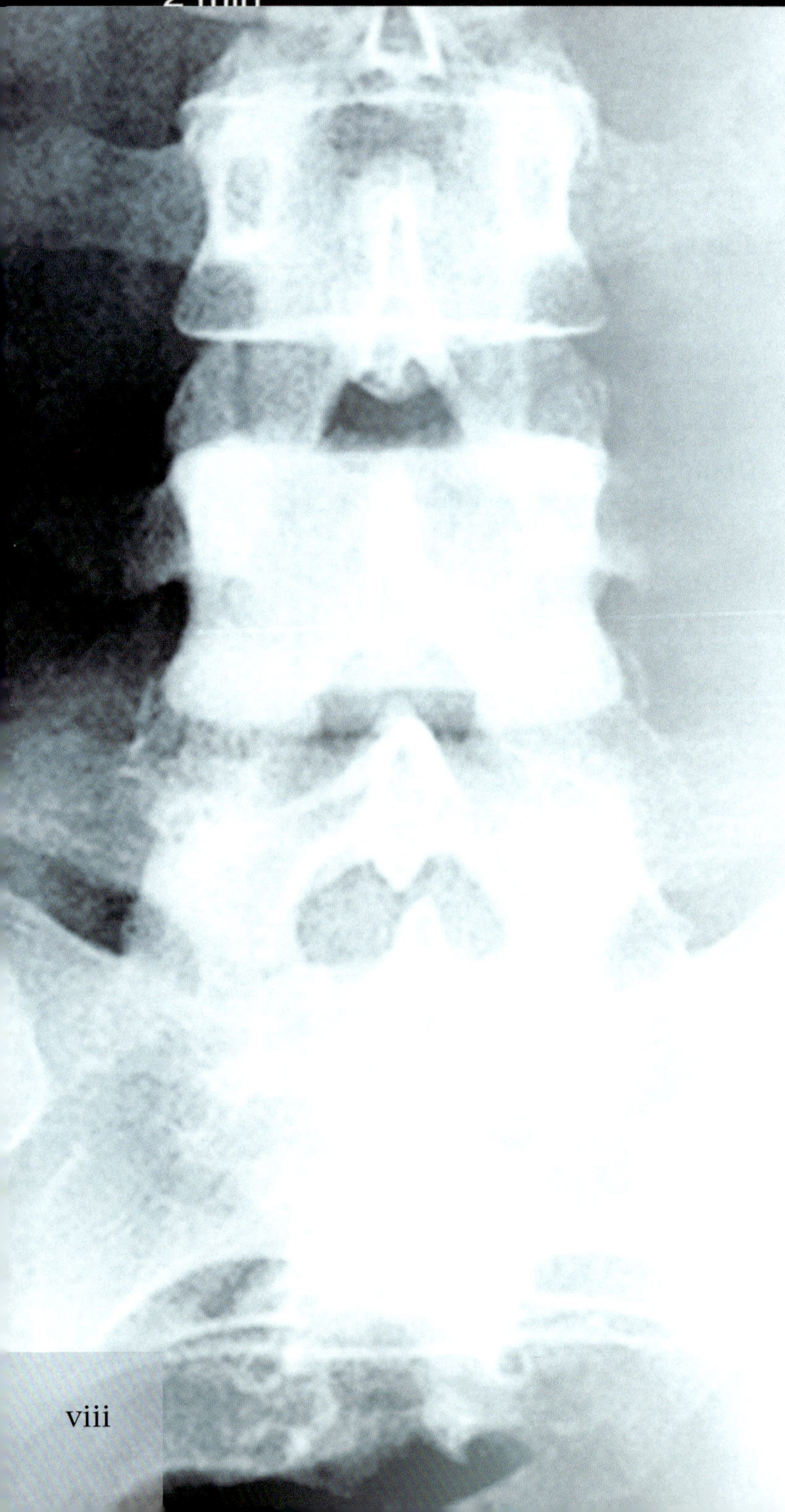

Since the publication of the first edition of *Diagnostic Imaging: Nuclear Medicine*, the world of nuclear medicine and molecular imaging has continued to rapidly evolve. PET/CT remains the most substantial advancement in the field in recent times, with PET/CT volumes continuing to climb. New PET/CT radiopharmaceuticals and time-of-flight technology have both become more mainstream. Astounding leaps have occurred in equipment such as with the incredible integrated PET/MR systems. Awareness of radiation dose to the patient has moved to the forefront of consciousness, and advances in software and detector equipment have helped dramatically lower radiation exposure. At the same time, many new therapies, radiotracers, and techniques push the boundaries of what is possible, showing the enduring importance of nuclear medicine in patient care.

The second edition reflects the changes seen in practice. Careful attention has been paid to the recent revisions in radioiodine therapy guidelines for cancer and hyperthyroidism. New chapters have been added, which cover the use of Ra-223 for the treatment of painful prostate cancer bone metastases and the use of I-123 ioflupane (DaTscan) for the diagnosis of parkinsonian syndromes. F-18 NaF PET/CT assessment for the bones is now thoroughly covered, including its indication for nonaccidental trauma in children. In addition, many of the popular quick reference tables have been added. These include easy-to-use tables in the completely updated pulmonary embolism chapter and differential diagnosis tables such as in the musculoskeletal chapters.

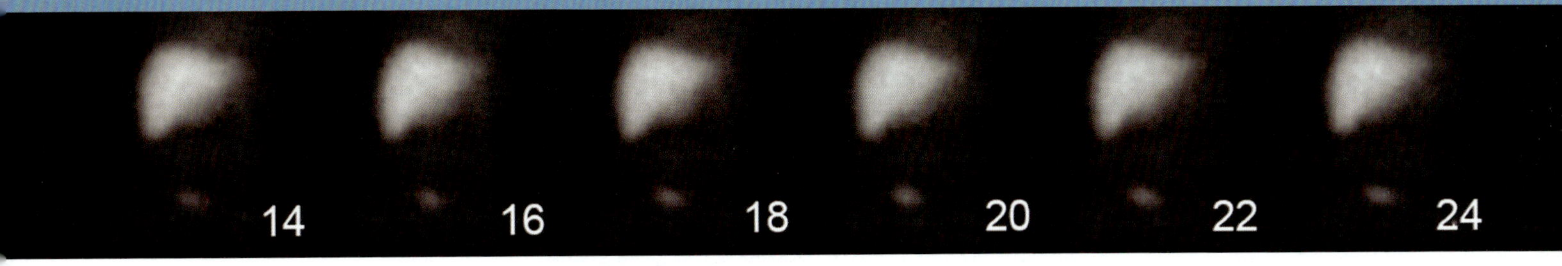

In order to make this text a more complete reference and study tool, new chapters have been dedicated to nuclear medicine physics and Nuclear Regulatory Commission (NRC) guidelines. In fact, all study guide topics listed for the American Board of Radiology board exam are fully covered. A radiopharmaceutical table now provides a critical overview, covering key parameters of the important agents currently in use. While these items are especially valuable for the physician preparing to undergo recertification or certification, they are also useful for the practitioner in the field.

Certainly, this edition continues to build on the successful philosophy of its predecessor. The topic-based format allows the reader to rapidly approach cases from the most practical standpoint. Incredible images illustrate the spectrum of disease, highlight potential pitfalls in the differential diagnosis, and outline critical anatomy. Each section contains multiple new images, maintaining the high standards expected from the *Diagnositc Imaging* series. Bulleted text describes all the details needed, from the level of the novice to that of the expert, but keeps the focus of each section sharp. Expanded sections have been added to better cover image interpretation and exam protocol advice, making this edition even more useful as a reference in the clinic.

We are especially proud of the team assembled to compile this text. They are a group of dedicated nuclear medicine physicians and nuclear radiologists who are also gifted teachers. Under the leadership of Dr. Paige Bennett (formerly Clark) of Wake Forest University Health Sciences and Dr. Umesh Oza of Baylor University, the text continues to be carefully edited and thoughtfully developed. In short, *Diagnostic Imaging: Nuclear Medicine, Second Edition*, continues to be a must-have for any practioner in the field.

Janis Petrik O'Malley, MD

Professor of Radiology
Director, Division of Molecular Imaging and Therapeutics
University of Alabama at Birmingham School of Medicine
Birmingham, Alabama

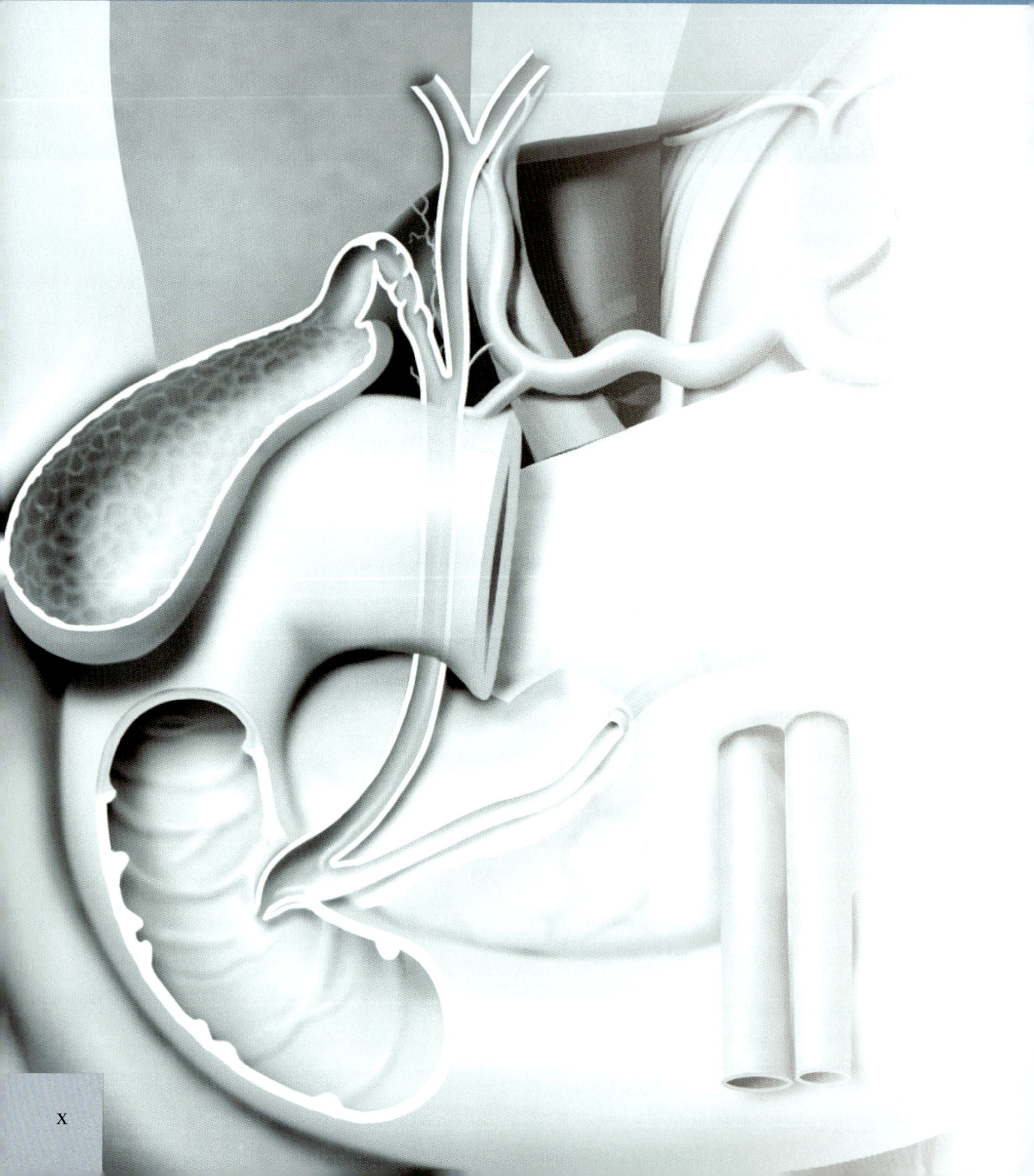

Acknowledgements

Text Editors
Nina I. Bennett, BA
Sarah J. Connor, BA
Tricia L. Cannon, BA
Terry W. Ferrell, MS
Lisa A. Gervais, BS
Karen E. Concannon, MA, PhD

Image Editors
Jeffrey J. Marmorstone, BS
Lisa A. M. Steadman, BS

Medical Editors
Philippe A. Tirman, MD
Whitney J. Morgan, MD

Illustrations
Richard Coombs, MS
Lane R. Bennion, MS
Laura C. Sesto, MA

Art Direction and Design
Tom M. Olson, BA
Laura C. Sesto, MA

Lead Editor
Arthur G. Gelsinger, MA

Production Coordinators
Angela M. G. Terry, BA
Rebecca L. Hutchinson, BA

ELSEVIER

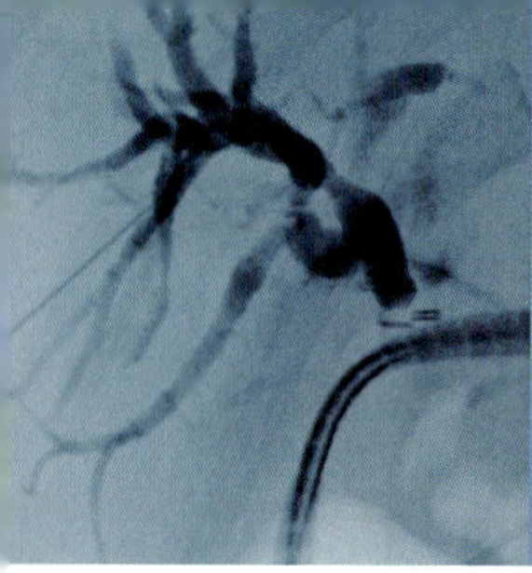

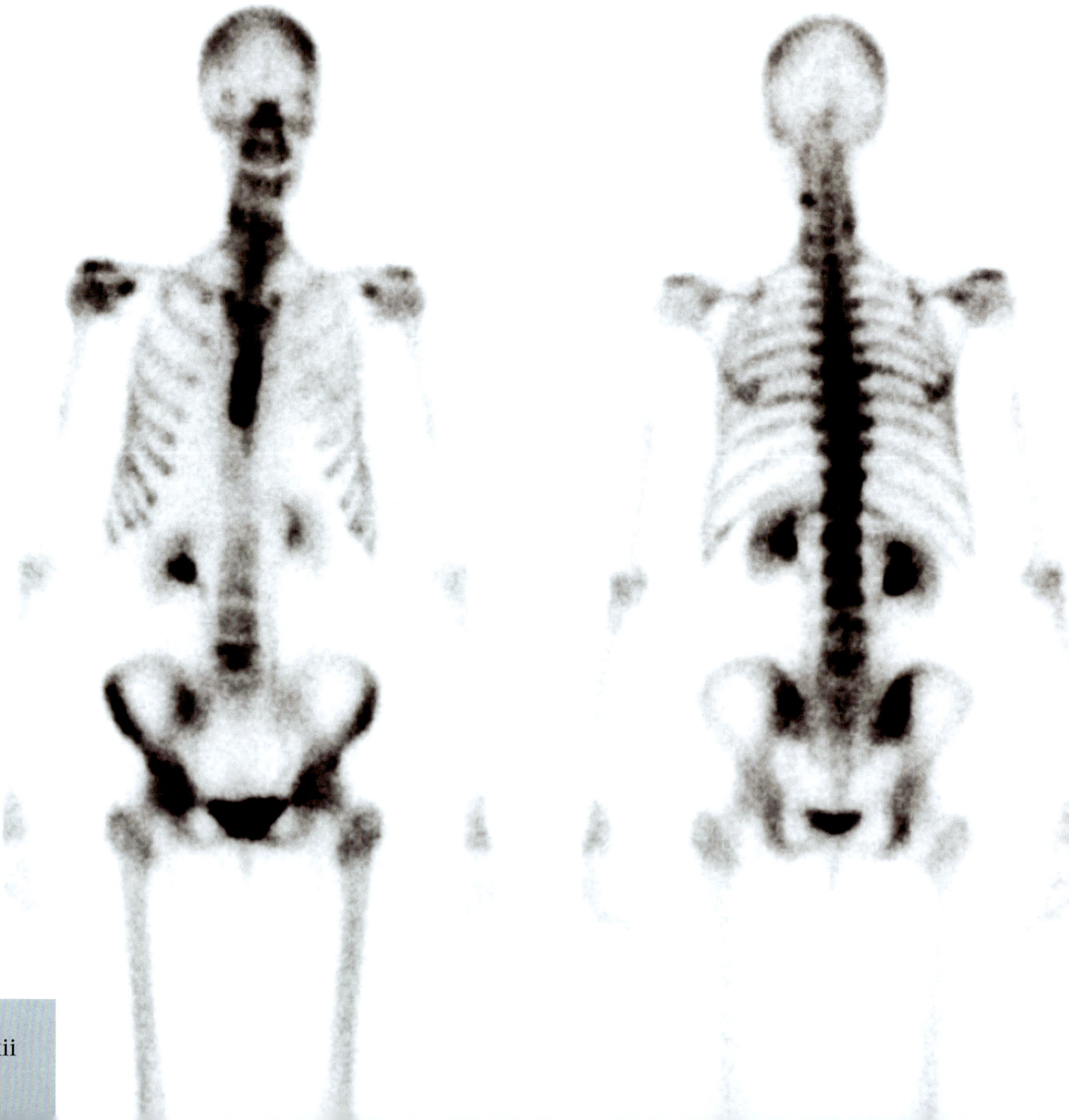

Sections

TABLE OF CONTENTS

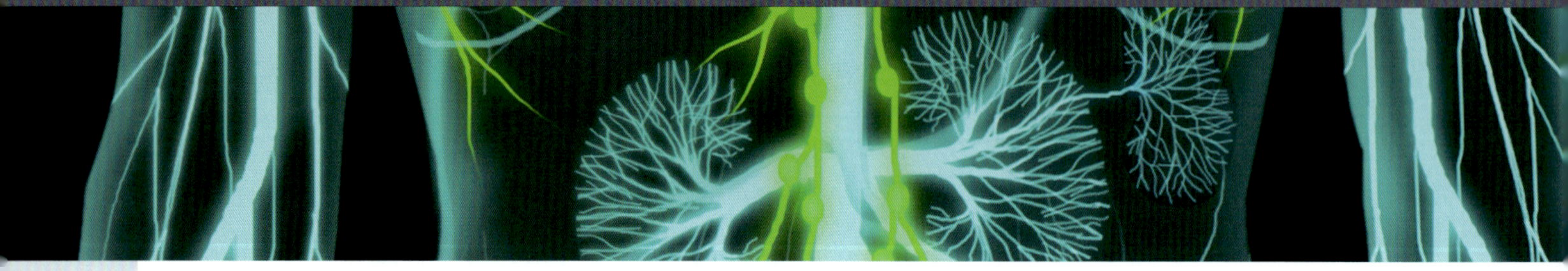

TABLE OF CONTENTS

TABLE OF CONTENTS

TABLE OF CONTENTS

TABLE OF CONTENTS

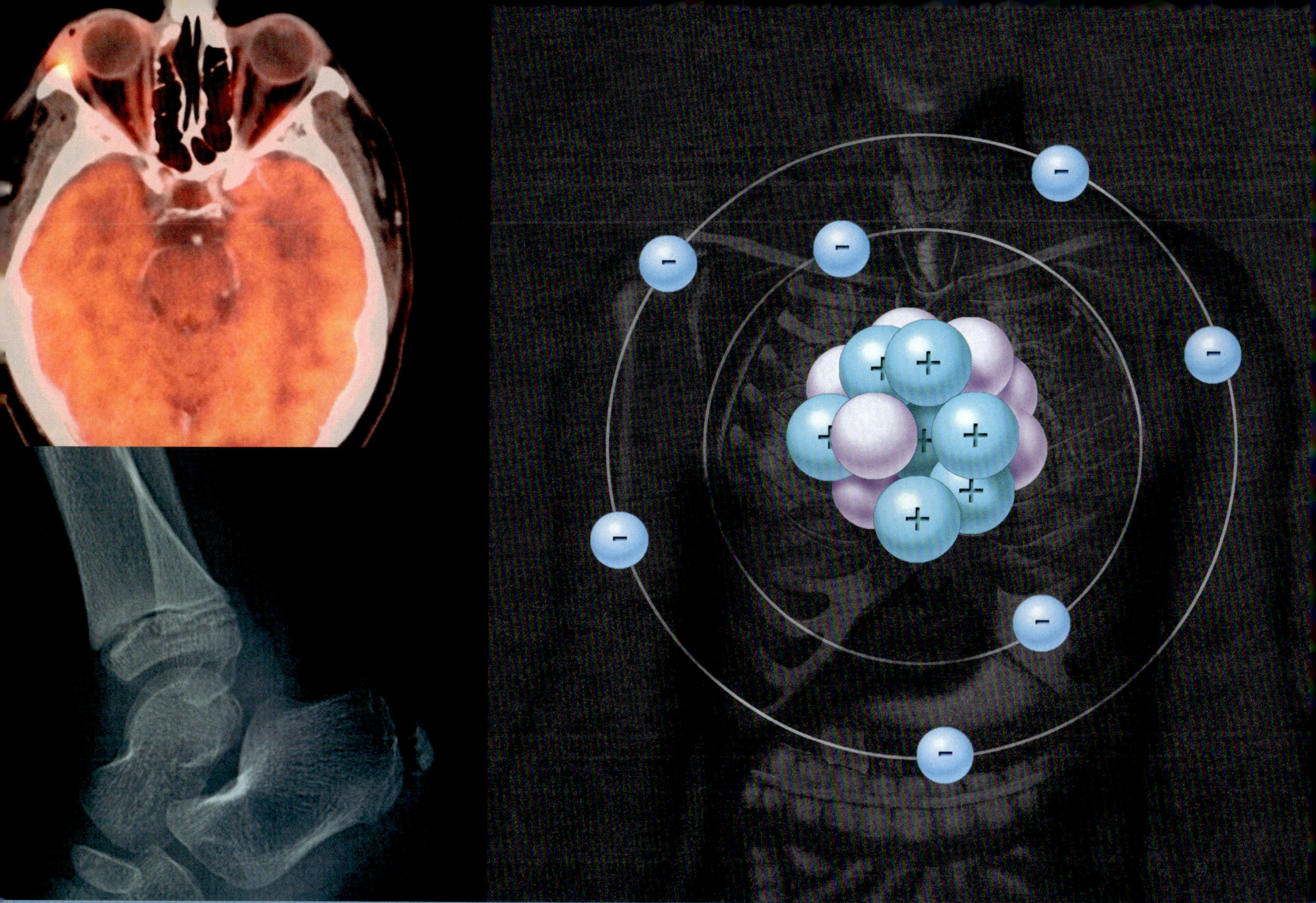

Diagnostic Imaging

Nuclear Medicine

SECOND EDITION

SECTION 1
Cardiac

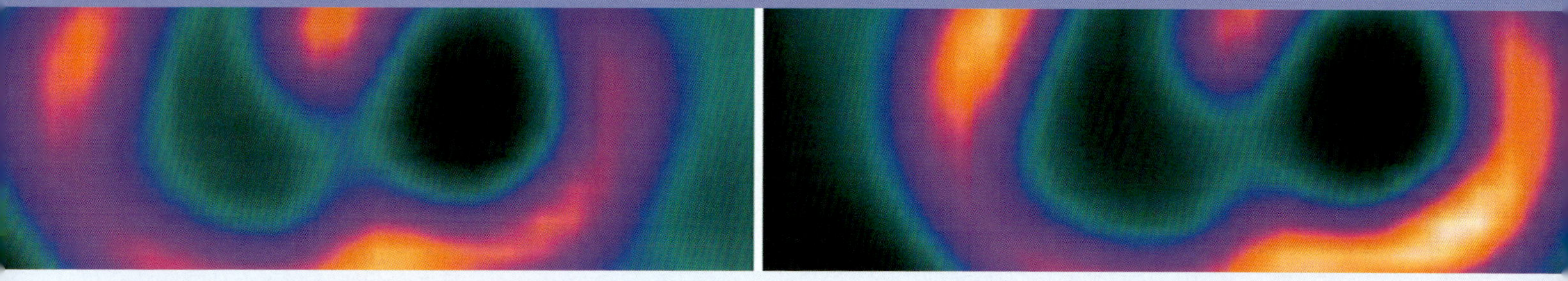

Introduction

Function and Coronary Artery Disease

Nuclear Cardiac Imaging

Nuclear cardiology encompasses studies that diagnose and risk stratify coronary artery disease, myocardial infarction and hibernation, left ventricular function, and detection of right-to-left shunt.

Myocardial perfusion imaging evaluates myocardial perfusion at rest and stress, diagnosing regional or global ischemia and myocardial infarction. In 1 meta-analysis of ~ 39,000 patients, patients with normal or low-risk patterns (e.g., mild reversible perfusion abnormalities in 1 vascular territory) on myocardial perfusion imaging had a 0.6% rate of cardiac death or myocardial infarction per year. In patients with moderate or severe reversible perfusion defects, the cardiac event rate was 6% per year, a much higher rate compared with low-risk or normal scans.

Myocardial perfusion imaging provides risk stratification in symptomatic and asymptomatic patients. Patients at high risk for coronary artery disease include those with diabetes mellitus, hyperlipidemia, hypertension, and a family history of coronary artery disease. If patients with risk factors are asymptomatic, myocardial perfusion imaging provides additional clinical information predicting cardiac events. For example, in asymptomatic diabetic patients with moderate or large perfusion defects, the event rate is 2.4% per year compared with a 0.4% per year event rate in patients with mildly abnormal or normal perfusion scans.

Evidence of severe disease on myocardial perfusion imaging correlates with an annual death rate of 2.9% to 4.2%. Evidence of high-risk disease includes 2-vessel reversible perfusion defects, transient ischemic dilatation (signifying global subendocardial ischemia), and lung uptake on Tl-201 studies.

Stress protocols with myocardial perfusion imaging are tailored to the clinical situation. Exercise stress protocol utilizing the modified Bruce protocol is used when possible. Note that with myocardial perfusion imaging, exercise stress tests are less valuable in patients with left bundle branch block, as this can cause a false-positive reversible perfusion defect in the septum. Pharmacologic stress protocols can be utilized in those patients unable to exercise. Vasodilator stress agents such as adenosine, regadenoson, and dipyridamole are most commonly used, followed by dobutamine if vasodilator stress is contraindicated.

Assessment of myocardial viability can be performed using Tl-201 and F-18 FDG PET/CT. In patients found to have underperfused yet viable or hibernating myocardium, regional wall motion is expected to improve after revascularization. One meta-analysis of ~ 3,000 patients with viable segments showed a 79% reduction in annual mortality after revascularization.

Nuclear cardiac imaging also has a role in risk stratification and management of patients with heart failure. Left ventricular function can be assessed using gated acquisitions of left ventricular function on myocardial perfusion imaging or with Tc-99m-labeled red blood cells (also called MUGA). Left ventricular ejection fractions using MUGA have been shown to have less inter- and intraobserver variability than other modalities, making it especially useful in serial determinations in patients undergoing chemotherapy.

Finally, when anatomic evaluation fails to diagnose a suspected right-to-left cardiac shunt, an indirect method of diagnosis can be obtained using nuclear medicine. If extrapulmonary localization of the pulmonary perfusion tracer Tc-99m MAA occurs, a right-to-left cardiac shunt is diagnosed.

Imaging Protocols

Myocardial Ischemia and Infarction

Cardiac radiotracers are taken up by the myocardium in proportion to cardiac blood flow. Images are obtained at rest and stress, then compared. Perfusion defects at stress that are not present at rest constitute inducible ischemia. Fixed perfusion defects at stress and rest signify myocardial infarction &/or myocardial hibernation.

Imaging protocols include single- and dual-isotope studies with Tc-99m-based perfusion agents &/or Tl-201 or PET/CT perfusion studies using Rb-82. Imaging with single-photon radiopharmaceuticals and gamma cameras is much more available clinically and less expensive than PET/CT myocardial perfusion imaging. In general, imaging with Tl-201 is used less commonly due to poorer imaging characteristics and dosimetry considerations as compared to Tc-99m-based radiopharmaceuticals.

Myocardial Viability

Myocardial viability can be assessed though Tl-201 rest-redistribution studies and F-18 FDG PET/CT. Tl-201 employs traditional gamma camera technology, 1 dose of radiopharmaceutical, and requires limited patient preparation. F-18 FDG PET/CT imaging of anaerobic glycolysis in hibernating, nonperfused myocardium is common, but requires recent meal and endogenous insulin response or exogenous insulin administration prior to F-18 FDG administration and PET/CT imaging. In addition, the F-18 FDG PET/CT data must be compared with a resting nuclear myocardial perfusion study, either a Tc-99m-based perfusion agent or Tl-201.

LV Function

Left ventricular function can be assessed with left ventriculography using Tc-99m-labeled red blood cells (traditionally called a MUGA scan) or gated myocardial perfusion scintigraphy, usually performed to diagnose cardiac ischemia. End-diastolic and end-systolic counts or volumes are utilized to calculate the left ventricular ejection fraction. Visual analysis of both types of studies allows for visual and quantitative analysis of regional and global left ventricular wall motion.

Right-to-Left Cardiac Shunt

To diagnose a suspected right-to-left cardiac shunt, a Tc-99m MAA pulmonary perfusion study is performed, with anterior and posterior images over the head, chest, and abdomen. In cases of right-to-left shunt, Tc-99m MAA will be present in the brain, lungs, and kidneys.

Practice Guidelines

The American Society of Nuclear Cardiology publishes clinical guidelines and quality standards for appropriate use, imaging, and reporting of nuclear cardiology studies. Content can be found online at www.asnc.org.

Selected References

1. Society of Nuclear Medicine and Molecular Imaging. ACR-SNMMI-SPR Practice Guideline for the Performance of Cardiac Scintigraphy. https://www.snmmi.org/ClinicalPractice/content.aspx?ItemNumber=6414#Cardio. Published October 1, 2009. Accessed July 31, 2015

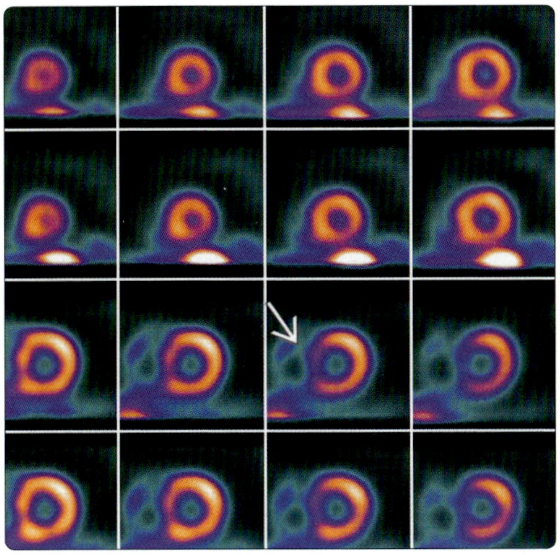

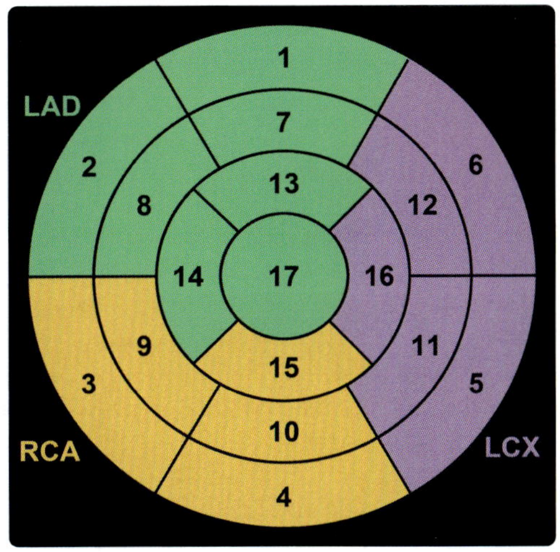

(Left) *This myocardial perfusion scan shows short-axis images of the left ventricle at stress (top) and rest (bottom). Note decreased activity in the membranous septum* ➔*, a normal finding.* **(Right)** *This graphic shows a short-axis bull's-eye of the left ventricle depicting the 17 segments and the associated vascular supply. These segments are used when reporting nuclear cardiology studies.*

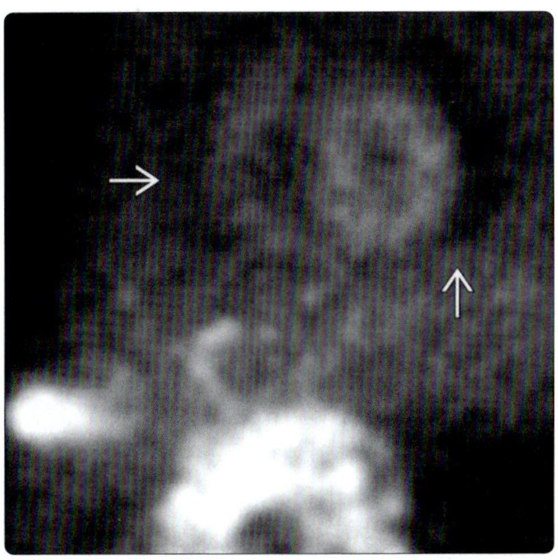

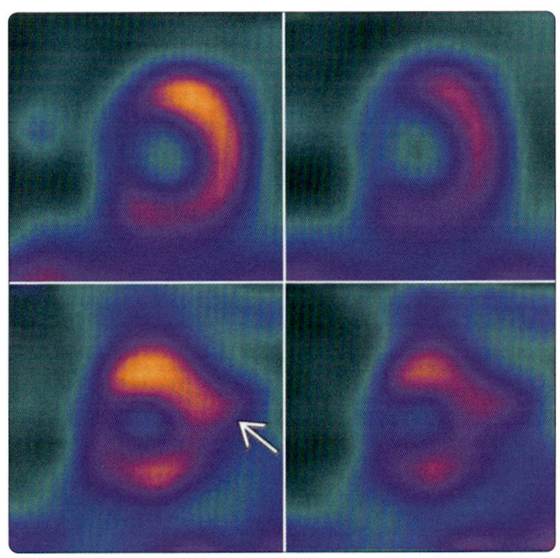

(Left) *Left anterior oblique raw image from a myocardial perfusion scan shows a photopenic defect around the heart* ➔*, corresponding to a pericardial effusion.* **(Right)** *Short-axis myocardial perfusion scan at stress (top) and rest (bottom) shows the "hurricane" sign* ➔*, an artifact caused by patient motion during the rest image acquisition.*

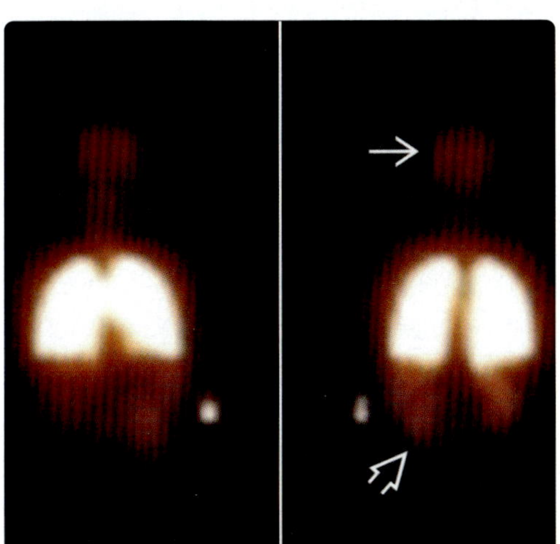

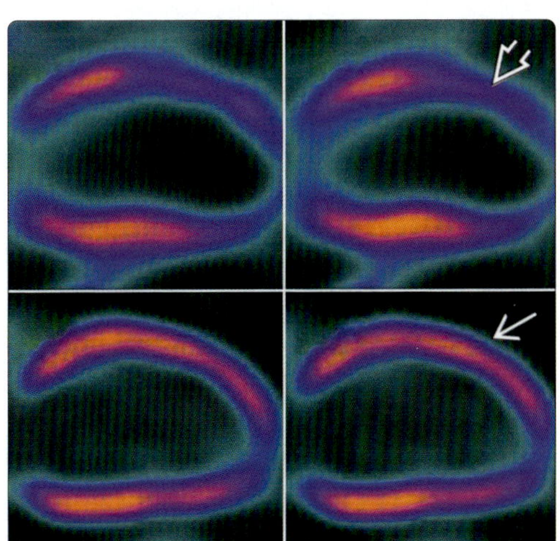

(Left) *Anterior and posterior Tc-99m MAA shunt study shows brain* ➔ *and kidney* ➔ *uptake, signifying a right-to-left cardiac shunt.* **(Right)** *Vertical long-axis F-18 FDG PET cardiac viability study shows uptake* ➔ *in a segment of hibernating myocardium* ➔ *on perfusion imaging. Revascularization of this region should improve myocardial contractility.*

KEY FACTS

IMAGING

- Multiple-gated cardiac blood pool acquisition (MUGA)
  - Low inter- and intraobserver variability (< 5%)
  - High reproducibility
- Radiopharmaceutical
  - 15-25 mCi (555-925 MBq) Tc-99m pertechnetate autologous labeled red blood cells (RBCs) IV
  - In vitro RBC labeling: Highest binding of radionuclide (~ 98%)
  - In vivo RBC labeling: > 80% binding
  - ROIs drawn around left ventricle
    - End systole, end diastole, and background
  - Heart must be in regular rhythm for optimal imaging
  - If background drawn over spleen or aorta, ejection fraction (EF) spuriously high
  - If background drawn over stomach or outside body, EF spuriously low
  - High unbound Tc-99m pertechnetate with recent transfusion, renal failure, heparin therapy, some chemotherapy, other medications

DIAGNOSTIC CHECKLIST

- Evaluate raw images (cine) for study quality
  - Counts, labeling, gating, views
- Compare qualitative estimation of left ventricular ejection fraction with quantitative calculation
- Comparison with previous studies important: Regions of interest should be similar
- Evaluate
  - Pericardial silhouette
  - Chamber sizes
  - Hypo/akinesis
  - Filling defects
  - Aneurysm
  - Ejection fraction

(Left) *Left anterior oblique multiple-gated cardiac blood pool acquisition (MUGA) shows the right ventricle, pulmonary artery, aorta, and left ventricle.* **(Right)** *Left anterior oblique MUGA shows region of interest (ROI) analysis: End diastole, end systole, and background ROIs.*

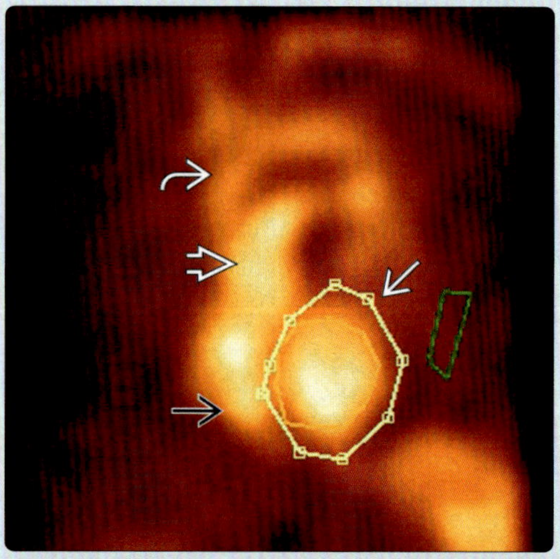

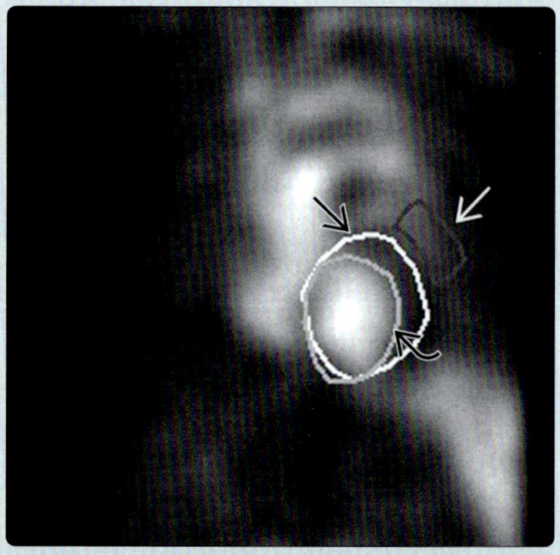

(Left) *Amplitude image demonstrates the degree or magnitude of contraction of the left ventricle. The red area contracts the most.* **(Right)** *Phase image demonstrates the sequence of contraction of the heart, with the right and left ventricles showing similar colors since they contract simultaneously.*

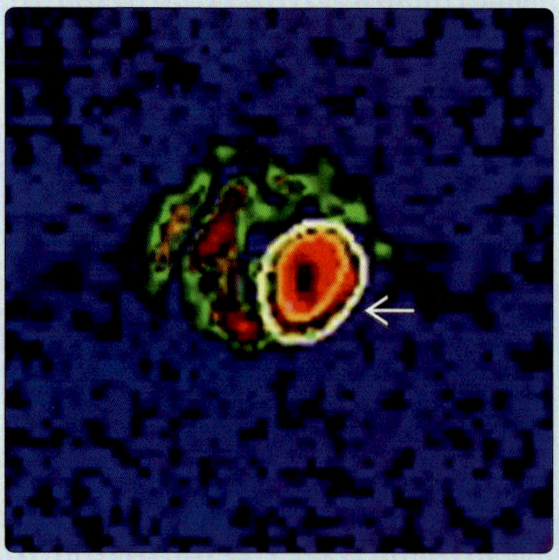

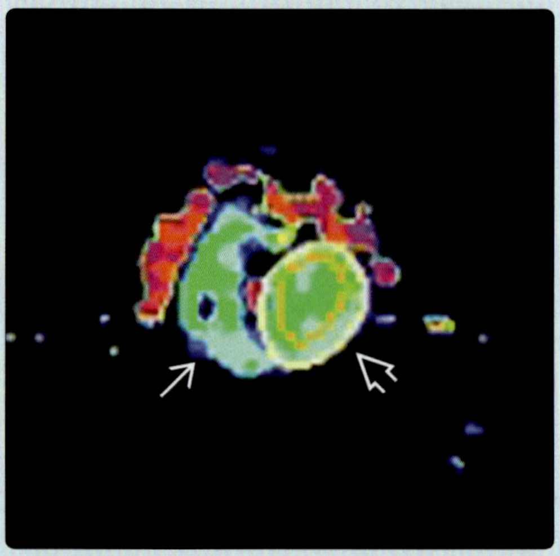

IMAGING

Imaging Recommendations

- Best imaging tool
  - Multiple-gated cardiac blood pool acquisition (MUGA)
  - Tc-99m labeled autologous red blood cells (RBCs)
    - Images obtained over heart
    - Analysis of counts at end diastole and end systole → left ventricular (LV) ejection fraction (EF)
  - Low inter- and intraobserver variability (< 5%)
  - High reproducibility
  - Excellent correlation with cardiac catheterization ventriculography (r = 0.94)
- Protocol advice
  - Patient prep: None
  - Radiopharmaceutical: 15-25 mCi (555-925 MBq) Tc-99m pertechnetate autologous labeled RBCs IV
    - In vitro RBC labeling
      - Highest binding of radionuclide (~ 98%)
      - Safety issues with reinjection of blood products
      - Contraindicated if heparin allergy
    - In vivo RBC labeling: > 80% binding
    - High unbound Tc-99m pertechnetate levels with recent transfusion, renal failure, heparin therapy, some chemotherapy, other medications
  - Dosimetry
    - Organ receiving largest radiation dose: Heart
  - Image acquisition
    - Patient supine
    - ECG gating
      - 16-32 frames per R-R interval
    - Planar images: LEAP/high-resolution collimator
    - Matrix: 64 x 64
    - Each image acquired for 300K counts or 5 min
    - Anterior view: 45° shallower than best septal LAO
      - Shows anterolateral and apical LV; right atrium and right ventricle
    - Best septal view LAO: Angle chosen that best shows septum between right and left ventricles
      - Shows septal, anterolateral, posterolateral LV
    - Left lateral/LPO: 45° greater than best septal LAO
      - Shows inferior, apical, anterolateral LV
    - Caudal angulation ± slanted collimator: May help separate ventricular from atrial blood pool
    - Image processing
      - Evaluate raw images (cine) for study quality: Counts, labeling, gating, views
  - Region of interest (ROI) analysis
    - ROIs drawn around LV: End systole, end diastole, and background
      - Manual, automatic, or semiautomatic ROI placement available
      - Avoid drawing background over spleen or aorta; EF will be spuriously high
      - Avoid drawing background over empty stomach or outside body; EF will be spuriously low
      - Background ~ 1/3 size of end diastole

Artifacts and Quality Control

- Heart must be in regular rhythm for optimal imaging
  - Irregular heartbeats rejected
    - Optimal: ≤ 10% irregular beats
    - Ejection fraction results less reliable if ≥ 30% irregular beats

DIFFERENTIAL DIAGNOSIS

Ischemic Dilated Cardiomyopathy

- Cardiovascular
  - Regional wall motion abnormalities in coronary artery distribution most common

Nonischemic Dilated Cardiomyopathy

- Toxic cardiomyopathy induced by chemotherapy
  - Serial LVEFs most common MUGA indication
- Also: Stress-induced, infectious, genetic, peripartum, sarcoid, autoimmune, cirrhosis, end-stage renal disease

DIAGNOSTIC CHECKLIST

Image Interpretation Pearls

- Compare qualitative estimation of LVEF with quantitative calculation
  - Reprocessing may be necessary if discrepancy
- Comparison with previous studies important: ROIs should be similar
  - Reprocessing may be necessary if discrepancy

Reporting Tips

- Cardiac morphology
  - Chamber sizes
  - Ventricular wall thickness
  - Pericardial silhouette
  - Filling defects
- Systolic function
  - Qualitative
    - Global LV function
    - Regional LV function
      - Hypo/akinesis, aneurysm
- Ejection fraction
  - Qualitative: Estimate from cine loop
  - Quantitative: ROI analysis of counts and calculation
    - LVEF (%): [End diastolic counts - background counts] - [end systolic counts - background counts] / [end diastolic counts - background counts] x 100
- Phase image: Shows sequence of contraction of atria and ventricles
- Amplitude image: Shows magnitude of contraction of atria and ventricles
- Right ventricular EF
  - Qualitative and quantitative analysis as with LVEF

SELECTED REFERENCES

1. American College of Radiology. ACR–SNM–SPR Practice Guideline for the Performance of Cardiac Scintigraphy, Resolution 14. http://snmmi.files.cms-plus.com/docs/Cardiac_Scintigraphy_1382731812393_3.pdf. Revised 2009. Accessed July 9, 2014

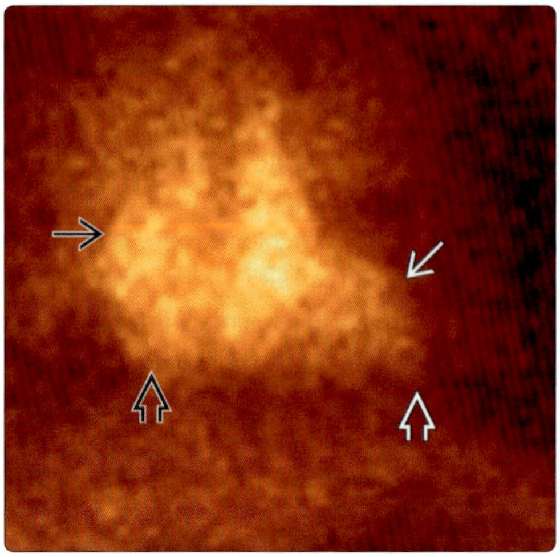

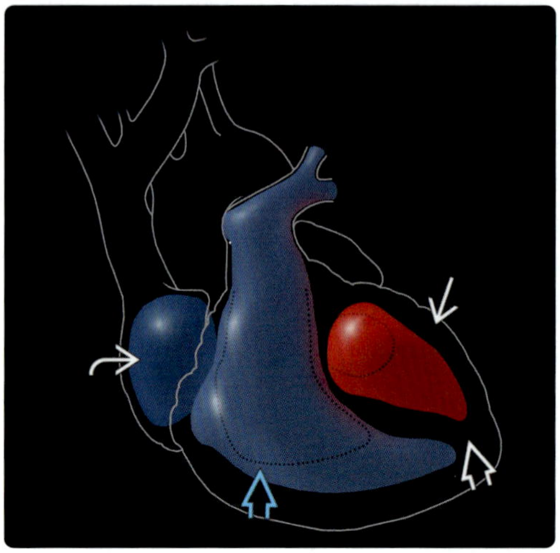

(Left) *Anterior MUGA shows right atrium ➙, right ventricle ➙, anterolateral left ventricle ➙, and left ventricular apex ➙.* **(Right)** *Anterior graphic of the heart shows right atrium ➙, right ventricle ➙, anterolateral left ventricle ➙, and left ventricular apex ➙.*

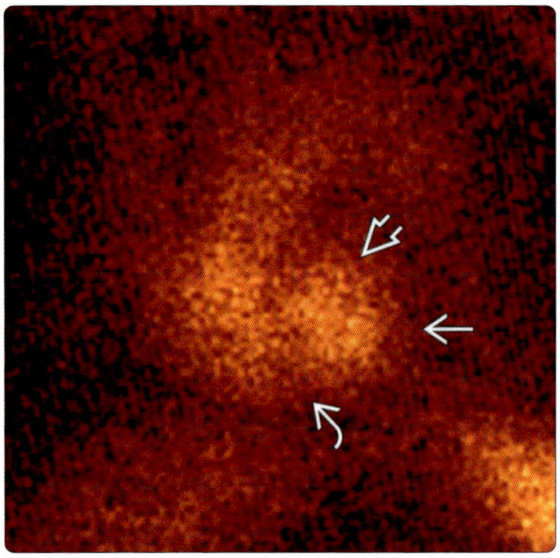

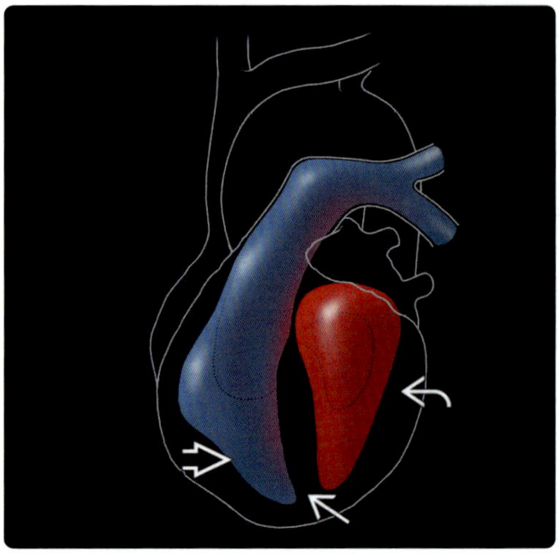

(Left) *Left anterior oblique MUGA shows septum ➙, anterolateral left ventricle ➙, and posterolateral left ventricle ➙. Also called the best septal view, this image is commonly obtained at 45°. Caudal tilt can also assist in obtaining best view of septum.* **(Right)** *Left anterior oblique graphic of the heart shows right ventricle ➙, septum ➙, and left ventricle ➙.*

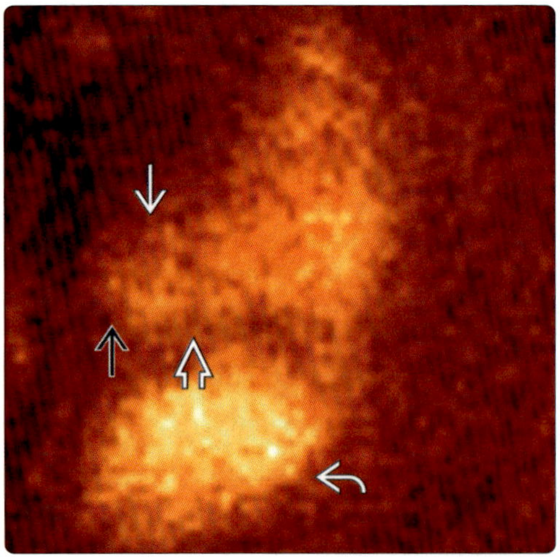

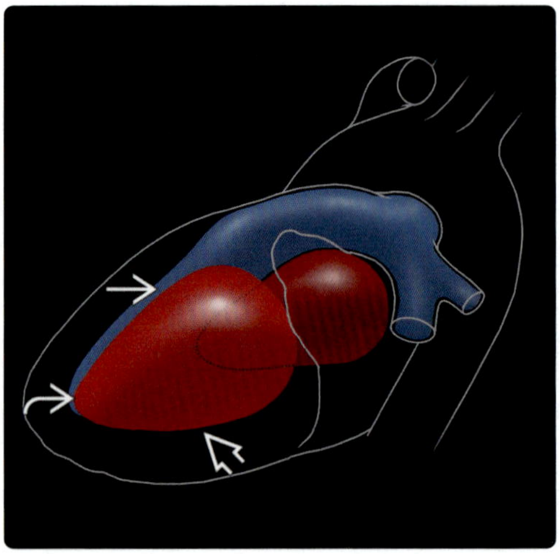

(Left) *Left posterior oblique MUGA shows inferior ➙, apical ➙, and anterolateral ➙ left ventricle. Note splenic ➙ activity, normal physiologic uptake on Tc-99m pertechnetate RBC studies.* **(Right)** *Left posterior oblique graphic of the heart shows inferior ➙, apical ➙, and anterolateral ➙ left ventricle.*

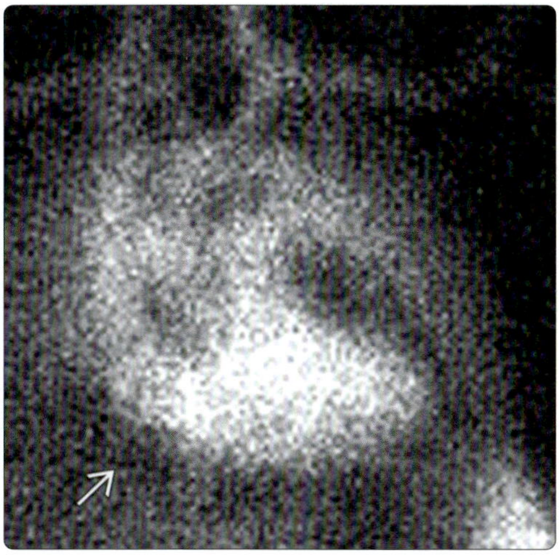

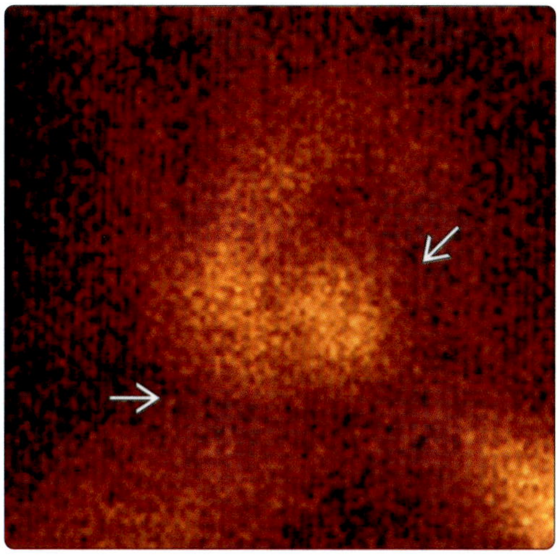

(Left) *Anterior MUGA shows a large photopenic defect* ➡ *surrounding the heart.* **(Right)** *Left anterior oblique MUGA in the same patient shows the photopenic defect* ➡ *around the heart, a large pericardial effusion.*

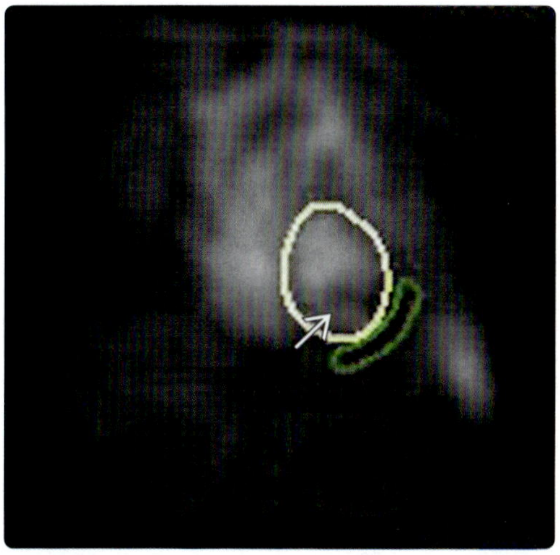

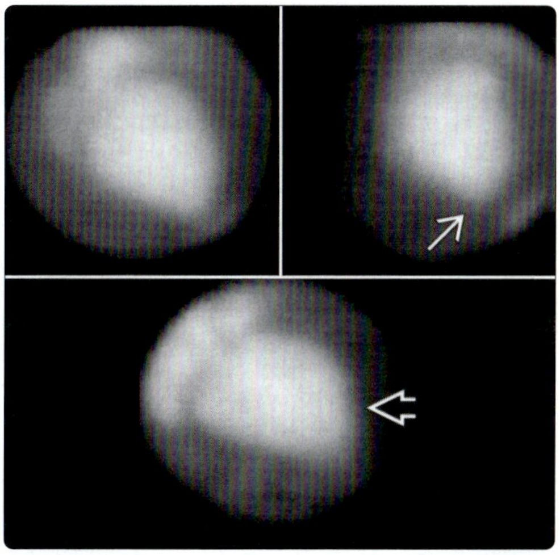

(Left) *Left anterior oblique MUGA shows a filling defect* ➡ *in the left ventricular apex. The differential diagnosis includes mass lesions and thrombus. Note that medical devices such as pacemakers and postmastectomy tissue expanders can cause artifactual filling defects on MUGA; however, these tend to be in different locations depending on the angle of imaging.* **(Right)** *This MUGA shows dilated left ventricle* ➡ *and LV dyskinesis* ➡ *apparent on end-systolic images, a small LV aneurysm.*

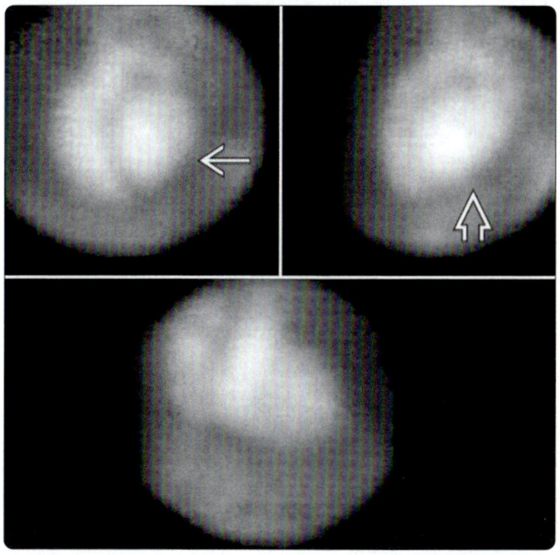

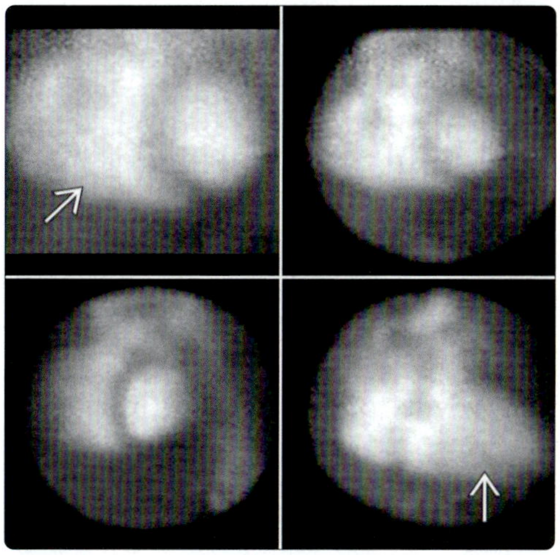

(Left) *This MUGA demonstrates dilated left ventricle and global hypokinesis, evidenced by minimal excursion between end diastole* ➡ *and end systole* ➡ *in a patient with chemotherapy-induced cardiomyopathy.* **(Right)** *This MUGA shows severe biventricular enlargement* ➡ *in a patient with viral-induced cardiomyopathy.*

Myocardial Infarction and Ischemia

KEY FACTS

DIAGNOSTIC CHECKLIST

- Raw images
  - May identify artifacts, extracardiac tracer uptake (cancer, infection, bowel), infiltration
- Study quality
  - Comment if excessive motion, poor radiotracer uptake/infiltration, technical error
- Artifacts
  - Motion, scatter, reconstruction, attenuation
- Adequacy of stress modality
  - Exercise or pharmacologic
- Perfusion images: Qualitative analysis
  - LV chamber size: Normal vs. dilated
  - 17 segment model: Describe stress/rest perfusion
  - Transient ischemic dilatation (TID): Dropout of endocardial border on stress
- Perfusion images: Quantitative analysis
  - 17 segment model: Each segment scored on 5-pt scale
  - Summed difference score: < 4 = normal; 4-8 = mildly abnormal; 9-13 = moderately abnormal; > 13 = severely abnormal
  - TID ratio: 1.12-1.36 positive for TID
- Gated images: Ejection fraction and wall motion
  - Brightening and endocardial excursion = normal
  - Hypokinesis/akinesis if photopenia, lack of endocardial excursion
  - Lower limits of normal EF for MPI: 45%
  - EF overestimated if small heart size
- Conclusion
  - Positive or negative for inducible ischemia
  - Positive or negative for myocardial infarction (± peri-infarct ischemia)
    - Consider possibility of hibernating myocardium, need for viability study
  - LV function: EF and wall motion

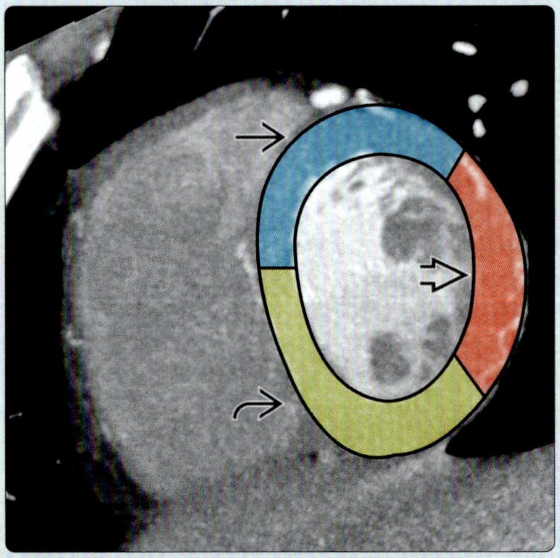

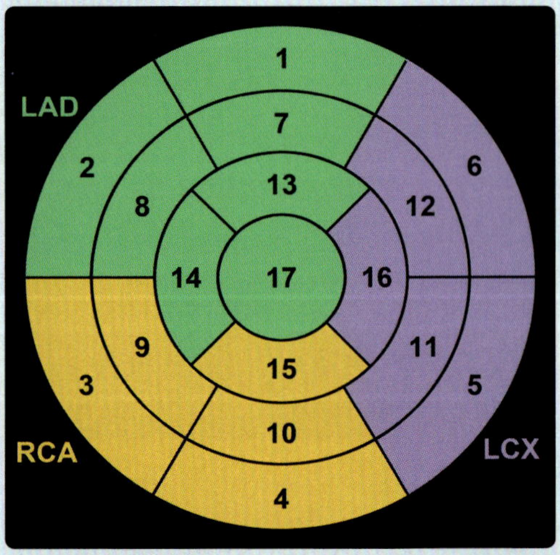

(Left) *Short axis view of the left ventricle on CT shows vascular territories supplying the myocardium. The left anterior descending artery supplies the anterior and septal walls ➡. The left circumflex artery supplies the lateral wall ⇨. The right coronary artery supplies the inferior and inferoseptal walls ↷.* **(Right)** *Drawing of short axis 17-segment model shows bull's-eye view of the heart for quantitative analysis.*

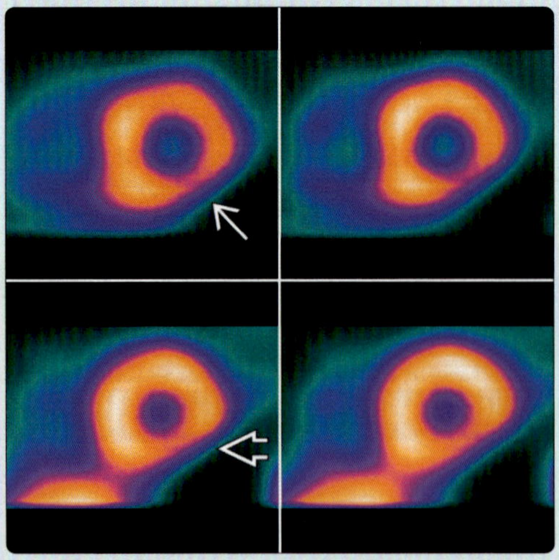

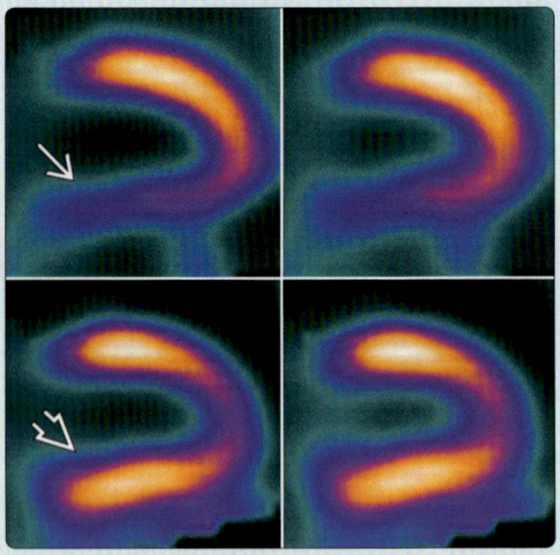

(Left) *Short axis MPI shows decreased activity in the inferolateral wall on rest ➡, which is more pronounced on stress ➡ images, signifying inferolateral infarction with peri-infarct ischemia. Note the perfusion defect appears flat.* **(Right)** *Vertical long axis MPI shows inferior wall before attenuation correction ➡ on SPECT/CT. After attenuation correction, counts in the inferior wall ➡ are no longer artifactually decreased by diaphragmatic/soft tissue attenuation in this obese patient.*

IMAGING

General Features

- Best diagnostic clue
  - Myocardial perfusion imaging (MPI)
    - Usually Tc-99m-based perfusion agent that localizes to myocardium
      - Radiotracer injected at rest, then image
      - Radiotracer injected at stress, then image
      - Rest and stress images compared
    - Myocardial ischemia: Perfusion defect evident on stress images, normal perfusion on rest images
    - Acute myocardial infarction (AMI): Perfusion defect on MPI with injection within 2 hrs of pain episode
    - Chronic myocardial infarction: Fixed perfusion defect on rest and stress images
    - Hibernating myocardium: Fixed perfusion defect on rest/stress images, normal on viability images
- Location
  - Anterior/septal wall: Left anterior descending (LAD) artery
  - Lateral wall: Circumflex artery
  - Inferior wall: Posterior descending artery (PDA)
    - Right coronary artery (RCA) in 85% (right dominant)
    - Continuation of circumflex in 15% (left dominant)
  - Apex: Usually from LAD, but variable

Imaging Recommendations

- Protocol advice
  - Patient preparation
    - Review for contraindications to stress test, pregnancy
    - Mostly required for stress portion of test
      - NPO for 4 hrs prior to stress test
      - No caffeine 12 hrs prior to pharmacologic stress
  - Radiopharmaceutical
    - Tc-99m sestamibi or Tc-99m tetrofosmin
      - Dose: 10-40 mCi (370 MBq to 1.4 GBq)
      - 1-day protocol: Up to 40 mCi (1.4 GBq) (10 mCi [370 MBq] for rest, 30 mCi [1.1 GBq] for stress)
      - 2-day protocol (patients > 250-275 lbs): 25-30 mCi (925 MBq to 1.1 GBq) for both rest and stress, 1 day apart
      - Dosimetry: Colon (sestamibi) and gallbladder wall (tetrofosmin) receive largest radiation dose
      - 6 hrs t1/2
    - Thallium-201 chloride
      - Dose: 2-4 mCi (74-148 MBq)
      - Rest images on dual-tracer MPI
      - Stress-rest images on Tl-201 only MPI
      - Redistribution imaging for viability
      - Long t1/2 (73 hrs) leads to higher dose than Tc-99m-based agents
      - Dosimetry: Kidneys receive largest radiation dose
    - Rb-82
      - Dose: 2D PET: 40-60 mCi (1.4-2.2 GBq); 3D PET: 10-20 mCi (370-740 MBq) BGO system; 30-40 mCi (1.1-1.4 GBq) LSO system
      - Generator produced
      - 75 sec t1/2
      - Cost-effective PET tracer for high-volume centers
      - Pharmacologic stress utilized due to short t1/2
      - Dosimetry: Kidneys receive largest radiation dose
    - N-13 ammonia
      - Dose: 15-25 mCi (555-925 MBq)
      - PET perfusion agent
      - Cyclotron produced (on-site due to 9.8 min t1/2)
      - Dosimetry: Urinary bladder receives largest radiation dose
  - Image acquisition: Tc-99m sestamibi and Tc-99m tetrofosmin
    - Patient position: Supine, upright/semiupright
    - Injection to imaging time: 15-60 min
    - Time between rest/stress injections: 30 min to 4 hrs
    - Collimator: Low energy, high resolution
    - 180° planar acquisition: Preferred if no attenuation correction (better spatial resolution, higher contrast, less attenuation)
    - SPECT and SPECT/CT: Preferred in obese patients, allows attenuation correction
    - Matrix: 64 x 64
    - Step and shoot or continuous acquisition
    - 60-64 projections; 20-25 sec per projection
    - ECG gate stress only or rest and stress
    - 8 frames/cycle standard
    - 140 keV with 15-20% window
  - Image acquisition: Tl-201
    - Similar to Tc-99m-based tracers, except
      - 70-80 keV with 15-20% window
      - 64 projections
      - Stress-rest MPI: Image 10 min after injection for stress images; rest (redistribution) images at 3-4 hrs
      - Rest only for dual-tracer MPI: Image 10 min after injection for rest images; utilize Tc-99m-based radiotracer for stress
      - Viability: Image 10 min after injection for rest images; redistribution (viability) images at 3-4 hrs
  - Image acquisition: Rb-82 and N-13 ammonia PET/CT
    - Rb-82: Image acquisition starts 1-1.5 min after injection, 5-10 min acquisition
    - N-13 ammonia: Image acquisition starts 4-5 min after injection, 10-15 min acquisition
    - Attenuation correction from CT for large patients
  - Image processing
    - Reconstruction using filtered backprojection or iterative reconstruction
    - Stress images usually displayed on top row, rest images on bottom row

Artifacts and Quality Control

- Motion artifact
  - Hurricane sign: Counts outside epicardial border on short axis
  - Blurred endocardial border
  - Lateral wall blurring
- Scatter artifact
  - Counts scatter into inferior wall due to high bowel activity
- Reconstruction artifact
  - Photopenia in inferior wall from high bowel activity
  - Photopenia at 11 o'clock position on short-axis views on rest and stress

- Attenuation
  - Soft tissue attenuation causing fixed defects
  - Misregistration of attenuation correction map and perfusion data

DIFFERENTIAL DIAGNOSIS

Myocardial Infarction

- Normal apical thinning
- Left ventricular hypertrophy: Fixed lateral wall defect
- Soft tissue attenuation of photons: Breast (anterior wall), diaphragm (inferior wall)
- Septal hypokinesis common in absence of MI, especially after coronary artery bypass graft surgery
- Decreased activity in lateral wall on N-13 ammonia PET can be seen in healthy controls
- Myocardial hibernation: Myocardium with little/no perfusion, but viable due to anaerobic glycolysis
  - 25% of fixed defects are viable on viability studies

Myocardial Ischemia

- Artifactual perfusion defects on stress only (e.g., bowel activity on stress images, shift of overlying soft tissue)
- Left bundle branch block: Functional septal reversibility with exercise stress (false-positive)

Other Vascular Disease

- Vasospastic disease (Prinzmetal angina)
- Microvascular disease (e.g., diabetes mellitus, syndrome X)

PATHOLOGY

General Features

- Etiology
  - Ruptured coronary artery plaque disrupts myocardial blood supply
    - Myocardial necrosis begins in 20-30 min, spreading from subendo- to epicardium
  - Risk factors
    - Hyperlipidemia, diabetes mellitus, hypertension, obesity, cigarette smoking, family history

CLINICAL ISSUES

Demographics

- Age
  - Men: Usually > 45 yrs
  - Women: > 55 yrs

DIAGNOSTIC CHECKLIST

Consider

- Myocardial infarction
  - Fixed perfusion defect, regional wall motion abnormality
  - Peri-infarct ischemia can cause chest pain
- Myocardial ischemia
  - Reversible perfusion defect on rest and stress images, no regional wall motion abnormality

Reporting Tips

- Raw images
  - Review to identify artifacts, extracardiac radiotracer uptake (breast/lung cancer, lymphoma, infection)
- Study quality
  - Comment if excessive motion, poor radiotracer uptake/infiltration, technical error
- Artifacts
  - Describe if present: Motion, scatter, reconstruction, attenuation
- Adequacy of stress modality
  - Exercise: Discuss percent age-predicted max heart rate achieved
  - Vasodilators: If infused and radiotracer injected per protocol, assume adequate stress
- Perfusion images
  - Qualitative analysis
    - LV chamber size: Normal vs. dilated
    - 17 segment model: Describe perfusion defects on stress and rest using these segments
    - Transient ischemic dilatation (TID): Dropout of endocardial border on stress
  - Quantitative analysis
    - Quantitative perfusion analysis
      - Computer generation of segmental perfusion scores in each of 17 segments on a 5-point scale at stress and rest (0 = normal, 4 = absent)
      - Summed stress score (SSS): Analysis of resting and stress-induced perfusion defects
      - Summed rest score (SRS): Analysis of resting perfusion defects
      - Summed difference score (SDS): SSS minus SRS; a measure of stress-induced ischemia
      - SDS: < 4 = normal; 4-8 = mildly abnormal; 9-13 = moderately abnormal; > 13 = severely abnormal
    - TID ratio: 1.12-1.36 correlates with multivessel disease
      - TID = endocardial volume at stress / endocardial volume at rest
- Gated images
  - Wall motion
    - Normal if brightening and endocardial excursion on gated slice images
    - Hypokinesis/akinesis if photopenia, lack of endocardial excursion
  - Ejection fraction
    - Lower limits of normal for MPI: 45%
    - Overestimated if small heart size
- Conclusion
  - Positive or negative for inducible ischemia
  - Positive or negative for myocardial infarction (± peri-infarct ischemia)
    - Consider possibility of hibernating myocardium, need for viability study
  - LV function: EF and wall motion

SELECTED REFERENCES

1. American College of Radiology. ACR-SNMMI-SPR Practice Guideline for the Performance of Cardiac Scintigraphy. http://snmmi.files.cms-plus.com/docs/Cardiac_Scintigraphy_1382731812393_3.pdf. Revised October 1, 2009. Accessed July 18, 2014
2. Struass et al. SNM Procedure Guideline for Myocardial Perfusion Imaging 3.3. http://snmmi.files.cms-plus.com/docs/Myocardial20Perfusion20Imaging203.3.pdf. June 14, 2008. Accessed July 18, 2014
3. Dorbala S et al: SNMMI/ASNC/SCCT guideline for cardiac SPECT/CT and PET/CT 1.0. J Nucl Med. 54(8):1485-507, 2013

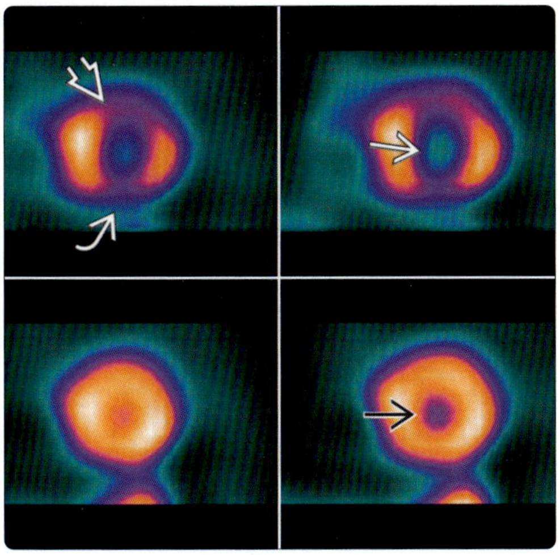

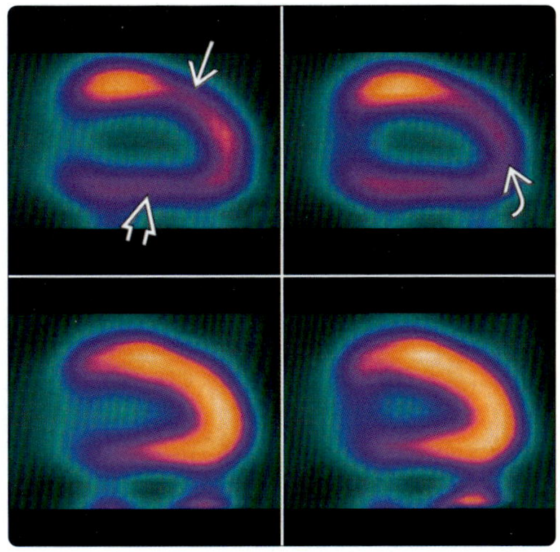

(Left) *Short axis MPI shows transient ischemic dilatation. Note normal endocardial border on rest, which appears to enlarge on stress. This high-risk finding is due to reversible subendocardial ischemia and suggests multivessel disease. Note also the anterior and inferior perfusion defects at stress.* **(Right)** *Vertical long axis MPI views (same patient) show enlarged endocardial border and severe stress-induced perfusion defects involving the anterior wall, inferior wall, and apex. Resting images below are normal.*

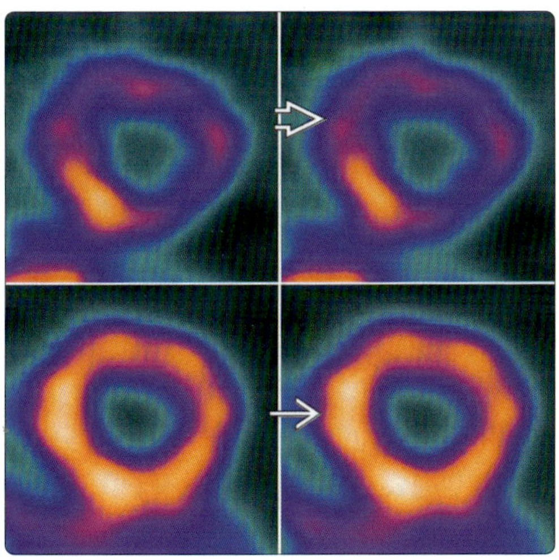

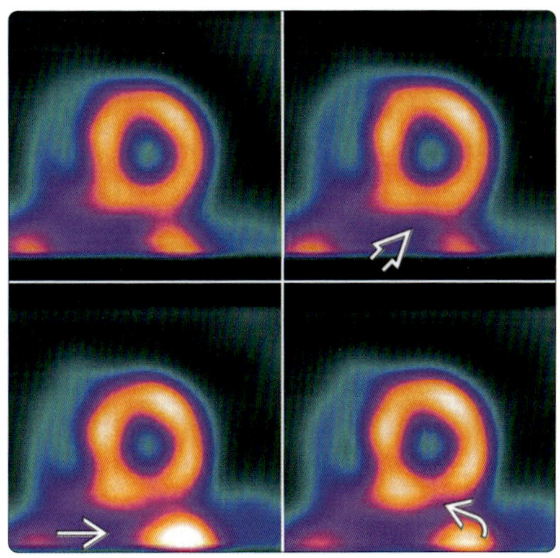

(Left) *Short axis MPI views in an obese patient show heterogeneous myocardium due to poor counts. The top row is prior to CT attenuation correction. The bottom row is after CT attenuation correction.* **(Right)** *Short axis MPI shows high activity in adjacent bowel. Note the adjacent inferior wall shows decreased counts on rest and normal counts on stress. The bowel activity caused decreased counts in the inferior wall due to reconstruction artifact.*

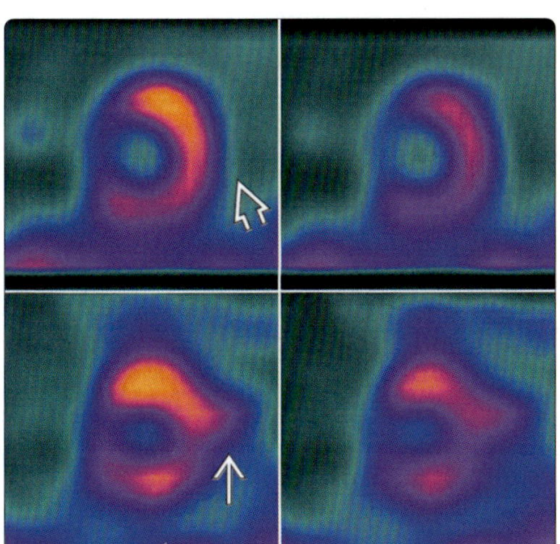

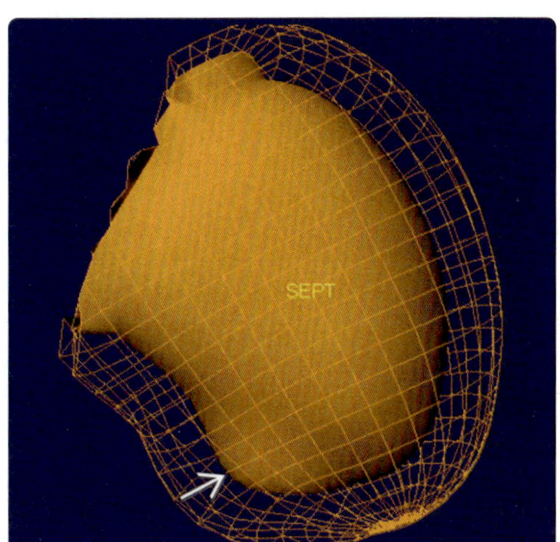

(Left) *Short axis MPI shows extracardiac activity extending from the left ventricle due to patient motion, called the hurricane sign. With motion correction, the hurricane sign disappeared.* **(Right)** *3D MPI rendering of the left ventricle at end systole shows a dilated left ventricle with dyskinesis at the inferoseptum, an apical aneurysm.*

(Left) *Short axis MPI shows multivessel coronary disease. Anteroseptal and inferolateral perfusion defects are more evident on stress compared with rest images.* **(Right)** *Horizontal long axis MPI in the same patient shows lateral inducible ischemia.*

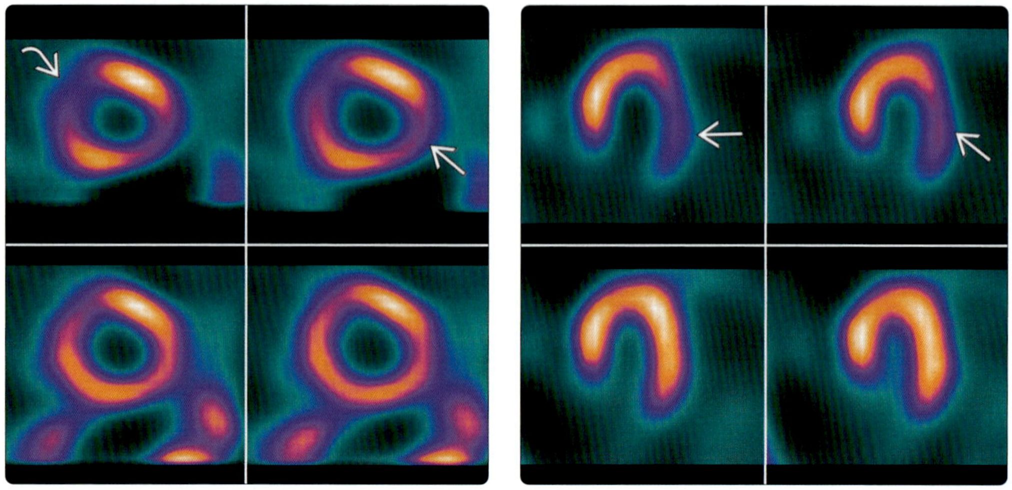

(Left) *Short axis MPI bull's-eye computer analysis in the same patient shows multivessel inducible ischemia in the anteroseptum, apical, and inferolateral walls on stress imaging.* **(Right)** *Short axis MPI bull's-eye computer analysis in the same patient at rest shows virtually normal perfusion.*

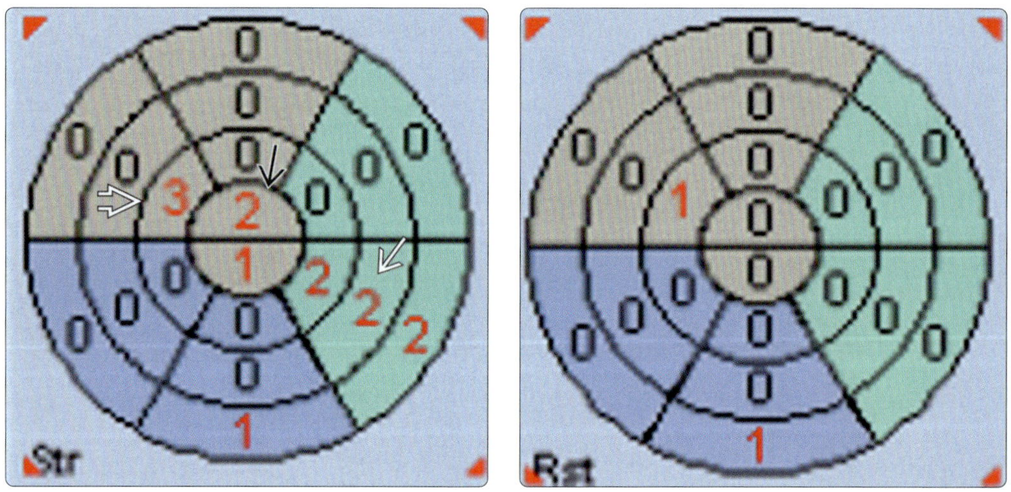

(Left) *3D view of MPI raw images shows normal myocardial radiotracer uptake.* **(Right)** *3D view of MPI raw images in the same patient who presented for follow-up MPI shows normal myocardial uptake and a large photopenic defect surrounding the heart, a pericardial effusion.*

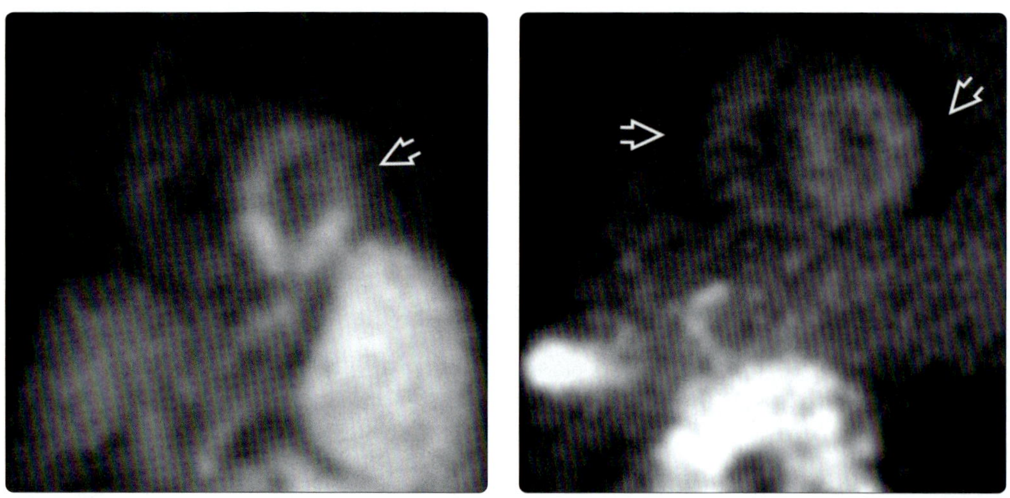

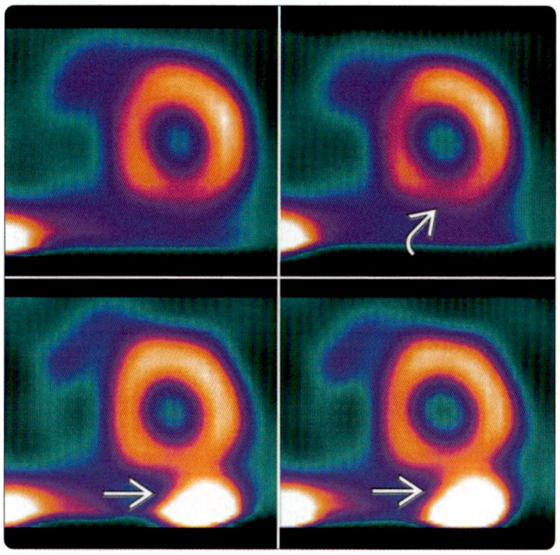

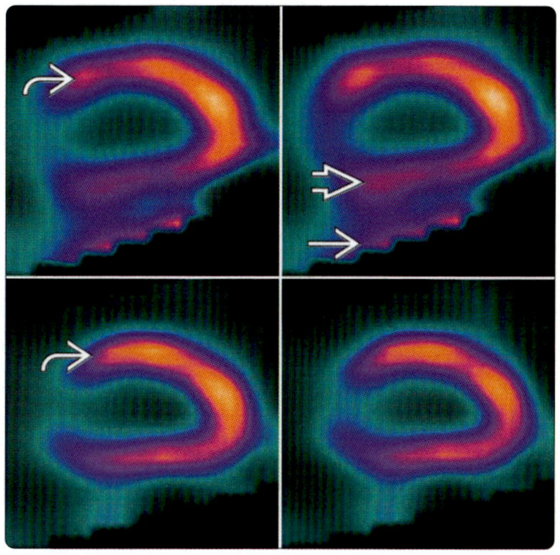

(Left) *Short axis MPI shows high counts in the bowel due to normal radiotracer excretion. Note the relatively diminished perfusion in the inferior wall on repeat image, confirming artifactual scatter of counts into the inferior wall.* **(Right)** *Vertical long axis MPI shows anterior inducible ischemia. Note high counts in bowel on stress images (hidden by computer processing). Coronary artery catheterization showed no inferior wall disease, suggesting reconstruction artifact reduced counts in this area on stress images.*

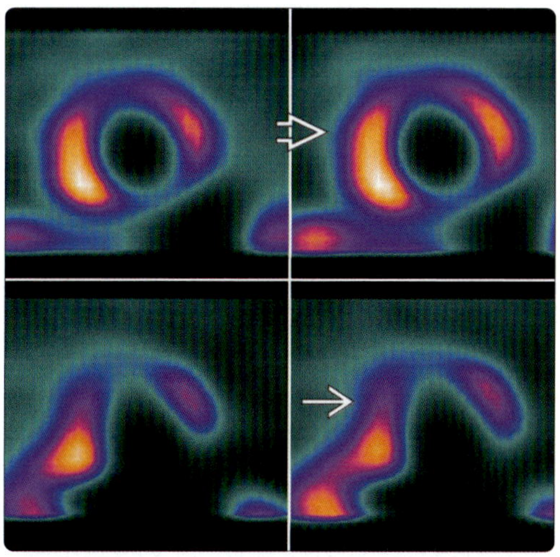

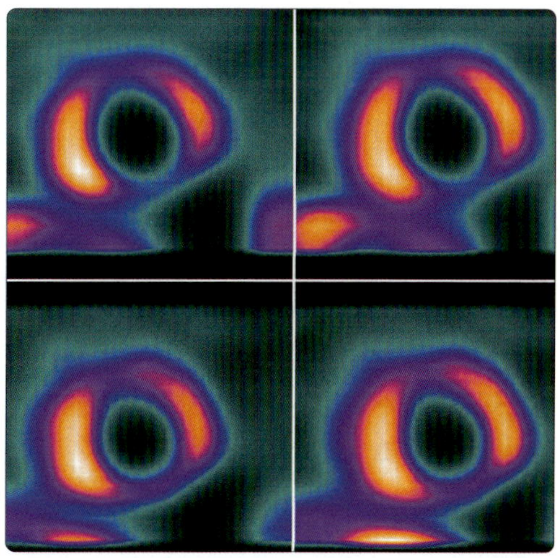

(Left) *Short axis MPI shows decreased counts in the left ventricle on stress that appear to improve on rest.* **(Right)** *Short axis MPI in the same patient with arms up during both rest and stress acquisitions show similar perfusion patterns. Note that the images must be obtained with similar patient positioning to avoid introduction of artifacts.*

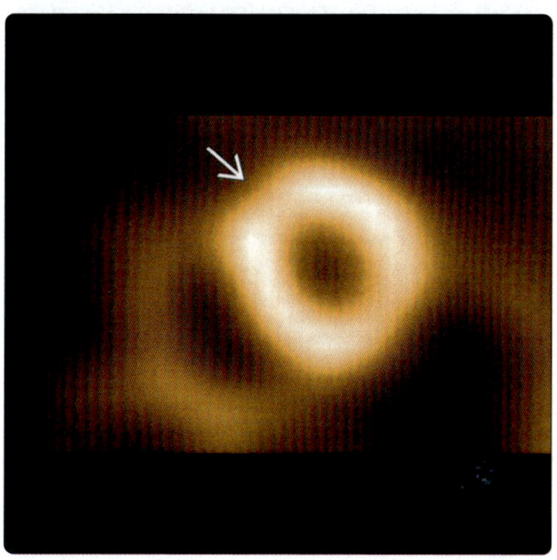

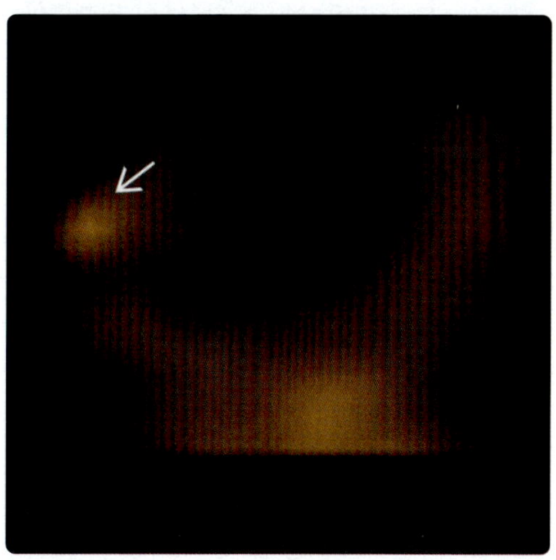

(Left) *Sagittal MPI raw images in an 86-year-old woman with atypical chest pain show normal myocardial uptake.* **(Right)** *Sagittal MPI raw images in the same patient show abnormal uptake in the left breast, a possible breast cancer. Mammographic correlation is necessary for this finding.*

Myocardial Viability

KEY FACTS

TERMINOLOGY

- Myocardial viability evaluation
  - Detection of myocardial hibernation or stunning vs. necrosis/infarction in patients with ischemic cardiomyopathy

IMAGING

- Tc-99m/Tl-201 myocardial perfusion scintigraphy
  - Viability present in 25% of regions called infarction
  - Viability present in up to 50% of patients with infarcted segments
- Perfusion-PET mismatch
  - Myocardial uptake of radioactive glucose analog compared with myocardial uptake of perfusion radiotracer (Tc-99m perfusion agent or Tl-201)
  - Anaerobic glucose utilization in underperfused myocardium = viability
- Tl-201 SPECT viability
  - Rest-redistribution mismatch
  - Delayed myocardial uptake in regions of underperfused myocardium = viability

TOP DIFFERENTIAL DIAGNOSES

- Myocardial hibernation
  - Chronic myocardial dysfunction due to chronically decreased myocardial perfusion (chronic total occlusions)
  - Regions of abnormal perfusion will show F-18 FDG utilization or redistribution on Tl-201
- Myocardial stunning
  - Temporary myocardial dysfunction due to short-term underperfusion or lack of perfusion to myocardium
  - Regions of abnormal perfusion will show F-18 FDG utilization or redistribution on Tl-201
- Myocardial infarction
  - Myocardial necrosis and remodeling (scar)
  - Regions of abnormal perfusion will show lack of F-18 FDG utilization or lack of redistribution on Tl-201

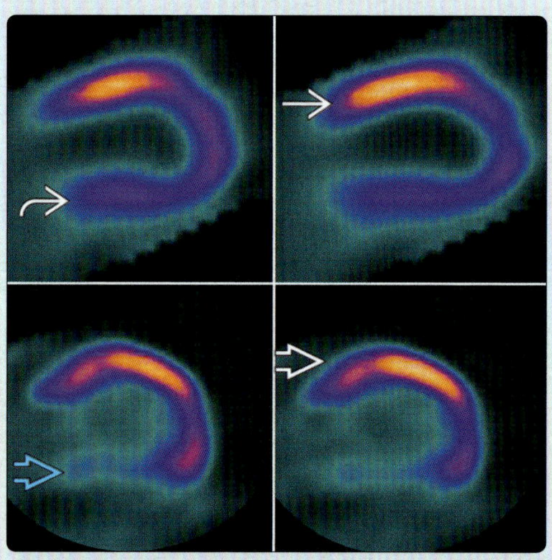
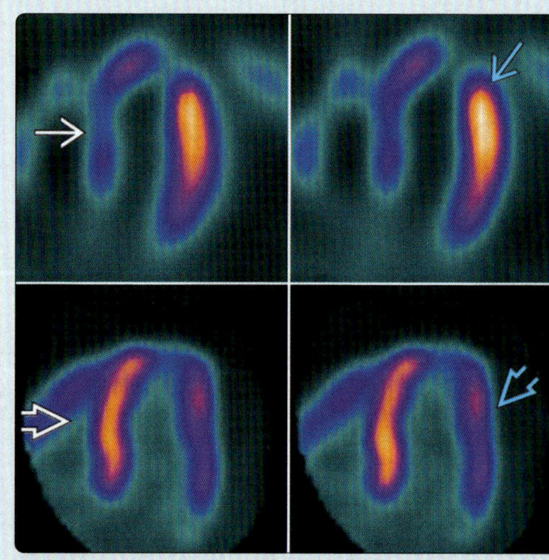

(Left) *Vertical long axis F-18 FDG PET viability shows normal perfusion in the anterior wall → with associated glucose metabolism →. This confirms glucose is an available substrate for hypoperfused inferior wall →, which does not show viability on PET →.* **(Right)** *Horizontal long axis F-18 FDG PET viability shows hypoperfused septum → with glucose utilization →, signifying viability. Note that the normally perfused lateral wall → is not utilizing glucose →, signifying free fatty acids are being utilized.*

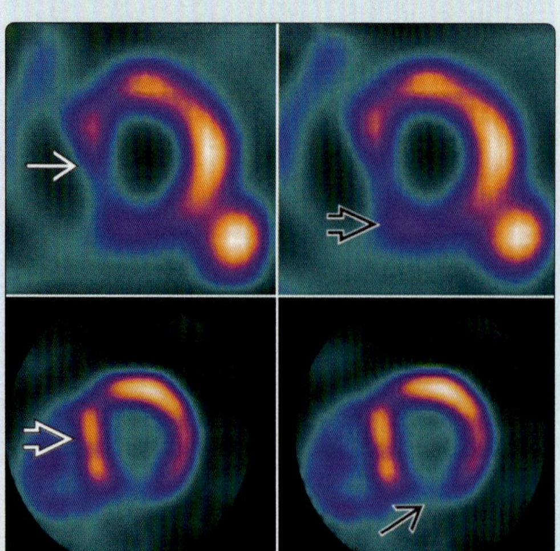
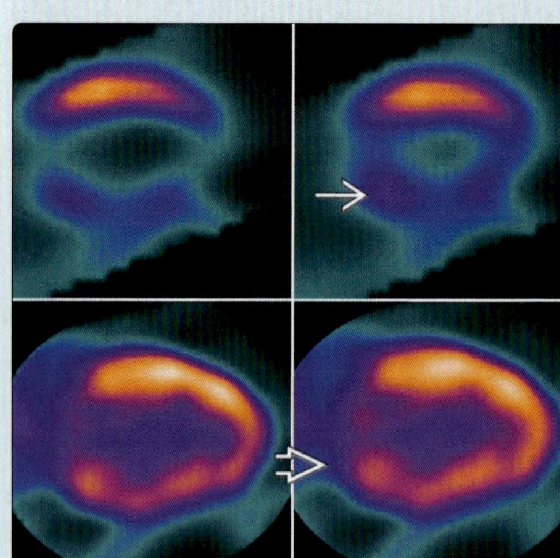

(Left) *Short axis F-18 FDG PET viability shows hypoperfused septum → that is utilizing glucose →, signifying viability. Note the inferior myocardial infarction → that is not viable →.* **(Right)** *Vertical long axis F-18 FDG PET viability shows inferior wall perfusion → and glucose metabolism → mismatch. This suggests that the inferior wall will improve in contractility after revascularization.*

TERMINOLOGY

Definitions

- Myocardial viability evaluation
  - Detection of myocardial hibernation or stunning vs. necrosis/infarction in patients with ischemic cardiomyopathy
    - Myocardial hibernation
      - Chronic myocardial dysfunction due to chronically decreased myocardial perfusion
    - Myocardial stunning
      - Temporary myocardial dysfunction due to short-term underperfusion or lack of perfusion to myocardium
  - Regions of hibernating/stunned myocardium likely to show improved contractility after revascularization

IMAGING

Nuclear Medicine Findings

- Tc-99m/Tl-201 myocardial perfusion scintigraphy
  - Viability present in 25% of regions called infarction
  - Viability present in up to 50% of patients with infarcted segments
- F-18 FDG PET viability
  - Perfusion-PET mismatch
    - Myocardial uptake of radioactive glucose analog compared with myocardial uptake of perfusion radiotracer (Tc-99m perfusion agent or Tl-201)
    - Anaerobic glucose utilization in underperfused myocardium = viability
- Tl-201 SPECT viability
  - Rest-redistribution mismatch
    - Myocardial uptake of Tl-201 at rest compared with delayed myocardial uptake (redistribution)
    - Delayed myocardial uptake in regions of underperfused myocardium = viability
      - > 10% increase in tracer uptake on redistribution images = viability
    - Comparison of Tl-201 uptake in underperfused segments to normally perfused segments
      - ~ 90% of segments with > 80% uptake of normal segments show functional improvement after revascularization
      - ~ 55% of segments with 50-60% uptake of normal segments show functional improvement after revascularization

Imaging Recommendations

- Protocol advice
  - F-18 FDG PET viability
    - Patient preparation
      - Obtain resting myocardial perfusion SPECT prior to F-18 FDG PET scan
      - Fast 6-12 hrs prior to F-18 FDG PET scan
      - F-18 FDG PET performed in presence of elevated insulin level (postprandial/post insulin administration)
      - Oral glucose loading (25-100 g) followed by blood glucose check at 45-90 min
      - Administer 1-5 units of insulin (sliding scale) depending on blood glucose level
    - Radiopharmaceutical
      - 5-15 mCi (185-555 MBq) F-18 FDG
      - Injection after glucose load/insulin administration
    - Dosimetry
      - Critical organ: Urinary bladder
    - Image acquisition
      - Imaging performed at ~ 60 mins after F-18 FDG injection
      - CT for attenuation correction
      - 3-10 min imaging time
    - Image processing
      - Match F-18 FDG PET images with myocardial perfusion SPECT images using dedicated myocardial perfusion scintigraphy software
  - Tl-201 viability
    - Patient preparation
      - None
    - Radiopharmaceutical
      - 2-4 mCi (74-148 MBq) Tl-201
    - Dosimetry
      - Critical organ: Testes, thyroid
    - Image acquisition
      - 10 min after injection; 4 &/or 24 hr images
      - LEAP collimator
      - SPECT/CT with CT for attenuation correction
      - Long imaging times recommended to enhance counting statistics on Tl-201 rest imaging
    - Image processing
      - Match rest images to redistribution images using dedicated myocardial perfusion scintigraphy software

Artifacts and Quality Control

- F-18 FDG PET viability
  - Severe type-II diabetes mellitus
    - Can have no F-18 FDG myocardial uptake despite insulin
    - Tl-201 preferred
  - Attenuation correction
    - Misregistration of attenuation map can cause artifactually increased or decreased counts
    - Attenuation correction recommended to decrease artifactual perfusion defects in inferior (diaphragm), anterior (breast) walls
  - SPECT perfusion
    - Overlapping bowel activity can add to counts in inferior wall, mimicking normal perfusion
- Tl-201 viability
  - Poor count statistics/artifacts due to obesity
    - Use attenuation correction
  - Movement during imaging
    - Motion correct or reimage
  - SPECT perfusion
    - Overlapping bowel activity can add to counts in inferior wall, mimicking normal perfusion
    - Attenuation correction recommended to decrease artifactual perfusion defects in inferior (diaphragm), anterior (breast) walls
  - Attenuation correction

- Misregistration of attenuation map can cause artifactually increased or decreased counts
  - Improper imaging time
    - Inadequate time for redistribution on Tl-201 imaging (image at both 4 and 24 hr after injection to increase sensitivity for viability)

DIFFERENTIAL DIAGNOSIS

Myocardial Hibernation

- Chronic myocardial dysfunction due to chronically decreased myocardial perfusion (chronic total occlusions)
- Regions of abnormal perfusion will show F-18 FDG utilization or redistribution on Tl-201

Myocardial Stunning

- Temporary myocardial dysfunction due to short-term underperfusion or lack of perfusion to myocardium
- Regions of abnormal perfusion will show F-18 FDG utilization or redistribution on Tl-201

Myocardial Infarction

- Myocardial necrosis and remodeling (scar)
- Regions of abnormal perfusion will show lack of F-18 FDG utilization or lack of redistribution on Tl-201

PATHOLOGY

Microscopic Features

- Myocardial viability requires
  - Sarcolemmal membrane integrity
  - Preserved metabolic activity
  - Adequate myocardial perfusion

CLINICAL ISSUES

Presentation

- Most common signs/symptoms
  - Heart failure
    - Regional &/or global wall motion abnormalities
    - Fatigue
    - Dyspnea
    - Physical activity limitations
  - Chronic total occlusions
    - Chest pain in up to 50%
    - ~ 12% heart failure

Demographics

- Age
  - 50-59 yrs: 8 per 1,000
  - 80-89 yrs: 66-79 per 1,000
- Epidemiology
  - USA: 5.1 million people have heart failure (2006)
  - Chronic total occlusions: 33-52% prevalence in patients with coronary artery disease

Natural History & Prognosis

- Patients with viable myocardium
  - Benefit from revascularization
  - If untreated, risk of cardiac death or nonfatal MI is increased
- Patients with nonviable myocardium
  - Increased morbidity and mortality with revascularization
- Viability testing most important in patients with heart failure
  - 50% of patients with heart failure: Death within 5 years
  - Revascularization: Decreases morbidity and mortality where viable myocardium is present

Treatment

- Revascularization with coronary artery bypass grafting
  - Older patients
  - Left main coronary artery disease
  - Diabetes mellitus
  - Triple vessel disease
- Revascularization with cardiac catheterization and percutaneous coronary intervention
  - Younger patients
  - Normal renal function
  - Lower risk coronary artery disease

DIAGNOSTIC CHECKLIST

Consider

- F-18 FDG PET viability
  - If no F-18 FDG activity in heart, consider improper patient preparation
- Tl-201 viability
  - Consider using Tl-201 in patients with severe type-II diabetes mellitus
    - Lack of F-18 FDG uptake can be due to severe insulin resistance
  - False-negative Tl-201 scans often due to imaging too early after tracer injection
    - If 4 hr images negative, repeat at 24 hrs
    - 24 hr images most sensitive
- CT attenuation correction for F-18 FDG PET/CT and SPECT/CT tracers to reduce soft tissue artifacts
  - Note that misregistration of attenuation map can cause artifacts as well

SELECTED REFERENCES

1. Society of Nuclear Medicine and Molecular Imaging. ASNC-SCCT-SNMMI Guideline for Cardiac SPECT/CT and PET/CT 1.0. http://snmmi.files.cms-plus.com/docs/ASNC_SCCT_SNMMI%20Guideline%20for%20Cardiac%20SPECT-CT%20and%20PET-CT.pdf. Created November 15, 2012. Accessed July 31, 2015
2. Society of Nuclear Medicine and Molecular Imaging. ACR-SNMMI-SPR Practice Guideline for the Performance of Cardiac Scintigraphy. http://snmmi.files.cms-plus.com/docs/Cardiac_Scintigraphy_1382731812393_3.pdf. Created October 1, 2009. Accessed July 31, 2015
3. Hoebers LP et al: Contemporary overview and clinical perspectives of chronic total occlusions. Nat Rev Cardiol. 11(8):458-69, 2014
4. Sogbein OO et al: New SPECT and PET radiopharmaceuticals for imaging cardiovascular disease. Biomed Res Int. 2014:942960, 2014
5. Arrighi JA et al: Multimodality imaging for assessment of myocardial viability: nuclear, echocardiography, MR, and CT. Curr Cardiol Rep. 14(2):234-43, 2012
6. Fefer P et al: Current perspectives on coronary chronic total occlusions: the Canadian Multicenter Chronic Total Occlusions Registry. J Am Coll Cardiol. 59(11):991-7, 2012
7. Strauss HW et al. Myocardial Perfusion Imaging 3.3. SNM, 2008

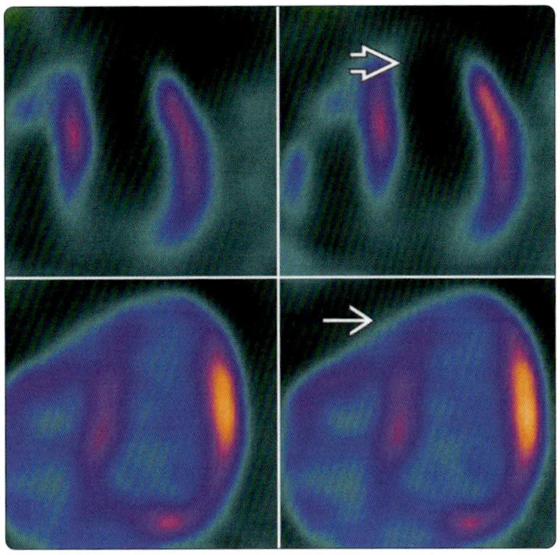

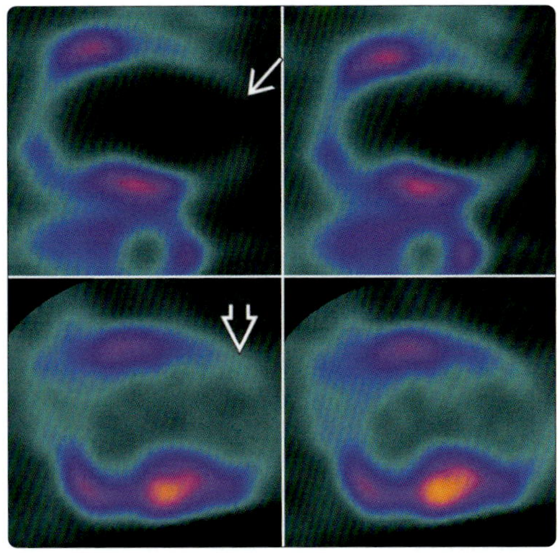

(Left) *Horizontal long axis F-18 FDG PET viability shows matched perfusion and glucose metabolism defects in the apex, signifying nonviable myocardial infarction.* **(Right)** *Vertical long axis F-18 FDG PET viability shows a large apical myocardial infarction that is not metabolizing glucose .*

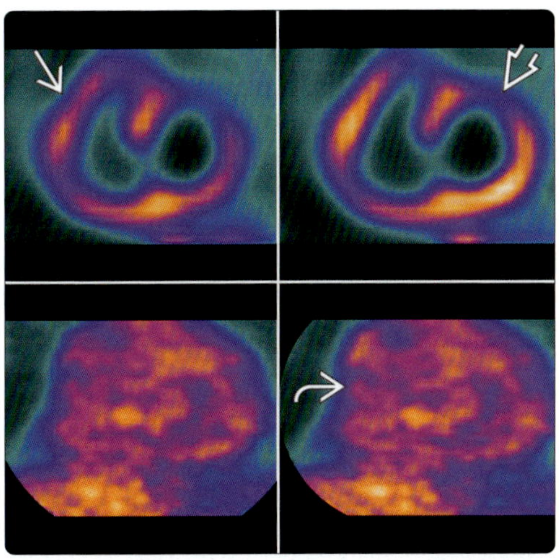

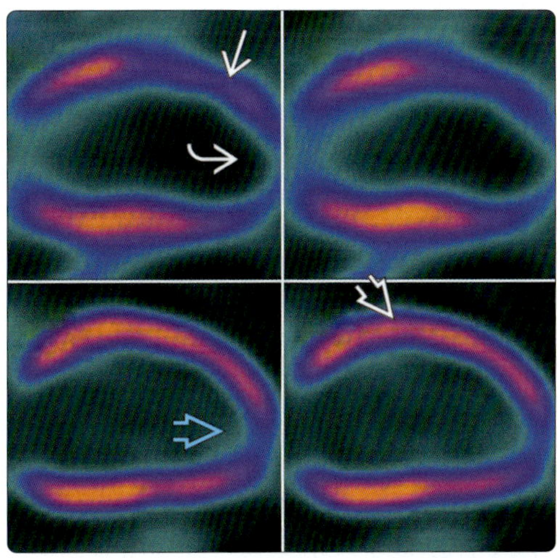

(Left) *Short axis F-18 FDG PET viability shows an enlarged right ventricle and an anterolateral perfusion defect . Note only blood pool activity , which may signify poor patient preparation or anterolateral nonviability. In highly insulin-resistant patients, the heart may not take up glucose despite viability.* **(Right)** *Vertical long axis F-18 FDG PET viability shows decreased anterior and apical perfusion. The anterior wall shows glucose metabolism, whereas the apex does not.*

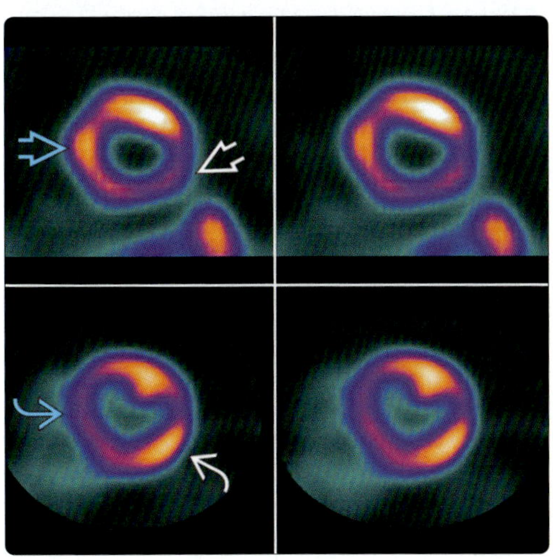

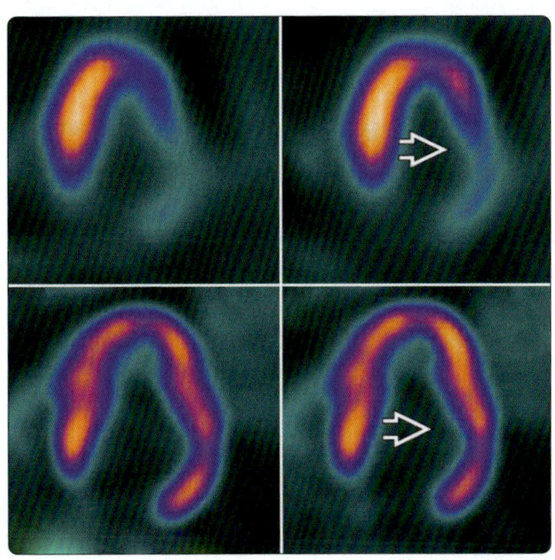

(Left) *Short axis F-18 FDG PET viability shows abnormal inferolateral perfusion with a high level of glucose metabolism , consistent with myocardial viability. Note the normal septum is not utilizing glucose but is still utilizing free fatty acids as an energy substrate.* **(Right)** *Horizontal long axis F-18 FDG PET viability shows viable, underperfused lateral wall .*

Right-to-Left Shunt

KEY FACTS

TERMINOLOGY

- Right-to-left shunt: Abnormal shunting of blood through cardiovascular and pulmonary system, bypassing the pulmonary capillary circulation
  - Can allow venous to arterial emboli, causing ischemia to multiple organs (e.g., brain, bowel)

IMAGING

- Tc-99m MAA pulmonary perfusion scan
  - Abnormal uptake within brain and kidneys confirms shunting of Tc-99m MAA administered intravenously
  - Tc-99m MAA should localize only in brain and kidneys with shunt
  - Must be differentiated from extrapulmonary uptake of free Tc-99m pertechnetate
    - Tc-99m can dissociate from MAA (resulting in free Tc-99m pertechnetate) due to lack of quality control in pharmacy and radiotracer handling
    - Free Tc-99m pertechnetate is also visualized in thyroid gland, salivary glands and gastric mucosa
  - Use reduced MAA particle count (100,000-200,000) in case of suspected shunt, pulmonary hypertension, pregnancy or pediatric patient
  - Can quantitate the degree of shunt if desired
    - Right-to-left shunt % = (total body counts - lung counts)/(total body counts x 100)

DIAGNOSTIC CHECKLIST

- Always scrutinize VQ scans for unexpected incidental uptake within brain or kidneys
- If uptake in kidneys, must look for brain or thyroid/salivary uptake
- Brain images: Most sensitive indicator of right-to-left shunt
- Nuclear medicine findings are not specific for location of shunt

(Left) *Anterior VQ scan shows normal uptake within lungs. There is no extrapulmonary uptake (brain or renal) to suggest a right-to-left shunt ➡.* **(Right)** *VQ scan shows expected uptake within the lungs on both anterior and posterior projections. Unexpected uptake within the kidneys bilaterally suggests either right-to-left shunt or free pertechnetate ➡.*

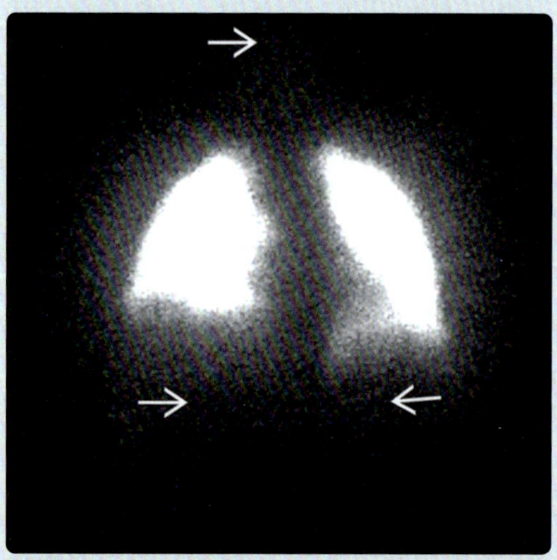

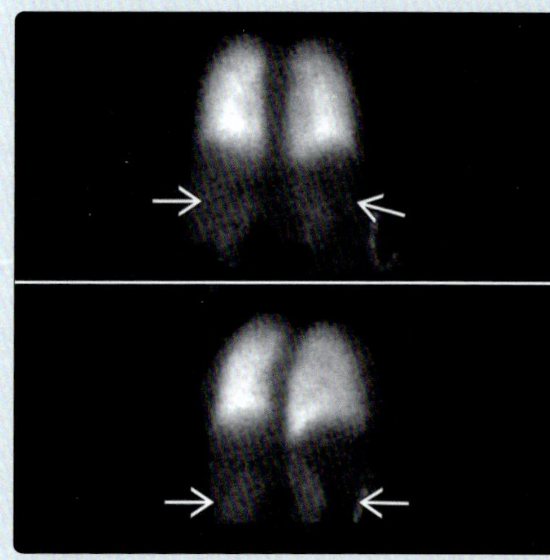

(Left) *VQ scan shows unexpected uptake within both brain ➡ and bilateral kidneys ➡ confirming presence of a right-to-left shunt.* **(Right)** *VQ scan shows unexpected uptake within both kidneys ➡ and thyroid tissue ➡ consistent with free pertechnetate rather than a right-to-left shunt.*

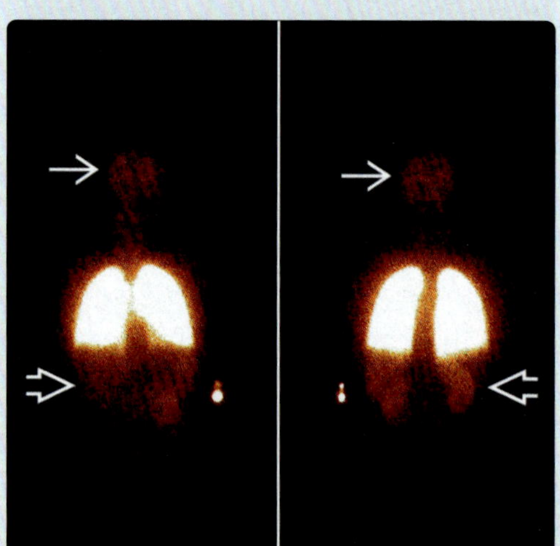

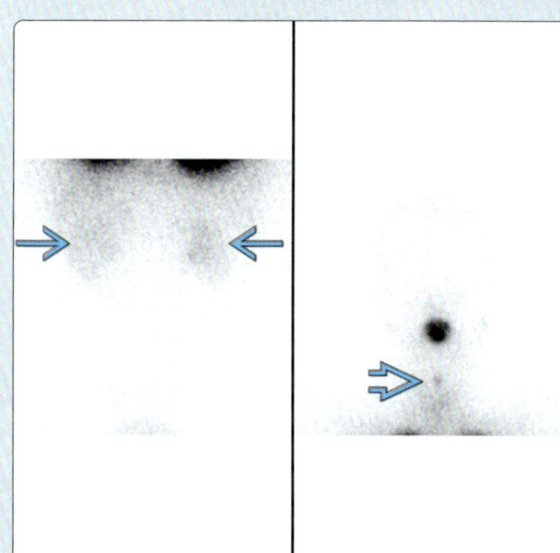

TERMINOLOGY

Definitions

- Right-to-left shunt: Abnormal shunting of blood through cardiovascular and pulmonary system, bypassing pulmonary capillary circulation
  - Can allow venous to arterial emboli, causing ischemia to multiple organs (e.g., brain, bowel)

IMAGING

Nuclear Medicine Findings

- Tc-99m MAA pulmonary perfusion scan
  - Abnormal uptake within brain and kidneys confirms shunting of Tc-99m MAA administered intravenously
    - Tc-99m MAA should localize only in brain and kidneys with shunt
  - Must be differentiated from extrapulmonary uptake of free Tc-99m pertechnetate
    - Tc-99m can dissociate from MAA (resulting in free Tc-99m pertechnetate) due to lack of quality control in pharmacy and radiotracer handling
    - Free Tc-99m pertechnetate is also visualized in thyroid gland, salivary glands, and gastric mucosa
  - May be incidental finding on V/Q scan for suspected pulmonary embolism

Protocol Advice

- Radiopharmaceutical
  - Tc-99m MAA
  - Use reduced MAA particle count (100,000-200,000) in case of suspected shunt, pulmonary hypertension, pregnancy, or pediatric patient
    - If shunt present, particles bypass pulmonary capillary bed initially and become trapped in brain/kidneys
    - Makes critical organs (brain, kidneys) at risk of unanticipated radiation exposure
  - IV injection in upper extremity sufficient
    - Can inject indwelling line but not through port or any filtered line because will filter out MAA particles
- Dose
  - Adults: 1-4 mCi (37-148 MBq) of Tc-99m MAA, ~ 200,000-700,000 particles
  - Children: 0.03 mCi/kg with minimum of 0.4 mCi
- Dosimetry
  - Adults: Largest radiation dose to lungs 0.067 mGy; effective dose 0.011 mSv
  - Pediatrics (5 year old): Largest radiation dose to lungs 0.21 mGy; effective dose 0.038 mSv
- Image acquisition
  - LEAP collimator
  - In addition to anterior/posterior planar images of lungs, posterior images of kidneys and anterior/posterior of brain
    - Brain images: Most sensitive indicator of right-to-left shunt
- Image processing
  - Can quantitate degree of shunt if desired
    - Right-to-left shunt % = (systemic counts/whole-body counts x 100%) = ([whole-body counts - lung counts]/whole- body counts) x 100%

DIFFERENTIAL DIAGNOSIS

Intracardiac Right-to-Left Shunts

- Adults
  - Atrial septal defect or patent foramen ovale
- Children
  - Atrial septal defect, patent foramen ovale, ventricular septal defect, or more complex congenital defects

Extracardiac Right-to-Left Shunts

- Pulmonary
  - Arteriovenous malformation (AVM)
    - Enlarge with time, most typically do not present until adulthood
    - May be single or multiple, simple or complex
      - Hereditary hemorrhagic telangiectasia (a.k.a. Osler-Weber-Rendu) syndrome: Multiple systemic AVMs
- Anomalous systemic venous return
  - Left superior vena cava (if communication with left atrium)

Acquired Shunts

- Hepatopulmonary syndrome (develop pulmonary AVMs)
- Post-traumatic/surgical

Free Tc-99m Pertechnetate

- Tc-99m pertechnetate can dissociate from MAA (resulting in free Tc-99m pertechnetate) due to lack of quality control in pharmacy and radiotracer handling
- Free Tc-99m pertechnetate also demonstrates uptake within kidneys
- Also shows uptake within thyroid &/or salivary glands, gastric mucosa

DIAGNOSTIC CHECKLIST

Image Interpretation Pearls

- Always scrutinize VQ scans for unexpected incidental uptake within brain or kidneys
- If uptake in kidneys, must look for brain or thyroid/salivary uptake
  - If brain uptake also noted, consistent with right-to-left shunt
  - If thyroid/salivary, gastric mucosa uptake also noted, free Tc-99m pertechnetate rather than shunt
- Nuclear medicine findings are not specific for location of shunt

SELECTED REFERENCES

1. Society of Nuclear Medicine and Molecular Imaging. SNMMI Procedure Standard for Lung Scintigraphy 4.0. http://snmmi.files.cms-plus.com/docs/Lung_Scintigraphy_V4_Final.pdf. Created July 19, 2011. Accessed July 31, 2015
2. Ito K et al: Cut-off value for normal versus abnormal right-to-left shunt percentages using (99m)Tc-macroaggregated albumin. Nucl Med Commun. 32(10):936-40, 2011
3. MacDonald A et al: Infrequently performed studies in nuclear medicine: Part 1. J Nucl Med Technol. 36(3):132-43; quiz 145, 2008
4. Graves MW et al: Scintigraphic diagnosis of a right to left shunt in end-stage lung disease. Respir Med. 97(5):549-54, 2003
5. Sugiyama M et al: Scintigraphic evaluation of small pulmonary right-to-left shunt and therapeutic effect in pulmonary arteriovenous malformation. Clin Nucl Med. 26(9):757-60, 2001

SECTION 2

Central Nervous System

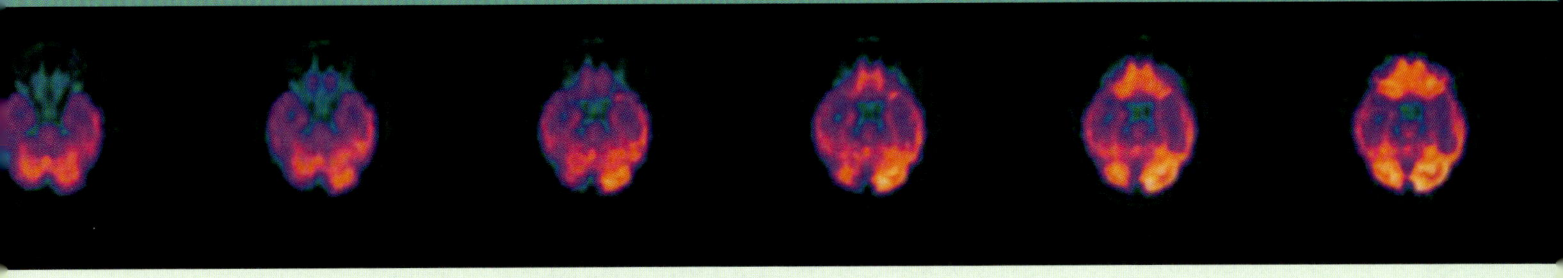

Introduction

Cerebrospinal Fluid

Dementia

Infection and Inflammation

Movement Disorders

Vascular

Introduction

Nuclear medicine central nervous system (CNS) scans continue to evolve, with applications in brain perfusion, metabolism, biomarker expression, and CSF flow. For example, in patients with mild cognitive impairment or dementia, a frontal- or posterior-predominant pattern on F-18 FDG PET/CT or Tc-99m HMPAO or ECD SPECT can direct medical therapy. Recent advances include imaging agents for molecular biomarkers of CNS disease, such as amyloid in Alzheimer disease or loss of dopamine transporter in Parkinson disease.

In patients with intractable seizures and nonlocalizing EEG, ictal and nonictal brain perfusion SPECT scans can be compared to find a seizure focus. Nuclear medicine physicians play an important role in analysis of seizure studies, often utilizing post-processing software for the most sensitive and specific analysis of this data. In one study of unilateral temporal lobe epilepsy and SPECT, correct lateralization with ictal SPECT occurred in 97% of patients.

Although brain death is a clinical diagnosis, confirmation of brain death with a nuclear brain perfusion study becomes necessary in the presence of confounding factors and is often useful for families when considering organ donation. As these situations often require, brain perfusion studies can be performed quickly at the bedside in the intensive care unit.

Nuclear CSF flow studies remain a valuable problem-solving tool in patients with symptoms of CSF shunt malfunction, CSF leak, and hydrocephalus, providing a sensitive imaging modality with whole-body imaging capability. In general, these studies provide additional sensitivity and specificity when compared to anatomic imaging alone.

MR and CT have for the most part replaced nuclear medicine for imaging brain tumors, ischemia, and vascular compromise. However, recognition of these patterns on nuclear CNS imaging remains useful to narrow differential diagnoses and problem-solve in complicated cases.

Dementia

Standard brain perfusion imaging studies use SPECT imaging in conjunction with Tc-99m HMPAO or Tc-99m ECD. These tracers are very similar and imaging can take place 45-90 minutes after injection. The patient's head can be restrained to avoid motion. F-18 FDG is a PET tracer that measures glucose metabolism in the brain and has largely surpassed SPECT for diagnosing an etiology for dementia. F-18 FDG requires patient preparation of fasting for 4-6 hours and no IV fluids that contain dextrose. Furthermore, patients need to be in a quiet, dark room with little noise in order to limit regional brain activation.

When evaluating patterns of dementia on F-18 FDG PET/CT or SPECT, it is important to keep in mind normal brain distribution of the radiotracer. For example, Alzheimer disease would show decreased activity in the posterior cingulate gyrus, precuneus, posterior temporal/parietal lobes, and, in later stages, the frontal lobes. However, there should be preservation of the basal ganglia, sensory motor strip, and occipital lobe. Given the better images obtained through PET imaging, F-18 FDG PET has largely overtaken SPECT for differentiating between different types of dementia.

The recent introduction of amyloid imaging into clinical practice allows physicians to directly evaluate for the presence of amyloid plaque in patients with dementia, a hallmark of Alzheimer disease. Amyloid PET imaging visualizes amyloid plaques following injection of F-18 florbetapir, F-18 flutemetamol, or F-18 florbetaben. In contrast to F-18 FDG, no fasting is necessary and blood glucose is not measured. All amyloid tracers are taken up in the white matter in normal and abnormal patients, but only patients with amyloid plaques have uptake in the gray matter. Hallmarks of a positive amyloid exam include loss of gray-white matter differentiation &/or focal gray matter uptake exceeding white matter uptake. Positive exams should be interpreted with caution because 10-20% of the cognitively normal elderly population is positive for amyloid plaques. Amyloid PET imaging can be used to definitively rule out Alzheimer disease in cognitively impaired patients.

Brain Death

Brain death studies typically use Tc-99m HMPAO or Tc-99m ECD to visualize perfusion in the brain. Lateral and anterior images are taken to visualize both the anterior and posterior fossa. Skull activity is often present and can be suppressed with a tourniquet. For determination of brain death, the findings either show activity in the brain or not. Complete absence of brain activity within the brain indicates no cerebral blood flow. Any activity within the calvarium means that there is some area of brain that is still perfusing and this would be negative for brain death. However, prognosis of these patients is often dismal, especially when only a small area of brain demonstrates perfusion.

Dopamine Transporter (DaT) Imaging

I-123 ioflupane (FP-CIT, DaTscan) measures the presence of dopamine transporter in the basal ganglia, which is decreased in Parkinson disease, atypical parkinsonism syndromes, or Lewy body disease. The radiotracer localizes to the dopamine transporters in the basal ganglia. Preparation includes blocking thyroid uptake with cold iodine (Lugol or SSKI). SPECT images are obtained 3-6 hours post tracer injection. Normal activity in the head of the caudate and putamen leads to a comma-shaped area of uptake on axial images. Loss of dopamine transporter in abnormal scans occurs preferentially in the putamen, resulting in a period-shaped area of uptake corresponding to the head of the caudate, with reduced or absent activity in the putamen. Caution must be taken to ensure patients are not on any medications that compete with the tracer and can artificially reduce normal activity in the basal ganglia.

CSF Flow Studies

Nuclear imaging is a sensitive modality for studying CSF flow and can be helpful to detect CSF leaks, evaluate a CSF shunt for patency, or to demonstrate normal pressure hydrocephalus. In all these studies, In-111 or Tc-99m diethylenetriamine pentaacetic acid (DTPA) is administered directly into the CSF. For shunt evaluation, tracer is injected into the shunt reservoir. For other CSF studies, tracer is injected into the spinal canal. Images are subsequently taken to evaluate CSF flow via normal tracks, or, in the case of a shunt study, drainage into the distal site, such as the peritoneal cavity, pleura, or atrium.

Selected References

1. Shivamurthy VK et al: Brain FDG PET and the diagnosis of dementia. AJR Am J Roentgenol. 204(1):W76-85, 2015
2. Nasrallah IM et al: Multimodality imaging of Alzheimer disease and other neurodegenerative dementias. J Nucl Med. 55(12):2003-11, 2014

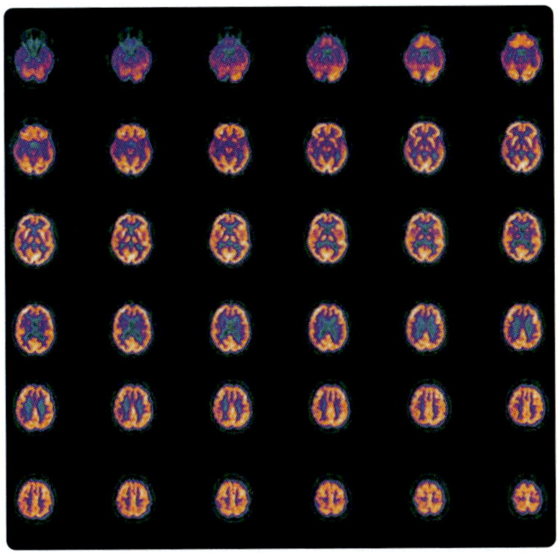

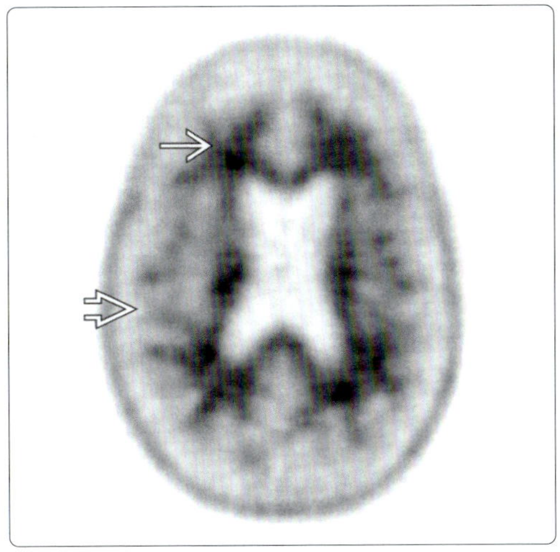

(Left) *Normal distribution of F-18 FDG PET demonstrates symmetric uptake in the brain without any hypometabolism in areas associated with dementia.* **(Right)** *Normal F-18 florbetapir PET shows physiologic white matter activity ➔ without significant uptake in the gray matter ➔, where amyloid plaques would be present in an abnormal study.*

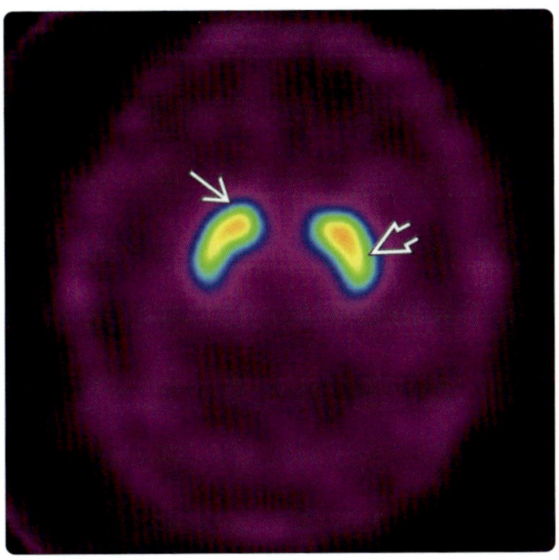

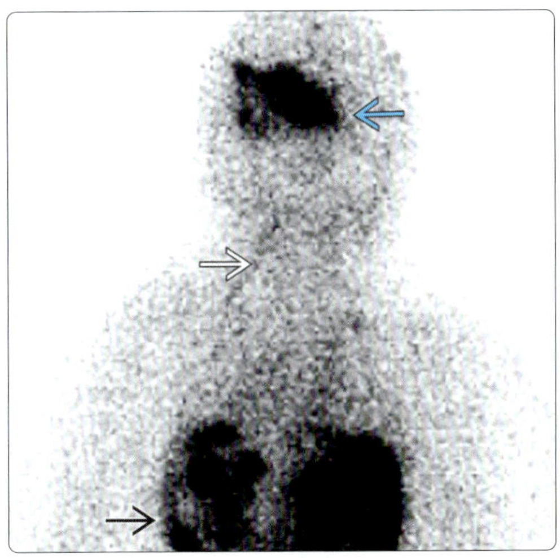

(Left) *Normal I-123 ioflupane SPECT demonstrates comma-shaped uptake that corresponds to the dopamine transporters located in the head of the caudate nucleus ➔ and putamen ➔. Abnormal images would have decreased or absent activity.* **(Right)** *Anterior Tc-99m DTPA ventriculoperitoneal shunt patency study shows a patent shunt. Activity is seen retrograde in the lateral ventricle ➔ as well as antegrade in the shunt tubing ➔ and peritoneal cavity ➔.*

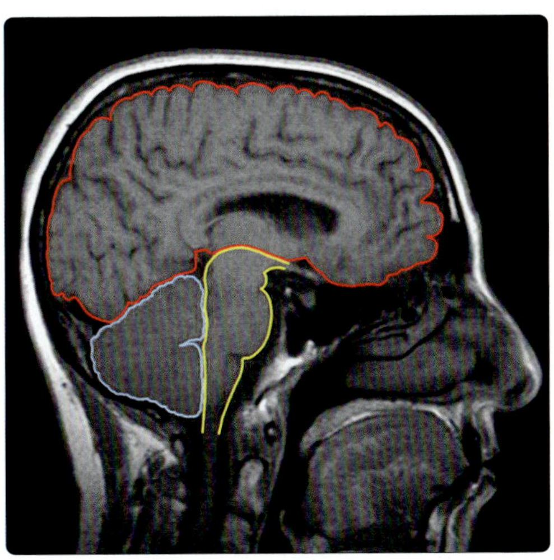

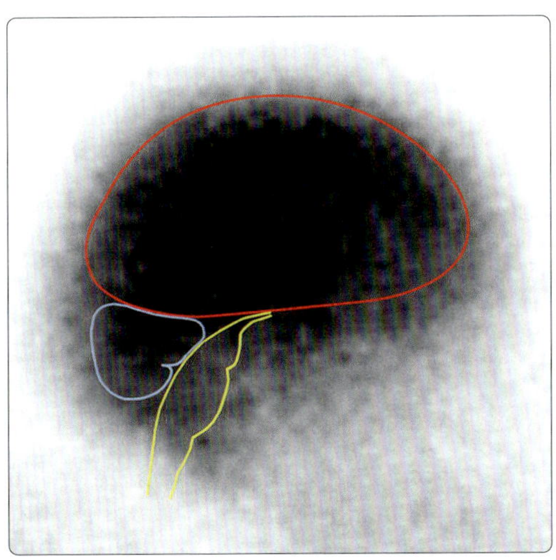

(Left) *Coronal MR demonstrates the cortex (red), cerebellum (blue), and brainstem (yellow). These areas should be completely devoid of tracer in an exam consistent with brain death.* **(Right)** *Lateral Tc-99m HMPAO brain perfusion scan shows gross approximation of where the cerebral cortex (red), cerebellar (blue), and brainstem (yellow) activity are located. This study shows normal brain perfusion.*

CSF Leak Evaluation

KEY FACTS

IMAGING

- Cerebrospinal fluid (CSF) outside expected location on radioisotope cisternography CSF imaging
  - Nose, nasopharynx, paranasal sinuses, temporal bone or ear, along spinal canal
- Imaging
  - In-111 or Tc-99m diethylenetriamine pentaacetic acid (DTPA) administered intrathecally
  - Gamma camera imaging to visualize leak at 2, 6, 12, and 24 hours after injection
  - Positive scan if activity outside expected location of CSF
  - SPECT may increase sensitivity
- Pledget analysis
  - Pledgets counted in gamma well counter in glass tubes
  - Pledgets with highest counts indicate possible leak site
  - Pledget counts considered positive if > 1.5x blood counts

PATHOLOGY

- Microscopic tears in dura
- Basilar skull fracture, paranasal sinus fracture

CLINICAL ISSUES

- Clear fluid in nose, nasopharynx, eustachian tube, temporal bone, ear, or along spinal canal
- Postural headaches exacerbated by sitting up
- Postural headaches relieved by lying down
- Lumbar puncture demonstrates low CSF pressure
- If no resolution in 1-2 weeks from conservative measures, invasive repair indicated

DIAGNOSTIC CHECKLIST

- If bladder or kidney visualized on radioiosotope CSF study, inadequate tracer injection due to dose extravasation
- Activity in stomach on radioisotope CSF study indicates rhinorrhea due to swallowing of leaked tracer
- Consider combining tracer with CT contrast and utilizing both nuclear imaging and CT cisternography

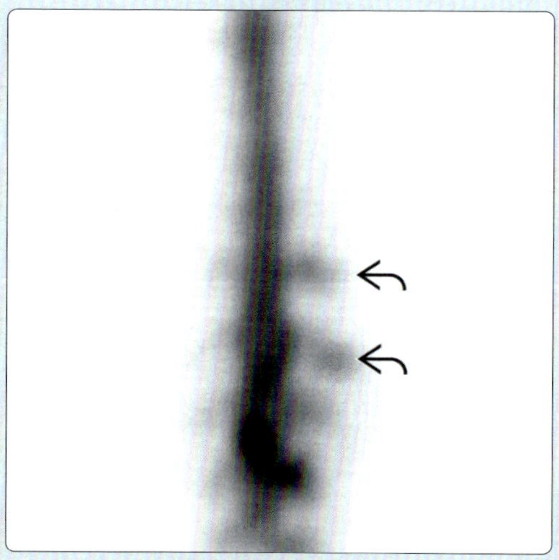
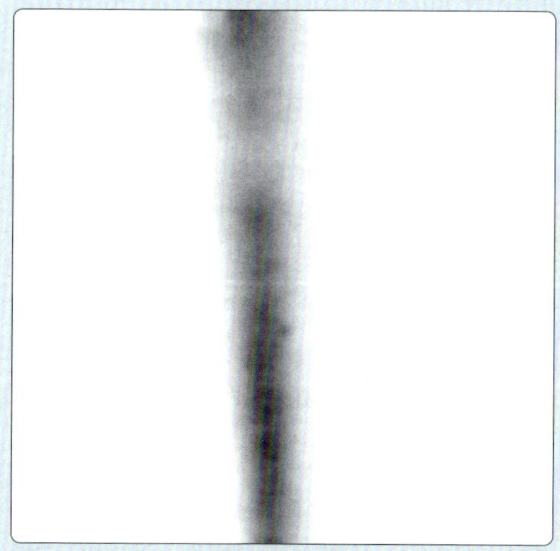

(Left) *Posterior Tc-99m DTPA cisternogram of the thoracic spine in a patient with headaches and low cerebrospinal fluid (CSF) pressure demonstrates tracer extravasation into extradural space, consistent with a dural tear.* **(Right)** *Similar posterior Tc-99m DTPA cisternogram in a patient with a negative scan demonstrates tracer confined to the dural space.*

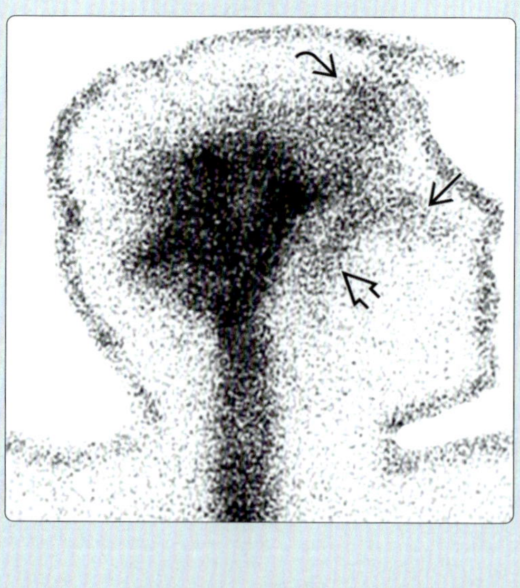
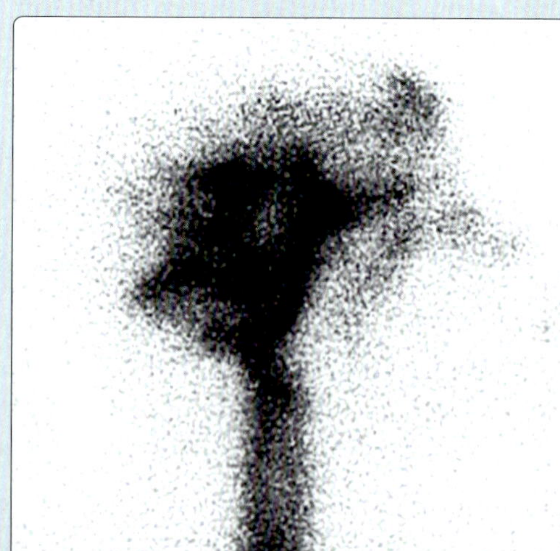

(Left) *Tc-99m DTPA cisternogram shows right lateral with surface anatomy drawn with point source. Cribriform plate leak results in activity in frontal sinus, nose, and nasopharynx.* **(Right)** *Tc-99m DTPA cisternogram shows the same patient but without surface anatomy map. Cribriform plate leak results in activity in frontal sinus, nose, and nasopharynx.*

TERMINOLOGY

Definitions

- Escape of cerebrospinal fluid (CSF) from normal CSF space
  - Post-traumatic, iatrogenic, congenital, or spontaneous
  - CSF rhinorrhea, CSF otorrhea, CSF otorhinorrhea, CSF fistula, rhinoliquorrhea, pseudomeningocele
  - Causes spontaneous intracranial hypotension (SIH), intracranial hypotension (IH), CSF hypovolemia

IMAGING

General Features

- Best diagnostic clue
  - Visualization of CSF outside expected location on radioisotope cisternography CSF imaging
    - Nose, nasopharynx, paranasal sinuses, temporal bone, ear, along spinal canal
    - Cribriform plate (most common site of traumatic CSF leak), ethmoid cells, frontal sinus, or frontoethmoidal complex
    - Varies from scant activity to profuse flow

Nuclear Medicine Findings

- Radioisotope cisternography CSF imaging
  - Highly specific
  - Nasal pledgets placed in nasal cavity and control pledget for lacrimal secretions placed under inferior nasal turbinate
  - In-111 or Tc-99m diethylenetriamine pentaacetic acid (DTPA) administered intrathecally
  - Gamma camera imaging to visualize leak at 2, 6, 12, and 24 hrs after injection of isotope
  - Pledgets scanned in glass tube during intervals
    - Pledgets with high count rates indicate possible leak site(s)
  - In positive study, radioactivity in pledgets significantly higher than level in concurrent blood sample
    - Nose or ear pack counts more sensitive than imaging
    - Pack counts considered positive if > 1.5x blood counts
    - Positive pack counts confirm leak despite negative images
  - Can be used to detect low volume or intermittent leaks
  - Positive scan if activity outside expected location of CSF

Imaging Recommendations

- Best imaging tool
  - In-111 DTPA radioisotope cisternography CSF imaging
    - Useful for serial images over time
    - CSF is labeled with ~ 0.5 mCi (18.5 MBq) In-111 DTPA by intrathecal injection
    - Tracer injection done carefully to avoid leakage of tracer out of injection site
    - Penetrate dura with needle bevel parallel to longitudinal plane of dural fibers
    - Keep patient in Trendelenburg for 5 min after tracer injection before removing needle
    - Mixing tracer with metrizamide prior to injection will cause metrizamide to act as transport vehicle, bringing tracer to potential leak site sooner for intracranial level leaks and facilitating combined nuclear and CT imaging
  - Tc-99m DTPA radioisotope cisternography CSF imaging
    - Useful for overpressure technique as imaging characteristics of Tc-99m better than In-111
    - Note: Off-label use for CSF imaging
  - CSF counting
    - Nose is packed and packs removed and counted
    - Packs should not be removed if possible until tracer is seen on images bathing area of clinical concern
    - Simultaneous blood sample should be drawn when nasal pledgets are removed to compare pledget count levels with blood levels of tracer
    - Pledget counts should classically be at least 1.5x blood levels to call positive
- Protocol advice
  - Patient preparation
    - Pledgets should be placed under direct visualization by ENT surgeon with consistent protocol
      - 6 nasal pledgets: 3 on each side at anterior, middle, and posterior locations or near superior meatus, middle meatus, and near cribriform plate
      - Pledgets should be clearly labeled
      - Ear pledgets should be placed if CSF otorrhea suspected
    - Tracer can be injected with normal pressure or CSF overpressure (injection of artificial CSF or Elliott's B solution)
    - Normal pressure technique: Leaked tracer appears more slowly; place pledgets after tracer reaches basal cisterns if possible
    - Overpressure technique: Leaked tracer appears quickly; place pledgets prior to tracer injection; imaging started earlier
      - Requires infusion pump, manometer (transient headache common)
      - Stop infusion if pressure > 500 cc H_2O or headache
  - Radiotracer
    - 0.5 mCi (18.5 MBq) In-111 DTPA by intrathecal injection
    - 1 mCi (37 MBq) sterile Tc-99m DTPA
  - Dosimetry
    - Spinal cord receives highest dose
  - Imaging protocol
    - Tracer can be injected alone or mixed with CT contrast for combined CT imaging and to aid in gravity flow
    - External radioactive markers or flood source aid anatomic orientation
    - Tracer monitored by preliminary images until bathes area of clinical concern, then images obtained
    - SPECT may ↑ sensitivity
    - With overpressure technique, imaging can be completed in < 1 hour
    - With normal pressure technique, imaging should start at 1-2 hrs, continue until 6-8 hrs or longer if necessary
    - Early and continuous imaging for spinal leaks
    - Medium-energy collimator if In-111 used
  - Pledget analysis
    - Pledget should be removed anterior, then middle, then posterior to avoid contaminating one pledget with another

- Venous blood sample drawn immediately before or after pledget removal, red cells sedimented by centrifugation
- 100 μL of serum counted in gamma well counter, along with pledgets (each in separate tube)
- Remove excess nasal mucus from surface of pledget prior to weighing and counting
- Weigh pledget before placement and before counting to establish fluid volume (1 g = 1 mL)
- Abnormal result: Counts in pledget > 1.5x counts in equal volume serum

DIFFERENTIAL DIAGNOSIS

Artifact

- Patient head motion during imaging
- Tracer contamination on patient's skin
- CSF rhinorrhea: Localization to particular side sometimes difficult since fluid can cross, flow from both nostrils

PATHOLOGY

General Features

- Etiology
  - Microscopic tears in dura
  - Basilar skull fracture, paranasal sinus fracture
  - Spontaneous, congenital, idiopathic
  - Complication of skull, sinus, or pituitary surgery
  - Complication of lumbar puncture
  - Postinfectious
  - Vigorous exercise or violent coughing, rupture of arachnoid diverticulum
- Genetics
  - 20% of spontaneous CSF leaks have minor skeletal features of Marfan syndrome
- Associated abnormalities
  - Subdural hematoma, connective tissue disorders, spina bifida

CLINICAL ISSUES

Presentation

- Most common signs/symptoms
  - Clear fluid observed in nose, nasopharynx, eustachian tube, temporal bone or ear, or along spinal canal
  - Reservoir sign
    - CSF leak accentuated by flexion of head
      - May indicate presence of fistula
  - Postural headaches exacerbated by sitting up
  - Postural headaches relieved by lying down
  - Lumbar puncture demonstrates low CSF pressure
- Other signs/symptoms
  - Lab tests of leaking fluid identify as CSF
  - Symptoms of meningitis, recurrent meningitis, encephalopathy
  - Conductive hearing loss, cranial nerve palsies, visual disturbances, anosmia
- Clinical profile
  - Onset of postural headache after surgery, trauma or lumbar puncture

Demographics

- Age
  - Peak: 30-40 years
- Gender
  - F:M = 2:1 for spontaneous CSF leaks
- Epidemiology
  - Risk factors for spontaneous leaks
    - Obesity, middle age, female

Natural History & Prognosis

- Can be intermittent or persistent
  - Traumatic
    - Usually resolves in 1 week
  - Nontraumatic
    - May persist for years
- Most leaks resolve spontaneously within several months
- Some leaks will persist
  - Continued symptoms include persistent headache, CSF hypotension, meningitis without repair
- Prognosis excellent, although deaths have been reported
  - Complications include pneumocephalus or meningitis

Treatment

- Conservative treatment
  - Bed rest
    - Head elevation, hydration
  - Avoid activity that increases pressure
    - Nose blowing, sneezing, coughing
    - Bowel movements: Stool softeners
- If no resolution in 1-2 weeks from conservative measures, invasive repair indicated
  - Lumbar drain or repeated lumbar puncture
  - Autologous blood patch/epidural blood patch (EBP) where blood clot used to seal leak
  - Endoscopic, intracranial, or extracranial repair depending on site, size, and nature of dural defect
- As an alternative to surgical therapy, fibrin sealant/glue can also be used to seal defect
- Epidural saline infusion

DIAGNOSTIC CHECKLIST

Consider

- Combining tracer with CT contrast and utilizing both nuclear imaging and CT cisternography
- Chemical, immunoelectrophoretic analysis of discharge
  - High glucose
  - β2-transferrin protein (most sensitive and specific)
  - β-trace protein

Image Interpretation Pearls

- If bladder or kidney visualized, inadequate tracer injection due to dose extravasation
- Activity in stomach indicates rhinorrhea due to swallowing of leaked tracer

SELECTED REFERENCES

1. Esposito F et al: Graded repair of cranial base defects and cerebrospinal fluid leaks in transsphenoidal surgery. Neurosurgery. 60(4 Suppl 2):295-303; discussion 303-4, 2007

CSF Leak Evaluation

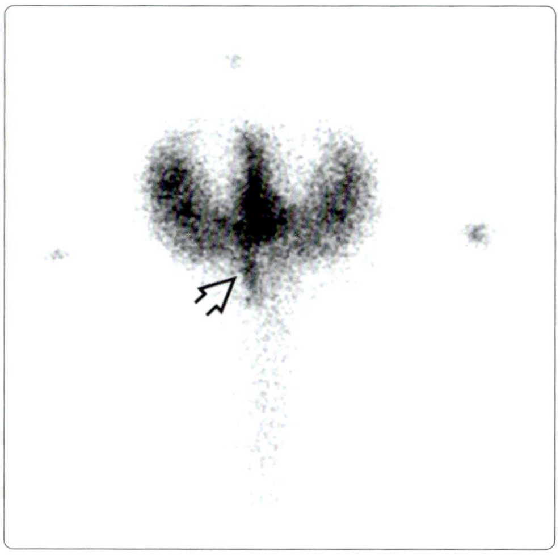

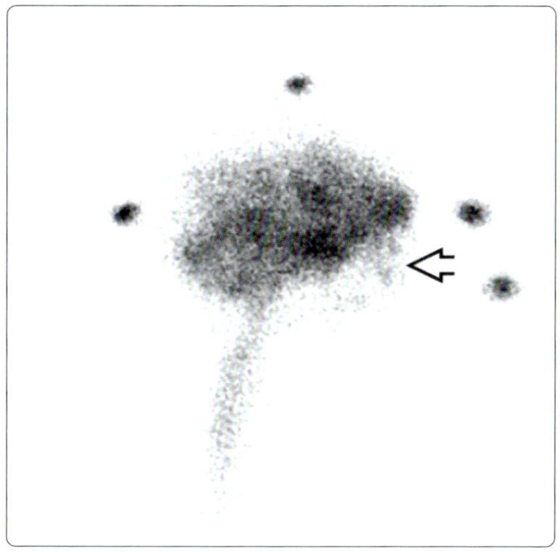

(Left) *Anterior CSF leak evaluation shows tracer extending below the skull base ⇨ into the right nasopharynx in this patient post sinus surgery.* **(Right)** *Right lateral CSF leak evaluation in the same patient shows the abnormal activity ⇨ below the skull base. Pledget counts were 500x plasma.*

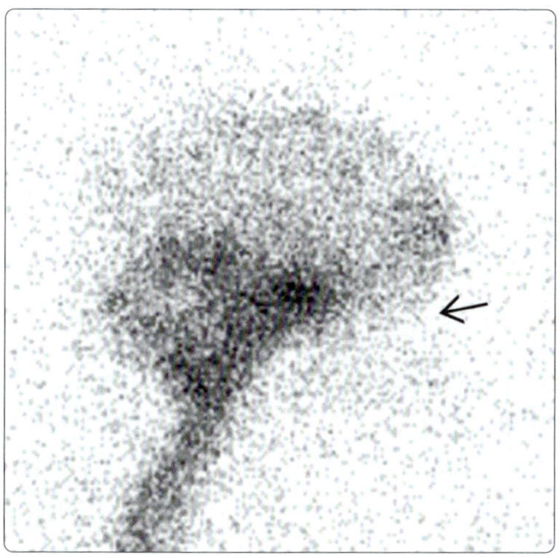

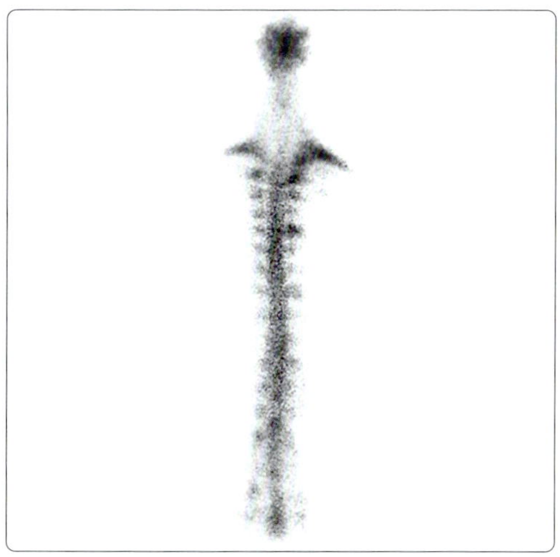

(Left) *Right lateral CSF leak evaluation shows no activity below the level of the skull base → despite pledget counts 200x greater than plasma. This is not uncommon.* **(Right)** *Posterior Tc-99m DTPA cisternogram in a patient with thoracolumbar dural tear and low CSF pressure shows extent of subarachnoid and extradural space. Site of such tears is difficult to find.*

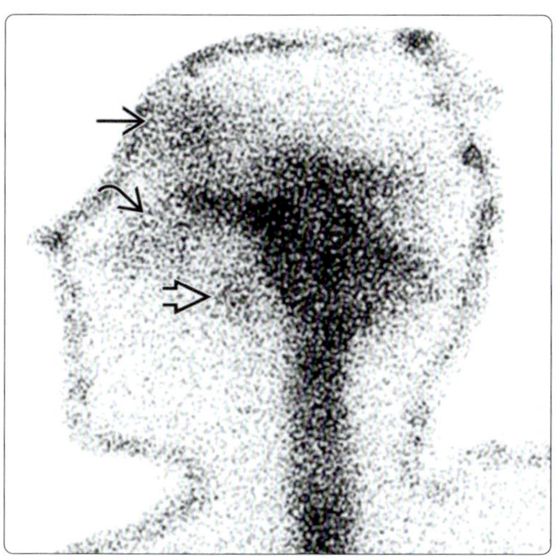

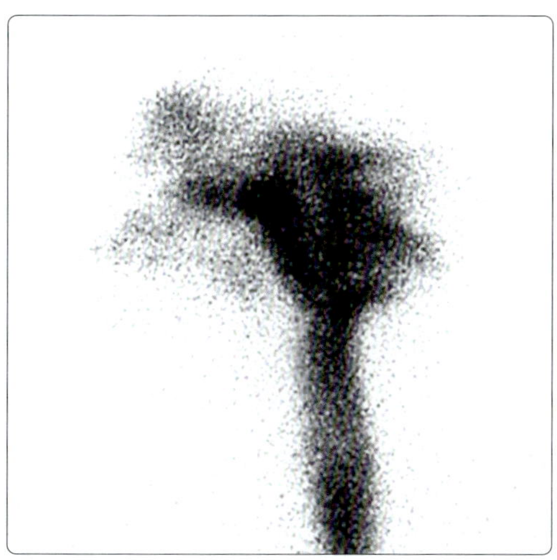

(Left) *Left lateral Tc-99m DTPA overpressure CSF study with surface anatomy shows leak from posterior frontal sinus resulting in activity in frontal sinus →, nose ↷, and pharynx ⇨.* **(Right)** *Left lateral CSF leak evaluation radionuclide of the same patient is shown without surface map.*

CSF Shunt Patency

KEY FACTS

IMAGING

- In-111 or Tc-99m DTPA ventricular shunt study
  - 25-gauge needle is used to puncture reservoir
  - 0.35 mL of patient CSF is aspirated into syringe containing radiotracer
  - Tracer and CSF flushed back into reservoir
  - While injecting, apply finger pressure on scalp overlying distal tubing to prevent forced injection of DTPA into distal tubing
  - Planar gamma camera images often sufficient
  - SPECT/CT to evaluate inconclusive findings
- Rapid passage of radiotracer through distal tip indicates shunt patency
- Clearance t1/2 from reservoir with patent distal shunt tip is usually 1-7.5 min
- For ventriculoperitoneal shunt, activity should diffuse freely throughout peritoneum and not be loculated

TOP DIFFERENTIAL DIAGNOSES

- **Shunt occlusion**
  - Proximal occlusion more common in children
  - Absence of ventricular reflux of radiotracer into ventricles after manual compression of tubing where it leaves reservoir suggests intracranial tip obstruction
  - Omentum can obstruct distal tip in ventriculoperitoneal shunts
  - Distal peritoneal catheter obstruction is more common in adults and leads to accumulation of CSF fluid near distal shunt tip
- **Shunt tubing**
  - Shunt tubing can become disconnected or kinked
  - Discontinuous tubing may still function due to epithelialization of track, reaching distal catheter site
  - If nonfunctioning, radiotracer activity will widen at area of discontinuity, will not reach distal catheter

(Left) *Lateral projection 5 min following injection of Tc-99m DTPA into the posterior shunt reservoir ➡ shows retrograde passage of radiotracer into the lateral ventricle ⮕.* **(Right)** *Ventriculoperitoneal (VP) shunt catheter is shown originating in the ventricle ➡ and connecting to the reservoir ➡ and valve ➡, which connects to the distal catheter which terminates in the peritoneum ➡.*

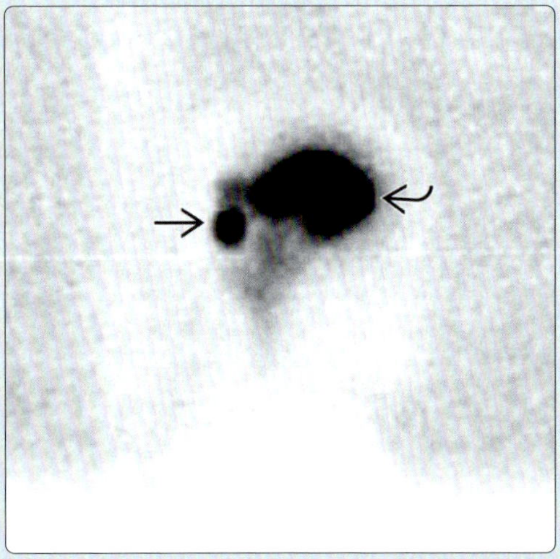

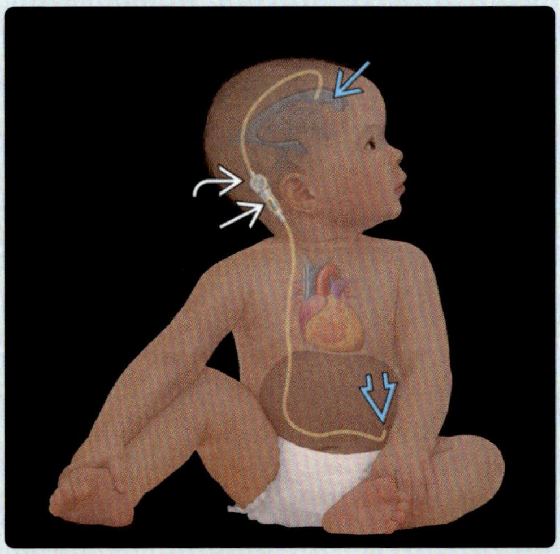

(Left) *Sagittal SPECT/CT demonstrates Tc-99m DTPA confined to the CSF space and lack of tracer outside, indicating shunt occlusion.* **(Right)** *Anterior planar image following injection of Tc-99m DTPA demonstrates a patent VP shunt. Activity is seen retrograde in the lateral ventricle ➡ as well as antegrade in the shunt tubing ➡ and peritoneal cavity ➡.*

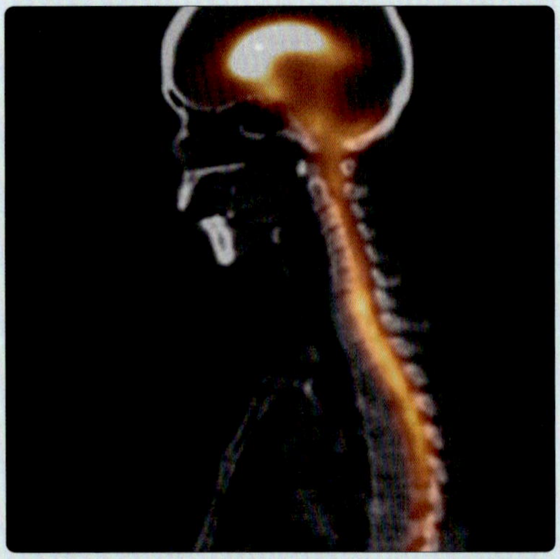

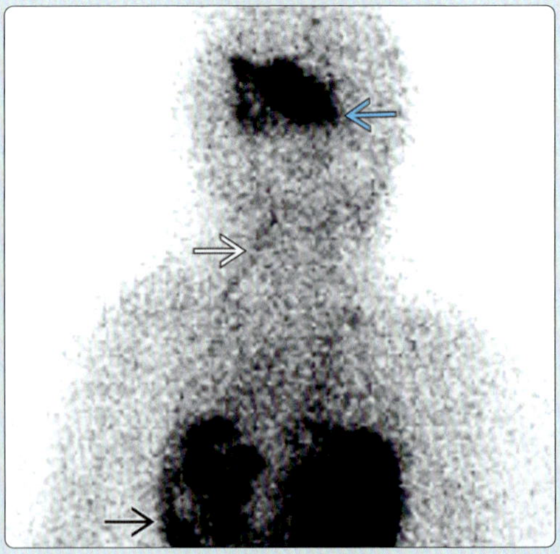

TERMINOLOGY

Definitions

- Cerebrospinal fluid (CSF) shunt: Surgically inserted drain that routes excess CSF in ventricles to a site where it is absorbed or collected
  - Proximal catheter is positioned in ventricular system
  - Reservoir with valve is located underneath scalp
  - Distal catheter ends in draining space
    - Ventriculoperitoneal (VP) shunt
      - Peritoneal cavity preferred since distal site has considerably better absorptive capacity and accessibility
    - Ventriculopleural (VPL) shunt
    - Ventriculoatrial (VA) shunt
- Endoscopic 3rd ventriculostomy
  - New alternative to shunting
  - Small opening in floor of 3rd ventricle allows free flow of intraventricular CSF into subarachnoid space
  - Used in patients with uncomplicated noncommunicating hydrocephalus caused by aqueductal stenosis or space-occupying lesions
  - Low infection risk
  - Symptoms gradually resolve (weeks to months)

IMAGING

Imaging Recommendations

- Best imaging tool
  - Screen with radiographs first to assess discontinuous shunt tubing
  - In-111 or Tc-99m DTPA ventricular shunt study
    - Rapid passage of radiotracer through distal tip indicates shunt patency
    - Clearance t1/2 from reservoir with patent distal shunt tip is usually 1-7.5 min
    - For ventriculoperitoneal shunt, activity should diffuse freely throughout peritoneum and not be loculated
    - Radionuclide study is superior to MR flow studies of shunt system
    - Exam has high sensitivity and specificity for shunt obstruction
- Protocol advice
  - Patient preparation
    - Patient supine
    - Sterile prep of shunt reservoir
  - Radiopharmaceutical
    - 0.5 mCi (18.5 MBq) sterile Tc-99m DTPA
    - 0.5 mCi (18.5 MBq) In-111 DTPA
    - 25-gauge needle is used to puncture reservoir
    - Opening pressures may be measured if clinically indicated
    - While injecting, apply finger pressure on scalp overlying distal tubing to prevent forced injection of DTPA into distal tubing
  - Image acquisition
    - Low-energy all-purpose collimator with Tc-99m DTPA or medium-energy collimator with In-111 DTPA
    - Serial planar anterior images usually taken at 1 min intervals for up to 20 min to monitor flow of CSF through shunt
      - Lateral images of head can also be obtained to visualize reflux into ventricles
      - Extend imaging to chest or abdomen, depending on location of distal shunt tip
    - Static abdominal images obtained after flow (up to 24 hrs) to assess diffusion of radionuclide material throughout abdominal cavity and rule out focal collection of fluid
    - SPECT/CT to evaluate inconclusive findings
    - Patient may sit up between images to simulate normal daily positioning for CSF flow

DIFFERENTIAL DIAGNOSIS

Shunt Occlusion

- Proximal occlusion more common in children
- Absence of ventricular reflux of radiotracer into ventricles after manual compression of tubing where it leaves reservoir suggests proximal tip obstruction
- Omentum can obstruct distal tip in ventriculoperitoneal shunts
- Distal peritoneal catheter obstruction is more common in adults and leads to accumulation of CSF fluid near distal shunt tip and may cause a peritoneal CSF pseudocyst

Shunt Tubing

- Tubing can become disconnected, migrate, or become kinked
  - Discontinuous tubing may still function due to epithelialization of track, reaching distal catheter site
  - If nonfunctioning, radiotracer activity will widen at area of discontinuity, will not reach distal catheter

CLINICAL ISSUES

Presentation

- Most common signs/symptoms
  - Acute shunt dysfunction
    - Headache, nausea, vomiting, irritability, seizures, lethargy, stupor, or coma
  - Chronic shunt dysfunction
    - Neuropsychological signs, increased head size, changes in feeding pattern, developmental delay, decline in mental status or level of consciousness, cranial nerve palsies, and bulging fontanelles

SELECTED REFERENCES

1. Nigim F et al: Shunting for hydrocephalus: analysis of techniques and failure patterns. J Surg Res. 191(1):140-7, 2014
2. Stone JJ et al: Revision rate of pediatric ventriculoperitoneal shunts after 15 years. J Neurosurg Pediatr. 11(1):15-9, 2013
3. Gonda DD et al: Ventriculoperitoneal shunting versus endoscopic third ventriculostomy in the treatment of patients with hydrocephalus related to metastasis. Surg Neurol Int. 3:97, 2012
4. Sivaganesan A et al: Neuroimaging of ventriculoperitoneal shunt complications in children. Pediatr Radiol. 42(9):1029-46, 2012
5. Kharkar S et al: Radionuclide shunt patency study for evaluation of suspected ventriculoperitoneal shunt malfunction in adults with normal pressure hydrocephalus. Neurosurgery. 64(5):909-16; discussion 916-8, 2009
6. Ouellette D et al: Additive value of nuclear medicine shuntograms to computed tomography for suspected cerebrospinal fluid shunt obstruction in the pediatric emergency department. Pediatr Emerg Care. 25(12):827-30, 2009
7. Vernet O et al: Radionuclide shuntogram: adjunct to manage hydrocephalic patients. J Nucl Med. 37(3):406-10, 1996
8. Estrada K: Notes on Nuclear Medicine Imaging (2008)

(Left) *Ventriculoatrial (VA) shunt catheter is shown originating in the ventricle and connecting to the reservoir and valve, which connects to the distal catheter which terminates in the atrium.* **(Right)** *Ventriculopleural (VPL) shunt catheter is shown originating in the ventricle and connecting to the reservoir and valve, which connects to the distal catheter which terminates in the pleural cavity.*

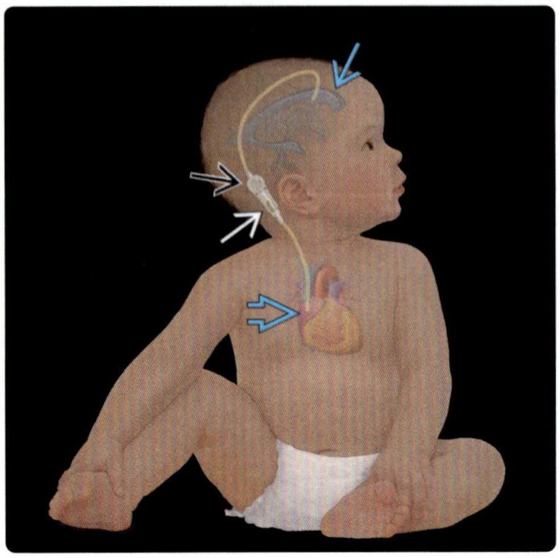

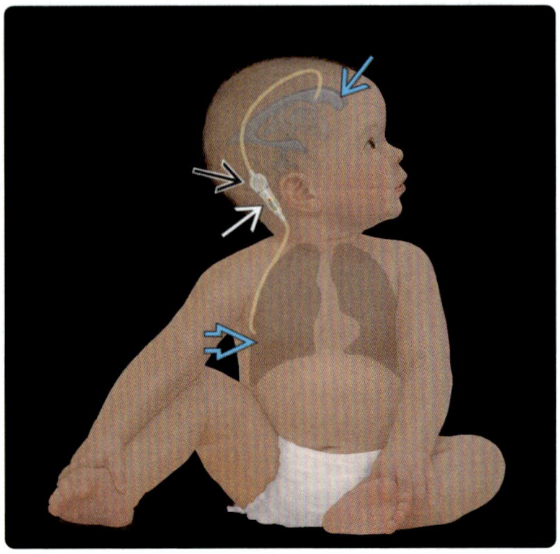

(Left) *Anterior planar image 45 min after Tc-99m DTPA injection shows tracer flowing freely into the shunt tubing and into the pleural space, indicating a patent VPL shunt.* **(Right)** *Anterior planar image 45 min after Tc-99m DTPA injection shows tracer flowing freely into the shunt tubing and into the peritoneal space, indicating a patent VP shunt.*

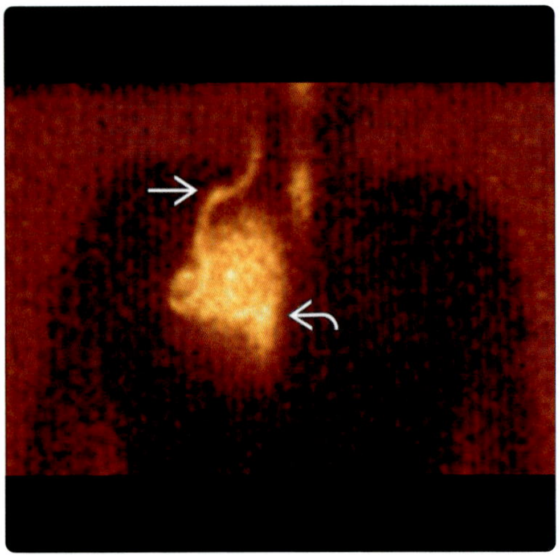

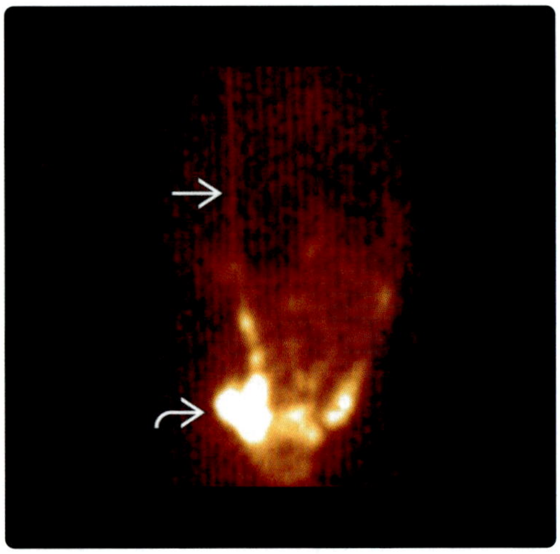

(Left) *Anterior planar image of the abdomen 4 hrs after Tc-99m DTPA injection shows tracer in the shunt tubing, but only a small amount is seen exiting the distal tip, indicating trapped fluid and compromised shunt flow.* **(Right)** *Lateral SPECT MIP 3 hrs after Tc-99m DTPA injection shows tracer confined to the CSF, indicating obstructed shunt.*

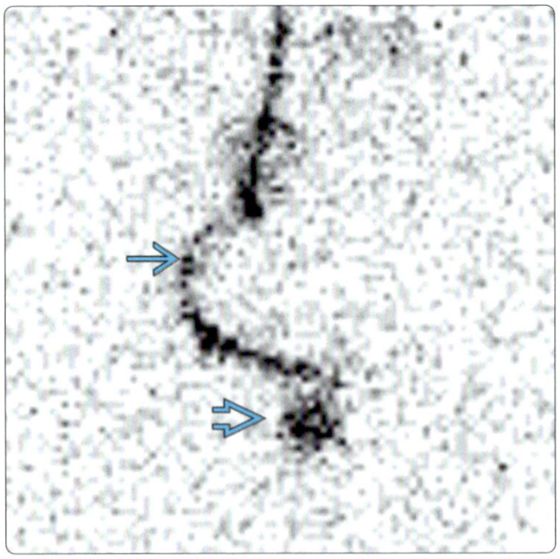

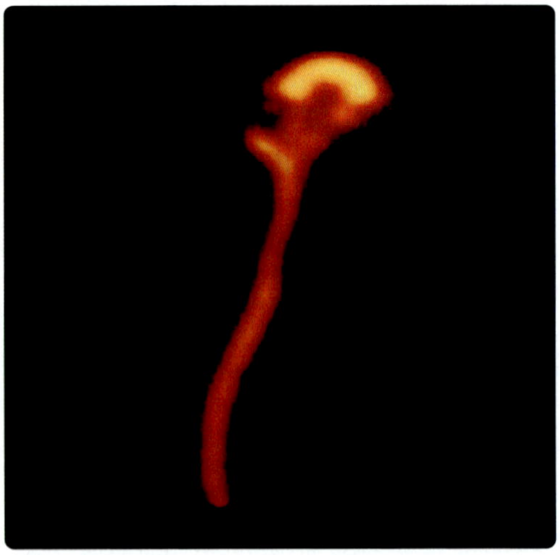

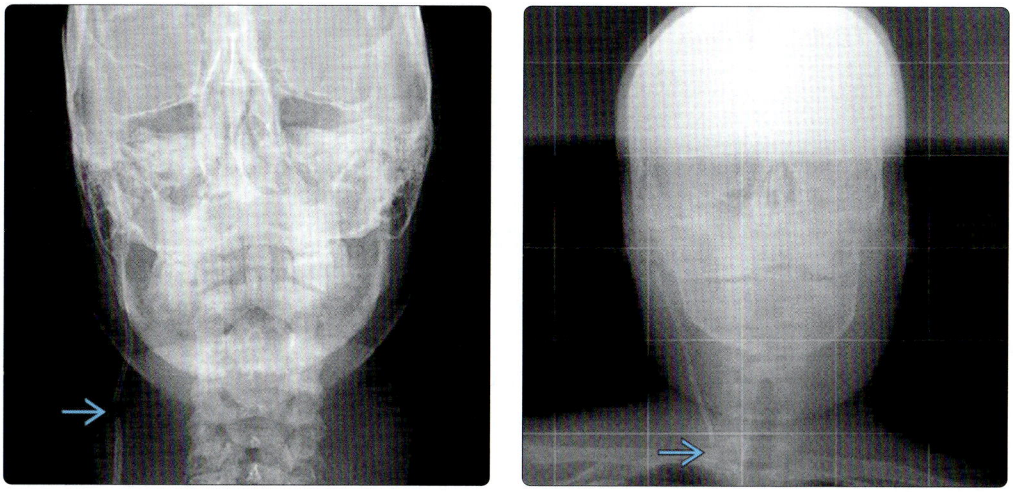

(Left) *AP skull radiograph demonstrates a discontinuity in the VP shunt catheter* ➔. **(Right)** *AP skull radiograph of a different patient also demonstrates a discontinuity in the VP shunt catheter* ➔.

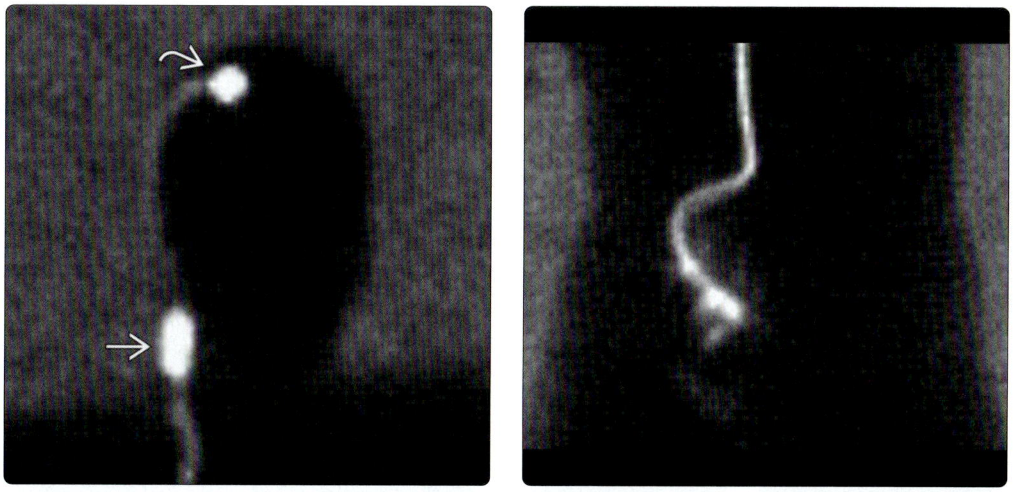

(Left) *Anterior shunt study after injection of tracer into the reservoir* ➔ *is shown. Tracer flows distally and widens at the area of the catheter discontinuity, but continues to flow inferiorly, indicating unobstructed flow* ➔. **(Right)** *Planar abdominal image 10 min after tracer injection in the same patient demonstrates unobstructed flow into peritoneal cavity. Later images demonstrated free tracer dissemination.*

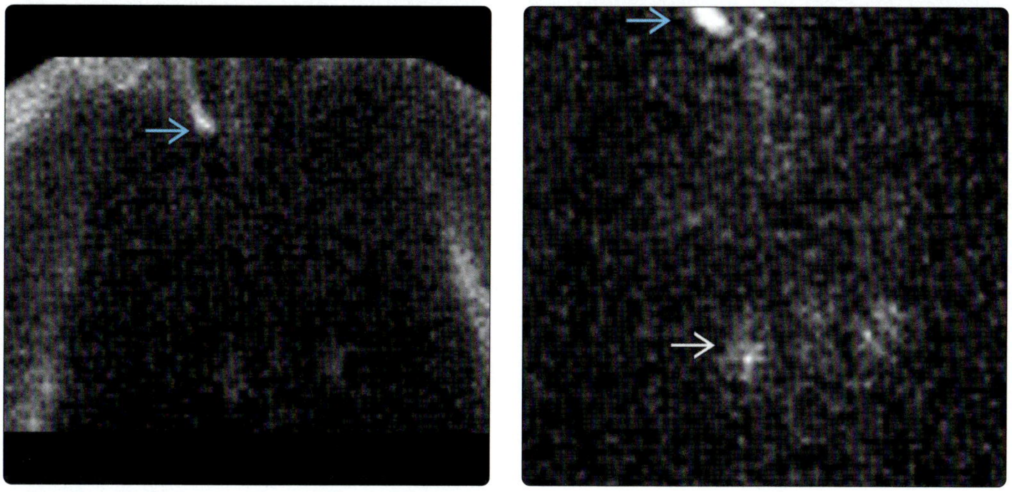

(Left) *Anterior shunt study in the same patient shows tracer abruptly ending at the area of the catheter discontinuity* ➔, *indicating obstructed flow.* **(Right)** *Planar abdominal image 60 min after tracer injection in the same patient demonstrates no tracer beyond the point of the catheter obstruction* ➔, *indicating obstruction. Slight activity is seen in kidneys* ➔ *secondary to reabsorption of tracer in the CNS.*

Normal Pressure Hydrocephalus

KEY FACTS

TERMINOLOGY

- Normal pressure hydrocephalus (NPH): Ventriculomegaly out of proportion to sulcal enlargement in setting of normal cerebrospinal fluid (CSF) pressure

IMAGING

- In-111 DTPA radionuclide cisternography
  - Used in patients in whom MR is contraindicated and CT is equivocal
  - Protocol
    - Intrathecal injection of In-111 DTPA
    - Obtain planar images with gamma camera immediately after injection and at 4, 24, and 48 hrs
  - Normal study
    - 1 hr: Radiotracer reaches basal cisterns
    - 2-6 hrs: Radiotracer reaches Sylvian fissures
    - 12 hrs: Radiotracer reaches cerebral convexities
    - 24 hrs: Radiotracer reaches superior sagittal sinus and is absorbed by arachnoid villi
    - Normally no radiotracer enters ventricles, although transient activity in ventricles at 4 hrs is still considered normal
  - NPH
    - Radiotracer activity in ventricles at ≥ 24 hrs
    - Absence of radiotracer activity in cerebral convexities by 24 hrs
  - SPECT/CT can help confirm ventricular activity

CLINICAL ISSUES

- Symptoms: Gait disturbance, urinary incontinence, dementia
- Treatment: Ventriculoperitoneal shunt

DIAGNOSTIC CHECKLIST

- Ventricular dilation on anatomic imaging may be solely due to cerebral atrophy
- Classic finding of NPH on radionuclide cisternography
  - Prominent ventricular activity at 24 hrs with absent activity over convexities

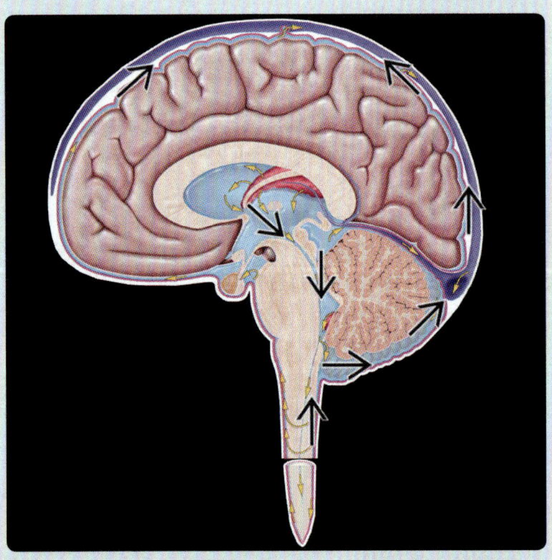

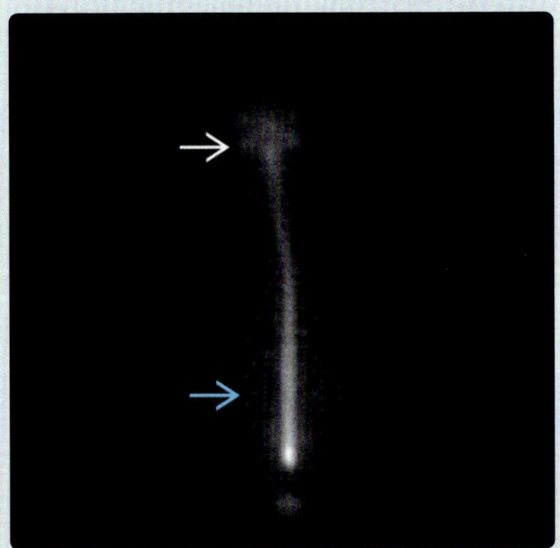

(Left) *Sagittal graphic of the brain shows CSF spaces in blue. Note direction of CSF flow from ventricular system to top of brain ⇨ where it is absorbed into venous system by arachnoid granulations.* **(Right)** *Posterior radionuclide cisternography in a normal patient immediately after lumbar puncture and injection of radiotracer confirms intrathecal placement ⇨. Basilar cisterns ➡ are evident.*

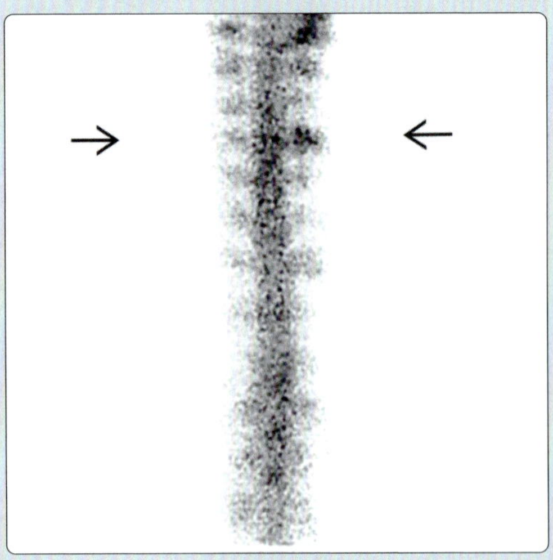

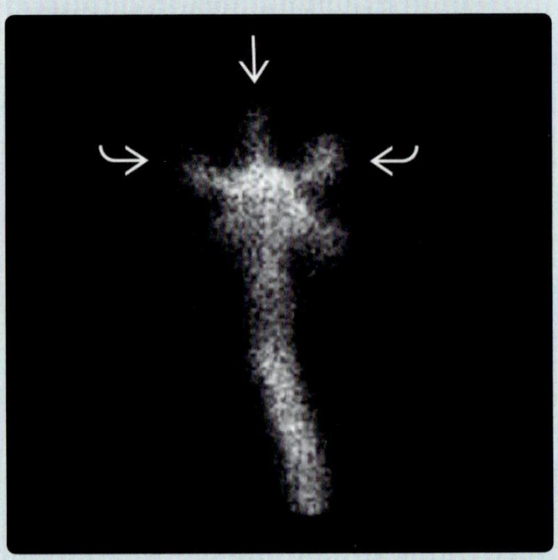

(Left) *Posterior radionuclide cisternography shows epidural injection of In-111 DTPA. Note the classic Christmas tree appearance ⇨ of radiotracer in the epidural space surrounding the thecal sac and spinal nerve roots.* **(Right)** *Anterior radionuclide cisternography at 4 hrs shows normal trident appearance of radiotracer in the anterior interhemispheric fissure ➡ and Sylvian fissures ➥.*

TERMINOLOGY

Abbreviations

- Normal pressure hydrocephalus (NPH)

Definitions

- Ventriculomegaly out of proportion to sulcal enlargement in setting of normal cerebrospinal fluid (CSF) pressure

IMAGING

Nuclear Medicine Findings

- In-111 DTPA radionuclide cisternography
  - Advantages
    - Provides physiologic information about CSF flow
    - Useful in patients who cannot receive MR or in whom CT is nondiagnostic (equivocal findings on CT)
    - May help determine who may benefit from ventriculoperitoneal (VP) shunt (controversial)
  - Disadvantages
    - Radiation
    - Time consuming
  - Normal study
    - 1 hr: Radiotracer reaches basal cisterns
    - 2-6 hrs: Radiotracer reaches Sylvian fissures
      - Trident sign: Activity in anterior interhemispheric fissure and Sylvian fissures resembles trident
    - 12 hrs: Radiotracer reaches cerebral convexities
    - 24 hrs: Radiotracer reaches superior sagittal sinus and is absorbed by arachnoid villi
    - No radiotracer activity should be seen in ventricles, although transient activity in ventricles at 4 hrs is still considered normal
  - NPH
    - 24-48 hrs: Ventricular activity is present and no activity is seen in cerebral convexities
      - Heart configuration: Appearance of radiotracer activity in lateral ventricles on anterior view
      - Comma (also c-shaped) configuration: Appearance of radiotracer activity in lateral ventricles on lateral views
      - Butterfly configuration: Appearance of radiotracer activity in lateral ventricles on posterior view
    - Radiotracer activity in lateral ventricles at 24 hrs or later is abnormal and consistent with diagnosis of NPH
    - Radiotracer activity not present in cerebral convexities by 24 hrs is abnormal and suggestive of NPH
  - CSF movement patterns on cisternography
    - Type I: Radiotracer activity in cerebral convexities at 24 hrs
      - Normal or noncommunicating hydrocephalus
    - Type II: Delayed activity in cerebral convexities at 24 hrs without ventricular activity
      - Cerebral atrophy or aging
    - Type IIIa: Radiotracer activity in cerebral convexities at 24 hrs with early transient ventricular activity
      - Indeterminate (can be seen with noncommunicating hydrocephalus, developing or resolving communicating hydrocephalus, or cerebral atrophy)
    - Type IIIb: No radiotracer activity in cerebral convexities at 24 hrs with early transient ventricular activity
      - Suggestive of NPH (communicating hydrocephalus)
    - Type IV: No radiotracer activity in cerebral convexities at 24 hrs with persistent ventricular activity
      - Suggestive of NPH (communicating hydrocephalus)

Other Modality Findings

- MR
  - First-line imaging to diagnose NPH
  - Findings include ventriculomegaly out of proportion to sulcal enlargement, hyperintense lesions in deep and periventricular white matter, and flow void in cerebral aqueduct
  - Contraindications include hardware incompatible with MR and claustrophobia
- CT
  - Shows ventriculomegaly out of proportion to sulcal enlargement

Imaging Recommendations

- Protocol advice
  - In-111 DTPA radionuclide cisternography
    - Radiopharmaceutical: In-111 diethylenetriaminepentaacetic acid (DTPA)
      - t1/2: 67 hrs (2.8 days)
      - Tc-99m DTPA not used due to short t1/2 and lack of FDA approval for intrathecal injection
      - keV: 173 and 247
      - Gamma emitter
      - Non-lipophilic
      - Not metabolized
      - Absorbed by arachnoid villi
    - Dosimetry
      - Spinal cord, brain, kidneys, bladder receive largest radiation dose
    - Patient preparation: Same as for any lumbar puncture (LP) except need radiotracer prepared ahead of time
    - Intrathecal injection of 0.5 mCi (18.5 MBq) In-111 DTPA
      - LP usually performed fluoroscopically by neuroradiologist and radiotracer injected by nuclear medicine physician
      - Need appropriate cleanup and disposal of equipment/trash due to radioactivity
      - Avoid contaminating patient's skin with radiotracer
    - Image acquisition
      - Planar &/or SPECT/CT with gamma camera
      - Low- or medium-energy, parallel hole collimator
      - Immediate anterior planar imaging to confirm intrathecal placement (bring portable gamma camera to LP suite or transport patient to nuclear medicine department)
      - 4, 24, and 48 hr planar images of head: Anterior, posterior, both laterals
      - 24 hr SPECT/CT images of head if ventricular activity equivocal on planar imaging

DIFFERENTIAL DIAGNOSIS

Alzheimer Dementia

- Ventriculomegaly with sulcal enlargement

- Small hippocampi
- Type II or IIIa CSF flow pattern on cisternography
- Dementia most pronounced clinical symptom

Normal Aging

- Type II CSF flow pattern on cisternography

Noncommunicating Hydrocephalus

- Type I CSF flow pattern on cisternography
- Usually diagnosed on MR

PATHOLOGY

General Features

- Etiology
  - Causes
    - Idiopathic (50%)
    - Secondary (50%)
      - Subarachnoid hemorrhage or subdural hematoma
      - Meningitis or encephalitis
      - Leptomeningeal carcinomatosis
      - Head trauma
      - Brain radiation
      - Neurosurgery
  - Pathophysiology
    - Impaired CSF resorption by arachnoid villi causes communicating hydrocephalus
    - Traditional theory: Increased resistance to CSF outflow
    - Newer theory: Increased pulsations in intracranial pressure has been suggested as potential mechanism
    - Dysfunctional CSF dynamics without increase in intracranial pressure

CLINICAL ISSUES

Presentation

- Most common signs/symptoms
  - Heterogeneous triad: Gait abnormality, urinary incontinence, dementia
    - All 3 present in only 10% of patients
    - Gait abnormality may manifest as magnetic gait, frontal ataxia, or gait apraxia
    - Urinary urgency usually precedes incontinence
    - Dementia usually manifests with frontal lobe symptoms such as apathy, lack of concentration and inattention, and psychomotor slowing
  - Symptom severity is related to CSF levels of neurofilament protein, a marker of neuronal degeneration
- Clinical profile
  - Reversible cause of dementia

Demographics

- Age
  - Most common in patients > 60 years of age
  - Idiopathic form of NPH tends to present in elderly
  - Secondary NPH can present at earlier age
- Gender
  - M = F

Natural History & Prognosis

- Natural course: Continuing cognitive and motor decline, akinetic mutism, and eventual death
- Potentially reversible cause of dementia when shunted, although gait symptoms are usually most predominant
- Some patients worsen after shunting

Treatment

- Ventricular shunt (most commonly ventriculoperitoneal)
  - Predictors of positive response to shunting
    - Patient < 75 years old
    - Early symptoms (mild gait abnormality and urinary urgency)
    - Known history of intracranial infection or bleeding (nonidiopathic NPH)
    - Gait abnormality as dominant clinical symptom
    - Absence of central atrophy or ischemia
    - Prominent CSF flow void
    - Response to CSF removal trial
- After shunt surgery
  - Variable outcome amongst studies, likely due to differing patient selection criteria

DIAGNOSTIC CHECKLIST

Consider

- Whether ventricular dilation is solely due to atrophy

Image Interpretation Pearls

- Classic finding of NPH on radionuclide cisternography
  - Prominent ventricular activity at 24 hrs with absent activity over convexities

SELECTED REFERENCES

1. Thut DP et al: ^{111}In-DTPA cisternography with SPECT/CT for the evaluation of normal pressure hydrocephalus. J Nucl Med Technol. 42(1):70-4, 2014
2. Ghosh S et al: Diagnosis and prognosis in idiopathic normal pressure hydrocephalus. Am J Alzheimers Dis Other Demen. 29(7):583-9, 2014
3. Virhammar J et al: Preoperative prognostic value of MRI findings in 108 patients with idiopathic normal pressure hydrocephalus. AJNR Am J Neuroradiol. 35(12):2311-8, 2014
4. Ziessman HA et al: Nuclear Medicine: The Requisites. 4th edition. Saunders; 2014
5. Qvarlander S et al: Pulsatility in CSF dynamics: pathophysiology of idiopathic normal pressure hydrocephalus. J Neurol Neurosurg Psychiatry. 84(7):735-41, 2013
6. Williams MA et al: Diagnosis and management of idiopathic normal-pressure hydrocephalus. Neurol Clin Pract. 3(5):375-385, 2013
7. Mettler FA et al: Essentials of Nuclear Medicine Imaging. 6th edition. Saunders; 2012
8. Marmarou A et al: Diagnosis and management of idiopathic normal-pressure hydrocephalus: a prospective study in 151 patients. J Neurosurg. 102(6):987-97, 2005

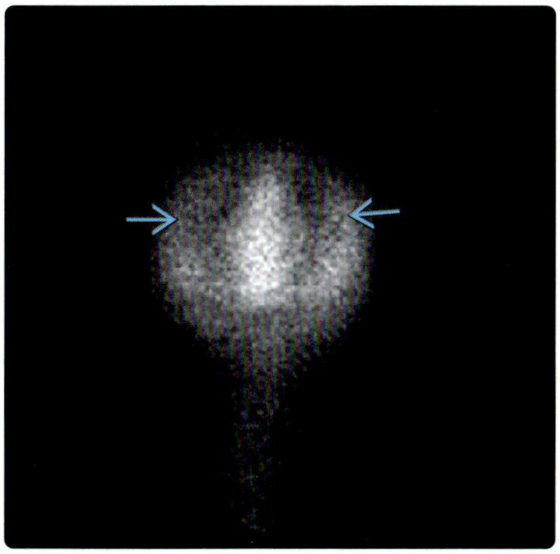

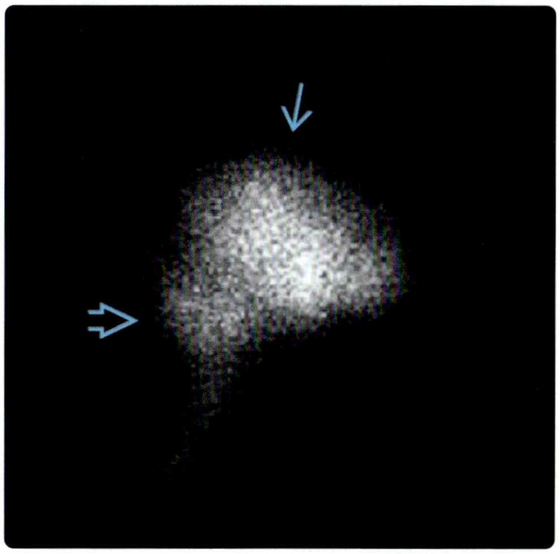

(Left) *Anterior radionuclide cisternography at 24 hrs demonstrates photopenia in the region of the lateral ventricles, a normal finding.* **(Right)** *Right lateral radionuclide cisternography at 24 hrs in a normal patient demonstrates no ventricular activity. Activity is present in the cerebral convexities as well as the suprasellar and basal cisterns.*

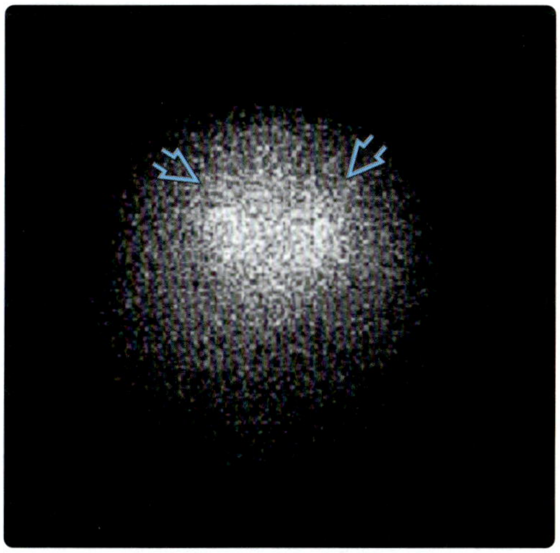

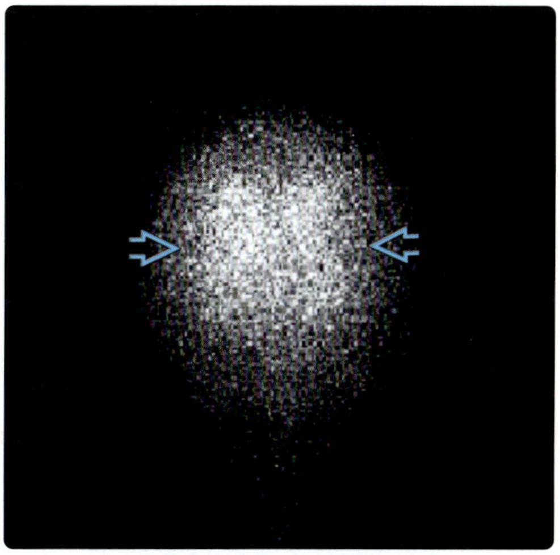

(Left) *Anterior radionuclide cisternography at 24 hrs in a patient with normal pressure hydrocephalus demonstrates activity in the lateral ventricles, showing a heart-shaped appearance.* **(Right)** *Posterior radionuclide cisternography at 24 hrs in a patient with normal pressure hydrocephalus at demonstrates activity in the lateral ventricles, giving them a butterfly-shaped appearance.*

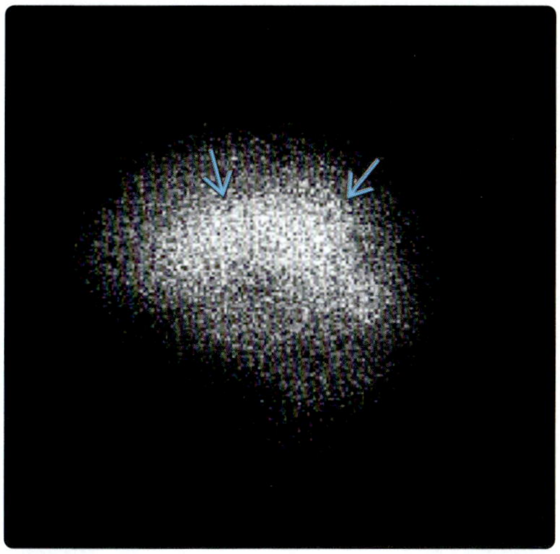

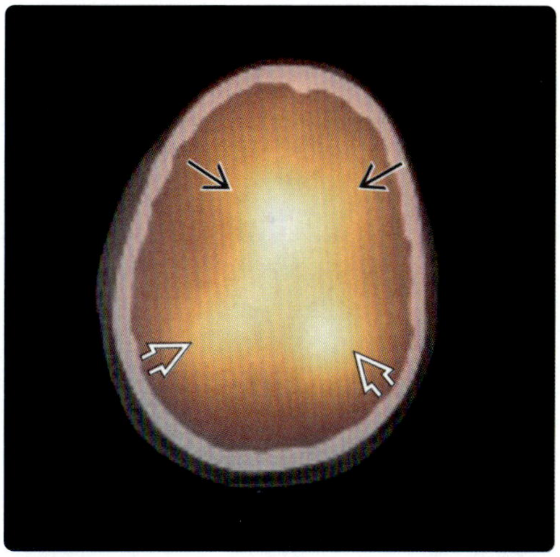

(Left) *Left lateral radionuclide cisternography at 24 hrs in a patient with normal pressure hydrocephalus demonstrates activity in the lateral ventricles, which have a "C" or comma-shaped appearance.* **(Right)** *Axial radionuclide cisternography SPECT/CT at 24 hrs in a patient with normal pressure hydrocephalus confirms activity in the lateral ventricles: Frontal horns and occipital horns.*

KEY FACTS

TERMINOLOGY

- Alzheimer disease (AD)
  - Progressive neurodegenerative disease of brain of unknown etiology generally characterized by impairments in episodic memory and other cognitive domains
  - Likely related to amyloid-beta (Aβ) and tau aggregation leading to synaptic dysfunction, neuronal/glial cell death

IMAGING

- Amyloid PET
  - Increased brain amyloid gray matter on PET is early biomarker in AD and appears prior to clinical symptoms
  - Absence of amyloid plaque rules out AD in patients with dementia
  - Positive amyloid PET scans do not in themselves diagnose AD and must be correlated with clinical symptoms
  - 10-20% of cognitively normal adult population has positive amyloid PET scans of uncertain significance
  - Decreased gray-white matter differentiation in at least 2 regions or single area of focally increased gray matter uptake are signs of positive florbetapir study
- F-18 FDG PET
  - Glucose hypometabolism in parietotemporal and posterior cingulate cortices; usually bilaterally symmetrical
  - Glucose hypometabolism continues to worsen with disease progression
- SPECT
  - 2nd-line study if PET is not available/reimbursed
- MR
  - Atrophy of medial temporal lobe structures (entorhinal cortex, hippocampus), visible as early as MCI

(Left) *Axial F-18 florbetapir PET in a patient with mild cognitive impairment (MCI) demonstrates homogeneous uptake throughout the brain, without clear distinction between gray ⇨ and white ➡ matter, consistent with heavy β-amyloid deposition in gray matter, which is seen in AD.* **(Right)** *Axial F-18 florbetapir PET demonstrates characteristic physiologic uptake in the white matter ➡, but no significant uptake in the gray matter ⇨. This clear distinction indicates no detectable amyloid deposition.*

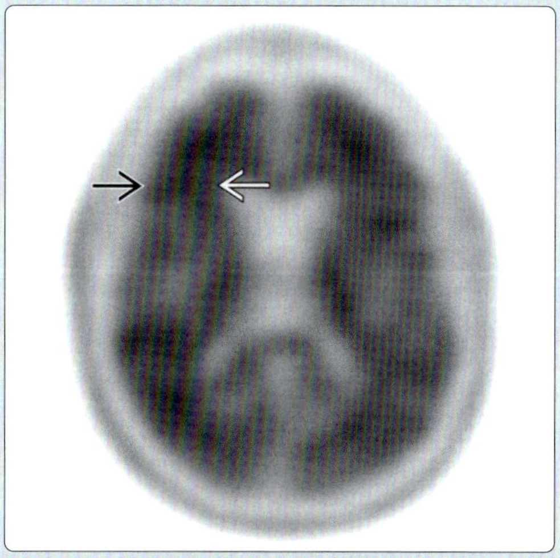

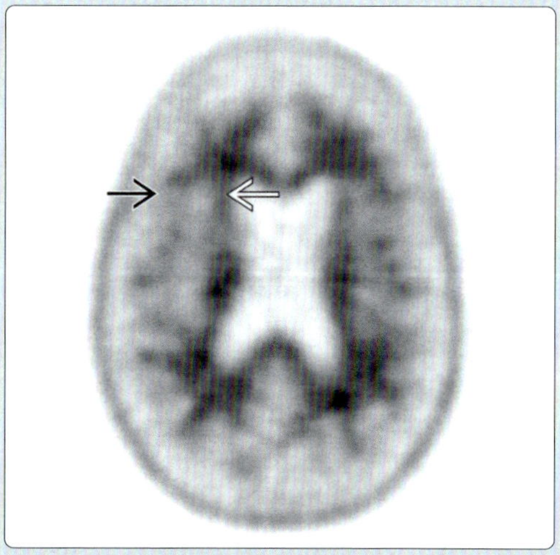

(Left) *Axial graphic at a similar level illustrates the presence of amyloid plaques in the cerebral gray matter ➡. These plaques bind tracer and make it difficult to distinguish between gray and white matter.* **(Right)** *In contrast, normal brain does not have amyloid plaques present in the gray matter ➡ and therefore only shows nonspecific white matter uptake on F-18 florbetapir PET.*

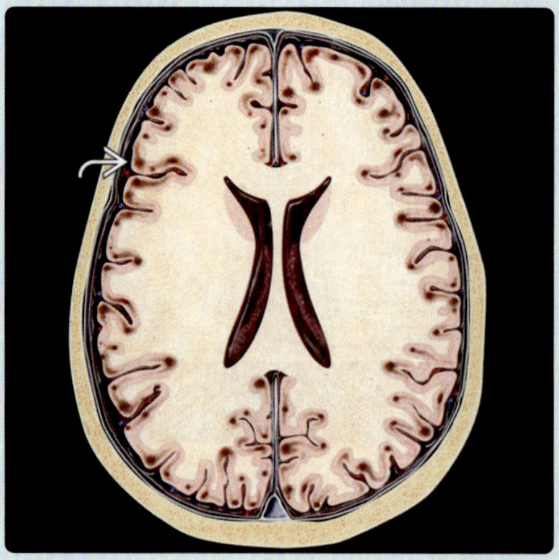

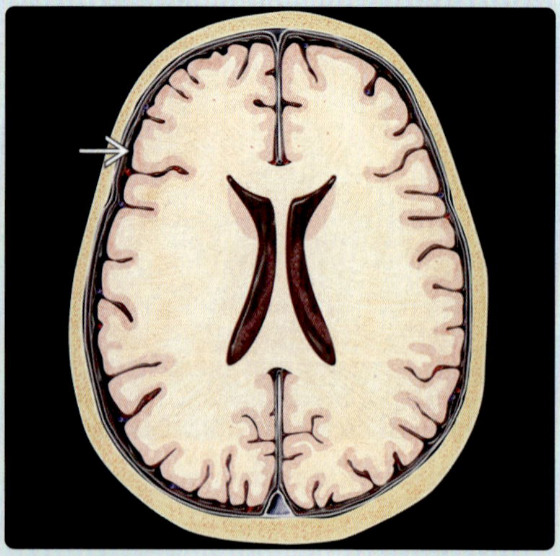

TERMINOLOGY

Definitions

- Alzheimer disease (AD)
  - Progressive neurodegenerative brain disease generally characterized by impairments in episodic memory and other cognitive domains
  - Likely related to amyloid-beta (Aβ) and tau aggregation leading to synaptic dysfunction, neuronal/glial cell death
  - Role of imaging
    - Early detection of preclinical AD
    - Diagnosis of AD with clinical presentation and other biomarkers
    - Differential diagnosis between AD and other causes of dementia

IMAGING

General Features

- Best diagnostic clue
  - Preclinical AD
    - Amyloid PET positive
    - Mild characteristic F-18 FDG PET hypometabolism in select areas
    - Early MR changes
  - Early AD
    - Amyloid PET positive
    - F-18 FDG PET and MR abnormalities become more evident
  - Late AD
    - Amyloid and F-18 FDG PET grossly positive
    - More extensive atrophy present (CT/MR)

Nuclear Medicine Findings

- Amyloid PET Imaging
  - F-18 florbetapir, flutemetamol, and florbetaben tracers are FDA approved
  - Increased brain amyloid in gray matter on PET
    - Early biomarker in AD, prior to clinical symptoms
    - Changes generally seen prior to F-18 FDG PET/MR abnormalities
  - Absence of amyloid plaque rules out AD in patients with dementia
  - Positive amyloid PET scans do not in themselves diagnose AD and must be correlated with clinical symptoms
  - 10-20% of cognitively normal adult population has positive amyloid PET scans (uncertain significance)
  - Interpretation of amyloid PET images
    - View in black-on-white background at high contrast levels
      - View axial images first
      - Coronal and sagittal views for confirmation of findings
    - Cerebellum gray-white differentiation is baseline for discerning normal gray matter from physiologic tracer retained in white matter
    - Signs of amyloid deposition
      - Decreasing cortical gray-white differentiation compared to cerebellar gray-white differentiation
      - Increasing gray matter uptake in temporal, parietal, and frontal cortices
      - Uptake in posterior cingulate gyrus and precuneus (may be early deposition sign)
      - F-18 florbetapir: Decreased gray-white matter differentiation in at least 2 regions or single area of focally increased gray matter uptake = positive
      - Occipital gray matter is less often amyloid positive
  - Artifacts and pitfalls
    - Severely diminished gray matter volume in AD patients may make abnormal exam appear normal due to contoured cortex
    - View fused PET/CT images as supplement to evaluate uptake relative to white and gray matter
    - Highest transaxial images above orbits often have diminished gray-white matter differentiation, even in normal patients
- F-18 FDG PET
  - General F-18 FDG uptake patterns
    - Mild cognitive impairment (MCI)
      - Medial temporal lobe hypometabolism: Most sensitive marker for predicting MCI
    - Early AD
      - Relative reduction in activity in parietal, temporal lobes and posterior cingulate gyri
      - Usually symmetric
      - Posterior cingulate cortex hypometabolism: Most sensitive marker for predicting MCI → AD
    - Early and advanced AD
      - Sparing of sensory motor cortex, basal ganglia, thalamus, primary visual cortex
    - Advanced AD
      - Progression of findings present in early AD
      - Usually symmetric
      - Frontal lobe hypometabolism
      - Moderate to severe atrophy
  - F-18 FDG PET most accurate when read in conjunction with quantitation software that compares F-18 FDG uptake in patient against uptake from normal database
  - SPECT with Tc-99m HMPAO or Tc-99m ECD has similar appearance as PET, but ↓ resolution and sensitivity

MR Findings

- T1WI, T2WI
  - Atrophy of medial temporal lobe structures (entorhinal cortex, hippocampus), visible as early as MCI
  - Rates of whole brain and hippocampal atrophy may be used to monitor progression of neurodegeneration
  - Often with coexisting microvascular disease and white matter hyperintensities

Imaging Recommendations

- Best imaging tool
  - Amyloid PET best for ruling out AD
  - Amyloid and F-18 FDG PET can help to differentiate between AD and other causes of dementia (frontotemporal dementia, Lewy body dementia)
  - PET may be used in early diagnosis of preclinical AD
  - Correlate imaging results with clinical picture and other biomarkers of AD
- Protocol advice

- Amyloid PET
  - Patient preparation
    - Patient needs to lie still for 20-30 min, so immobilization techniques may be necessary
  - Radiopharmaceutical
    - F-18 florbetapir (Amyvid)
    - F-18 flutemetamol (Vizamyl)
    - F-18 florbetaben (Neuraceq)
  - Dose: 10 mCi (370 MBq)
  - Dosimetry: Gallbladder wall receives highest dose, followed by intestines
  - Image acquisition
    - Depends largely on available PET scanner
    - CT typically used for attenuation correction; older PET scanners may use separate source (such as Ge-68/68-Ga) for transmission scan
    - Imaging begins 30-60 min after injection
    - 20-30 min static images typically done in clinical setting
    - Matrix: Transaxial 128 x 128 or 256 x 256
    - Pixel size: 2-4 mm
    - Filtered back projection or iterative reconstruction
- F-18 FDG PET
  - Patient preparation
    - Patient should fast, stop IV fluids containing dextrose, stop parenteral feeding for 4-6 hrs
    - Blood sugar should be < 150-200 mg/dL
    - Patient should be placed in quiet, dimly lit room prior to and after injection for 30 min
  - Radiopharmaceutical: F-18 FDG
  - Dose: 5-20 mCi (185-740 MBq)
  - Dosimetry: Urinary bladder receives largest dose
  - Image acquisition: 30-60 min after injection
- SPECT
  - 2nd-line study if PET is not available/reimbursed
  - Patient preparation
    - Place patient in quiet, dimly lit room prior to and after injection for 30 min
  - Radiopharmaceutical
    - Tc-99m exametazime (HMPAO)
    - Tc-99m bicisate (ethyl cystine dimer [ECD])
  - Dose: 15-30 mCi (555 MBq to 1.1 GBq)
  - Dosimetry
    - Tc-99m HMPAO: Kidneys receive highest dose
    - Tc-99m ECD: Bladder wall receives highest dose
  - Image acquisition
    - Optimal imaging time for Tc-99m HMPAO: 90 min post injection
    - Optimal imaging time for Tc-99m ECD: 45 min post injection

DIFFERENTIAL DIAGNOSIS

Vascular Dementia (Multi-Infarct Dementia)

- Impaired blood supply to brain regions
- 2nd most common cause of dementia
- Global atrophy with diffuse white matter lesions/infarcts that generally correlate with cognitive symptoms

AD Mixed Dementia

- AD and vascular dementia

Lewy Body Disease

- Commonly presents with hallucinations, sleep disturbances, and parkinsonian motor features
- F-18 FDG PET hypometabolism in occipital cortex distinguishes from AD

Frontotemporal Dementia

- Commonly presents with personality and behavioral changes
- Atrophy of frontal and anterior temporal lobes
- F-18 FDG PET hypometabolism primarily in frontal and anterior temporal lobes distinguishes from AD mixed dementia
- Composed of characteristic features of more than 1 type of dementia; commonly includes AD

Creutzfeldt-Jakob Disease

- Rapidly fatal, prion-related disease with impairments in cognition and behavioral changes
- MR DWI: Hyperintensity in striatum, cingulum, neocortex

Progressive Supranuclear Palsy

- Signs and symptoms of dementia, plus gait, balance and eye movement abnormalities

Corticobasal Degeneration

- Progressive disorder of nerve cell loss/atrophy (cerebral cortex and basal ganglia)
- Cognitive dysfunction and movement disorders

Causes of Reversible Dementia

- Normal pressure hydrocephalus
- Hypothyroidism
- Infections: Neurosyphilis, HIV
- Trauma (e.g., chronic subdural hematoma)
- Tumor, other mass lesions
- Depression
- Vitamin B12 deficiency

Other Neurodegenerative Disease

- Parkinson disease
- Huntington disease

PATHOLOGY

General Features

- Etiology
  - Most likely combination of genetic, lifestyle, and environmental factors
  - Probable role of Aβ and tau in pathogenesis
  - Accumulation of extracellular amyloid plaques contribute to disrupted synaptic communication and neuronal death
  - Accumulation of intracellular tau tangles contribute to disruption of nutrient and molecular transfer and neuronal death
- Genetics
  - Early-onset, familial AD
    - Single-gene mutation
      - Amyloid precursor protein (APP) gene on chromosome 21
      - Presenilin 1 (*PSEN1*) gene on chromosome 14
      - Presenilin 2 (*PSEN2*) gene on chromosome 1

- Results in formation of abnormal proteins involved in APP
  - May contribute to production of harmful forms of Aβ and Aβ-related pathology
- Late-onset, sporadic AD
  - Significant risk is related to apolipoprotein E (ApoE) gene on chromosome 19
  - ApoE plays role in cholesterol transport and Aβ maintenance
  - ApoE exists as 3 alleles (e2, e3, e4) with each individual carrying 2 copies
  - ApoE-e4 allele is present in 20-30% of USA population and confers increased risk for AD development
  - 40-65% of individuals with AD carry at least 1 copy of e4 allele

CLINICAL ISSUES

Presentation

- Most common signs/symptoms
  - Significant impairment in memory and cognition
  - Mood and personality changes
- Clinical profile
  - Preclinical AD
    - Amyloid PET turns positive during this period
    - No noticeable symptoms of AD with early AD brain changes (up to 20 years before symptoms)
  - MCI due to AD
    - Change in cognition within 1 or more cognitive domains with functional independence intact
  - Possible AD
    - Significant cognitive/behavioral symptoms
      - Must represent change from prior status
      - Must interfere with functional ability
      - In presence of sudden onset &/or another disorder that could cause similar symptoms, like cerebrovascular disease
  - Probable AD
    - Insidious change of cognitive/behavioral symptoms that interferes with functional ability
      - Not in presence of another disorder that could cause similar symptoms
  - Visual variant of AD
    - Impaired visuospatial skills without memory complaints

Demographics

- Epidemiology
  - Estimated 5.2 million Americans affected by AD
  - Most common cause of dementia (60-80% of cases)
  - Prevalence
    - ~ 11% of adults ≥ 65 years
    - ~ 32% of adults ≥ 85 years

Treatment

- No current disease-modifying treatment for AD
- Cholinesterase inhibitors may delay worsening of cognitive symptoms for 6-12 months
- NMDA inhibitors may temporarily delay worsening of symptoms

DIAGNOSTIC CHECKLIST

Key Imaging Findings

- Preclinical AD
  - Amyloid PET positive
  - F-18 FDG PET hypometabolism
  - Early MR changes
- Early AD
  - PET/MR abnormalities become more evident
- Late AD
  - F-18 FDG and amyloid PET grossly positive
  - More extensive atrophy present on CT/MR

SELECTED REFERENCES

1. Thies W et al: 2013 Alzheimer's disease facts and figures. Alzheimers Dement. 9(2):208-45, 2013
2. Hyman BT et al: National Institute on Aging-Alzheimer's Association guidelines for the neuropathologic assessment of Alzheimer's disease. Alzheimers Dement. 8(1):1-13, 2012
3. Jack CR Jr: Alzheimer disease: new concepts on its neurobiology and the clinical role imaging will play. Radiology. 263(2):344-61, 2012
4. Herholz K et al: Clinical amyloid imaging in Alzheimer's disease. Lancet Neurol. 10(7):667-70, 2011
5. McKhann GM et al: The diagnosis of dementia due to Alzheimer's disease: recommendations from the National Institute on Aging-Alzheimer's Association workgroups on diagnostic guidelines for Alzheimer's disease. Alzheimers Dement. 7(3):263-9, 2011
6. Sperling RA et al: Toward defining the preclinical stages of Alzheimer's disease: recommendations from the National Institute on Aging-Alzheimer's Association workgroups on diagnostic guidelines for Alzheimer's disease. Alzheimers Dement. 7(3):280-92, 2011
7. Vitali P et al: Diffusion-weighted MRI hyperintensity patterns differentiate CJD from other rapid dementias. Neurology. 76(20):1711-9, 2011
8. Frisoni GB et al: The clinical use of structural MRI in Alzheimer disease. Nat Rev Neurol. 6(2):67-77, 2010

(Left) *Axial F-18 florbetapir PET in a patient with MCI demonstrates homogeneous uptake throughout the brain, without clear distinction between gray and white matter, consistent with heavy β-amyloid deposition in gray matter, which is seen in AD.* **(Right)** *Axial F-18 florbetapir PET shows uptake in the white matter but no significant uptake in the gray matter throughout, especially in the precuneus, indicating no detectable amyloid deposition.*

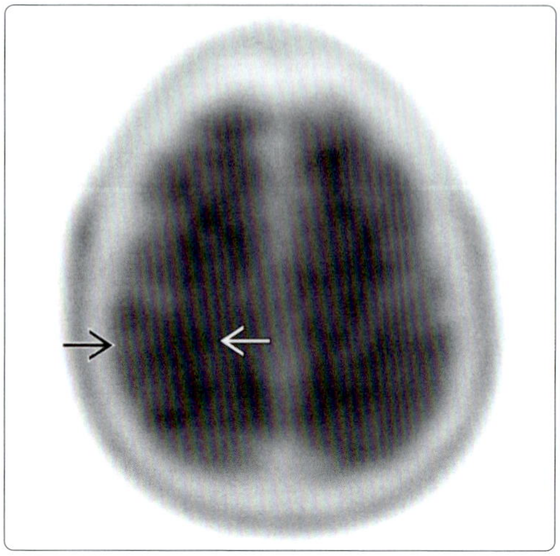

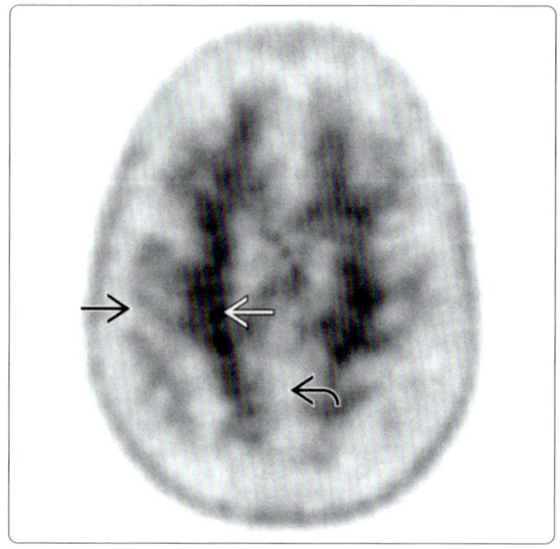

(Left) *More inferior axial F-18 florbetapir PET in the same patient shows homogeneous uptake throughout the brain, without clear distinction between gray and white matter in the temporal lobe, consistent with heavy β-amyloid deposition in gray matter, which is seen in AD.* **(Right)** *More inferior axial F-18 florbetapir PET in the same patient demonstrates characteristic uptake in the white matter, but no significant uptake extending in the gray matter, indicating no detectable amyloid deposition.*

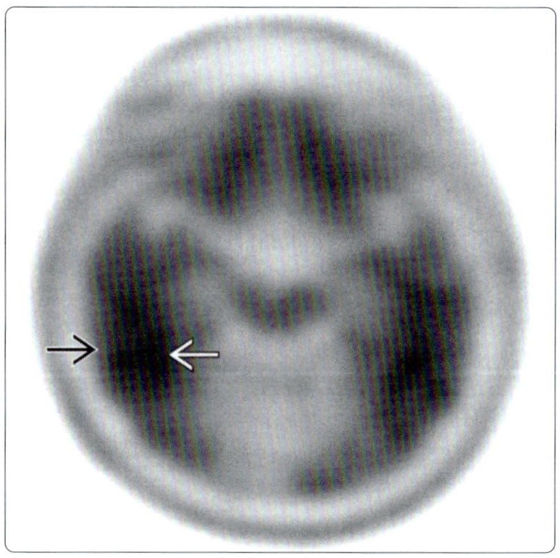

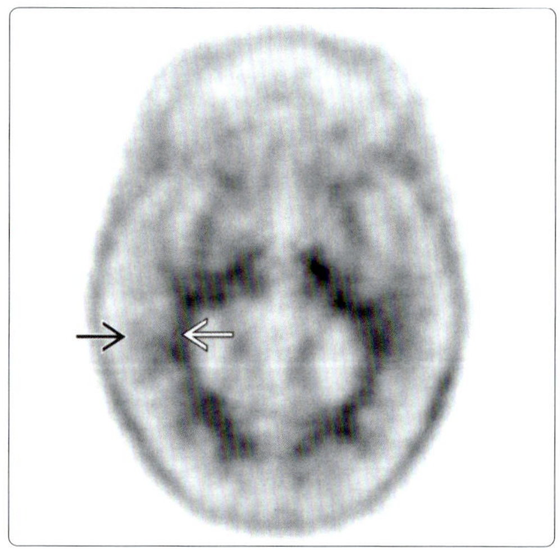

(Left) *More inferior F-18 florbetapir PET in the same patient shows homogeneous uptake in the temporal lobe gray matter. However, the cerebellum maintains a clear distinction between gray and white matter, which is expected even in patients with significant amyloid deposition. Therefore, the cerebellum is used as a reference for gray/white distinction in all patients.* **(Right)** *More inferior axial F-18 florbetapir PET in the same patient again demonstrates clear cerebellar gray and white differentiation.*

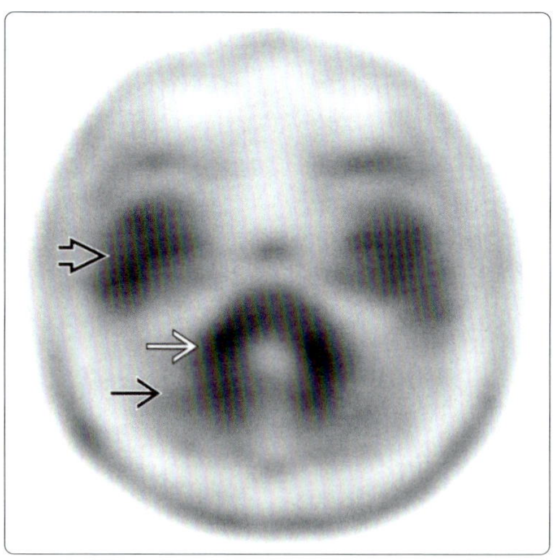

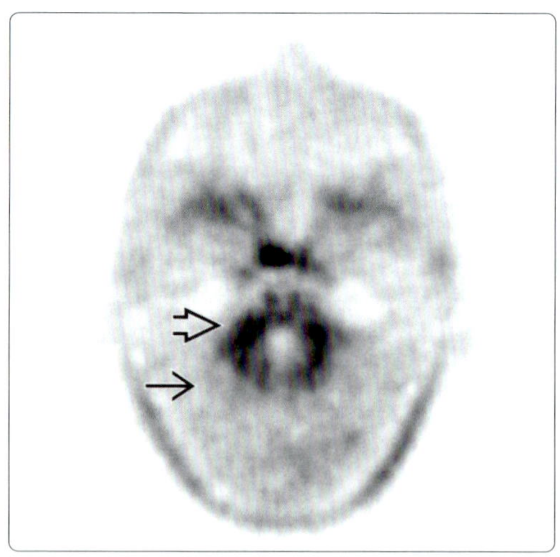

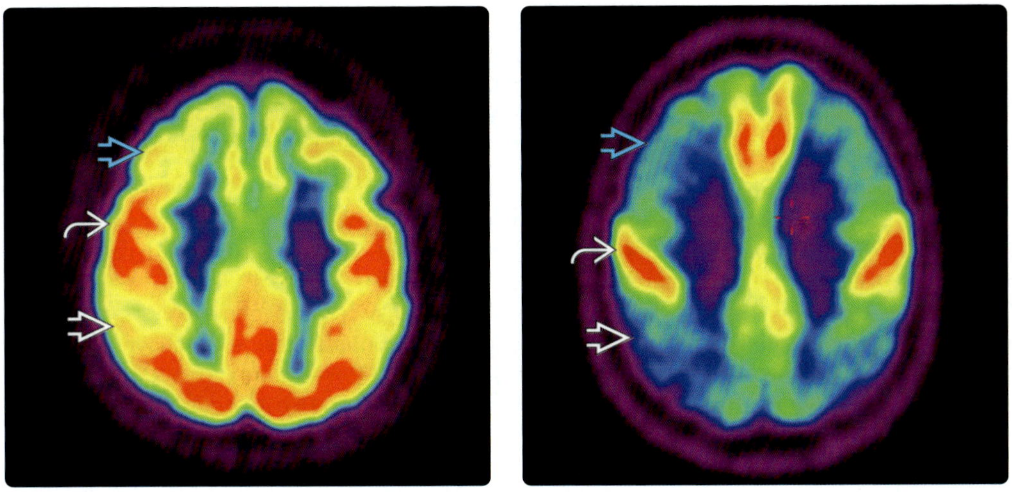

(Left) *Axial F-18 FDG PET in an elderly patient with mild dementia shows AD findings of reduced metabolism in the posterior parietal and frontal cortices. Importantly, there is sparing of the sensorimotor region.* **(Right)** *Axial F-18 FDG PET in a patient with late-stage AD demonstrates severely reduced metabolism in the posterior parietal and frontal cortices. Importantly, there is characteristic sparing of the sensorimotor region.*

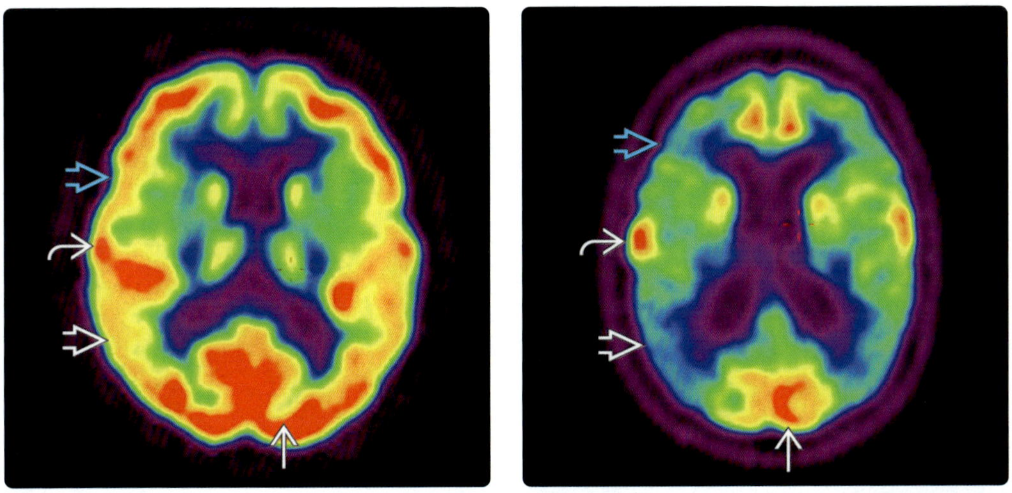

(Left) *More inferior axial F-18 FDG PET in the same patient shows further evidence of hypometabolism of the posterior parietal and frontal cortices. Importantly, there is characteristic sparing of the sensorimotor region and visual cortex.* **(Right)** *More inferior axial F-18 FDG PET in the same patient shows severe hypometabolism of the posterior parietal and frontal cortices. Importantly, there is sparing of the sensorimotor region and visual cortex.*

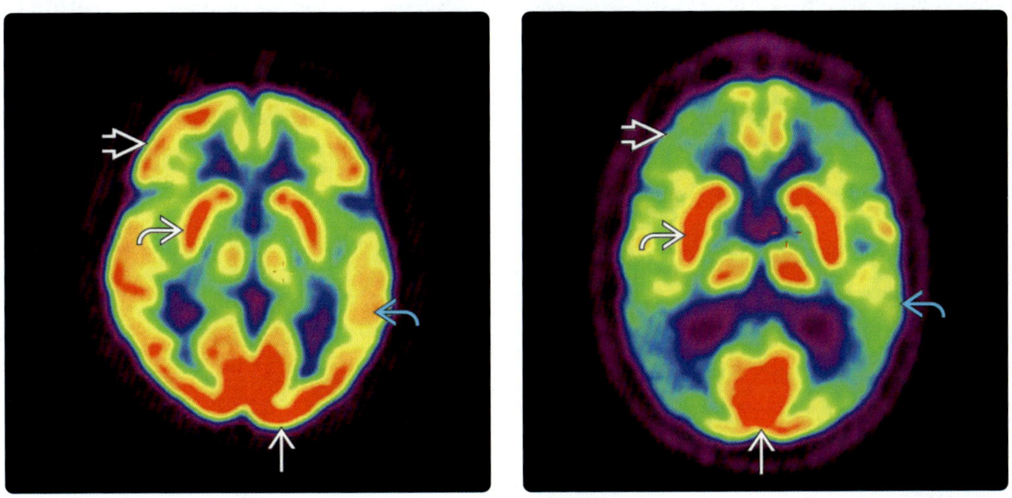

(Left) *More inferior axial F-18 FDG PET in the same patient shows hypometabolism of the temporal and frontal cortices. Importantly, there is sparing of the basal ganglia and visual cortex.* **(Right)** *More inferior axial F-18 FDG PET in the same patient shows severe hypometabolism of the temporal and frontal cortices. Importantly, there is characteristic sparing of the basal ganglia and visual cortex.*

Frontotemporal Dementia

KEY FACTS

TERMINOLOGY

- Frontotemporal dementia (FTD): Progressive neurodegenerative disorder of frontal/anterior temporal lobes

IMAGING

- F-18 FDG PET
  - Helps differentiate between FTD and other causes of dementia
  - May be used in early diagnosis
  - Glucose hypometabolism
    - First in frontal lobes
    - Progresses to include regions of temporal/parietal lobes
  - Occurs before atrophy visually evident on CT/MR
- Tc-99m HMPAO SPECT
  - Similar pattern of frontal hypoperfusion as F-18 FDG PET
  - Potentially less sensitive than F-18 FDG PET

PATHOLOGY

- Heterogeneous pathological and clinical subtypes
- Pathological subtypes of FTD are classified based upon pattern of protein accumulation in groups encompassing disorders of frontotemporal lobar degeneration
- Etiology uncertain, but associated with 3 major protein aggregates

CLINICAL ISSUES

- Progressive changes in behavior, personality, language and other cognitive functions
- Insidious onset of behavioral and cognitive dysfunction
- More significant behavioral, language, executive functioning impairment than memory
- No current disease-modifying treatment for FTD

(Left) *Axial F-18 FDG PET shows findings associated with FTD: Predominant frontal* ➡ *and temporal lobe hypometabolism. These changes occur prior to CT or MR changes.* **(Right)** *Axial CT shows classic morphological changes of frontotemporal dementia. Note predominant frontal* ➡ *and temporal lobe atrophy bilaterally.*

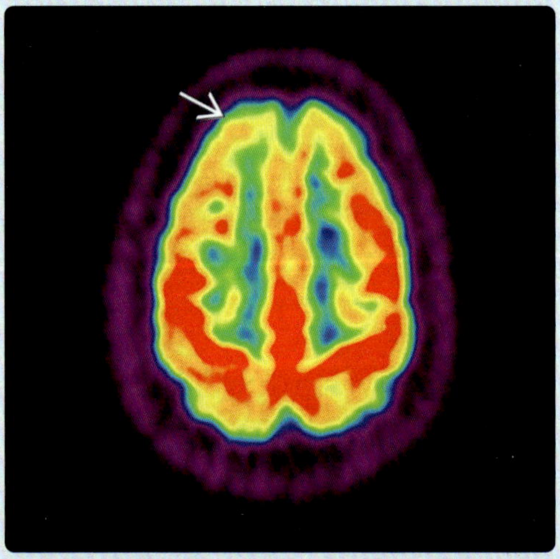

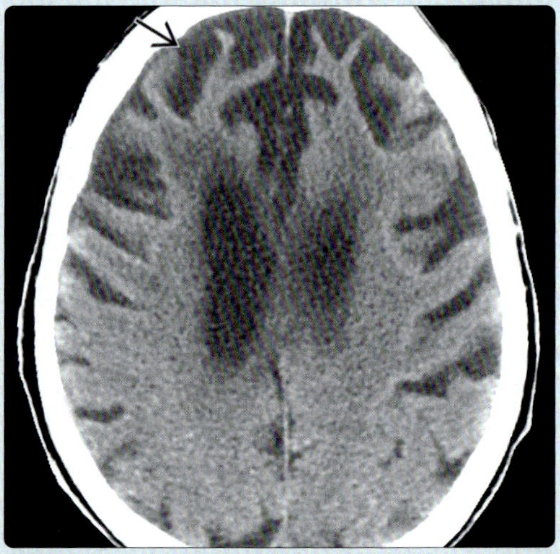

(Left) *Axial F-18 FDG PET shows findings associated with FTD: Predominant frontal* ➡ *and temporal lobe hypometabolism.* **(Right)** *Axial FDG PET/CT in the same patient shows predominately frontal hypometabolism in purple/blue areas* ➡, *signifying regions with a z-score > 2, or 2 standard deviations less than expected in normal controls.*

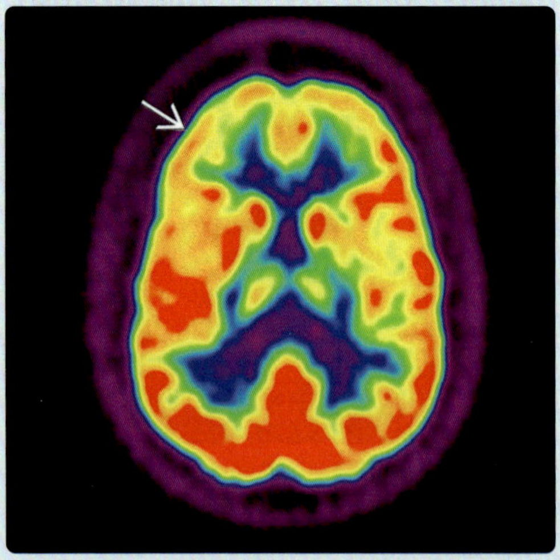

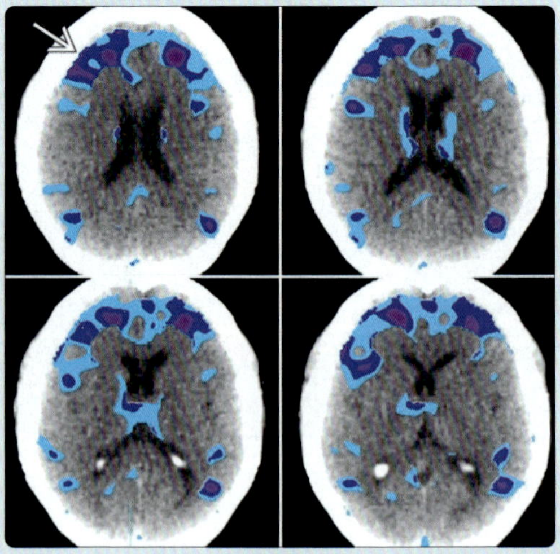

TERMINOLOGY

Abbreviations

- Frontotemporal dementia (FTD)

Definitions

- Progressive neurodegenerative disorder of frontal/anterior temporal lobes
  - Commonly characterized by behavioral/personality changes and impairments in other cognitive domains leading to functional decline
  - Previously referred to as Pick disease
    - Now only used to describe pathologically confirmed cases with Pick bodies

IMAGING

Imaging Recommendations

- Best imaging tool
  - F-18 FDG PET helps to differentiate between FTD and other causes of dementia, e.g., Alzheimer disease (AD) and Lewy body disease (DLB)
  - PET/SPECT may be used in early diagnosis
  - Correlates with disease progression
  - CT/MR documents atrophy of mainly frontal/temporal lobe structures
    - Look for reversible causes of dementia, e.g., normal pressure hydrocephalus
- F-18 FDG PET
  - Patient preparation
    - Patient should fast, stop IV fluids containing dextrose, and stop parenteral feeding for 4-6 hours
    - Blood sugar should be < 150-200 (mg/dL)
    - Patient should be placed in quiet, dimly lit room prior to and after injection (30 min)
  - Radiopharmaceutical: F-18 FDG
  - Dose: 5-20 mCi (185-740 MBq)
  - Dosimetry: Urinary bladder receives largest dose
  - Image acquisition: Image 30-60 min after injection
- SPECT
  - 2nd-line study if F-18 FDG PET is not available/reimbursed
  - Patient preparation
    - Patient should be placed in quiet, dimly lit room prior to and after injection (30 min)
- Radiopharmaceutical
  - Tc-99m exametazime (HMPAO)
  - Tc-99m ethyl cysteinate dimer (ECD)
- Dose: 15-30 mCi (555 MBq to 1.1 GBq)
- Dosimetry
  - Tc-99m HMPAO: Kidneys receive highest dose
  - Tc-99m ECD: Bladder wall receives highest dose
- Image acquisition
  - Optimal imaging time for Tc-99m HMPAO: 90 min post injection
  - Optimal imaging time for Tc-99m ECD: 45 min post injection

Nuclear Medicine Findings

- F-18 FDG PET/CT
  - Glucose hypometabolism first in frontal lobes with progression to include regions of temporal/parietal lobes
    - Anterior cingulate cortex, frontal insula, caudate nuclei, thalamus may also have hypometabolism bilaterally
    - Relative sparing of motor cortex
    - Hemispheric metabolic asymmetry may be present
  - Occurs before atrophy visually evident on CT/MR
  - Most sensitive diagnostic tool currently available
  - Glucose hypometabolism worsens with disease progression
  - May be used to distinguish between FTD and AD
    - AD shows hypometabolism in posterior cingulate/temporoparietal regions
  - Attenuation correction CT can show
    - Preferential atrophy of frontal/temporal lobes
    - Increased CSF space surrounding medial temporal lobes
    - Enlargement of lateral ventricles
- Tc-99m HMPAO SPECT
  - Pattern is similar to F-18 FDG PET, with decreased radiotracer activity in frontal/temporal lobes
    - SPECT generally has less sensitivity and quantitative potential compared to PET
  - More sensitive than structural MR in detecting early changes

Artifacts and Quality Control

- Immobilize patient's head to decrease motion, attenuation correction artifacts

DIFFERENTIAL DIAGNOSIS

Alzheimer Disease

- Most common cause of dementia generally leading to impairments in episodic memory and other cognitive domains
- Related to aggregation of amyloid-β and τ proteins
- Early F-18 FDG hypometabolism in parietotemporal and posterior cingulate cortices and positivity on amyloid PET

Vascular Dementia

- 2nd most common cause of dementia
- Caused by impaired blood supply to brain regions
- Global atrophy with diffuse white matter lesions (infarcts)
- Lesions generally correlate with cognitive symptoms

Dementia With Lewy Bodies

- Commonly presents with hallucinations, sleep disturbances, and parkinsonian motor features
- F-18 FDG PET hypometabolism in occipital cortex

Corticobasal Degeneration

- Commonly presents with significant extrapyramidal symptoms, visual/spatial and cognitive impairment
- Asymmetric cortical atrophy (left > right) in frontal and parietal structures, especially within superior parietal lobe
- Bilateral atrophy of basal ganglia

Progressive Supranuclear Palsy

- Characterized by impairments in gait/balance, supranuclear ophthalmoplegia (impaired downward gaze), behavioral/personality changes, parkinsonism, and dementia
- Atrophy of structures within midbrain and basal ganglia

Psychiatric Illness

- Bipolar disorder, schizophrenia, obsessive compulsive disorder

Reversible Dementia

- Mass lesions (brain tumor), head trauma, normal pressure hydrocephalus, vitamin B12 deficiency, hypothyroidism, infections (neurosyphilis, Lyme disease)

Other Neurodegenerative Disease

- Amyotrophic lateral sclerosis, Parkinson disease, Huntington disease

PATHOLOGY

General Features

- Etiology
  - Heterogeneous pathological and clinical subtypes
  - Pathological subtypes of FTD are classified based upon pattern of protein accumulation in groups encompassing disorders of frontotemporal lobar degeneration
  - Etiology uncertain, but associated with 3 major protein aggregates
    - Tau (microtubule-associated protein)
    - TDP-43 (transactive response DNA binding protein of 43kD)
    - FUS (tumor-associated protein; fused in sarcoma)
- Genetics
  - Autosomal dominant inheritance in 10-25% of FTD cases
  - Positive family history of FTD is only known risk factor
    - 30-50% of individuals with behavioral variant FTD have positive family history
- Associated abnormalities
  - May overlap with
    - Motor neuron disease (amyotrophic lateral sclerosis)
    - Parkinsonian syndromes (corticobasal syndrome and progressive supranuclear palsy)

CLINICAL ISSUES

Presentation

- Most common signs/symptoms
  - Progressive changes in behavior, personality, language and other cognitive functions
    - Memory loss
    - Disinhibition
    - Emotional blunting, apathy
    - Irritability
    - Loss of sympathy/empathy
    - Stereotyped compulsive behavior
    - Hyperorality (changes in eating behavior)
- Clinical profile
  - FTD is comprised of 2 categories and 3 main clinical syndromes
    - Behavioral variant FTD
      - Most common accounting for approximately 1/2 of cases
      - Progressive decline in social function with personality changes, often associated with a lack of inhibition
      - Associated with (symmetrical/right) frontal and anterior temporal dysfunction
    - Language presentation (primary progressive aphasia)
      - Progressive decline in language relative to other cognitive domains
      - Subdivided into semantic dementia (SD) and progressive non-fluent aphasia (PNFA)
      - SD: Associated with (left) anterior temporal dysfunction; fluent speech with deterioration in semantic memory and single-word comprehension
      - PNFA: Associated with (left) frontotemporal dysfunction; preserved single-word comprehension with apraxia and expressive agrammatism

Demographics

- Age
  - Mean age of onset: 50-60 years
  - Approximately 10% > 70 years
  - Younger onset than AD, which is generally > 65 years

Natural History & Prognosis

- Insidious onset of behavioral and cognitive dysfunction
- More significant behavioral, language, executive functioning impairment than memory
- Slowly progressive, with eventual functional impairment
- Median survival ~ 8-10 years after diagnosis; varies widely based upon underlying pathology

Treatment

- No current disease-modifying treatment for FTD

SELECTED REFERENCES

1. Josephs KA et al: Neuropathological background of phenotypical variability in frontotemporal dementia. Acta Neuropathol. 122(2):137-53, 2011
2. Piguet O et al: Behavioural-variant frontotemporal dementia: diagnosis, clinical staging, and management. Lancet Neurol. 10(2):162-72, 2011
3. Seelaar H et al: Clinical, genetic and pathological heterogeneity of frontotemporal dementia: a review. J Neurol Neurosurg Psychiatry. 82(5):476-86, 2011
4. Zhang Y et al: White matter damage in frontotemporal dementia and Alzheimer's disease measured by diffusion MRI. Brain. 132(Pt 9):2579-92, 2009
5. Diehl-Schmid J et al: Decline of cerebral glucose metabolism in frontotemporal dementia: a longitudinal 18F-FDG-PET-study. Neurobiol Aging. 28(1):42-50, 2007

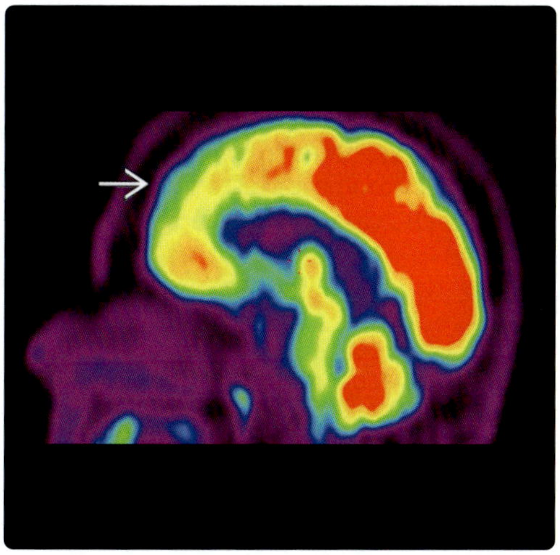

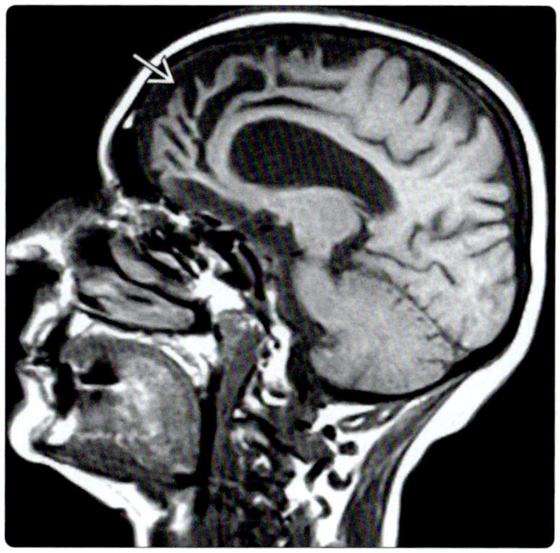

(Left) *F-18 PET findings associated with frontotemporal dementia include predominant frontal* ➡ *and temporal lobe hypometabolism. CT in this patient was normal (not shown). These changes occur prior to CT or MR changes.* **(Right)** *MR shows classic morphological changes of advanced frontotemporal dementia. Note predominant frontal* ➡ *lobe atrophy. There was also temporal lobe atrophy bilaterally (not shown).*

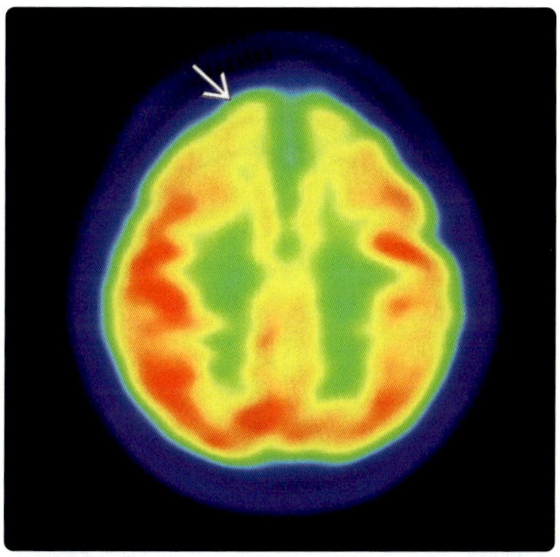

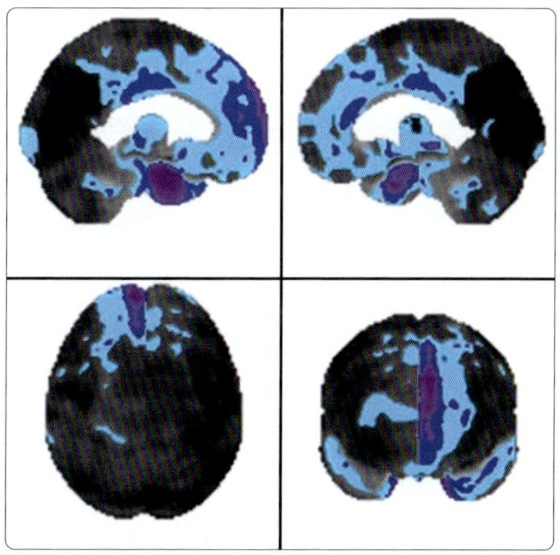

(Left) *Axial F-18 FDG PET demonstrates predominantly frontal hypometabolism* ➡ *in a patient with a normal CT scan.* **(Right)** *F-18 FDG PET with 3D stereotaxic surface projections (SSP) (top: Medial; bottom: Superior and anterior) illustrates the Z-score maps of a patient suspected to have FTD, with hypometabolism in the frontal and anterior temporal lobes (blue/purple).*

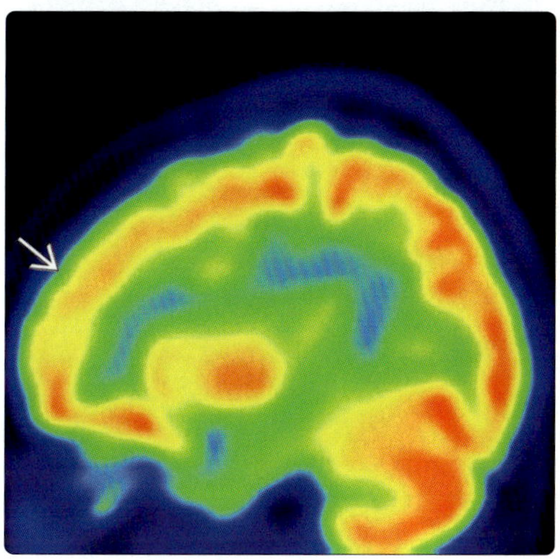

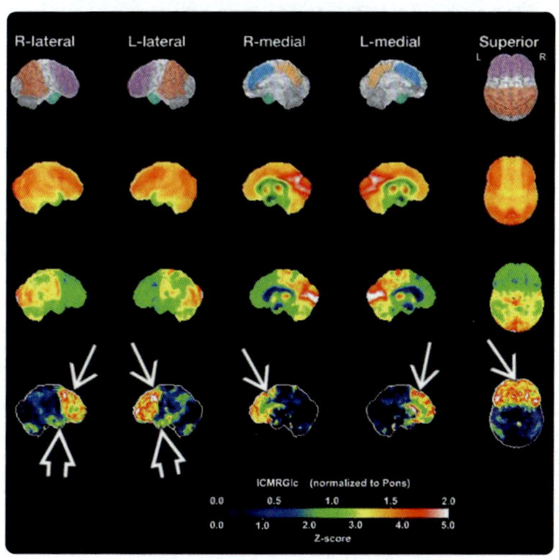

(Left) *Sagittal F-18 FDG PET of the same patient demonstrates predominantly frontal hypometabolism* ➡. **(Right)** *F-18 FDG PET shows SSP reference maps (1st row), elderly control map of glucose metabolism (2nd row), and patient's glucose metabolism (3rd row), which demonstrates strikingly diminished metabolism in the frontal and temporal lobes. Z-score map (4th row) illustrates areas of hypometabolism (compared to normal controls) in the frontal* ➡ *and temporal lobe* ➡. *(Courtesy University of Utah Medical Center.)*

Lewy Body Disease

KEY FACTS

TERMINOLOGY

- Progressive neurodegenerative disease characterized by parkinsonism, visual hallucinations, fluctuations in cognition (alertness/attention) and other cognitive impairments leading to functional decline

IMAGING

- Low dopamine transporter uptake in basal ganglia on SPECT
- Significant occipital lobe glucose hypometabolism relative to Alzheimer disease (AD)
- Dopamine transporter (I-123 FP-CIT) SPECT
- Diffuse Lewy body disease (LBD) and Parkinson disease (PD) demonstrate low dopamine transporter and uptake uptake in putamen, ± preservation in caudate head
- May aid in diagnosis between LBD and AD
- F-18 FDG PET
  - Generalized glucose hypometabolism with significant occipital lobe hypometabolism

TOP DIFFERENTIAL DIAGNOSES

- Parkinson disease and Parkinson disease dementia (PDD)
- Alzheimer disease

PATHOLOGY

- Undetermined cause; likely related to combination of genetic, lifestyle, and environmental factors
- Significant amount of LBD cases involves comorbid Alzheimer pathology

CLINICAL ISSUES

- Parkinsonism
- Fluctuating cognition especially in attention/alertness
- Recurrent visual hallucinations
- Progressive impairment of cognition with motor complications leading to a loss of functional independence
- No current disease-modifying treatment for LBD

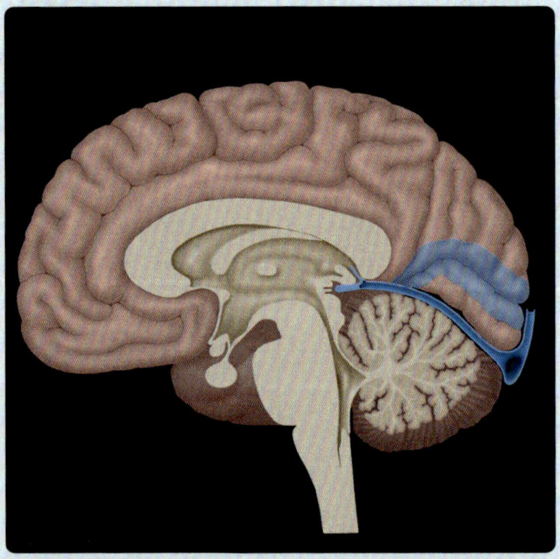

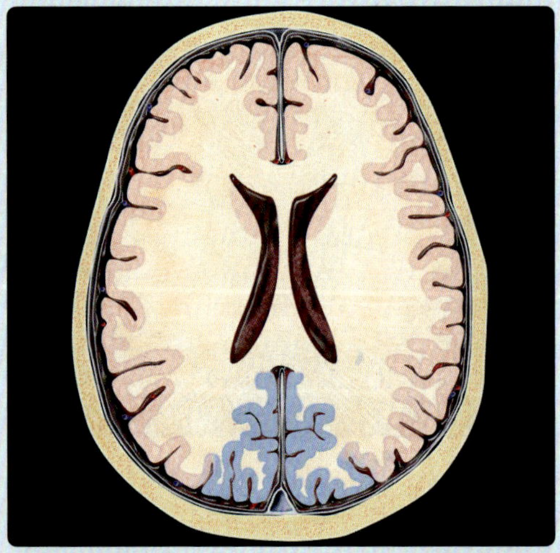

(Left) *Sagittal graphic of the brain depicts the territory of the primary visual cortex in the occipital lobe (blue) that is decreased in Lewy body disease (LBD) on F-18 FDG PET.* **(Right)** *Transaxial graphic of the brain outlines the occipital lobe in blue.*

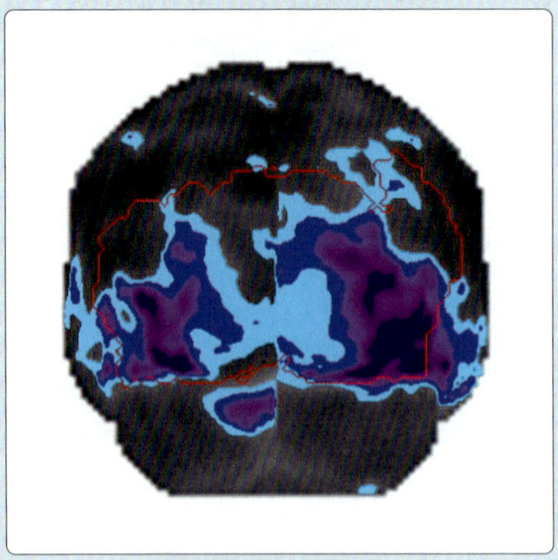

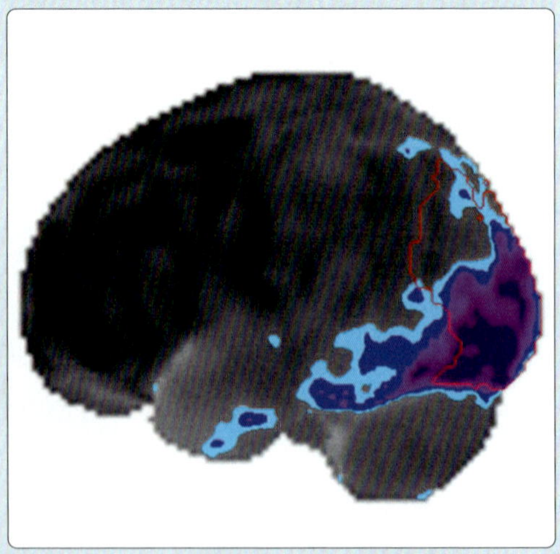

(Left) *Posterior image from an F-18 FDG PET scan with quantitative mapping shows decreased activity posteriorly (blue/purple), predominantly in the occipital lobe (red outline).* **(Right)** *Left lateral surface image with quantitative mapping of areas in the same patient shows decreased activity posteriorly (blue/purple), predominantly in the occipital lobe (red outline). These findings are typical for LBD.*

TERMINOLOGY

Abbreviations

- Lewy body disease (LBD)
- Lewy body variant of Alzheimer disease (LBV)

Synonyms

- LBD is commonly referred to as dementia with Lewy bodies

Definitions

- Progressive neurodegenerative disease of brain characterized by parkinsonism, visual hallucinations, fluctuations in cognition (alertness/attention) and other cognitive impairments leading to functional decline

IMAGING

General Features

- Best diagnostic clue
  - Low dopamine transporter uptake in basal ganglia on SPECT
  - Significant occipital lobe glucose hypometabolism relative to Alzheimer disease (AD)
  - Relative sparing of atrophy within medial temporal lobe structures
- Location
  - Cortical, subcortical, and brainstem structures; midbrain, basal ganglia, occipital lobe

Imaging Recommendations

- Best imaging tool
  - Dopamine transporter (DaT) SPECT with I-123 FP-CIT (ioflupane)
    - Binds reversibly to dopamine transporter (DaT) predominantly in presynaptic striata
    - Normal uptake of tracer is in head of caudate and putamen
    - LBD and PD both demonstrate low uptake in putamen ± preservation in caudate head
    - Abnormal DaT imaging suggestive feature for LBD diagnosis
    - DaT imaging differentiates between LBD (abnormal DaT) and AD (normal DaT)
    - Cannot reliably distinguish between other disorders with parkinsonism
  - F-18 FDG PET
    - Generalized glucose hypometabolism with significant occipital lobe hypometabolism
      - Occipital lobe involvement may help distinguish from AD-like pattern of hypometabolism
      - Similar hypometabolic pattern seen in PD and PDD
    - Medial temporal lobe hypometabolism less severe than in AD
- Protocol advice
  - I-123 FP-CIT (Ioflupane)
    - Patient preparation
      - Patient should be off all interfering dopaminergic medications
      - Pretreat with thyroid blocker (oral potassium solution, Lugols) 1 hour before tracer injection
      - Pregnancy category C: It is unknown whether I-123 ioflupane can cause fetal damage or early termination of pregnancy
    - Radiopharmaceutical: I-123 ioflupane
    - Dose: 3-5 mCi (111-185 MBq)
    - Dosimetry: Striata receives highest radiation exposure, followed by bladder, bowel and lungs (assuming thyroid is blocked)
    - Image acquisition: 3-6 hours after injection
  - F-18 FDG PET
    - Patient preparation
      - Patient should fast, stop IV fluids containing dextrose, stop parenteral feeding for 4-6 hours
      - Blood sugar should be 150-200 mg/dL
      - Patient should be placed in quiet, dimly lit room prior to and after injection for 30 min
    - Radiopharmaceutical: F-18 FDG
    - Dose: 5-20 mCi (185-740 MBq)
    - Dosimetry: Urinary bladder receives largest dose
    - Image acquisition: 30-60 min after injection

DIFFERENTIAL DIAGNOSIS

Parkinson Disease (PD) and PD Dementia (PDD)

- Neurodegenerative disease that often presents with cogwheel rigidity, shuffled gate, pill-rolling tremor at rest, akinesia
- Shares similar Lewy body-related neuropathology to LBD
- Dementia may develop, but generally 10 years after diagnosis of motor symptoms
  - PDD: PD cases where dementia is diagnosed 1 year after onset of motor symptoms

Alzheimer Disease

- Most common cause of dementia
- Impairments in episodic memory and other cognitive domains
- Related to aggregation of amyloid-β and τ proteins
- Early F-18 FDG hypometabolism in parietotemporal and posterior cingulate cortices
- F-18 FDG PET hypometabolism spares occipital visual cortex
- Positive on amyloid PET

Vascular Dementia

- 2nd most common cause of dementia
- Caused by impaired blood supply to brain regions
- Global atrophy with diffuse white matter lesions (infarcts)
- Lesions generally correlate with cognitive symptoms

Frontotemporal Dementia (FTD)

- Commonly presents with personality and behavioral changes
- Atrophy of frontal and anterior temporal lobes
- F-18 FDG PET hypometabolism primarily in frontal/anterior temporal lobes

PATHOLOGY

General Features

- Etiology
  - Undetermined cause; likely related to combination of genetic, lifestyle, and environmental factors

- Probable role for abnormal processing of α-synuclein (SYN) protein
- Individuals that have at least 1 first-degree relative with family history of LBD/other dementia may have increased risk for development of LBD
- Associated abnormalities
  - Significant amount of LBD cases involves comorbid Alzheimer pathology
    - LBD is diagnosed when dementia is present before or concurrently with parkinsonian features

Gross Pathologic & Surgical Features

- Relative preservation of total brain volume relative to other dementias
- Increased volume of lateral ventricles relative to healthy controls
- Decreased pigmentation within substantia nigra (midbrain) and loci cerulei (pons)

CLINICAL ISSUES

Presentation

- Most common signs/symptoms
  - Parkinsonism
  - Fluctuating cognition especially in attention/alertness
  - Recurrent visual hallucinations
- Other signs/symptoms
  - REM sleep behavior disorder
  - Severe neuroleptic sensitivity
  - Low dopamine transporter uptake in basal ganglia (SPECT/PET)
  - Repeated falls/syncope
  - Hallucinations (other than visual)
  - Depression
  - Severe autonomic dysfunction
- Clinical profile
  - 3 main types of dementia related to continuum of Lewy body clinicopathology
    - Diffuse Lewy body disease
      - Dementia with diffuse cortical LB pathology
      - No other significant pathology (minimal plaques/tangles)
    - Parkinson disease with dementia
      - PD patients diagnosed with dementia 1 year after onset of motor symptoms
      - Onset of dementia in PD is generally 10 years after motor symptoms
    - Lewy body variant of Alzheimer disease
      - Pathology consistent with cortical LB and AD-like pathological changes (amyloid plaques/neurofibrillary tangles)
      - Most common presentation, occurring in an estimated 70% of LBD cases

Natural History & Prognosis

- Progressive impairment of cognition with motor complications leading to loss of functional independence
  - Core features include fluctuating cognition with impact on alertness/attention, visual hallucinations, and features of parkinsonism
- Memory loss is less prominent early symptom in LBD, but may develop with progression of disease
  - Significant distinction from AD, where memory is common early symptom

Treatment

- No current disease-modifying treatment for LBD
- Several therapies may help alleviate common symptoms
- Levodopa can be used for some motor symptoms
- Cholinesterase inhibitors may be used for some cognitive symptoms

DIAGNOSTIC CHECKLIST

Image Interpretation Pearls

- SPECT/PET have value in diagnosis and distinguishing between other dementias
- Occipital lobe hypometabolism and normal mediotemporal uptake distinguish LBD from AD

SELECTED REFERENCES

1. Siderowf A et al: PET imaging of amyloid with Florbetapir F 18 and PET imaging of dopamine degeneration with 18F-AV-133 (florbenazine) in patients with Alzheimer's disease and Lewy body disorders. BMC Neurol. 14(1):79, 2014
2. Ishii K: PET Approaches for Diagnosis of Dementia. AJNR Am J Neuroradiol. Epub ahead of print, 2013
3. Colloby SJ et al: Neuropathological correlates of dopaminergic imaging in Alzheimer's disease and Lewy body dementias. Brain. 135(Pt 9):2798-808, 2012
4. Treglia G et al: Diagnostic performance of myocardial innervation imaging using MIBG scintigraphy in differential diagnosis between dementia with lewy bodies and other dementias: a systematic review and a meta-analysis. J Neuroimaging. 22(2):111-7, 2012
5. Kantarci K et al: Dementia with Lewy bodies and Alzheimer disease: neurodegenerative patterns characterized by DTI. Neurology. 74(22):1814-21, 2010
6. Mrak RE et al: Dementia with Lewy bodies: Definition, diagnosis, and pathogenic relationship to Alzheimer's disease. Neuropsychiatr Dis Treat. 3(5):619-25, 2007
7. Weisman D et al: Dementia with Lewy bodies. Semin Neurol. 27(1):42-7, 2007
8. Whitwell JL et al: Focal atrophy in dementia with Lewy bodies on MRI: a distinct pattern from Alzheimer's disease. Brain. 130(Pt 3):708-19, 2007
9. Bozzali M et al: Brain tissue damage in dementia with Lewy bodies: an in vivo diffusion tensor MRI study. Brain. 128(Pt 7):1595-604, 2005
10. McKeith IG et al: Diagnosis and management of dementia with Lewy bodies: third report of the DLB Consortium. Neurology. 2005 Dec 27;65(12):1863-72. Epub 2005 Oct 19. Review. Erratum in: Neurology. 65(12):1992, 2005
11. Minoshima S et al: Alzheimer's disease versus dementia with Lewy bodies: cerebral metabolic distinction with autopsy confirmation. Ann Neurol. 50(3):358-65, 2001
12. Barber R et al: MRI volumetric study of dementia with Lewy bodies: a comparison with AD and vascular dementia. Neurology. 54(6):1304-9, 2000
13. Hu XS et al: 18F-fluorodopa PET study of striatal dopamine uptake in the diagnosis of dementia with Lewy bodies. Neurology. 55(10):1575-7, 2000

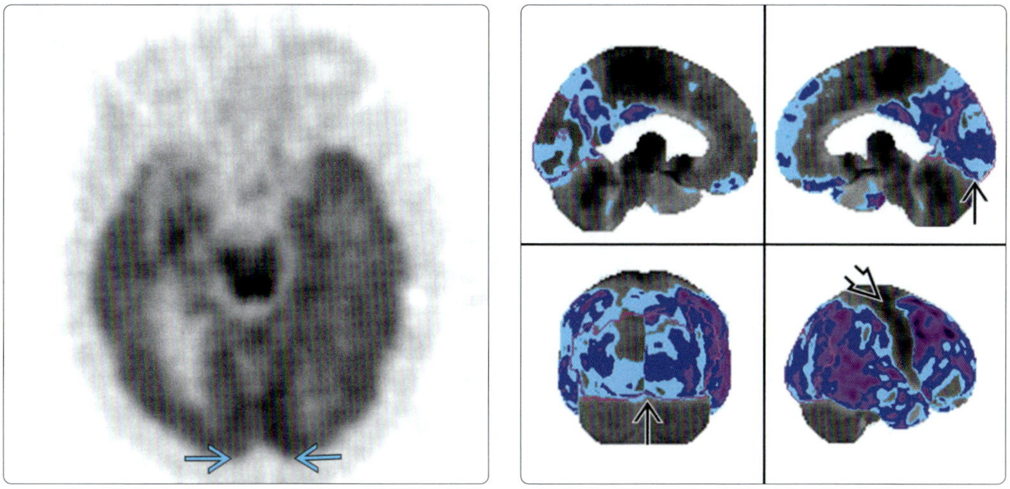

(Left) *Axial F-18 FDG PET of advanced LBD demonstrates decreased activity throughout the cortex, including the occipital lobe* ➡. **(Right)** *Surface images with quantitative mapping of areas showing decreased metabolism in patients with LBD demonstrate decreased activity in the posterior cingulate gyrus, precuneus and temporal lobes (blue/purple) with sensorimotor sparing* ➡*. In contrast to AD, there is decreased activity in the posterior visual areas in the occipital lobe* ➡.

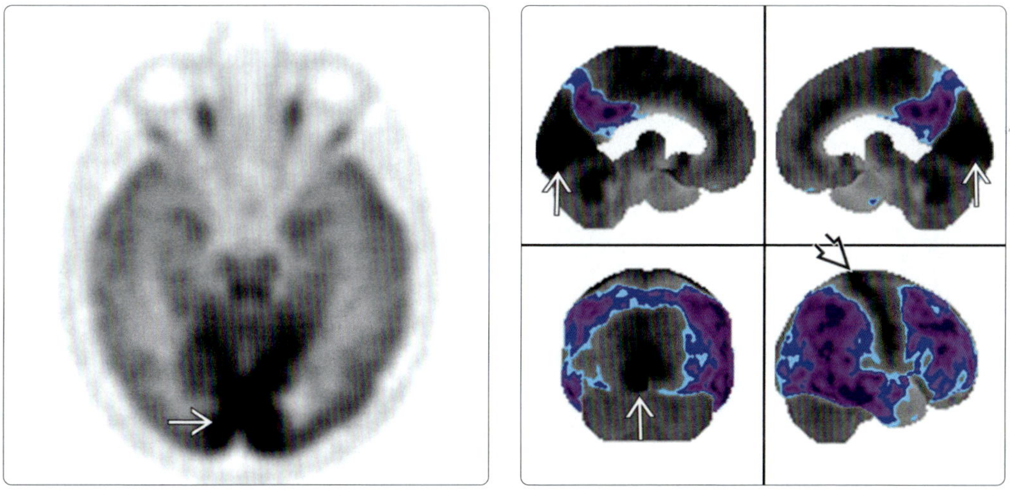

(Left) *Axial F-18 FDG PET of advanced AD demonstrates decreased activity throughout the cortex, with sparing of the occipital lobe* ➡*, which distinguishes it from LBD.* **(Right)** *Surface images with quantitative mapping show decreased metabolism in a patient with AD. There is characteristic hypometabolism (with sparing of the sensorimotor cortex* ➡*). In contrast to LBD, there is significant sparing of the posterior visual areas in the occipital lobe* ➡.

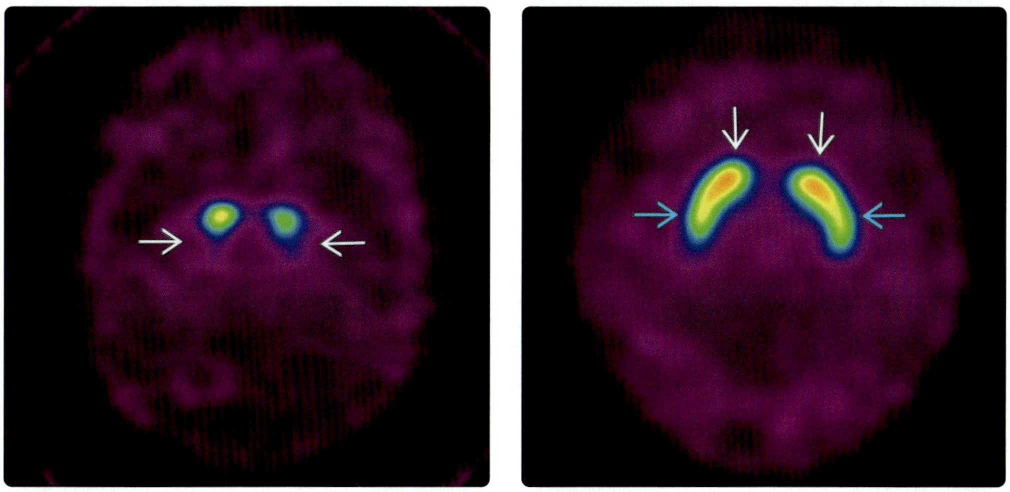

(Left) *I-123 ioflupane image demonstrates significant abnormally decreased activity in the putamen bilaterally* ➡. **(Right)** *I-123 ioflupane image demonstrates normal symmetric activity in the head of the caudate* ➡ *and putamen bilaterally* ➡.

Multi-Infarct Dementia

KEY FACTS

TERMINOLOGY

- Impairments in cognition and behavior affecting functional status due to pathologic changes resulting from various vascular insults throughout brain

IMAGING

- Multifocal or focal infarcts involving cortical gray matter, subcortical white matter, and other structures
- Generally involve cerebral hemispheres, thalamus, basal ganglia
- Glucose hypometabolism in multifocal (scattered) pattern of cortical with subcortical regions
- Altered pattern depending on subtype (i.e., strategic infarct dementia vs. multi-infarct dementia)
- May be used in differential diagnosis between vascular dementia (VaD) and Alzheimer disease (AD)
- Amyloid PET imaging does not demonstrate gray matter amyloid deposition
- SPECT with Tc-99m HMPAO or Tc-99m ECD shows similar asymmetrically decreased perfusion

PATHOLOGY

- Vascular-related lesions leading to loss of brain function
- Chronic small vessel insults > large vessel infarcts

CLINICAL ISSUES

- Significant heterogeneity in clinical presentation depending on location, type, and size of vascular lesion
- Overt disease: Cognitive impairment due to clinically evident vascular event (i.e., stroke)
- Covert disease: Insidious process of vascular insults (clinically silent strokes)
- 2nd most common cause of dementia after AD

(Left) *Axial graphic of the brain shows multifocal infarcts involving the cortical gray matter and subcortical white matter bilaterally.* **(Right)** *Coronal FLAIR MR of a 72-year-old woman demonstrates FLAIR signal abnormality in the periventricular and subcortical white matter (leukoaraiosis). This finding is consistent with a small vessel ischemic etiology.*

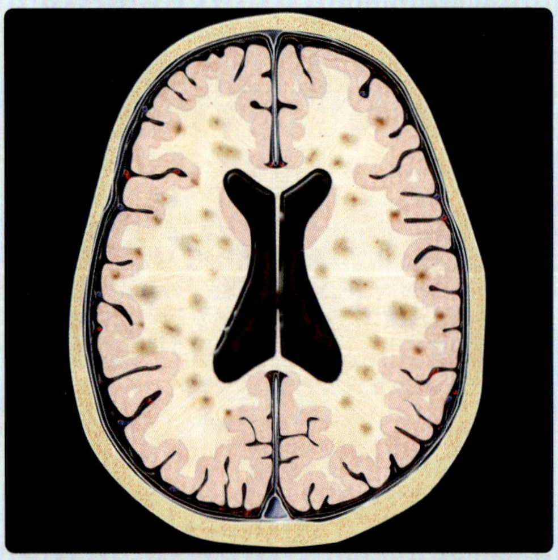

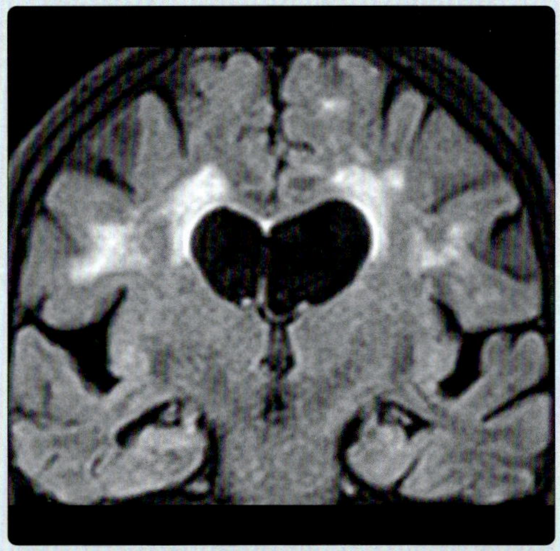

(Left) *F-18 FDG PET in an elderly patient presenting with dementia demonstrates bilateral areas of hypometabolism* ➔, *consistent with vascular dementia (VaD).* **(Right)** *F-18 FDG PET of a different patient presenting with dementia demonstrates more unilateral areas of hypometabolism* ➔ *and globally decreased F-18 FDG uptake, also consistent with VaD.*

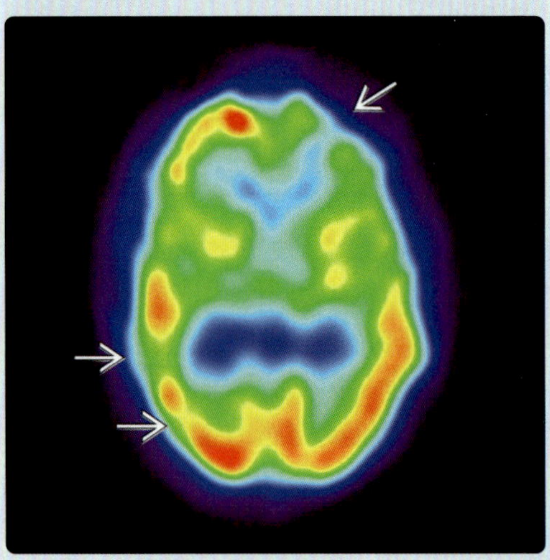

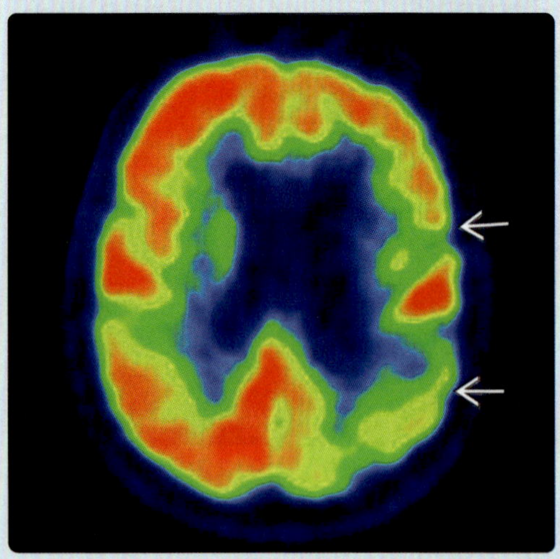

TERMINOLOGY

Definitions

- Impairments in cognition and behavior affecting functional status due to pathologic changes resulting from various vascular insults throughout brain
- Vascular cognitive impairment (VCI) is more comprehensive term incorporating vascular dementia (VaD) as well as other vascular-related cognitive impairment, including mild cognitive impairment due to vascular disease

IMAGING

General Features

- Best diagnostic clue
  - Multifocal or focal infarcts involving cortical gray matter, subcortical white matter, and other structures
  - Generally involve cerebral hemispheres, thalamus, basal ganglia
  - Bilateral > unilateral

Nuclear Medicine Findings

- F-18 FDG PET/CT
  - Glucose hypometabolism in multifocal (scattered) pattern of cortical with subcortical regions
    - Altered pattern depending on subtype (i.e., strategic infarct dementia vs. multi-infarct dementia)
    - Hypometabolism often in clinically affected areas: Correlate with other clinical findings
  - May be used in differential diagnosis between VaD and Alzheimer disease (AD)
    - AD pattern: Hypometabolism in bilateral parietotemporal with posterior cingulate cortices: Extension to frontal/occipital
    - VaD may have hypometabolism in subcortical areas, which are spared in AD
- Amyloid PET imaging does not demonstrate gray matter amyloid deposition
- SPECT with Tc-99m HMPAO or Tc-99m ECD shows similar asymmetrically decreased perfusion

Imaging Recommendations

- Best imaging tool
  - F-18 FDG PET may aid in differential diagnosis
  - MR to see vascular insults and look for potential reversible causes of dementia
- Protocol advice
  - F-18 FDG PET
    - Patient preparation
      - Patient should fast, stop IV fluids containing dextrose, stop parenteral feeding for 4-6 hrs
      - Blood sugar should be < 150-200 mg/dL
      - Patient should be placed in quiet, dimly lit room prior to and after injection for 30 min
    - Radiopharmaceutical: F-18 FDG
    - Dose: 5-20 mCi (185-740 MBq)
    - Dosimetry: Urinary bladder receives largest dose
    - Image acquisition: 30-60 min after injection

DIFFERENTIAL DIAGNOSIS

Alzheimer Disease

- Early F-18 FDG hypometabolism in parietotemporal and posterior cingulate cortices

Dementia With Lewy Body

- F-18 FDG PET hypometabolism in occipital cortex

Normal Pressure Hydrocephalus

- Dilated ventricles on CT or MR

Frontotemporal Dementia (FTD)

- F-18 FDG PET hypometabolism primarily in frontal and anterior temporal lobes

Causes of Reversible Dementia

- Normal pressure hydrocephalus, vitamin B12 deficiency, hypothyroidism, depression, mass lesions (brain tumor), infections (neurosyphilis, HIV), trauma (chronic subdural hematoma)

PATHOLOGY

General Features

- Vascular-related lesions leading to loss of brain function
- Chronic small vessel insults > large vessel infarcts

Risk Factors

- History of myocardial infarction/coronary artery disease, stroke/transient ischemic attack (TIA)
- Atherosclerosis, hypertension, hyperlipidemia, atrial fibrillation
- Diabetes, obesity, smoking, advanced age

CLINICAL ISSUES

Presentation

- Significant heterogeneity in clinical presentation depending on location, type, and size of vascular lesion
- Other: Seizures, bladder incontinence, gait disturbance, and additional focal abnormalities
- Overt disease: Cognitive impairment due to clinically evident vascular event (i.e., stroke)
- Covert disease: Insidious process of vascular insults (clinically silent strokes)

Demographics

- 2nd most common cause of dementia after AD

DIAGNOSTIC CHECKLIST

Image Interpretation Pearls

- Heterogeneous F-18 FDG activity without any pattern indicative of VaD
- Lesions can include basal ganglia and other areas typically spared in other diseases

SELECTED REFERENCES

1. Iadecola C: The pathobiology of vascular dementia. Neuron. 80(4):844-66, 2013
2. Ishii K: PET Approaches for Diagnosis of Dementia. AJNR Am J Neuroradiol. Epub ahead of print, 2013
3. Risacher SL et al: Neuroimaging biomarkers of neurodegenerative diseases and dementia. Semin Neurol. 33(4):386-416, 2013

KEY FACTS

IMAGING

- Abscess
  - Usually: Peripheral hypermetabolism with central hypometabolism on F-18 FDG PET/CT
- *Toxoplasma gondii*
  - Toxoplasmosis is hypometabolic on F-18 FDG PET/CT
  - Lymphoma is hypermetabolic on F-18 FDG PET/CT
- Encephalitis
  - CNS inflammation, most common etiology is viral (e.g., herpes simplex encephalitis)
    - Acute: Hypermetabolism on F-18 FDG PET/CT
    - Subacute: May be isointense to gray matter on F-18 FDG PET/CT
    - Chronic, nonactive: Hypometabolic on F-18 FDG PET/CT

TOP DIFFERENTIAL DIAGNOSES

- Abscess
  - Focal pyogenic infection (bacterial, fungal, parasitic)
- Encephalitis
  - Atypical infectious encephalitis: Any location
  - Herpes simplex encephalitis: Parenchymal infection caused by herpes simplex virus type 1 (HSV-1)
    - Medial temporal and inferior frontal lobes; cingulate gyrus and contralateral temporal lobe highly suggestive
  - Rasmussen encephalitis: Chronic, unilateral brain inflammation; etiology unclear
  - Limbic encephalitis
    - Rare paraneoplastic syndrome associated with primary tumor, often lung
    - Imaging may be indistinguishable from herpes simplex encephalitis on MR and F-18 FDG PET/CT
- Toxoplasmosis
  - Opportunistic infection in immunocompromised patients

(Left) *Coronal F-18 FDG PET shows hypermetabolic activity in the left temporal lobe ⇨ and basal ganglia ⇨, typical for acute herpes simplex encephalitis.* **(Right)** *Coronal T1 C+ MR in the same patient shows enhancement of the left temporal lobe ➡ and basal ganglia ➡, corresponding to hypermetabolism on PET.*

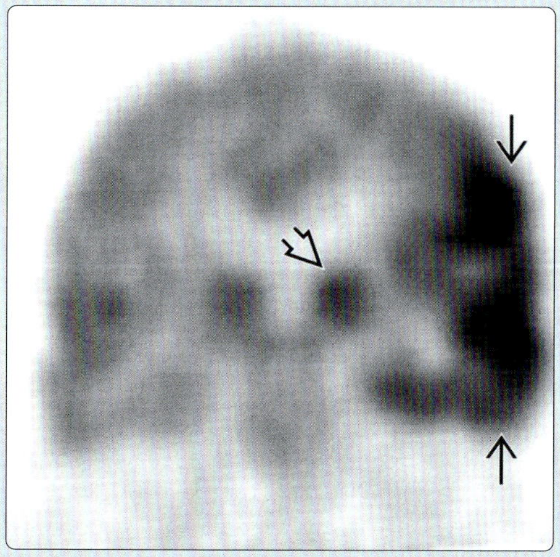

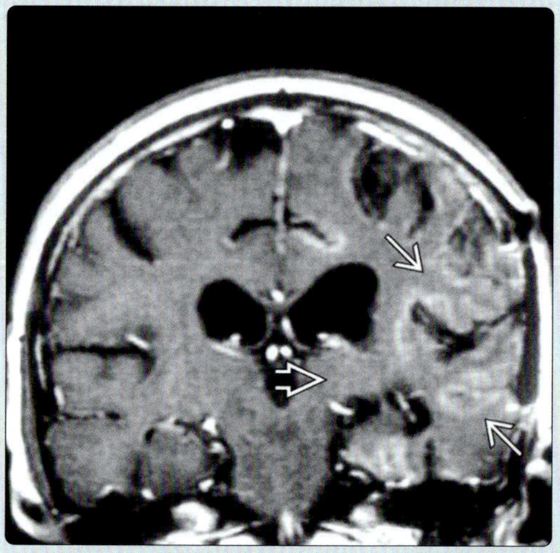

(Left) *Axial F-18 FDG PET shows a ring of hypermetabolism in the left parietal lobe ⇨. In an HIV-positive patient, this would be most consistent with lymphoma. Infection with toxoplasmosis would be hypometabolic.* **(Right)** *Axial F-18 FDG PET in a patient with Rasmussen encephalitis shows diffuse right hemispheric hypometabolism ⇨. Late in the disease, diffuse hemicerebral atrophy occurs.*

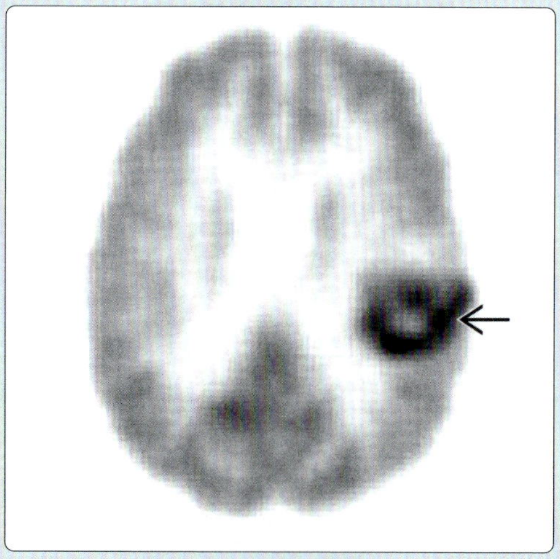

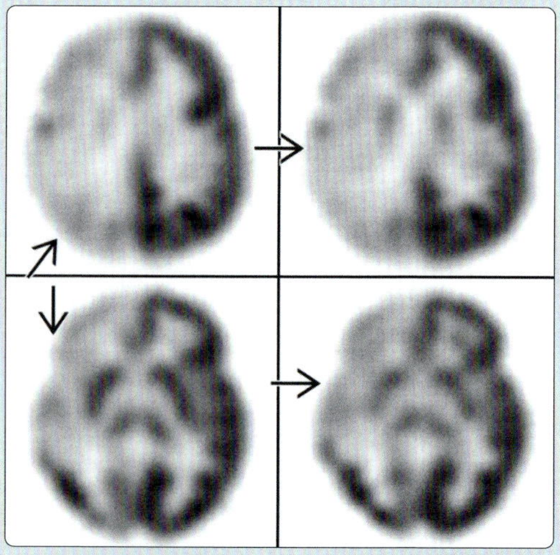

IMAGING

Nuclear Medicine Findings

- PET
  - Abscess
    - Focal CNS infection (bacterial, fungal, parasitic etiologies)
      - Usually: Peripheral hypermetabolism with central hypometabolism on F-18 FDG PET/CT
    - *Toxoplasma gondii*
      - Common opportunistic infection in HIV/AIDS patients
      - Appears as ring-enhancing lesion on CT/MR; differential diagnosis is toxoplasmosis vs. lymphoma
      - Toxoplasmosis is hypometabolic on F-18 FDG PET/CT
      - Lymphoma is hypermetabolic on F-18 FDG PET/CT
  - Encephalitis
    - CNS inflammation; most common etiology is viral (e.g., herpes simplex encephalitis)
      - Acute: Hypermetabolism on F-18 FDG PET/CT
      - Subacute: May be isointense to gray matter on F-18 FDG PET/CT
      - Chronic, nonactive: Hypometabolic on F-18 FDG PET/CT

Imaging Recommendations

- Best imaging tool
  - MR best for diagnosing brain abscess and encephalitis; however, false-negatives can occur in 1st few days of opportunistic infection, herpes simplex encephalitis
  - F-18 FDG PET/CT can be used for problem-solving in unclear cases after MR/CT
  - Abscess and encephalitis may be an incidental finding on F-18 FDG PET/CT
- Protocol advice
  - F-18 FDG PET/CT
    - Patient preparation
      - Patient should fast, stop IV fluids containing dextrose, and stop parenteral feeding for 4-6 hours
      - Blood sugar should be < 150-200 (mg/dL)
      - Patient should be placed in quiet, dimly lit room prior to and after injection (30 min)
    - Radiopharmaceutical: F-18 FDG
    - Dose: 5-20 mCi (185-740 MBq)
    - Dosimetry: Urinary bladder receives largest dose
    - Image acquisition: Image 30-60 min after injection

DIFFERENTIAL DIAGNOSIS

Abscess

- Focal pyogenic infection (bacterial, fungal, parasitic)
- Primarily gray-white junction, supratentorial, also atypical locations
- MR/CT: Depending on acuity, enhancing ring with central low density and peripheral edema
  - Ring enhancement = capsular stage

Encephalitis and Cerebritis

- Brain inflammation caused by various pathogens, most commonly viral
- Atypical infectious encephalitis: Any location
- Herpes simplex encephalitis: Parenchymal infection caused by herpes simplex virus type 1 (HSV-1)
  - Medial temporal and inferior frontal lobes; cingulate gyrus and contralateral temporal lobe highly suggestive
  - Limbic system most typically (temporal lobes, insula, subfrontal, cingulate gyri)
  - Cerebral convexities, asymmetrical, basal ganglia often spared, atypical in children
  - Children atypical: Primarily cerebral hemispheres
  - Usually bilateral; can be asymmetrical
- Rasmussen encephalitis (RE): Chronic, unilateral brain inflammation; etiology unclear
  - Unilateral cerebral atrophy
    - Initially focal involvement, then hemispheric
    - When hemispheric, worse precentral and inferior frontal
- Limbic encephalitis
  - Rare paraneoplastic syndrome associated with primary tumor, often lung
  - Imaging may be indistinguishable from herpes simplex encephalitis on MR and F-18 FDG PET/CT
  - Subacute symptom onset (weeks to months) vs. acute in herpes simplex encephalitis

Toxoplasmosis

- Opportunistic infection in immunocompromised patients
- Most common cause of CNS mass lesion in HIV patients
- Reported to have low uptake on F-18 FDG PET/CT
- Negative F-18 FDG PET/CT study may differentiate from CNS lymphoma

DIAGNOSTIC CHECKLIST

Image Interpretation Pearls

- Ring-enhancing lesions on MR: Toxoplasmosis vs. lymphoma
  - Can be useful for equivocal or problematic cases on MR/CT to differentiate toxoplasmosis vs. lymphoma, particularly in HIV-positive patients
  - Toxoplasmosis: Hypometabolic on F-18 FDG PET/CT
- Can help determine acuity of CNS infection/inflammation
  - Acute: Hypermetabolic on F-18 FDG PET/CT
  - Chronic: Hypometabolic on F-18 FDG PET/CT

SELECTED REFERENCES

1. Floeth FW et al: 18F-FET PET Differentiation of Ring-Enhancing Brain Lesions. J Nucl Med. 47(5):776-782, 2006
2. Lee BY et al: FDG-PET findings in patients with suspected encephalitis. Clin Nucl Med. 29(10):620-5, 2004
3. Scheid R et al: Serial 18F-fluoro-2-deoxy-D-glucose positron emission tomography and magnetic resonance imaging of paraneoplastic limbic encephalitis. Arch Neurol. 61(11):1785-9, 2004
4. Fiorella DJ et al: (18)F-fluorodeoxyglucose positron emission tomography and MR imaging findings in Rasmussen encephalitis. AJNR Am J Neuroradiol. 22(7):1291-9, 2001
5. Kassubek J et al: Limbic encephalitis investigated by 18FDG-PET and 3D MRI. J Neuroimaging. 11(1):55-9, 2001
6. Leonard JR et al: MR imaging of herpes simplex type 1 encephalitis in infants and young children: a separate pattern of findings. AJR Am J Roentgenol. 174(6):1651-5, 2000
7. Hoffman JM et al: FDG-PET in differentiating lymphoma from nonmalignant central nervous system lesions in patients with AIDS. J Nucl Med. 34(4):567-75, 1993
8. Hanson MW et al: FDG-PET in the selection of brain lesions for biopsy. J Comput Assist Tomogr. 15(5):796-801, 1991

Parkinson Disease

KEY FACTS

TERMINOLOGY

- Chronic, progressive brain disorder characterized by loss of dopaminergic neurons that leads to tremors at rest, rigidity, slowed movements, and gait

IMAGING

- Loss of dopaminergic neurons on I-123 FP-CIT (ioflupane)
- Dopamine transporters typically decreased for all Parkinson syndromes (Parkinson disease [PD] and atypical parkinsonism syndromes [APS])
- I-123FP-CIT confirms loss of dopaminergic neurons
- Sensitivity > 90% for differentiating PD and essential tremor
- Normal scans demonstrate comma-shaped uptake on axial images
- Abnormal scans demonstrate period-shaped uptake on axial images, indicating more pronounced loss of uptake in putamen
- Abnormal uptake may be initially detected in contralateral putamen relative to clinical symptoms
- Patient should be off all interfering dopaminergic medications
- Pretreat with thyroid blocker (oral potassium solution, Lugol) 1 hr before tracer injection
- Image acquisition: 3-6 hrs after injection
- Loss of dopaminergic neurons on I-123 FP-CIT
- Relatively normal F-18 FDG PET in PD

TOP DIFFERENTIAL DIAGNOSES

- Multiple system atrophy (MSA)
- Progressive supranuclear palsy (PSP)
- Dementia with Lewy bodies (DLB)
- Corticobasal degeneration (CBD)

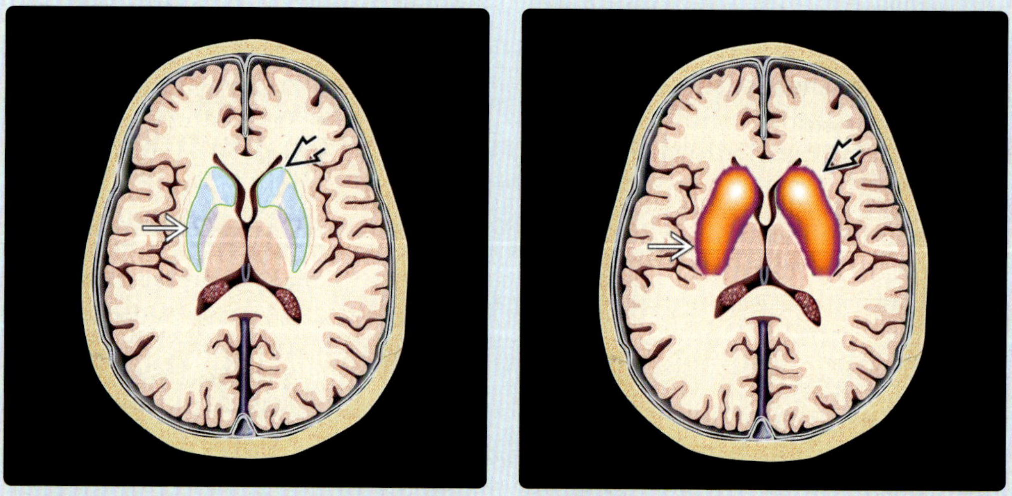

(Left) *Graphic demonstrates brain anatomy and an area of uptake (blue) in the head of the caudate ⇨ and putamen ➡.* **(Right)** *Normal uptake (orange) is shown overlaid on the head of the caudate ⇨ and putamen ➡.*

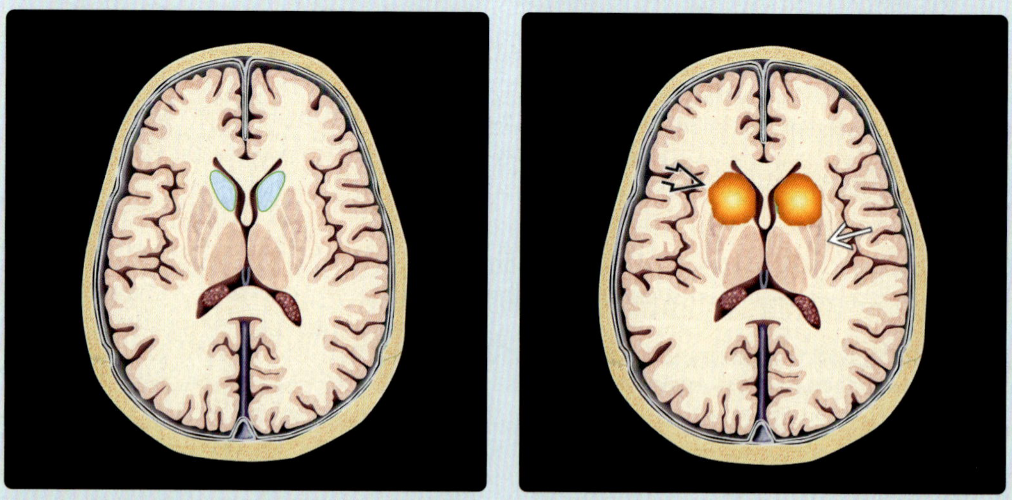

(Left) *Graphic demonstrates brain anatomy and an area of uptake (blue) in the head of the caudate.* **(Right)** *Abnormal uptake (orange) is shown overlaid on the head of the caudate ⇨ but not in the expected area of the putamen ➡.*

TERMINOLOGY

Abbreviations

- Parkinson disease (PD)

Definitions

- Chronic, progressive brain disorder characterized by loss of dopaminergic neurons that leads to tremors at rest, rigidity, slowed movements, and gait

IMAGING

General Features

- Best diagnostic clue
  - Loss of dopaminergic neurons on I-123 FP-CIT (ioflupane)
  - Relatively normal F-18 FDG PET/CT
    - Distinct abnormal patterns in atypical parkinsonism syndromes (APS)

Imaging Recommendations

- Best imaging tool
  - Dopamine transporter SPECT (I-123 FP-CIT)
    - Molecular imaging agent that binds to dopamine transporters located on presynaptic nigrostriatal axons
    - Dopamine transporters typically decreased for all Parkinson syndromes (PD and APS)
    - Dopamine transporters are located in putamen and caudate nucleus
    - I-123 FP-CIT confirms loss of dopaminergic neurons
    - Sensitivity > 90% for differentiating PD and essential tremor
    - May be symmetric or asymmetric
    - Differentiates PD and APS from essential tremor and drug-induced parkinsonism
    - PD and APS demonstrate decreased activity in putamen and caudate
    - Does **not** differentiate PD from APS or between APSs
    - Image interpretation
      - Normal scans demonstrate comma-shaped uptake on axial images
      - Abnormal scans demonstrate period-shaped uptake on axial images indicating more pronounced loss of uptake in putamen
      - Abnormal uptake may be initially detected in contralateral putamen relative to clinical symptoms
      - Abnormal patterns
        - Asymmetric putamen activity
        - Symmetrically absent putamen activity with preservation of caudate
        - Absent putamen activity with significantly decreased caudate uptake
  - F-18 FDG PET/CT
    - Shows patterns of neuronal dysfunction that are particular to specific parkinsonian syndromes
    - Only approved by FDA for dementia, use for parkinsonism syndromes is off-label
    - Typically normal in PD
      - Preserved F-18 FDG PET/CT in basal ganglia differentiates PD from parkinsonian syndromes
- Protocol advice
  - I-123 FP-CIT (ioflupane)
    - Patient should be off all interfering dopaminergic medications
      - Cocaine, amphetamines, and methylphenidate severely decrease binding
      - Ephedrine and phentermine may decrease binding
      - Bupropion, fentanyl, and some anesthetics may decrease binding
    - Patient preparation
      - Pretreat with thyroid blocker (400 mg of oral potassium solution or single dose of Lugol solution) 1 hr before tracer injection
      - Pregnancy category C: Unknown whether I-123 can cause fetal damage or early termination of pregnancy
    - Radiopharmaceutical: I-123 FP-CIT (ioflupane)
    - Dose: 3-5 mCi (111-185 MBq) intravenously
    - Dosimetry: Striata receives highest radiation exposure, followed by bladder, bowel, and lungs (assuming thyroid is blocked)
    - Image acquisition: 3-6 hrs after injection
      - SPECT or SPECT/CT acceptable but attenuation correction is recommended
      - Photopeak should be set to 159 keV ± 10%
      - 128 x 128 matrix is recommended
  - F-18 FDG PET/CT
    - Patient preparation
      - Patient should fast, stop IV fluids containing dextrose, stop parenteral feeding for 4-6 hrs
      - Blood sugar should be 150-200 mg/dL
      - Patient should be placed in quiet, dimly lit room prior to and after injection for 30 min
    - Radiopharmaceutical: F-18 FDG
    - Dose: 5-20 mCi (185-740 MBq)
    - Dosimetry: Urinary bladder receives largest dose
    - Image acquisition: 30-60 min after injection

Artifacts and Quality Control

- Certain medications can significantly alter scan appearance and should be discontinued/documented
- Ensure patient is off competing medications if activity is diffusely low

DIFFERENTIAL DIAGNOSIS

Atypical Parkinsonian Syndromes

- Multiple system atrophy (MSA)
  - Family of neurodegenerative disorders
  - Includes olivopontocerebellar atrophy, Shy-Drager syndrome, striatonigral degeneration
  - Symptoms include parkinsonism, ataxia, and autonomic dysfunction
    - Cerebellar dominant (MSA-C) and parkinsonian dominant (MSA-P)
  - F-18 FDG PET
    - MSA-P shows decreased putamen activity
    - MSA-C shows decreased activity in cerebellum
  - Amyloid PET negative
  - I-123 FP-CIT SPECT positive
- Progressive supranuclear palsy (PSP)
  - Symptoms include parkinsonism, bradykinesia, rigidity, postural instability, dysphagia, dysarthria

- F-18 FDG PET/CT
  - Decreased F-18 FDG activity in basal ganglia, frontal lobes, anterior cingulate, midbrain
- Amyloid PET negative
- Ioflupane SPECT positive
- Dementia with Lewy bodies (DLB)
  - Symptoms include dementia, visual hallucinations, parkinsonism
  - F-18 FDG PET/CT shows generalized reduced cortical FDG uptake
    - Decreased uptake most pronounced in occipital and posterior parietal regions
  - Amyloid PET is positive in > 50% of patients
  - I-123 FP-CIT SPECT positive
- Corticobasal degeneration (CBD)
  - Cognitive/behavioral symptoms precede movement dysfunction
  - Symptoms include akinesia, rigidity, dystonia, apraxia, executive dysfunction, aphasia
  - Patients do not respond to levodopa
  - F-18 FDG PET/CT
    - Relative decreased activity in contralateral cortex and basal ganglia
    - May be caused by increased ipsilateral uptake
  - Amyloid PET negative
  - I-123 FP-CIT SPECT positive, typically asymmetric and decreased contralateral to symptoms

Benign Essential Tremor

- Negative I-123 FP-CIT SPECT

Vascular Parkinsonism

- Negative I-123 FP-CIT SPECT

Drug-Induced Parkinsonism

- Negative I-123 FP-CIT SPECT

PATHOLOGY

General Features

- Parkinson disease accounts for over 70% of parkinsonian patients
- Loss of dopaminergic neurons
  - Affected neurons project from substantia nigra (midbrain) to putamen and caudate
  - Putamen typically affected earlier and more severely
  - Symptoms begin to show after about 50% of neurons are affected

CLINICAL ISSUES

Presentation

- Most common signs/symptoms
  - Rigidity, tremor, bradykinesia, postural imbalance

Demographics

- Prevalence of about 1% in adults over 65

DIAGNOSTIC CHECKLIST

Image Interpretation Pearls

- I-123 FP-CIT SPECT differentiates between diseases related to dopamine loss (PD and APS) and those that mimic them clinically (benign tremor and vascular parkinsonism)
- F-18 FDG PET/CT may play role in differentiating between PD and APS

Reporting Tips

- Reporting scheme in literature
  - Normal: 2 comma-shaped areas of uptake
  - Abnormal grade 1: Asymmetric uptake (normal [comma shape] on one side and abnormal [period shape] on other side)
  - Abnormal grade 2: Abnormal (period shape) reduced putamen activity bilaterally
  - Abnormal grade 3: Markedly reduced uptake bilaterally

SELECTED REFERENCES

1. Broski SM et al: Structural and functional imaging in parkinsonian syndromes. Radiographics. 34(5):1273-92, 2014
2. Bajaj N et al: Clinical utility of dopamine transporter single photon emission CT (DaT-SPECT) with (123I) ioflupane in diagnosis of parkinsonian syndromes. J Neurol Neurosurg Psychiatry. 84(11):1288-95, 2013
3. Djang DS et al: SNM practice guideline for dopamine transporter imaging with 123I-ioflupane SPECT 1.0. J Nucl Med. 53(1):154-63, 2012
4. Brooks DJ: Imaging approaches to Parkinson disease. J Nucl Med. 51(4):596-609, 2010
5. Tang CC et al: Differential diagnosis of parkinsonism: a metabolic imaging study using pattern analysis. Lancet Neurol. 9(2):149-58, 2010
6. Booij J et al: Dopamine transporter imaging with [(123)I]FP-CIT SPECT: potential effects of drugs. Eur J Nucl Med Mol Imaging. 35(2):424-38, 2008
7. Eckert T et al: FDG PET in the differential diagnosis of parkinsonian disorders. Neuroimage. 26(3):912-21, 2005
8. Marek K et al: [123I.] Neurology. 57(11):2089-94, 2001
9. Seil FJ et al: Reorganization of organotypic cultures of mouse cerebellum exposed to cytosine arabinoside: a timed ultrastructural study. J Comp Neurol. 313(2):193-212, 1991
10. FDA prescribing information for DaTscan Website. http://www.accessdata.fda.gov/drugsatfda_docs/nda/2011/022454sOrig1s000Lbl.pdf

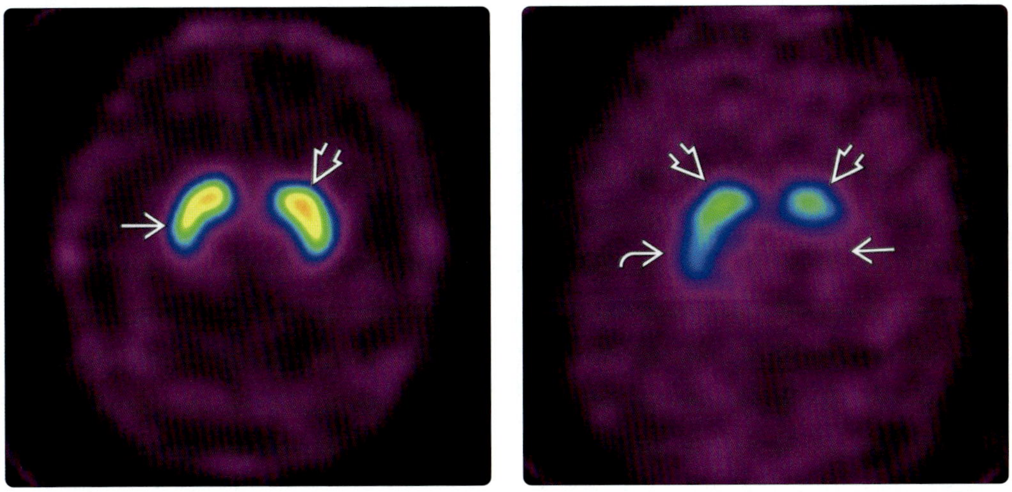

(Left) *Axial I-123 FP-CIT SPECT shows normal putamen activity and caudate activity. These finding are not consistent with Parkinson disease (PD) or atypical parkinsonism syndromes (APS).* **(Right)** *Axial I-123 FP-CIT SPECT shows absent left putamen activity, preserved but decreased right putamen activity, and preserved caudate activity. These finding are consistent with PD or APS.*

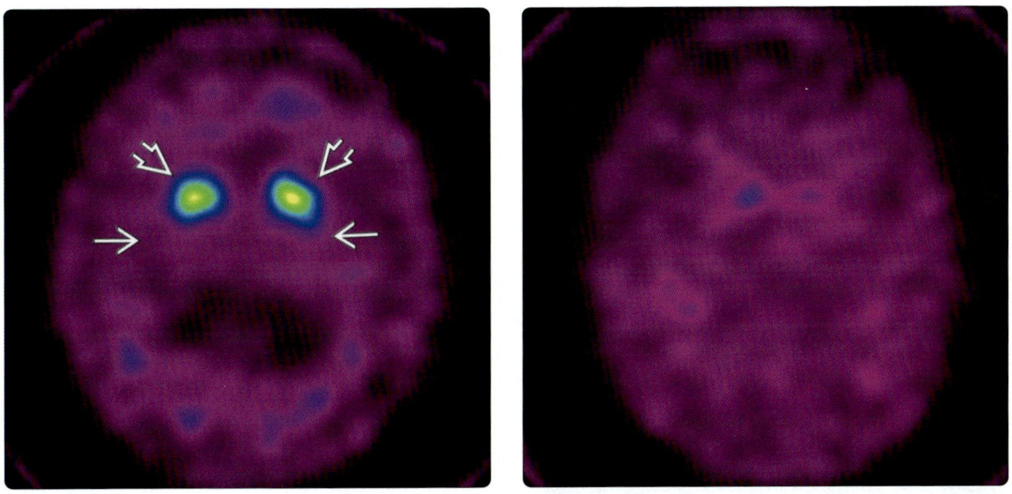

(Left) *Axial I-123 FP-CIT SPECT shows absent bilateral putamen activity and preserved caudate activity. These finding are consistent with PD or APS.* **(Right)** *Axial I-123 FP-CIT SPECT shows absent bilateral putamen activity and almost absent caudate activity. These finding are consistent with PD or APS if patient was not on any interfering medications.*

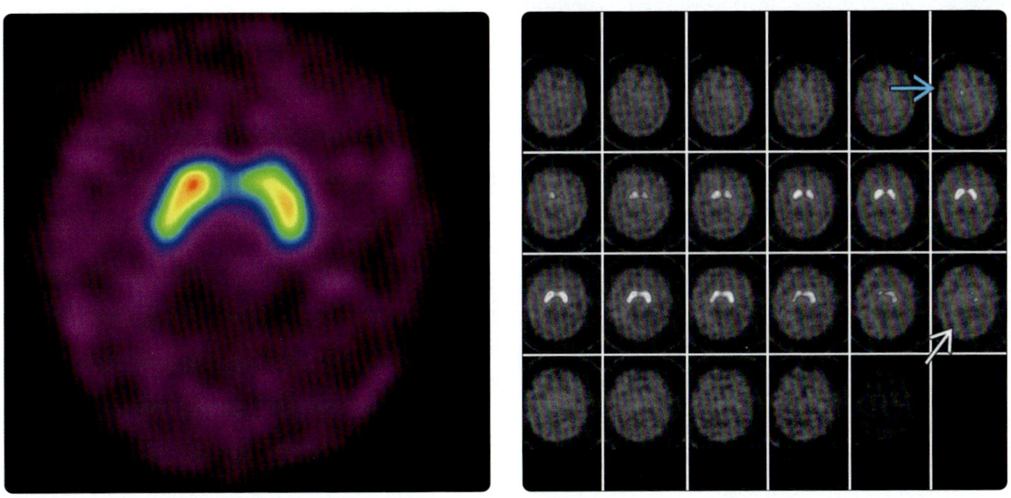

(Left) *Axial I-123 FP-CIT SPECT shows bilateral comma-shaped appearance consistent with a normal study. Note the slight asymmetry between sides, which may be secondary to head positioning.* **(Right)** *Axial I-123 FP-CIT SPECT images of the same patient from superior to inferior demonstrate full appearance of caudate heads and putamen.*

Brain Death

KEY FACTS

TERMINOLOGY

- Legal definition of brain death
  - Irreversible cessation of circulatory and respiratory functions
  - Irreversible cessation of all functions of entire brain, including brainstem
  - Primarily a clinical diagnosis
- Ancillary studies used when clinical picture equivocal &/or to shorten length of observation period
- Brain death diagnosis important for organ donation status
- Imaging may confirm brain death but does not substitute for clinical criteria

IMAGING

- Nuclear medicine brain death study
  - Evaluate for presence or absence of cerebral blood flow &/or brain parenchymal uptake
  - In many states, must assess cerebral blood flow to both supra- and infratentorial brain
    - Cerebral cortex, cerebellum, brainstem
- **Brain parenchyma scintigraphy**
  - Tc-99m exametazime (HMPAO), Tc-99m ethyl cysteinate dimer (ECD)
  - Delayed images are usually definitive for presence or absence of cerebral blood flow
- **Normal cerebral uptake**
  - Uptake in all portions of brain
- **Abnormal cerebral uptake**
  - Patchy areas of absent or diminished uptake
- **Absent cerebral uptake**
  - No uptake in all portions of brain
  - Hot nose sign
- **Reporting recommendations**
  - Cerebral &/or cerebellar perfusion absent or present
  - Cerebral &/or cerebellar perfusion present although abnormal (discuss specific regions of uptake/lack of uptake)

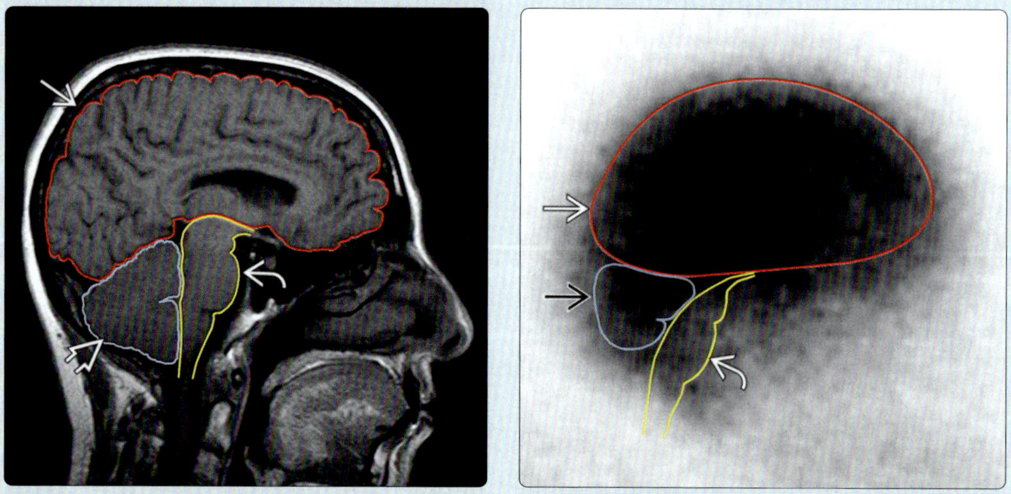

(Left) *Coronal MR demonstrates the cortex (red), cerebellum (blue), and brainstem (yellow).* **(Right)** *Lateral Tc-99m HMPAO shows gross approximation of where the cerebral cortex (red), cerebellar (blue), and brainstem (yellow) activity are located.*

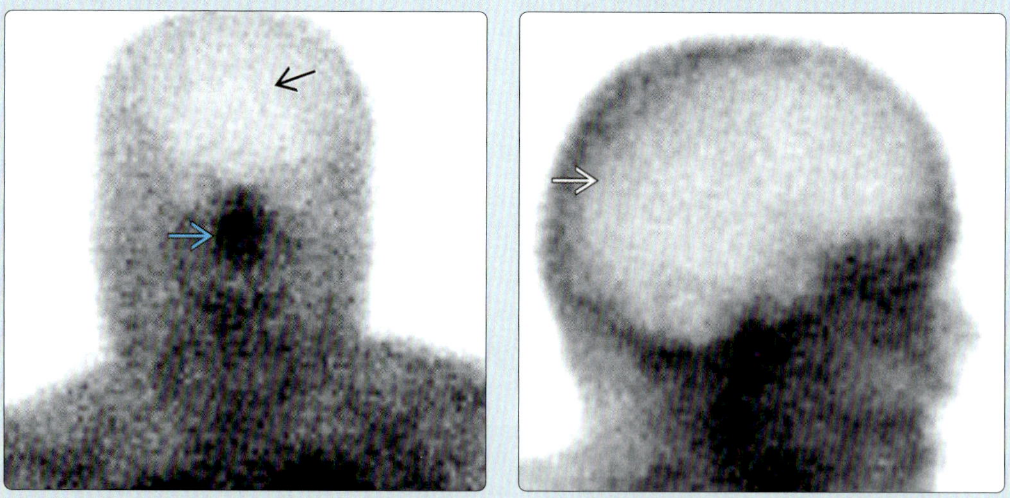

(Left) *Anterior image of a patient injected with Tc-99m HMPAO demonstrates no visible brain activity, consistent with brain death. Note the hot nose sign.* **(Right)** *Lateral image of the same patient demonstrates no visible brain activity, consistent with brain death.*

TERMINOLOGY

Definitions

- Legal definition of brain death
  - Irreversible cessation of circulatory and respiratory functions
  - Irreversible cessation of all functions of entire brain, including brainstem
- Most facilities require 2 independent clinical confirmations of brain death
- Primarily a clinical diagnosis
  - Ancillary studies used when clinical picture equivocal &/or to shorten length of observation period
- Brain death diagnosis important for organ donation status
- Imaging may confirm brain death but does not substitute for clinical criteria

IMAGING

General Features

- Best diagnostic clue
  - Nuclear medicine brain death study
    - Evaluate for presence or absence of cerebral blood flow &/or brain parenchymal uptake
    - In many states, must assess cerebral blood flow to both supra- and infratentorial brain
      - Cerebral cortex
      - Cerebellum
      - Brainstem

Nuclear Medicine Findings

- **Brain parenchyma scintigraphy**
  - Tc-99m exametazime (HMPAO), Tc-99m ethyl cysteinate dimer (ECD)
  - Lipophilic radiotracers that localize to brain parenchyma in proportion to blood flow
  - Delayed images are usually definitive for presence or absence of cerebral blood flow
  - Allows assessment of cerebrum, cerebellum, brainstem
  - Does not require bolus technique
  - Tc-99m HMPAO preferred since it accumulates in brain parenchyma within 2 min and takes several hrs before significant redistribution
  - **Normal cerebral uptake**
    - Uptake in all portions of brain
  - **Abnormal cerebral uptake**
    - Patchy areas of absent or diminished uptake
  - **Absent cerebral uptake**
    - No uptake in all portions of brain
    - Hot nose sign
      - Early increased activity in nasopharyngeal region on anterior view
      - Increased intracranial pressure leads to shunting of blood from internal carotids to external carotid system
      - Nonspecific sign secondary to false-positives
- **Brain nuclear angiogram**
  - Flow radiotracers: Tc-99m DTPA or Tc-99m pertechnetate
  - Older technique
  - Only allows assessment of anterior brain circulation
    - May not meet legal requirements of brainstem or posterior fossa assessment
  - Requires good bolus technique and adequate cardiac output
  - **Normal cerebral perfusion**
    - Angiographic phase
      - Trident sign: Early simultaneous visualization of the paired anterior cerebral arteries (ACAs) and each middle cerebral artery (MCA)
    - Blood pool phase
      - Visualization of venous sinuses but not brain
  - **Abnormal cerebral perfusion**
    - Angiographic phase
      - May see asymmetrical flow or incomplete trident
    - Blood pool phase
      - May see uptake in epidural hematoma, choroid plexus (Tc-99m pertechnetate uptake), or areas of blood brain barrier breakdown
  - **Absent cerebral perfusion**
    - Angiographic phase
      - Absence of trident; empty light bulb sign; hot nose sign
    - Blood pool phase
      - Delayed images may visualize venous sinuses from centrally draining scalp perforators
      - Lack of superior sagittal sinus activity helps confirm lack of cerebral perfusion

Imaging Recommendations

- Protocol advice
  - Patient preparation
    - Tourniquet encircling head can diminish scalp blood flow
  - Radiopharmaceutical
    - Brain parenchyma: Tc-99m HMPAO or Tc-99m ECD
    - Brain blood flow: Tc-99m DTPA or Tc-99m pertechnetate, but not recommended
  - Dose
    - Brain parenchyma: 15-20 mCi (555-740 MBq) for adults; 0.3 mCi/kg for children
    - Brain blood flow: Up to 30 mCi (1.1 GBq)
  - Dosimetry
    - Brain parenchyma agents: Kidneys and bladder receive highest radiation dose
    - Brain blood flow agents: Not recommended
      - Tc-99m DTPA: Bladder wall receives highest dose
  - Image acquisition
    - Gamma camera with field of view large enough to image entire head and neck
    - Portable gamma camera useful for bedside imaging in ventilated patient in intensive care unit
    - Flow images
      - Brain parenchyma: Image acquisition starting at time of radiotracer injection and ending well after venous phase
      - 1-3 sec per frame for at least 60 sec
      - Brain angiogram: Tracer flow should be observed from level of carotids to skull vertex
    - Static planar images
      - Brain parenchyma: Anterior and lateral planar views should be obtained after at least 20 min

- Brain angiogram: Anterior, posterior, and lateral view
- Chin slightly tucked on lateral view to allow visualization of posterior fossa
- SPECT
  - May be obtained in addition to flow and planar images with brain parenchyma tracers
  - Allows better visualization of perfusion to posterior fossa and brainstem structures
  - More difficult than bedside planar images with portable gamma camera
- Reporting recommendations
  - Cerebral and cerebellar perfusion absent
  - Cerebral and cerebellar perfusion present
  - Cerebral and cerebellar perfusion present, although abnormal (discuss specific regions of uptake/lack of uptake)
- If equivocal, may repeat exam with 2x dose in 6 hrs or regular dose in 24 hrs

Artifacts and Quality Control

- Inadequate preparation or instability of radiotracer may result in agent that fails to show uptake in brain
- Tracer can accumulate in superior sagittal sinus and thus be mistaken as sign of cerebral arterial flow
- Infiltration of tracer at injection site can lead to inadequate radiotracer in vascular space
- Hyperemic scalp structures can mimic brain parenchyma uptake

DIFFERENTIAL DIAGNOSIS

Diffuse Cerebral Edema

- Reversible causes (drug overdose, status epilepticus) can mimic brain death clinically

Increased Blood Flow to Scalp

- Head trauma/ecchymosis (compare with CT)
- Cerebrospinal fluid shunts and intracranial pressure transducers

Other Brain Death Mimics

- Locked-in syndrome, neuromuscular blockade, high spinal cord injury, massive MCA infarct

PATHOLOGY

General Features

- Etiology
  - Severe cell swelling leads to increased intracranial pressure (ICP)
  - Markedly elevated ICP decreases cerebral blood flow
  - If ICP > end-diastolic pressure in cerebral arteries, diastolic reversal occurs
  - If ICP > systolic pressure, blood flow ceases

Gross Pathologic & Surgical Features

- Markedly swollen brain with severely compressed sulci
- Bilateral descending transtentorial herniation
  - Downward displacement of diencephalon
  - Grooving of temporal lobes by tentorial incisura

CLINICAL ISSUES

Presentation

- Most common signs/symptoms
  - Profound coma (GCS = 3), "known cause," absence of brainstem reflexes, apnea
- Clinical profile
  - Clinical diagnosis of brain death highly reliable if examiners are experienced, use established clinical criteria
  - Ancillary studies include brainstem auditory evoked responses (BAER), EEG, radionuclide brain study, transcranial Doppler US, MR/MRA, CT angiography and CT perfusion study

Natural History & Prognosis

- Brain death usually followed by somatic death within few days
- No set guidelines exist for observation period but usually 6-24 hrs
- Brainstem-level responses and spinal reflexes may be present at first but sequentially fade out

DIAGNOSTIC CHECKLIST

Consider

- Prior to study
  - Quality control on Tc-99m HMPAO and ECD are important as poor tag negates study
  - Focused history, including head trauma, surgery, possibility of hypothermia or drug overdose, review of anatomic imaging
- Brain nuclear angiogram agents (Tc-99m pertechnetate, Tc-99m DTPA)
  - Successful anterior (posterior occasionally) flow sequence critical; consider viewing dynamically
  - 5-30 min delayed posterior (anterior) plus lateral
- Brain parenchyma agents (Tc-99m HMPAO, Tc-99m ECD)
  - Flow sequence not critical
  - Planar anterior and lateral images at 10-20 min or longer
  - Images often performed on portable gamma camera in intensive care unit
  - SPECT is more sensitive but not necessary

SELECTED REFERENCES

1. Donohoe KJ et al: SNM practice guideline for brain death scintigraphy 2.0. J Nucl Med Technol. 40(3):198-203, 2012
2. Wijdicks EF et al: Evidence-based guideline update: determining brain death in adults: report of the Quality Standards Subcommittee of the American Academy of Neurology. Neurology. 74(23):1911-8, 2010
3. Booth CM et al: Is this patient dead, vegetative, or severely neurologically impaired? Assessing outcome for comatose survivors of cardiac arrest. JAMA. 291(7):870-9, 2004
4. Belber CJ: Brain death documentation: analysis and issues. Neurosurgery. 53(4):1009; author reply 1009, 2003
5. Conrad GR et al: Scintigraphy as a confirmatory test of brain death. Semin Nucl Med. 33(4):312-23, 2003
6. Donohoe KJ et al: Procedure guideline for brain death scintigraphy. J Nucl Med. 44(5):846-51, 2003
7. Flowers WM Jr et al: Accuracy of clinical evaluation in the determination of brain death. South Med J. 93(2):203-6, 2000

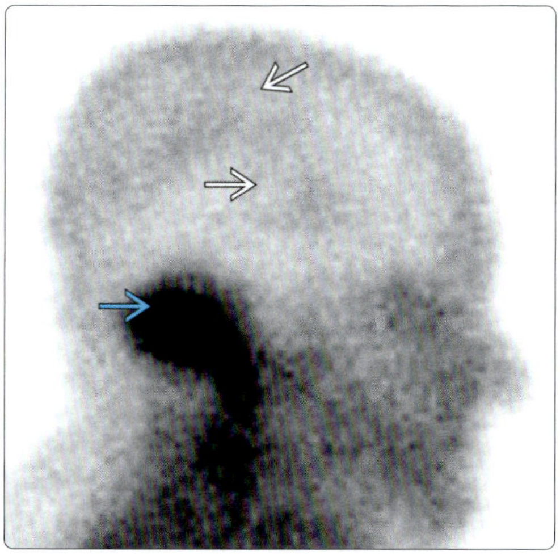

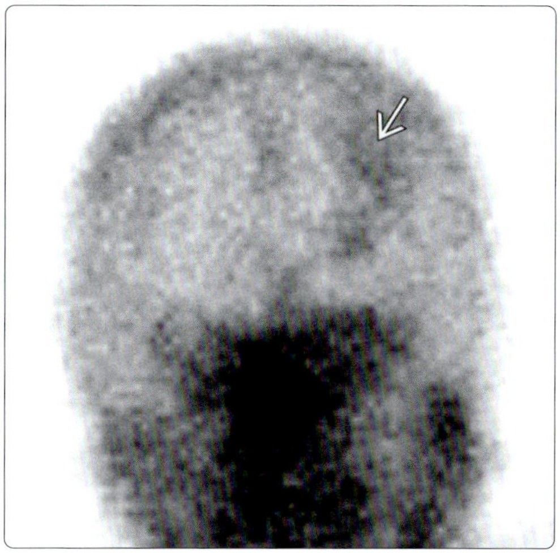

(Left) *Lateral image of a patient injected with Tc-99m HMPAO demonstrates minimal visible brain activity* ➡*, which is not consistent with brain death, although prognosis is grim. Furthermore, there is intense uptake in the infratentorial region* →*, which may be cerebellar activity.* **(Right)** *Anterior image of the same patient demonstrates minimal visible brain activity* ➡*, which is not consistent with brain death, although prognosis is grim.*

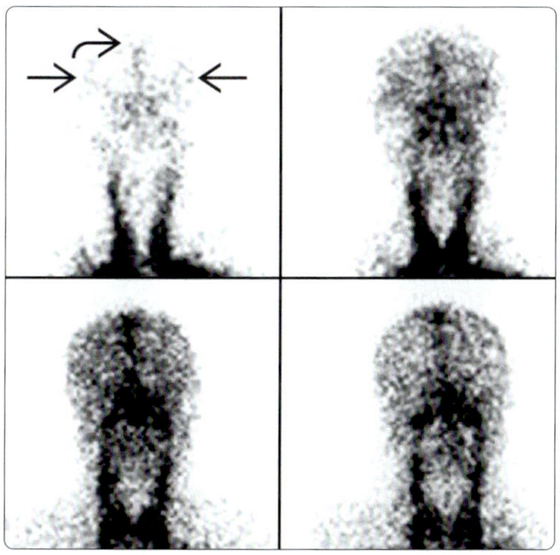

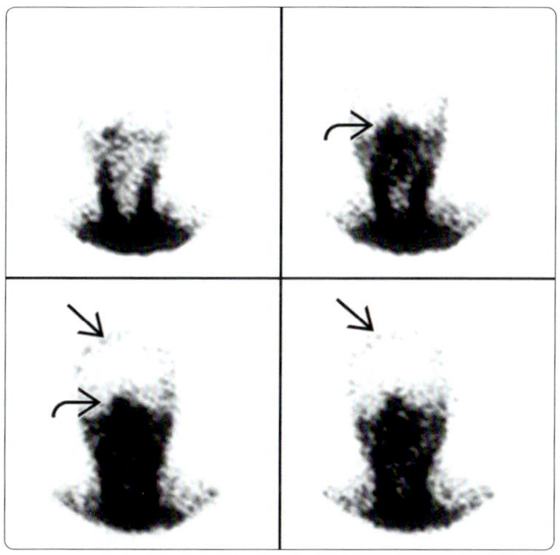

(Left) *Normal cerebral blood flow scan in the angiographic phase demonstrates normal trident sign consisting of middle cerebral* → *and paired anterior cerebral* ↪ *arteries.* **(Right)** *Tc-99m pertechnetate scan in the angiographic phase shows absence of trident sign with shunting of blood to scalp (empty light bulb sign)* → *and to central face (hot nose sign)* ↪*.*

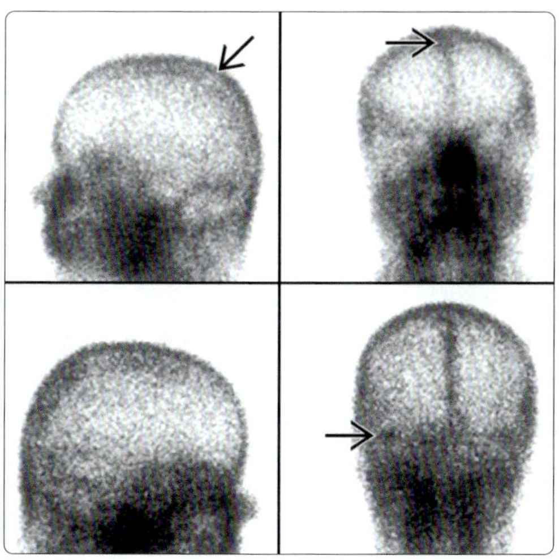

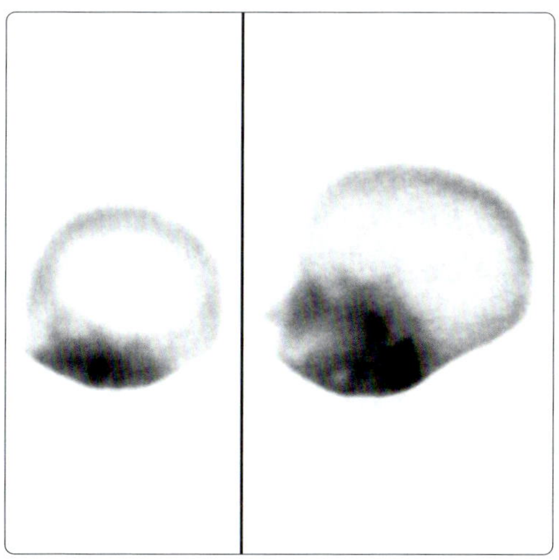

(Left) *Tc-99m pertechnetate blood pool study shows normal venous sinus activity* →*. There is no activity in the brain itself (this is normal).* **(Right)** *Tc-99m blood pool study in the same patient with no definite venous sinus activity suggests (but does not confirm) brain death.*

Cerebrovascular Ischemia

KEY FACTS

IMAGING

- Assessment of functional cerebrovascular reserve in chronic stenotic occlusive disease
  - Tc-99m ECD/HMPAO SPECT with Diamox challenge
    - Diamox is a carbonic anhydrase inhibitor that crosses the blood brain barrier and increases pCO_2, which leads to increased blood flow in normal vessels
    - Vessels that are already maximally vasodilated due to stenosis will show decreased uptake
  - 1 g Diamox (acetazolamide) IV, wait 30 min before injecting tracer
  - If patient is allergic to sulfonamide, cross-reactivity possible but unlikely; has been given in patients with sulfonamide allergy without adverse reactions
  - Decrease sensory input and motor activity for 30 min prior to and 30 min after injection (patient sits in quiet room with eyes closed)
- Preoperative assessment prior to temporal lobectomy for epilepsy
  - Wada test with Tc-99m ECD/HMPAO SPECT
    - Injection of sodium amobarbital to anesthetize cerebral hemisphere to determine dominant hemisphere for speech/memory prior to surgery
    - Injection of Tc-99m HMPAO during sodium amobarbital infusion with subsequent SPECT imaging to evaluate for collateral circulation resulting in amobarbital crossover to contralateral cerebral hemisphere
- Preoperative assessment prior to carotid sacrifice
  - Balloon occlusion test (BOT) with Tc-99m ECD/HMPAO SPECT
    - BOT coupled with SPECT to assess regional blood flow prior to carotid artery sacrifice
  - With balloon inflated, inject 20-30 mCi (740 MBq to 1.1 GBq) ECD or HMPAO peripherally
  - Ideally, allow balloon occlusion for 15 min prior to injection (if patient asymptomatic) to allow collateral vascular dilation

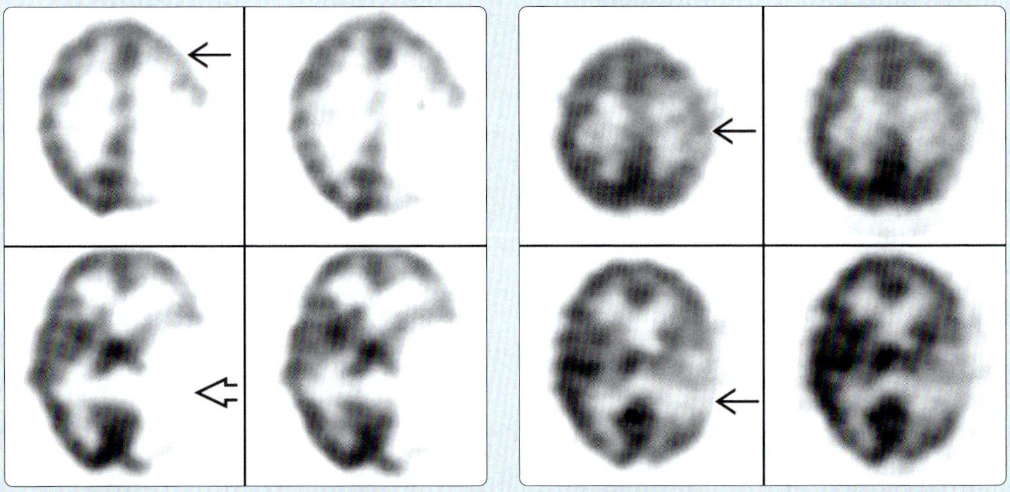

(Left) *Axial Tc-99m HMPAO SPECT in conjunction with balloon occlusion of left ICA test to assess collateral adequacy shows good collateral flow from ACA territory → but poor collateral to PCA and MCA territories ⇨.* **(Right)** *Axial Tc-99m HMPAO SPECT in the same patient shows some baseline decrease in the compromised territory →, likely due to mass effect from base of skull tumor.*

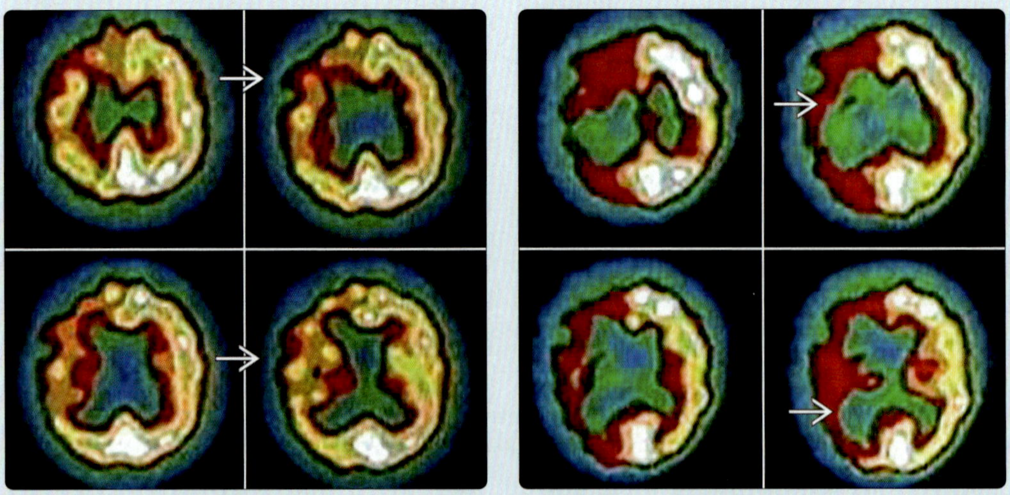

(Left) *Baseline axial Tc-99m HMPAO SPECT shows mild decreased perfusion in right cerebral hemisphere ➡ in a patient with known right carotid occlusion.* **(Right)** *Tc-99m HMPAO SPECT with Diamox challenge in the same patient shows lack of functional vascular reserve on the right ➡, indicative of at-risk brain parenchyma.*

TERMINOLOGY

Definitions

- Decrease or interruption of blood supply to brain

IMAGING

Nuclear Medicine Findings

- Tc-99m ECD/HMPAO SPECT with Diamox challenge: Assessment of functional cerebrovascular reserve in chronic stenotic occlusive disease
  - Images obtained with Diamox
    - Diamox is a carbonic anhydrase inhibitor that crosses the blood brain barrier and increases pCO_2, which leads to increased blood flow in normal vessels
    - Vessels that are already maximally vasodilated due to stenosis will show decreased uptake
  - Decreased activity in brain positive for inducible ischemia if same region normal baseline SPECT
  - Diamox-only SPECT shows increased sensitivity over non-Diamox SPECT for detection of ischemic regions of clinical significance
- Wada test with Tc-99m ECD/HMPAO SPECT: Preoperative assessment prior to temporal lobectomy for epilepsy
  - Injection of sodium amobarbital to anesthetize a cerebral hemisphere to determine dominant hemisphere for speech/memory prior to surgery
  - Simultaneous injection of Tc-99m ECD/HMPAO with subsequent SPECT imaging used to evaluate for collateral circulation resulting in amobarbital crossover to contralateral cerebral hemisphere
- Balloon occlusion test (BOT) with Tc-99m ECD/HMPAO SPECT: Preoperative assessment prior to carotid sacrifice
  - Carotid sacrifice may be done for large en bloc surgical resection of skull base tumors or treatment of intracranial aneurysms
  - BOT coupled with SPECT to assess regional blood flow prior to carotid artery sacrifice
  - BOT with SPECT typically requires 15-30 min occlusion time and transport of patient to multiple image suites
  - If decreased activity in region on BOT, consider baseline study to compare
- Tc-99m ECD/HMPAO SPECT: Postinterventional assessment
  - Spasm or postinterventional vascular compromise: Decreased uptake
  - Prediction of hyperperfusion syndrome following carotid and other bypass procedures: Increased uptake
- Tc-99m ECD/HMPAO SPECT: Cerebral infarction in problem or equivocal cases
  - Assessment of penumbra at risk for extension of infarction: Decreased perfusion surrounding region of infarction
  - Assessment of subacute infarction: Small amounts of perfusion in regions of suspected infarction may support salvage procedure

Imaging Recommendations

- Protocol advice
  - Patient preparation
    - Baseline SPECT
      - Avoid caffeine, alcohol, or other drugs known to affect cerebral blood flow
      - Patient sits in quiet room with no stimulus
    - Diamox challenge
      - 1 g Diamox (acetazolamide) IV, wait 30 min before injecting tracer
      - If patient allergic to sulfonamide, cross-reactivity possible, but unlikely; has been given in patients with sulfonamide allergy without adverse reactions
      - Decrease sensory input and motor activity for prior to and 30 min after injection (patient sits in quiet room with eyes closed)
    - Balloon occlusion test
      - With balloon inflated, inject 20-30 mCi (740 MBq to 1.1 GBq) ECD or HMPAO peripherally
      - Ideally, allow balloon occlusion for 15 min prior to injection (if patient asymptomatic) to allow collateral vascular dilation
      - Ideally, leave balloon inflated for 10-15 min after injection of tracer (if patient asymptomatic) to allow localization of tracer
  - Radiopharmaceutical
    - Tc-99m exametazime (HMPAO)
    - Tc-99m ethyl cysteinate dimer (ECD)
  - Dose: 15-30 mCi (555 MBq to 1.1 GBq)
  - Dosimetry
    - Tc-99m HMPAO: Kidneys receive highest dose
    - Tc-99m ECD: Bladder wall receives highest dose
  - Image acquisition
    - SPECT ± CT
    - Tc-99m HMPAO: 90 min post injection
    - Tc-99m ECD: 45 min post injection

DIAGNOSTIC CHECKLIST

Consider

- On provocative studies, such as Diamox challenge brain SPECT and balloon occlusion test brain SPECT, perform baseline SPECT only if provocative study positive
- Avoid Diamox challenge brain SPECT within 3 days of acute stroke or recent intracranial hemorrhage
- Diamox can provoke migraines in patients with history of migraines

SELECTED REFERENCES

1. Sorteberg A: Balloon occlusion tests and therapeutic vessel occlusions revisited: when, when not, and how. AJNR Am J Neuroradiol. 35(5):862-5, 2014
2. Vagal AS et al: The acetazolamide challenge: techniques and applications in the evaluation of chronic cerebral ischemia. AJNR Am J Neuroradiol. 30(5):876-84, 2009
3. Hori M et al: The magnetic resonance Matas test: Feasibility and comparison with the conventional intraarterial balloon test occlusion with SPECT perfusion imaging. J Magn Reson Imaging. 21(6):709-14, 2005
4. Lampl Y et al: Prognostic significance of blood brain barrier permeability in acute hemorrhagic stroke. Cerebrovasc Dis. 20(6):433-7, 2005
5. Maulaz A et al: Selecting patients for early stroke treatment with penumbra images. Cerebrovasc Dis. 20 Suppl 2:19-24, 2005
6. Ueda T et al: Single-photon emission CT imaging in acute stroke. Neuroimaging Clin N Am. 15(3):543-51, x, 2005
7. Latchaw RE et al: Guidelines and recommendations for perfusion imaging in cerebral ischemia: A scientific statement for healthcare professionals by the writing group on perfusion imaging, from the Council on Cardiovascular Radiology of the American Heart Association. Stroke. 34(4):1084-104, 2003

SECTION 3

Gastrointestinal

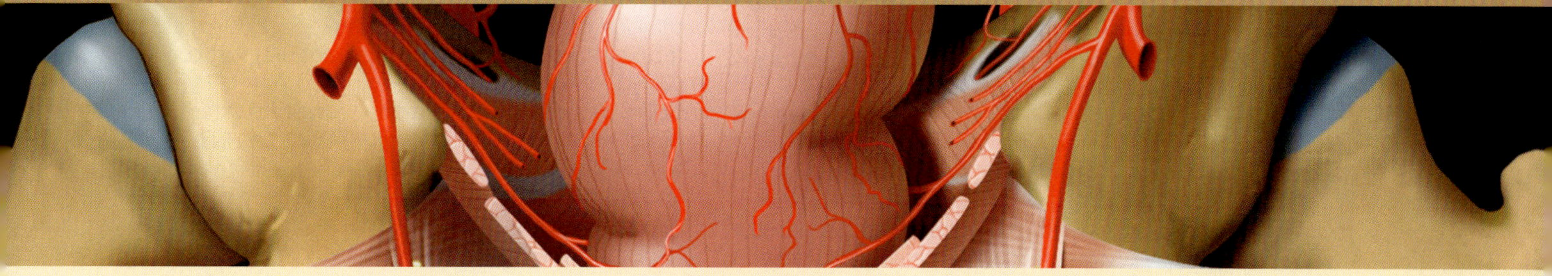

Introduction

Hepatobiliary

Gastrointestinal

Infection and Inflammation

Spleen

Introduction

Nuclear gastrointestinal imaging comprises functional studies of the stomach, liver, gallbladder, and spleen, as well as localizing the source of GI bleeding and abdominopelvic infection. These studies provide a useful adjunct to anatomic imaging in complicated cases and are often the standard of care for optimal clinical management in patients with chronic abdominal pain, occult infection, and GI bleeding.

Imaging Protocols

Gastric Emptying

Symptoms of postprandial nausea, bloating, and abdominal pain can be caused by gastric emptying that is too fast or too slow. In patients with gastroparesis, gastric emptying studies using Tc-99m sulfur colloid in a standardized egg sandwich meal can confirm the diagnosis as well as evaluate the efficacy of prokinetic agents. Interestingly, in one study, 23% of patients with suspected gastroparesis actually showed rapid gastric transit on a nuclear gastric emptying study, even though they had not undergone a surgery that could cause dumping syndrome. Recent studies suggest abnormal emptying of solids &/or liquids can cause symptoms of gastroparesis. A dual-radiotracer technique (Tc-99m sulfur colloid in an egg sandwich and In-111 DTPA in water) is now being performed, showing coincident solid and liquid emptying during the same four-hour study. Liquid gastric emptying studies are used in pediatric patients with feeding difficulties/failure to thrive and in adult and pediatric patients with feeding tubes. The value of these studies often lies in determining when a patient's stomach empties, so that feeding schedules can be optimized to the appropriate times.

Biliary Patency and Function

In patients with acute right upper quadrant (RUQ) pain, ultrasound can have a sensitivity as low as 54% for acute cholecystitis. Assessing patency of the cystic duct and common bile duct using Tc-99m IDA derivatives offers valuable clinical information early in the disease course, when outcomes can be optimized with early cholecystectomy. Patients with chronic intermittent RUQ pain and a patent biliary system can have acalculous cholecystopathy or gallbladder dyskinesia. Defined as a gallbladder ejection fraction 35-38% on hepatobiliary scan, patients with gallbladder dyskinesia can be triaged to laparoscopic cholecystectomy with symptomatic relief 94-98% of the time.

After laparoscopic cholecystectomy, the incidence of bile leak can be as high as 3%. Hepatobiliary scans become useful in patients with postoperative pain to diagnose biliary leak or biloma. In addition, enterogastric bile reflux, a complication of gallbladder and gastric surgery that causes postoperative abdominal pain, can be seen on hepatobiliary scan.

Liver and Spleen Imaging

Although anatomic imaging with US, CT, and MR characterizes the vast majority of abdominal lesions, a small percentage remain indeterminate. To avoid liver biopsy, Tc-99m IDA derivatives, Tc-99m sulfur colloid, and Tc-99m red blood cell (RBC) scans can diagnose focal nodular hyperplasia, hepatic adenomas, and hemangiomas, particularly in lesions > 2 cm. Similarly, ectopic splenic tissue can be diagnosed, avoiding biopsy if confused with cancer recurrence and directing surgery in patients with recurrent idiopathic thrombocytopenic purpura post splenectomy. Radiotracer-based localization of splenic tissue remains important in infants with certain congenital anomalies, as ultrasound can be inconclusive and insensitive. In these patients, the presence or absence of splenic tissue directs antibiotic therapy and offers information on projected lifespan.

GI Bleeding

After hemodynamic stabilization, the ultimate clinical management of lower GI bleeding requires bleeding site localization and subsequent intervention, most commonly with colonoscopy. However, colonoscopy requires a cleansing bowel preparation and has poor visibility in cases of brisk GI bleed. In patients with intermittent or active GI bleeding, Tc-99m RBC scans diagnose the site of bleeding as well as immediately direct intervention (e.g., coiling of blood vessels at a time when angiography is likely to be positive). In one large study, arteriography for GI bleeding was found to have a sensitivity of only 41%. When Tc-99m RBC scan and arteriography are used together, the sensitivity of arteriography increases to 61-72%.

Abdominal Infection and Inflammation

Nuclear medicine imaging of inflammation and infection surveys the entire body in one study and is often used in patients with occult bacteremia and sepsis, fever of unknown origin, and suspected postsurgical abscess. These studies are particularly valuable in postoperative patients whose anatomic imaging can be inconclusive or suggests multifocal sites of infection that need clinical intervention, such as drainage. In outpatients, the signs and symptoms of intraabdominal infections can overlap and the physical exam can be inconclusive. In patients with inflammatory bowel disease (IBD), nuclear medicine can assess disease activity and direct therapy.

- F-18 FDG PET/CT: Often the fastest and least expensive whole-body survey in the inpatient setting, focal uptake in inflammation and infection is easily identified with this high-resolution scan, accompanied by CT localization; images are obtained one hour after F-18 FDG administration
- Tc-99m HMPAO WBC: Provides whole-body images from relatively low dose of Tc-99m radiotracer; often used to diagnose infection in children, in extremities, and to confirm active IBD; images are obtained within four hours after readministration of labeled WBCs; given ideal imaging characteristics of Tc-99m, SPECT/CT images are superior to those performed using In-111 WBCs
- In-111 WBC: Traditional whole-body WBC scan; provides images 24 hours after readministration of WBCs; especially useful in conjunction with Tc-99m MDP bone scans to evaluate for osteomyelitis in bone that has undergone trauma or surgery; remains useful as whole-body infection survey
- Ga-67 citrate: Provides information on inflammation/infection 24-48 hours after injection; traditionally used in patients with fever of unknown origin, it is sensitive for lymphoma as well as granulomatous infections and occult abscess; superior sensitivity to WBC scans in suspected vertebral osteomyelitis

Selected References

1. Middleton ML et al: Planar scintigraphic imaging of the gastrointestinal tract in clinical practice. Semin Nucl Med. 42(1):33-40, 2012

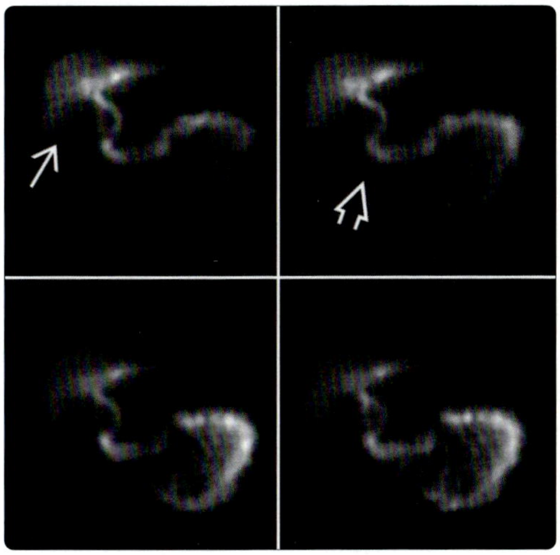

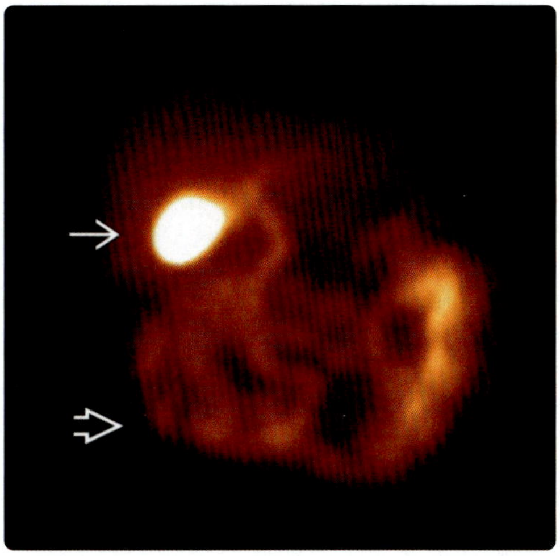

(Left) *Anterior Tc-99m HIDA hepatobiliary scan in a patient post cholecystectomy shows normal hepatic uptake ➡ and biliary-to-bowel transit ➡ without a bile leak.* **(Right)** *Anterior Tc-99m HIDA hepatobiliary scan in a patient with right upper quadrant pain shows normal gallbladder ➡ and bowel ➡ activity.*

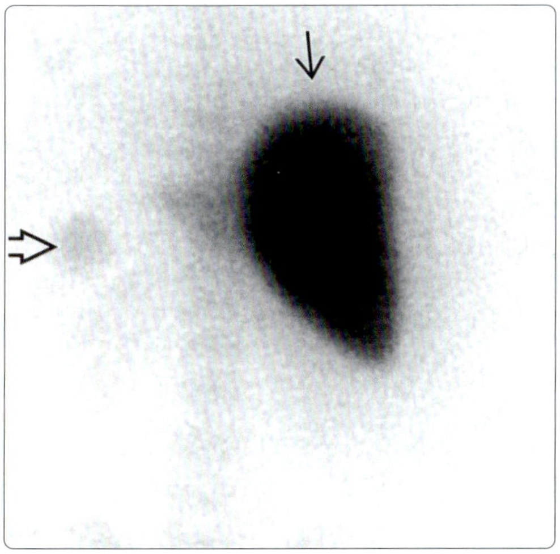

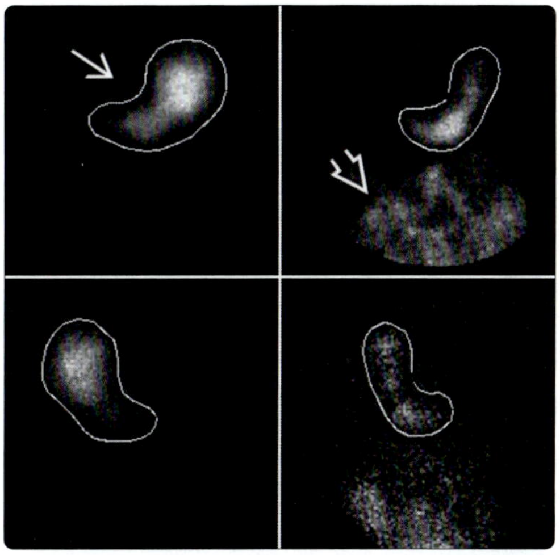

(Left) *Posterior Tc-99m sulfur colloid liver spleen scan in a patient post splenectomy for idiopathic thrombocytopenic purpura with recurrent thrombocytopenia shows normal uptake in the liver ➡ and a splenule ➡.* **(Right)** *Anterior (top) and posterior (bottom) Tc-99m sulfur colloid gastric emptying scan shows over 50 % emptying of the stomach ➡ into the bowel ➡ at 60 minutes, suggestive of rapid gastric transit. Rapid gastric transit and gastroparesis have similar symptoms.*

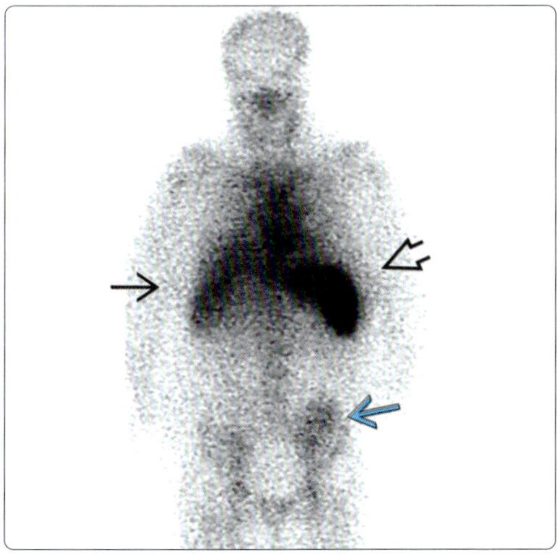

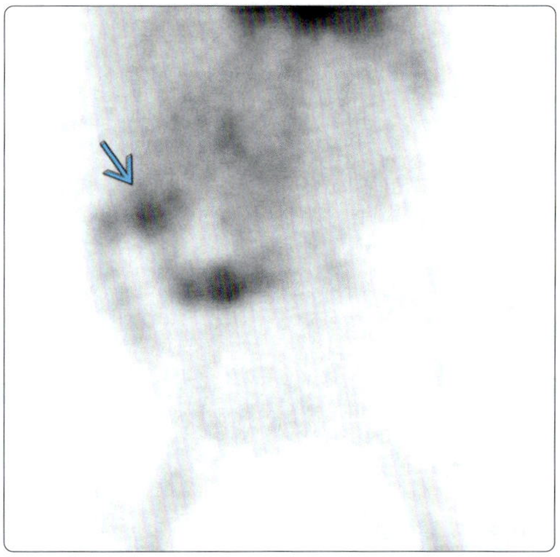

(Left) *Anterior In-111 WBC scan in a hospitalized patient with bacteremia shows normal biodistribution, with uptake in spleen ➡ greater than liver ➡. Note also the physiologic uptake in a transplant kidney ➡.* **(Right)** *Anterior Tc-99m labeled RBC scan in a patient with GI bleeding originating near the hepatic flexure shows abnormal activity ➡ within the lumen of the colon.*

KEY FACTS

IMAGING

- Tc-99m IDA hepatobiliary scintigraphy
  - Normal: Gallbladder (GB) filling and biliary-to-bowel transit within 1 hr
  - Acute cholecystitis: No GB filling on post-morphine or 4 hr images
  - Low-grade common bile duct (CBD) obstruction: Delayed biliary-to-bowel transit > 1 hr and < 24 hrs
  - High-grade CBD obstruction: No biliary-to-bowel transit on hepatobiliary scintigraphy > 24 hrs
  - Rim sign: Hepatic retention of tracer due to adjacent inflammation around GB fossa with no GB filling
  - Bile leak: Indicative of GB perforation ± fistulization

DIAGNOSTIC CHECKLIST

- Causes of false-negative hepatobiliary scan: Acute cholecystitis
  - Bowel loop simulating GB (especially duodenal bulb)
  - 15% of acute acalculous cholecystitis has visualization of GB
  - Bile leak due to GB perforation
  - Congenital anomaly simulating GB
  - Renal excretion of radiotracer
- Causes of false-negative hepatobiliary scan: High-grade CBD obstruction
  - Low-grade, partial, or intermittent CBD obstruction
    - Poor clearance from biliary ducts and delayed transit into small bowel > 60 min
    - Small or transient stones in CBD
    - Normal lab values
- Cause of false-positive hepatobiliary scan: Hepatic dysfunction
  - Marked soft tissue background and blood pool activity with severe liver dysfunction
  - Can mimic CBD obstruction
  - Can mimic acute cholecystitis, delayed images at 18-24 hrs can decrease false-positives

(Left) *Graphic shows the gallbladder (GB), cystic duct, common hepatic duct, common bile duct (CBD), sphincter of Oddi, and second portion of the duodenum.* **(Right)** *Graphic shows the GB, cystic duct, and mid CBD with an impacted calculus.*

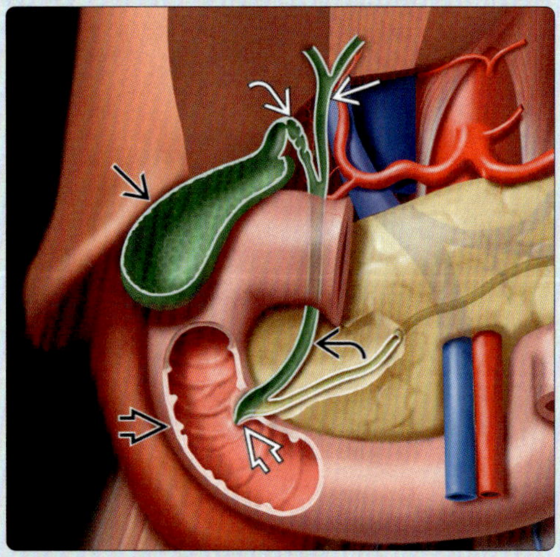

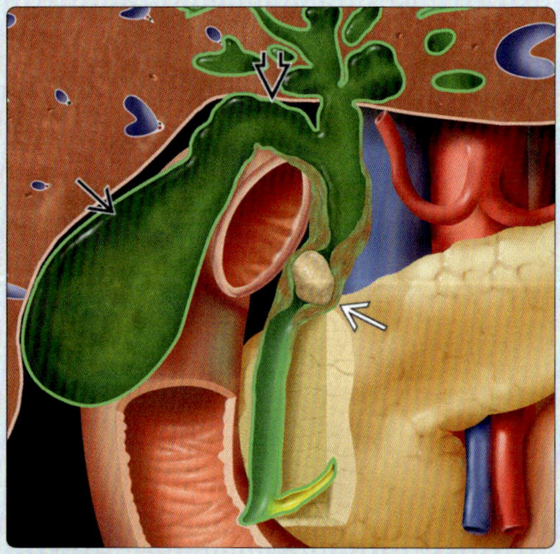

(Left) *Normal hepatobiliary scintigraphy study shows. GB, cystic duct and CBD. Note faint radiotracer in the liver and bowel.* **(Right)** *MRCP 3D reconstruction of the biliary system in patient post cholecystectomy is shown. Left and right intrahepatic ducts, CBD, second portion of duodenum, gallstone in the distal CBD.*

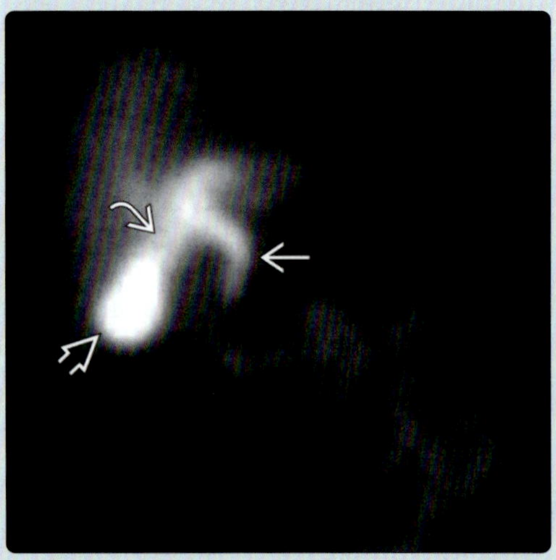

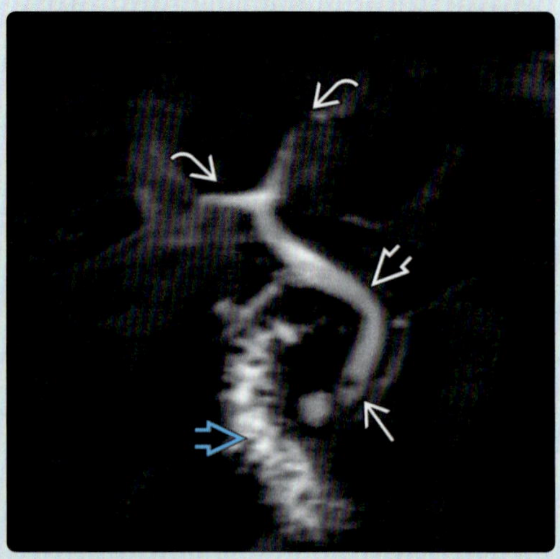

IMAGING

General Features

- Best diagnostic clue
  - Tc-99m IDA hepatobiliary scintigraphy
    - Normal
      - Radiotracer taken up by liver
      - Radiotracer progresses through intrahepatic/extrahepatic biliary ducts
      - Gallbladder (GB) filling and biliary-to-bowel transit within 1 hr
    - Acute cholecystitis
      - Acute calculous cholecystitis (ACC): No GB visualization on hepatobiliary scintigraphy due to cystic duct obstruction secondary to gallstone impaction
      - Acute acalculous cholecystitis (AAC): No GB visualization on hepatobiliary scintigraphy secondary to cystic duct obstruction not related to gallstones
      - Absence of GB filling in 1st hr of imaging
      - No GB visualization despite IV morphine sulfate administration or delayed 4 hr images
      - Partial GB filling in 15% of AAC cases
    - Low-grade common bile duct (CBD) obstruction
      - Delayed biliary-to-bowel transit > 1 hr but < 24 hrs
    - High-grade CBD obstruction
      - Delayed biliary-to-bowel transit on hepatobiliary scintigraphy > 24 hrs
      - Persistent hepatogram
    - Angiographic phase
      - Hyperemic blush in GB fossa represents GB inflammation
      - Abscess or gangrene in 36% of patients with hyperemia
    - Rim sign
      - Hepatic retention of tracer due to adjacent inflammation around GB fossa with no GB filling
      - Seen within 1st hr of imaging
      - Although radiotracer clears from liver, rim sign persists on delayed images
      - Seen in 20% of acute cholecystitis cases
      - Almost 50% of cases with rim sign have complicated cholecystitis
        - GB ulceration/necrosis
        - Fibrinous exudate/empyema
        - Gangrene
        - Perforation
    - Bile leak
      - Indicative of GB perforation ± fistulization

Imaging Recommendations

- Best imaging tool
  - Acute cholecystitis
    - Tc-99m IDA hepatobiliary scintigraphy sensitivity: 92%
    - Abdominal ultrasound (AUS) sensitivity: 73%
    - Tc-99m IDA scan + AUS sensitivity: 98%
  - High-grade CBD obstruction
    - Tc-99m IDA hepatobiliary scintigraphy
      - Sensitivity: 97%
      - Specificity: 90%
- Protocol advice
  - Patient preparation
    - Fasting > 2 hrs but < 24 hrs
    - Premedication with cholecystokinin (CCK) if > 24 hr fasting or parenteral nutrition
      - 0.02 mcg/kg of CCK over 30-60 min
      - 15-30 min before radiotracer administration
    - Recent opioid administration can yield false-positive: Delay study for 4 t1/2 of opioid
    - Hyperbilirubinemia: Hepatic uptake of mebrofenin higher than with disofenin; use if bilirubin > 30 mg/dL
  - Radiopharmaceutical
    - Iminodiacetic acid (IDA) derivate
      - Tc-99m mebrofenin/disofenin 3-5 mCi (111-185 MBq)
      - Hyperbilirubinemia: May increase dose (6-10 mCi [222-370 MBq])
  - Imaging acquisition
    - Patient supine
    - Image over abdomen
    - Large field-of-view camera equipped with low-energy all-purpose or high-resolution collimator
    - Matrix: 128 x 128
    - Angiographic phase x 1 min (4 sec/frame)
    - Dynamic acquisition (1 frame/min) for 60 min
      - May also take static images at 15-30 min intervals up to 60 min
    - Delayed images as necessary
      - If small bowel is present but no GB within 60 min
        - Morphine sulfate 0.04 mg/kg or standard 2 mg dose IV over 2-3 min and additional imaging up to 60 min to evaluate for GB uptake
        - If morphine contraindicated, 4 hr delayed images to evaluate for GB uptake
    - If GB is present but no small bowel within 60 min
      - Continue delayed imaging up to 24 hr to evaluate for biliary-to-bowel transit
      - Oral fatty meal or IV CCK infusion to contract GB if no contraindication
  - Dosimetry
    - GB wall receives highest dose
  - Imaging processing
    - Frame-by-frame snapshot of angiographic phase shows blood flow
    - Frame-by-frame snapshot helps localize when GB fills

Artifacts and Quality Control

- Duodenal bulb activity could mimic GB (false-negative)
  - Right lateral view to confirm anterior location of GB
  - Left anterior oblique to separate GB from duodenal bulb
  - Oral administration of 8 oz of water to wash out radiotracer in duodenum
- Dilated cystic duct simulating GB
  - Lateral view can be useful
  - SPECT/CT for better anatomic evaluation
- Hepatic dysfunction
  - Marked soft tissue background and blood pool activity with severe liver dysfunction
  - Can mimic CBD obstruction

- Delayed images at 18-24 hrs can decrease false-positives for acute cholecystitis
- Right lateral decubitus
  - Facilitates tracer entry into bowel
- When discordant or equivocal result of AAC or ACC
  - Tc-99m HMPAO white blood cell (WBC) scan
    - Wait 24 hrs after hepatobiliary scan to inject
    - Inject Tc-99m HMPAO WBCs 1-2 hrs before imaging
  - In-111 WBC scan
    - Can inject In-111 WBCs immediately after Tc-99m IDA
    - Image at 24 hrs

DIFFERENTIAL DIAGNOSIS

CBD Obstruction

- Severe liver dysfunction
  - Review lab values
  - Acute viral or nonviral hepatitis
  - Acute on chronic liver disease
- Opioid medication
  - Contracts sphincter of Oddi
- Sphincter of Oddi dysfunction
  - Suspected when biliary-to-bowel transit is present but > 60 min
- Intrahepatic cholestasis
- Biliary atresia
  - Pediatric population

Acute Calculous and Acalculous Cholecystitis

- Congenital biliary abnormalities
  - Intrahepatic GB
  - GB agenesis
- Severe illness
  - Shock/sepsis
- GB torsion
  - Rotation of GB on its mesentery along axis of cystic duct and cystic artery
  - Peak incidence in patients 65-75 years of age
  - Rare
- Chronic cholecystitis
  - Severe chronic GB dysfunction &/or dyskinesia ± cholelithiasis
- Extrinsic/intrinsic GB compression
  - Abscess
  - Cholangiocarcinoma
  - Compressive abdominal tumor (hepatocellular carcinoma, lymphoma, gastrointestinal stromal tumor, adenopathy)
- Postcholecystectomy
  - Unclear prior surgery
- Severe liver dysfunction
  - Review lab values
  - Acute viral or nonviral hepatitis
  - Acute on chronic liver disease
- Improper patient preparation
  - < 2 hr fasting
    - Postprandial GB contractions prevent tracer accumulation and visualization
  - > 24 hr fasting
    - May result in atonic, distended, or sludge-filled GB

PATHOLOGY

General Features

- Acute calculous cholecystitis
  - Etiology
    - Cystic duct obstruction secondary to gallstone impaction
    - Vascular congestion, edema, and infiltration of polymorphonuclear leukocytes into GB wall
  - Risk factors
    - Obesity
    - > 40 years of age
    - Rapid weight loss
    - Female
    - Pregnancy
    - Diabetes mellitus
    - Hemolytic disease
    - Total parenteral nutrition
    - Postmenopausal estrogens
    - Ceftriaxone
  - Epidemiology
    - 10-20% of Americans have gallstones
    - Each year up to 3% of patients with gallstones experience biliary colic
    - Acute cholecystitis will develop in about 20% of this population
- Acute acalculous cholecystitis
  - Etiology
    - Primary mechanism
      - Seeding GB wall with bacteria, ischemia/reperfusion, or effects of eicosanoid proinflammatory mediators
    - Intrinsic obstruction
      - Secondary to bile/sludge or obstructive inflammatory material
      - Reduced GB motility secondary to prolonged fasting/parenteral nutrition &/or opiate treatment
    - Extrinsic obstruction
      - Abscess/adenopathy
      - Fibrosis
  - Risk factors
    - Diabetes mellitus
    - Elderly
    - Immunocompromised status
    - Sepsis
    - Multiorgan dysfunction
    - Hypovolemia/shock
    - Bowel ischemia/vasculitis
- Common bile duct obstruction
  - Etiology
    - Lithiasis
      - Pre/post cholecystectomy
    - Neoplastic process from biliary, pancreatic, or liver origin
      - Jaundice; often painless
    - Iatrogenic
      - Post cholecystectomy
    - Inflammatory stricture
      - Primary cholangitis
    - Parasite

      - Ascariasis lumbricoides
      - Clonorchis sinensis
      - Fasciola hepatica
    - Others
      - Hemobilia
      - Duodenal diverticulum
      - Choledochal cyst
  - Risk factors
    - Same risk factors as acute calculous cholecystitis
    - Recent laparoscopic cholecystectomy
    - Foreign travel, gastrointestinal neoplasm, ulcerative colitis

Staging, Grading, & Classification

- CBD obstruction grading
  - Very strong predictors
    - Presence of CBD stone on transabdominal ultrasound
    - Clinical acute cholangitis
    - Bilirubin > 4 mg/dL (68 micromol/L)
  - Strong predictors
    - CBD dilatation on US > 6 mm (in patient with GB)
    - Bilirubin 1.8-4 mg/dL (31-68 micromol/L)
  - Moderate predictors
    - Abnormal liver biochemical tests other than bilirubin
    - Age > 55 yrs
    - Clinical gallstone pancreatitis
- High risk (> 50% of probability of having CBD obstruction)
  - At least 1 very strong predictor &/or both strong predictors
- Intermediate risk (10-50% of probability of having CBD obstruction)
  - 1 strong predictor &/or at least 1 moderate predictor
- Low risk (< 10% of probability of having CBD obstruction)
  - No predictors

CLINICAL ISSUES

Natural History & Prognosis

- Acute calculous cholecystitis
  - Untreated disease can progress to severe complications
- Acute acalculous cholecystitis
  - Morbidity and mortality of 35-40%
  - High incidence of gangrene, GB perforation and abscess
- High-grade CBD obstruction
  - Untreated disease can progress to cholangitis (mortality: 20-30%)
- Low-grade CBD obstruction
  - Asymptomatic or chronic right upper quadrant pain
  - Increased risk of pancreatitis

Treatment

- Acute cholecystitis
  - Prompt laparoscopic cholecystectomy
  - Open approach used for patients with perforation, pericholecystic abscess or empyema
  - Percutaneous US-guided cholecystostomy for critical/unstable patients
  - Antibiotics and supportive therapy
- High-grade CBD obstruction
  - Associated acute cholangitis
    - Antibiotic and supportive therapy
  - High-risk patient
    - ERCP followed by elective cholecystectomy
  - Intermediate-risk patient
    - Preoperative: Confirmation of lithiasis by endoscopic ultrasound/MRCP
      - Positive: ERCP
      - Negative: Elective cholecystectomy
    - Intraoperative: Confirmation of lithiasis by laparoscopic US/cholangiography
      - Negative: Laparoscopic cholecystectomy
      - Positive: Laparoscopic CBD exploration or postoperative ERCP
  - Low-risk patient
    - Laparoscopic cholecystectomy
      - No intraoperative cholangiography needed
- Low-grade CBD obstruction
  - If symptomatic: Elective cholecystectomy

DIAGNOSTIC CHECKLIST

Image Interpretation Pearls

- Mimics of acute cholecystitis on hepatobiliary scan
  - Bowel loop simulating GB (especially duodenal bulb)
  - 15% of AAC has visualization of GB (false negative)
  - Bile leak due to GB perforation
  - Congenital anomaly simulating GB
  - Renal excretion of radiotracer
- Mimics of high-grade CBD obstruction on hepatobiliary scan
  - Low-grade, partial, or intermittent CBD obstruction
    - Poor clearance from biliary ducts and delayed transit into small bowel > 60 min
    - Small or transient stones in CBD
    - Normal lab values

SELECTED REFERENCES

1. ACR-SNMMI-SPR Practice Guideline for Hepatobiliary Scintigraphy 4.0. http://snmmi.files.cms-plus.com/docs/Hepatobiliary_Scintigraphy_V4.0b.pdf. Published August 23, 2010. Accessed July 10, 2014
2. Kaoutzanis C et al: Abdominal ultrasound versus hepato-imino diacetic acid scan in diagnosing acute cholecystitis--what is the real benefit? J Surg Res. 188(1):44-52, 2014
3. Lambie H et al: Tc99m-hepatobiliary iminodiacetic acid (HIDA) scintigraphy in clinical practice. Clin Radiol. 66(11):1094-105, 2011
4. Ziessman HA: Nuclear medicine hepatobiliary imaging. Clin Gastroenterol Hepatol. 8(2):111-6, 2010
5. Ziessman HA: Acute cholecystitis, biliary obstruction, and biliary leakage. Semin Nucl Med. 33(4):279-96, 2003

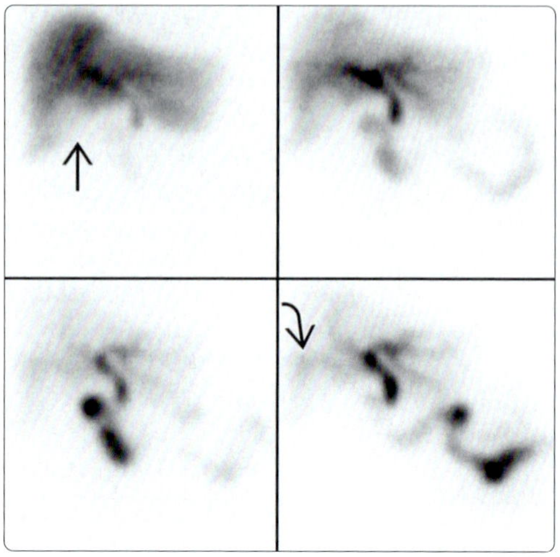
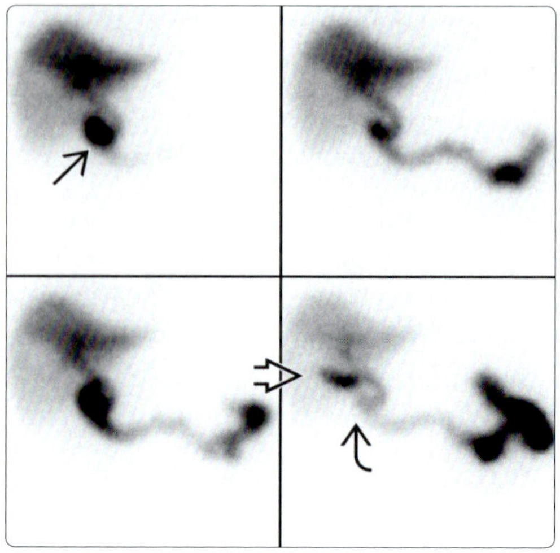

(Left) *Hepatobiliary scan in a patient with acute cholecystitis shows no activity in the GB on post-morphine images →. A rim sign → is evident on delayed images, signifying hyperemia.* **(Right)** *The duodenal bulb → mimics GB filling on early hepatobiliary scintigraphy images. Over time, the radiotracer moves from the bulb. At 45 min, the GB is identified → and radiotracer has washed out of the duodenal bulb →.*

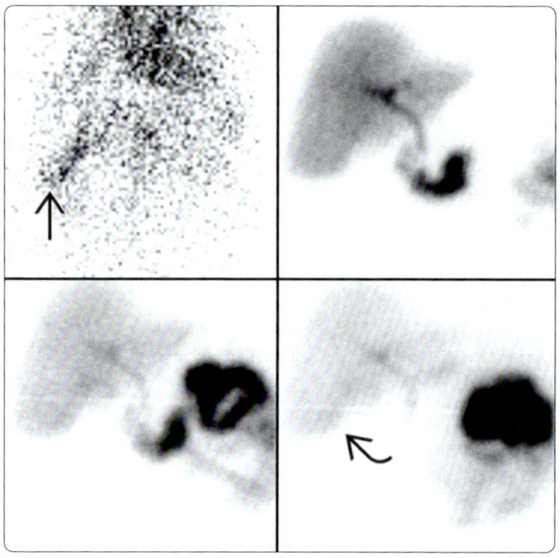
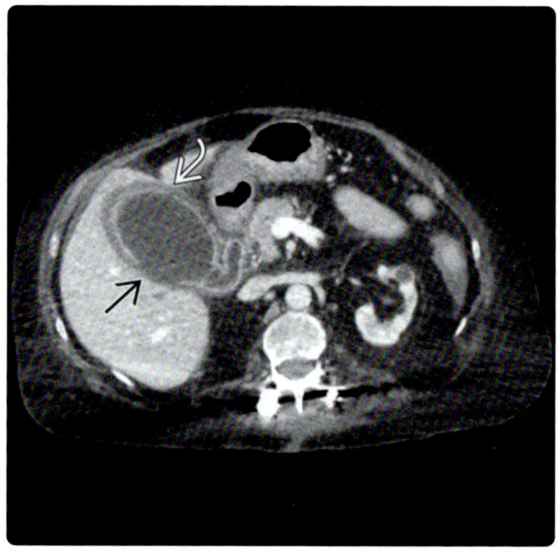

(Left) *Hepatobiliary scintigraphy shows GB fossa blush → on angiographic phase and a rim sign →. The GB was not visualized in this patient with acute acalculous cholecystitis.* **(Right)** *Axial CECT in the same patient shows marked GB and cystic duct wall enhancement →. Note the lack of enhancement in the posterior GB wall consistent with necrosis →, increasing risk of perforation.*

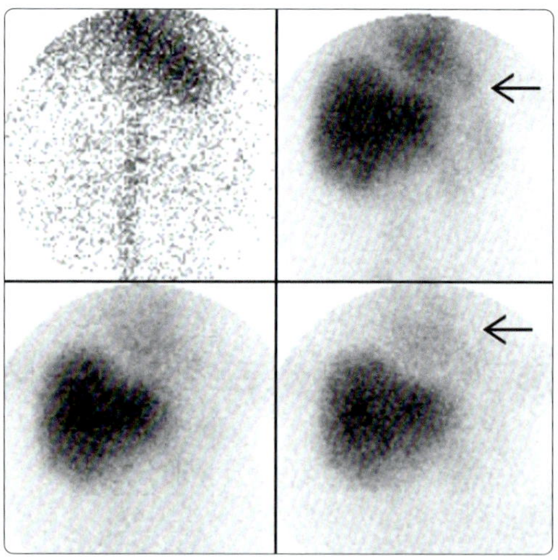
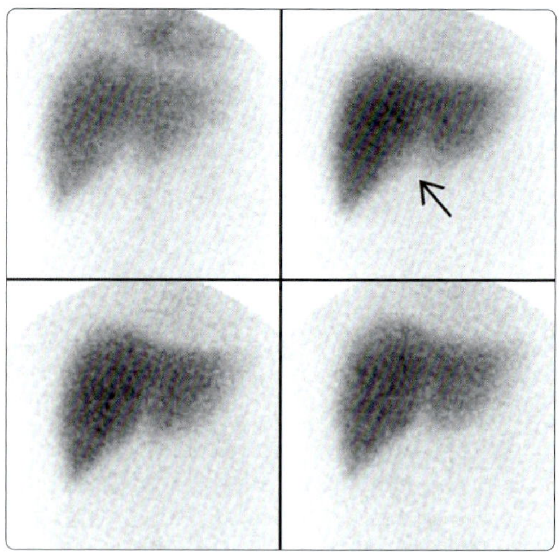

(Left) *Hepatobiliary scintigraphy shows abnormal blood flow with poor hepatic uptake of radiotracer. At 1 hr and 24 hr, blood pool activity remains high →. These findings suggest severe hepatic dysfunction and limit the evaluation of acute cholecystitis.* **(Right)** *Hepatobiliary scintigraphy shows persistent hepatogram → with no GB or small bowel activity on 24 hr images, consistent with high-grade CBD obstruction.*

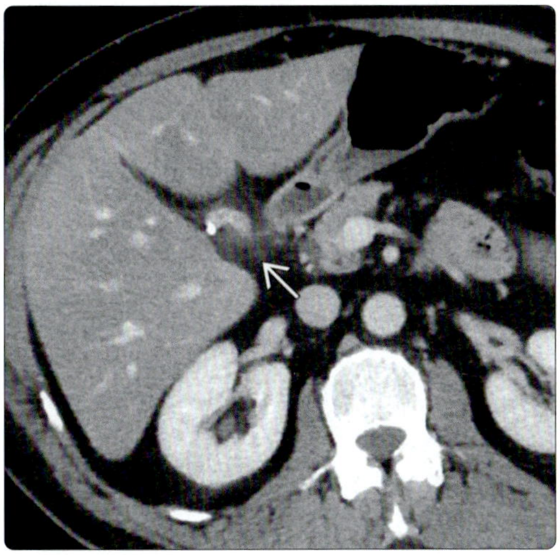

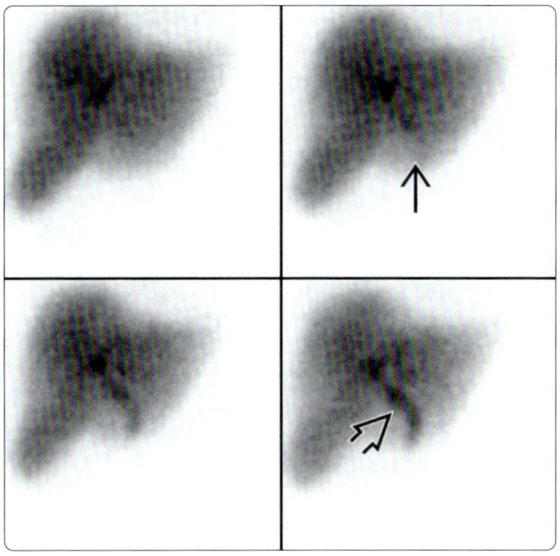

(Left) *Axial CECT in a patient post cholecystectomy shows enhancement of the cystic stump and pericystic fat stranding suggestive of cholangitis. No stones are identified.* **(Right)** *Hepatobiliary scintigraphy in the same patient shows activity in the CBD. On 24 hr delayed images, the entire CBD is evident, but lack of bowel activity suggests high-grade CBD obstruction. MRCP confirmed distal choledocholithiasis.*

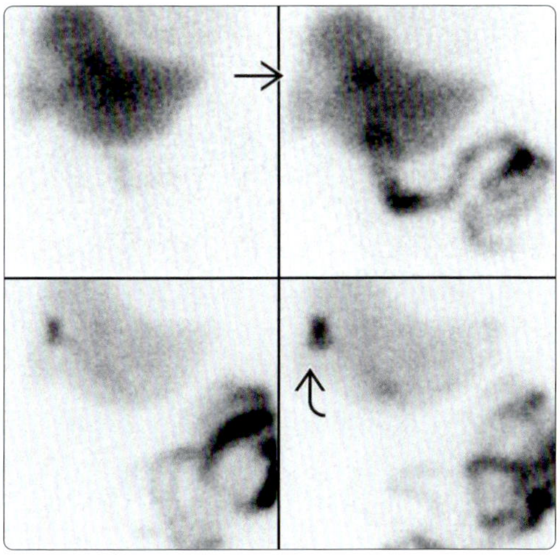

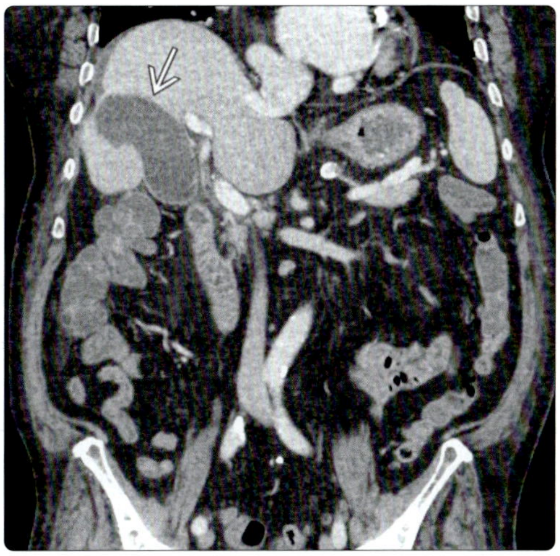

(Left) *Hepatobiliary scintigraphy shows photopenic defect in the liver parenchyma. On later images, activity is evident in this region suggestive of intrahepatic GB.* **(Right)** *Coronal CECT in the same patient shows the intrahepatic GB.*

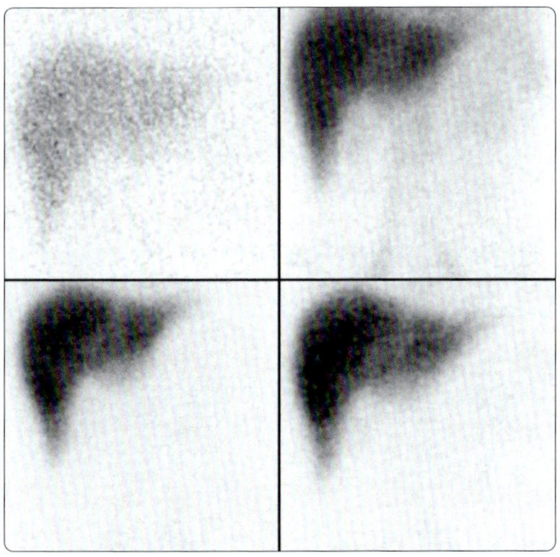

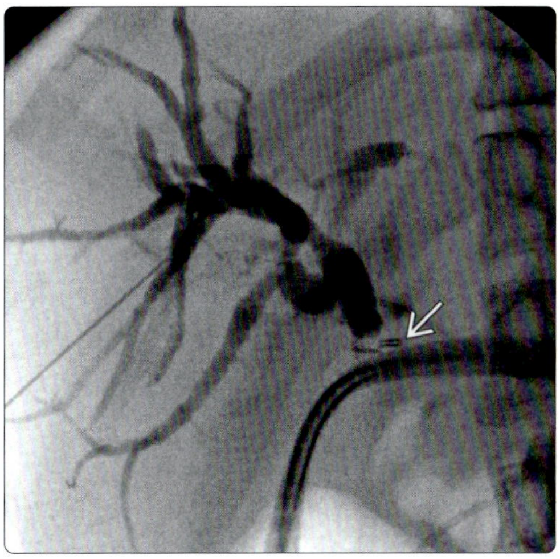

(Left) *Hepatobiliary scintigraphy in a patient post cholecystectomy with hyperbilirubinemia shows no biliary-to-bowel transit to 24 hrs of imaging. Retained gallstones in the CBD are suspected.* **(Right)** *Cholangiogram in the same patient shows a CBD clip and no gallstones.*

(Left) *Hepatobiliary scintigraphy shows heterogeneous filling of the GB with central photopenia. Enterogastric reflux of bile is also evident.* **(Right)** *Axial CT shows a fundal GB mass with pericholecystic stranding, consistent with primary neoplasm.*

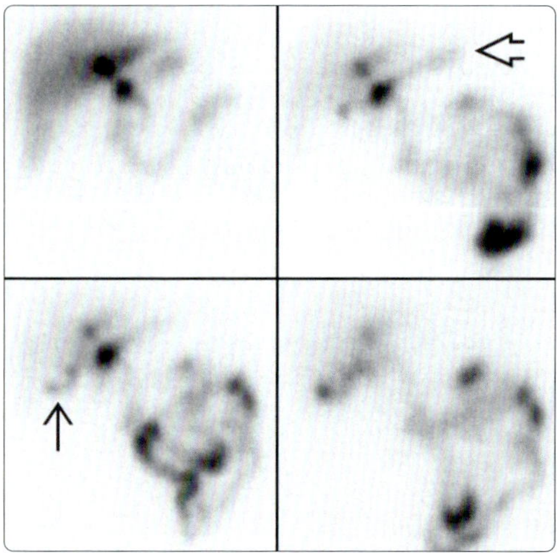

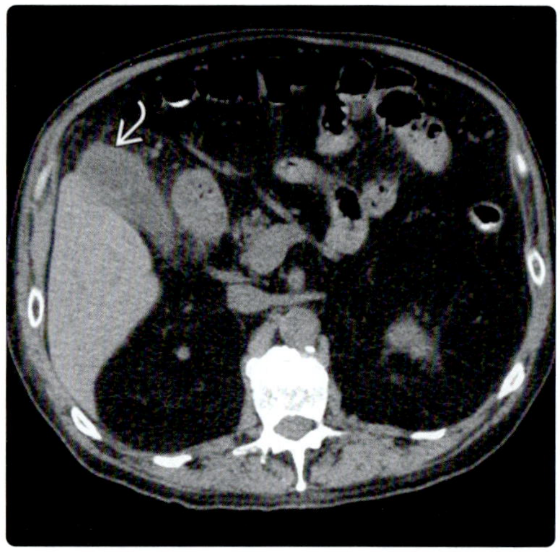

(Left) *Hepatobiliary scintigraphy shows abnormal pattern of GB filling, possibly a congenital anomaly or choledochal cyst.* **(Right)** *Coronal CT in the same patient confirms a partially septated, bilobed GB.*

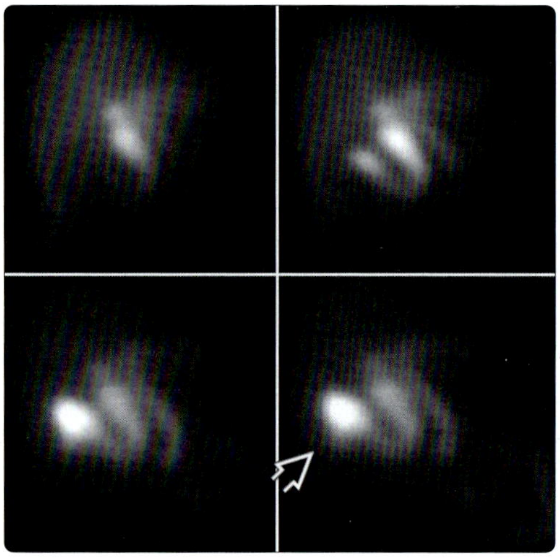

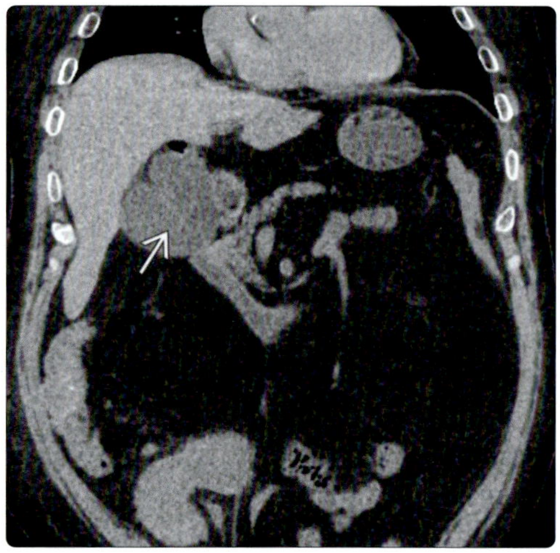

(Left) *Hepatobiliary scintigraphy shows progressive accumulation of activity inferior to the left hepatic lobe and normal biliary-to-bowel transit.* **(Right)** *Axial CECT in the same patient correlates with GB. Note the malrotated kidney as well.*

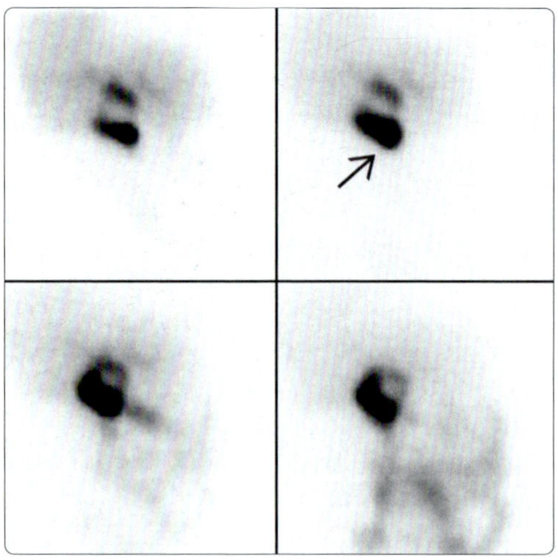

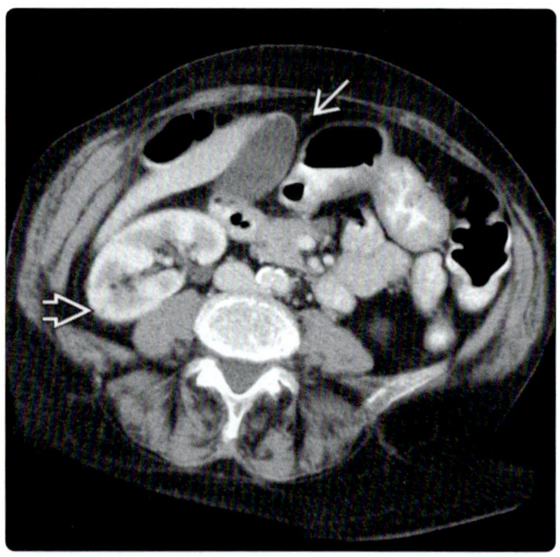

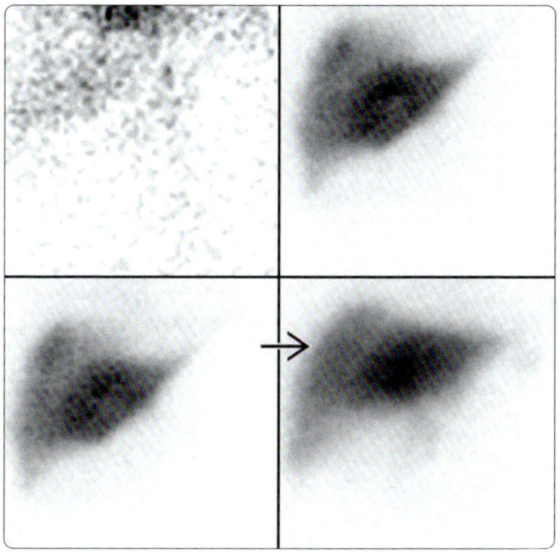

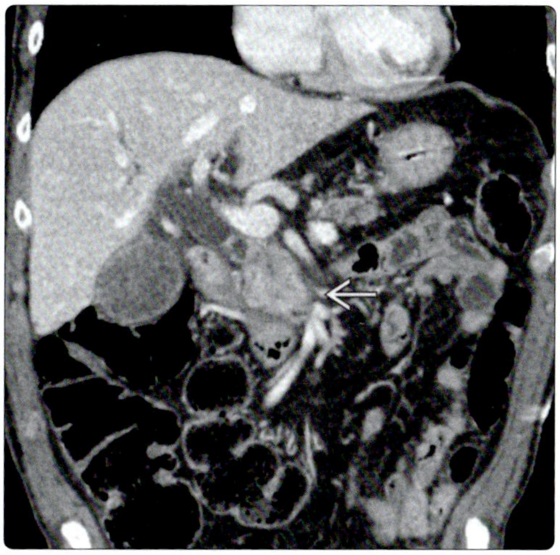

(Left) *Hepatobiliary scintigraphy shows normal angiogram and persistent hepatogram* → *with no GB or bowel activity on images to 12 hrs, suggestive of high-grade CBD obstruction in a patient with marked jaundice.* **(Right)** *Coronal CECT in the same patient shows a pancreatic head mass* ➡ *obstructing the distal CBD.*

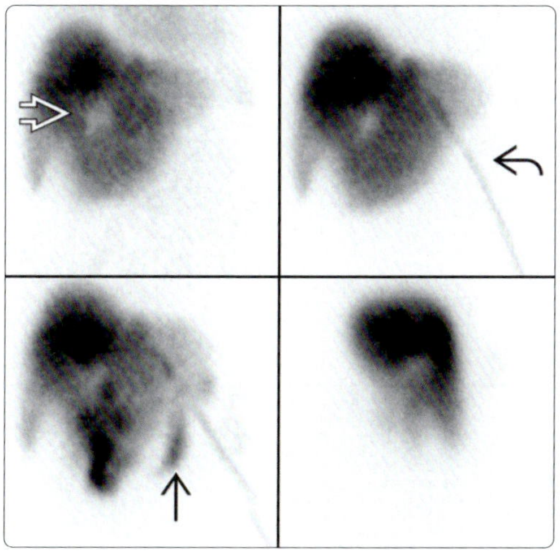

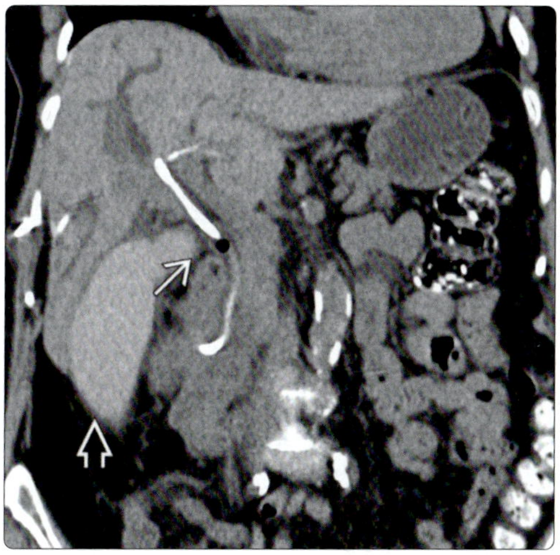

(Left) *Hepatobiliary scintigraphy in a patient with a pancreatic mass shows central photopenic defect* ➡*, a large liver metastasis. Note left intrahepatic biliary drain* ↶*. Small bowel* → *is identified on delayed images confirming patency of the CBD stent. Photopenic GB fossa on delayed images suggests either acute cholecystitis or tumor involvement of the cystic duct.* **(Right)** *Coronal CT in the same patient shows CBD stent* ➡ *and distended GB without tumor involvement* ➡*.*

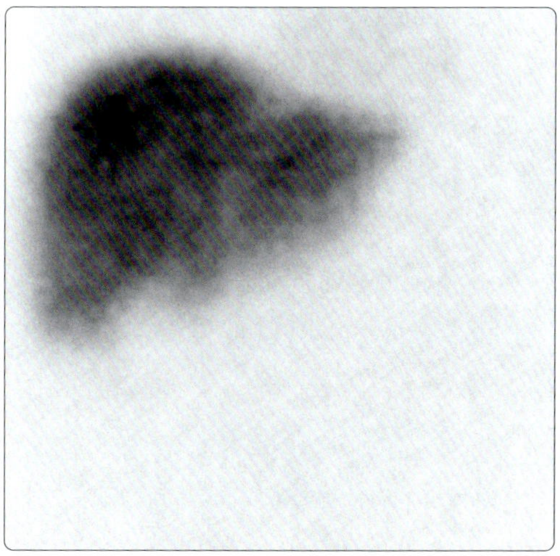

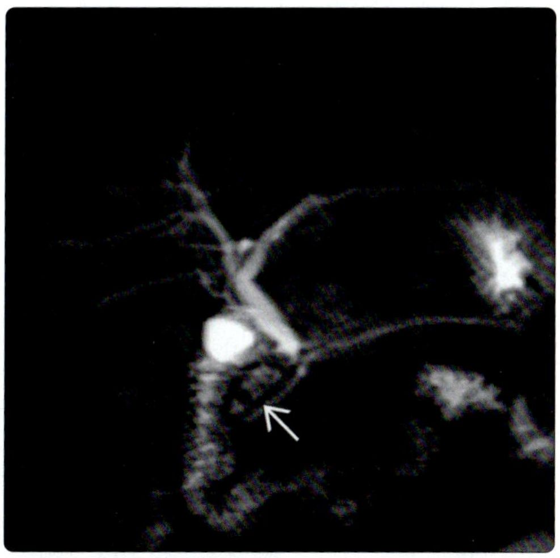

(Left) *Hepatobiliary scintigraphy in a patient post laparoscopic cholecystectomy is shown. No small bowel is visualized on 24 hr delayed static image. High-grade CBD obstruction is suspected.* **(Right)** *MRCP reconstruction in the same patient shows choledocholithiasis* ➡*.*

Biliary Leak

KEY FACTS

TERMINOLOGY

- Biliary leak: Focal collection or free flow of bile into abdomen, usually postsurgical complication

IMAGING

- Tc-99m IDA hepatobiliary scintigraphy: Radiotracer outside normal biliary system or small bowel
  - Abnormal activity usually starts in GB fossa, porta hepatis, near cystic stump as biloma
  - Reappearing liver sign: As radiotracer decreases in liver parenchyma over time, focal leak projecting over liver increases over time
  - Radiotracer can track inferior to right hepatic lobe → right paracolic gutter/Morison pouch, over liver dome, or freely into peritoneum
  - Near biliary enteric anastomosis after liver transplant
  - Bile may flow through surgical drainage tubes
  - Bile may spread to retroperitoneum
  - Bile may spread to dependent portions of pelvis
- Fluid collections on US, CT are nonspecific
  - Cannot differentiate bile leak from seroma/abscess
- Static images at 2-4 hrs, 24 hrs (slow leak)
  - Include drains/bags to detect slow leak
  - Include pelvis
- Oblique, lateral
  - Localize abnormalities in anteroposterior plane
- Right lateral decubitus
  - Facilitates tracer pooling away from central bile duct and enteric system

DIAGNOSTIC CHECKLIST

- SPECT/CT for anatomic correlation
  - Prior enterobiliary anastomosis
  - Complex surgical procedures
  - Multiple fluid collections
- If no leak, note that enterogastric reflux of bile can also cause abdominal pain post cholecystectomy

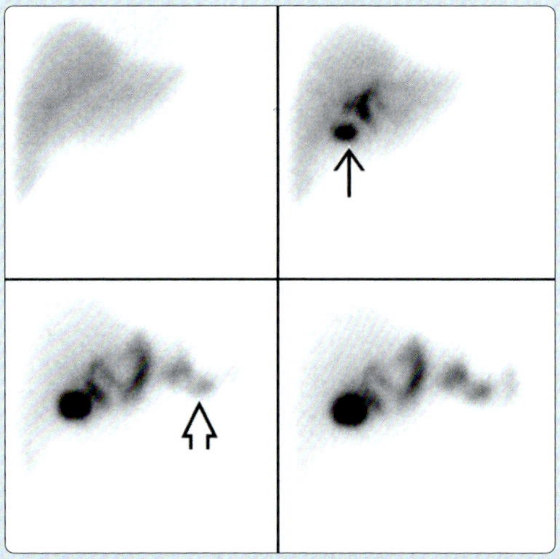

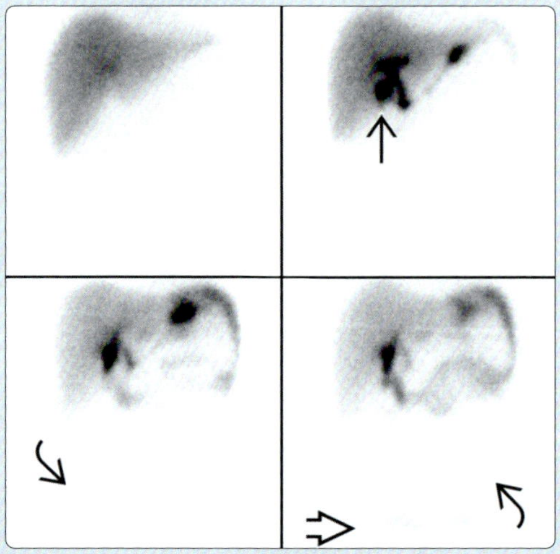

(Left) *In a patient post cholecystectomy, progressive accumulation of radiotracer in the gallbladder (GB) fossa ➙ suggests biloma. On delayed images, this activity traverses the left upper abdomen ⇨.* **(Right)** *In a patient post cholecystectomy, bile leakage starts in the GB fossa ➙ and moves to the bilateral paracolic gutters ➘ and the pelvis ⇨.*

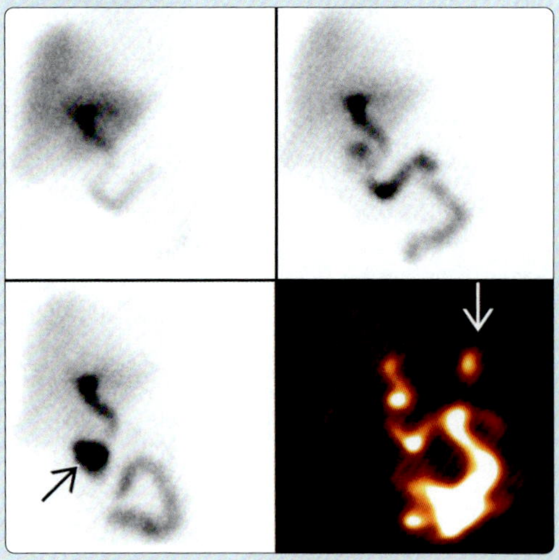

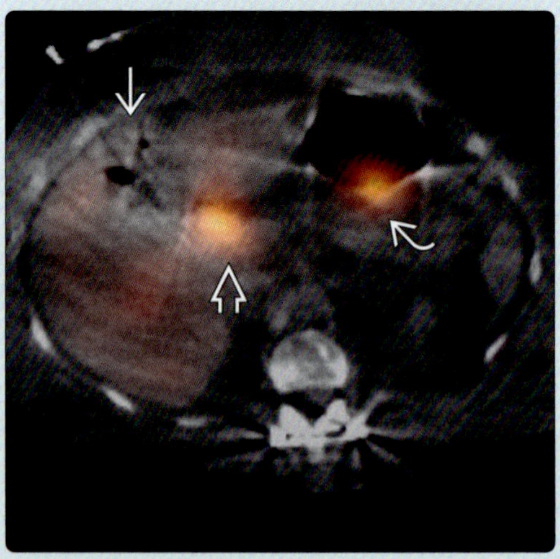

(Left) *A patient post cholecystectomy underwent hepatobiliary scintigraphy. Activity near the GB fossa ➙ could represent a bile leak or duodenal activity. On SPECT, accumulation of radiotracer in the left upper quadrant ➡ suggests enterogastric reflux.* **(Right)** *Axial fused SPECT/CT in the same patient shows air-fluid collection without radiotracer, confirming no bile leak ➡. The activity on the scintigraphy represents the duodenum ➡ and enterogastric reflux ➘.*

TERMINOLOGY

Definitions

- Focal collection or free flow of bile into abdomen
  - Usually postsurgical complication

IMAGING

General Features

- Best diagnostic clue
  - Tc-99m IDA hepatobiliary scintigraphy: Radiotracer found outside normal biliary system or small bowel
    - Abnormal activity usually starts in gallbladder (GB) fossa, porta hepatis, near cystic stump as biloma
    - Reappearing liver sign: As radiotracer decreases in liver parenchyma over time, focal leak projecting over liver increases over time
    - Radiotracer can track inferior to right hepatic lobe → right paracolic gutter/Morison pouch, over liver dome, or freely into peritoneum
    - Near biliary enteric anastomosis after liver transplant
    - Bile may flow through surgical drainage tubes
    - Bile may spread to retroperitoneum
    - Bile may spread to dependent portions of pelvis

Imaging Recommendations

- Best imaging tool
  - Tc-99m IDA hepatobiliary scintigraphy
    - Fluid collections on US, CT are nonspecific; cannot differentiate bile leak from seroma/abscess
- Protocol advice
  - Patient preparation
    - None
    - Physician should know
      - Surgical history
      - Location and number of abdominal drains
      - Location of fluid collection(s) on CT or US
      - Severity of liver dysfunction or hyperbilirubinemia
  - Radiopharmaceutical
    - Iminodiacetic acid (IDA) derivatives
      - Tc-99m mebrofenin/disofenin: 3-5 mCi (111-185 MBq) IV
  - Imaging acquisition
    - Patient supine
    - Large field-of-view camera with low-energy all-purpose collimator
    - Matrix: 128 x 128
    - Image over abdomen
      - Angiographic phase x 1 min (4 sec/frame)
      - Dynamic acquisition (1 frame/min) for 60 min
      - Static images at 2-4 hr, 24 hr for slow leak
    - Image over pelvis on delayed static images
    - SPECT/CT for anatomic correlation if prior enterobiliary anastomosis, complex surgical procedures, or multiple fluid collections
  - Dosimetry
    - Biliary system receives highest radiation dose
  - Additional nuclear medicine imaging options
    - Oblique, lateral: Localize abnormalities in anteroposterior plane
    - Right lateral decubitus: Facilitates tracer pooling away from central bile duct and enteric system
    - SPECT/CT decreases false-positive studies
    - Include drains/bags on delayed images

DIFFERENTIAL DIAGNOSIS

Afferent Bowel Loop

- Surgical history (Billroth II, Roux-en-Y) important

Midgut Malrotation

- May mimic extravasation in subhepatic region

Variant Anatomy

- Choledochal cyst

PATHOLOGY

General Features

- Etiology
  - Most often postprocedural: Cholecystectomy or liver transplant
  - Blunt or penetrating trauma to right upper quadrant/epigastrium
  - Gangrenous gallbladder with perforation

CLINICAL ISSUES

Presentation

- Most common signs/symptoms
  - Fever, right upper quadrant pain, hyperbilirubinemia

Treatment

- Small, slow leaks
  - Conservative therapy
- Larger leaks
  - Surgical revision
  - Endoscopic placement of transpapillary stent
  - Percutaneous transhepatic biliary drainage

DIAGNOSTIC CHECKLIST

Image Interpretation Pearls

- Delayed images at 24 hrs including drains/bags to detect slow leak
- SPECT/CT is useful to decrease false-positives in cases of anatomic complexity or several fluid collections
- If no leak, note that enterogastric reflux can also cause abdominal pain post cholecystectomy

SELECTED REFERENCES

1. Melamud K et al: Biliary imaging: multimodality approach to imaging of biliary injuries and their complications. Radiographics. 34(3):613-23, 2014
2. Arun S et al: Added value of SPECT/CT over planar Tc-99m mebrofenin hepatobiliary scintigraphy in the evaluation of bile leaks. Nucl Med Commun. 34(5):459-66, 2013
3. Al Sofayan MS et al: Nuclear imaging of the liver: is there a diagnostic role of HIDA in posttransplantation? Transplant Proc. 41(1):201-7, 2009

(Left) *Hepatobiliary scintigraphy confirms prompt radiotracer activity in a percutaneous GB fossa drain and receptacle bag post cholecystectomy. Note the normal activity in the small bowel.* **(Right)** *In a patient post cholecystectomy with percutaneous GB fossa drain, normal radiotracer progression through the biliary system and the small bowel is evident. Subtle activity in GB fossa could represent the cystic duct stump. On a 2-hour image, radiotracer in the drain signifies bile leak.*

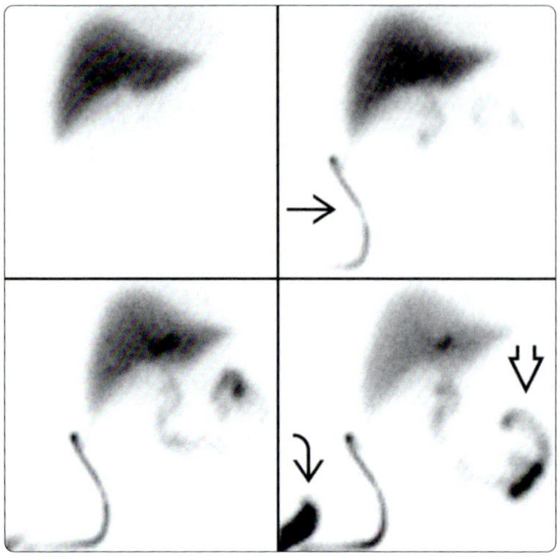

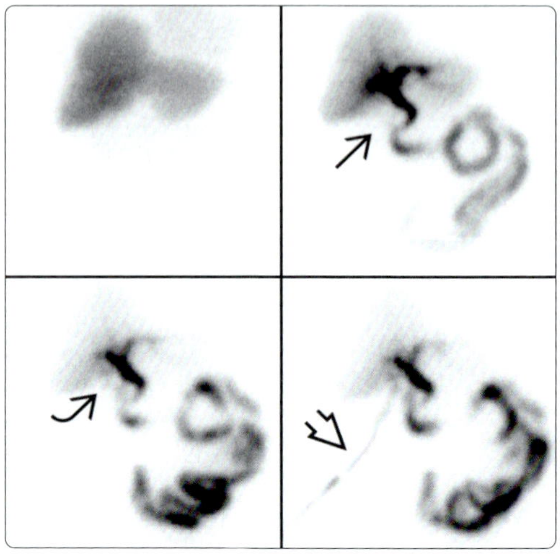

(Left) *In a patient with enterojejuno anastomosis, focal activity in GB fossa is suspicious for a bile leak. However, it seems to connect to the small bowel.* **(Right)** *Coronal fused SPECT/CT in the same patient shows that the GB fossa activity is an afferent loop of the enterojejuno anastomosis that extends inferiorly. No bile leak is identified.*

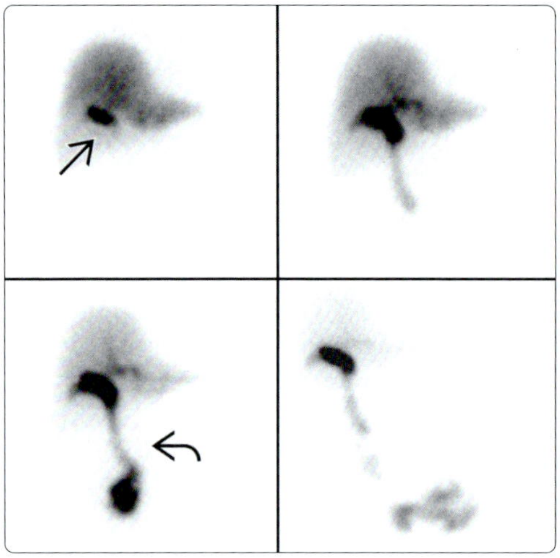

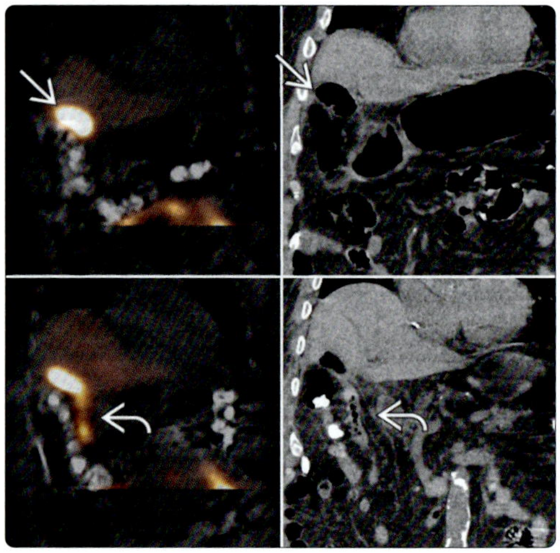

(Left) *A patient with right upper quadrant pain underwent hepatobiliary scintigraphy. Activity accumulates in the GB fossa and spreads to the right paracolic region. However, the radiotracer moves to the left upper quadrant in a pattern that suggests intraluminal transit of tracer through the colon.* **(Right)** *A delayed static image in the same patient shows activity within the colon, confirming a cholecystocolonic fistula.*

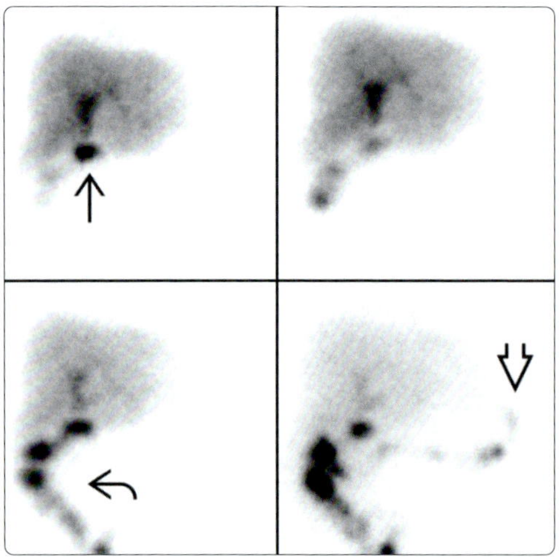

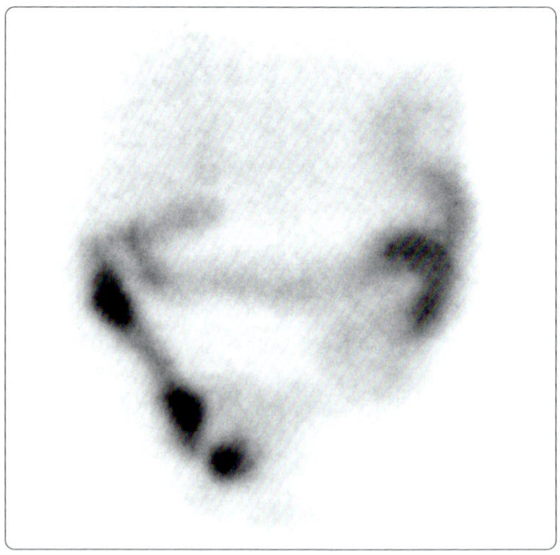

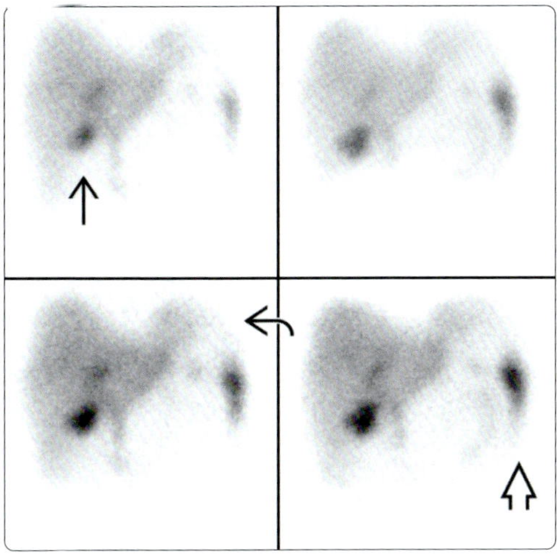

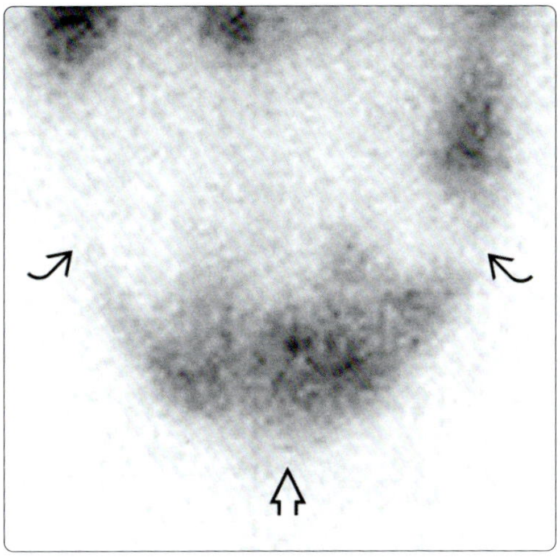

(Left) *Activity in the GB fossa is evident with foci of activity in the left upper quadrant and the left paracolic gutter in a patient post cholecystectomy with suspected bile leak.* **(Right)** *A delayed static image of the lower abdomen and pelvis in the same patient shows activity in the bilateral paracolic gutters and the pelvis, signifying a bile leak.*

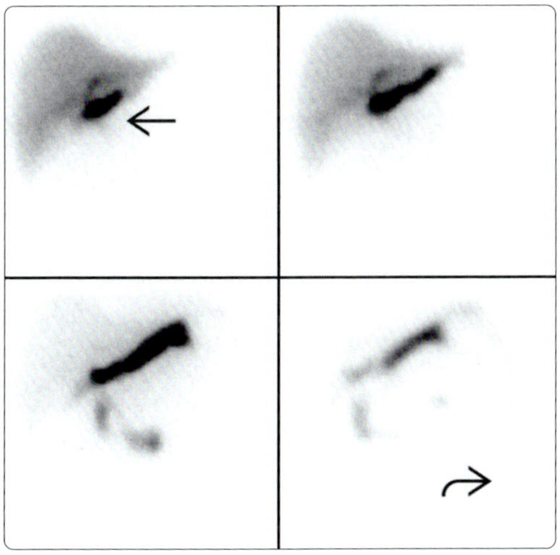

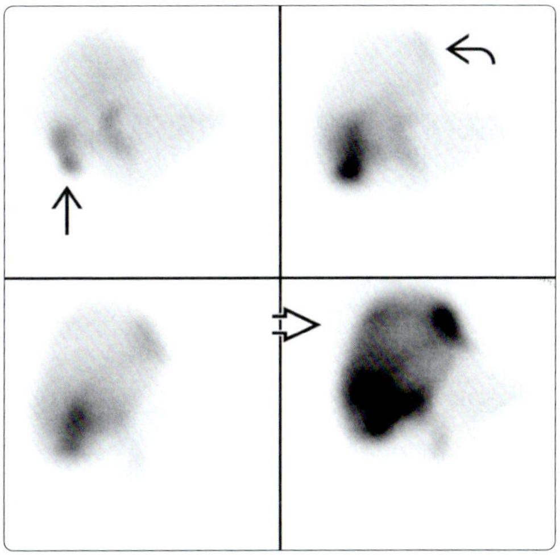

(Left) *A patient with blunt abdominal trauma had free fluid in the abdomen on CT. On hepatobiliary scintigraphy, radiotracer accumulates inferior to the left hepatic lobe and the left paracolic gutter, confirming bile leak.* **(Right)** *Reappearing liver sign is shown in a patient with bile leak. Activity appears in GB fossa and spreads superiorly, accumulating into the perihepatic spaces. Note that hepatic activity clears over time, and then seems to reappear.*

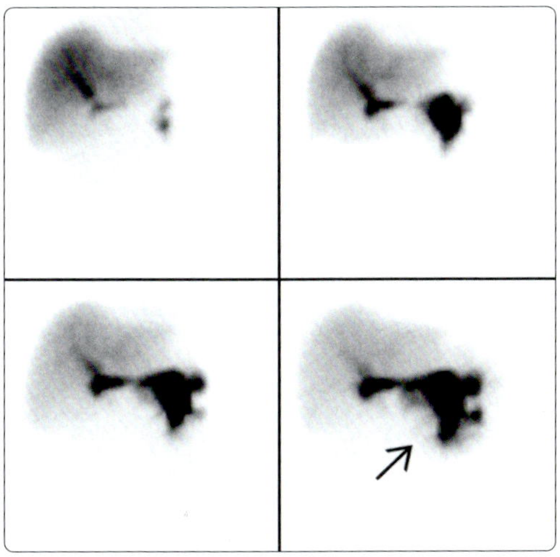

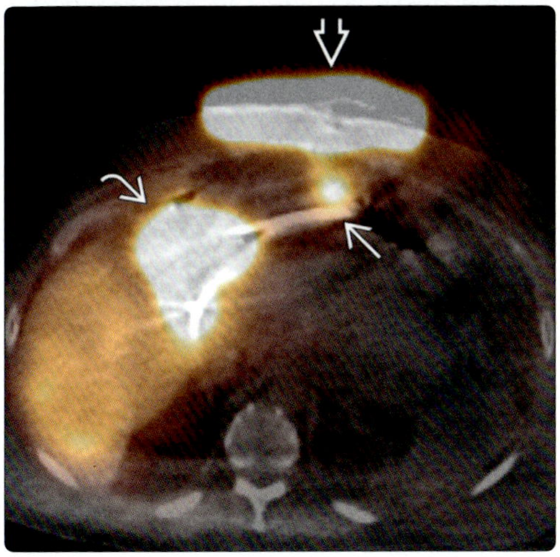

(Left) *In a patient post liver transplant, radiotracer accumulates in the mid abdomen.* **(Right)** *Axial fused SPECT/CT in the same patient shows a biliary enterocutaneous fistula. Radiotracer tracked from the porta hepatis through the abdominal cavity and saturated the laparotomy bandages.*

Functional Hepatobiliary Disease

KEY FACTS

TERMINOLOGY

- Chronic calculous cholecystitis
  - Decreased GBEF in presence of cholelithiasis
- Chronic acalculous cholecystitis/GB dyskinesia
  - Decreased GBEF in absence of cholelithiasis
- Sphincter of Oddi dysfunction
  - Delayed biliary-to-bowel radiotracer transit

IMAGING

- Chronic cholecystitis
  - Tc-99m IDA hepatobiliary scintigraphy with calculated GBEF after cholecystokinin (CCK) IV infusion
    - Infusion of IV CCK at 0.02 µg/kg for 60 min with normal GBEF > 38%
    - Infusion of IV CCK at 0.015 µg/kg for 45 min with images at 60 min with normal GBEF > 40%
- Sphincter of Oddi dysfunction
  - Delayed biliary-to-bowel transit > 30 min
  - Time of biliary visualization > 15 min
  - Prominent biliary tree

TOP DIFFERENTIAL DIAGNOSES

- Acute cholecystitis
- Liver dysfunction
- Contraindicated medication
- Partial common bile duct obstruction
- Cyst duct syndrome (rare)

DIAGNOSTIC CHECKLIST

- Rule out contraindicated drugs that can affect GBEF
- LAO or right lateral view sometimes needed to separate bowel from GB
- Enterogastric reflux of bile on hepatobiliary scan can be cause of epigastric/RUQ pain
- Patient with normal GBEF may become abnormal over period of years
- GBEF normal range depends on CCK infusion protocol; SNMMI recommends infusion of 45-60 min

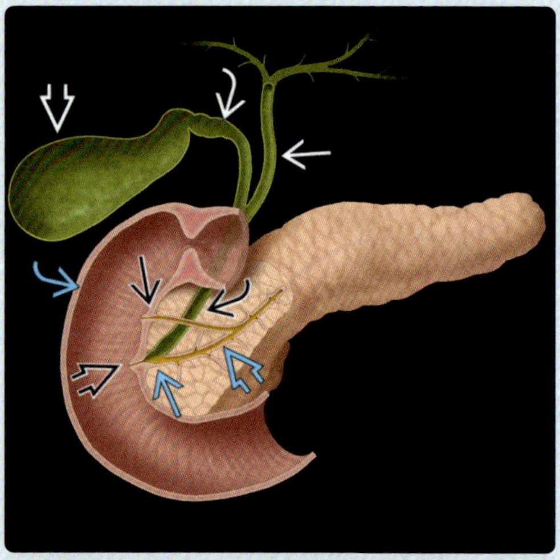

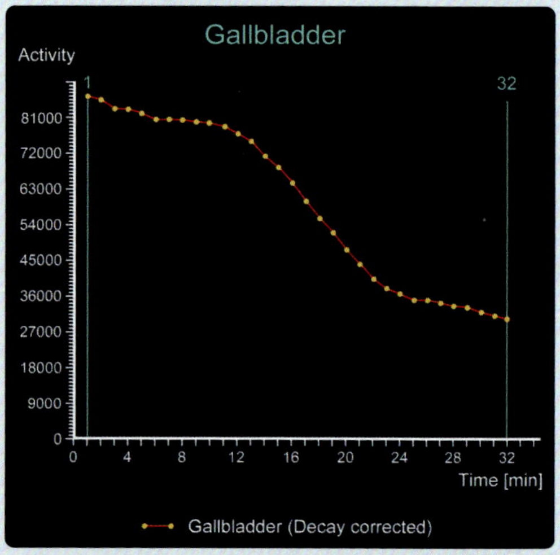

(Left) *Graphic shows gallbladder, cystic duct, common hepatic duct, common bile duct, main pancreatic duct of Wirsung, accessory pancreatic duct of Santorini (terminates in the minor papilla), hepatopancreatic sphincter of Oddi, hepatopancreatic ampulla of Vater, and duodenum.* **(Right)** *30 min CCK infusion protocol shows normal GBEF > 35%.*

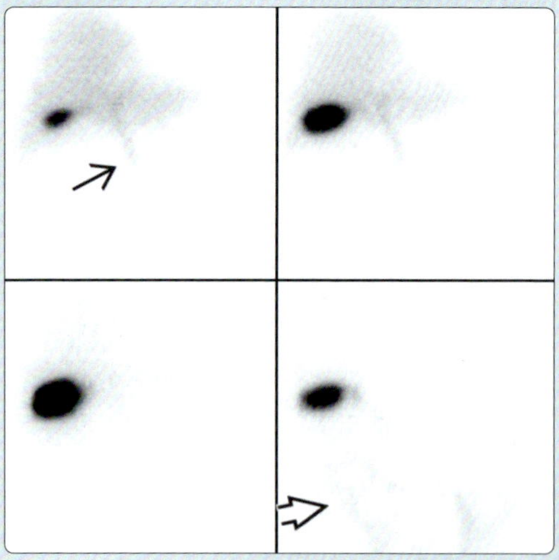

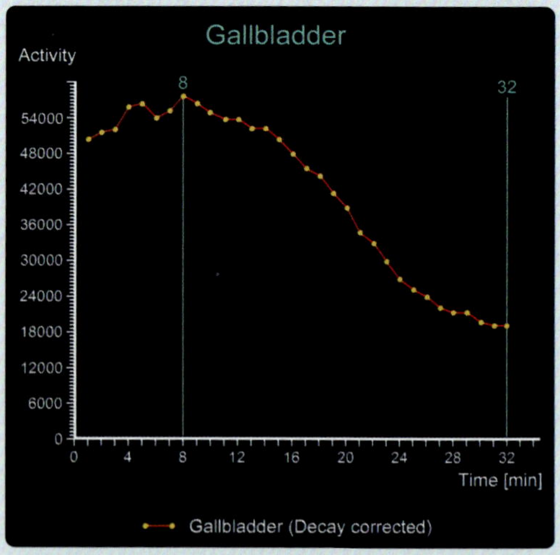

(Left) *Hepatobiliary scan shows common bile duct (CBD) at 20 min. The CBD remains visible without passage of radiotracer into the small bowel for 120 min. Finally, after CCK infusion, small bowel is seen.* **(Right)** *Normal GBEF with 30 minute protocol CCK infusion is shown. Abnormal retention of radiotracer in the CBD is concerning for sphincter of Oddi dysfunction (SOD) vs. partial CBD obstruction.*

TERMINOLOGY

Definitions

- Chronic calculous cholecystitis
  - Decreased gallbladder ejection fraction (GBEF) in presence of cholelithiasis
- Chronic acalculous cholecystitis/GB dyskinesia
  - Decreased GBEF in absence of cholelithiasis
- Sphincter of Oddi dysfunction (SOD)
  - Delayed biliary-to-bowel radiotracer transit

IMAGING

General Features

- Best diagnostic clue
  - Chronic cholecystitis
    - Delayed GB filling > 60 min
    - Delayed biliary-to-bowel transit > 60 min
    - Calculated GBEF < 38%
  - SOD
    - Delayed biliary-to-bowel transit > 30 min
    - Time of biliary visualization > 15 min
    - Prominent biliary tree
    - Sensitivity 49%, specificity 78%

Imaging Recommendations

- Best imaging tool
  - Tc-99m IDA hepatobiliary scintigraphy with calculated GBEF after cholecystokinin (CCK) IV infusion
- Protocol advice
  - Patient preparation
    - Discontinue medications that inhibit GB contraction
      - Opiates
      - Benzodiazepines
      - Progesterone
      - Ethanol
      - Octreotide
      - Indomethacin
      - Nicotine
      - Nifedipine
      - Pirenzepine
      - Theophylline
      - Atropine
    - Discontinue medication that contracts sphincter of Oddi
      - Neostigmine
      - Morphine; opiate antagonist (naloxone) can be used for reversal if necessary
    - NPO > 2 hr, < 24 hr
    - CCK contraindication
      - Pregnancy
      - Allergy
  - Radiopharmaceutical
    - Tc-99m mebrofenin/disofenin: 3-5 mCi (111-185 MBq) IV
  - Imaging acquisition to investigate chronic cholecystitis
    - Patient supine
    - Large field-of-view camera with low-energy all-purpose collimator
    - Matrix: 128 x 128
    - Image over abdomen
    - Angiographic phase x 1 min (4 sec/frame)
    - Dynamic acquisition (1 frame/min) for 60 min
  - CCK protocol
    - If GB filling and bowel activity is seen by 45-60 min, GBEF can be calculated
    - Best-validated reference database, which resulted in least variability of reference values, recommends
      - Infusion of IV CCK at 0.02 μg/kg for 60 min with normal GBEF > 38%
      - Infusion of IV CCK at 0.015 μg/kg for 45 min with images at 60 min with normal GBEF > 40%
    - Using immediate pre-CCK image and last post-CCK images, regions of interest (ROIs) are drawn around GB and adjacent liver (background)
    - GBEF (%) = [(net GBmax) - (net GBmin) / GBmax] x 100
    - Motion correction should be applied if needed
    - Fatty meal often used as alternative to CCK; however, it is not reproducible and normal gastric emptying is needed
  - Additional nuclear medicine imaging options
    - Left anterior oblique, right lateral to separate GB from duodenal bulb before drawing ROI to calculate GBEF

DIFFERENTIAL DIAGNOSIS

Acute Cholecystitis

- Lack of GB filling
- Patient with acute onset or acute on chronic right upper quadrant pain
- Abnormal lab values
  - Elevated white blood cells
  - Mild elevation in serum aminotransferases, amylase, &/or mild hyperbilirubinemia

Contraindicated Medication

- Opiates are most common interaction
  - Naloxone can be used to reverse opiate agonist

Liver Dysfunction

- Can delay GB filling &/or transit to small bowel
- GBEF could be underestimated either with severe hepatic dysfunction or any severe illness

Cyst Duct Syndrome (Rare)

- Cystic duct narrowing caused by chronic inflammation and fibrosis, or cyst ductal kinking

Partial Common Bile Duct Obstruction

- Could simulate SOD
- US or MRCP/labs should be considered if obstruction suspected
- Patient may have history of recurrent pancreatitis
- Other causes of distal partial CBD obstruction can mimic SOD
  - Pancreatic tumor
  - Ampulla of Vater tumor

PATHOLOGY

General Features

- Etiology
  - Chronic calculous cholecystitis

- In presence of gallstones, inflammatory changes in GB wall produce abnormal GB contraction and decreased GBEF
- Chronic acalculous cholecystitis
  - In absence of gallstones, inflammatory changes in GB wall produce abnormal GB contraction and decreased GBEF
- Gallbladder dyskinesia
  - Poor GB contractility that results in decreased GBEF, without evidence of inflammatory changes in GB wall
  - Pathophysiology uncertain/hormonal
  - Abnormal CCK release, reduced GB CKK receptor sensitivity/density
- Sphincter of Oddi dysfunction
  - Known as postcholecystectomy syndrome
  - Causes recurrent biliary pain in 10% of patients post cholecystectomy
  - GB acts as reservoir to release pressure from CBD, and subsequent GB resection makes symptoms evident
  - Symptoms possibly present before GB resection but obscured due to associated GB dysfunction
  - Structural
    - Inflammatory changes, strictures, fibrosis, adenomyosis, or muscular hypertrophy
  - Functional
    - Pathophysiology uncertain: Hormonal or neurologic disturbance
    - Confirm by sphincter of Oddi manometry
- Risk factors
  - Chronic calculous cholecystitis
    - Obesity
    - > 40 years old
    - Rapid weight loss
    - Pregnancy
    - Female
  - Chronic acalculous cholecystitis
    - Diabetes mellitus
    - Cirrhosis
    - Myotonic dystrophy
    - Irritable bowel syndrome
    - Celiac disease
    - Obesity
  - SOD
    - Prior ERCP or procedure
    - Inflammatory bowel disease
    - Post cholecystectomy

CLINICAL ISSUES

Treatment

- Chronic calculous/acalculous cholecystitis
  - Selective laparoscopy cholecystectomy
- SOD
  - Patients with positive Rome III criteria, abnormal liver test, and dilated CBD
    - ERCP and endoscopy sphincterotomy
  - Patient with positive Rome III criteria, either abnormal liver enzymes or dilated CBD
    - Should have sphincter of Oddi manometry (SOM) to confirm dysfunction prior to endoscopic sphincterotomy
  - Patient with positive Rome III criteria, normal liver enzymes and normal CBD
    - Poor correlation with SOM and response to sphincterotomy
    - Clinical follow-up to rule out other causes
- Rome III criteria
  - Clinical criteria to diagnose GB &/or SOD
  - All of the following conditions must be met
    - Pain located in epigastrium &/or right upper quadrant
    - Episodes last 30 min or longer
    - Recurrent symptoms occur at different intervals (not daily)
    - Pain builds up to steady level
    - Moderate to severe pain that interrupts patient's daily activities or leads to urgent care for relief
    - Pain not relieved by bowel movements
    - Pain not relieved by postural changes
    - Pain not relieved by antacids
    - Exclusion of other structural disease that would explain symptoms

DIAGNOSTIC CHECKLIST

Consider

- Enterogastric reflux can be seen on hepatobiliary scan and be cause of epigastric or RUQ pain

Image Interpretation Pearls

- LAO or right lateral view sometimes needed before drawing ROI to separate bowel from GB

Reporting Tips

- Review patient medications to rule out contraindicated drugs that can affect GBEF
- GBEF normal range depends on CCK infusion protocol; SNMMI recommends longer infusion of 45-60 min
- Patient with normal GBEF may progress to abnormal GBEF over period of years

SELECTED REFERENCES

1. Ziessman HA: Hepatobiliary Scintigraphy in 2014. J Nucl Med. 55(6):967-975, 2014
2. Santhosh S et al: Quantitative cholescintigraphy with fatty meal in the diagnosis of sphincter of Oddi dysfunction and acalculous cholecystopathy. Indian J Gastroenterol. 31(4):186-90, 2012
3. Ziessman HA: Functional hepatobiliary disease: chronic acalculous gallbladder and chronic acalculous biliary disease. Semin Nucl Med. 36(2):119-32, 2006
4. Sostre S et al: A noninvasive test of sphincter of Oddi dysfunction in postcholecystectomy patients: the scintigraphic score. J Nucl Med. 33(6):1216-22, 1992

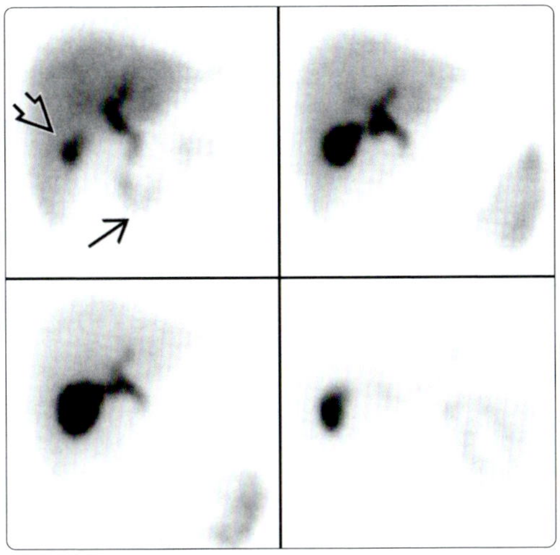

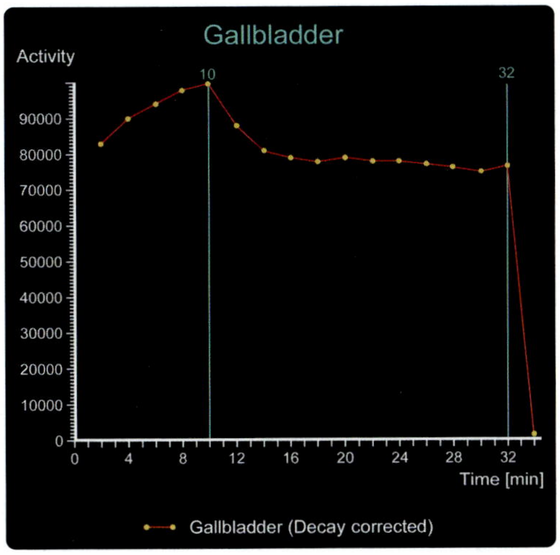

(Left) *There is a qualitative impression of normal GBEF. Small bowel is seen by 15 min, and GB filling is seen by 10 min.* **(Right)** *GBEF with 30 minute CCK infusion protocol in the same patient is abnormally low at 24%. This may be a false-positive and could be normal with a longer infusion time of 1 hr.*

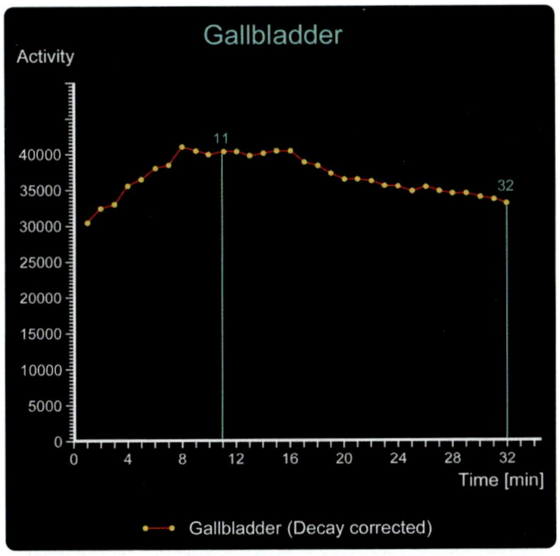

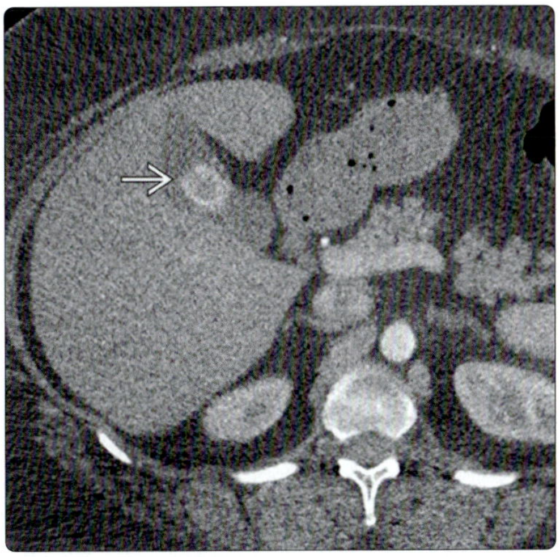

(Left) *30 minute CCK infusion protocol shows markedly abnormal GBEF (< 35%).* **(Right)** *Axial CECT in the same patient shows cholelithiasis, favoring the diagnosis of chronic calculous cholecystitis.*

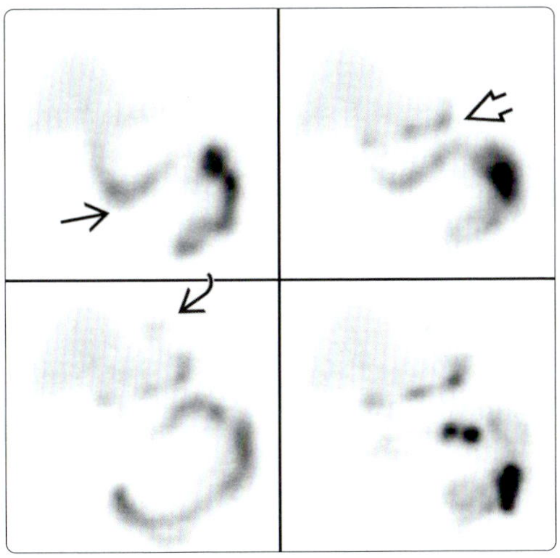

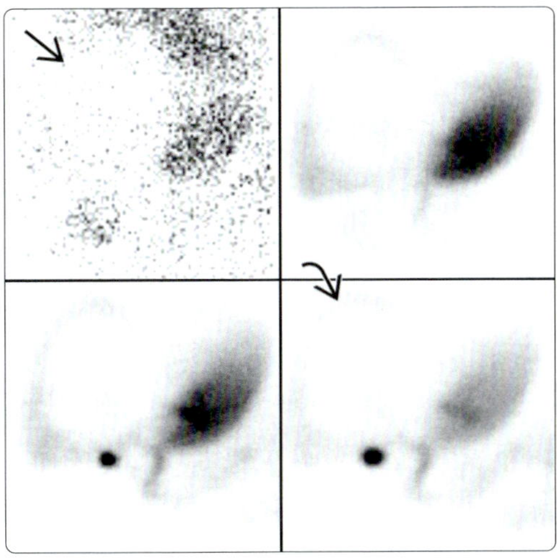

(Left) *Patient with suspected SOD shows normal biliary-to-bowel transit in < 5 min and marked enterogastric reflux extending superiorly to an outpouching, likely a hiatal hernia.* **(Right)** *Patient with right upper quadrant pain shows a large defect on flow images during entire examination. The patient had normal GBEF and biliary-to-bowel transit. Hepatic masses consistent with metastases were evident on US.*

Benign Solid Liver Lesions

KEY FACTS

TERMINOLOGY

- Hemangioma: Benign liver tumor that arises from endothelial cells
- Focal nodular hyperplasia (FNH): Benign tumor believed to be hyperplastic response to anomalous artery or vascular insult
- Hepatic adenoma: Liver tumor that arises from epithelial cells with very low malignant potential

IMAGING

- **Focal nodular hyperplasia**
  - Tc-99m IDA scintigraphy
    - Typical findings (~ 90% of FNH lesions): Focal activity > liver parenchyma, better seen with lesions > 2 cm
  - Tc-99m sulfur colloid (SC) scintigraphy
    - Focal activity ≥ liver parenchyma in ~ 2/3 of cases; 1/3 show low uptake
- **Hepatic hemangioma**
  - Focal area of activity > liver parenchyma that increases over time on Tc-99m red blood cell (RBC) scintigraphy
- **Hepatic adenoma**
  - Always photopenic on Tc-99m HIDA, Tc-99m SC, or Tc-99m RBC scintigraphy

TOP DIFFERENTIAL DIAGNOSES

- Hepatocellular carcinoma (HCC) or metastatic disease
- Regenerative nodules
- Superior vena cava syndrome
- Budd-Chiari syndrome, hepatic venous occlusive disease

DIAGNOSTIC CHECKLIST

- Tc-99m IDA scan or Tc-99m SC scan when IV contrast contraindicated for anatomic imaging (CT/MR)
- SPECT/ CT can help with multiple lesions, lesion near main vessels, &/or size 1-2 cm

(Left) *Axial CT angiogram incidentally revealed 2 enhancing lesions, incompletely characterized, that are possibly hemangiomas.* **(Right)** *Axial RBC scintigraphy SPECT in the same patient demonstrates increased focal uptake above the liver background at 1 hour, confirming the diagnosis of multiple hepatic hemangiomas. Note the inferior vena cava, spleen, and aorta.*

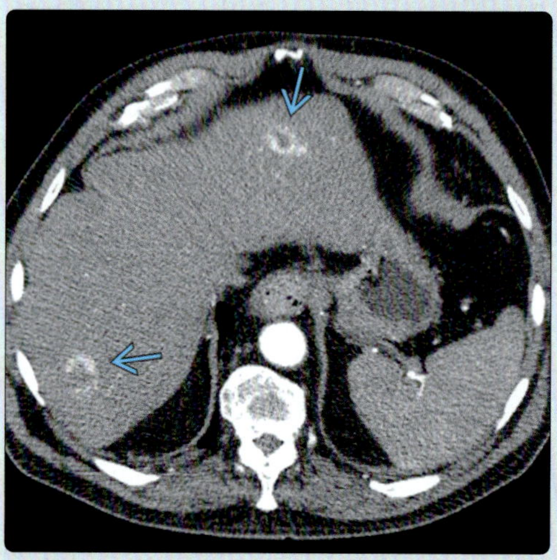

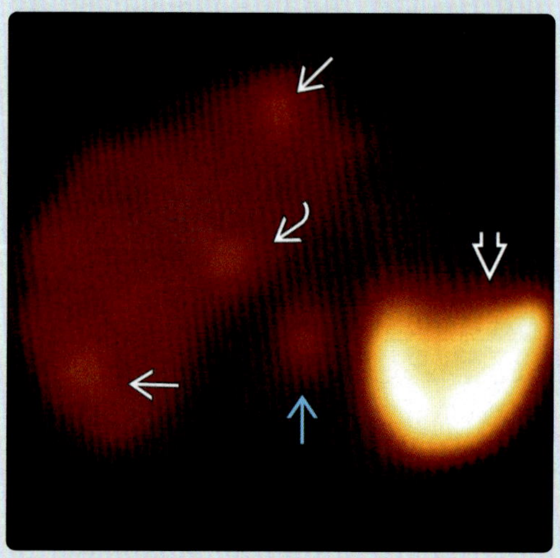

(Left) *Axial Tc-99m IDA SPECT in a patient with right upper quadrant pain shows focal increased uptake above the liver background, likely focal nodular hyperplasia.* **(Right)** *Axial T1 FS MR in the same patient shows an enhancing lesion in the posterior right hepatic lobe with a central scar that is consistent with focal nodular hyperplasia.*

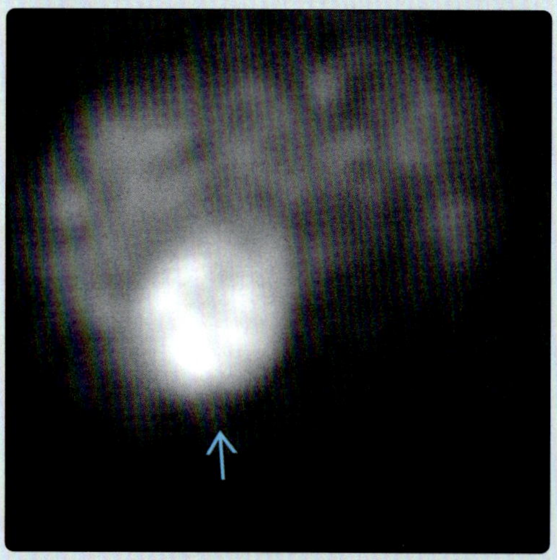

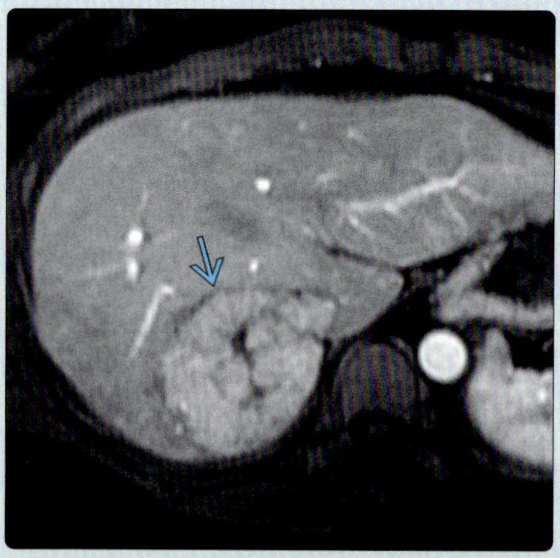

TERMINOLOGY

Definitions

- Benign solid liver lesions
  - Hemangioma: Benign liver tumor that arises from endothelial cells
  - Focal nodular hyperplasia (FNH): Benign tumor believed to be hyperplastic response to anomalous artery

IMAGING

Nuclear Medicine Findings

- Nuclear medicine used for diagnosis when IV contrast contraindicated for anatomic imaging (CT/MR)
- **FNH**
  - Tc-99m IDA scintigraphy
    - Typical findings (~ 90% of FNH lesions): Focal activity > liver parenchyma, better seen with lesions > 2 cm
    - Early visualization with persistent tracer/delayed washout
    - More accurate than Tc-99m sulfur colloid (SC) scan
  - Tc-99m SC scintigraphy
    - Presence of functioning Kupffer cells allows Tc-99m SC accumulation
    - Focal activity ≥ liver parenchyma in ~ 2/3 of cases; 1/3 show low uptake
    - Lesions iso- or hyperintense when compared to liver parenchyma do not require biopsy
- **Hepatic hemangioma**
  - Focal area of activity > liver parenchyma that increases over time on Tc-99m red blood cell (RBC) scintigraphy
  - Photopenic on angiographic phase images
  - Specificity = 99% with lesion > 2 cm, not adjacent to main liver vessels

Imaging Recommendations

- Protocol advice
  - **Tc-99m IDA scintigraphy**
    - Patient preparation
      - □ None
    - Radiopharmaceutical
      - □ 3-5 mCi (111-185 MBq) Tc-99m mebrofenin/disofenin
    - Dosimetry
      - □ Biliary system receives highest radiation dose
    - Imaging acquisition
      - □ Patient supine
      - □ Large FOV camera with low-energy all-purpose (LEAP) collimator
      - □ 128 x 128 matrix
      - □ Image over abdomen
      - □ Angiographic phase x 1 min (4 sec/min)
      - □ Static anterior and posterior images at 15, 30, and 60 min if needed
      - □ SPECT/CT if needed for better localization, multiple lesions, &/or size 1-2 cm
  - **Tc-99m sulfur colloid (SC) scintigraphy**
    - Patient preparation
      - □ Review liver function and presence of portal hypertension, which can alter uptake and biodistribution of radiotracer
    - Radiopharmaceutical
      - □ 4-6 mCi (198-222 MBq) Tc-99m SC
      - □ Particle size: 01-1 μm
      - □ Optimal accumulation in 5-10 min; could be delayed with liver failure or portal hypertension (20-30 min)
    - Dosimetry
      - □ Liver receives largest radiation dose
    - Imaging acquisition
      - □ Patient supine
      - □ Large FOV camera LEAP collimator
      - □ 128 x 128 matrix
      - □ Angiographic phase x 1 min (4 sec/min)
      - □ Static anterior and posterior images at 10-20 min
      - □ SPECT/CT if needed for better localization, multiple lesions, &/or size 1-2 cm
  - **Tc-99m RBC scintigraphy**
    - Patient preparation
      - □ Inquire about heparin allergy (used in labeling process)
      - □ Rule out hemolysis (can decrease percentage of labeled RBCs)
    - Radiopharmaceutical
      - □ 20-25 mCi (740-925 MBq) Tc-99m pertechnetate to label RBCs
    - Dosimetry
      - □ Heart receives largest radiation dose
    - Imaging acquisition
      - □ Patient supine
      - □ Image abdomen
      - □ LEAP collimator
      - □ 128 x 128 matrix
      - □ Anterior flow study (1-5 sec/frame x 1 min)
      - □ Static planar anterior and posterior images at 30, 60, and 120 min
      - □ SPECT/CT if needed for better localization, multiple lesions, lesion near main vessels, &/or size 1-2 cm

DIFFERENTIAL DIAGNOSIS

Hepatic Adenoma

- Liver tumor that arises from epithelial cells; very low malignant potential, risk of hemorrhage
- Always photopenic on Tc-99m IDA, Tc-99m SC, or Tc-99m labeled RBC scan

Hepatocellular Carcinoma or Metastatic Disease

- Tc-99m IDA: Initially cold to ≥ 1 hr; delayed fill-in can be seen (bile lakes)
- Tc-99m RBC scan: Could have increased flow without increasing activity over time

Regenerative Nodules

- Can show increased uptake on Tc-99m SC scan

Superior Vena Cava Syndrome

- Redistribution of Tc-99m SC to left lobe secondary to collateralization
  - Focal hepatic hot spot sign: Focally increased Tc-99m SC uptake in segment IV

Budd-Chiari Syndrome, Hepatic Venous Occlusive Disease

- Tc-99m SC accumulates normally in caudate lobe secondary to drainage by inferior vena cava; remaining liver parenchyma is decreased

PATHOLOGY

General Features

- Etiology
  - Focal nodular hyperplasia
    - Postulated to arise from vascular malformation, probably by dysregulation of angiopoietin genes with subsequent blood hyperperfusion leading to secondary hyperplastic area of liver parenchyma
    - Multiple FNH syndrome: 2 or more FNH in combination with liver hemangiomas, vascular malformations, &/or intracranial tumor
    - 2-5 lesions in 30% (> 5 lesions rare)
    - Multiple FNH also described in Klippel-Trenaunay and von Recklinghausen syndromes
  - Hemangioma
    - Uncertain etiology
    - Most likely originate from congenital vascular malformation or hamartoma that subsequently increases in size

CLINICAL ISSUES

Presentation

- Most common signs/symptoms
  - Focal nodular hyperplasia
    - Usually asymptomatic, incidental finding
    - Occasional hepatomegaly, abdominal mass, fullness
  - Hemangioma
    - Usually asymptomatic, incidental finding
    - Giant hemangioma > 4 cm are symptomatic in 40% of cases
      - Fullness, mild discomfort

Demographics

- Epidemiology
  - Focal nodular hyperplasia
    - Incidence: 3% of normal population by large autopsy series
    - Usually 3rd or 4th decades, rarely infantile or childhood
    - F > M (8:1/12:1)
    - Right lobe > left (2:1)
  - Hemangioma
    - Incidence: 0.4-20% depending on autopsy studies
    - Usually 3rd to 5th decades
    - F > M (6:1)
    - Right lobe > left

Natural History & Prognosis

- Focal nodular hyperplasia
  - Usually benign course
  - May cause pain secondary to mass effect
  - Rarely hemorrhage (2-3%); hemoperitoneum
  - Infarction unusual
  - No malignant potential
  - Can grow during pregnancy or with oral contraceptives
  - Complete radiologic involution has been reported in handful of cases
- Hemangioma
  - Usually benign course
  - Complications
    - Rupture: With size 5-10 cm, incidence < 4%, mortality 70-80% (decreased to 36% for patients who receive STAT surgery)
    - Thrombosis
    - Sclerosis
    - Can grow during pregnancy or with oral contraceptives
    - Uncommon complications: Kasabach-Merritt syndrome and Bornman-Terblanche-Blumgart syndrome

DIAGNOSTIC CHECKLIST

Consider

- Tc-99m IDA or Tc-99m SC scan when IV contrast material for CT/MR contraindicated
- SPECT/ CT can help with multiple lesions, lesion near main vessels, &/or size 1-2 cm

Image Interpretation Pearls

- Focal nodular hyperplasia
  - Tc-99m IDA scintigraphy
    - Typical findings (~ 90% FNH lesions): Focal activity > liver parenchyma, better seen with lesions > 2 cm
  - Tc-99m sulfur SC scintigraphy
    - Focal activity ≥ liver parenchyma in approximately 2/3 of cases; 1/3 show low uptake
    - Liver cirrhosis can produce colloid shift to spleen and bone marrow, decreasing sensitivity of Tc-99m SC for detection of focal liver lesions
    - 1/3 of FNH photopenic on Tc-99m SC scan
- Hepatic hemangioma
  - Focal area of activity > liver parenchyma that increases over time on Tc-99m labeled RBC scintigraphy

SELECTED REFERENCES

1. Margonis GA et al: Benign Solid Tumors of the Liver: Management in the Modern Era. J Gastrointest Surg. ePub, 2015
2. Yedibela S et al: Management of hemangioma of the liver: surgical therapy or observation? World J Surg. 37(6):1303-12, 2013
3. Schmidt E et al: Varying appearance of focal nodular hyperplasia in nuclear medicine imaging. Clin Nucl Med. 33(1):71-3, 2008
4. Huynh LT et al: The typical appearance of focal nodular hyperplasia in triple-phase CT scan, hepatobiliary scan, and Tc-99m sulfur colloid scan with SPECT. Clin Nucl Med. 30(11):736-9, 2005
5. Steiner D et al: Diagnosis of focal nodular hyperplasia with hepatobiliary scintigraphy using a modified SPECT technique. Clin Nucl Med. 28(2):136-7, 2003

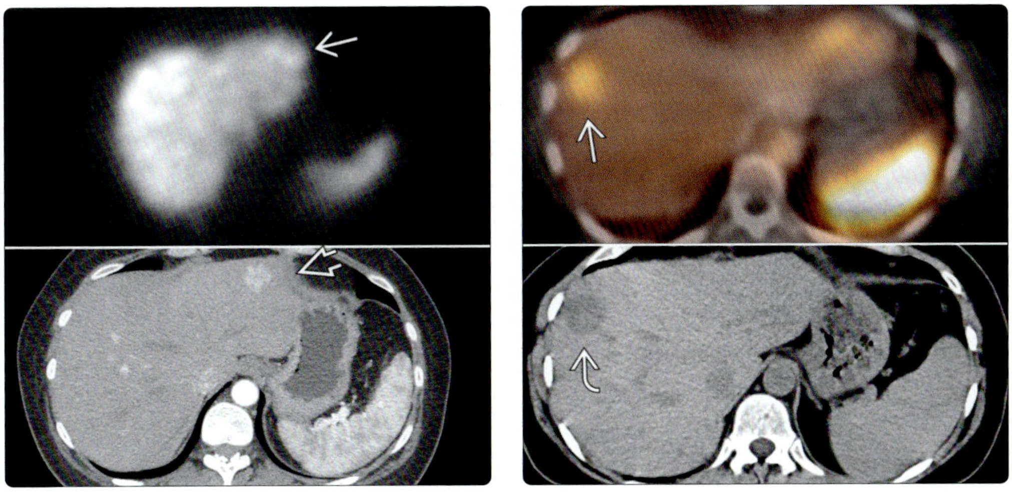

(Left) *Axial Tc-99m SC SPECT shows normal background uptake → in the left hepatic lobe, suggesting FNH as diagnosis of the arterial enhancing lesion → on the axial CECT scan.* **(Right)** *Axial Tc-99m RBC fused SPECT/CT in a patient with colon cancer and renal failure demonstrates a focal area of increased activity → above liver background in the right hepatic lobe, corresponding to the lesion → on axial NECT scan, confirming the diagnosis of hemangioma.*

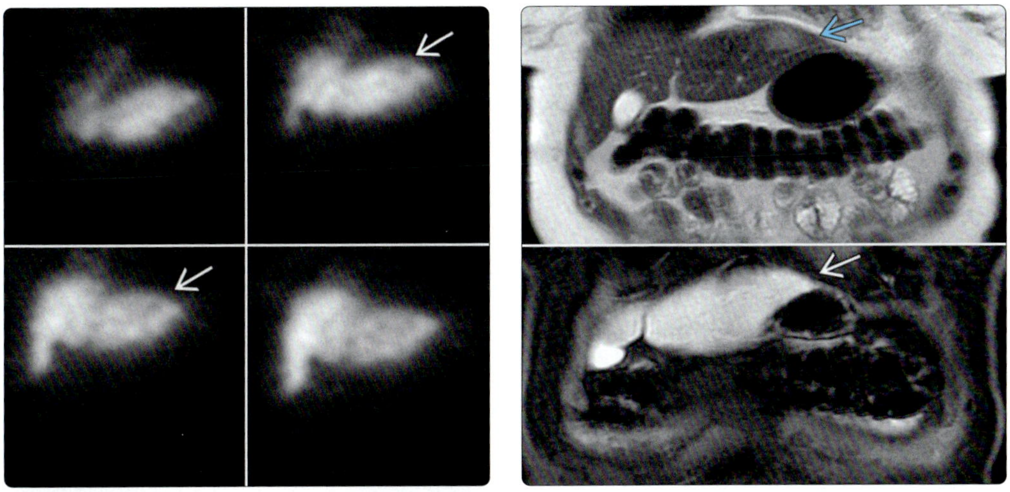

(Left) *Coronal Tc-99m SC SPECT in a patient with a hepatic mass on ultrasound shows a photopenic lesion → in the left hepatic lobe.* **(Right)** *Coronal T2-weighted MR in the same patient shows a hyperintense lesion → that demonstrates enhancement at 20 minutes → with hepatobiliary contrast agent, making the diagnosis of FNH.*

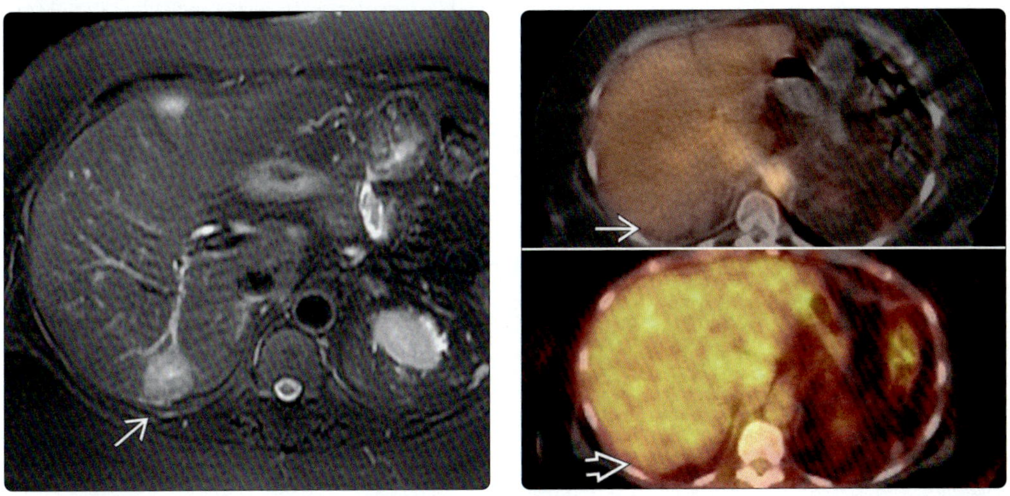

(Left) *Axial T2 FS MR in a patient with breast cancer shows a hepatic lesion →, favored to represent a sclerosing hemangioma.* **(Right)** *Tc-99m RBC fused SPECT/CT in the same patient shows background level activity → in the lesion that did not increase over time. On the axial F-18 FDG PET/CT, the lesion is not FDG-avid, → favoring the diagnosis of sclerosing hemangioma over metastasis.*

Gastrointestinal Bleed Localization

KEY FACTS

IMAGING

- GI bleed scintigraphy
  - Focal activity distinct from vasculature or organ
  - Focal activity increases over time and moves within tubular structure
  - If focal activity persists and does not move over time, likely not GI bleed
- Upper GI bleed
  - Esophagus, stomach, proximal duodenum
- Small bowel bleed
  - Centrally located
  - Serpiginous pattern
  - Less common than colorectal bleed
- Colorectal bleed
  - Peripheral, elongated pattern
  - Well-defined haustrations
  - Rectal bleed: Lateral or postvoid images helpful
- Delayed imaging (e.g., 24 hr static image) not useful for localization
  - May show interval bleeding in GI tract
  - Usually unable to determine origin due to antegrade/retrograde peristalsis in interval

DIAGNOSTIC CHECKLIST

- Celiac artery
  - Lower 1/3 of esophagus, stomach, 1st and 2nd parts of duodenum
  - Pancreas, spleen, liver, biliary system
- Superior mesenteric artery
  - 2nd part of duodenum to distal 1/3 of transverse colon
- Inferior mesenteric artery
  - Distal 1/3 of transverse colon to proximal rectum
- Internal iliac artery
  - Middle and inferior rectum

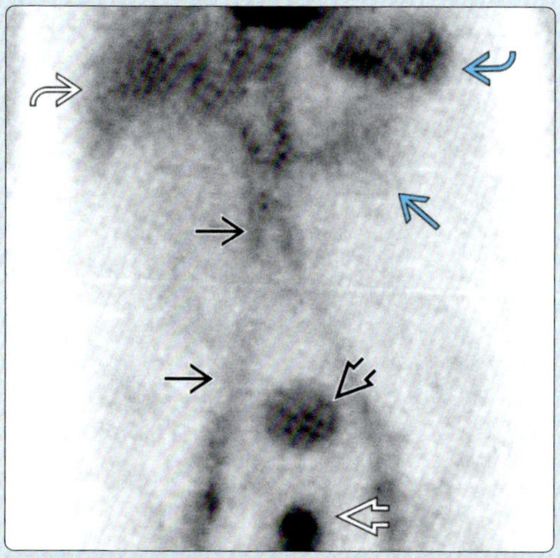
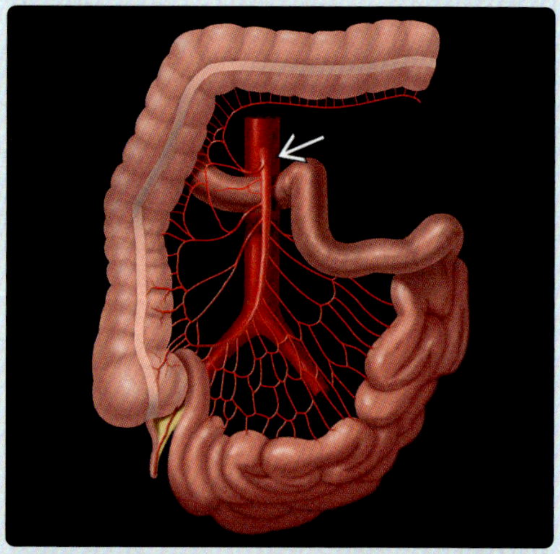

(Left) *Normal structures are shown on anterior Tc-99m RBC scintigraphy. Blood pool in the heart is visible at top center. Note liver and spleen, faint gastric uptake, abdominal aorta, inferior vena cava and iliac vessels, urinary bladder, and genitalia.* **(Right)** *Coronal graphic shows bowel supplied by superior mesenteric artery, from the 2nd part of the duodenum to the distal 1/3 of the transverse colon.*

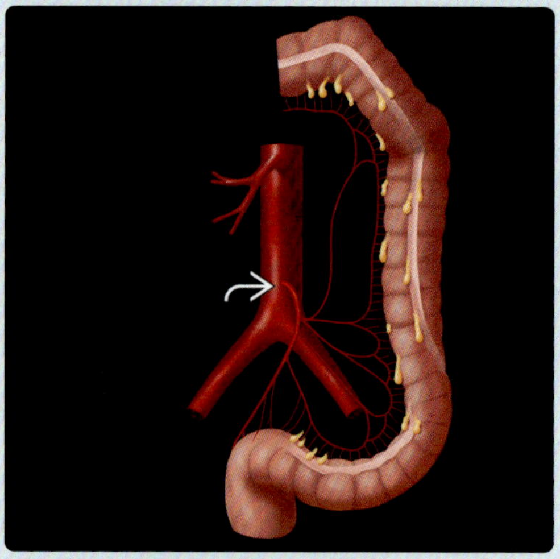
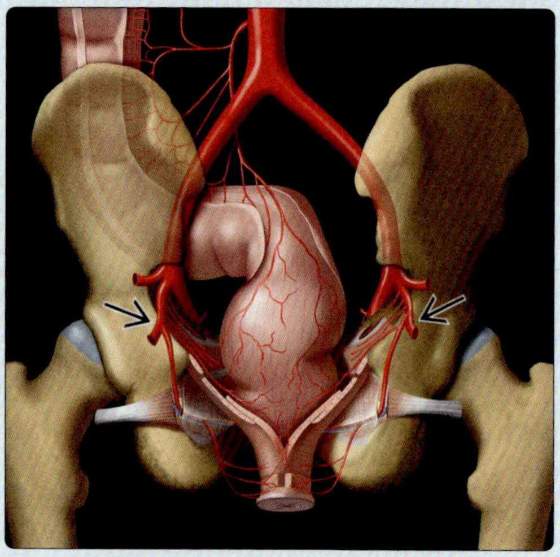

(Left) *Coronal graphic shows bowel supplied by the inferior mesenteric artery, from the distal 1/3 of the transverse colon to the proximal rectum.* **(Right)** *Coronal posterior graphic shows the middle and inferior rectum, supplied by branches of the internal iliac artery.*

TERMINOLOGY

Definitions

- Localization of GI bleed origin on scintigraphy to direct angiographic/endoscopic intervention or selective surgery
  - Tc-99m red blood cells (RBCs)
  - Tc-99m sulfur colloid (SC)

IMAGING

General Features

- Best diagnostic clue
  - Focal activity distinct from normal vascular structure or solid organ
  - Activity increases over time and moves within tubular structure
  - If activity persists and does not move over time, likely not GI bleed
- Location
  - Upper GI bleed: Proximal to ligament of Treitz
    - Celiac artery
      - Lower 1/3 of esophagus, stomach, 1st and 2nd parts of duodenum
      - Pancreas, spleen, liver, biliary system
  - Lower GI bleed: Distal to ligament of Treitz
    - Superior mesenteric artery
      - 2nd part of duodenum to distal 1/3 of transverse colon
      - Pancreas
    - Inferior mesenteric artery
      - Distal 1/3 of transverse colon to proximal rectum (above dentate line)
    - Internal iliac artery
      - Middle and inferior rectum (below dentate line)
- Detection rates
  - 83% of active hemorrhage detected by 90 min
  - Positive when bleeding rate exceeds 0.05-0.1 cc/min
  - Minimum of 3-5 cc blood required to localize

Nuclear Medicine Findings

- Tc-99m labeled red cell scintigraphy
  - Focal activity distinct from normal vascular structure or organ
  - Blush on flow images may be evident
  - Dynamic images demonstrate large vs. small bowel pattern
  - Anterograde or retrograde transit due to peristalsis
  - Upper GI bleed
    - Varices and esophageal bleed usually detected on upper endoscopy
    - Gastric bleeding may be confused with free pertechnetate uptake and excretion by gastric mucosa
      - Image of uptake in thyroid may be useful to confirm free Tc-99m pertechnetate
    - Scintigraphy useful prior to endoscopic intervention with intermittent bleeding
  - Small bowel bleed
    - Centrally located
    - Serpiginous pattern
    - Less common than colorectal bleed
  - Colorectal bleed
    - Peripheral, elongated pattern
    - Well-defined haustrations
    - Rectal bleed: Lateral or postvoid images useful
  - Pitfalls
    - Normal accumulation of Tc-99m RBCs
      - Blood pool of abdominopelvic vessels
      - Superficial abdominal vessels
      - Spleen
      - Liver
      - Kidney: Normal, ptotic or pelvic kidney
      - Enlarged uterus/fibroid
      - Urinary bladder
      - Genitalia
    - Poor RBC label leads to free Tc-99m pertechnetate in bowel or urinary system
    - Delayed imaging (e.g., 24 hr static) not useful for localization
      - May show interval bleeding in GI tract
      - Usually unable to determine origin due to antegrade/retrograde peristalsis in interval

Imaging Recommendations

- Best imaging tool
  - Tc-99m RBC scintigraphy
    - Useful in intermittent bleeding
    - One injection can monitor bleeding over several hrs (up to 24)
    - Sensitivity higher than Tc-99m sulfur colloid (SC) with in vitro labeling
    - Poor labeling or hemolysis can decrease sensitivity
    - Heparin used in labeling kit
    - Patients with hemolysis syndromes (e.g., thalassemia) may have poor tag
  - Tc-99m SC scintigraphy
    - No need to manipulate blood products
    - Useful in patients with heparin allergy
    - Window for detection after injection ~ 1 hr
    - Not as useful for intermittent bleeding
    - Liver and spleen uptake may obscure splenic or hepatic flexure source
- Protocol advice
  - Patient preparation
    - Inquire about heparin allergy
  - Radiopharmaceutical
    - 1st line: 8-12 mCi (296-444 MBq) Tc-99m pertechnetate labeled RBCs
    - 2nd line: 10-15 mCi (370-555 MBq) Tc-99m sulfur colloid (SC)
  - Dosimetry
    - Tc-99m RBCs: Heart receives largest radiation dose
    - Tc-99m SC: Spleen receives largest radiation dose
  - Image acquisition
    - Patient supine
    - Image abdomen and pelvis
    - Collimator: LEAP or diverging (if portable)
    - 128 x 128 matrix
    - Anterior flow study (1-5 sec/frame x 1 min)
    - Dynamic anterior images; 10-60 sec/frame

- Generally image 60-90 min; up to several hrs if Tc-99m RBCs
- Lateral or post-void view for rectal bleeding/confirmation of genitourinary activity
- Image processing
  - Frame-by-frame snapshot helps localize exact origin of bleed
  - Cine loop viewing to increase sensitivity of bleed detection

DIFFERENTIAL DIAGNOSIS

Distal Esophageal Bleed

- Dilated esophageal varices in distal esophagus

Gastric Bleed

- Gastroesophageal or upper abdomen portosystemic shunt and varices
- Gastritis/hyperemia
- Gastric uptake of free Tc-99m pertechnetate with secretion into small bowel can mimic GI bleed

Small Bowel Bleed

- Abdominal aortic aneurysm
- External abdominal wall bleeding/wound
- Free Tc-99m pertechnetate in renal collecting system
- Hemobilia
- Solid organ bleeding

Colorectal Bleed

- Free Tc-99m pertechnetate in urinary bladder
- Normal genitourinary uptake
- Solid organ bleeding

PATHOLOGY

General Features

- Etiology
  - Upper GI bleed
    - Duodenal ulcer (24%)
    - Gastric erosions (23%)
    - Gastric ulcer (21%)
    - Varices (10%)
    - Mallory-Weiss tear (7%)
    - Esophagitis (6%)
    - Neoplasm (3%)
    - Other (11%)
  - Lower GI bleed
    - Diverticulosis (42%)
    - Colitis (29%)
    - Ischemia (18%)
    - Anorectal (16%)
    - Postpolypectomy (13%)
    - Neoplasia (11%)
    - Angiodysplasia (3%)

CLINICAL ISSUES

Demographics

- Epidemiology
  - More common over age 65
  - Annual incidence (2006)
    - Principal diagnosis in 182 per 100,000 persons hospitalized
  - Cause of over 16,000 inpatient deaths per year

Treatment

- Angiographic intervention
  - Procedure of choice if patient hemodynamically unstable
  - Positive scintigraphy increases chance of positive angiography and intervention (goal is within 30 min of positive scan)
  - Successful if patient is actively bleeding at time of study
    - > 0.5 cc/min for mesenteric angiography
    - > 5-7 cc/min for nonselective aortic angiography
  - Interventional: Embolotherapy (foam and coils) for upper and lower GI bleed
  - Transjugular intrahepatic portosystemic shunt for esophageal/gastric varices
- Endoscopic intervention
  - Mechanical: Clips, balloons, sutures
  - Thermal: Laser photocoagulation and electrocoagulation
- Surgical intervention
  - Scintigraphic localization allows partial or selective bowel resection
  - Prevents unsuspected small bowel bleed from being missed at operation
  - Negative scintigraphy may indicate no need for surgical intervention

DIAGNOSTIC CHECKLIST

Reporting Tips

- Specific site of origin most effectively directs interventional angiography to offending arterial supply
  - Celiac: Lower 1/3 of esophagus, stomach, 1st and 2nd parts of duodenum
  - SMA: 2nd part of duodenum to distal 1/3 of transverse colon
  - IMA: Distal 1/3 of transverse colon to proximal rectum
  - Internal iliac: Middle and inferior rectum
- Notify referring physician of positive GI bleed scintigraphy ASAP to facilitate minimally invasive therapeutic interventions while patient still bleeding

SELECTED REFERENCES

1. ACR-SNMMI-SPR Practice Guideline for the Performance of Gastrointestinal Scintigraphy. http://snmmi.files.cms-plus.com/docs/GI_Scintigraphy_1382731852503_4.pdf Published October 1, 2010. Accessed May 6, 2014
2. Howarth DM: The role of nuclear medicine in the detection of acute gastrointestinal bleeding. Semin Nucl Med. 36(2):133-46, 2006
3. Strate LL: Lower GI bleeding: epidemiology and diagnosis. Gastroenterol Clin North Am. 34(4):643-64, 2005
4. Levy R et al: Retrospective study of the utility of nuclear scintigraphic-labeled red cell scanning for lower gastrointestinal bleeding. ANZ J Surg. 73(4):205-9, 2003
5. Zuckier LS: Acute gastrointestinal bleeding. Semin Nucl Med. 33(4):297-311, 2003
6. Ponzo F et al: Tc-99m sulfur colloid and Tc-99m tagged red blood cell methods are comparable for detecting lower gastrointestinal bleeding in clinical practice. Clin Nucl Med. 27(6):405-9, 2002
7. Meller J et al: [Improved detection of gastrointestinal bleeding sites with 99mTc market autologous erythrocytes and continuous dynamic scintigraphy with cine-mode display.] Chirurg. 71(3):292-9, 2000

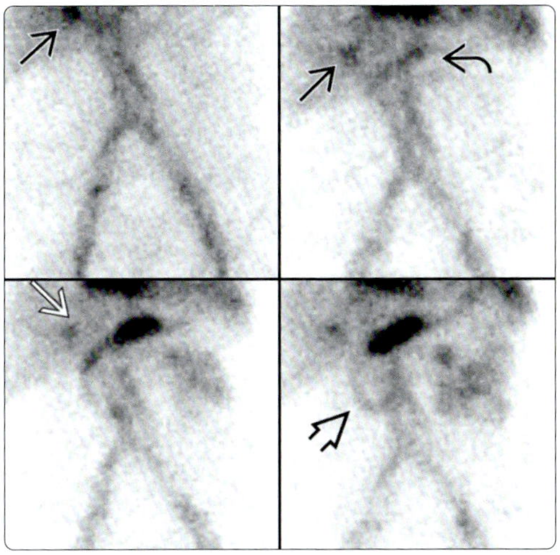

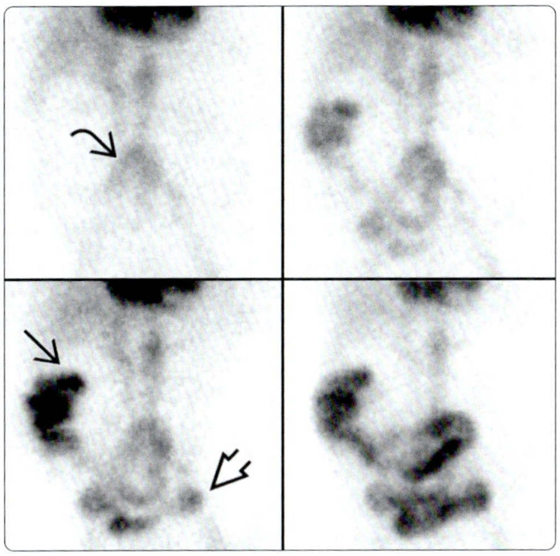

(Left) *Anterior Tc-99m RBC scintigraphy shows activity → that moves distally into proximal duodenum → and small bowel →, consistent with gastric source of bleeding. Note persistent focal increased activity in liver →. A hemangioma was evident on CT (not shown).* **(Right)** *Anterior Tc-99m RBC scintigraphy shows bleeding in lower abdomen → that moves in a serpiginous fashion retrograde and antegrade into cecum → and ileum →, consistent with small bowel origin.*

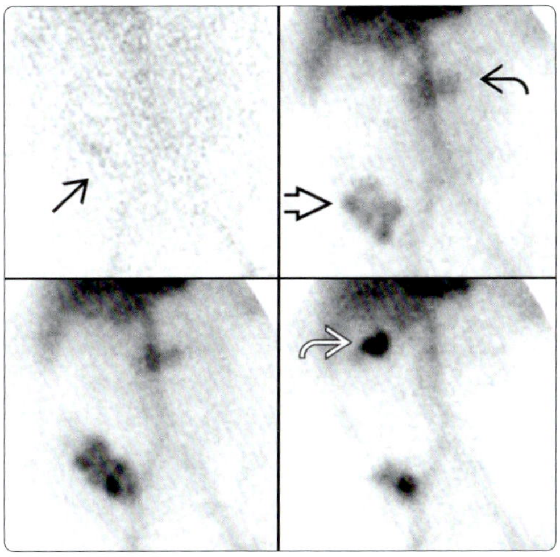

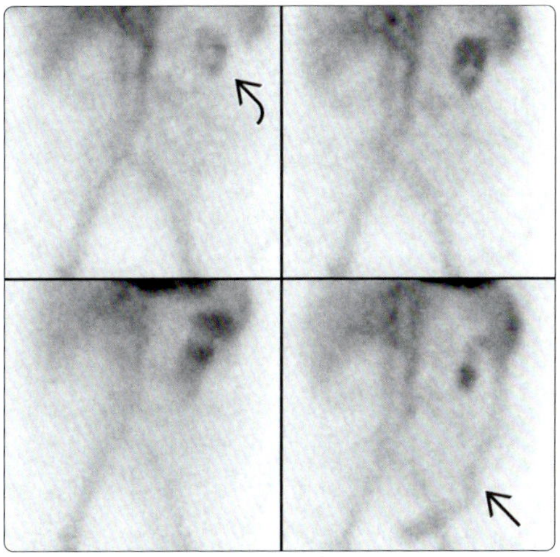

(Left) *Anterior Tc-99m RBC scintigraphy shows bleed originating in cecum → on flow and dynamic → images. Peristalsis moves the Tc-99m RBCs to transverse colon → and hepatic flexure →.* **(Right)** *Anterior Tc-99m RBC scintigraphy shows bleed origination in splenic flexure →, which moves distally in a peripheral, elongated pattern to sigmoid colon →.*

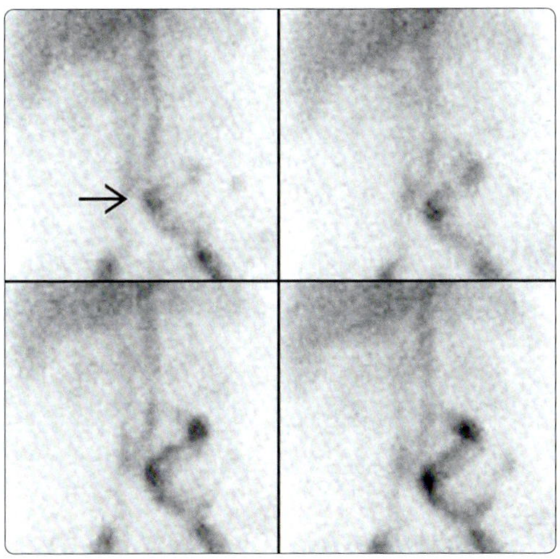

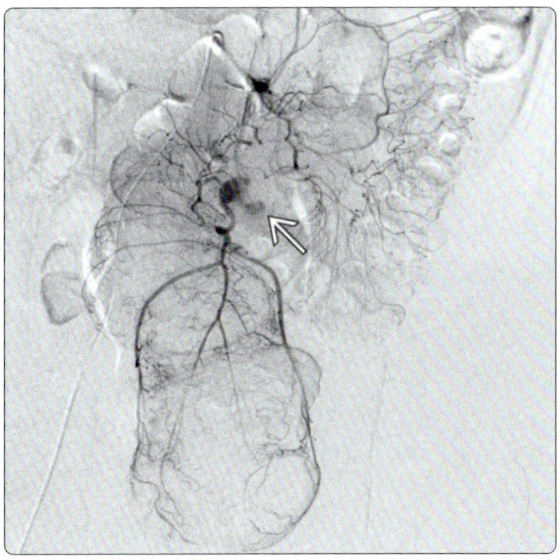

(Left) *Anterior Tc-99m RBC scintigraphy shows bleed originating in sigmoid colon → with retrograde and antegrade peristalsis.* **(Right)** *Selective anterior arteriography of sigmoid artery in the same patient confirms active extravasation →, likely diverticular bleeding. Embolization was successfully performed.*

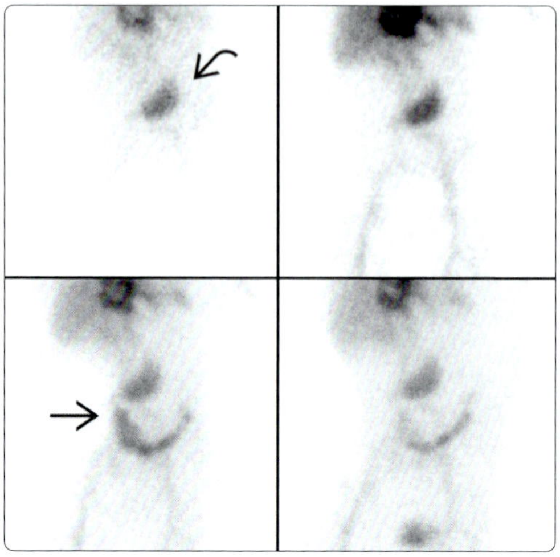

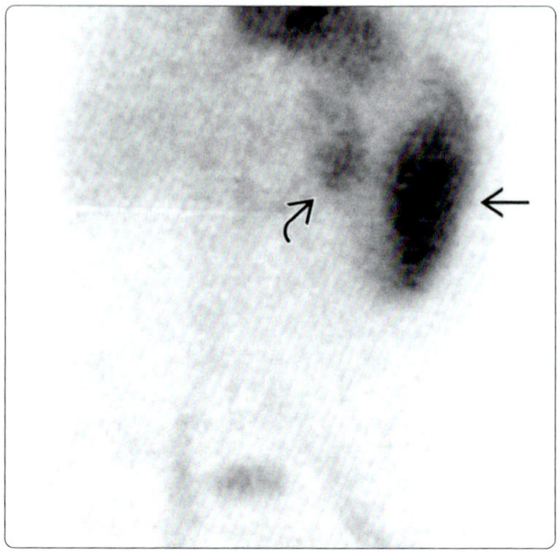

(Left) *Anterior Tc-99m RBC scintigraphy shows central abdomen activity in this patient's known abdominal aortic aneurysm. Note tubular accumulation of RBCs consistent with sigmoid bleeding origin.* **(Right)** *Anterior Tc-99m RBC scintigraphy shows splenomegaly and varices in a patient with cirrhosis.*

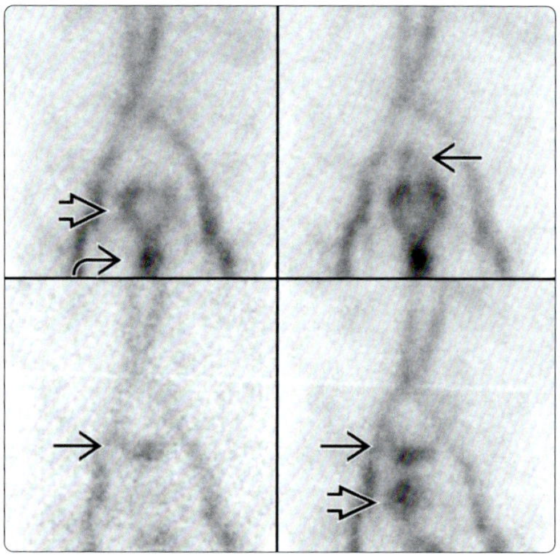

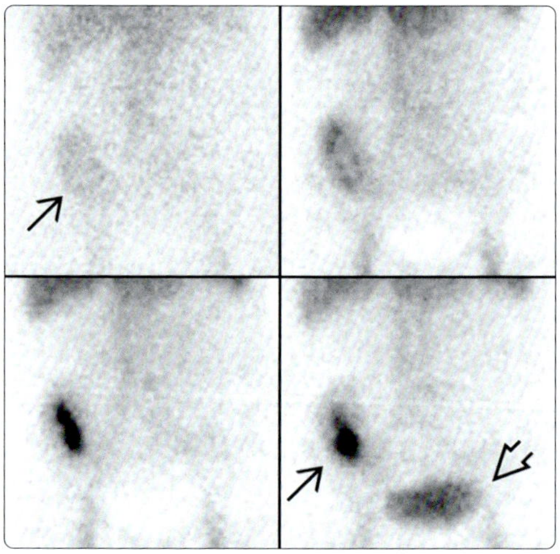

(Left) *Anterior Tc-99m RBC scintigraphy shows radiotracer in a catheterized urinary bladder and normal genital activity. Focal activity superior to urinary bladder persists after bladder drained, with origin in rectosigmoid colon.* **(Right)** *Anterior Tc-99m RBC scintigraphy shows focal activity in RLQ that increases over time in a pelvic transplant kidney and urinary bladder. Note that activity that does not move in a tubular pattern over time is likely not a GI bleed.*

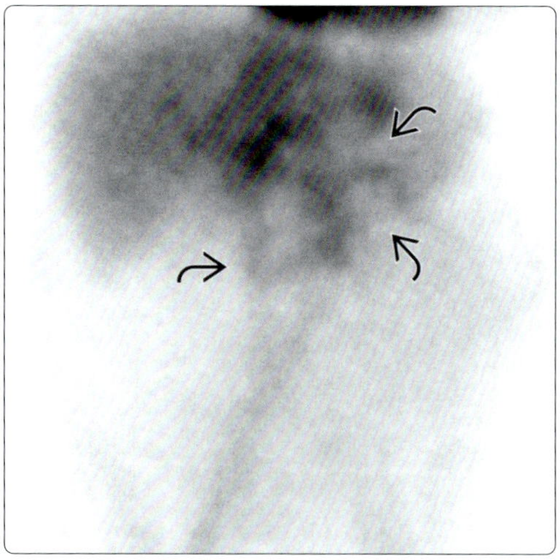

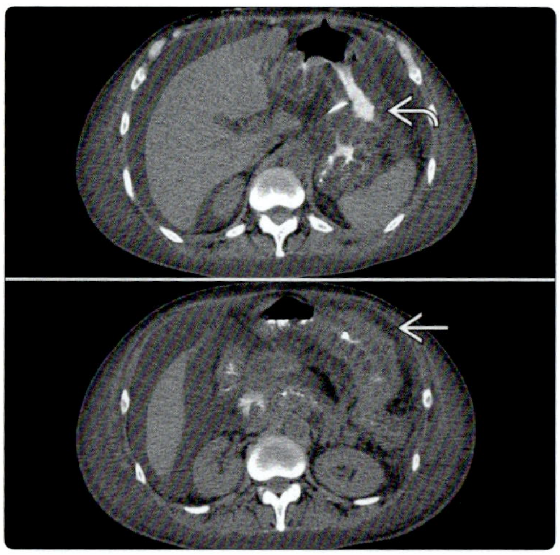

(Left) *Anterior Tc-99m RBC scintigraphy shows activity in the upper abdomen that appears diffuse and without distal progression, most consistent with hyperemia.* **(Right)** *Axial CT in the same patient shows marked edema of gastric and transverse colon wall.*

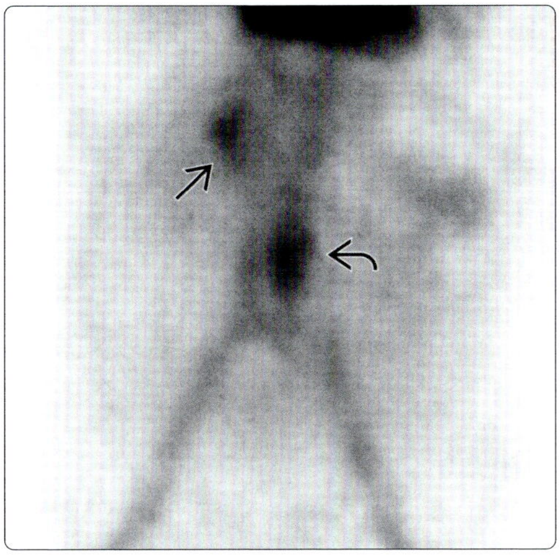

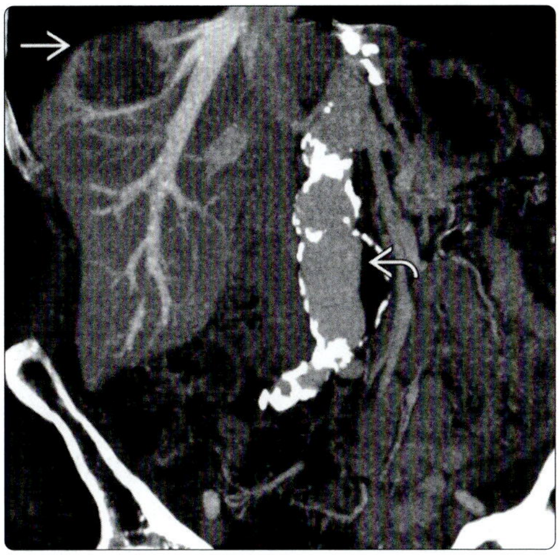

(Left) *Anterior Tc-99m RBC scintigraphy shows focal static activity in an infrarenal abdominal aneurysm. Another static focus in RUQ represents a hypervascular liver mass.* **(Right)** *Coronal CECT in the same patient shows a fusiform infrarenal abdominal aneurysm with extensive atherosclerosis. A hypervascular liver mass with capsular enhancement is consistent with hepatocellular carcinoma.*

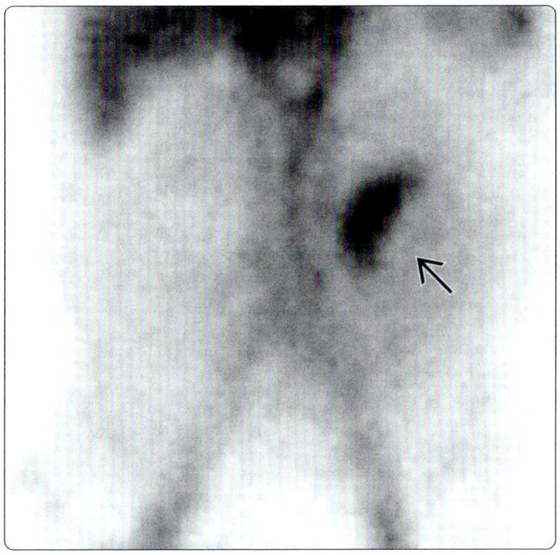

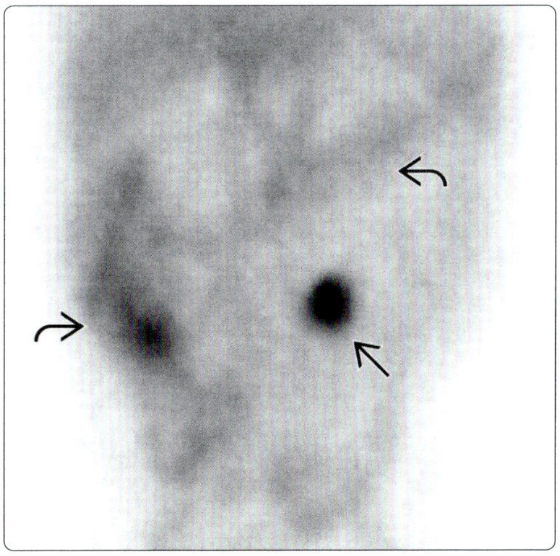

(Left) *Anterior Tc-99m RBC scintigraphy shows static focal activity over left flank that increased over time but did not move (a superficial abdominal wound). No acute bleed was identified in 90 min of study.* **(Right)** *Delayed anterior image at 18 hrs in the same patient shows abdominal wall wound in addition to activity in colon, confirming interval intraluminal bleeding. Delayed interval images are not useful as they do not localize site of origin of bleed.*

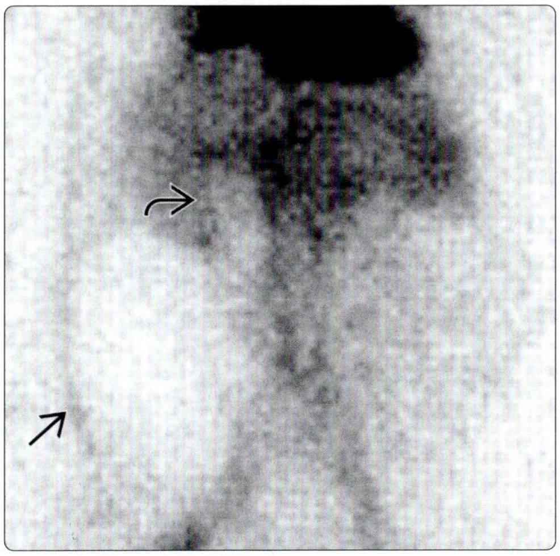

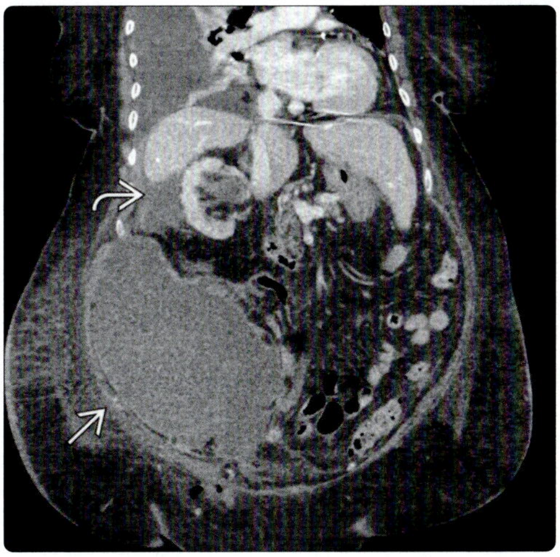

(Left) *Anterior Tc-99m RBC scintigraphy shows hematomas, one in right flank and one retroperitoneal. No acute bleeding was identified.* **(Right)** *Coronal CECT in the same patient shows a perinephric space hematoma and a large hematoma in the right lower quadrant, complications of renal radiofrequency ablation.*

Gastric Emptying

KEY FACTS

TERMINOLOGY

- Solid gastric emptying mostly due to peristaltic pump
  - Solid curve analysis
    - Phase 1 (lag phase): Retained in gastric fundus, transported to antrum where diluted, ground (~ 60 min post ingestion)
    - Phase 2: Antropyloric wave-like contractions dilute, empty into duodenum
- Liquid emptying mostly due to pressure pump
  - Liquid curve analysis
    - Empties directly into duodenum, no lag phase

IMAGING

- Gastric emptying scintigraphy (GES): Adults
  - Normal solid retention
    - 2 hrs: < 60%
    - 4 hrs: 0-10%
  - 4-hr retention: Greatest specificity in diagnosis of delayed gastric emptying
- Normal liquid retention
  - 1 hr: < 50%
- Rapid gastric transit of solids
  - < 70% at 30 min &/or < 30% at 60 min
  - Or < 50% retention at 1 hr

CLINICAL ISSUES

- Gastroparesis
  - Nausea, vomiting, early satiety, bloating, abdominal pain
- Rapid gastric transit (dumping syndrome)
  - Early begins 15-30 min after meal: Nausea, vomiting, bloating, cramping, diarrhea, dizziness, fatigue
  - Late begins 1-3 hrs after meal: Weakness, sweating, dizziness

DIAGNOSTIC CHECKLIST

- Evaluate images for pulmonary aspiration/GERD
- Stomach region of interest should be similar throughout study, exclude duodenal bulb/small bowel

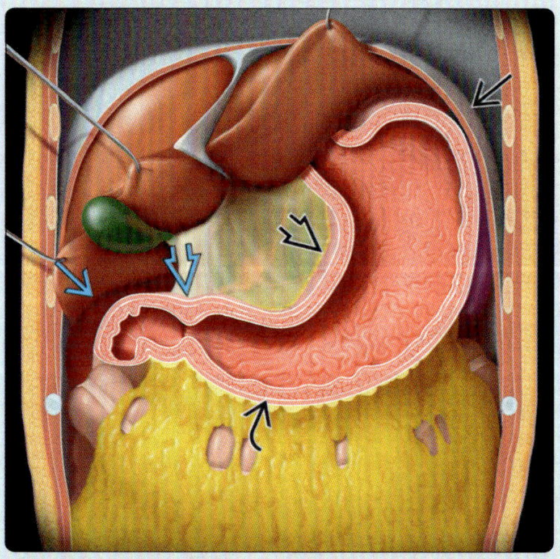

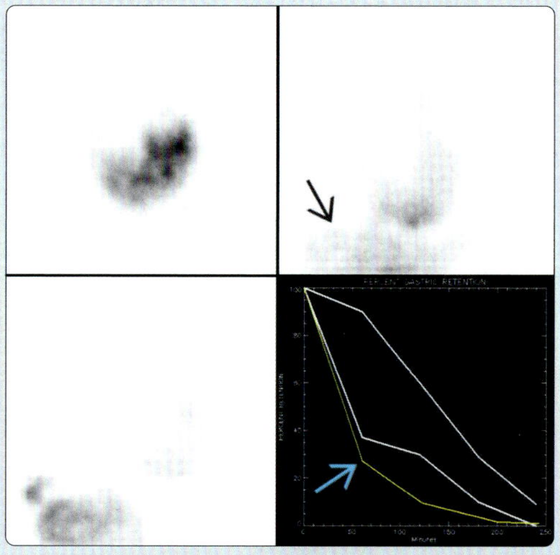

(Left) *Coronal graphic shows gastric anatomy: Gastric fundus, body, antrum, and pylorus. Note duodenal bulb.* **(Right)** *Solid gastric emptying study in a patient with postprandial nausea and flushing shows that > 70% of the meal is in the small bowel at 60 min, suggestive of dumping syndrome.*

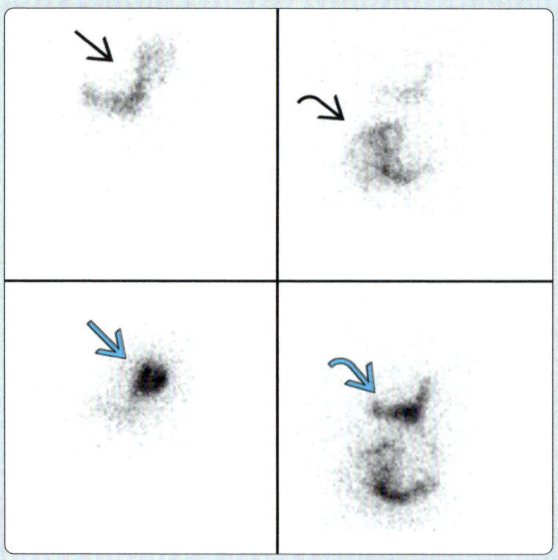

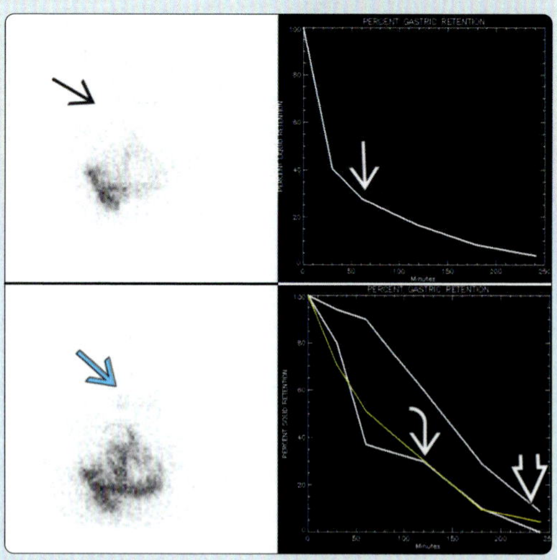

(Left) *Solid-liquid GES using Tc-99m sulfur colloid in an egg sandwich and In-111 in water is shown. The water is diffusely distributed in the stomach at 0 min; the solid meal is in the fundus. At 120 min, water is mostly in the small bowel, and the solid meal is in the gastric antrum and small bowel.* **(Right)** *At 240 min, both liquid and solid are out of the stomach. Normal gastric retention percentages are < 50% at 60 min for liquid and < 30% at 120 min and < 10% at 240 min for solid.*

TERMINOLOGY

Definitions

- **Normal gastric physiology**
  - Normal capacity of stomach varies 0.25-1.7 L
  - Solid emptying mostly due to peristaltic pump
    - Active contractile waves and pyloric opening
    - Solid curve analysis
      - Phase 1 (lag phase): Retained in gastric fundus, transported to antrum where diluted, ground (~ 60 min post ingestion)
      - Phase 2: Antropyloric wave-like contractions dilute, empty into duodenum
  - Liquid emptying mostly due to pressure pump
    - Global tonic stomach contractions and pyloric opening
    - Liquid curve analysis
      - Empties directly into duodenum, no lag phase
      - Depends on differential pressures between stomach and small bowel and pyloric opening (pressure pump)

IMAGING

General Features

- Gastric emptying scintigraphy (GES): Adults
  - Normal solid retention
    - 2 hrs: < 60%
    - 4 hrs: 0-10%
    - 4-hr retention: Greatest specificity in diagnosis of delayed gastric emptying
  - Normal liquid retention
    - 1 hr: < 50%
  - Rapid gastric transit of solids
    - < 70% at 30 min &/or < 30% at 60 min
    - Or < 50% retention at 1 hr
- Gastric emptying scintigraphy: Pediatrics
  - Normal values for infants/children vary in literature
  - GES with Tc-99m sulfur colloid in milk
    - Normal gastric retention at 1 hr
      - Infants: 36-78%; children: 42-56%

Imaging Recommendations

- Best imaging tool
  - Gastric emptying scintigraphy
    - Solid GES
      - Tc-99m sulfur colloid in egg sandwich or chicken livers/beef stew
    - Liquid GES
      - Tc-99m sulfur colloid in formula/milk/water
      - PO or via NG/gastrostomy tube
      - Often used to detect liquid residuals
    - Dual label GES (solid and liquid) combined
      - Tc-99m sulfur colloid in egg sandwich or chicken livers/beef stew + 150 μCi (5.5 MBq) In-111 diethylenetriamine pentaacetic acid (DTPA) in 120 mL of water
      - Studies suggest gastroparesis could be specific for solid &/or liquid, with similar symptoms
      - One study showed normal solid emptying with delayed liquid emptying, most often in nondiabetic
- Protocol advice
  - Patient preparation
    - NPO 4 hrs or past midnight
    - Solids: Patient should finish > 75% of meal
      - 118 mL (4 oz) of liquid egg whites + 2 slices of toasted white bread + 30 g of jelly or jam + 120 mL of water
      - If allergic to egg, use chicken liver/beef stew
    - Menstrual cycle: Can affect gastric emptying; days 1-10 most accurate
    - Tobacco and alcohol: Withhold for ~ 24 hrs
    - Diabetes mellitus: Glucose level should be < 200 mg/dL as hyperglycemia causes stomach not to empty
    - Prokinetic agents: Metoclopromide, tegaserod, domperidone, erythromycin
      - Stop 2 days prior to study unless assessing treatment response
    - Antikinetic agents: Opioids, antispasmodics
      - Stop 2 days prior to study
    - Other drugs that may affect gastric motility (should be stopped for 4 half-lives prior to study)
      - Atropine, nifedipine, progesterone, octreotide, theophylline, benzodiazepine, proton pump inhibitors, phentolamine
  - Radiopharmaceutical
    - 0.5-1 mCi (18-37 MBq)Tc-99m sulfur colloid for solid meal
    - 150 μCi (5.5 MBq) In-111 diethylenetriamine pentaacetic acid (DTPA) in water if solid + liquid study
    - Pediatric doses: No weight-based dose established
      - Tc-99 sulfur colloid for solid or liquid study minimum and maximum administered activity: 0.25 and 1 mCi (37 MBq)
  - Meal preparation
    - Egg sandwich: Mix Tc-99m sulfur colloid into 118 mL (4 oz) of liquid egg white
      - Cook eggs in microwave, stir until omelette consistency
    - Spread 30 g of jam/jelly on toasted bread
    - Serve with 120 mL of water
    - Liquid label: 150 μCi In-111 DTPA in 120 mL water; 0.5 mCi (18.5 MBq) Tc-99m sulfur colloid in milk/formula/water if liquid emptying measured separately
    - Chicken livers
      - Microwave chicken livers 1 min; add to beef stew; microwave another minute
  - Image acquisition
    - Time required to eat meal should be < 10 min; record any uneaten meal
    - Low-energy all-purpose collimator
    - Matrix: 128 x 128
    - Patient standing or sitting upright (same position for entire examination)
    - Anterior and posterior planar images for 60 sec
      - 1 minute after meal consumption and at 60, 120, 180, and 240 min
    - If bedridden patient, obtain left anterior oblique view over stomach at same time points as above
  - Image processing
    - Regions of interest (ROI) drawn around stomach on anterior and posterior images

- ROI should be similar on each frame
- ROI should avoid duodenal bulb, small bowel
- Use geometric mean to determine counts at each time point
  - Geometric mean of 2 numbers: Square root of their product

DIFFERENTIAL DIAGNOSIS

Gastroparesis

- Abnormal gastric retention without anatomic obstruction

Rapid Gastric Transit

- Rapid gastric emptying or dumping syndrome
- Similar symptoms as gastroparesis

Gastric Obstruction

- Abnormal biologic or foreign obstruction (e.g., bezoar)
- Gastric outlet obstruction (GOO)
  - Obstruction at level of pylorus
  - Partial GOO
    - Delayed emptying secondary to narrowing of pylorus, proximal duodenum or gastric antrum
    - Solid emptying typically more delayed than liquid

Large Type 3 or 4 Hiatal Hernia

- Intrathoracic proximal stomach or entire stomach can delay gastric emptying

Gastroesophageal Reflux Disease (GERD)

- Severe GERD can delay emptying, especially if dilated esophagus &/or hiatal hernia

PATHOLOGY

General Features

- Etiology
  - Gastroparesis
    - Incidence: 2.4 per 100,000 person-year (women specifically: 9.8 per 100,000 person-year)
    - Diabetics: 20-40% have gastroparesis
    - Etiology
      - Gastroparesis: Loss of Cajal interstitial cells: GI pacemaker, regulate motility & peristalsis
      - Diabetes mellitus or hyperglycemia > 200 mg/dL
      - Idiopathic
      - Postviral
      - Iatrogenic (medicine, surgery)
      - Neurological disease
      - Autoimmune intestinal dysmotility
      - Others: Paraneoplastic syndrome, mesenteric ischemia, scleroderma
  - Rapid gastric transit (dumping syndrome)
    - Early gastric dumping syndrome
      - Rapid onset, usually within 15-30 min
      - Water shifts from plasma to bowel with hypotension, sympathetic response
    - Late gastric dumping syndrome
      - 2-3 hrs after meal
      - Hyperglycemia → hyperisulinemia response, development of hypoglycemia
    - Etiology
      - 25-50% patients post gastric surgery
      - Nonsurgical causes: Diabetic neuropathy, amyloidosis, idiopathic neuropathy, Zollinger-Ellison, peptic ulcer disease
  - Partial GOO
    - Peptic ulcer disease, neoplasm, superior mesenteric artery syndrome

CLINICAL ISSUES

Presentation

- Most common signs/symptoms
  - Gastroparesis
    - Nausea, vomiting, early satiety, bloating, abdominal pain
  - Rapid gastric transit (dumping syndrome)
    - Patients can have early, late, or both types
    - Early begins 15-30 min after meal
      - Nausea, vomiting, bloating, cramping, diarrhea, dizziness, fatigue
    - Late begins 1-3 hrs after meal
      - Weakness, sweating, dizziness

Treatment

- Delayed gastric emptying
  - Conservative: Low-fat diet, frequent small meals, no undigestible fiber, liquefied, jejunal feeding tube in severe cases
  - Medical: Prokinetic agents (erythromycin, metoclopramide); antiemetic agents (antihistamines, phenothiazines, 5HT3 antagonists)
  - Diabetic gastroparesis: 75% resolved with prokinetics, glycemic control
- Gastric outlet obstruction
  - Pyloroplasty, gastrectomy, gastrojejunal bypass
- Rapid gastric transit (dumping syndrome)
  - Conservative: Dietary changes
  - Medical: Octreotide, precose, cholestyramine, proton pump inhibitors

DIAGNOSTIC CHECKLIST

Consider

- Left anterior oblique images in bedridden patients (less accurate than AP imaging with geometric mean calculation)
- Evaluate images for evidence of pulmonary aspiration/GERD
- Confirm ROI around stomach is similar throughout study, excludes duodenal bulb/small bowel

SELECTED REFERENCES

1. Cooper CJ et al: Rapid or normal gastric emptying as new supportive criteria for diagnosing cyclic vomiting syndrome in adults. Med Sci Monit. 20:1491-5, 2014
2. Shin AS et al: Diagnostic assessment of diabetic gastroparesis. Diabetes. 62(8):2667-73, 2013
3. Sachdeva P et al: Gastric emptying of solids and liquids for evaluation for gastroparesis. Dig Dis Sci. 56(4):1138-46, 2011
4. Ziessman HA et al: The added diagnostic value of liquid gastric emptying compared with solid emptying alone. J Nucl Med. 50(5):726-31, 2009
5. Couturier O et al: Gastric scintigraphy with a liquid-solid radiolabelled meal: performances of solid and liquid parameters. Nucl Med Commun. 25(11):1143-50, 2004

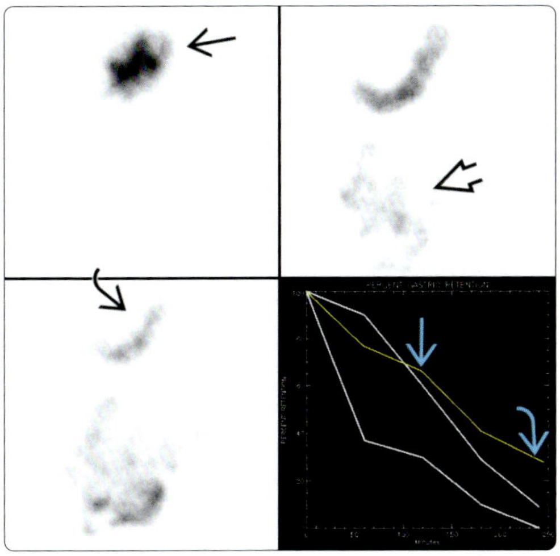

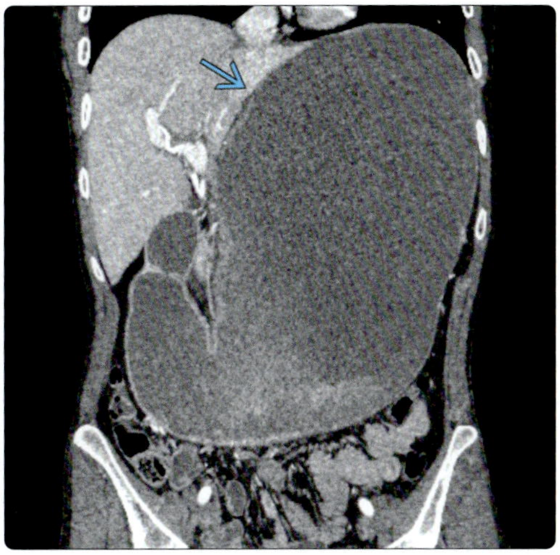

(Left) *Gastric emptying scan shows the meal in the gastric fundus at 0 min. Meal contents are evident in the small bowel at 120 min and the gastric retention is slightly elevated. At 240 min, the meal is evident in the stomach with abnormally high retention.* **(Right)** *This patient with superior mesenteric artery syndrome showed abnormally increased gastric retention times on gastric emptying scan. Coronal CT shows a markedly distended stomach.*

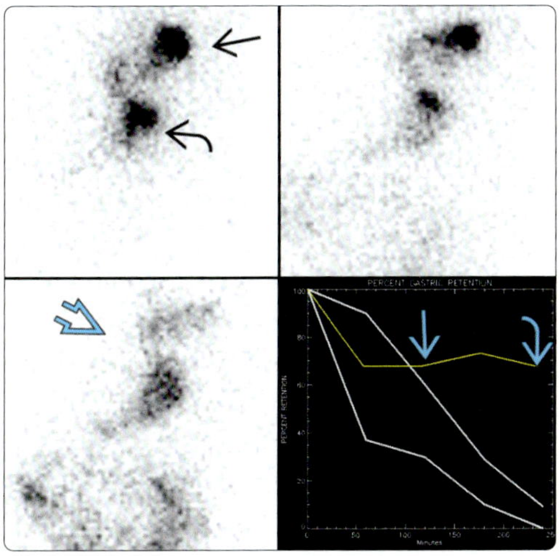

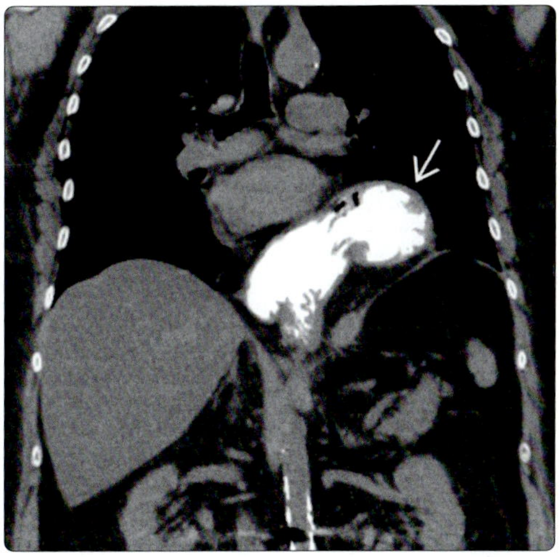

(Left) *Gastric emptying scan in a patient with a large hiatal hernia shows the intrathoracic and intrabdominal portions of the stomach. At 240 min, the meal remains evident in both portions of the stomach. Abnormally high retention at 120 and 240 min is evident.* **(Right)** *Coronal CT in the same patient shows a large sliding type 3 hiatal hernia.*

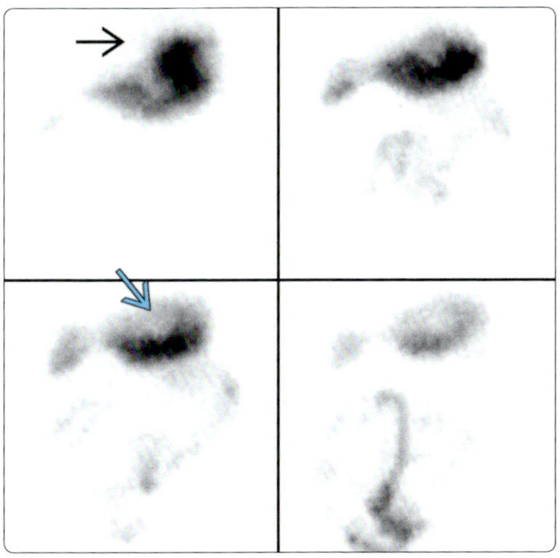

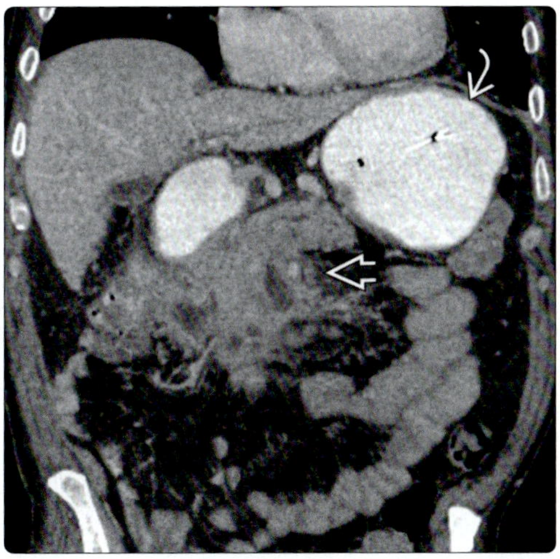

(Left) *Patient with weight loss and vomiting underwent gastric emptying scan, which shows marked retention throughout with a central photopenic defect.* **(Right)** *Coronal CT in the same patient shows a pancreatic mass causing partial outlet obstruction with severe retention of oral contrast in the stomach.*

Abdominal Infection and Inflammatory Disease

KEY FACTS

IMAGING

- Abdominal infection or inflammatory disease
  - Abnormal, focal uptake on 1 of several nuclear medicine studies
  - Uptake in infection and inflammation often greater than liver
  - Abnormal uptake persists or increases over time
- **In-111 WBC and Tc-99m HMPAO WBC scintigraphy**
  - Leukocytes that are labeled ex vivo remain functional, allowing migration to infection/inflammation
- **Gallium-67 scintigraphy**
  - Ga-67: Ferric ion analog that forms complexes with plasma transferrin, bound by intracellular lactoferrin in leucocytes, taken up by bacterial siderophores
- **F-18 FDG PET/CT**
  - Radioactive glucose analog utilized by activated leukocytes, inflammatory processes

DIAGNOSTIC CHECKLIST

- Choose most appropriate nuclear medicine scan given clinical history
  - Tc-99m HMPAO WBC scintigraphy in children to decrease radiation dose
  - Ga-67 scintigraphy
    - Spondylitis or discitis
    - Chronic (> 2 weeks) osteomyelitis/otitis
  - Add SPECT/CT to better localize abnormalities on WBC and Ga-67 scintigraphy
  - F-18 FDG PET/CT offers benefits over traditional nuclear medicine studies
    - No blood products required
    - Study can be completed faster than WBC and Ga-67 scintigraphy
    - Findings can be nonspecific, as with WBC and Ga-67 scintigraphy

(Left) *Anterior and posterior In-111 WBC scan shows normal biodistribution: Highest activity in the spleen →, followed by liver → and bone marrow →. Note the normal faint uptake in the lungs →.* **(Right)** *Anterior Ga-67 scan shows normal biodistribution: Highest activity in the lower large bowel →, followed by liver and spleen →, bone →, and lacrimal glands →. Note the faint renal and bladder uptake →.*

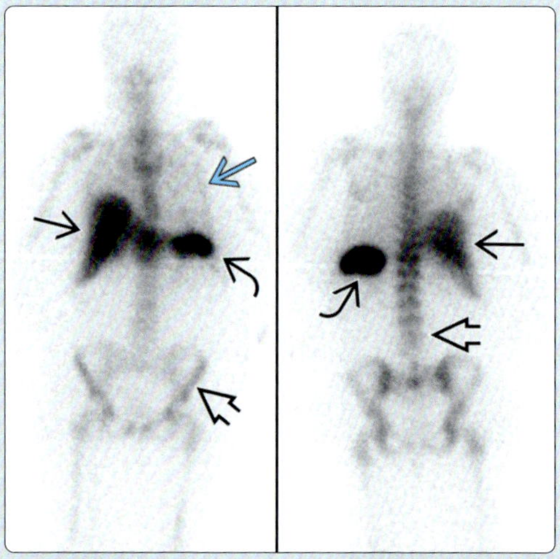

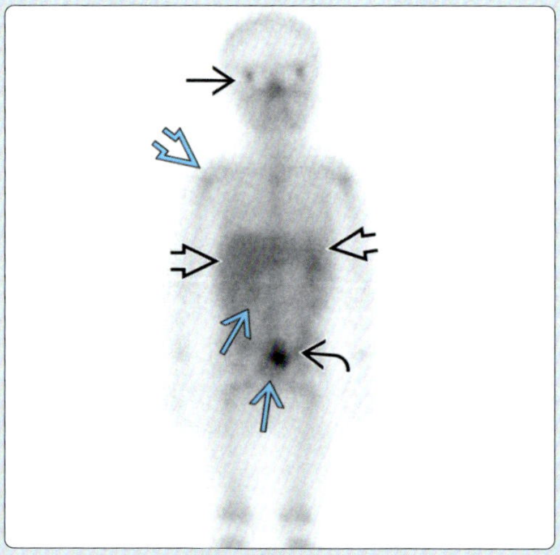

(Left) *Coronal CT shows polycystic kidney disease → in a patient with fever.* **(Right)** *Anterior and posterior In-111 WBC scans in the same patient show heterogeneous focal uptake in the right polycystic kidney →, denoting infected cysts.*

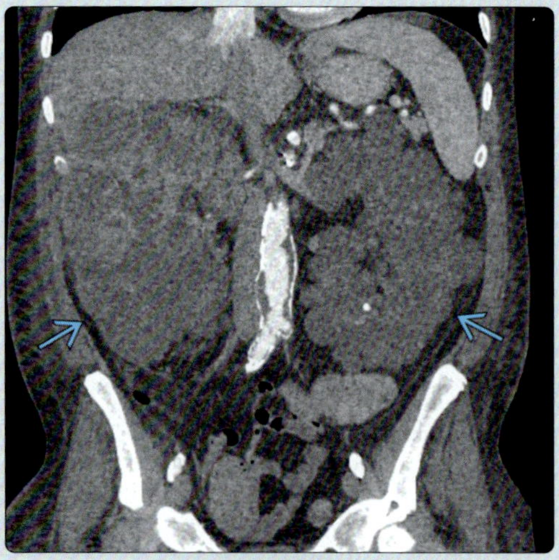

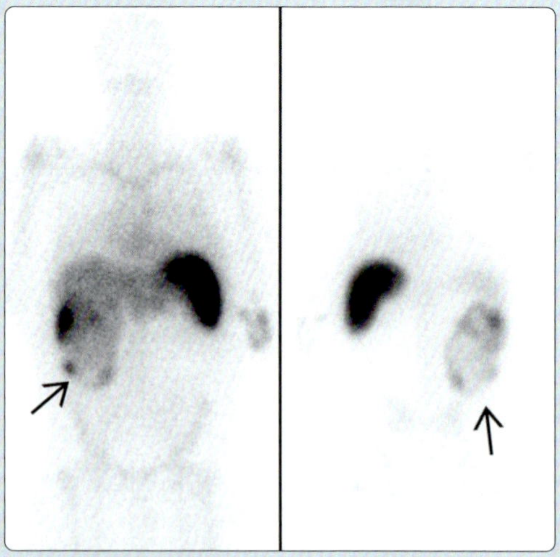

IMAGING

General Features

- Best diagnostic clue
  - Uptake in infection/inflammation often ≥ liver
  - Abnormal uptake persists or increases over time
  - Abnormal, focal uptake on 1 of several nuclear medicine studies

Nuclear Medicine Findings

- **In-111 WBC and Tc-99m HMPAO WBC scintigraphy**
  - Leukocytes that are labeled ex vivo remain functional, allowing migration to infection/inflammation
  - Normal biodistribution of In-111 WBC
    - Spleen > liver > bone marrow
  - Normal biodistribution of Tc-99m HMPAO WBC
    - 1-4 hours: Blood pool, spleen > liver, GI tract, kidneys, and bladder
    - After 4 hours: Bowel activity normal
  - Blood pool
    - Normal: Tc-99m HMPAO WBC shows marked blood pool; In-111 WBC shows faint activity
    - If focal > 24 hrs: Consider vasculitis, recent line placement, or infected graft
  - Lung
    - Diffuse uptake: Normal up to 18 hours
    - Diffuse uptake > 18 hours: Nonspecific, but can be seen in ARSD
    - Focal uptake > 18 hours: Pneumonia/abscess
  - Bowel
    - Faint activity in 1/3 of normal patients
    - Focal activity: Consider infection or inflammatory bowel disease (IBD)
      - IBD: Bowel activity on Tc-99m HMPAO WBC (early uptake, increasing activity at 2 and 4 hours)
    - Moderate/high activity that moves intraluminally over time
      - Epistaxis, pneumonia with cough (tagged WBCs swallowed and move through GI tract)
      - Gastrointestinal bleeding should also be considered
  - Kidneys and bladder
    - Abnormal if evident on In-111 WBC scan
      - Can have normal, low-level uptake in renal transplants
    - Mild/moderate activity on Tc-99m HMPAO WBC can be normal due to free Tc-99m
- **Gallium-67 (Ga-67) scintigraphy**
  - Ga-67: Ferric ion analog that forms complexes with plasma transferrin, bound by intracellular lactoferrin in leucocytes, taken up by bacterial siderophores
  - Normal biodistribution: Skeleton, liver > spleen, large intestine, lacrimal glands, nose
  - Kidney
    - Normal: Faint/diffuse uptake first 48 hours if no renal failure
    - Diffuse uptake > 48 hours: Possible nephritis or renal failure
    - Focal or patchy uptake > 48 hours: Abscess &/or pyelonephritis
- **F-18 FDG PET/CT**
  - Radioactive glucose analog utilized by activated leukocytes, inflammatory processes
  - Normal biodistribution: Brain, heart, liver > spleen, red marrow, bowel, kidneys, ureter, bladder

Imaging Recommendations

- Best imaging tool
  - **In-111 WBC scintigraphy**
    - Fever of unknown origin (FUO): > 38.3 °C for > 3 weeks, without source after 1 week of investigation
    - Cardiovascular infection
    - Abdominal abscess
    - Peritoneal cavity and retroperitoneal infection/abscess
    - Sensitivity decreased with chronic abscess &/or administration of antibiotics > 3 weeks
    - Immunosuppression or prolonged corticosteroids can decrease sensitivity
    - WBC count > 3,000 cells/mL ideal
  - **Tc-99m HMPAO WBC scintigraphy**
    - Pediatric patients, decreased radiation exposure
    - Acute cholecystitis
    - Inflammatory bowel disease
    - Extremity imaging (osteomyelitis)
    - Sensitivity decreased with chronic abscess &/or administration of antibiotics > 3 weeks
    - Immunosuppression or prolonged corticosteroids can decrease sensitivity
    - WBC count > 3,000 cells/mL ideal
  - **Ga-67 scintigraphy**
    - Immunosuppressed &/or neutropenic patient with fever; no minimum WBC count required
    - Spondylitis &/or discitis
    - Sarcoidosis/granulomatous disease, opportunistic/fungal infections
    - Nonsuppurative or lymphocyte-mediated infections
    - Chronic (> 2 weeks) osteomyelitis/otitis
    - FUO
    - Splenic abscess
    - Avoids handling/reinjection of blood products
  - **F-18 FDG PET/CT**
    - FUO
    - Osteomyelitis
    - Vasculitis/endograft infection
    - Splenic abscess
    - Neutropenic/immunocompromised patients (no minimum WBC count required)
    - Avoids handling/reinjection of blood products
- Protocol advice
  - **In-111 WBC and Tc-99m HMPAO WBC scintigraphy**
    - Leukocytes labeled with In-111 oxine or Tc-99m HMPAO
    - Patient preparation
      - WBC count > 3,000 cells/mL ideal
      - Heparin used in preparation; no heparin allergy
    - Radiopharmaceutical
      - **In-111 oxine:** Adult: 0.3-1 mCi (12-37 MBq); pediatric dose: 0.007-0.0135 mCi/kg
      - **Tc-99 m HMPAO:** Adult: 10-20 mCi (370-740 MBq); pediatric dose: 0.05 mCi/kg

- Quality assurance essential: Correct patient identification/handling blood products
- 60 mL syringe with 9 mL of acid-citrate-dextrose anticoagulant solution or heparin
- Add 50 mL of patient's blood to syringe (pediatrics: Minimum volume = 10-15 mL)
- Avoid shaking sample, high centrifugal force separation, temperatures > 70° F, or needles < 20-g to preserve leukocytes
- Labeled leukocytes should be administered within 1-4 hours of labeling
- Flush with normal saline; note that dextrose infusions on existing IVs can cause leukocyte clumping
- Imaging acquisition
  - In-111 WBC scan: 24 hours
    - Anterior and posterior whole-body survey with patient supine and medium-energy collimator; photopeak 173 and 247 KeV
  - Tc-99m HMPAO WBC scan: 1-4 hours
    - Anterior and posterior abdomen/pelvis with patient supine, or extremity images with low-energy all-purpose collimator; photopeak 140 KeV
  - Matrix: 128 x 128
  - SPECT/CT useful for 3D localization
- Dosimetry
  - Spleen receives largest radiation dose
- **Ga-67 scintigraphy**
  - Patient preparation
    - Recent blood transfusion, hemolysis, use of deferoxamine produces saturation of iron-binding transferrin sites and alters Ga-67 biodistribution
    - Administration of paramagnetic contrast agent Gd-DTPA, gadopentate within 24 hours can alter biodistribution (increased bone activity)
    - Laxatives/enemas can decrease bowel activity
  - Radiopharmaceutical: Ga-67
    - Adult: 5-10 mCi (185-370 MBq)
    - Pediatric: 0.04-0.07 mCi/ kg
  - Dosimetry
    - Lower large bowel receives highest radiation dose
- Imaging acquisition
  - Patient supine
  - 24-hour anterior/posterior whole-body scan
    - 48 and 72 hour images useful: Decrease background, evaluate normal bowel vs. abnormality
  - Large field-of-view gamma camera; photopeaks 93, 184 and 296 KeV (393 KeV not acquired)
  - Medium-energy parallel hole collimator
  - Matrix: 128 x 128
  - SPECT/CT useful for 3D localization
- **F-18 FDG PET/CT**
  - Similar protocol to oncologic indications

DIFFERENTIAL DIAGNOSIS

Acute Splenic/Hepatic Infarct &/or Hematoma

- Focal area of activity on WBC scan up to 7 days

Gastrointestinal Bleeding due to Bowel Ischemia or Infarct/Swallowed WBC due to Pneumonia or Epistaxis

- Mimics bowel inflammation on WBC scan

Splenosis/Polysplenia

- Focal upper abdominal uptake on WBC scan; correlate with anatomic images

Lymphoma/Acute Heterotopic Bone/Myositis

- Can be positive on WBC scan

Ostomy Sites/Catheter and Intravenous Lines

- Subtle to moderate uptake on WBC or Ga-67 scan

Renal Transplant

- Noninfected transplant can show faint, diffuse uptake on WBC and Ga-67 scan

Acute/Chronic Renal Failure and Nephritis

- Diffuse uptake on Ga-67 scan

Residual Bowel Activity

- Common on Ga-67 scan; delayed imaging or enema/laxative can decrease false-positives

Thymus

- Increased uptake in young patients on Ga-67 scan (thymic rebound post chemotherapy, or normal)

Tumor Lysis

- Focal uptake on Ga-67 scan due to radiation or chemotherapy

DIAGNOSTIC CHECKLIST

Consider

- Choose most appropriate nuclear medicine scan, given clinical history
- Tc-99m HMPAO WBC scintigraphy in children to decrease radiation dose
- Add SPECT/CT to better localize abnormalities on WBC and Ga-67 scintigraphy
- F-18 FDG PET/CT offers benefits over traditional nuclear medicine studies
  - No blood products required
  - Study can be completed faster than WBC and Ga-67 scintigraphy
  - Findings can be nonspecific, as with WBC and Ga-67 scintigraphy

SELECTED REFERENCES

1. Kouijzer IJ et al: FDG-PET in fever of unknown origin. Semin Nucl Med. 43(5):333-9, 2013
2. Love C et al: Radionuclide imaging of inflammation and infection in the acute care setting. Semin Nucl Med. 43(2):102-13, 2013
3. Auler MA et al: The role of nuclear medicine in imaging infection. Semin Roentgenol. 42(2):117-21, 2007
4. Love C et al: FDG PET of infection and inflammation. Radiographics. 25(5):1357-68, 2005
5. Charron M et al: Are 99mTc leukocyte scintigraphy and SBFT studies useful in children suspected of having inflammatory bowel disease? Am J Gastroenterol. 95(5):1208-12, 2000

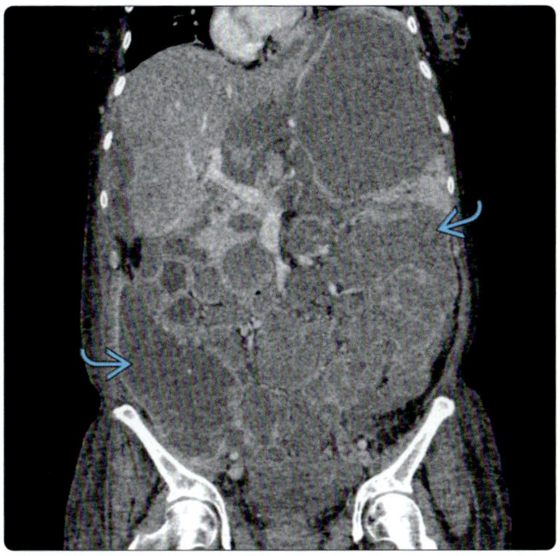

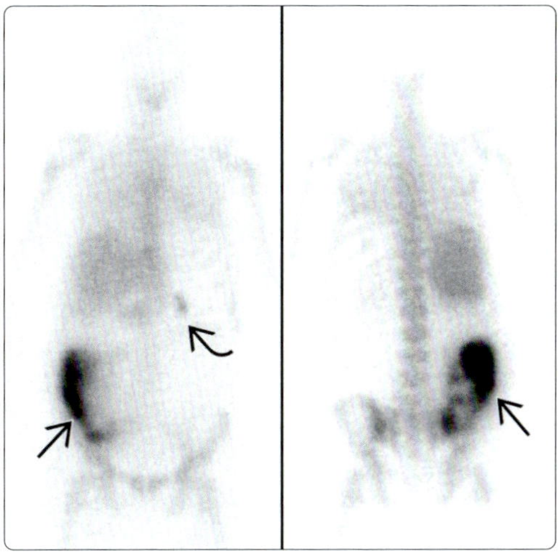

(Left) *Coronal enhanced CT scan shows fluid collections* ➔ *in a febrile patient with mucinous peritoneal carcinomatosis. The diagnosis of abscess by CT is challenging.* **(Right)** *Anterior and posterior In-111 WBC scans in the same patient show 2 infections: One in the mid abdomen* ➔ *and another in the right lower quadrant* ➔*. Note that the spleen is absent because the patient had a prior splenectomy.*

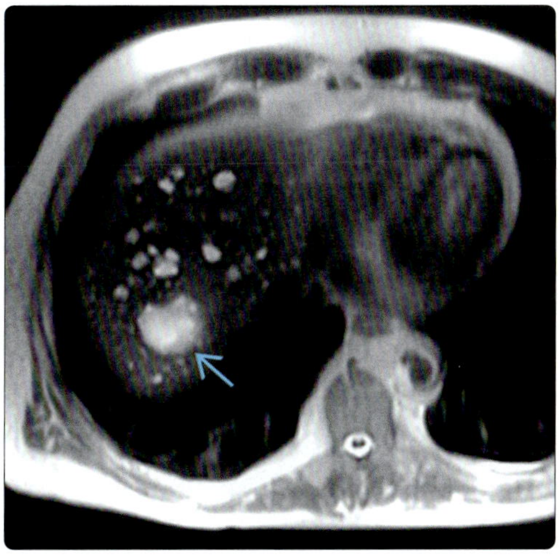

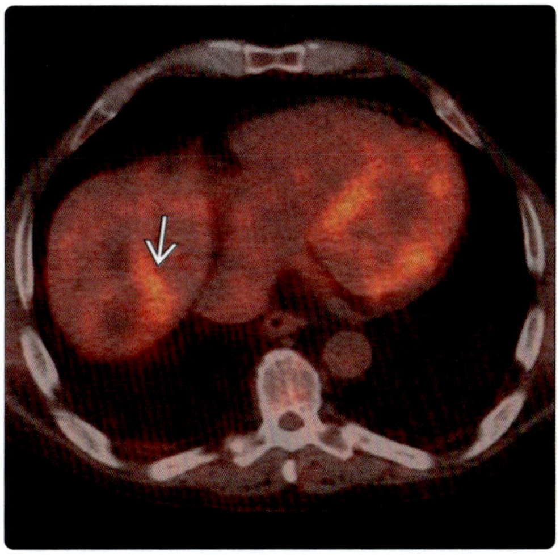

(Left) *Axial T2 MR shows an immunocompromised patient with fever, polycystic liver and kidney disease* ➔*. MR is inconclusive for infection.* **(Right)** *Axial fused F-18 FDG PET/CT in the same patient shows focal hepatic dome uptake* ➔ *consistent with liver abscess.*

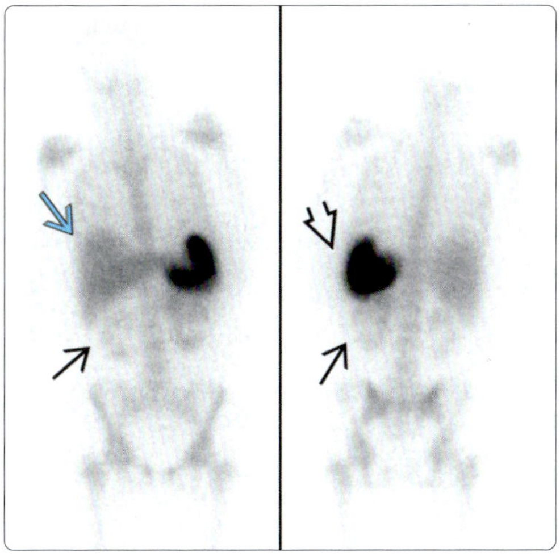

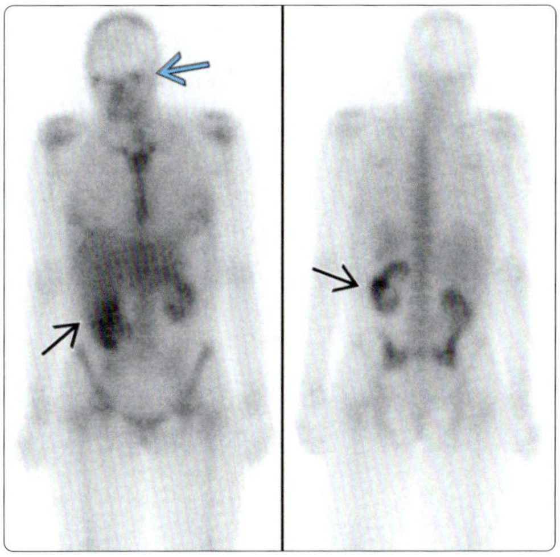

(Left) *Anterior and posterior In-111 WBC scans show bilateral renal patchy uptake, diagnostic of bilateral pyelonephritis* ➔*. Note normal spleen* ➔ *and liver* ➔ *uptake.* **(Right)** *Anterior and posterior Ga-67 scans show bilateral renal uptake at 48 hours in this patient with acute renal failure due to interstitial nephritis* ➔*. Note the normal lacrimal gland uptake* ➔*.*

(Left) *Anterior and posterior In-111 WBC scans show focal uptake in the posterior right hepatic lobe →, consistent with hepatic abscess.* **(Right)** *Anterior In-111 WBC scan shows diffuse uptake in the abdomen →. Bacterial peritonitis was evident on paracentesis.*

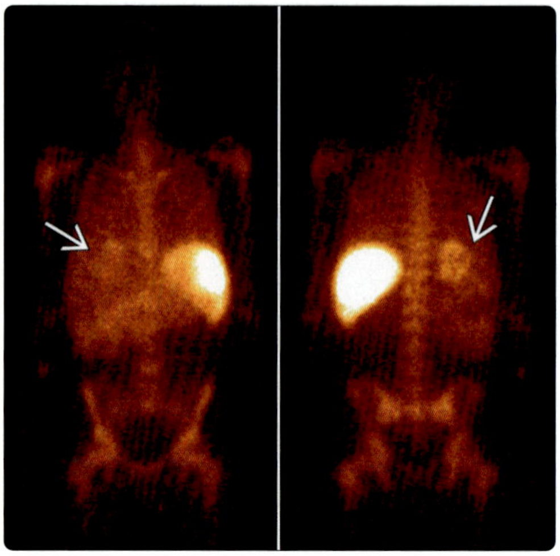

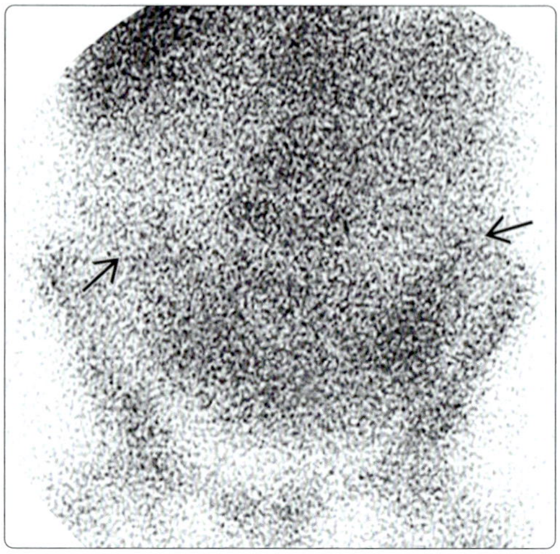

(Left) *Anterior In-111 WBC scan shows uptake in the right colon in this patient with colitis →. Right lateral image shows linear uptake → in laparotomy incision. Focal uptake in the left upper quadrant → represents residual spleen post splenectomy.* **(Right)** *Posterior Ga-67 scan shows focal uptake in the right hemiabdomen →, representing a psoas muscle abscess evident on follow-up CT.*

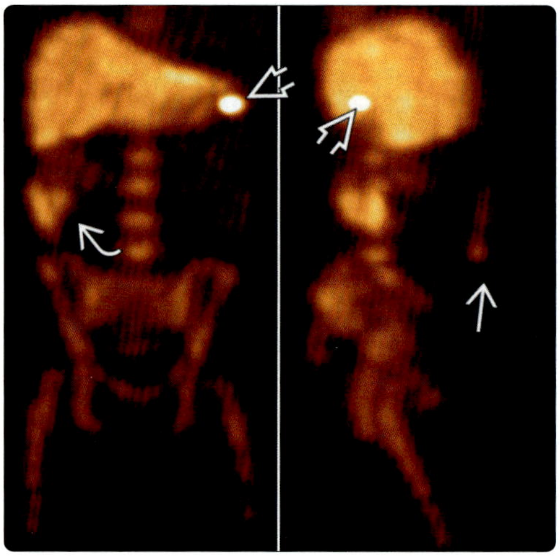

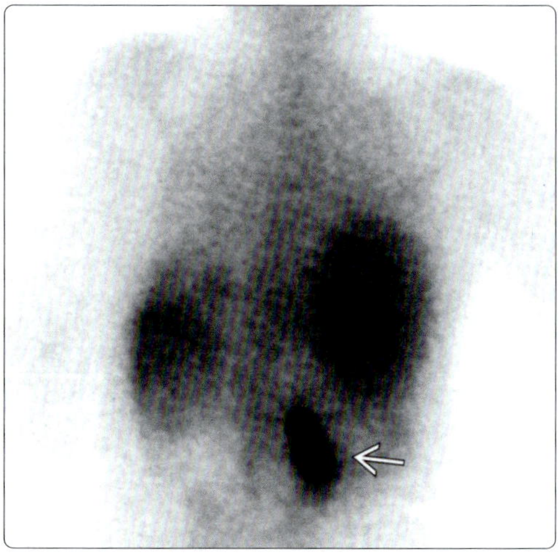

(Left) *Anterior Tc-99m HMPAO WBC scan in a patient with Crohn disease shows right lower quadrant uptake →, suspicious for disease flare. Note normal radiotracer excretion in the bladder → and faint blood pool activity →.* **(Right)** *Axial CT in the same patient shows acute sigmoiditis → with associated stricture and dilated proximal bowel →.*

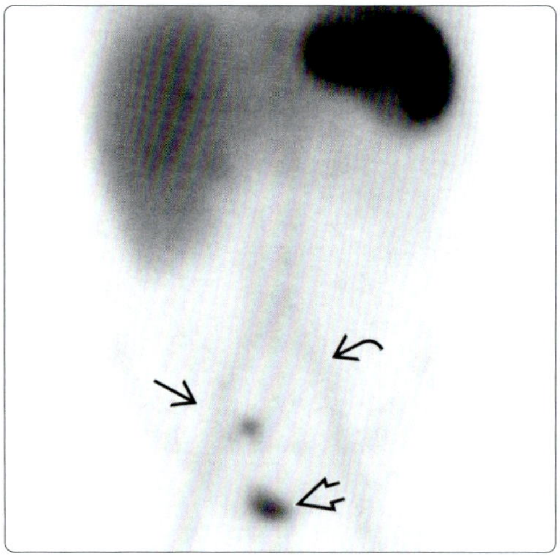

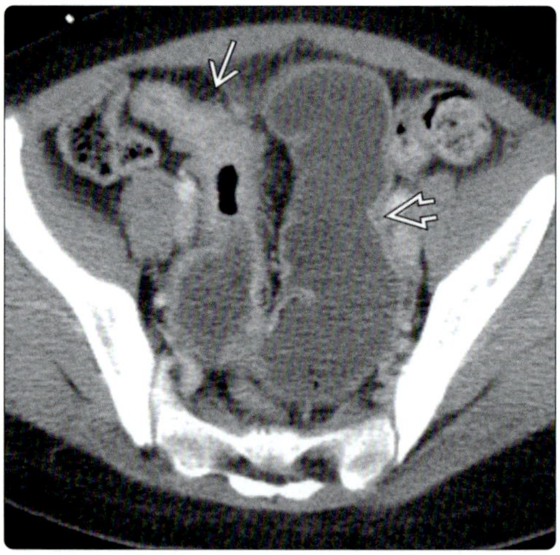

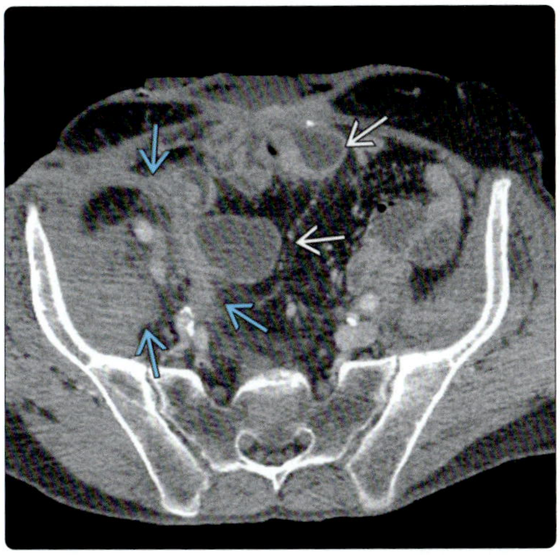

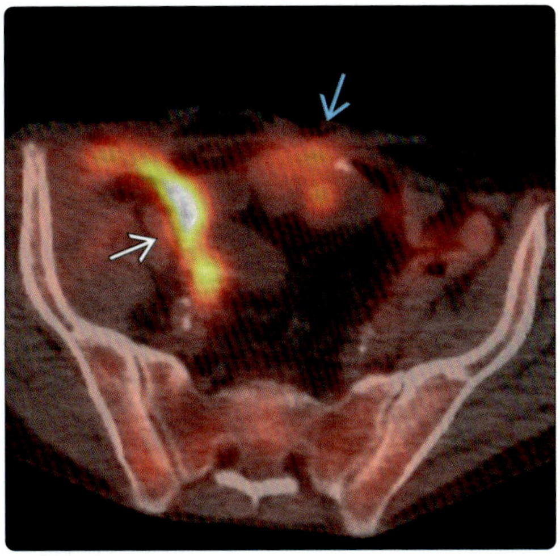

(Left) *Axial CT in an immunocompromised patient with fever of unknown origin shows fluid-filled loops of small bowel secondary to adhesions and areas of soft tissue stranding in the right pelvic side wall.* **(Right)** *Axial F-18 FDG PET/CT in the same patient was positive for right pelvic side wall uptake, consistent with infection. Note the normal small bowel uptake.*

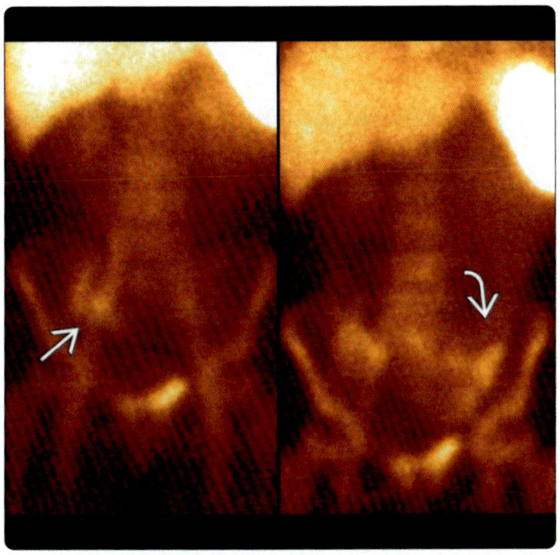

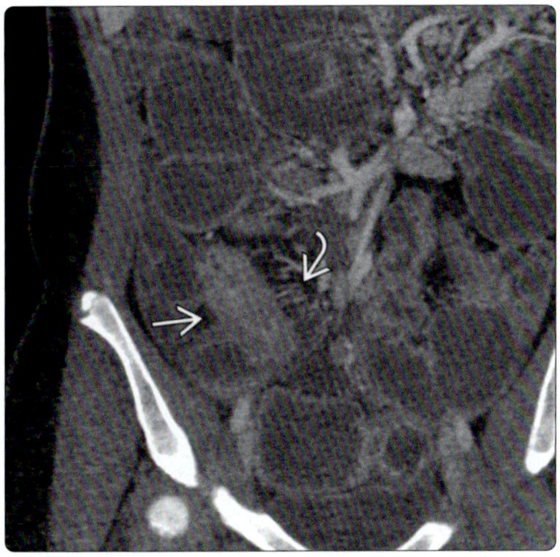

(Left) *Anterior Tc-99m HMPAO WBC scan in a patient with Crohn disease shows focal activity in the terminal ilium at 30 minutes, followed by a new area of uptake in the sigmoid colon at 2 hours.* **(Right)** *Coronal CT enterography in the same patient shows mural thickening and enhancement of the terminal ileum with fibrofatty proliferation and perivascular inflammatory changes of the mesentery (the comb sign), suggestive of flare. Mild thickening of the sigmoid colon was also evident (not seen in this image).*

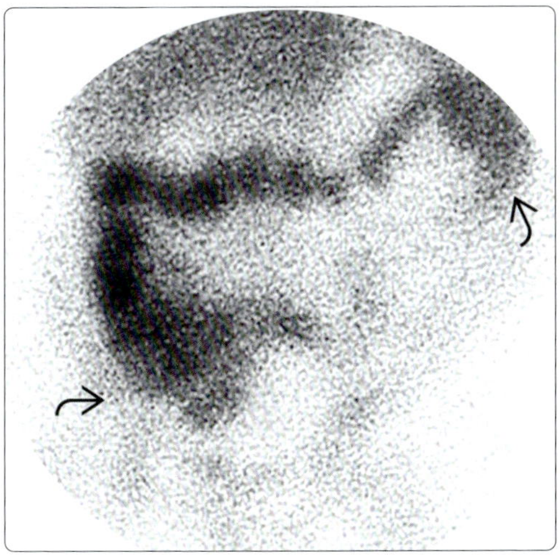

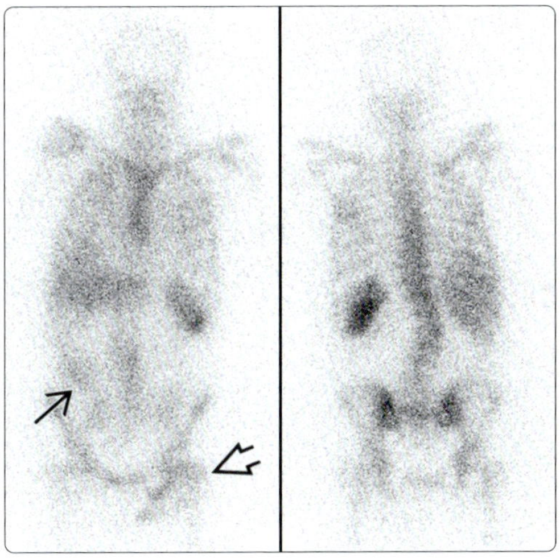

(Left) *Anterior In-111 WBC scan shows uptake in the colon that moved intraluminally over time, denoting an incidental active GI bleed.* **(Right)** *Anterior In-111 WBC scan in patient with low white blood count shows low-level activity throughout the normal biodistribution. Faint uptake was present in a postsurgical abscess and a left thigh hematoma. Low-level activity can also occur if the In-111 does not tag properly to the WBCs.*

Spleen Localization

KEY FACTS

IMAGING

- Tc-99m pertechnetate denatured RBC scan
  - Spleen culls heat-damaged RBCs from circulation
    - Insufficient RBC damage: Blood pool activity, little spleen accumulation
    - Excessive RBC damage: Hepatic uptake > splenic uptake
  - Spleen: Increased radiotracer uptake over time
  - Liver: Stable or decreased radiotracer uptake over time
  - SPECT or SPECT/CT often useful, especially with hepatic variants, small or multiple lesions
  - Must follow appropriate precautions for drawing and reinjecting blood products
- Tc-99m sulfur colloid liver-spleen scan
  - Similar activity in liver and spleen may be difficult to distinguish
  - Can compare with hepatobiliary scintigraphy to determine hepatic contours

TOP DIFFERENTIAL DIAGNOSES

- Splenectomy
  - Postsurgical absence of spleen
  - Splenules may be present
- Accessory spleen
  - Congenital focus of splenic tissue in addition to normal spleen
- Splenosis
  - Multiple foci of splenic tissue, often post-traumatic
- Wandering spleen
  - Abnormal peritoneal attachments unable to keep spleen in normal position
- Heterotaxy syndrome
  - Asplenia (53%)
  - Polysplenia (42%)
  - Single right-sided spleen (5%)
  - Normal left-sided spleen (rare)

(Left) *Axial CT shows a small nodule in the left subphrenic space ➡ in this patient post distal pancreatectomy and splenectomy due to pancreatic tumor, findings concerning for tumor recurrence.* **(Right)** *Axial fused Tc-99m pertechnetate SPECT denatured RBC scan in the same patient shows uptake in the nodule ➡, consistent with splenule.*

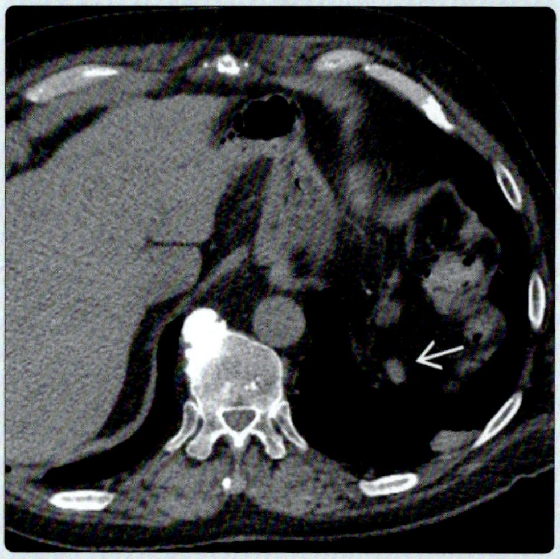

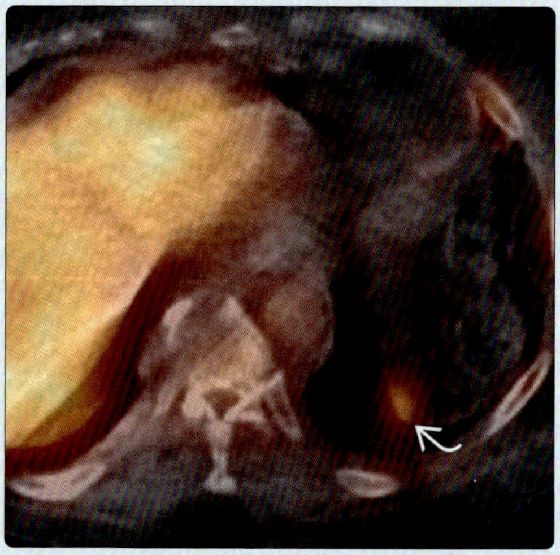

(Left) *Axial T2-weighted MR shows a solid mass in the pancreatic tail ➡ with similar intensity to splenic parenchyma ⇨.* **(Right)** *Axial Tc-99m sulfur colloid SPECT in the same patient shows marked uptake in the pancreatic mass ➡, consistent with intrapancreatic splenule.*

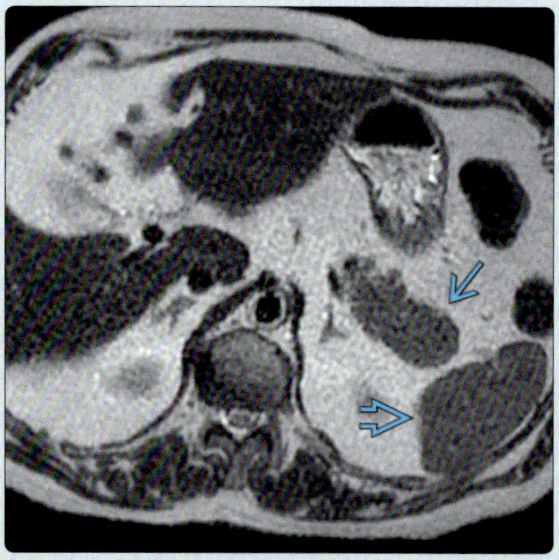

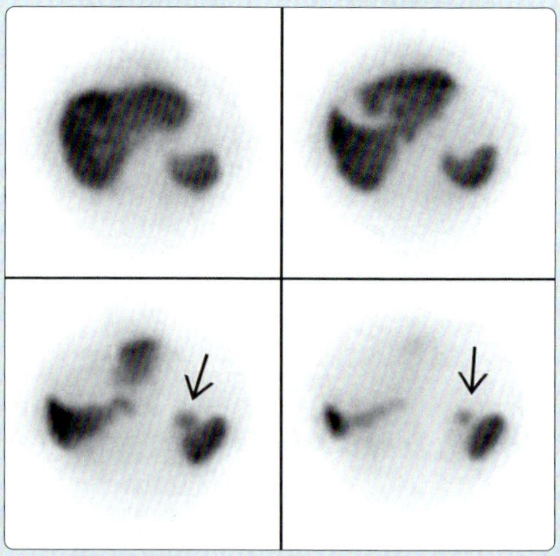

IMAGING

Nuclear Medicine Findings

- Tc-99m pertechnetate denatured RBC scan
  - Activity in splenic tissue increases over time due to accumulation of heat-damaged RBCs
    - Activity in liver is stable or decreases over time

Imaging Recommendations

- Tc-99m pertechnetate denatured RBC scan
  - Patient preparation
    - None
  - Radiopharmaceutical
    - Follow appropriate precautions for drawing and reinjecting blood products
    - Adult: Label 3 cc patient's blood with 15-30 mCi (555-1110 MBq) Tc-99m pertechnetate
    - Children: Label 3cc patient's blood with 0.2-0.4 mCi/kg (7-15 MBq/kg) Tc-99m pertechnetate
    - Heat-damage Tc-99m pertechnetate-labeled RBCs in water bath for 15 min at 49-50°C
    - Insufficient RBC damage: Blood pool activity, little spleen accumulation
    - Excessive RBC damage: Hepatic uptake > splenic uptake
    - After cooling to room temperature, administer heat-damaged autologous RBCs to patient IV
  - Dosimetry
    - Spleen receives largest dose
  - Image acquisition
    - Low-energy all-purpose parallel hole collimator
    - Posterior planar images for 3-5 min each at 15, 30, and 45 min after injection
    - SPECT or SPECT/CT
      - Used to define organ contours, especially with hepatic variants
      - Used for lesions less than 2-3 cm or multiple lesions
- Additional nuclear medicine imaging options
  - Tc-99m sulfur colloid liver-spleen scan
    - Similar activity in liver and spleen
    - May be compared to hepatobiliary scintigraphy, which defines hepatic contours
  - Hepatobiliary scintigraphy
    - Tc-99m HIDA scan defines hepatic contours
    - Early planar or SPECT images
    - Correlate with denatured RBC scan or Tc-99m sulfur colloid liver-spleen scan

DIFFERENTIAL DIAGNOSIS

Splenectomy

- Postsurgical absence of spleen
- Splenules may be present

Accessory Spleen

- Congenital focus of splenic tissue in addition to normal spleen, functions normally
- Most frequently just outside hilum of normal spleen, may be intrapancreatic

Splenosis

- Multiple foci of splenic tissue, often post-traumatic

Wandering Spleen

- Normal spleen, abnormal peritoneal attachments unable to keep spleen in normal position

Heterotaxy Syndrome

- Embryological mishap of aberrant lateralization of visceral organs and vena cavae, including splenic abnormalities
  - If present, spleen should be on same side as stomach due to mesenteric anatomy (correlate with gastric bubble on CXR)
- Splenic anomalies associated with heterotaxy
  - Asplenia (53%)
  - Polysplenia (42%)
  - Single right-sided spleen (5%)
  - Normal left-sided spleen (rare)

CLINICAL ISSUES

Presentation

- Most common signs/symptoms
  - Ectopic splenic tissue
    - Accessory spleen
      - Often incidental finding on anatomic imaging, may be confused with tumor
    - Ectopic splenic tissue
      - In patients post splenectomy for idiopathic thrombocytopenic purpura, may cause recurrent anemia, thrombocytopenia
      - Splenosis can occur in trauma patients
  - Asplenia
    - Immunologic and hematologic abnormalities
    - Up to 80% mortality in 1st year of life
  - Polysplenia
    - Functional asplenia with immunologic/hematologic abnormalities
    - Up to 60% mortality in 1st year of life

Treatment

- Asplenia or functional asplenia
  - Antibiotics against encapsulated organisms
- Idiopathic thrombocytopenic purpura
  - If medical management fails, splenectomy
  - Post splenectomy with recurrent thrombocytopenia: Excision of remaining splenic tissue

DIAGNOSTIC CHECKLIST

Image Interpretation Pearls

- Tc-99m pertechnetate denatured RBC scan
  - Splenic activity increases over time
  - Liver activity stable or decreases over time
  - SPECT/CT often useful, especially for characterization of small or multiple lesions or with hepatic variants
- Tc-99m sulfur colloid liver-spleen scan
  - Use SPECT/CT to distinguish spleen and liver as uptake similar in both

SELECTED REFERENCES

1. Applegate KE et al: Situs revisited: imaging of the heterotaxy syndrome. Radiographics. 19(4):837-52; discussion 853-4, 1999
2. Freeman JL et al: CT of congenital and acquired abnormalities of the spleen. Radiographics. 13(3):597-610, 1993

SECTION 4

Lymphatic and Vascular

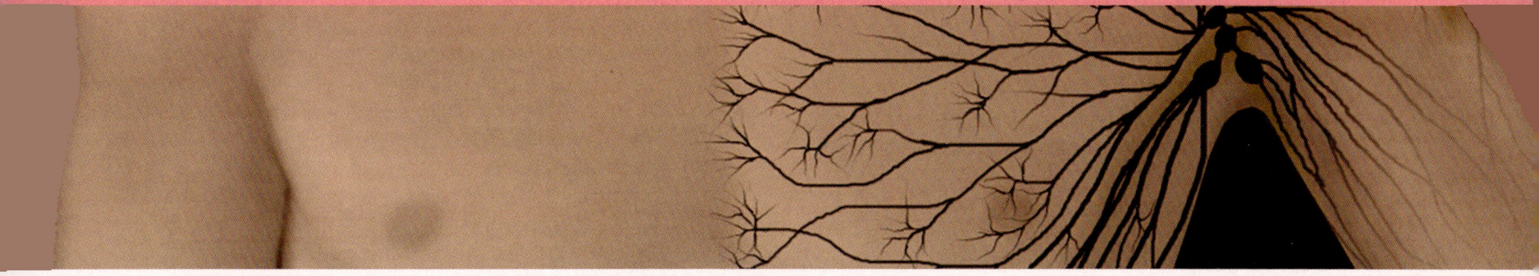

Introduction

Lymphatic

Vascular

Introduction

Nuclear vascular imaging has limited applications for monitoring disease activity in large vessel vasculitis and diagnosing vascular graft infections. These indications can be evaluated efficiently using F-18 FDG PET/CT, replacing the more cumbersome labeled WBC scan when appropriate. Sentinel lymph node mapping and lymphoscintigraphy direct the surgical approach for state-of-the-art staging in breast and skin cancers. In patients with lower extremity edema, lymphoscintigraphy provides a nuclear lymphangiogram with a streamlined procedure and imaging protocol.

Vascular Imaging

Large Vessel Vasculitis

F-18 FDG PET/CT can provide an assessment of disease activity in patients with large vessel vasculitis, an autoimmune-mediated inflammatory process. Homogeneously increased activity in the walls of large arteries indicates active disease, which decreases with effective treatment. This is especially useful when balancing the risks of potential untreated vasculitis (occlusion, rupture, hemorrhage) versus the side effects of immune-modulating drugs.

Vascular Graft Infection

Focal, heterogeneous, or asymmetrically increased graft uptake on F-18 FDG PET/CT or labeled WBC scan suggests vascular graft infection. Homogeneous, low-level uptake is a normal postoperative finding. In the inpatient setting, F-18 FDG PET/CT is a cost-effective, efficient indication for localization of infection. Compared with In-111 WBC scintigraphy, F-18 FDG PET/CT can be completed within 2 hours versus 24 hours, it has better resolution, does not require the reinjection of blood products, and is interpreted in a fashion similar to In-111 WBC scan. Tc-99m HMPAO WBC scans can also be performed with imaging 1-3 hours after injection of labeled WBCs, with better imaging characteristics compared to In-111 labeled WBCs.

Lymphatic Imaging

Sentinel Lymph Node Mapping

Sentinel lymph node mapping and biopsy provides valuable prognostic information, directs oncologic surgical and medical therapy, and decreases the morbidity associated with radical lymphadenectomy. Theoretically, a sentinel lymph node is the first to receive lymphatic drainage from a site of cancer. In practice, multiple lymph nodes within a lymph node basin as well as multiple lymph node basins can drain a single tumor site. Surgeons often remove 3-5 sentinel lymph nodes for a single tumor. As this procedure directs surgical management, a time-out procedure to confirm correct procedure, correct site &/or side of tumor (with marking of the injection site on the patient), and correct radiopharmaceutical is prudent. Although unusual, surgical cancellations have been caused by incorrect site injections due to unclear orders, patient &/or physician misidentification of the primary tumor site, miscommunication, as well as radiopharmaceutical mishaps (e.g., wrong radiotracer, inadequate tagging).

Due to the high rate of upper extremity lymphedema after axillary lymphadenectomy, the sentinel lymph node mapping procedure has become standard of care for patients with breast cancer to decrease morbidity. Clinical research shows that sentinel lymph node biopsy is > 90% accurate for regional nodal staging when compared with complete lymphadenectomy. As lymphatic drainage of the breast occurs in the ipsilateral axilla, intraoperative gamma probe detection of sentinel lymph nodes obviates the need for imaging.

Patients with primary melanoma at risk of regional lymph node metastases also undergo sentinel lymph node mapping. Sentinel lymph node mapping of skin cancer is more complicated than that of breast cancer. For example, a left arm melanoma may show sentinel lymph nodes in the epitrochlear and axillary nodal basins. A melanoma on the trunk can drain to either axillary or groin basins, in addition to subcutaneous in-transit lymph nodes. Particularly with truncal and head and neck cancers, unexpected drainage basins commonly appear on scintigraphy. Thus, this procedure requires comprehensive imaging of all potential lymph node basins as well as complete characterization of lymph nodes in multiple imaging planes prior to marking the sentinel lymph node preoperatively.

As the radiotracer is suspended in acidic solution, subcutaneous or intradermal injections can be painful. Subcutaneous lidocaine can be used prior to radiotracer injection of the breast. Intradermal lesions are more difficult to anesthetize and are often performed without local anesthesia. However, for example, in the case of midline vulvar tumors that require sentinel lymph node mapping, full sedation administered by certified physician/nursing staff or an anesthesiologist is required to alleviate the significant pain associated with radiotracer injection in this area. Similar thoughtful preparation is required on a case-by-case basis for tumors in other sensitive regions.

Lymphedema Evaluation

Lymphedema is caused by congenital or acquired lymphatic obstruction. Congenital absence or a decreased number of lymphatic channels occurs in familial and sporadic forms, and can be associated with genetic syndromes like Turner syndrome. Secondary lymphedema occurs due to tumor compression, lymphadenectomy, radiation therapy, and infections such as filariasis.

In patients with slowly progressive lower extremity edema, the differential diagnosis includes chronic venous insufficiency, generalized edematous states (e.g., heart or renal failure), and deep venous thrombosis. Tc-99m sulfur colloid lymphoscintigraphy can identify signs of lymphatic obstruction, such as dermal backflow, collateral or dilated lymphatic channels, or absent or asymmetric visualization of lymph nodes and lymphatic trunks.

This nuclear medicine study replaced lymphangiography, which was performed with contrast administration into the web spaces between fingers or toes, requiring 4 needle sticks per extremity. With lymphoscintigraphy, the radiotracer is injected subcutaneously in the distal dorsum of the hands or feet with only 1 injection per extremity. Although anesthetic cream or spray helps alleviate pain associated with the needle stick, the radiotracer is suspended in an acidic solution that causes pain in the subcutaneous tissues that topical anesthetics cannot reach. Reassuring the patient through the 1-2 minutes of discomfort is often sufficient; however, subcutaneous lidocaine can also be used.

Selected References

1. Duce V et al: Sentinel Node Mapping in Melanoma of the Back: SPECT/CT Helps Discriminate "True" and "False" in-Transit Lymph Nodes. Clin Nucl Med. ePub, 2015
2. Moncayo VM et al: Lymphoscintigraphy and Sentinel Nodes. J Nucl Med. 56(6):901-907, 2015

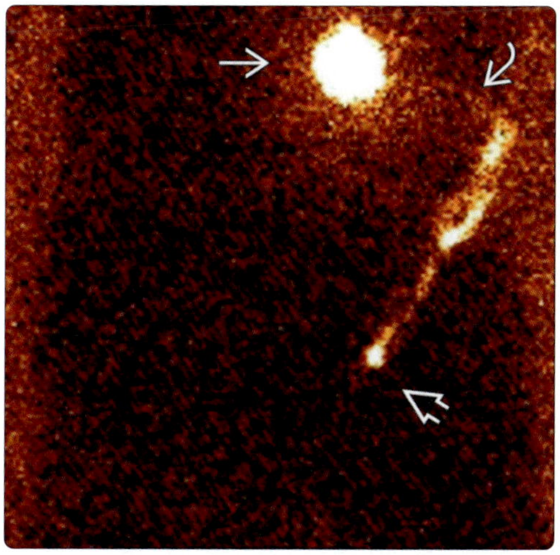

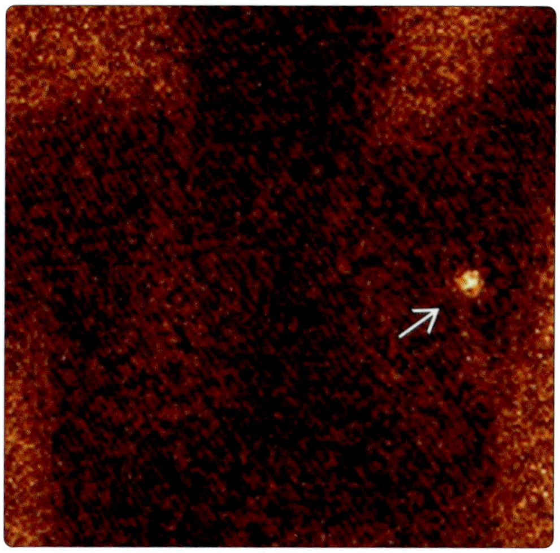

(Left) *Anterior Tc-99m filtered sulfur colloid lymphoscintigraphy in a patient with melanoma shows the peritumoral injection site on the left back* ➡, *the lymphatic channel* ➡ *within the flank, and a left groin sentinel lymph node* ➡. **(Right)** *Anterior lymphoscintigraphy in the same patient shows an axillary sentinel lymph node* ➡ *as well. Both sentinel lymph nodes were excised at surgery.*

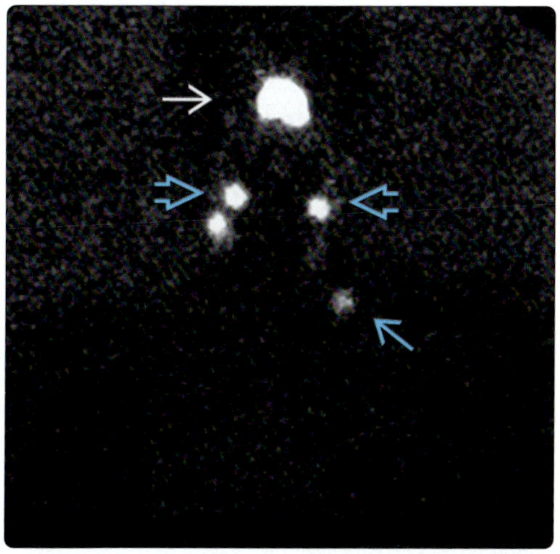

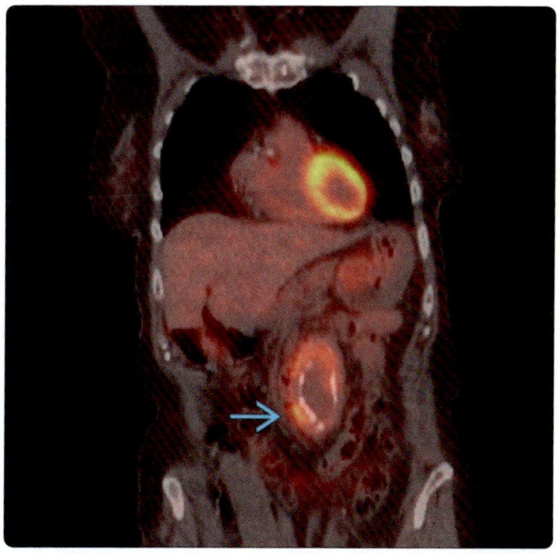

(Left) *Anterior lymphoscintigraphy in a patient with melanoma on the back of the head* ➡ *shows bilateral cervical sentinel lymph nodes* ➡ *as well as a left supraclavicular sentinel lymph node* ➡*. These were all excised at surgery.* **(Right)** *Coronal fused F-18 FDG PET/CT in a patient with fever and abdominal aortic aneurysm shows heterogeneously increased activity in the rind encompassing the aneurysm* ➡*, consistent with infection.*

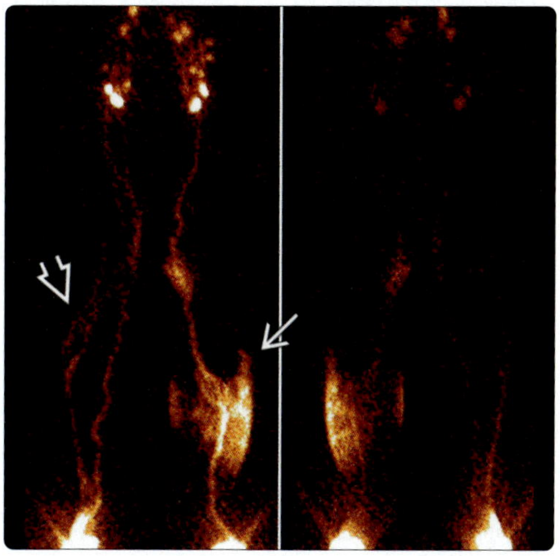

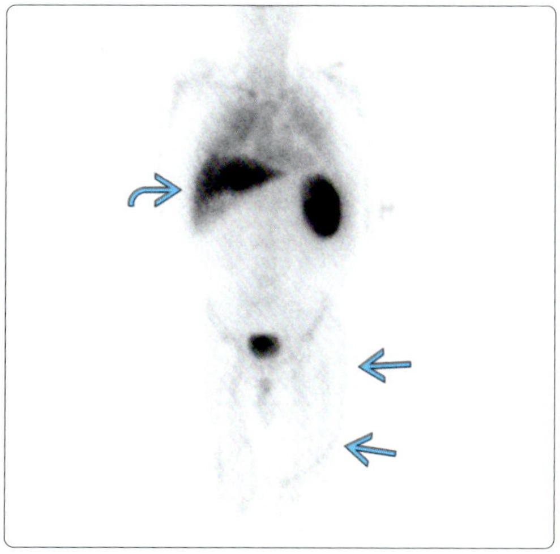

(Left) *Anterior (left) and posterior (right) lymphoscintigraphy in a patient with bilateral lower extremity edema shows dermal backflow* ➡ *of radiotracer into superficial lymphatics and lymphatic collateralization* ➡. **(Right)** *Anterior In-111 WBC scan in a patient with a left femoral artery bypass graft shows diffuse, low-level activity* ➡ *that is less than liver* ➡*, a common finding in noninfected grafts.*

KEY FACTS

IMAGING

- Tc-99m sulfur colloid lymphoscintigraphy
  - Standard diagnostic study of choice to guide differential diagnosis of extremity edema

TOP DIFFERENTIAL DIAGNOSES

- Primary lymphedema
  - Congenital or genetic causes resulting in pathologic development of lymphatic vessels
- Secondary lymphedema
  - Typically secondary to malignant conditions &/or treatments in developed world (most commonly breast cancer)
  - Filariasis is most common cause worldwide (nematode *Wucheria bancrofti*)
- Nonlymphatic causes of extremity edema
  - Chronic venous insufficiency
  - Generalized edematous state
  - Cellulitis (unilateral or bilateral)
  - Deep venous thrombosis

DIAGNOSTIC CHECKLIST

- Normal lymphatic drainage
  - Symmetric, bilateral lymphatic uptake of radiotracer
  - May not visualize radiotracer in normal lymphatic channels
  - Absence of signs present in lymphedema
- Lymphedema
  - Delayed uptake of radiotracer in extremity of interest despite exercise
  - Dermal backflow (stocking sign) in extremity
  - Presence of collateral &/or dilated lymphatic channels
  - Interruption of lymphatic channels
  - Absent or asymmetric visualization of lymph nodes, lymphatic trunks

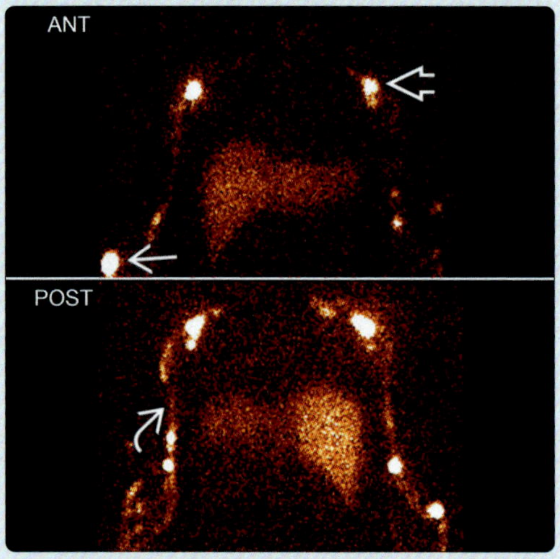

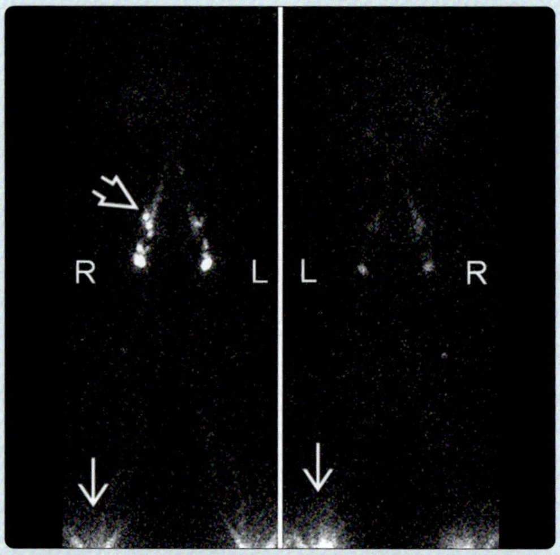

(Left) *Normal distribution of bilateral upper extremity Tc-99m sulfur colloid lymphoscintigraphy is shown. Note the site of injection ➔, axillary nodes ➔, and lymphatic channels within the upper arm ➔.* **(Right)** *Normal Tc-99m sulfur colloid lymphoscintigraphy of the bilateral lower extremities is shown. Note the injection sites ➔ and inguinal nodal chains ➔.*

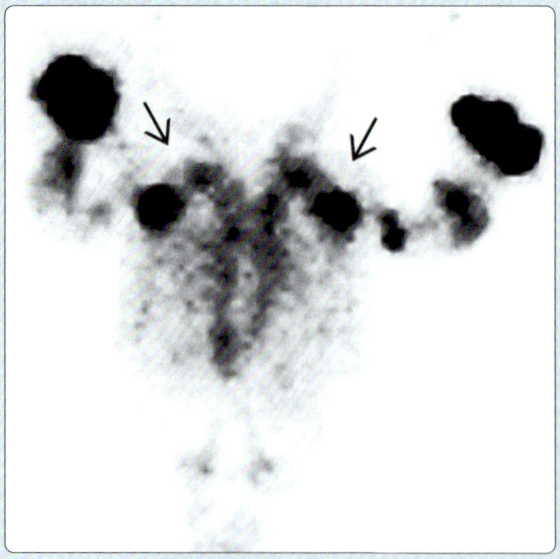

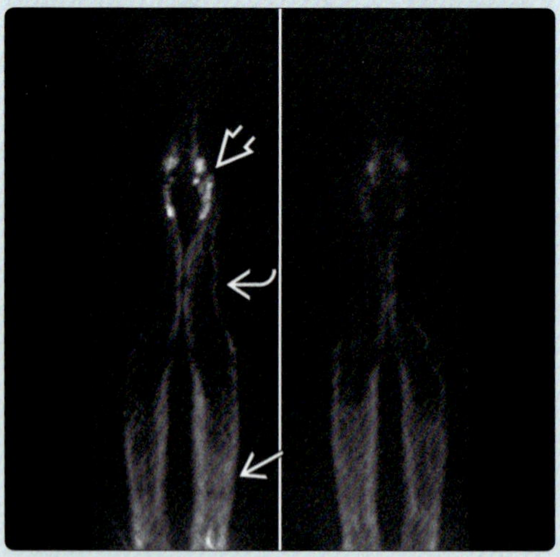

(Left) *Anterior Tc-99m sulfur colloid lymphoscintigraphy shows tracer pooling in distorted, dilated lymphatic channels ➔ in both upper extremities in a 4-month-old infant with congenital lymphedema.* **(Right)** *Tc-99m sulfur colloid lymphoscintigraphy of the lower extremities shows extensive dermal backflow ➔ of the lower calves and tracer within the deep lymph channels of the legs ➔ and deep inguinal nodes ➔ in a patient with history of lymphedema praecox.*

TERMINOLOGY

Definitions

- Abnormal accumulation of lymphatic fluid resulting in soft tissue edema secondary to impeded transport of lymph through lymphatic system

IMAGING

Nuclear Medicine Findings

- Tc-99m sulfur colloid lymphoscintigraphy
  - Standard diagnostic study of choice to guide differential diagnosis of extremity edema
  - Contrast lymphangiography fallen out of favor due to invasiveness, advent of CT and MR
  - Useful to map lymphatic drainage anatomy for surgical planning
  - Normal lymphatic drainage
    - Symmetric, bilateral lymphatic uptake of radiotracer
    - May not visualize radiotracer in normal lymphatic channels
    - Absence of signs present in lymphedema
  - Lymphedema
    - Delayed uptake of radiotracer in extremity of interest despite exercise
    - Dermal backflow (stocking sign) in extremity
    - Presence of collateral &/or dilated lymphatic channels
    - Interruption of lymphatic channels
    - Absent or asymmetric visualization of lymph nodes, lymphatic trunks

CT Findings

- Nonspecific skin thickening
- Subcutaneous reticulation/fluid accumulation
- May show evidence of prior mastectomy, lymphadenectomy
- Nodal metastases/dysfunction
- Lymphangitic carcinomatosis in extreme examples

MR Findings

- Nonspecific dermal thickening
- Circumferential skin edema
- Increased volume of subcutaneous tissue
- Honeycombing between muscle and skin
- May also elucidate primary etiology of poor lymphatic drainage

Imaging Recommendations

- Protocol advice
  - **Tc-99m sulfur colloid lymphoscintigraphy**
  - Patient preparation
    - Anesthetic cream on injection sites 1 hour prior to injection to reduce needle stick pain
    - Warn patient that radiotracer is suspended in acidic solution that will burn for 1-2 min after injection
  - Radiopharmaceutical
    - Subcutaneous injection of dorsum of both hands or feet (adjacent to metacarpo-/metatarsophalangeal joints)
    - Cleanse injection sites prior to injection
    - Tc-99m sulfur colloid, ideally filtered to particle size of 50-70 nm
      - 0.5-1 mCi (19-37 MBq) Tc-99m sulfur colloid in 0.4 mL for each extremity of interest
      - Tc-99m albumin colloid or Tc-99m human serum albumin can be used in lieu of sulfur colloid
      - Separate syringe and doses of similar activities for each injection site
      - Inject bilaterally to assess degree of asymmetry on images
    - After injection, extremity exercise (patient walks or squeezes rubber ball in hands for 5 min) to aid in lymphatic return
  - Dosimetry
    - No definite critical organ given small dose
    - No absolute contraindications
    - Pregnancy or breastfeeding are relative contraindications
      - Lymphedema is rarely medical emergency, so consider delaying study until after breastfeeding or delivery
  - Image acquisition
    - Low-energy, all-purpose collimator
    - Upper extremity
      - Image immediately after extremity exercise
      - Patient supine
      - Injection sites just out of FOV
      - Anterior and posterior images including both upper extremities and chest
    - Lower extremity
      - Image immediately after extremity exercise
      - Patient supine
      - Injection sites just out of FOV
      - Sweep of chest, abdomen, pelvis, and bilateral lower extremities in anterior and posterior projections
      - May repeat images at 1, 2, or 3 hours as needed
    - Imaging terminated once clinical question answered &/or liver uptake visualized
      - If liver uptake shown after locoregional soft tissue/nodal uptake, indicates tracer has had enough time to transit deep system adequately

DIFFERENTIAL DIAGNOSIS

Primary Lymphedema

- Congenital or genetic causes resulting in pathologic development of lymphatic vessels
  - Congenital causes more common than genetic
  - Primary classified by age at onset
    - Congenital lymphedema
      - Onset at birth up to age 2 years
    - Lymphedema praecox
      - Arises during puberty or pregnancy (up to 35 years)
    - Lymphedema tarda
      - Onset after 35 years (often upper extremity lymphedema)
- Similar imaging findings
- Key feature to differentiate primary lymphedema from generalized edematous state: Rate of capillary filtration is normal in patients with lymphedema

Secondary Lymphedema

- Result of other conditions or treatments
  - Typically secondary to malignant conditions &/or treatments in developed world (most commonly breast cancer)
    - Compression of lymphatics or nodes by tumor
    - Infiltration of lymphatic channels by tumor cells (lymphangitic carcinomatosis)
    - Lymphadenectomy
    - Radiation therapy
  - Filariasis is most common cause worldwide (nematode *Wucheria bancrofti*)

Nonlymphatic Causes of Extremity Edema

- Chronic venous insufficiency
- Generalized edematous state
  - Cardiogenic
  - Noncardiogenic edema (e.g., renal, hepatic failure)
- Cellulitis (unilateral or bilateral)
- Deep venous thrombosis

PATHOLOGY

General Features

- Etiology
  - Primary: Absent or decreased lymphatic channels
    - Congenital
    - Milroy disease
      - Autosomal dominant with high penetrance
      - Lymphedema can be present at birth
    - Syndrome-associated
      - Turner, Klippel-Trenaunay-Weber, Noonan, etc.
    - Lymphedema praecox
      - Onset of peripheral lymphedema at puberty to 35 years
      - Familial (Meige disease) or sporadic
    - Lymphedema tarda
      - Onset: > 35 years
  - Secondary: Acquired lymphatic obstruction
    - Iatrogenic
      - Lymph node dissection
      - Vascular surgery
      - Radiation therapy
    - Post-infectious (e.g., filariasis)
    - Tumor/lymphadenopathy → lymphatic obstruction
    - Chronic venous insufficiency

CLINICAL ISSUES

Presentation

- Most common signs/symptoms
  - Gradual onset of asymmetric swelling of affected limb
  - Recurrent soft tissue infection, deep venous thrombosis
  - Chronic lymphedema increases risk of lymphangiosarcoma
    - e.g., Stewart-Treves syndrome (post mastectomy)

Demographics

- Epidemiology
  - Sequelae of cancer therapy is most common cause in developed countries
  - Worldwide: Parasitic infection is most common cause (filariasis)

Treatment

- Extremity elevation
- Compression
- Massage
- Microsurgery
- Liposuction
- Hyperthermia
- Medications
  - e.g., diuretics, coumarin, antibiotics

DIAGNOSTIC CHECKLIST

Consider

- Injection of tracer in dorsum of hands/feet sufficient
  - Technique of injecting web spaces between fingers and toes obsolete
- Image patient after injection and extremity exercise

Image Interpretation Pearls

- Compare both extremities
- Dermal backflow abnormal
- Collateralization of lymphatic channels abnormal
- Absent, interrupted deep lymphatics abnormal

SELECTED REFERENCES

1. Notohamiprodjo M et al: MR lymphangiography at 3.0 T: correlation with lymphoscintigraphy. Radiology. 264(1):78-87, 2012
2. Infante JR et al: Lymphoscintigraphy for differential diagnosis of peripheral edema: diagnostic yield of different scintigraphic patterns. Rev Esp Med Nucl Imagen Mol. 31(5):237-42, 2012
3. Balci TA et al: Gall bladder visualization in lymphoscintigraphy. Lymphat Res Biol. 10(4):208-10, 2012
4. Cooper KL et al: Positron emission tomography (PET) and magnetic resonance imaging (MRI) for the assessment of axillary lymph node metastases in early breast cancer: systematic review and economic evaluation. Health Technol Assess. 15(4):iii-iv, 1-134, 2011
5. Jensen MR et al: Lymphoedema of the lower extremities–background, pathophysiology and diagnostic considerations. Clin Physiol Funct Imaging. 30(6):389-98, 2010
6. Tartaglione G et al: Intradermal lymphoscintigraphy at rest and after exercise: a new technique for the functional assessment of the lymphatic system in patients with lymphoedema. Nucl Med Commun. 31(6):547-51, 2010
7. Kerchner K et al: Lower extremity lymphedema update: pathophysiology, diagnosis, and treatment guidelines. J Am Acad Dermatol. 59(2):324-31, 2008
8. Scarsbrook AF et al: Pearls and pitfalls of radionuclide imaging of the lymphatic system. Part 2: evaluation of extremity lymphoedema. Br J Radiol. 80(951):219-26, 2007
9. Tiwari A et al: Differential diagnosis, investigation, and current treatment of lower limb lymphedema. Arch Surg. 138(2):152-61, 2003
10. Moshiri M et al: Using lymphoscintigraphy to evaluate suspected lymphedema of the extremities. AJR Am J Roentgenol. 178(2):405-12, 2002
11. British Nuclear Medicine Society Protocol for Lymphoscintigraphy
12. Use of Lymphoscintigraphy in the Management of Chronic Oedema - Journal of Lymphoedema

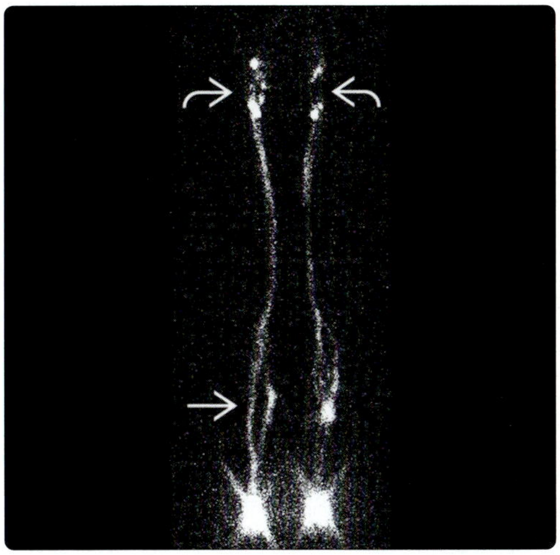

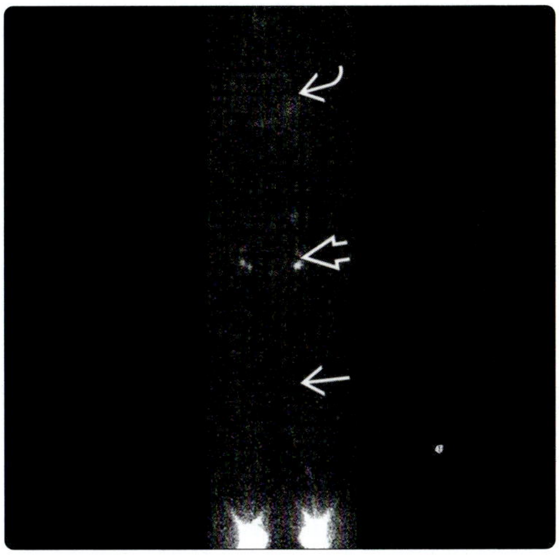

(Left) *Tc-99m sulfur colloid lymphoscintigraphy in the lower extremities of a lymphedema patient shows tortuous, collateralized lymphatics within the calves* ➡ *and deep inguinal lymph nodal uptake* ➡*.* **(Right)** *Tc-99m sulfur colloid lymphoscintigraphy of the lower extremities shows normal lymph channels of the legs* ➡*, inguinal nodes* ➡*, and uptake within a chylous left pleural effusion* ➡ *in this patient with chyloptysis.*

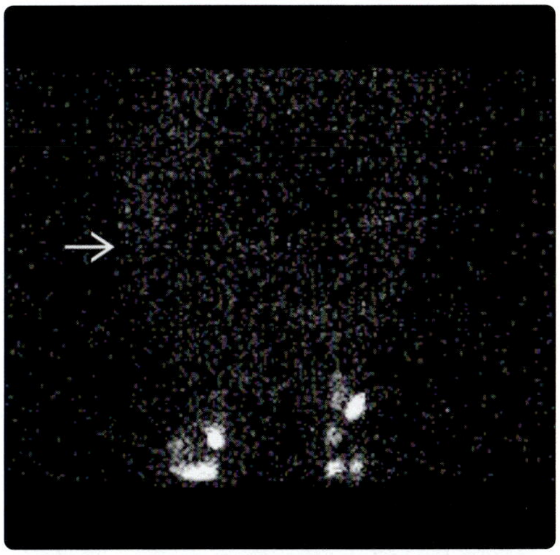

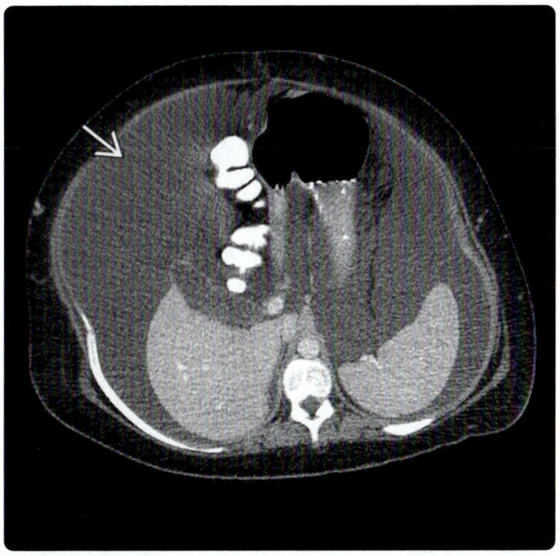

(Left) *Image centered over the abdomen in a patient with ascites undergoing Tc-99m sulfur colloid lymphoscintigraphy of the lower extremities shows amorphous abnormal activity within the central abdomen* ➡*.* **(Right)** *Axial CT of the same patient shows gross ascites* ➡ *under tension, which correlates with central abdominal tracer uptake on lymphoscintigraphy.*

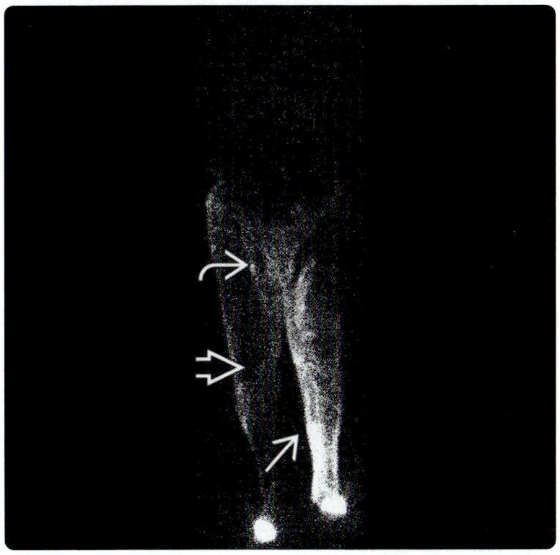

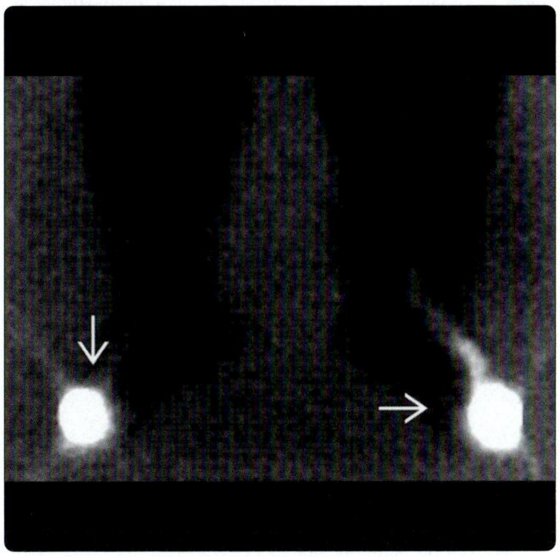

(Left) *Tc-99m sulfur colloid lymphoscintigraphy shows marked asymmetric bilateral dermal backflow* ➡*, tortuous lymphatic channels* ➡*, and scrotal edema* ➡*.* **(Right)** *Tc-99m sulfur colloid injection of bilateral webspaces* ➡ *is shown, obscuring the fine lymphatic anatomy of the feet, obviating the need for this historical approach. The dorsum of the feet should be injected instead.*

KEY FACTS

TERMINOLOGY

- Sentinel lymph node (SLN)
  - 1st lymph node(s) visualized in lymphatic drainage basin of malignancy
  - Most likely to have tumor cells before other nodes within similar drainage pathways
- Sentinel lymph node mapping
  - Tc-99m sulfur colloid taken up by lymphatic system to lymph node basin
  - Lymphoscintigraphic imaging may be performed to locate drainage basins (e.g., in patients with melanoma)
  - Intraoperative gamma probe detects gamma rays from SLN at surgery
  - Isosulfan blue dye injected during surgery; stains SLN blue for visual colocalization with radioactive SLN
  - Guides lymphadenectomy, radiation port planning, staging of malignancy
  - Reduces morbidity of locoregional radical lymphadenectomy (lymphedema, pain)

TOP DIFFERENTIAL DIAGNOSES

- Sentinel lymph nodes
  - Most commonly in typical ipsilateral lymph node basins
  - Can be in contralateral or aberrant lymph node basins
  - Includes subcutaneous in-transit lymph nodes
- False-negative sentinel lymph nodes
  - Lymph nodes infiltrated with tumor cannot function properly
  - ~ 20% of sentinel nodes with gross tumor at surgery may not visualize on Tc-99m sulfur colloid SLN mapping
- Skin, clothing, bedding contamination
  - May mimic SLN on lymphoscintigraphy
- Lymphatic valves and channels
  - Tc-99m sulfur colloid in lymphatic valves and channels will clear with time, while SLNs increase with time
  - Use orthogonal or oblique projections to differentiate linear lymphatic channels from discrete SLNs

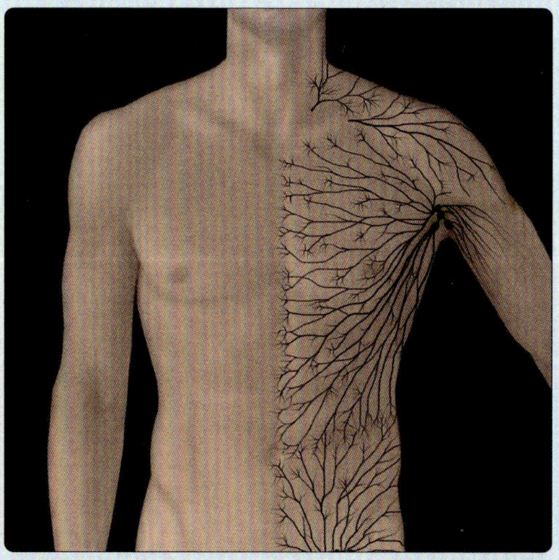

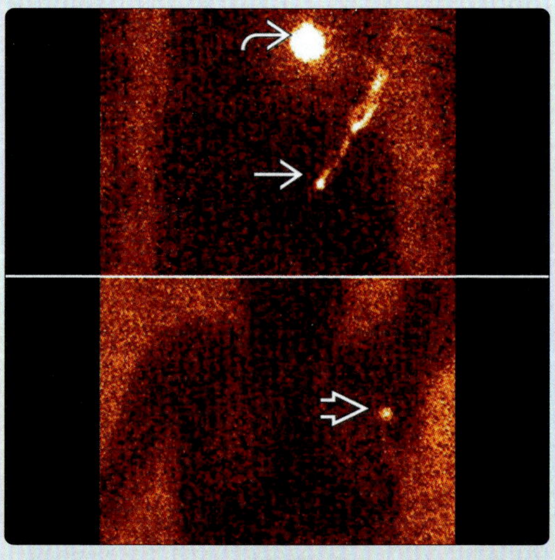

(Left) *Coronal graphic shows theoretical lymphatic drainage patterns for truncal lesions, also called Sappey's lines. Note that aberrant drainage patterns and subcutaneous in-transit sentinel lymph nodes (SLNs) are common, requiring complete imaging of all potential drainage basins, not just the ones that are expected.* **(Right)** *Anterior Tc-99m sulfur colloid lymphoscintigraphy following intradermal peritumoral injection of a melanoma ➲ demonstrates SLNs in both the left inguinal ➡ and left axillary ➡ drainage basins.*

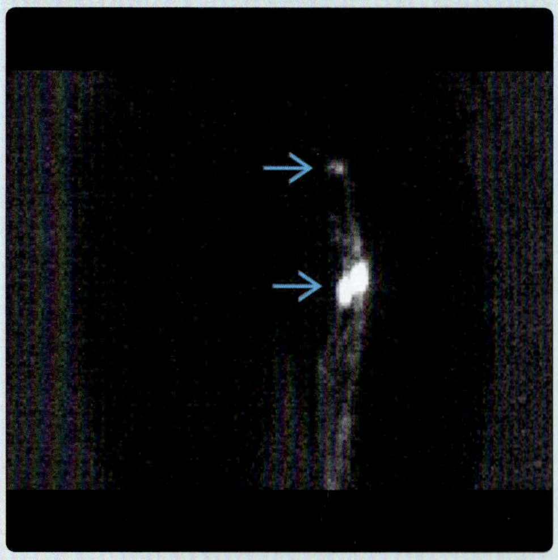

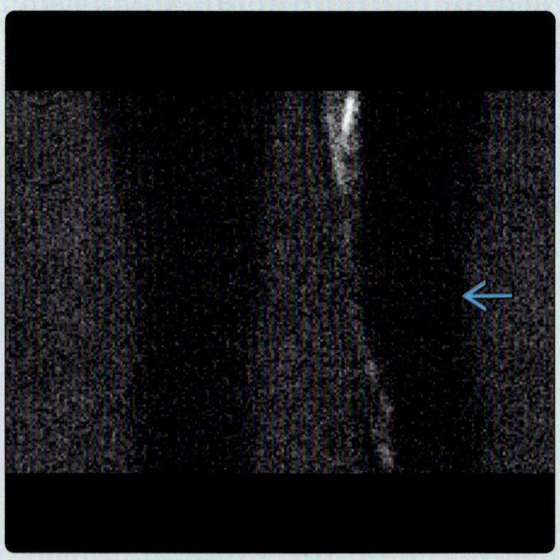

(Left) *Anterior Tc-99m sulfur colloid lymphoscintigraphy in patient with a left foot melanoma shows SLNs in the left groin ➡.* **(Right)** *Anterior lymphoscintigraphy in the same patient shows no sentinel lymph node in the left popliteal fossa ➡, another lymph node drainage basin for the distal lower extremity. Note that the antecubital fossa and axilla should both be imaged for distal arm lesions.*

TERMINOLOGY

Definitions

- Sentinel lymph node (SLN)
  - 1st lymph node(s) visualized in lymphatic drainage basin of malignancy
  - Most likely to have tumor cells before other nodes within similar drainage pathways
- Sentinel lymph node mapping
  - Tc-99m sulfur colloid injected at primary tumor site prior to surgery/therapy
    - Tc-99m sulfur colloid taken up by lymphatic system to lymph node basin
    - Lymphoscintigraphic imaging may be performed to locate drainage basins (e.g., in patients with melanoma)
    - Intraoperative gamma probe detects gamma rays from SLN at surgery
    - Isosulfan blue dye injected during surgery; stains SLN blue for visual colocalization with radioactive SLN
  - Mapping > 92% effective in locating SLN
    - Guides lymphadenectomy, radiation port planning, staging of malignancy
    - Truncal, head and neck tumors often require surgery at multiple lymphatic drainage basins
  - Used most commonly for melanoma and breast cancer
  - Reduces morbidity of locoregional radical lymphadenectomy (lymphedema, pain)

IMAGING

Nuclear Medicine Findings

- Tc-99m sulfur colloid SLN mapping
  - Focal increased activity in regional lymphatic bed that increases over time
    - 1 lymphatic bed can have multiple SLNs
  - Multiple lymphatic beds can drain a single tumor site
    - In the 1800s, an anatomist delineated theoretical drainage pattern for entire body (called Sappey's lines)
      - However, lymphatic drainage does not always follow Sappey's lines (especially with head & neck and truncal melanomas)
      - In-transit SLNs can be present in subcutaneous tissues outside lymph node basins
      - Radiation, surgery (biopsy, wide excisions), and bulky adenopathy can disrupt expected drainage patterns
- Locations
  - Head & neck cancer (including cutaneous malignancies)
    - Occipital, pre-auricular, anterior/posterior cervical, submandibular, supraclavicular, axillary are typical nodal basins
    - Lymph drainage pattern highly variable, multiple basins often present (especially for scalp lesions)
  - Cutaneous malignancies (e.g., melanoma, Merkel cell carcinoma)
    - Truncal
      - Lymph drainage pattern highly variable
      - Can have both cephalad and caudal drainage basins for single truncal lesions
      - Image neck, chest, abdomen, and pelvis to detect all possible SLN basins
      - Above L2 umbilical line, axillary drainage more common
      - Below L2 umbilical line, drainage to groin more common
    - Extremity
      - Arms: Epitrochlear and axillary nodes
      - Legs: Popliteal and inguinal nodes
  - Breast cancer
    - Ipsilateral axilla
    - Clinical significance of internal mammary SLN unclear
    - Images often not obtained, as axillary SLN easily detected by gamma probe and blue dye at surgery
  - Vulvar cancer
    - Inguinal, femoral, and iliac chain nodes

Imaging Recommendations

- Protocol advice
  - **Tc-99m sulfur colloid SLN mapping**
  - Radiopharmaceutical: Tc-99m sulfur colloid
    - Filtered sulfur colloid particles (50-100 nm) preferred for adequate lymphatic uptake in cutaneous malignancies
    - Unfiltered sulfur colloid particles used in patients with breast cancer
    - Injection often painful due to acidic radiopharmaceutical preparation: Subsides within 1-2 min
    - Other tracers (rarely used) include Tc-99m macroaggregated albumin (MAA), antimony sulfur colloid
  - Dose: 0.5-1 mCi (19-37 MBq) Tc-99m sulfur colloid
    - Injected intradermally for cutaneous malignancies
    - Subcutaneous areolar (or, alternately, peritumoral) injection for breast cancers
    - Injection can be performed day of or day before surgery
  - Dosimetry
    - Injection site absorbed dose < 925 mGy
    - Injected breast equivalent dose < 15 mSv
    - Patient effective dose < 0.56 mSv
  - Image acquisition
    - 5 minute planar static images with low-energy all-purpose parallel hole collimator
    - Anterior/posterior and lateral images of all possible lymphatic drainage sites
    - Lead shield over injection site may facilitate imaging of adjacent SLNs
    - On selected images, place sheet source behind patient to delineate body contours or outline body contour with point source
      - Note that sheet source can obscure superficial/neck SLNs
    - Head & neck and truncal tumors: Delayed imaging to 90 min may be useful to evaluate for additional drainage basins
    - For axillary nodes, image with arm behind head or out to side
    - Obtain lateral projections to localize focus in anteroposterior plane

- □ For example, a node that appears to be in axilla on anterior images may prove to be in-transit node on back in a patient with truncal melanoma
  - For head & neck tumors, image anterior/poster and lateral head, neck, axillae
- Localization of SLN on lymphoscintigraphy
  - Patient in position similar to surgery
  - View real time on p-scope: Set at 100% persistence, frequent manual reset
  - Localize SLN with radioactive marker: Capillary tube or cotton swab with Tc-99m pertechnetate (enclosed in test tube or other barrier to avoid site contamination)
  - Image SLN at 2 angles, mark over anticipated surgical approach
  - Once SLN localized with radioactive marker, mark with indelible marker
- Handheld gamma probe for intraoperative lymph node localization
  - Indelible mark from lymphoscintigraphy orients surgeon to nodal basin of SLN
  - Gamma probe detects radioactivity from SLN
  - Highest counts typically correlate with blue-dyed SLN
- Cutaneous malignancies
  - Perilesional intradermal injection: 4 quadrants vs. multiple perimeter injections both acceptable
    - □ Injection sites ~ 0.5 cm to 1 cm from lesion or scar
  - At least 3-4 injection sites at minimum
  - Avoid injecting into inflamed tissue as lymphatics in edematous tissue are altered
    - □ May not transport tracer/reveal actual SLN
  - Use gentle back pressure on syringe when withdrawing needle to prevent radiotracer contamination of patient/sheets/detector
    - □ Prevents artifacts and mistaken droplets of tracer for additional SLNs
- Breast cancer
  - Subareolar upper outer edge of areola: 1 injection; 85-100% effective
    - □ Gently massage injection site to assist transit of Tc-99m sulfur colloid into lymphatics
  - Periareolar (subdermal): 4 injections; 92-100% effective
  - Peritumoral (deep): 4 injections adjacent to solid tumor/biopsy site; ranges from 50-95% effective; sometimes (1-5%) adds additional drainage route such as internal mammary chain or supraclavicular
  - If peritumoral injection follows recent open excision biopsy: Ultrasound guidance to avoid injection into seroma/hematoma
  - Direct tumoral injection less common, more difficult to target but has similar results to above techniques
  - If nonpalpable primary tumor and peritumoral or intratumoral injection desired: Ultrasound or mammographic guidance
  - Use gentle back pressure on syringe when withdrawing needle to prevent squirting tracer onto patient/sheets/detector
    - □ Prevents artifacts and mistaken droplets of tracer for additional SLNs
- Vulvar malignancies
  - Similar to melanoma injection
  - Very painful procedure; consider anesthesia for patient

DIFFERENTIAL DIAGNOSIS

Sentinel Lymph Nodes

- Most commonly in typical ipsilateral lymph node basins
- Can be in contralateral or aberrant lymph node basins
- Includes subcutaneous in-transit lymph nodes

False-Negative Sentinel Lymph Nodes

- Lymph nodes infiltrated with tumor cannot function properly
- ~ 20% of sentinel nodes with gross tumor at surgery may not visualize on Tc-99m sulfur colloid SLN mapping

Skin, Clothing, Bedding Contamination

- May mimic SLN on lymphoscintigraphy

Lymphatic Valves and Channels

- Tc-99m sulfur colloid in lymphatic valves and channels will clear with time, whereas SLNs increase with time
- Use orthogonal or oblique projections to differentiate linear lymphatic channels from discrete SLNs

CLINICAL ISSUES

Presentation

- Most common signs/symptoms
  - Palpable enlarged lymph node may or may not be present
  - May have lymphatic obstruction (lymphedema) in cases of advanced nodal spread

DIAGNOSTIC CHECKLIST

Consider

- For truncal malignancy, image both axillae and inguinal regions due to variable drainage patterns
- For head & neck tumors, image anterior/posterior and lateral head, neck, axillae
- For patients with vulvar cancer, consider patient anesthesia during subcutaneous injections as they are very painful
- Utilize meticulous technique to avoid contaminating skin/clothing/sheets with radiotracer during injection to avoid false-positive nodes

SELECTED REFERENCES

1. Giammarile F et al: The EANM and SNMMI practice guideline for lymphoscintigraphy and sentinel node localization in breast cancer. Eur J Nucl Med Mol Imaging. 40(12):1932-47, 2013
2. Intenzo CM et al: Lymphoscintigraphy in cutaneous melanoma: an updated total body atlas of sentinel node mapping. Radiographics. 29(4):1125-35, 2009
3. Alazraki N et al: Procedure guideline for lymphoscintigraphy and the use of intraoperative gamma probe for sentinel lymph node localization in melanoma of intermediate thickness 1.0. J Nucl Med. 43(10):1414-8, 2002
4. Kern KA: Breast lymphatic mapping using subareolar injections of blue dye and radiocolloid: illustrated technique. J Am Coll Surg. 192(4):545-50, 2001
5. Yudd AP et al: Use of sentinel node lymphoscintigraphy in malignant melanoma. Radiographics. 19(2):343-53; discussion 354-6, 1999

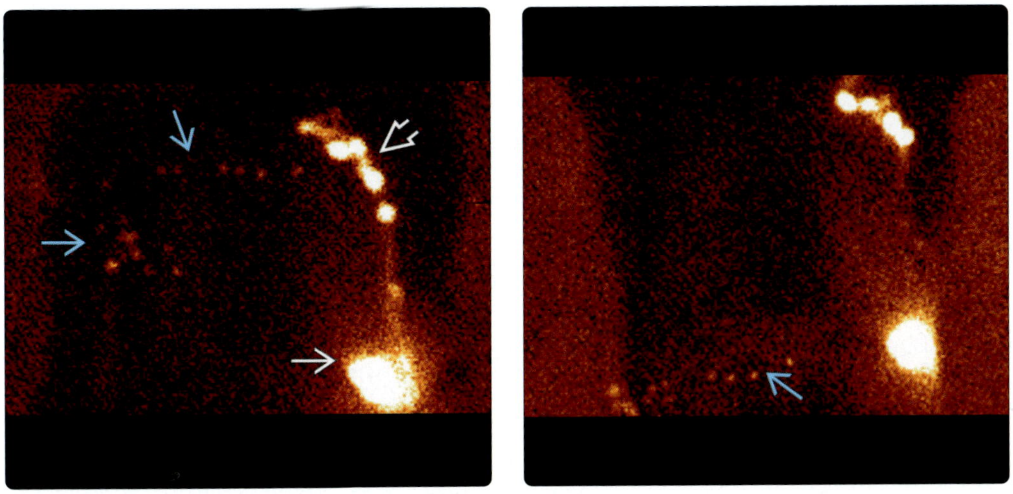

(Left) *Anterior Tc-99m sulfur colloid lymphoscintigraphy shows distal left arm injection site and left axillary sentinel lymph nodes. Indeterminate activity suggests in-transit nodes &/or aberrant drainage.* **(Right)** *Anterior Tc-99m sulfur colloid lymphoscintigraphy in the same patient after repositioning shows that the activity has changed locations, consistent with Tc-99m sulfur colloid contamination of the patient's gown during radiotracer injection.*

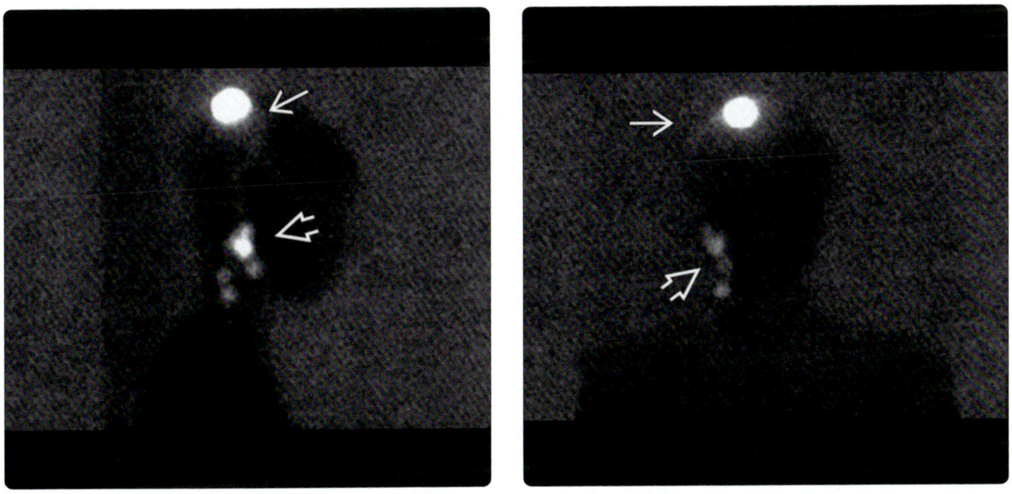

(Left) *Right lateral Tc-99m sulfur colloid lymphoscintigraphy of a scalp melanoma shows cervical chain SLNs.* **(Right)** *Anterior lymphoscintigraphy in the same patient shows the injection site and that the sentinel cervical chain nodes are on the right. Other potential drainage sites for this lesion include the left cervical chain, preauricular, posterior occipital, and supraclavicular.*

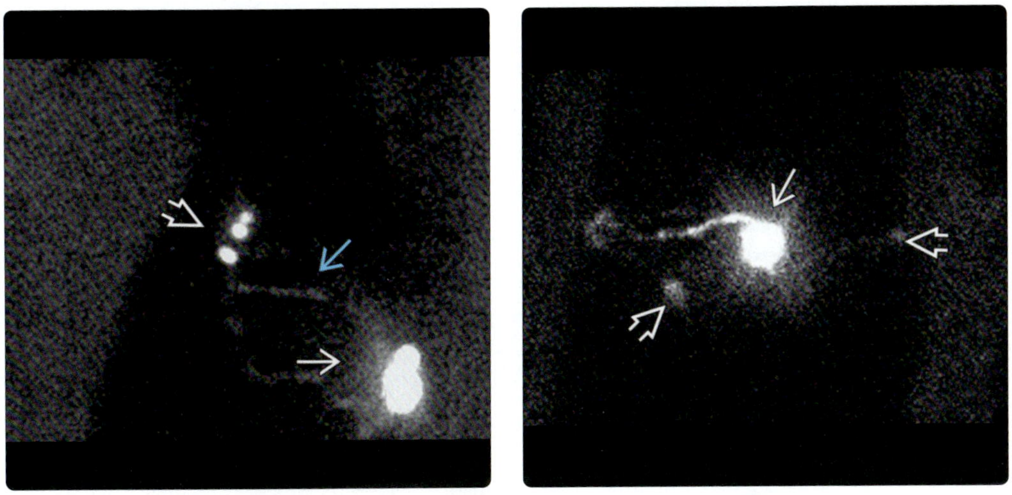

(Left) *Left lateral Tc-99m sulfur colloid lymphoscintigraphy in a patient with truncal melanoma shows the injection site and left axillary SLNs. Note radiotracer within the lymphatic channel. A low-level flood source outlines the patient.* **(Right)** *Anterior lymphoscintigraphy in a patient with vulvar cancer shows the injection site and bilateral inguinal sentinel lymph nodes.*

Large Vessel Vasculitis

KEY FACTS

TERMINOLOGY

- Large vessel vasculitis
  - Inflammation of aorta and major branch vessels due to T-cell response to unknown antigen

TOP DIFFERENTIAL DIAGNOSES

- Large vessel vasculitis
  - F-18 FDG PET/CT
    - Homogeneously increased activity in walls of large arteries (aorta, iliac, femoral, subclavian, carotid)
- Atherosclerosis
  - F-18 FDG PET/CT
    - Mild, heterogeneous activity, skipped regions
    - Intense activity: Ulcerated plaques
- Vascular thrombosis
  - F-18 FDG PET/CT
    - Increased activity in lumen, not vascular wall
- Vascular grafts
  - F-18 FDG PET/CT or In-111 WBC scintigraphy
    - Mild, diffuse activity
    - Intense, focal activity if infected
- Aneurysm
  - F-18 FDG PET/CT or In-111 WBC scintigraphy
    - Homogeneous activity
- Other causes of aortitis
  - Autoimmune (e.g., autoimmune arthritides, Cogan syndrome, systemic lupus erythematosus)
  - Infectious (e.g., syphilis)

CLINICAL ISSUES

- F-18 FDG PET/CT
  - Helps diagnose vasculitis when other imaging equivocal
  - Detects early disease much better than other modalities
  - Useful in ambiguous situations (e.g., when temporal biopsy negative but clinical suspicion remains high)
  - Useful for monitoring response to therapy: Hypermetabolic activity and extent of disease should decrease

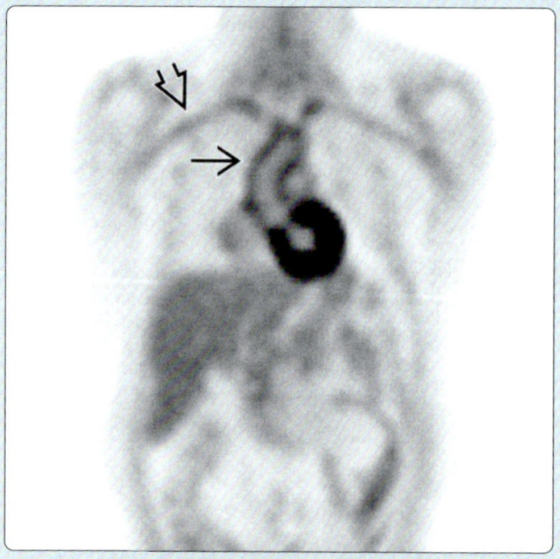
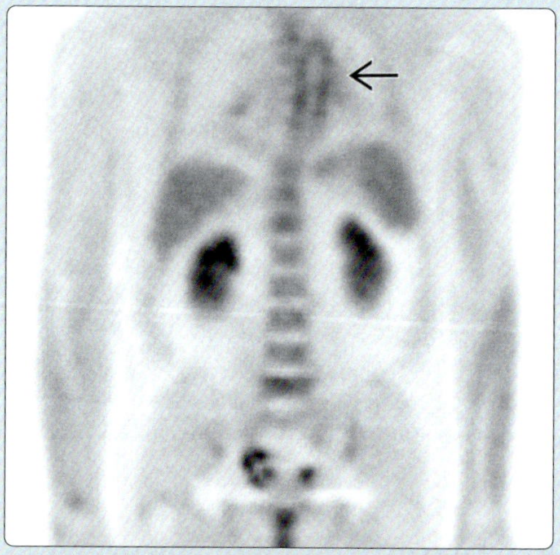

(Left) *Diffuse, homogeneously increased F-18 FDG uptake is shown in the ascending aorta and bilateral subclavian arteries in a patient with giant cell arteritis.* **(Right)** *Increased F-18 FDG uptake is shown in the descending aorta in a patient with giant cell arteritis.*

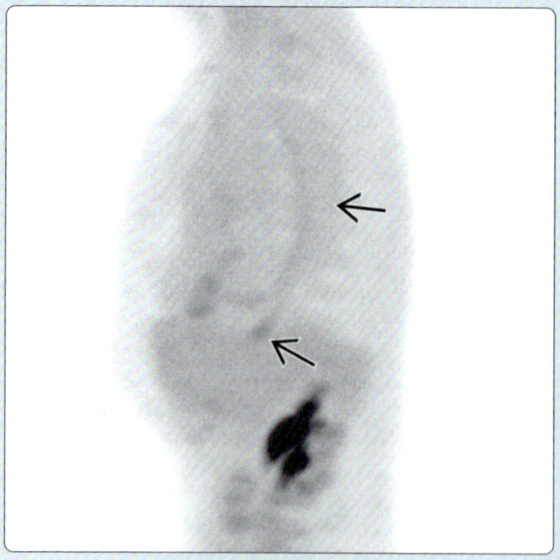
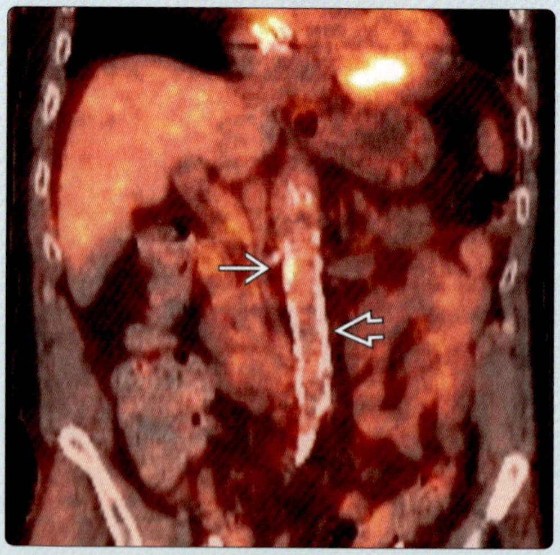

(Left) *Asymmetric heterogeneous F-18 FDG uptake is shown in the descending thoracic aorta in a patient with atherosclerosis.* **(Right)** *Focal F-18 FDG uptake in an atherosclerotic plaque is shown in the descending aorta of a patient with extensive atherosclerosis. Note the dense calcification of the atherosclerosis.*

TERMINOLOGY

Definitions

- Large vessel vasculitis: Inflammation of aorta and major branch vessels
  - Giant cell arteritis
    - Predominately affects Caucasians
    - Common cause of temporal arteritis
      - Temporal artery biopsy not sensitive for large vessel vasculitis, cannot differentiate between Takayasu and giant cell arteritis
  - Takayasu arteritis
    - More common in Asian or Indian patients

IMAGING

Imaging Recommendations

- Best imaging tool
  - F-18 FDG PET/CT
    - Homogeneously increased activity in walls of large arteries (aorta, iliac, femoral, subclavian, carotid)
    - Resolution of PET/CT scanner limits detection to larger arteries
    - Activity decreases with effective treatment
- Protocol advice
  - Image 3 hours post injection (blood pool activity cleared)
  - Low serum glucose (< 150 ng/dL) critical to minimize blood pool activity

Correlative Imaging Features

- CT angiography: Luminal irregularity (aneurysm, stenosis, occlusion, dilation)
- Ultrasound: Hypoechoic vascular halo
- MR: Wall thickening and edema

DIFFERENTIAL DIAGNOSIS

Large Vessel Vasculitis

- F-18 FDG PET/CT
  - Homogeneously increased activity in walls of large arteries (aorta, iliac, femoral, subclavian, carotid)

Atherosclerosis

- F-18 FDG PET/CT
  - Mild, heterogeneous activity, skipped regions
  - Intense activity: Ulcerated plaques

Vascular Thrombosis

- F-18 FDG PET/CT
  - Increased activity in lumen, not vascular wall

Vascular Grafts

- F-18 FDG PET/CT or In-111 WBC scintigraphy
  - Mild, diffuse activity
  - Intense, focal activity if infected

Aneurysm

- F-18 FDG PET/CT or In-111 WBC scintigraphy
- Homogeneous activity normal
  - Intense, focal activity if infected

Other Causes of Aortitis

- Autoimmune (e.g., autoimmune arthritides, Cogan syndrome, systemic lupus erythematosus)
- Infectious (e.g., syphilis)

PATHOLOGY

General Features

- Etiology
  - Inflammation caused by T-cell response to unknown antigen
- Associated abnormalities
  - Polymyalgia rheumatica: Present in 40% of patients with giant cell arteritis
    - F-18 FDG uptake in soft tissues of shoulders and hips if present

CLINICAL ISSUES

Presentation

- Most common signs/symptoms
  - Systemic: Fever, malaise, weight loss, night sweats, anorexia, depression
  - ↑ erythrocyte sedimentation rate, C-reactive protein
  - Temporal arteritis: Temporal tenderness, blindness, headache, scalp tenderness, jaw claudication
  - Giant cell arteritis/temporal arteritis identified as cause of fever of unknown origin in 17% of cases
  - Vascular occlusion symptoms (nonpalpable/asymmetric pulses, claudication), rupture, hemorrhage
  - Severe myalgias; neck, shoulder, pelvic muscle stiffness

Demographics

- Age
  - Giant cell arteritis: Most commonly > 50 years old
  - Takayasu arteritis: Most commonly < 50 years old
- Gender
  - Much more common in females for both Takayasu and giant cell arteritis

Natural History & Prognosis

- Untreated disease → severe vascular consequences due to occlusion, rupture, hemorrhage

Treatment

- High-dose corticosteroids

DIAGNOSTIC CHECKLIST

Consider

- F-18 FDG PET/CT
  - Helps diagnose vasculitis when other imaging equivocal
  - Detects early disease much better than other modalities
  - Useful in ambiguous situations (e.g., when temporal biopsy negative but clinical suspicion remains high)
  - Useful for monitoring response to therapy: Hypermetabolic activity and extent of disease should decrease

SELECTED REFERENCES

1. Fuchs M et al: The impact of 18F-FDG PET on the management of patients with suspected large vessel vasculitis. Eur J Nucl Med Mol Imaging. 39(2):344-53, 2012

Vascular Graft Infection

KEY FACTS

IMAGING

- F-18 FDG PET/CT
  - Normal
    - Diffuse, mild homogeneous uptake is normal finding and can persist for years, caused by inflammatory reaction to synthetic graft material
    - Hematomas or seromas can mimic abscess on CT but are relatively cold on PET/CT
  - Infection
    - Focal &/or inhomogeneous uptake greater than inactive muscle and fat, or greater than liver activity, is concerning for infection
    - Use of standardized uptake values (SUVs) has not been validated for graft infection
- Labeled WBC scintigraphy
  - Normal
    - Mild, homogeneous uptake along distribution of vascular graft is normally seen up to 1 year postop; however, can persist indefinitely
    - Most false-positives occur in early postoperative period due to cross labeling of platelets
  - Colonization
    - Moderately increased uptake along vascular graft inner surface, often patchy
  - Abscess or phlegmon
    - Focal, asymmetrical uptake along or near graft
    - Proximal and distal anastomoses most vulnerable to infection

DIAGNOSTIC CHECKLIST

- Age of graft important (homogeneous uptake normal if surgery < 1 year)
- Consider possibility of vascular thrombotic disease, most important cause of false-positives
- Focal or asymmetrical uptake on labeled WBC scan or F-18 FDG PET/CT is positive
- Other imaging modalities are often negative

(Left) *In-111 WBC scan shows focal increased uptake at the distal anastomosis ➔ in a patient with an aortobifemoral bypass, which is consistent with an infected graft.* **(Right)** *Axial CECT in the same patient shows graft irregularity ➔ at the anastomosis with surrounding stranding and inflammatory changes.*

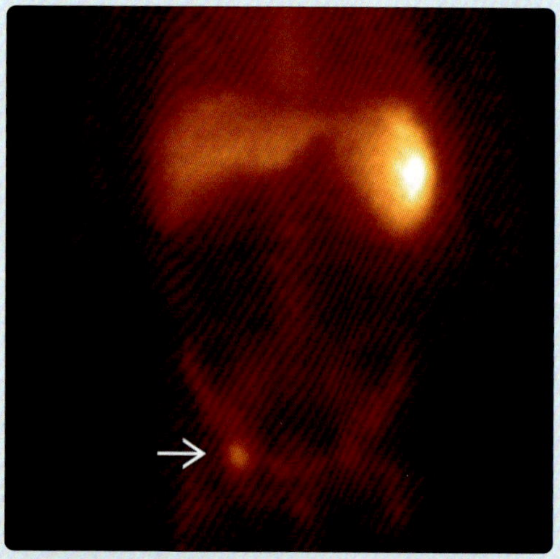

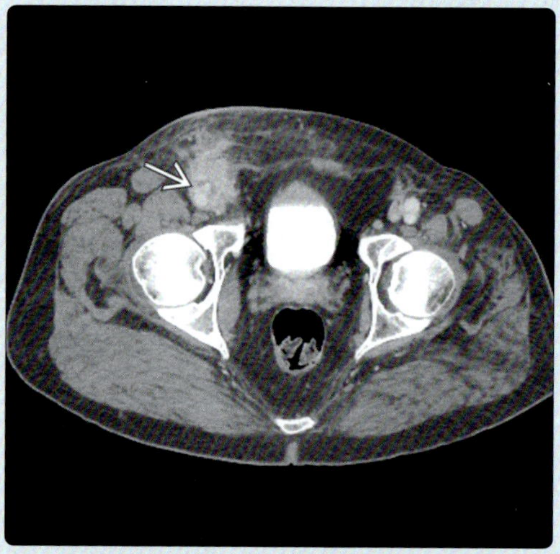

(Left) *In-111 WBC scan shows normal homogeneous uptake in a femoral to popliteal graft on the right ➔ and a external iliac to popliteal graft on the left ➔. Incidentally, note the increased uptake at the injection site ➔.* **(Right)** *Coronal F-18 FDG PET shows diffuse uptake in the soft tissues of the left extremity in a dialysis patient with cellulitis ➔. Focal uptake within the graft indicates thrombosis ➔. Incidentally, note enteritis ➔.*

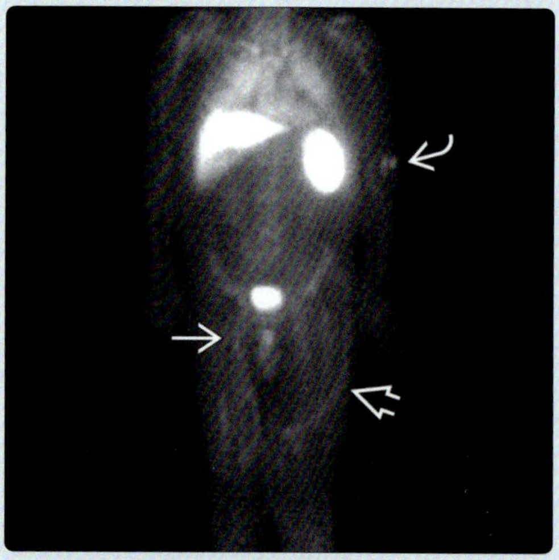

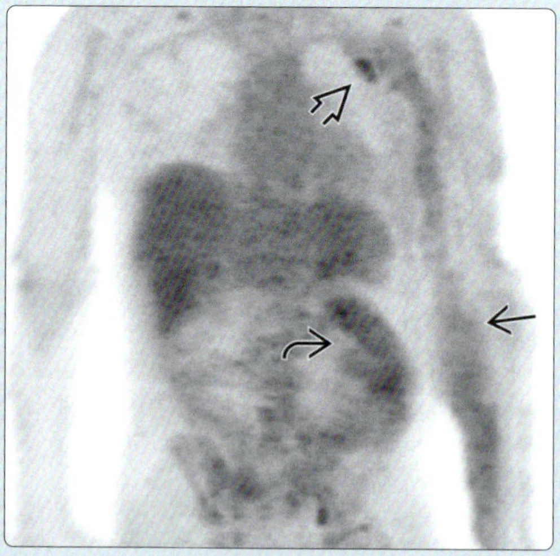

TERMINOLOGY

Definitions

- Common vascular grafts: Aortic or aortoiliac for aneurysm repair, peripheral grafts for dialysis access or peripheral arterial disease
  - Infected graft: Inflammatory change, phlegmon or abscess associated with bacterial ingrowth into or around vascular graft
  - Colonized graft: Bacteria living on graft without frank inflammation or invasion
  - Graft incorporation: Ingrowth of normal host cells into vascular graft creating pseudoendothelium
  - Graft disincorporation: Loss of host pseudoendothelium resulting in areas of bare graft

IMAGING

General Features

- Best diagnostic clue
  - Focal, asymmetric, markedly increased uptake/activity on labeled white blood cell (WBC) scan or F-18 FDG PET/CT
    - Proximal and distal anastomoses are most common sites of involvement
    - Along distribution of vascular graft

Nuclear Medicine Findings

- PET/CT
  - Normal
    - Diffuse mild, homogeneous uptake is normal finding and can persist for years, caused by inflammatory reaction to synthetic graft material
    - Hematomas or seromas can mimic abscess on CT but are relatively cold on F-18 PET/CT
  - Infection
    - Focal &/or inhomogeneous uptake greater than inactive muscle and fat, or greater than liver activity, is concerning for infection
    - Use of standardized uptake values (SUVs) has not been validated for graft infection
  - Vascular enteric fistula
    - Focal activity at site of infected fistula
    - Vascular enteric fistulas
      - Most common site: Where duodenum crosses aorta
      - Also: Between aorta and transverse colon; between descending colon and iliac graft
    - Uptake in bowel due to low-grade, intermittent bleeding
- Labeled leukocyte scintigraphy
  - Normal
    - Mild homogeneous uptake along distribution of vascular graft is normal up to 1 year postop, can persist indefinitely
    - Most false-positives occur in early postoperative period due to cross labeling of platelets
  - Colonization
    - Moderately increased uptake along vascular graft inner surface, often patchy
  - Abscess or phlegmon
    - Focal, asymmetrical uptake along or near graft
    - Proximal and distal anastomoses most vulnerable to infection
  - Vascular enteric fistulas
    - Focal increased uptake at site of fistula
    - Uptake in bowel due to low-grade, intermittent bleeding

Imaging Recommendations

- Protocol advice
  - In-111 WBC scintigraphy
    - Oblique views are helpful to separate vascular structures from adjacent bone marrow activity, often a problem in mid-lower lumbar spine and where external iliac vessels cross over pubic bones
    - Patient must have sufficient WBCs to be labeled (no leukopenia)
    - In-111 generally preferable to Tc-99m exametazime (HMPAO) leukocytes
  - Tc-99m HMPAO WBC scintigraphy
    - Tc-99m HMPAO leukocytes can be compromised by significant blood pool activity, which can obscure underlying lower grade infection
    - Imaging out to 24 hours is desirable
    - Improved SPECT imaging characteristics over In-111 leukocytes
  - F-18 FDG PET/CT
    - Improved spatial resolution and ability to define extent of infection compared to In-111 WBC scan
    - Several studies show high sensitivity in evaluation of prosthetic graft infection
    - Emerging role in evaluating infective endocarditis, including prosthetic valves
    - F-18 FDG uptake alone lacks specificity; when combined with CT specificity increases substantially
- Additional nuclear medicine imaging options
  - Tc-99m sulfur colloid marrow scan
    - May be necessary to determine if groin activity is bone marrow or vascular graft
    - Dual isotope imaging possible when used with In-111 labeled leukocytes, but not with Tc-99m labeled HMPAO leukocytes
- Correlative imaging features
  - CT or ultrasound may show fluid collection around infected graft, thickened graft, graft occlusion, or anastomotic aneurysm
    - Nonspecific and can be normal, even long after graft placement (lymphocele)
  - CT may show air around infected graft
    - Highly specific for infected graft but rarely seen
  - MR may show fluid collection and associated enhancement around graft
    - Fluid collection nonspecific; enhancement more specific
  - Vascular enteric fistula
    - Difficult to demonstrate by angiography and findings are often subtle on CT
    - Direct endoscopic imaging contraindicated because can worsen bleeding

DIFFERENTIAL DIAGNOSIS

Normal Blood Pool Activity

- More common with Tc-99m HMPAO WBCs than In-111 WBCs

Normal Vascular Graft Activity

- Common in recent postoperative period and may persist indefinitely, which can create false-positive results
- Infected graft differs in that it is intense, patchy, or asymmetric in uptake

Thrombus

- Labeled WBCs localize in acute arterial or deep venous thrombosis, increased uptake on F-18 FDG PET/CT

Normal Bone Marrow Activity in Close Proximity to Vascular Graft on In-111 WBCs

- Oblique images, SPECT/CT may resolve

Acute Aortic Syndrome

- Includes arterial dissection, unstable aneurysm, intramural hematoma
- Correlate with anatomic imaging

Atherosclerosis

- Inflammation in plaques causes uptake on F-18 FDG PET/CT and should be scattered throughout major vessels

PATHOLOGY

Gross Pathologic & Surgical Features

- Normal graft
  - Inner surface of graft initially consists of bare vascular graft material
  - During 1st postop year, cells grow into graft material creating pseudoendothelium
  - Grafts can be autologous (often saphenous vein) or synthetic (Dacron for large vessels; Gore-Tex/polytetrafluroethylene for medium vessels)
- In colonized grafts, organisms infect graft without frank invasion or destruction, and pseudoendothelium is lost, leaving bare areas of graft material
- Infected grafts can show abscess, phlegmon, aneurysm, or septic thrombus

Microscopic Features

- Labeled leukocyte preparations
  - Labeled cells include mixture (1/3 each) of white cells, red cells, and platelets
  - Because leukocytes are larger, bulk of labeled cellular material is leukocytes
- In normal grafts, initial bare graft is a nidus for platelet/mononuclear cell adhesion
  - Results in homogeneous uptake along vascular graft
  - Chronic low-level inflammation due to foreign material can cause normal uptake
- Colonization
  - Loss of pseudoendothelium results in exposed graft material, a nidus for adhesion of labeled cells
- Microbiology
  - Most common organism is *Staphylococcus*, often methicillin-resistant (MRSA)

CLINICAL ISSUES

Presentation

- Most common signs/symptoms
  - Low-grade fever, may be absent if chronic infection
  - Leukocytosis
  - May present with superficial surgical wound infection
  - Draining sinus or nonhealing wound common if graft is peripheral
- Other signs/symptoms
  - GI bleeding if there is vascular enteric fistula (rare)
  - Septic emboli to lower extremities
  - Pseudoaneurysm at distal anastomoses
  - Unusual signs/symptoms
    - Hypertrophic osteoarthropathy (may be unilateral)
    - Pretibial swelling

Natural History & Prognosis

- Graft infections only occur in up to 6% of cases; however, morbidity and mortality from graft infections is very high
  - Sepsis, septic emboli, and graft thrombosis occur with time
- Infection less common with endovascular stent grafts
- Grafts near groin, such as for aortobifemoral or femoropopliteal bypass, are at higher risk for infection

Treatment

- Complete surgical excision of infected graft with remote reconstruction is preferred treatment
- If graft is removed, revascularization is achieved with either in situ reconstruction or bypass revascularization at remote site
- Long-term antibiotics without surgery has high failure rate due to presence of foreign material and biofilms

DIAGNOSTIC CHECKLIST

Consider

- Age of graft (homogeneous uptake normal if surgery < 1 year)
- Possibility of vascular thrombotic disease, most important cause of false-positives

Image Interpretation Pearls

- Focal or asymmetrical uptake on labeled WBC scan or F-18 FDG PET/CT is positive
- Diffuse symmetrical uptake is usually normal
- Other imaging modalities are often negative
- Colonization can also cause uptake on leukocyte scan, due to inflammation and loss of pseudoendothelium inside graft

SELECTED REFERENCES

1. Haroon A et al: Role of fluorine 18 fluorodeoxyglucose positron emission tomography-computed tomography in focal and generalized infectious and inflammatory disorders. Clin Infect Dis. 54(9):1333-41, 2012
2. Bruggink JL et al: Current role of imaging in diagnosing aortic graft infections. Semin Vasc Surg. 24(4):182-90, 2011
3. Cavalcanti Filho JL et al: PET/CT and vascular disease: current concepts. Eur J Radiol. 80(1):60-7, 2011
4. Liberatore M et al: Clinical usefulness of technetium-99m-HMPAO-labeled leukocyte scan in prosthetic vascular graft infection. J Nucl Med. 39(5):875-9, 1998

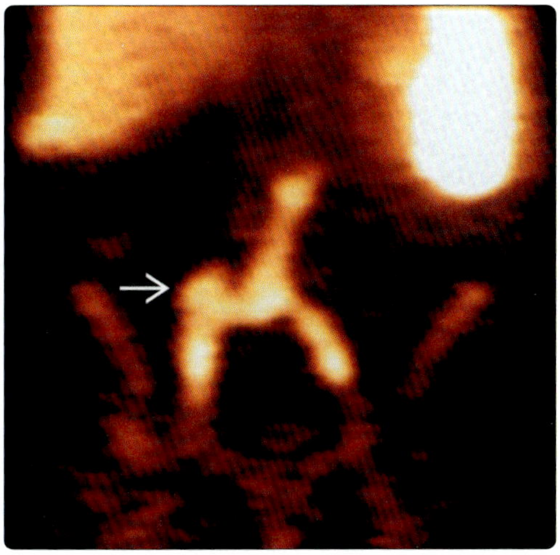
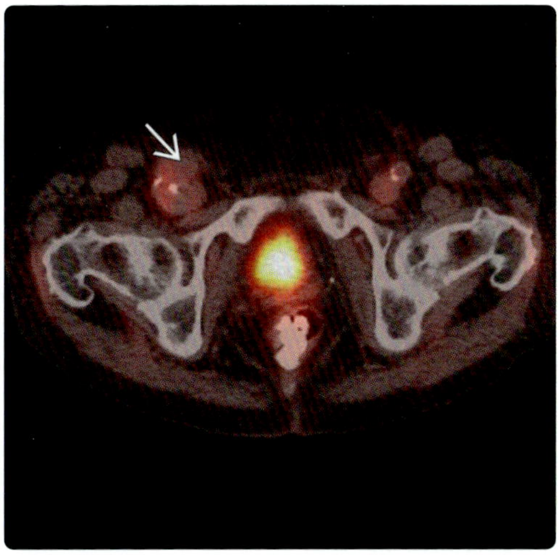

(Left) *Tc-99m HMPAO labeled leukocyte scan with coronal SPECT shows marked and asymmetrical uptake in an infected aortobiiliac graft. An abscess was also present in the proximal right iliac region* ➡. **(Right)** *Axial fused F-18 FDG PET/CT shows a noninfected pseudoaneurysm at the distal aspect of an aortoiliac bypass graft* ➡. *Note the lack of intense activity and normal mild activity in the graft. The anastomotic sites are vulnerable to aneurysm formation.*

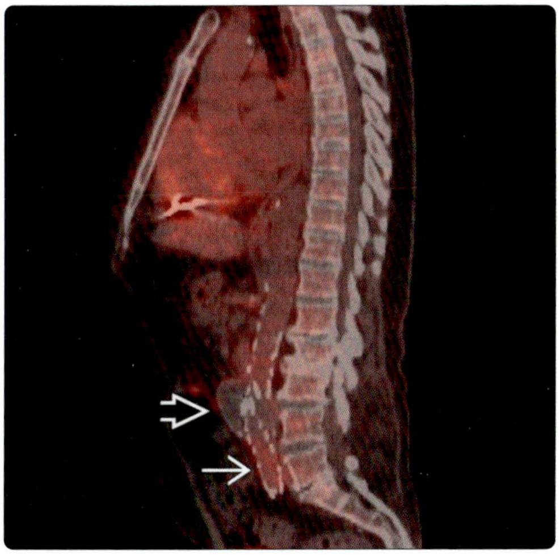
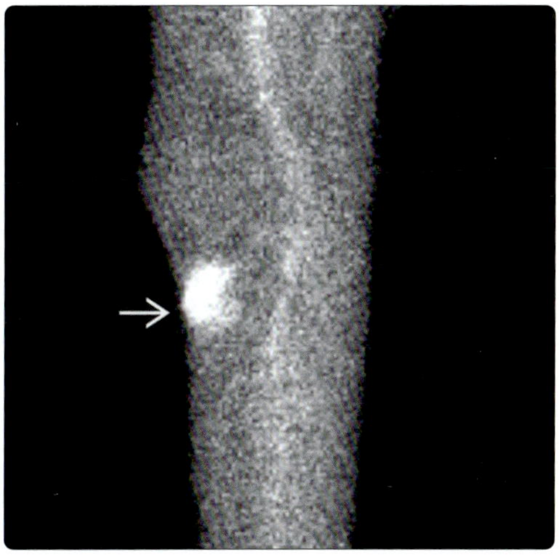

(Left) *Sagittal fused F-18 FDG PET/CT shows normal mild, diffuse homogeneous uptake* ➡ *in an endovascular graft placed for abdominal aortic aneurysm repair* ➡. **(Right)** *Tc-99m HMPAO labeled leukocyte scan shows increased uptake in an abscess inferolateral to the knee* ➡. *The collection is separate from the popliteal artery and endovascular graft.*

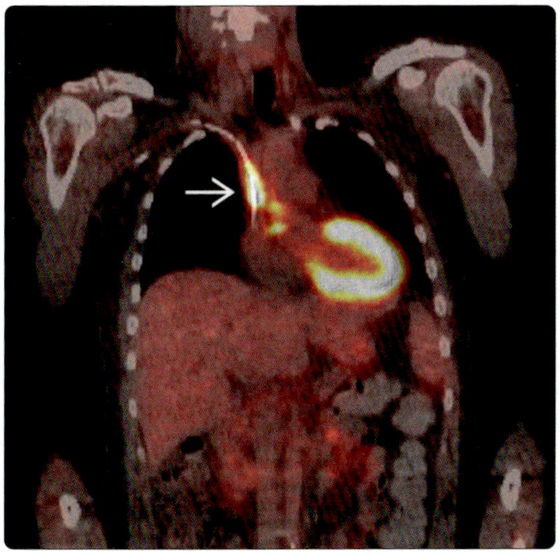
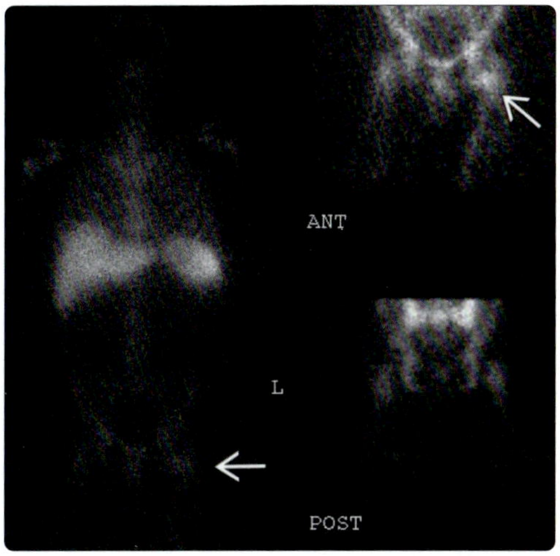

(Left) *Coronal fused F-18 FDG PET/CT shows a central venous catheter in the superior vena cava with increased activity at its distal aspect* ➡. *Differential diagnosis would include infection and thrombosis.* **(Right)** *In-111 WBC scan shows increased uptake at the left femoral anastomosis* ➡ *in a patient with an infected aortobifemoral bypass graft.*

SECTION 5

Musculoskeletal

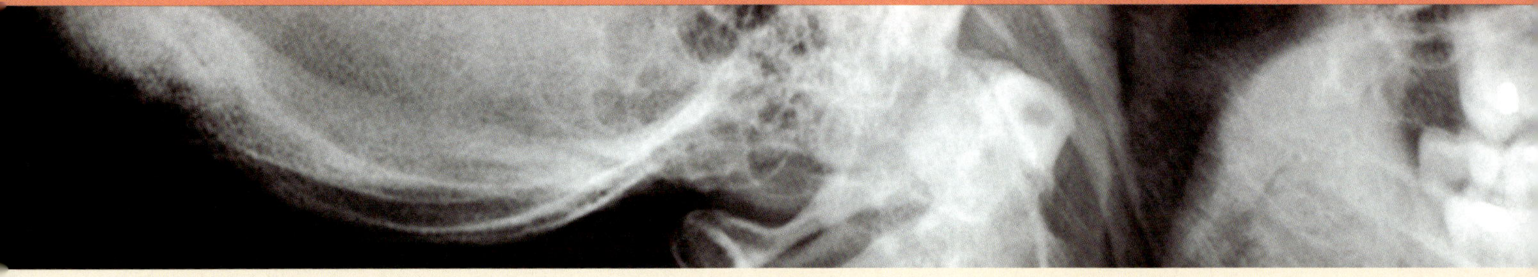

Introduction

Bone Tumors

Bone Dysplasias

Bone Mineral Density

Infection and Inflammation

Metabolic Disease

Trauma

Vascular

Introduction

Skeletal scintigraphy is one of the most common procedures performed in a nuclear medicine department. Patients are often referred for imaging in the setting of skeletal pain, trauma, vascular compromise of bone, malignancy, infection, arthritis, and prior orthopedic surgery/hardware placement. Imaging could be performed as a 3-phase protocol, limited imaging, whole-body imaging, &/or SPECT imaging. The two most common radiopharmaceutical agents used for imaging are Tc-99m MDP (Medronate) and Tc-99m HDP (TechneScan). Both are bone-seeking agents that undergo physicochemical adsorption (chemisorption) to the hydroxyapatite structure of bone tissue. Therefore, more uptake is seen in bone-forming pathology or growth regions of immature bone in the presence of osteoblasts. Uptake is dependent on blood flow to the bone and extraction efficiency (bone turnover).

During the initial 24 hours following intravenous injection of Tc-99m MDP, approximately 50% of the dose is retained in the skeleton, and approximately 50% is excreted in the urine. The critical organ is the urinary bladder wall. Clearance of radioactivity from the blood is rapid, with approximately 10% of the injected dose remaining at 1 hour, and less than 5% and 2% at 2 and 4 hours, respectively. This rapid clearance allows for early optimal imaging with elevated bone-to-background ratio. Normal uptake is homogeneous and most significant in the axial and proximal appendicular skeleton. Faint visualization of the kidneys is normal while the urinary bladder is visualized from normal excretion of tracer.

Detailed patient history is useful, including history of trauma, presence of hardware, bone surgeries, prior radiation and chemotherapy, recent pregnancy/breast feeding, dental issues/surgeries, prior bone scans, and correlative imaging. Laboratory values regarding serum tumor markers and markers of bone turnover should be reviewed. Additional history regarding past or current occupation and physical activities may be useful, as would whether the patient is right- or left-handed. Physical examination may be useful in the evaluation of extremity ulcers to correlate location of ulcer and findings on bone scan.

Patient preparation is an important part of nuclear medicine imaging. Generally, drinking at least 16 oz of water between radiopharmaceutical injection and imaging is recommended to maintain good hydration, which results in better target-to-background activity. The patient should also be informed of the protocols that may be utilized (3-phase, SPECT) and time needed for imaging. Prior to imaging, any removable metallic objects must be removed. Patient should be asked to void immediately prior to whole-body or pelvic imaging to reduce activity in the urinary bladder.

Delayed-phase imaging typically occurs 2-4 hours after radiopharmaceutical injection. Consider a longer time delay in patients with poor renal function or dehydration. Single head or dual head gamma cameras are used with the advantage of dual head being reduction in imaging time when performing whole-body sweeps in the anterior and posterior projection or planar static images needing both anterior and posterior views. Low-energy, high-resolution parallel hole collimators are preferred while pinhole or diverging collimators are helpful for troubleshooting and for imaging smaller osseous structures.

F-18 NaF PET bone scan has reemerged as a method to identify osseous metastatic disease, including localization and determination of extent of disease. The resolution and pharmacokinetics are far greater than Tc-99m-based bone agents and the total exam time is shorter. However, the radiation exposure to the patient is 68% greater with F-18 PET bone scan if 10 mCi (370 MBq) of F-18 is used. The mechanism of uptake is incorporation of fluoride ions into the bone matrix in sites of newly mineralizing bone, such as during growth, infection, malignancy (primary or secondary), after trauma, or during inflammation. During shortages of Tc-99m, F-18 PET bone scans offer an alternative for skeletal imaging.

Imaging Protocols

Whole-Body Imaging

The utility and advantage of bone scans over radiographs or MR is their ability to screen the entire skeletal system for disease. In patients with a known malignancy, a whole-body bone scan is performed in the anterior and posterior projections. Additional static images of the calvarium in lateral projections and images to fully include the upper extremities are often performed. Whole-body imaging is also important in looking for polyostotic disease in patients with fibrous dysplasia, Paget disease, histiocytosis, enchondromas, or osteochondromas. Similar utility is shown for multifocal joint-centered symptoms, screening all involved joints.

Limited Bone Scan

Planar regional images have better resolution than whole-body examinations. These limited bone scans are often used to address a very specific clinical question. For example, thoracic static views can be obtained to diagnosis an occult rib fracture. To address a specific sclerotic lesion on a radiograph or CT, a limited bone scan could be performed to assess the uptake of tracer associated with the lesion. However, a whole-body bone scan would be more useful to exclude a multifocal aggressive osseous process.

Three-Phase Bone Scan

The 3-phase bone scan offers sensitivity and specificity. The first phase addresses the degree of blood flow to the region of interest while the second phase evaluates the degree of hyperemia in the soft tissues and adjacent bone. Delayed phase determines the amount of bone formation occurring. One of the most common indications for a 3-phase bone scan is the evaluation of osteomyelitis in the setting of a diabetic foot ulcer, prior orthopedic fixation, or joint replacement. Noninfectious indications include evaluation and staging of complex regional pain syndrome and evaluating for avascular necrosis.

SPECT and SPECT/CT

SPECT imaging allows for better image contrast and precise lesion localization. In complex anatomical structures such as the spine, SPECT allows for greater accuracy in the determination of the source of abnormal activity in addition to lesion detection and characterization. SPECT is an added procedure rather than a stand-alone procedure in that whole-body images or limited bone scan are performed initially followed by SPECT imaging. SPECT/CT has even more advantage of lesion localization, but should be used judiciously in the context of radiation exposure.

Selected References

1. Brenner AI et al: The bone scan. Semin Nucl Med. 42(1):11-26, 2012

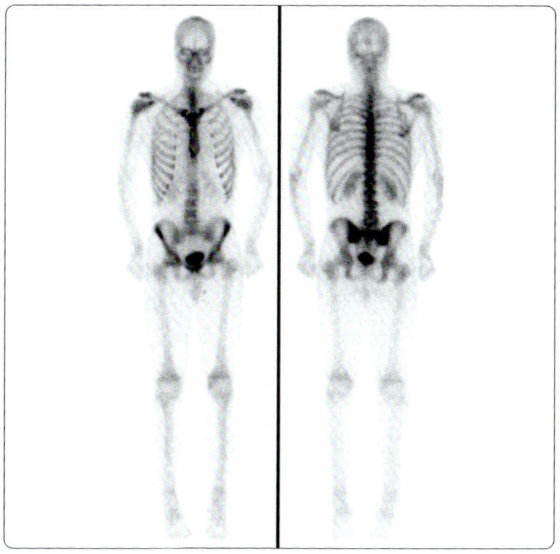

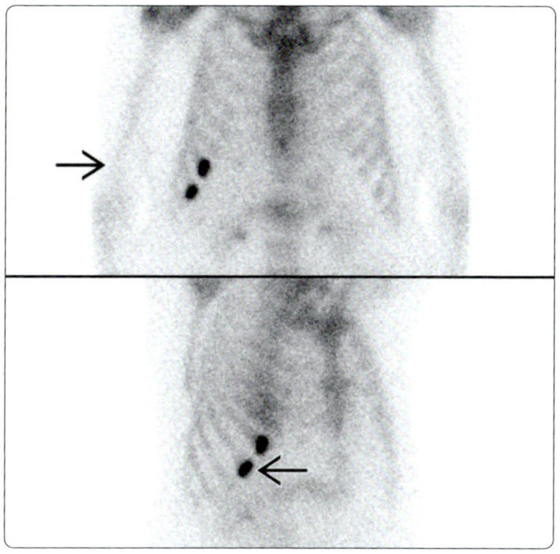

(Left) *Normal whole-body bone scan in the anterior and posterior projections shows faint visualization of the kidneys and normal excretion of tracer into the bladder.* **(Right)** *Limited bone scan of the thorax shows 2 contiguous round foci of activity in the right anterior 7th and 8th ribs →, most compatible with rib fractures near the costochondral junctions.*

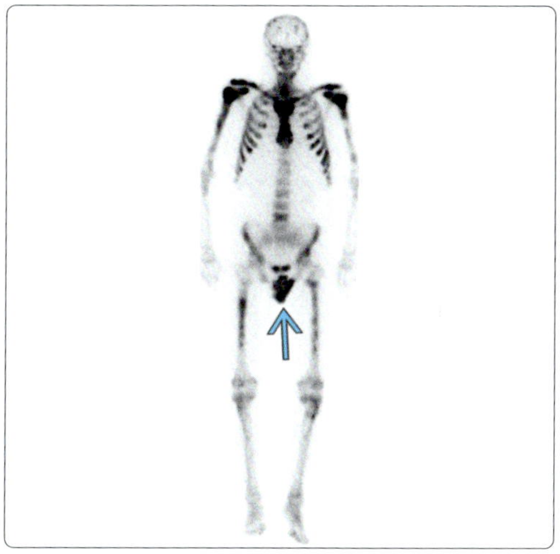

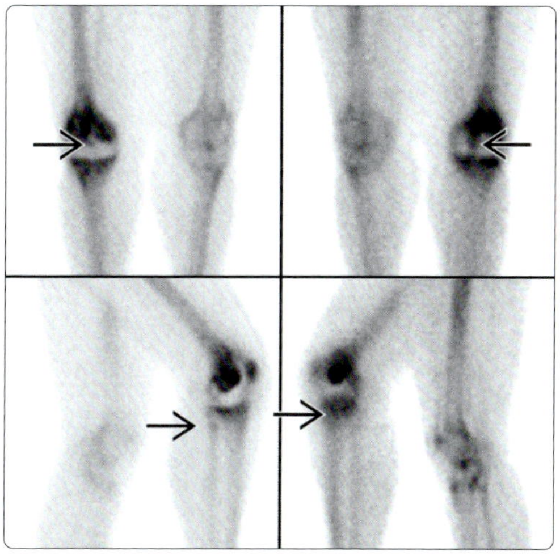

(Left) *Whole-body bone scan in the anterior projection shows widespread osseous activity throughout the axial and appendicular skeleton, most compatible with metastatic disease. Absent visualization of the kidneys make this a "superscan." There is contamination artifact over the lower pelvis →.* **(Right)** *Delayed-phase images from a 3-phase bone scan show periprosthetic uptake of tracer → involving the right knee arthroplasty. Findings are nonspecific and could represent aseptic loosening or an infected prosthesis.*

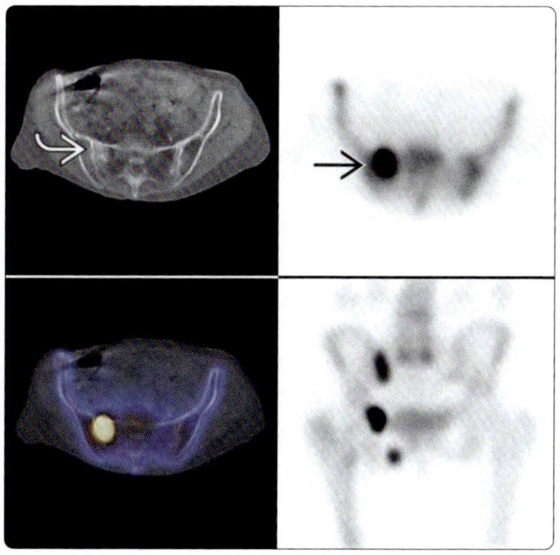

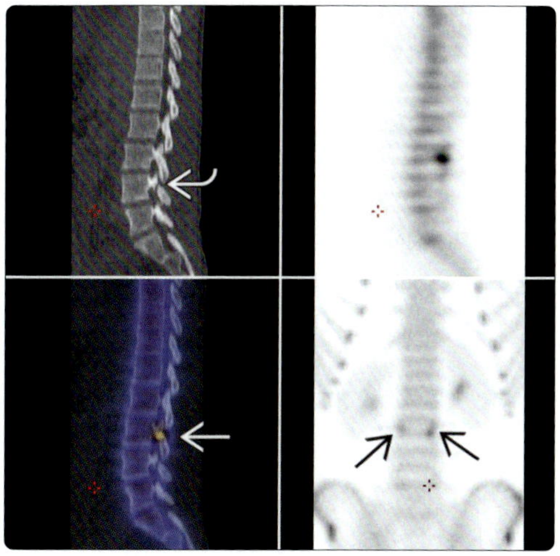

(Left) *SPECT/CT from a limited bone scan of the pelvis shows focal increased activity in the right sacrum →. There is focal sclerosis on the localization CT →. In the appropriate clinical setting, these findings are most compatible with a sacral insufficiency fracture.* **(Right)** *SPECT/CT MIP of the lumbar spine shows bilateral foci of activity in the lumbar spine →. Fusion image in the sagittal view shows 1 of the foci of activity → to localize to a defect → in the pars interarticularis of L3 vertebral body, compatible with spondylolysis.*

KEY FACTS

IMAGING

- Whole-body survey shows increased activity in primary malignant bone tumor & metastases in osteosarcoma, chondrosarcoma, & Ewing sarcoma
- Radiographic skeletal survey is more useful than bone scan in multiple myeloma secondary to lytic nature & often indolent disease
- Benign bones lesions mostly have variable appearance on bone scan & should always be correlated with other imaging
- Stage & assess response to therapy in malignant bone tumors with whole-body F-18 FDG PET/CT
- Large variances of uptake in benign bone tumors limits use of F-18 FDG PET/CT in clinical practice in evaluating benign bone tumors

CLINICAL ISSUES

- Osteochondroma is most common benign bone tumor
- Osteosarcoma is most common primary bone malignancy (excluding multiple myeloma), 35% of all primary bone malignancies

DIAGNOSTIC CHECKLIST

- Tc-99m MDP bone scan useful to identify polyostotic or metastatic lesions in osteosarcoma, chondrosarcoma, Ewing sarcoma
- Increased uptake between ribs on bone scan is concerning for osteosarcoma lung metastases
- Heterotopic ossification after surgery can be difficult to distinguish on bone scan from tumor recurrence
- Postsurgical change can show increased bone uptake on bone scan
- New uptake in area of benign lesions could represent fracture or malignant transformation

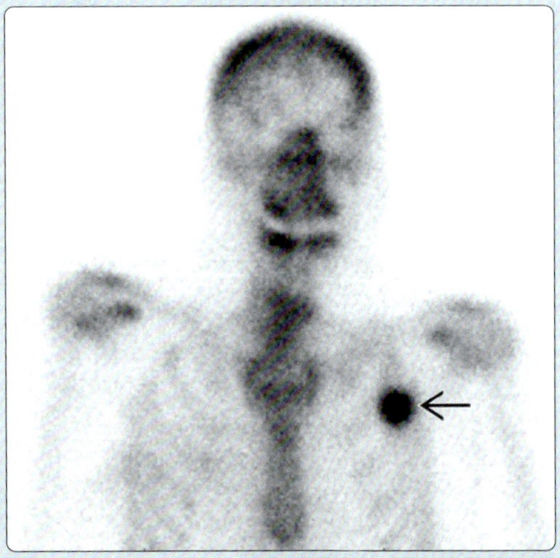

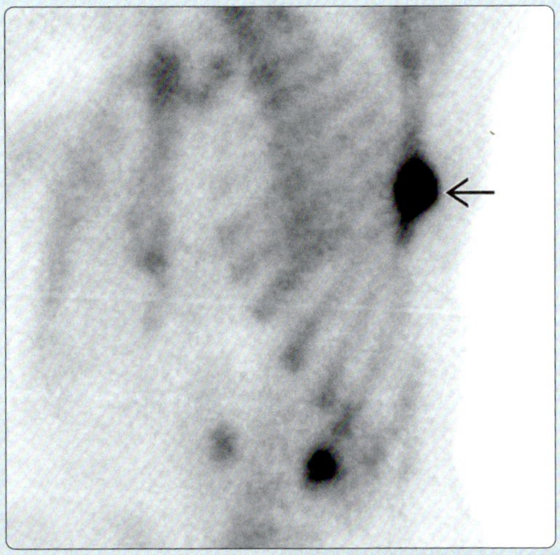

(Left) *Tc-99m MDP bone scan in the anterior projection shows uptake of tracer ➔ projecting over the left chest wall.* **(Right)** *Left anterior oblique view on the same patient shows focal activity ➔ to localize to the left scapula. This view is helpful when added to the anterior and posterior views to distinguish the scapular lesion from a rib or extraosseous lesion. The bone scan appearance is nonspecific, but was proven to be an osteosarcoma.*

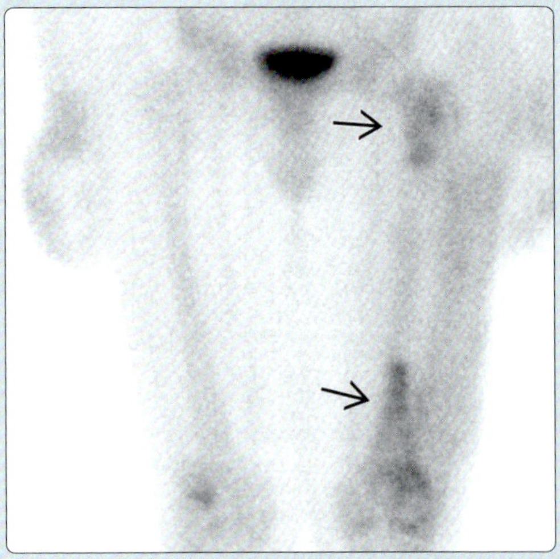

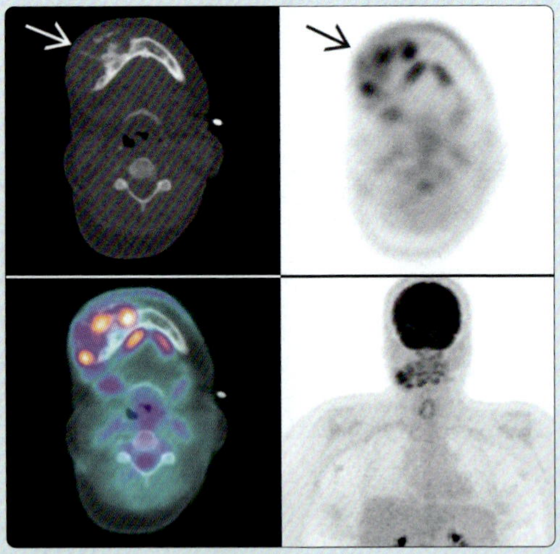

(Left) *Anterior Tc-99m bone scan in a patient with chondrosarcoma of the left femur status post resection and fixation shows increased uptake ➔ in the proximal and distal femur. Additional imaging would be necessary to differentiate between hardware induced uptake and skip metastasis.* **(Right)** *F-18 FDG PET/CT was performed on a patient for staging osteosarcoma of the right mandible ➔. Attenuation correction CT shows an expansile lesion ➔ with bone and soft tissue component.*

TERMINOLOGY

Bone Imaging and Dysplasias

- Malignant
  - **Hot**: Chondrosarcoma, Ewing sarcoma, osteosarcoma, metastases, adamantinoma
  - **Cold**: Multiple myeloma; metastases, purely lytic
- Benign
  - **Hot**: Paget disease, osteoblastoma, chondroblastoma, aneurysmal bone cyst, osteoid osteoma, giant cell tumor
  - **Isointense or mild**: Fibrous dysplasia, fibrous cortical defect, nonossifying fibroma, enchondroma
  - **Cold**: Enostosis, osteopathia striata, bone cyst
  - **Variable**: Osteochondroma/multiple hereditary exostoses, Langerhans cell histiocytosis, hemangioma

IMAGING

General Features

- Best diagnostic clue
  - Tc-99m MDP bone scan
    - Whole-body survey shows increased activity in primary malignant bone tumor & metastases in osteosarcoma, chondrosarcoma, & Ewing sarcoma
    - Multiple myeloma: Radiographic skeletal survey shows lytic lesions; bone scan not useful due to lytic nature & often indolent disease
    - Benign bones lesions mostly have variable appearance on bone scan
      - Primary diagnosis of benign bone tumor is by radiographs, CT, and MR
      - Utility of bone scan is to evaluate for multifocal disease or evaluate incidental sclerotic lesions on CT or radiographs
  - F-18 FDG PET/CT
    - Primary malignant osseous tumors (osteosarcoma, Ewing sarcoma, & chondrosarcoma) show intense uptake of tracer
      - Stage & assess response to therapy
    - Multiple myeloma: Increased activity in lytic bone lesion or extramedullary site
    - Large variances of uptake in benign bone tumors limits use of F-18 FDG PET/CT in clinical practice in evaluating benign bone tumors
- Location & skeletal scintigraphic appearance
  - Osteosarcoma
    - Typically long bone metaphyses, particularly distal femur; also proximal tibia and humerus
    - Axial involvement: Adults > children
    - Intense, often heterogeneous uptake on bone scan
  - Ewing sarcoma
    - Most often extremity long bones, particularly femur, & also pelvic bones; typically follows distribution of red marrow
    - Less common: Spine, hands, & feet
    - Intense more homogeneous uptake on bone scan
  - Chondrosarcoma
    - Bone scan uptake is usually intense & typically greater than low-grade chondrosarcoma
    - Central chondrosarcomas (~ 75%)
      - Arise within medullary cavity
      - Most common: Proximal femur, pelvic bones, proximal humerus
      - Precursor lesion: Enchrondroma (up to 40%)
    - Peripheral chondrosarcomas (~ 10%)
      - Arise from cartilage cap of preexisting osteochondroma
      - Most common: Pelvic bones & shoulder girdle
      - Precursor lesion: Osteochondroma
    - Dedifferentiated (~ 10%)
      - Common in pelvis, femur, proximal humerus, ribs
      - Can be intraosseous or extraosseous mass
      - Precursor lesion: Rarely in multiple osteochondromas & enchondromatosis
    - Clear cell (< 2%)
      - Epiphysis of long bones
    - Mesenchymal (< 2%)
      - Maxilla, mandible common
    - Periosteal chondrosarcomas (< 1%)
      - Very rare tumor that arises on surface of bones
      - Long bones most common site, particularly distal femur
  - Multiple myeloma
    - Plasma cells in bone marrow
    - Lytic lesions throughout skeleton
    - No role for bone scan
  - Adamantinoma
    - Anterior tibial cortex
    - Low-grade malignant lesion
    - Focal increased uptake
  - Osteoid osteoma
    - Cortically based lesion most commonly in femur, tibia, spine, hands, and feet
    - 3-phase positive with double density sign, intense central uptake, & moderate uptake in surrounding area
    - Delayed uptake in nidus secondary to presence of osteoblasts
  - Langerhans cell histiocytosis
    - Metaphysis & flat bones
      - Most often involves skull, mandible, pelvis, spine, ribs, & long bones
    - Solitary more common than multiple
    - Generally whole-body radiological skeletal survey preferred over bone scan
    - Bone scan useful to determine active lesions & response to therapy
  - Fibrous dysplasia
    - Medullary lesion
    - Monostotic: Femur, ribs, tibia, facial bones, & humerus
    - Polyostotic: Femur, tibia, pelvis, feet, ribs, facial bones, & lumbar spine
  - Giant cell tumors
    - Epiphyseal in location
    - Distal femur, proximal tibia, distal radius, sacrum, & proximal humerus
    - Increased tracer uptake peripherally with photopenia centrally (doughnut sign)
  - Aneurysmal bone cyst
    - Eccentrically in medullary cavity
    - Posterior elements of spine

 - Metaphysis of long bones
 - Upper & lower limbs, spine, & sacrum
 - Can show diffuse homogeneous uptake or peripheral uptake & central photopenia
- Hemangioma
 - Vertebral bodies & craniofacial bones
 - Variable uptake on bone scan: Normal/warm/cold
- Unicameral bone cyst
 - Centrally in medullary cavity
 - Majority in proximal humerus & femur
 - Can be cold defect or increased peripheral uptake & absent central activity
 - Fracture complication would show increased uptake
- Osteoblastoma
 - Posterior elements of spine & sacrum
 - Focal increased uptake, nonspecific
- Enchondroma
 - Typically solitary lesions in central medullary cavity
 - If solitary, more common in hand
 - Multiple lesions (Ollier disease & Maffucci syndrome)
 - Femur, tibia, humerus, hands, & feet
 - Mildly increased uptake in lesions that are large enough for gamma camera detection
 - Fractures can show change in uptake when following these lesions
 - Bone scan cannot reliably differentiate low-grade chondrosarcoma from enchondroma
- Fibrous cortical defect (FCD)/nonossifying fibroma (NOF)
 - Fibroxanthoma is also frequently used term for these tumors; lesions < 3 cm are called FCD, > 3 cm are called NOF
 - Cortically based lesion in metaphysis; tibia and femur most common
 - Usually no uptake or mild uptake in "healed" lesions that have filled with bone, and moderate uptake in "healing" lesions that are filling with normal bone
- Enostosis (bone island)/osteopoikilosis
 - Medullary in location
 - Can occur anywhere, but more often in pelvis, femurs, and ribs
 - Osteopoikilosis: Multiple enostoses near joints & predominantly in appendicular skeleton
 - Most bone islands have no uptake on bone scan; larger lesions may show very mild uptake
- Osteopathia striata
 - Dense linear striations in diaphyses & metaphyses of long & tubular bones
 - Parallel striations to long axis of bones
 - Iliac bones may show fan-shaped striations
 - No significant uptake on bone scan
- Chondroblastoma
 - Well-defined, osteolytic lesion with thin sclerotic rim located in epiphysis or apophyses of long bone
 - Femur, tibia, humerus, patella, and tarsal bones
 - Skeletally immature patient
 - Bone scan shows focal increased uptake
- Osteochondroma
 - Most common benign bone tumor
 - Most commonly in long bones of upper & lower extremity: Femur, tibia, humerus
 - Metaphyseal location with cortical & medullary bone continuous with underlying bone
 - Hereditary multiple exostoses is characterized by development of multiple osteochondromas
 - Uptake on bone scan is directly correlated with degree of enchondral bone formation

PATHOLOGY

Staging, Grading, & Classification

- Osteosarcoma & chondrosarcoma (Musculoskeletal Tumor Society)
 - Stage I: Low-grade, localized tumors
 - Stage II: High-grade, localized tumors
 - A or B designation for inside vs. outside bone, respectively
 - Stage III: Metastatic tumors
- Ewing sarcoma (& all other malignant bone tumors) can be staged with AJCC staging system
- Multiple myeloma (International staging system)
 - Stage I: Serum beta-2 microglobulin < 3.5 mg/L & albumin level ≥ 3.5 g/dL
 - Stage II: Beta-2 microglobulin level between 3.5 and 5.5 **or** albumin < 3.5 and beta-2 microglobulin < 3.5
 - Stage III: Serum beta-2 microglobulin > 5.5

DIAGNOSTIC CHECKLIST

Consider

- Tc-99m MDP bone scan
 - Identify metastatic lesions in osteosarcoma, chondrosarcoma, Ewing sarcoma
 - Not useful for tumor margins or soft tissue component
 - Not useful for multiple myeloma
 - Evaluate bone pain with SPECT if planar bone scan normal
- F-18 FDG PET/CT
 - Useful for staging primary bone malignancies
 - Degree of uptake often corresponds with tumor grade in chondrosarcoma
 - Has been shown to predict therapeutic response in osteosarcoma & Ewing sarcoma
 - Full inspiration CT has better sensitivity for small lung nodules than F-18 FDG PET/CT
 - Increased activity in lytic lesion or extramedullary sites of multiple myeloma

Image Interpretation Pearls

- Increased uptake between ribs on bone scan is concerning for osteosarcoma lung metastases
 - Oblique & lateral views help differentiate soft tissue vs. bone lesions
- Postsurgical change can show increased uptake
- Heterotopic ossification after surgery can be difficult to distinguish on bone scan from tumor recurrence
- New uptake in area of benign lesions could represent fracture or malignant transformation

SELECTED REFERENCES

1. Costelloe CM et al: FDG PET/CT of primary bone tumors. AJR Am J Roentgenol. 202(6):W521-31, 2014

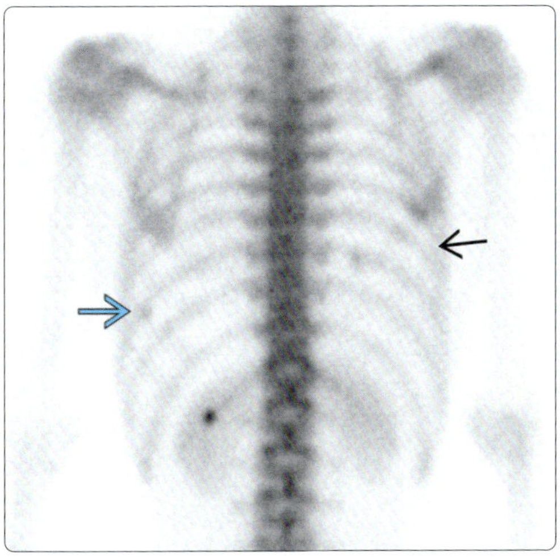

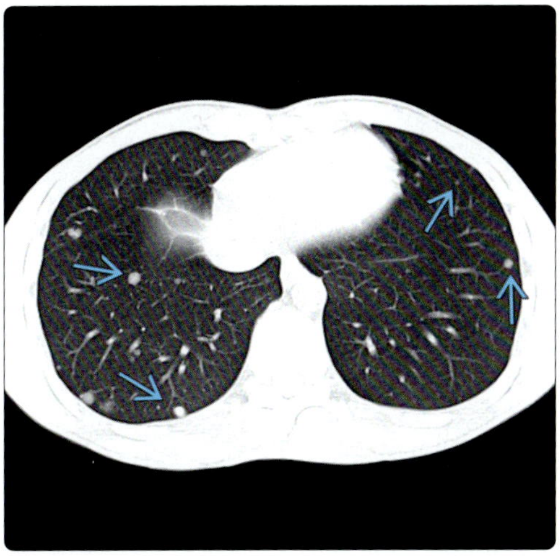

(Left) *Posterior view of the thorax from a Tc-99m MDP bone scan shows evidence of lung metastasis in a patient with primary osteosarcoma. Increased uptake between the ribs is concerning for lung metastasis. This scan shows uptake in the right mid-lung field medially* → *and left lower lung field laterally* →. *Lung metastasis is very common at presentation in patients with osteosarcoma.* **(Right)** *Transaxial CT of the same patient shows multiple bilateral pulmonary metastasis* →.

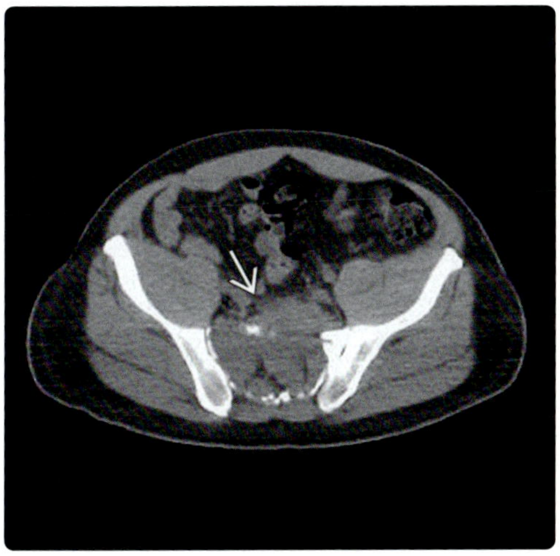

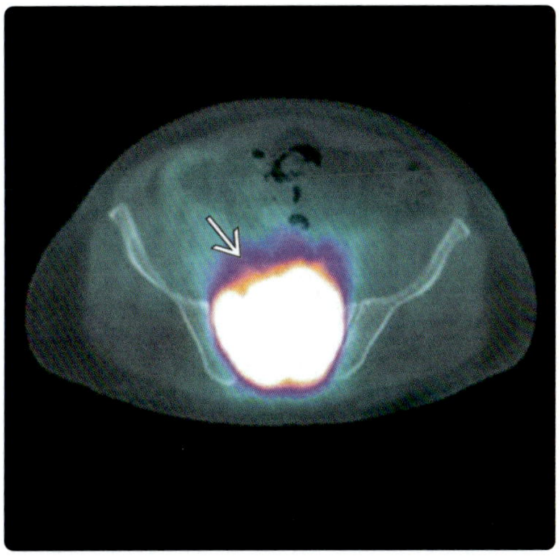

(Left) *Transaxial CT through the pelvis shows a large destructive soft tissue mass* → *in the sacrum in this patient with clinical findings of multiple myeloma.* **(Right)** *Fused F-18 FDG PET/CT at the same level shows intense uptake* → *within this lesion that is compatible with an active myelomatous lesion (plasmacytoma).*

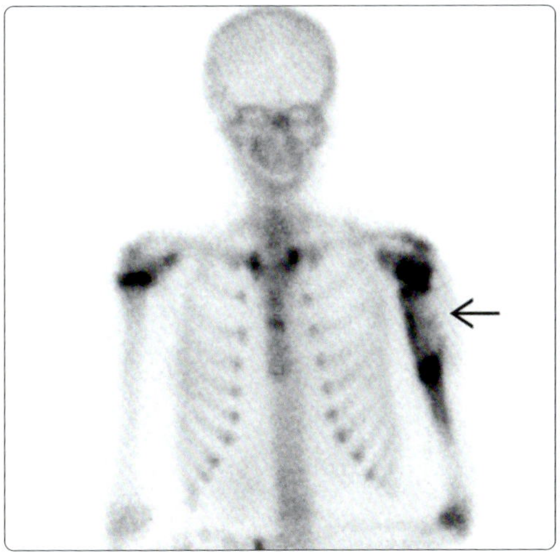

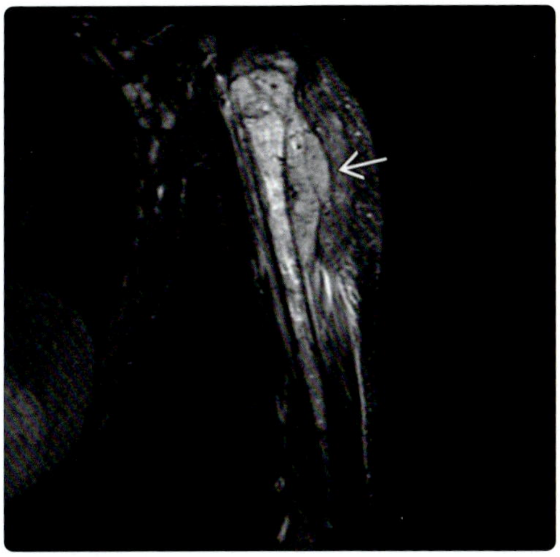

(Left) *A skeletally immature patient presents with a left humeral mass. Anterior Tc-99m bone scan shows a long segment lesion in the left humerus* → *with slight heterogeneous uptake. The scintigraphic findings are nonspecific, but no other lesions are shown.* **(Right)** *Corresponding STIR MR in the coronal plane shows a large aggressive lesion in the humerus with involvement of the adjacent soft tissues* →. *Findings are compatible with a Ewing sarcoma. MR imaging allows better lesion extent evaluation.*

(Left) *Enchondroma of the right femur ⇨ is shown on a whole-body bone scan in the anterior and posterior projection. Scattered arthritic/degenerative changes are shown without evidence for polyostotic disease.* **(Right)** *AP radiograph of the right distal femur shows a ring and arc matrix lesion ➡ in the distal femoral diaphysis spanning approximately 9 cm in the craniocaudal dimension. This is consistent with an enchondroma.*

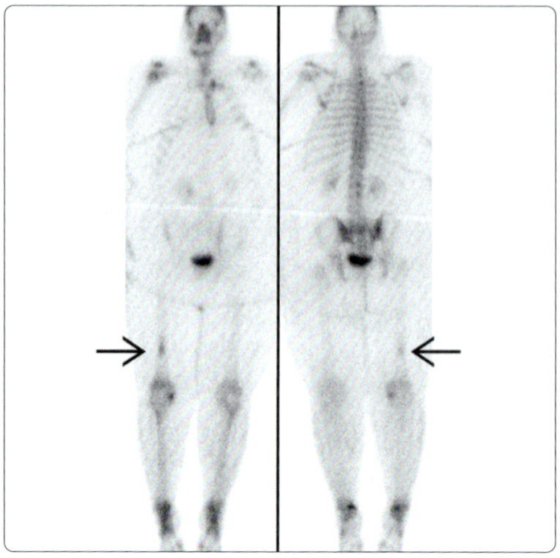

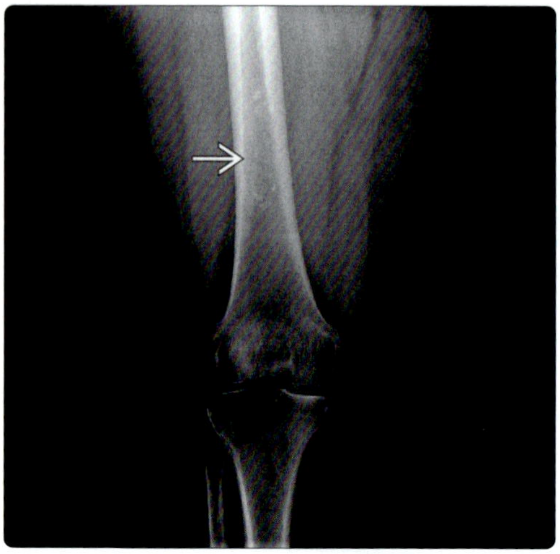

(Left) *Anterior bone scan in a skeletally immature patient shows a focus of increased activity ⇨ within the right mandible in patient with biopsy-proven giant cell tumor (GCT).* **(Right)** *Transaxial NECT (bone window) of the same patient shows an expansile lesion with mixed soft tissue heterogeneity and wispy septations ➡ within the right parasymphyseal region and body of the mandible.*

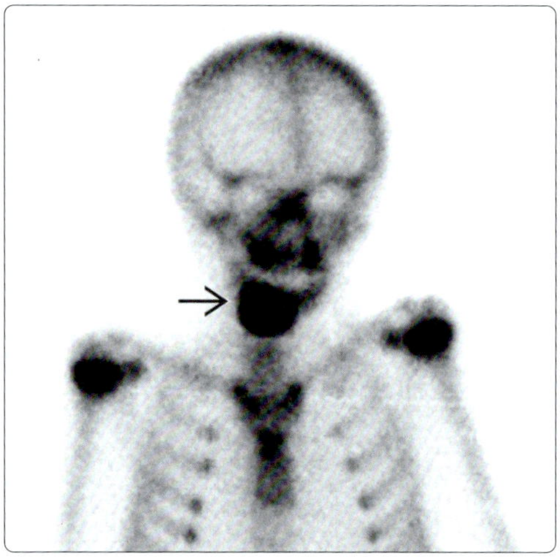

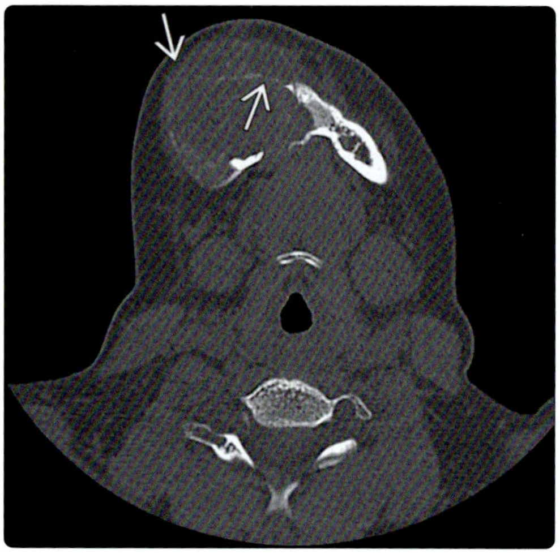

(Left) *Anterior and posterior whole-body bone scan in a patient with known GCT shows focal increased uptake in the left lateral femoral condyle ⇨.* **(Right)** *AP radiograph of the left knee in the same patient shows a lytic expansile lesion ➡ in the lateral femoral condyle that is compatible with a GCT.*

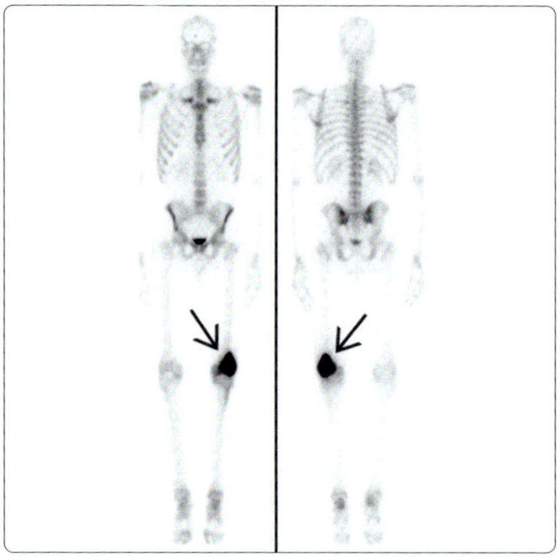

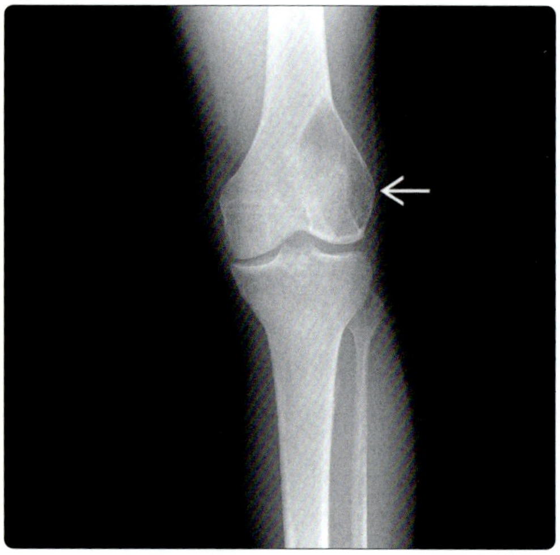

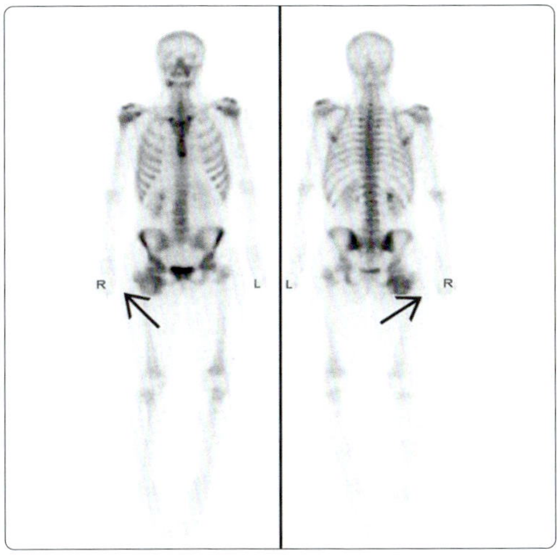

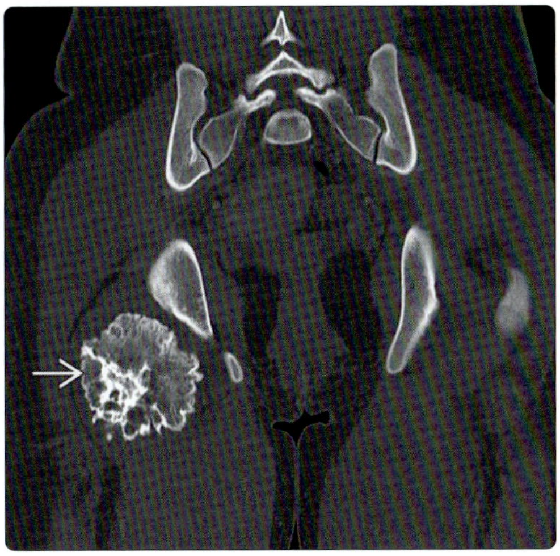

(Left) *Whole-body anterior and posterior bone scan shows a large region of uptake involving the right proximal femur* ⇨. *The uptake appears to extend beyond the expected cortical margins of the proximal femur. No polyostotic disease is shown.* **(Right)** *Coronal CT in the same patient shows an exophytic mass* ➡ *with contiguous cortex and a medullary cavity with the femoral neck (not shown). Findings are compatible with a solitary osteochondroma.*

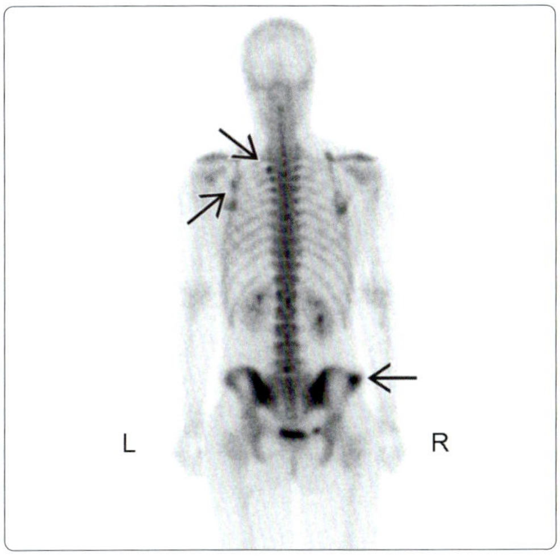

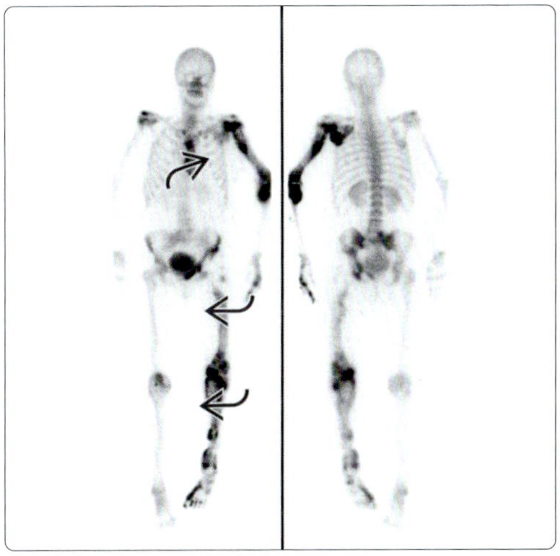

(Left) *Posterior bone scan shows multiple foci* ⇨ *of activity involving the right iliac crest, posterior left 3rd rib, and left scapula. These findings were proven to be multiple hereditary exostoses.* **(Right)** *Whole-body anterior and posterior bone scan shows multiple long segment lesions with predominant left-sided involvement. Deformities of the left upper and lower extremities are also shown* ↷. *These findings are most compatible with polyostotic fibrous dysplasia.*

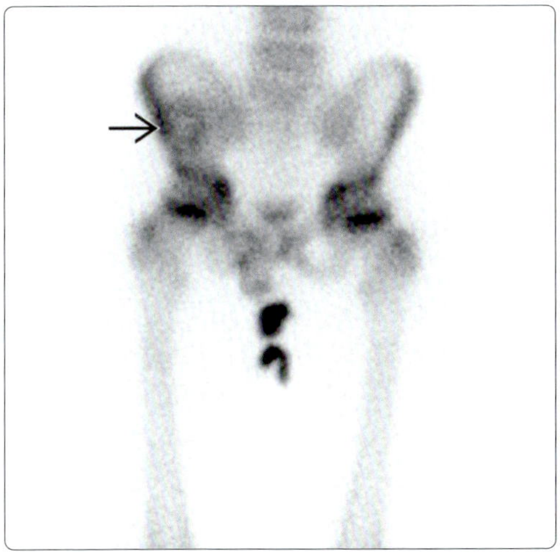

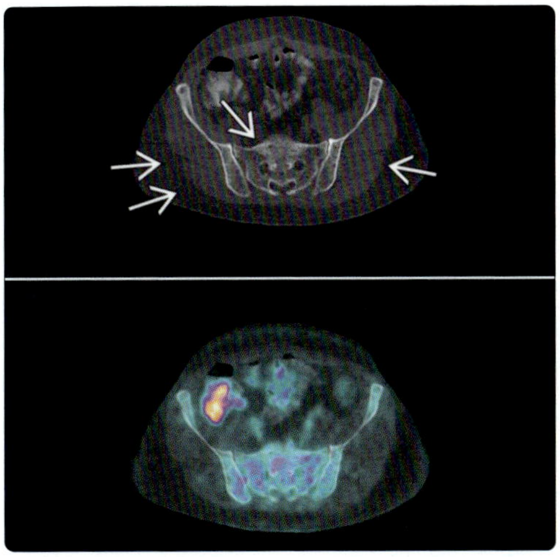

(Left) *Right iliac osteoid osteoma* ⇨ *is shown on this anterior static bone scan. Typically, the nidus would show intense uptake with less intense uptake in the surrounding sclerosis, creating a double density sign.* **(Right)** *F-18 FDG PET/CT for assessment of treatment response in a patient with multiple myeloma shows innumerable lytic lesions* ➡ *in the pelvic bones and sacrum without significant F-18 FDG uptake. These findings are most compatible with treated multiple myeloma.*

KEY FACTS

IMAGING

- Whole-body bone scan
  - Focal increased uptake on bone scan
    - Most metastases show ↑ tracer accumulation on bone scan, indicating cortical remodeling
    - Multifocal lesions in random distribution in areas of accelerated osteoblastic remodeling
      - Only 15% of solitary lesions on bone scan are metastases (spine is most common site)
      - Solitary rib lesion often benign (~ 10% metastases)
      - Solitary skull lesions often benign (can be seen in ~ 10% of patients without metastases)
  - Focal photopenia on bone scan
    - Usually aggressive, overwhelmingly osteolytic/osteoclastic tumors
    - 80% of photopenic lesions are metastases in cancer patients
    - Differential diagnosis: Radiotherapy (multiple adjacent vertebrae), bone infarct (sickle cell disease), avascular necrosis
  - Superscan
    - Disseminated bone lesions with diffusely increased skeletal activity, relative absence of renal and soft tissue activity
  - Flare phenomenon
    - Mixed response bone scan post-therapy: Some lesions resolved, some stable, some new
    - Increased conspicuity and number of lesions can occur due to healing and osteoblastic remodeling by 4-6 weeks post therapy
  - False-negative bone scan
    - Tumors confined to marrow may have no significant cortical remodeling and may not be visualized on bone scan

(Left) *Lateral oblique bone scan in a patient with breast cancer shows increased uptake in the skull base, indicative of metastasis.* **(Right)** *Posterior bone scan in a patient with breast cancer shows the typical elongated appearance of multiple rib metastases. Note multiple vertebral metastases.*

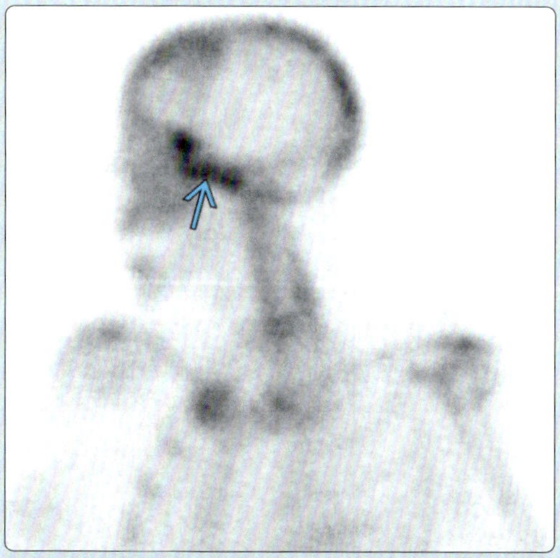

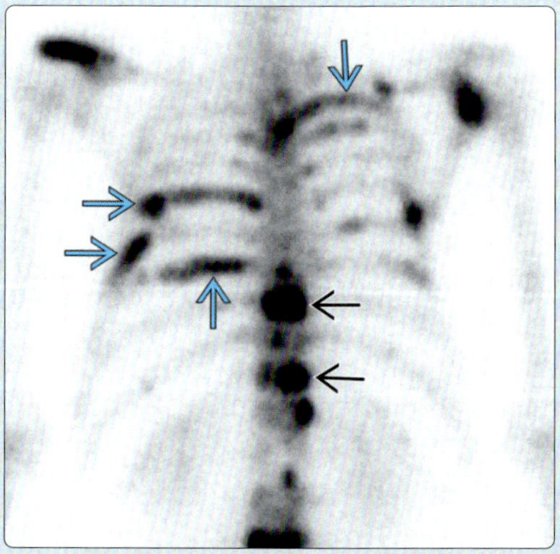

(Left) *Posterior bone scan in a patient with sebaceous carcinoma of the forehead shows focal increased uptake in multiple adjacent ribs, consistent with rib fractures. The exact location of the additional area of focal uptake in a rib or inferior angle of the scapula is difficult to determine due to overlapping anatomy.* **(Right)** *Posterior bone scan with the arm abducted confirms the location of increased uptake in the inferior angle of scapula. Chest CT showed healing fracture.*

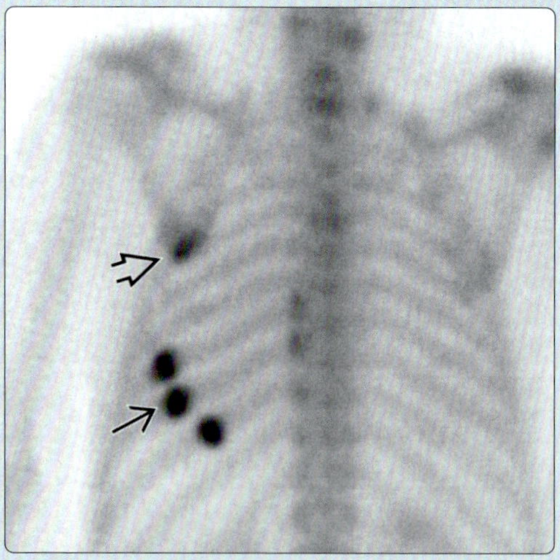

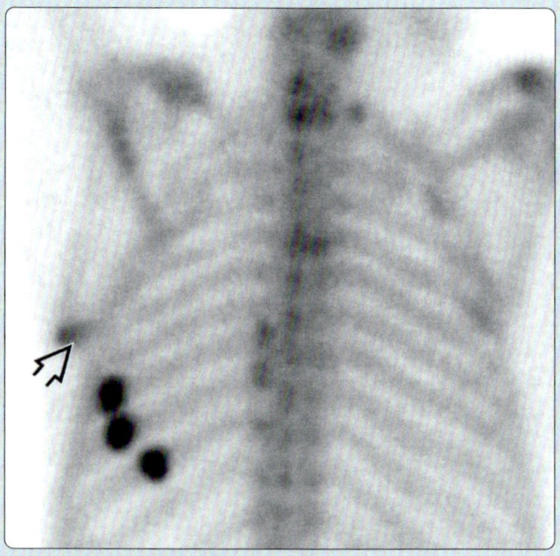

IMAGING

General Features

- Best diagnostic clue
  - Whole-body bone scan
    - Multifocal lesions in random distribution in areas of accelerated osteoblastic remodeling
    - Most metastases show ↑ tracer accumulation on bone scan, indicating cortical remodeling
- Location
  - Ribs, spine, pelvis, appendicular bones (esp. proximal femora and humeri), sternum, calvarium
  - Randomly distributed (vs. patterns of trauma, metabolic bone disease, or other benign process)
  - Especially areas of red marrow
  - Less common distally in long bones
- Typical appearance of osteoblastic metastases
  - Multiple scattered bone lesions
    - Predilection for red marrow (axial and proximal appendicular skeleton)
    - Lesions in distal long bones uncommon
  - Only 15% of solitary lesions on bone scan are metastases (spine is most common site)
    - Exception: 80% of solitary sternal lesions in breast cancer patients are metastatic
    - Vertebrae: Asymmetric, focal uptake (not confined to endplate), involvement of pedicle suggestive of metastasis
  - Solitary rib lesion often benign (~ 10% metastases)
    - Ribs: Long, linear uptake suggestive of metastasis, may be expansile
  - Solitary skull lesions often benign (can be seen in ~ 10% of patients without metastases)
- Photopenic metastases
  - Usually aggressive, overwhelmingly osteolytic/osteoclastic tumors
  - 80% of photopenic lesions are metastases in cancer patients
  - Renal cell carcinoma, thyroid carcinoma, poorly differentiated anaplastic tumors, myeloma
    - Occasionally lung, breast, neuroblastoma
  - Differential diagnosis: Radiotherapy (multiple adjacent vertebrae), bone infarct (sickle cell disease), avascular necrosis
- Superscan
  - Disseminated bone lesions with diffusely increased skeletal activity, relative absence of renal and soft tissue activity
  - Breast and prostate cancers most common
- Flare phenomenon
  - Mixed response bone scan post therapy: Some lesions resolved, some stable, some new
  - Increased conspicuity and number of lesions can occur due to healing and osteoblastic remodeling by 4-6 weeks post therapy
  - Do not confuse with disease progression; bone pain may also increase during flare
  - Exercise caution in interpretation for ~ 3-6 months: Activity declines and tends to resolve thereafter
  - F-18 FDG PET/CT can help distinguish treatment-induced flare and tumor response from progression
- False-negative bone scan
  - Tumors confined to marrow may have no significant cortical remodeling and may not be visualized on bone scan
  - Multiple myeloma, anaplastic neoplasms, renal cell carcinoma, thyroid carcinoma, neuroblastoma, histiocytosis, reticulum cell sarcoma

Imaging Recommendations

- Best imaging tool
  - **Whole-body bone scan**
    - For diagnosis of skeletal metastases, staging, restaging, assessment, and monitoring response to therapy
    - Most efficient imaging modality, allows whole-body evaluation with single study
    - SPECT/CT may be added for 3D and anatomic evaluation
    - Sensitivity 80-90%, better than plain radiograph or CT but somewhat nonspecific
    - Plain film correlation for ambiguous or solitary lesions; additional evaluation with diagnostic CT or MR as necessary
- Protocol advice
  - Whole-body bone scan
    - Patient preparation
      - □ Hydrate patient prior to and during the procedure to improve target to background activity
      - □ Patient should urinate prior to imaging
    - Radiopharmaceutical: Tc-99m methylene diphosphonate (MDP) or Tc-99m hydroxymethylene diphosphonate (HDP)
      - □ Inject tracer in extremity away from sites of interest to prevent false-positive results due to endovascular pooling, venous valvular adherence
    - Dose: Adults: 20-30 mCi (740 MBq to 1.1 GBq) Tc-99m MDP or HDP IV; markedly obese adults: 0.3-0.35 mCi/kg (11-13 MBq/kg)
      - □ Pediatric dose: 0.25-0.3 mCi/kg (9-11 MBq/kg), minimum: 0.5-1.0 mCi (2-4 MBq)
    - Image acquisition
      - □ Delayed (skeletal phase) images at 2-5 hrs after tracer injection
      - □ Delayed (6-24 hrs) images may be helpful in patients with poor cardiac output, renal insufficiency, or urinary retention
      - □ Energy window: 20% centered at 140 KeV
      - □ Continuous whole-body scan: Determine count rate (usually anterior chest), adjust scanning speed to obtain > 1.5 million counts for anterior or posterior planar whole-body image
      - □ Spot images: 1st spot view of axial skeleton (usually chest) for 500,000 to 1 million counts, remainder spot views acquired for same time
    - Special views
      - □ Oblique views of ribs (lateral rib lesions, underlying renal activity)
      - □ Postvoid pelvic spot view: If bladder activity overlaps pelvic bones

Skeletal Metastases: Tracer Uptake Patterns on Bone Scan

Hot Lesions	Cold Lesions	Isointense Lesions
Breast cancer	Renal cell carcinoma	Renal cell carcinoma
Lung cancer	Thyroid carcinoma	Thyroid carcinoma
Prostate cancer	Anaplastic neoplasms	Anaplastic neoplasms
Transitional cell carcinoma	Neuroblastoma	Neuroblastoma
Colorectal cancer		Multiple myeloma
Medulloblastoma		Reticulum cell sarcoma
Osteosarcoma		Histiocytosis
Neuroendocrine tumors (carcinoid)		Leukemia, lymphoma
Lymphoma		

    - □ Sit on detector view: Evaluation of pelvic lesions (especially in patients with prostate cancer), urinary bladder activity overlapping bones, and patient unable to void completely
    - □ Thorax with arm abducted and adducted to differentiate rib and scapular activity
    - □ SPECT and SPECT/CT: Helpful for evaluation of suspicious lesions within pelvis and spine
- Additional nuclear medicine imaging techniques
  - **F-18 NaF PET/CT**
    - Highly sensitive bone-seeking PET tracer; greater sensitivity and better spatial resolution than bone scan
    - Better pharmacokinetics with 2x greater bone uptake and faster blood clearance
    - Adult dose: 5-10 mCi (185-370 MBq) IV, for markedly obese adults: 10 mCi (370 MBq)
    - Pediatric dose: 0.06 mCi/kg (2.22 MBq/kg), range: 0.5-5 mCi (18.5-185 MBq)
  - **F-18 FDG PET/CT**
    - More sensitive and specific as compared to Tc-99m MDP/HDP bone scan for osteolytic lesions (e.g., non-small cell lung cancer, lymphoma)
    - Reveals marrow lesions in F-18 FDG-avid disease prior to cortical involvement (often before bone scan becomes positive)
    - Limited sensitivity for osteoblastic or some slow-growing lesions

DIFFERENTIAL DIAGNOSIS

Degenerative Processes, Arthropathies

- Acromioclavicular & sternoclavicular joints, intervertebral disc spaces, facet joints (esp. lower cervical/lumbar spine), knees, 1st carpometacarpal joints, and small joints of feet

Healing Fracture or Bone Injury

- Usually focal rather than infiltrative or elongated
- Exclude pathologic fracture on correlative imaging

Physiologic Activity

- Nasopharynx, calvarium, sacroiliac joints, excreted tracer in urinary tract
- Growth plates in skeletally immature patient
  - May obscure underlying metastatic disease such as neuroblastoma; look for asymmetry

Primary Bone Tumors

- Lymphoma, myeloma, enchondroma, osteoma, fibrous dysplasia

Avascular Necrosis, Osteonecrosis, Infarct

- Femoral and humeral heads, knees

Metabolic Disease, Infection, or Inflammation

- Brown tumor of hyperparathyroidism
- Orthopedic hardware complications
- Periodontal disease
- Paget disease

CLINICAL ISSUES

Presentation

- Most common signs/symptoms
  - Pain most common symptom
  - Typical presentation: History of primary malignancy and bone pain in absence of (or with trivial) corresponding insult
  - Bone pain without known primary (15%)
  - Lesion noted incidentally on conventional imaging
  - Abnormal alkaline phosphatase elevation
    - Present in ~ 50% of patients

DIAGNOSTIC CHECKLIST

Image Interpretation Pearls

- Suspicious for metastases: Increased tracer localization in lesions not attributable to trauma, degenerative changes, or physiologic activity
- Photopenic lesions are suspicious for highly aggressive lesions, marrow fibrosis (often post radiation), or marrow replacement (hemangioma)
- Single lesions may be difficult to categorize, necessitating additional imaging

SELECTED REFERENCES

1. Davila D et al: Evaluation of Osseous Metastasis in Bone Scintigraphy. Semin Nucl Med. 45(1):3-15, 2015
2. Cheung FH: The practicing orthopedic surgeon's guide to managing long bone metastases. Orthop Clin North Am. 45(1):109-19, 2014
3. Mick CG et al: Molecular imaging in oncology: (18)F-sodium fluoride PET imaging of osseous metastatic disease. AJR Am J Roentgenol. 203(2):263-71, 2014

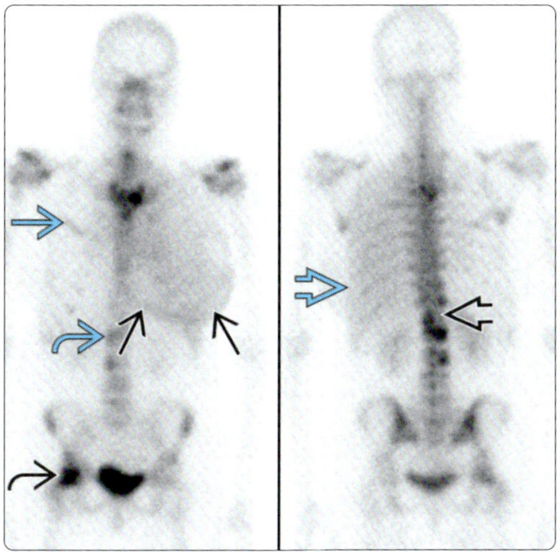

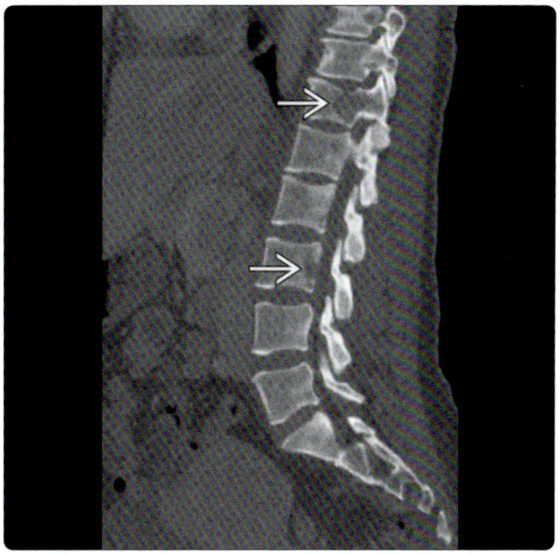

(Left) *Anterior and posterior bone scan in a patient with breast cancer shows increased uptake in the left breast, multiple skeletal metastases, and mild diffuse increased uptake in malignant pleural disease posteriorly. Note both the increased and decreased tracer uptake in spine metastases. Note also uptake in the rib, spine, and right femur.* **(Right)** *Sagittal CT MRP reconstruction in the same patient shows multiple lytic spine metastases.*

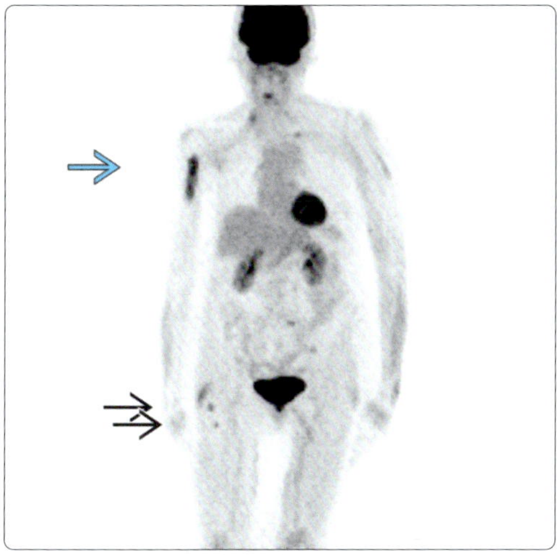

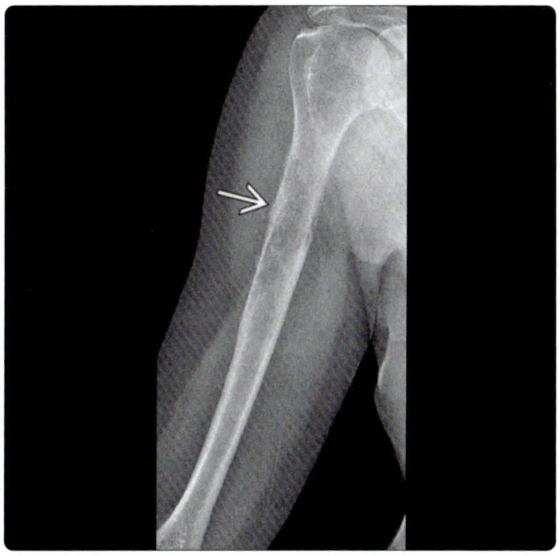

(Left) *Anterior F-18 FDG PET MIP in a patient with breast cancer shows linear increased tracer uptake in the right proximal humerus, indicative of metastasis. Note 2 small foci of increased uptake in the right proximal femur, indicative of additional sites of metastases.* **(Right)** *Anterior radiograph of the right humerus in the same patient shows a lytic lesion corresponding to increased uptake on bone scan consistent with metastasis.*

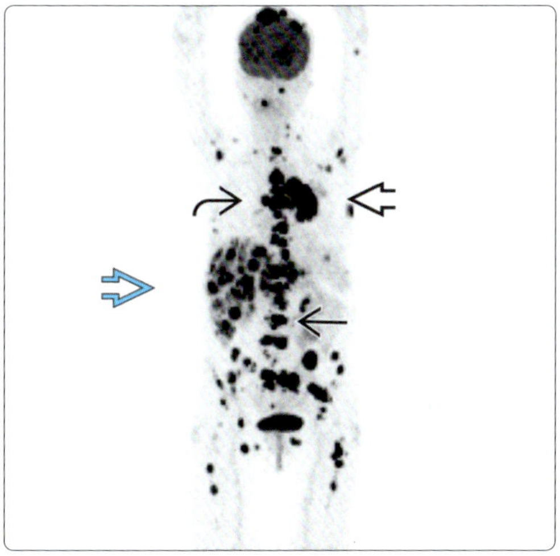

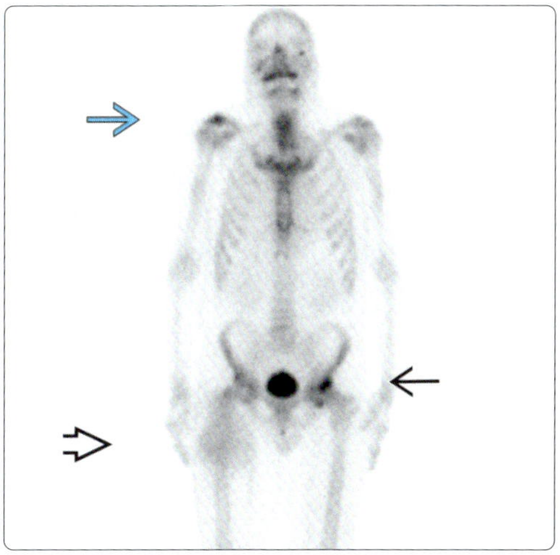

(Left) *Anterior F-18 FDG PET shows large hypermetabolic left parahilar lung cancer with hypermetabolic mediastinal lymph nodes, liver, and skeletal metastases.* **(Right)** *Anterior bone scan in a patient with myxoid liposarcoma shows subtle, ill-defined increased tumor uptake in the right proximal thigh. Incidental degenerative uptake is noted in the left hip joint and right acromioclavicular joint.*

(Left) *Anterior and posterior bone scan in a patient with breast cancer shows increased tracer uptake in the sternum and thoracic vertebra, indicative of metastases.* **(Right)** *Anterior and left lateral F-18 NaF PET in the same patient shows increased tracer uptake in the sternum, multiple thoracic and lumbar vertebrae, right ilium, and both pubis, indicative of metastases. Note higher sensitivity of F-18 NaF PET as compared to bone scan.*

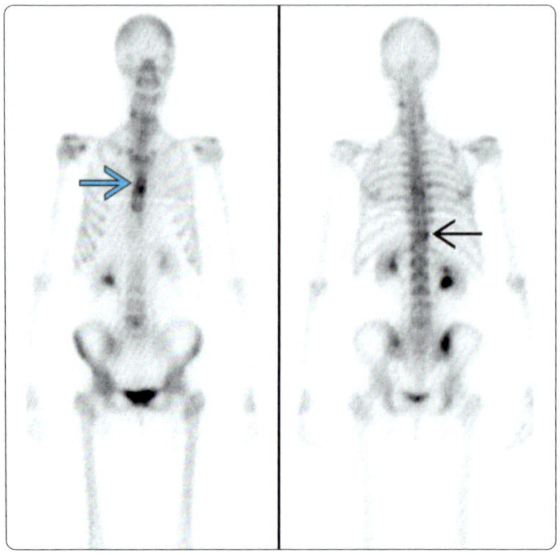

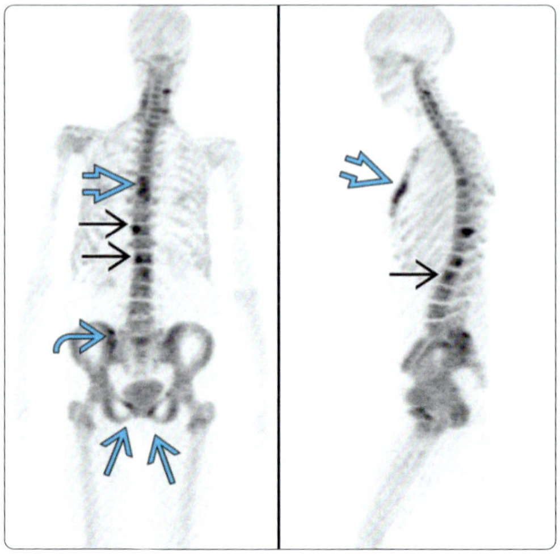

(Left) *Normal anterior and posterior bone scan is shown in a patient with breast cancer.* **(Right)** *Anterior and left lateral F-18 FDG PET in the same patient shows multiple skeletal and extraskeletal metastases. Uptake in a left breast mass, spine metastases, and left axillary lymph nodes is evident.*

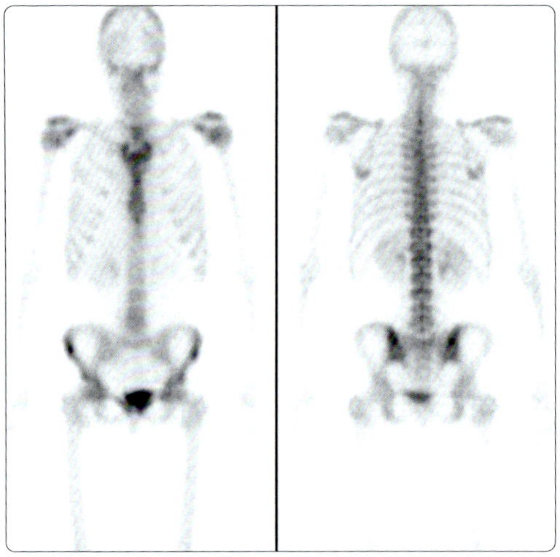

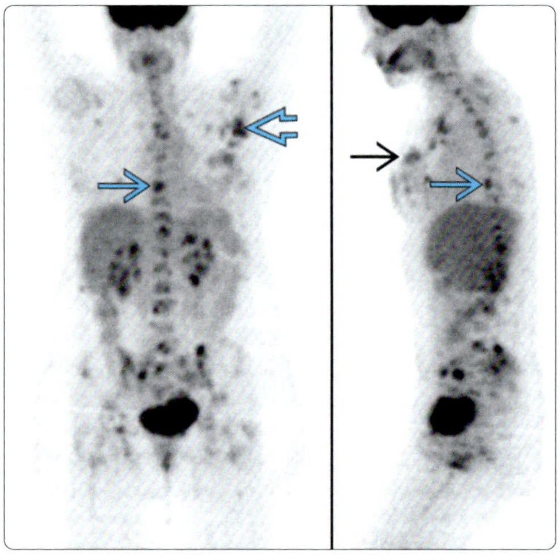

(Left) *Anterior and posterior bone scan in a patient with breast cancer shows multiple skeletal metastases. Note uptake in the spine and rib.* **(Right)** *Anterior and posterior bone scan in the same patient shows increased conspicuity of skeletal metastases after chemotherapy, consistent with flare phenomenon. Note the spine, rib, and pelvic metastases.*

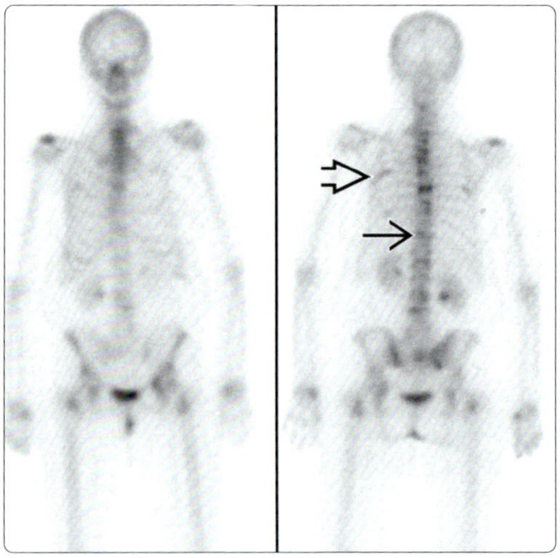

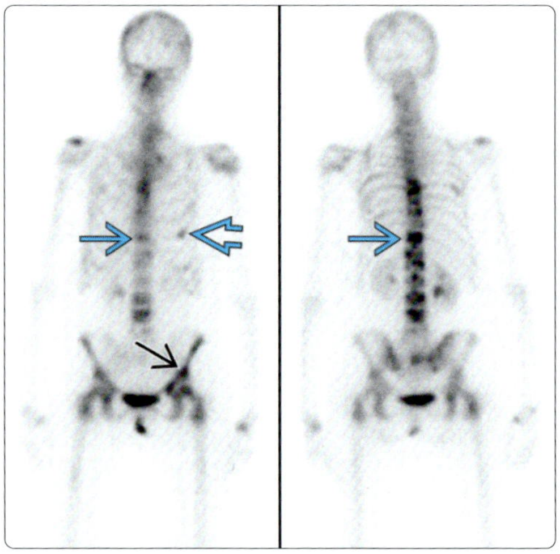

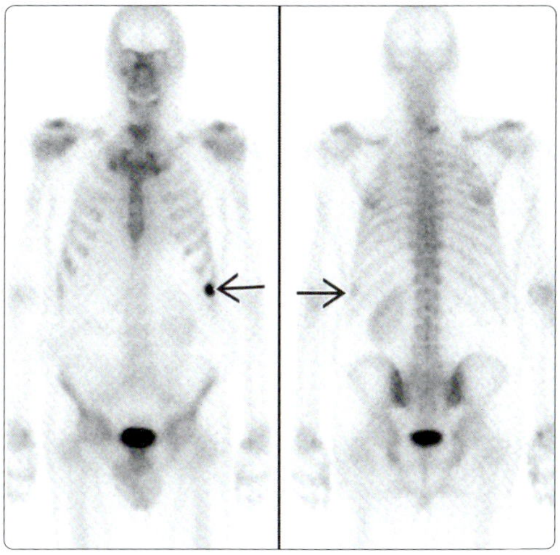

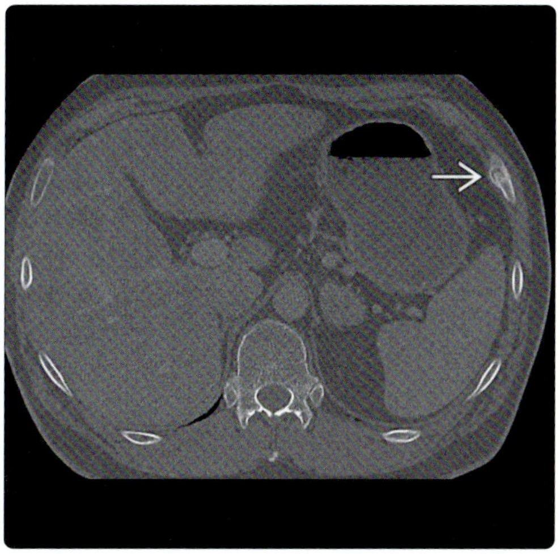

(Left) *Anterior and posterior bone scan in a patient with renal cell carcinoma shows a solitary focus of increased tracer uptake in the anterior end of the left 8th rib* ➙. **(Right)** *Axial CT in the same patient shows that focal increased uptake on bone scan corresponds to a subacute rib fracture* ➙.

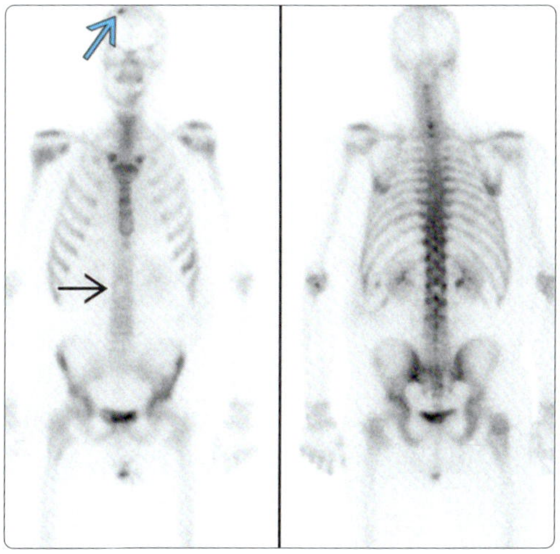

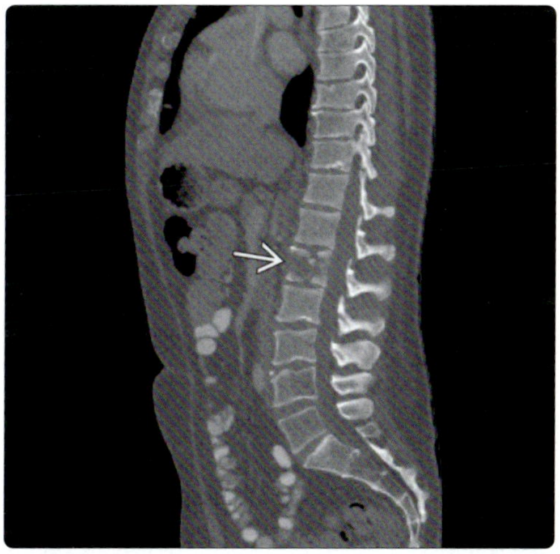

(Left) *Anterior bone scan in a patient with chondroblastic osteosarcoma shows focal increased tracer uptake in the skull* ➙*, consistent with metastasis. Note photopenic spine metastasis* ➙*. These are difficult to visualize on bone scan, and multiple additional lytic metastases could not be visualized.* **(Right)** *Sagittal CT in the same patient shows a lytic lesion with pathological fracture in the L1 vertebral body* ➙ *corresponding to photopenic spine metastasis.*

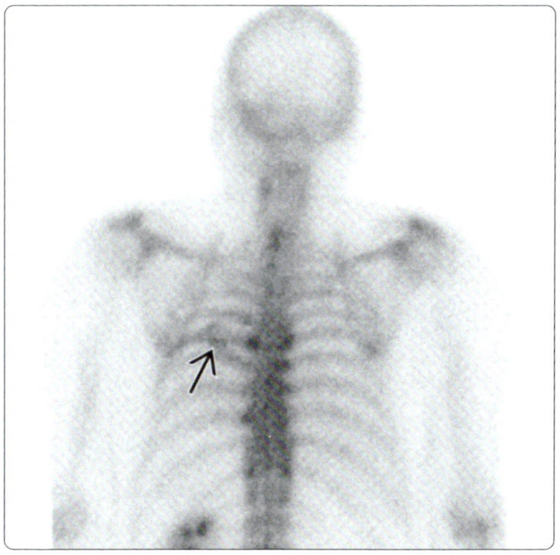

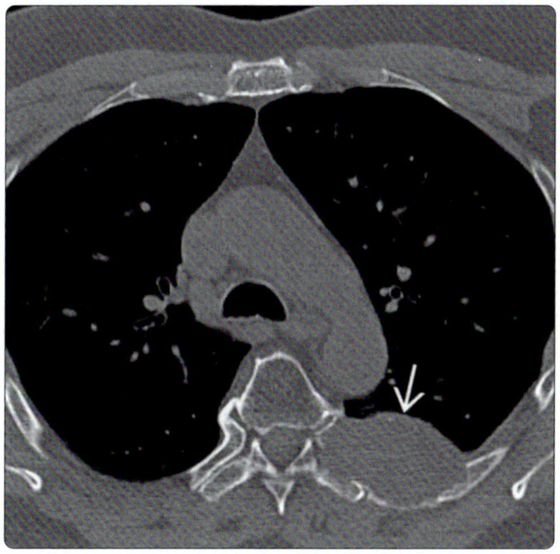

(Left) *Posterior bone scan shows central decreased and peripheral mildly increased tracer uptake in a lytic expansile rib metastasis* ➙ *from renal cell carcinoma. Renal cell carcinoma metastases can be cold on bone scan.* **(Right)** *Axial CT in the same patient shows a large large lytic expansile metastasis in the left 6th rib* ➙.

Fibrous Dysplasia

KEY FACTS

TERMINOLOGY

- Fibrous dysplasia (FD): Fibrous tissue replaces normal medullary spaces
  - Monostotic: Ribs > femur > facial bones
  - Polyostotic: Diaphyseal or metaphyseal femur > tibia > pelvis > foot > ribs, skull, facial bones
  - Craniofacial: Bones of sinuses > temporal, occipital
  - Cherubic: Bilateral maxilla and mandible, symmetric

IMAGING

- Tc-99m MDP bone scan
  - Variable uptake, useful to evaluate extent of disease
- F-18 FDG PET
  - Variable uptake
- Ga-67 scintigraphy
  - Increased activity in FD

TOP DIFFERENTIAL DIAGNOSES

- Paget disease
- Osteogenesis imperfecta
- Bone tumors
- Neurofibromatosis

CLINICAL ISSUES

- Usually benign/self-limiting
- < 1% malignant degeneration
- Most polyostotic in patients < 15 years
- Monostotic often in patients > 30 years

DIAGNOSTIC CHECKLIST

- Significantly increased activity on bone scan with acute pain
  - Pathologic fracture
  - Malignant degeneration
    - Osteosarcoma > fibrosarcoma > malignant fibrous histiocytoma > chondrosarcoma

(Left) *Lateral radiograph of the left femur shows an expansile, lucent lesion ➔ in the diaphysis. There is no cortical disruption or internal matrix. Mild scalloping of the anterior cortex is present ➦.* **(Right)** *Anterior radiograph of the left femur in the same patient shows an expansile, lucent lesion ➔ in the diaphysis. No internal matrix or soft tissue mass is present. The cortex appears intact.*

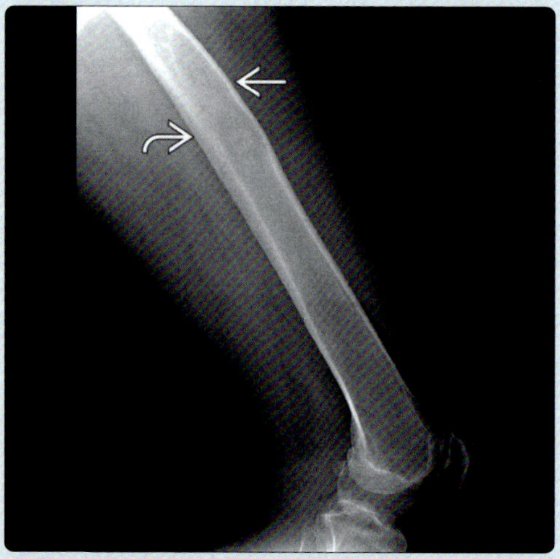

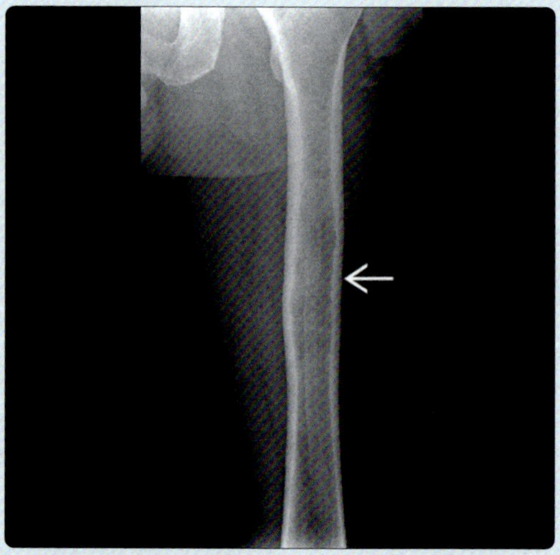

(Left) *Anterior bone scan in the same patient shows mildly increased activity ➔ in the left proximal femoral diaphysis. Otherwise arthritic/degenerative type of uptake is noted in the remainder of the skeleton. There is no scintigraphic evidence for polyostotic disease.* **(Right)** *Lateral static image of the left femur in the same patient shows mildly increased activity ➔ in the left proximal diaphysis. Joint centered degenerative uptake is shown in the knees.*

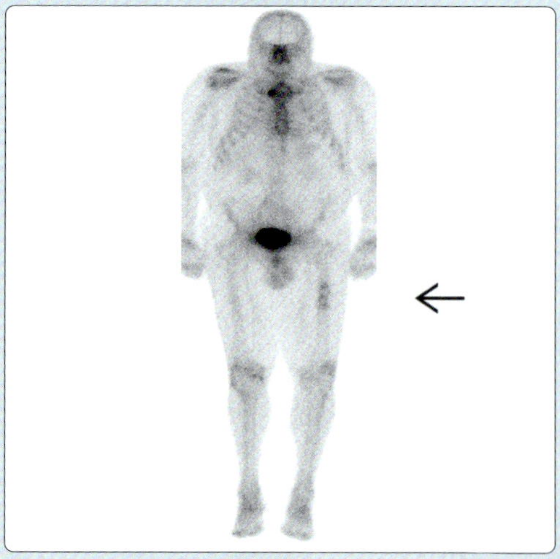

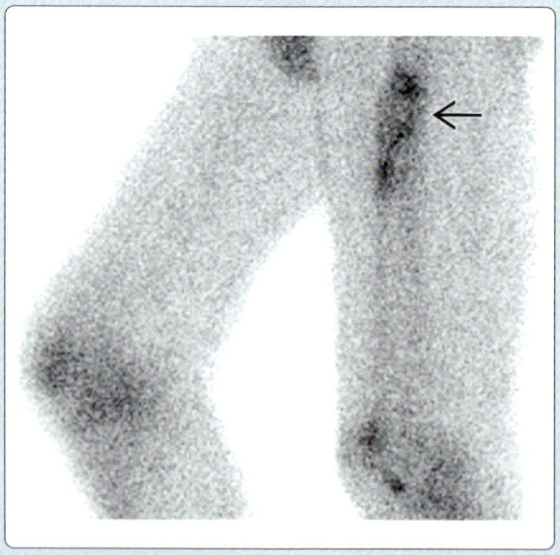

TERMINOLOGY

Abbreviations

- Fibrous dysplasia (FD)

Synonyms

- Lichtenstein-Jaffe disease
- Osteitis fibrosa disseminata
- Fibrous osteodystrophy

Definitions

- Fibrous tissue replaces normal medullary spaces
  - Weaker than normal bone
  - At risk for pain, pathologic fracture, bone deformity
- Usually an incidental finding

IMAGING

General Features

- Location
  - Eccentric lesion, but not in cortex
  - Monostotic
    - Ribs > femur > facial bones
  - Polyostotic
    - Diaphyseal or metaphyseal femur > tibia > pelvis > foot > ribs, skull, facial bones
  - Craniofacial
    - Bones of sinuses > temporal, occipital
  - Cherubic
    - Bilateral maxilla and mandible, symmetric

Nuclear Medicine Findings

- Ga-67 scintigraphy
  - Can show increased activity in FD
  - Not indicated for FD, typically incidental finding
- Tc-99m MDP bone scan
  - Uptake variable
  - Best utility: Identify monostotic vs. polyostotic FD
  - May identify (sensitive) subtle lesions not radiographically apparent
  - Specificity too low to diagnose FD with bone scan
  - Increased activity in pathologic fracture
- F-18 FDG PET/CT
  - Variable uptake may be based on active fibroblasts
  - May mimic osseous metastasis
  - Cannot reliably predict sarcomatous transformation
  - SUV cannot be used to diagnose FD
    - Localization CT images may be more useful to characterize lesion as FD

Radiographic Findings

- Lucent tumor-like lesion
- Medullary-based lesion
- Can be slightly eccentric
- Homogeneous appearance
- ± expansion
- Endosteal scalloping
- Dense sclerotic margin = rind sign
- Typically ellipsoid
- No periosteal reaction
- Radiolucent, ground-glass appearance
- Patient < 2 years of age does not have ground-glass appearance, rather streaked heterogeneous appearance
- Disruption of cortex in association with soft tissue mass at location of preexisting FD worrisome for malignant degeneration

CT Findings

- Intramedullary mass
- Expansile
- No mineral cortex typically
  - On occasion may have foci of cartilage
- No associated soft tissue mass
- Active lesions enhance
- Useful to define extent of individual lesions particularly in facial bones
- Exclude soft tissue mass

MR Findings

- Variations in cellular components account for their variable MR appearance
- Homogeneous ↓ T1
- Intermediate to high on T2
- Heterogeneous enhancement after gadolinium administration

Imaging Recommendations

- Protocol advice
  - Tc-99m MDP bone scan
    - Whole-body imaging key to establish monostotic vs. polyostotic disease
    - Planar spot images of known or suspected lesions
    - Consider SPECT/CT in skull/face and feet for optimal localization
    - 3-phase bone scan can be positive in all 3 phases
      - Not typically indicated in FD

DIFFERENTIAL DIAGNOSIS

Paget Disease

- Lytic, osteogenic, then sclerotic, flame-shaped, extending toward diaphysis

Osteogenesis Imperfecta

- Deformed, often curvaceous, long bones with moderate diaphyseal uptake

Bone Tumors

- Primary tumors; metastases mimic polyostotic FD

Neurofibromatosis

- Intramedullary lesions rare
- Smooth-bordered café au lait spots (coast of California)
  - McCune-Albright café au lait spots (jagged edges similar to coast of Maine)

PATHOLOGY

General Features

- Etiology
  - Developmental anomaly rather than neoplasm
  - Normal bone marrow replaced by fibroosseous tissue
    - Classically described as marrow replaced by Chinese characters

- Woven bone layers with fibrous tissue
- Gross appearance is firm, solid, white mass replacing medullary cavity
- Microscopic findings include irregular spindles of woven bone, usually nonmineralized, scattered throughout fibrocellular matrix
- Cartilage formation may occur
- Degree of haziness on radiography directly correlates with underlying histopathology
  - More radiolucent lesions have predominantly fibrous elements
  - More radiopaque lesions contain greater proportion of woven bone
- Genetics
  - Sporadic FD: No well-documented case of vertical transmission from parent to offspring
  - Linked to genetic mutation of 20q13.2-13.3
  - Cherubism: Autosomal dominant, variable
  - No environmental factors associated with disease
- Associated abnormalities
  - Calvarial and facial asymmetry, exophthalmos
  - Craniofacial form
    - Leontiasis ossea → leonine facies
  - Femur
    - Coxa vara (shepherd's crook)
  - McCune-Albright syndrome
    - FD
    - Café au lait spots (jagged edges similar to coast of Maine)
    - Endocrinopathy
      - Precocious puberty
      - Hyperthyroidism
      - Acromegaly
      - Cushing syndrome
  - Mazabraud syndrome
    - Single or multiple intramuscular myxomas with fibrous dysplasia; rare
  - Associated with aneurysmal bone cysts (ABC)

CLINICAL ISSUES

Presentation

- Most common signs/symptoms
  - Pain, pathologic fracture
    - Repetitive fractures at same site
    - More often pathologic fracture if associated ABC exists
  - Bone enlargement, expansion, deformity
  - Cranial nerve impingement
  - Most small lesions asymptomatic, incidentally noted
  - Pediatric patients often present with fracture or limp
    - < 2 years old

Demographics

- Age
  - Most polyostotic < 15 years
  - Monostotic often > 30 years

Natural History & Prognosis

- Usually benign/self-limiting
- < 1% malignant degeneration
  - Rapid expansion of preexisting FD lesion in association with pain

DIAGNOSTIC CHECKLIST

Consider

- Significantly ↑ activity on bone scan with acute pain
  - Pathologic fracture
  - Malignant degeneration
    - Osteosarcoma > fibrosarcoma > malignant fibrous histiocytoma > chondrosarcoma
- SPECT/CT in skull/face and feet for optimal localization

SELECTED REFERENCES

1. Bousson V et al: Fibrous dysplasia and McCune-Albright syndrome: imaging for positive and differential diagnoses, prognosis, and follow-up guidelines. Eur J Radiol. 83(10):1828-42, 2014
2. Bloem JL et al: Bone and soft tissue tumors of hip and pelvis. Eur J Radiol. 81(12):3793-801, 2012
3. Hsu W et al: Radionuclide imaging in the diagnosis and management of orthopaedic disease. J Am Acad Orthop Surg. 20(3):151-9, 2012
4. Sandhu SV et al: Clinicoradiologic perspective of a severe case of polyostotic fibrous dysplasia. J Oral Maxillofac Pathol. 16(2):301-5, 2012
5. Zhang Y et al: Multiple metastasis-like bone lesions in scintigraphic imaging. J Biomed Biotechnol. 2012:957364, 2012
6. Amit M et al: Fibrous dysplasia of the sphenoid and skull base. Otolaryngol Clin North Am. 44(4):891-902, vii-viii, 2011
7. Ihde LL et al: Sclerosing bone dysplasias: review and differentiation from other causes of osteosclerosis. Radiographics. 31(7):1865-82, 2011
8. Cook GJ et al: Miscellaneous indications in bone scintigraphy: metabolic bone diseases and malignant bone tumors. Semin Nucl Med. 40(1):52-61, 2010
9. Dumitrescu CE et al: McCune-Albright syndrome. Orphanet J Rare Dis. 3:12, 2008
10. Leet AI et al: Current approach to fibrous dysplasia of bone and McCune-Albright syndrome. J Child Orthop. 1(1):3-17, 2007
11. Fitzpatrick KA et al: Imaging findings of fibrous dysplasia with histopathologic and intraoperative correlation. AJR Am J Roentgenol. 182(6):1389-98, 2004
12. Nakahara T et al: Use of bone SPECT in the evaluation of fibrous dysplasia of the skull. Clin Nucl Med. 29(9):554-9, 2004
13. Zhibin Y et al: The role of radionuclide bone scintigraphy in fibrous dysplasia of bone. Clin Nucl Med. 29(3):177-80, 2004
14. Aoki J et al: FDG PET of primary benign and malignant bone tumors: standardized uptake value in 52 lesions. Radiology. 219(3):774-7, 2001

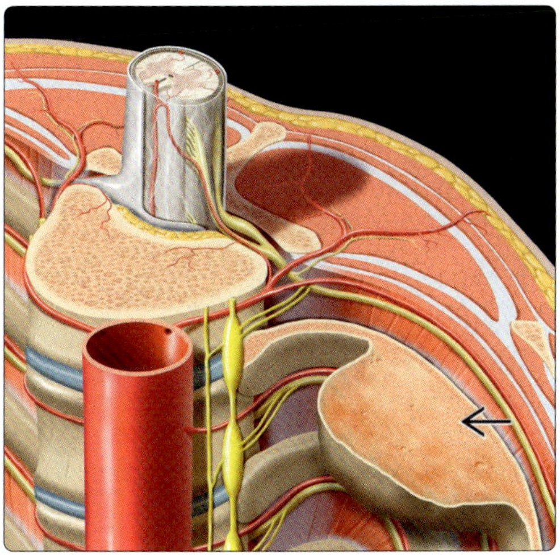

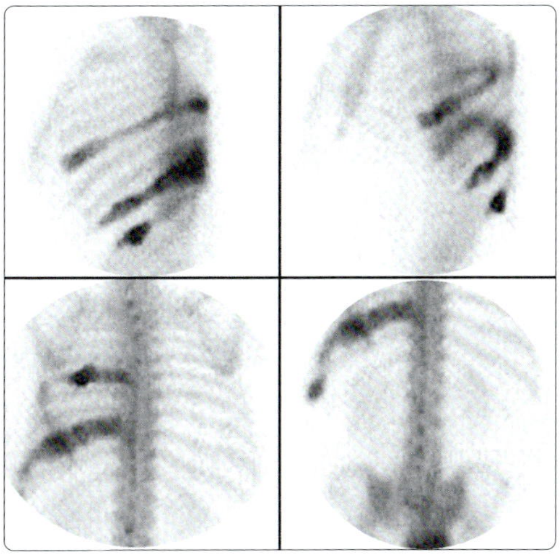

(Left) *Graphic of fibrous dysplasia involving a posterior rib shows intact cortex, intramedullary location, and expansile appearance →.* **(Right)** *Multiple spot images of the ribs show long segment activity in a slightly expanded appearance of the ribs. The findings are in keeping with polyostotic FD.*

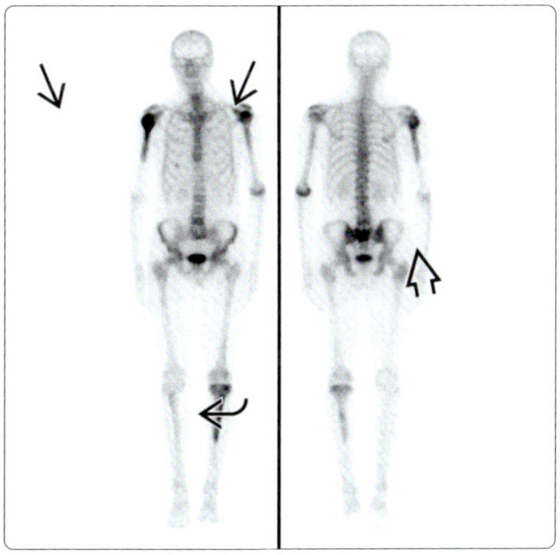

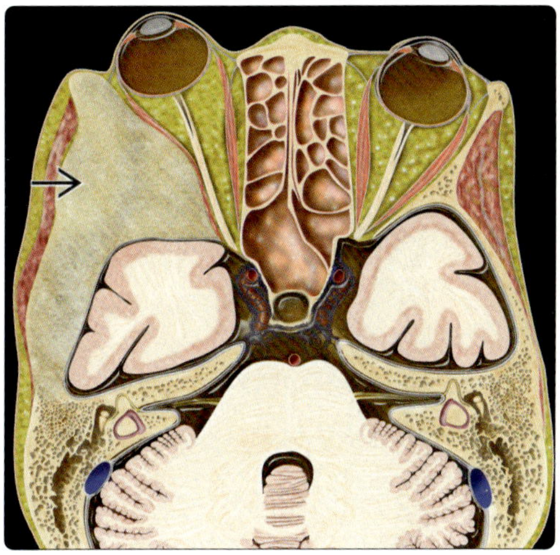

(Left) *Anterior and posterior whole-body bone scan shows multifocal long segment lesions involving the bilateral humeri → and left tibia →. A lesion in the sacrum is also noted →. Findings are compatible with polyostotic fibrous dysplasia.* **(Right)** *Graphic of fibrous dysplasia of the right sphenoid bone shows an intramedullary location and expansile appearance →. If bilateral, the presentation is often referred to as "cherubism."*

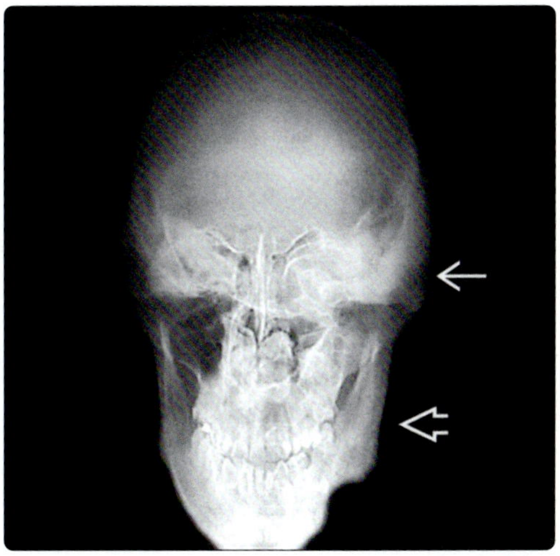

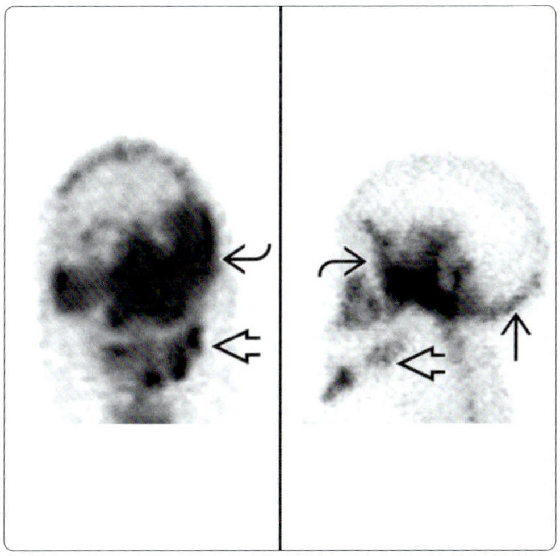

(Left) *AP radiograph of the skull and facial bones shows ground-glass density and expansion of the temporal bone → and mandible →.* **(Right)** *Anterior and lateral images of the calvarium in the same patient show increased activity in the left skull base →, temporal bone →, and mandible →. Combined with the radiographic findings, these findings are compatible with craniofacial FD.*

KEY FACTS

TERMINOLOGY

- Paget disease (PD) of bone; osteitis deformans; osteoporosis circumscripta (skull)
- Active disease begins with osteolytic phase followed by sclerotic or mixed active phase; inactive or quiescent phase demonstrates sclerotic lesions
- Although thickened, abnormal bone weaker and bone deformity or fracture common

IMAGING

- Intense activity & expansile appearance of entire affected bone on bone scan
- Pelvis (30-75%) > vertebra (30-75%) > skull (25-65%) > proximal long bones (esp. femur)
- Intensely ↑ bone scan uptake can be seen in all areas of active disease even before radiographic change
- Uptake may be particularly intense in lytic phase
- Typically involves whole bone
- Inactive or quiescent phase should show no increased uptake
- Osteoporosis circumscripta may show uptake only at margins of lesion
- Worsening lesion on bone scan raises possibility of superimposed primary or metastatic tumor
- After therapy for PD, bone scan may normalize, but often activity in lesion becomes heterogeneous

CLINICAL ISSUES

- Malignant degeneration rare (generally < 1%)

DIAGNOSTIC CHECKLIST

- Bone scan most sensitive test to detect PD
- Whole-body bone scan used to assess extent of PD
- Focal increased activity over background of affected bone: Consider fracture, malignant degeneration

(Left) *Anterior planar bone scan of a 76-year-old man shows diffuse increased uptake of tracer throughout the entire right femur ➔ typical of PD.* **(Right)** *Corresponding radiograph in the same patient shows marked cortical thickening and coarsened trabeculae ➔ throughout the proximal femur typical of PD.*

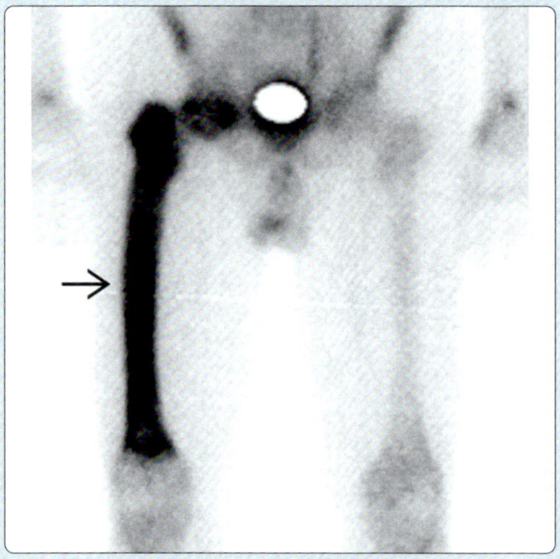

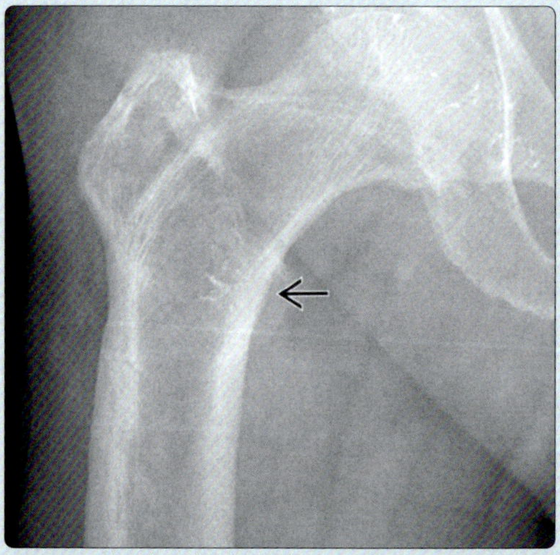

(Left) *Classic cotton wool skull uptake ➡ is shown in this bone scan of an elderly patient with Paget disease.* **(Right)** *Corresponding radiograph of this patient shows diffuse involvement of the skull.*

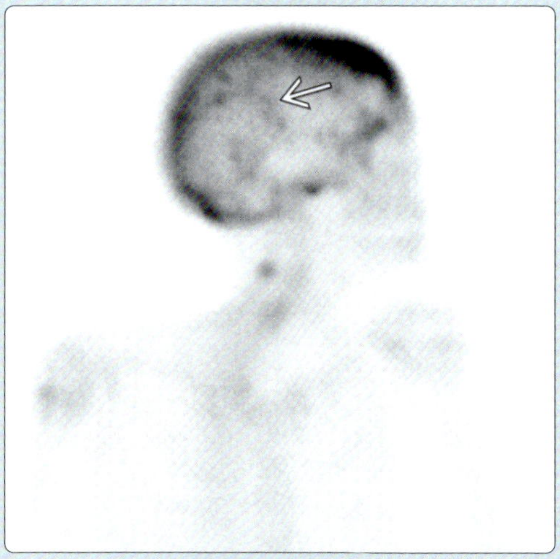

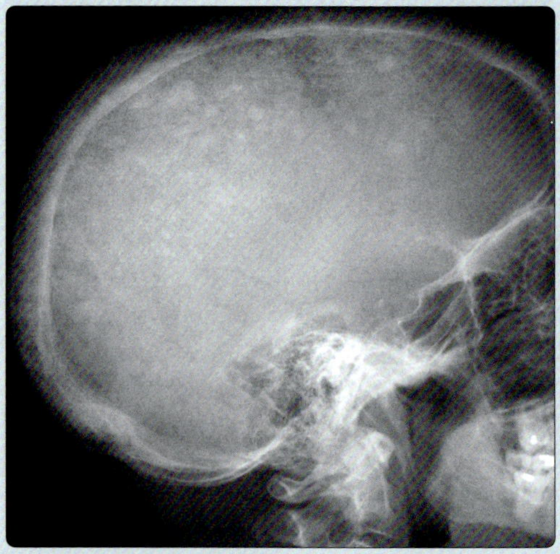

TERMINOLOGY

Abbreviations

- Paget disease (PD)

Synonyms

- Osteitis deformans; osteoporosis circumscripta (skull)

Definitions

- Disorder of abnormal/excessive bone remodeling characterized by coarse trabeculae, sclerosis, and expansion of one or more bones
- Active disease begins with osteolytic phase followed by sclerotic or mixed active phase; inactive or quiescent phase demonstrates sclerotic lesions
- Although thickened, abnormal bone is weaker and bone deformity or fracture is common

IMAGING

General Features

- Best diagnostic clue
  - Intense activity & expansile appearance of entire affected bone on bone scan
- Location
  - Predominantly axial skeleton, proximal femur
    - Pelvis (30-75%) > vertebra (30-75%) > skull (25-65%) > proximal long bones (esp. femur)
    - May affect any bone
    - Ribs, fibula, hands, feet uncommon
  - Polyostotic > monostotic (10-35%)
- Morphology
  - Lytic phase often → large, geographic lesion
  - Sclerotic or mixed phase: Coarse, thick trabeculae in expanded bone

Nuclear Medicine Findings

- Bone scan
  - Intensely ↑ uptake can be seen in all areas of active disease even before radiographic change
    - Uptake may be particularly intense in lytic phase
    - Typically involves whole bone
    - Inactive or quiescent phase should show no increased uptake
    - Osteoporosis circumscripta may show uptake at margins of lesion
  - Angiographic images from 3-phase bone scan show increased blood flow with intensity closely correlating with level of disease activity
  - Disease deterioration or recurrence often found on bone scan before lab value changes
  - Worsening lesion on bone scan raises possibility of superimposed primary or metastatic tumor
    - Cold region may appear if malignant lesion becomes necrotic
  - After therapy for PD, bone scan may normalize, but often activity in lesion becomes heterogeneous
- Labeled leukocyte scintigraphy
  - PD can cause increased uptake in absence of infection; Tc-99m sulfur colloid marrow map can confirm presence of expanded bone marrow
  - Photopenic defects can also occur with PD (hypocellularity with sclerosis)
- Ga-67 scintigraphy
  - Currently, not typically utilized for PD
  - Uptake usually of similar intensity to bone scan
  - Occasionally more accurate than bone scan alone in monitoring for malignant transformation
    - Development of malignancy will show ↑ accumulation compared to bone scan uptake
- PET
  - F-18 FDG PET/CT can show increased uptake, but cannot reliably distinguish malignant transformation
  - F-18 NaF PET bone scan can be used for semiquantitative analysis and serial follow-up

Radiographic Findings

- Skull: Osteoporosis circumscripta, focal cotton wool densities, and cranial thickening, esp. in frontal bone, with inner and outer table involvement
  - Cementomas in mandible and maxilla may affect teeth
- Spine: Picture frame vertebra or ivory vertebra; compression fracture; PD typically involves both body and posterior elements of same level
- Pelvis: Iliopubic/ilioischial thickening, unilateral extensive lesion common, acetabuli protrusio
- Long bones: Epiphyseal predominance with advancing wedge or flame-shaped osteolysis, deformity common

CT Findings

- Bone CT
  - Characteristic patterns similar to radiographs: Lysis then irregular coarsened trabeculae, expansile lesion

MR Findings

- Useful for evaluating neurological complications of disease or malignant degeneration
- Normal marrow signal until disease very advanced; mildly increased T1 and low T2 signal, unless tumor or fracture present, causing contrast enhancement or ↑ signal on T2WI

Imaging Recommendations

- Best imaging tool
  - Bone scan most sensitive modality for whole-body skeletal survey
    - Diagnose PD, extent of disease, and active/quiescent disease

DIFFERENTIAL DIAGNOSIS

Bone Metastases

- Most frequently differential concern encountered in work-up of PD
- Can mimic lytic or sclerotic phases of PD; intense uptake on bone scan can create falsely expanded appearance of bone

Primary Bone Tumor

- Primary bone tumors such as osteosarcoma and chondrosarcoma typically show markedly increased uptake on bone scan
- Benign tumors, i.e., giant cell tumor, aneurysmal bone cyst, and enchondromas are focal with mild uptake
- Radiographic correlation often diagnostic

Fibrous Dysplasia (FD)

- Benign developmental disorder leading to fibroosseous tissue replacing medullary spaces of one or more bones
- Favored sites of FD: Ribs, skull, femur
  - Rib and distal extremity involvement more common than in PD; spine and pelvic FD less common
- Bone scan: Moderate to intense radiotracer accumulation
- F-18 FDG PET/CT: Usually negative or minimal activity
- Presentation usually differs from PD: Young adults/teens, may be associated with cutaneous café au lait spots and endocrine abnormalities
- FD has widely variable radiographic appearance

PATHOLOGY

General Features

- Etiology
  - Proposed viral or slow viral etiology (controversial)
  - Some relation to paramyxovirus described; measles-like particles and respiratory syncytial virus antigens both found in some cases
- Genetics
  - Up to 40% have positive family history; 15-20% have first-degree relative affected
  - Certain genetic mutations such as 1/p62 found in familial form and some sporadic cases
- Associated abnormalities
  - Metastases may coexist; possibly increased blood flow causes increased susceptibility
  - Malignant degeneration
  - Giant cell tumors: Lytic lesions usually in facial bones
  - Plasma cell myeloma possibly associated

Microscopic Features

- Giant osteoclasts with more numerous nucleoli and intranuclear inclusion bodies → osteolysis
- Osteoblasts recruited for compensatory bone formation → deposition of disorganized lamellar bone
- Marrow spaces fill with fibrous connective tissue, blood vessels → hypervascularity
- Hypocellularity may ensue → regions of sclerotic bone only

CLINICAL ISSUES

Presentation

- Most common signs/symptoms
  - Asymptomatic in ~ 90%
  - Painful extremities, bowing long bones, 2° osteoarthritis
  - Neurological complications: Deafness, spinal cord compression
  - High-output CHF: Likely due to hyperemia in affected bones rather than arteriovenous malformations as previously thought
- Laboratory findings
  - ↑ serum alkaline phosphatase, ↑ urinary and serum hydroxyproline
    - Levels usually reflect disease status
    - Lower levels in patients with monostotic PD
  - Ca^{2+}, phosphorus and acid phosphatase usually normal

Demographics

- Age
  - Rare < 40 years, incidence increases with age
- Gender
  - M > F (1.8:1)
- Epidemiology
  - Incidence varies with geography: Greater in some cold climate countries and populations with ancestors from Great Britain and rare in Asia and Scandinavia

Natural History & Prognosis

- Many patients asymptomatic, requiring no treatment
- Lasting remission may be achieved
- Malignant degeneration rare (generally < 1%)
  - While risk low, it is ↑ in widespread disease (up to 5-10%)
  - 1° tumors: Osteosarcoma (50-60%) > fibrosarcoma (20-25%) > chondrosarcoma (10%)
  - Investigate worsening pain and soft tissue mass or developing lytic area, especially if previously sclerotic

Treatment

- Bisphosphonates (e.g., alendronate) first line
  - Binds onto bone matrix and inhibits osteoclast number and demineralization
- Calcitonin may be used to inhibit bone reabsorption; inhibitory effects on osteoclasts often incomplete
- Plicamycin (Mithracin): Inhibits RNA synthesis and osteoclast action; side effects common (renal/liver failure, bone marrow suppression)
- Osteotomy or surgical decompression of vertebral disease may be required for severe cases

DIAGNOSTIC CHECKLIST

Consider

- Bone scan most sensitive test to detect PD
- Whole-body bone scan used to assess extent of PD
- Focal increased activity over background of affected bone: Consider fracture, malignant degeneration
- Bone metastases vs. PD
  - New sites in patient with longstanding PD suggest metastatic disease
  - Radiographic, MR, biopsy correlation may be necessary to distinguish PD from metastases

SELECTED REFERENCES

1. Ralston SH et al: Pathogenesis of Paget disease of bone. Calcif Tissue Int. 91(2):97-113, 2012
2. Cortis K et al: Imaging Paget's disease of bone–from head to toe. Clin Radiol. 66(7):662-72, 2011
3. Theodorou DJ et al: Imaging of Paget disease of bone and its musculoskeletal complications: review. AJR Am J Roentgenol. 196(6 Suppl):S64-75, 2011
4. Layfield R: The molecular pathogenesis of Paget disease of bone. Expert Rev Mol Med. 9(27):1-13, 2007

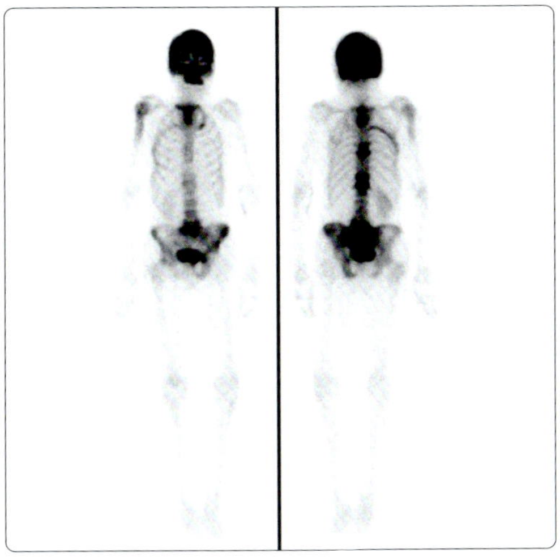

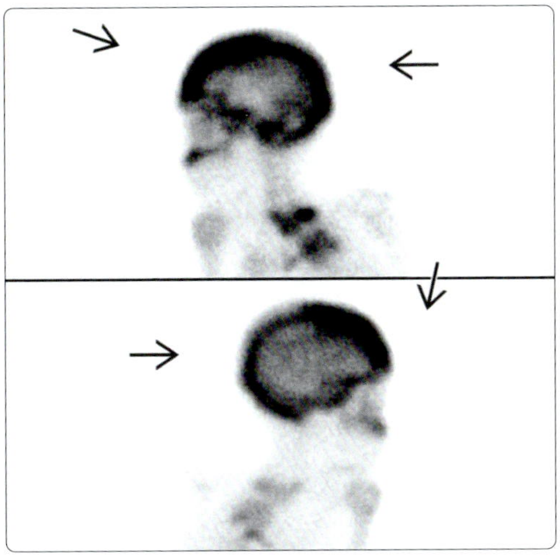

(Left) *Anterior and posterior whole-body bone scan shows multiple sites of pagetoid changes throughout the axial and appendicular skeleton.* **(Right)** *Lateral skull views of the same patient show increased activity along the calvarium →.*

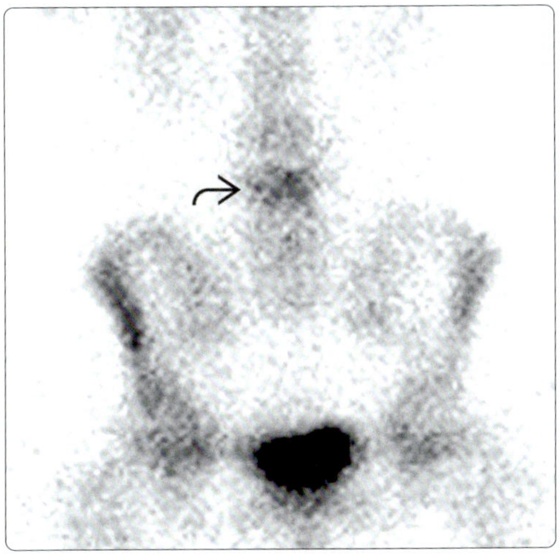

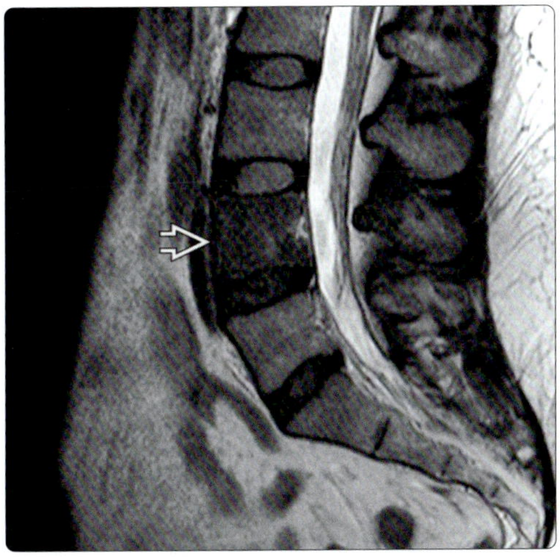

(Left) *Anterior bone scan shows minimal uptake in L4 vertebral body ↗ in a patient with stable, treated PD.* **(Right)** *Sagittal T2 MR of the same patient shows low signal in L4 vertebra ⇨, typical of advanced or treated PD.*

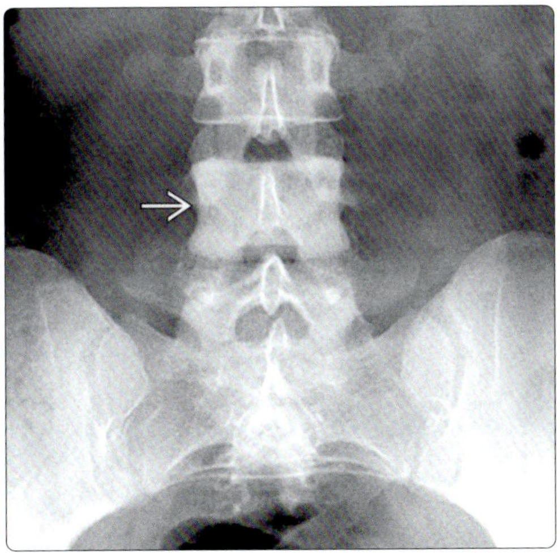

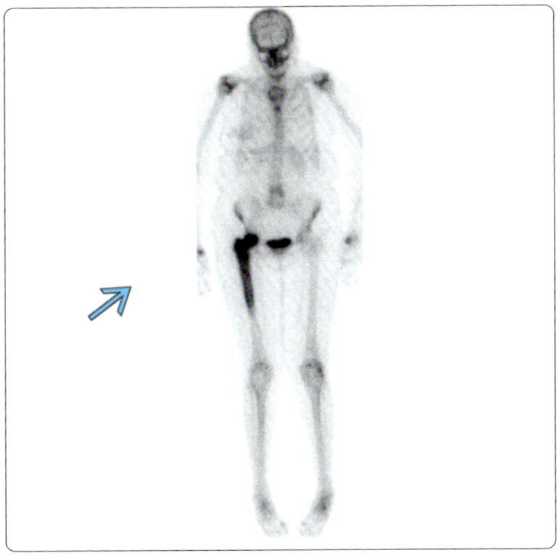

(Left) *AP radiograph shows diffuse sclerosis of L4 → causing a mild ivory vertebra appearance typical of PD. (Courtesy R. Lopez, MD.)* **(Right)** *Anterior whole-body bone scan shows increased activity in the right proximal → femur with a leading edge in a V-shape distally, compatible with monostotic PD.*

KEY FACTS

TERMINOLOGY

- Osteopenia
  - Bone density that is not normal but also not as low as osteoporosis
  - According to WHO criteria, osteopenia is defined as BMD lying 1.0-2.5 standard deviations below average value for young healthy women (T-score of -1.0 < -2.5 SD)
- Osteoporosis
  - Systemic skeletal disease characterized by low bone mass and microarchitectural deterioration of bone tissue with consequent increase in bone fragility and susceptibility to fracture
  - According to WHO criteria, osteoporosis is defined as BMD lying 2.5 standard deviations or more below average value for young healthy women (T-score of < -2.5 SD)

IMAGING

- Dual x-ray absorptiometry (DXA) is considered current gold standard for osteoporosis diagnosis and fracture risk prediction

DIAGNOSTIC CHECKLIST

- T-scores are reported for postmenopausal women and men aged 50 and older
- Z-scores are reported for premenopausal women and men under age of 50
- 1/3 radius used in obese patients, those with primary hyperparathyroidism, or if spine or hip cannot be measured or correctly interpreted
- Changes in BMD from one scan to another must exceed least significant change to be considered statistically significant

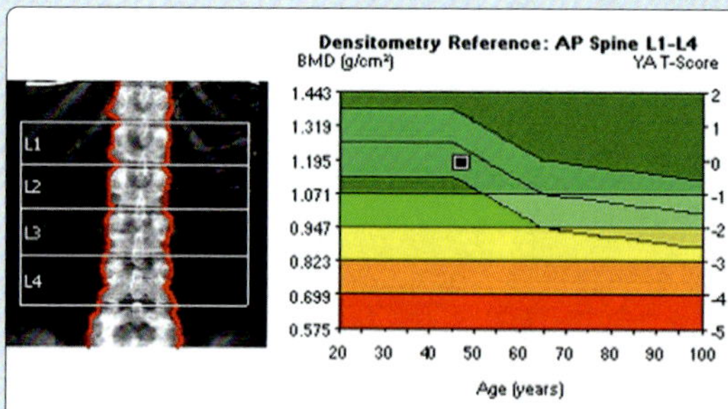

Region	BMD (g/cm²)	Young-Adult (%)	Young-Adult T-Score	Age-Matched (%)	Age-Matched Z-Score
L1	1.192	104	0.4	100	0.0
L2	1.178	97	-0.3	93	-0.8
L3	1.221	100	0.0	96	-0.5
L4	1.138	94	-0.6	89	-1.1
L1-L4	1.180	99	-0.1	94	-0.6

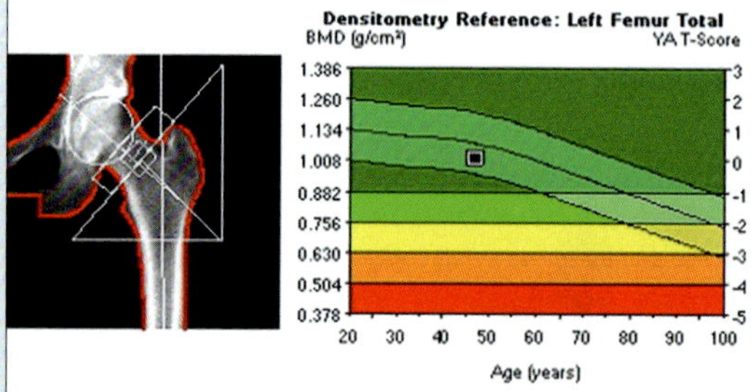

Region	BMD (g/cm²)	Young-Adult (%)	Young-Adult T-Score	Age-Matched (%)	Age-Matched Z-Score
Neck	0.980	94	-0.4	92	-0.6
Total	1.015	101	0.1	94	-0.5

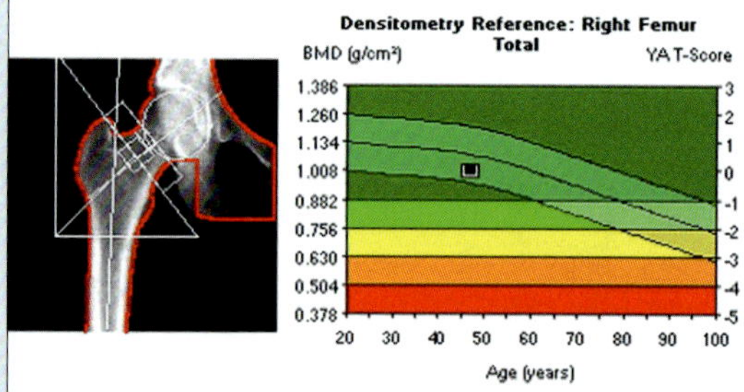

Region	BMD (g/cm²)	Young-Adult (%)	Young-Adult T-Score	Age-Matched (%)	Age-Matched Z-Score
Neck	0.939	90	-0.7	88	-0.9
Total	1.004	100	0.0	93	-0.6

Normal DXA of the spine and hips in a premenopausal woman is shown. The total spine Z-score is -0.1 and both hips are greater than -1.0.

TERMINOLOGY

Definitions

- Osteopenia
  - Bone density that is not normal, but also not as low as osteoporosis
    - According to WHO criteria, osteopenia is defined as BMD lying 1.0-2.5 standard deviations below average value for young healthy women (T-score -1.0 < -2.5 SD)
- Osteoporosis
  - Osteoporosis-related bone loss occurs when bone resorption exceeds bone formation
    - Peak bone mass occurs in the 20s
    - Bone loss increases with age and after menopause
  - Systemic skeletal disease characterized by low bone mass and microarchitectural deterioration of bone tissue with consequent increase in bone fragility and susceptibility to fracture
    - According to World Health Organization (WHO) criteria, osteoporosis is defined as BMD lying 2.5 standard deviations or more below average value for young healthy women (T-score < -2.5 SD)
- T-score
  - Calculated by taking difference between patient's measured BMD and mean BMD of healthy young adults, matched for gender and ethnic group, and expressing difference relative to young adult population SD
- Z-score
  - Compared with mean BMD expected for healthy subject matched for age, gender, and ethnic origin

IMAGING

General Features

- Best diagnostic clue
  - Dual x-ray absorptiometry (DXA)
    - Considered current gold standard for diagnosis of osteoporosis and fracture risk prediction
- Location
  - Lumbar spine and hip
  - 1/3 radius used in obese patients, those with primary hyperparathyroidism, or if spine or hip cannot be measured or correctly interpreted

Radiographic Findings

- Bone mass loss of 30-50% detected on radiography

CT Findings

- Quantitative CT (QCT)
  - Uses calibration phantom to determine volumetric BMD from Hounsfield units
    - Advantage over DXA is ability to evaluate cancellous bone and not cortical bone
    - Avoids soft tissue calcifications
    - Higher cost than DXA and more radiation to hip than DXA

Ultrasonographic Findings

- Quantitative ultrasound (QUS) measurements of BMD have been developed, but only measure peripheral bones (calcaneus, phalanges, etc.)
  - More portable, less expensive, and nonionizing as compared to DXA

Imaging Recommendations

- Best imaging tool
  - DXA
    - Considered current gold standard for diagnosis of osteoporosis and fracture risk prediction
      - Large, expensive equipment that is not portable and has ionizing radiation
    - Positioning spine straight and centered in field with inclusion of lowest vertebra with ribs and inferiorly to pelvic brim
    - Positioning of hip involves straightening femur with 15–25° of internal rotation, placing long axis of femoral neck perpendicular to x-ray beam, and is confirmed by little or no lesser trochanter seen on scan

Artifacts and Quality Control

- Degenerative disease in spine and hips may falsely elevate BMD
- Compression deformity in lumbar spine may falsely elevate BMD
- Systemic disease such as osteomalacia may underestimate bone mass
- Obesity, overlying metallic hardware, soft tissue calcifications, prior barium sulfate administration, scoliosis, and vertebral anomalies may also confound BMD measurements

PATHOLOGY

Staging, Grading, & Classification

- According to WHO, osteoporosis is defined by bone densitometry as T-score < -2.5
- According to WHO, osteopenia is defined by bone densitometry as T-score -1 to -2.5
- WHO fracture risk (FRAX) is assigned based on clinical risk factors, bone mineral density, and mortality data to quantify patient's 10-year probability of hip or major osteoporotic fracture
  - Uses only BMD of femoral neck
  - Country specific
  - Include risk factors of age, sex, low body mass index, prior fracture after age 50, parental history of hip fracture, smoking history, past or current use of corticosteroids, alcohol intake, other secondary causes of osteoporosis, and rheumatoid arthritis
    - Previous vertebral or hip fracture is the most important predictor of fracture risk
  - To reduce fracture risk, recommend treating patients with FRAX 10-year risk scores of ≥ 3% for hip fracture or ≥ 20% for major osteoporotic fracture

CLINICAL ISSUES

Demographics

- Epidemiology
  - 75 million people affected in US, Japan, and Europe
    - 10 million affected in US alone and 34 million are at risk

- Lifetime risk for wrist, hip, or vertebral fracture estimated to be 30-40%
- Osteoporotic fracture costs are in the tens of billions of dollars

Natural History & Prognosis

- 8.9 million fractures worldwide are due to osteoporosis
- Morbidity and mortality increase with fractures in elderly

Treatment

- Bisphosphonates
- Selective estrogen receptors modulators
- Hormone replacement
- Strontium
- Calcium and vitamin D supplementation

Risk Factors for Osteoporosis

- Genetic or constitutional
  - White or asian ethnicity
  - Family (maternal) history of fractures
  - Small body frame and long hip axis length
  - Premature menopause (<45 years) and late menarche
- Lifestyle
  - Nulliparity
  - Prolonged secondary amenorrhea
  - Smoking
  - Excessive alcohol intake
  - Inactivity
  - Prolonged immobilization
  - Prolonged parenteral nutrition
  - Low body weight
- Medical disorders
  - Anorexia nervosa
  - Malabsorption
  - Primary hyperparathyroidism
  - Thyrotoxicosis
  - Primary hypogonadism
  - Prolactinoma
  - Hypercortisolism
  - Rheumatoid arthritis
  - Chronic obstructive lung disease
  - Chronic neurological disorders
  - Chronic renal failure
  - Type I diabetes mellitus
  - Post transplantation
- Drugs
  - Chronic corticosteroid therapy
  - Excessive thyroid therapy
  - Anticoagulants
  - Chemotherapy
  - Gonadotropin-releasing hormone agonist or antagonist
  - Anticonvulsant
  - Chronic phosphate binding antacid use

DIAGNOSTIC CHECKLIST

Image Interpretation Pearls

- Evaluate for proper technique
  - For spine, patient should be centered on table and T12 to pelvic brim should be imaged
  - For hip, femur should be straight on table with 15-25º internal rotation and nonvisualization of lesser trochanter
- Assess for potential sources of error and artifact

Reporting Tips

- T-scores are reported for postmenopausal women and men aged 50 and older
- Z-scores are reported for premenopausal women and men under age of 50
  - Z-score of -2.0 or lower is below expected range for age
  - Z-score above -2.0 is within expected range for age
- Changes in BMD from one scan to another must exceed least significant change to be considered statistically significant
  - Least significant change is considered 2.8 times the precision error of technique

SELECTED REFERENCES

1. Pisani P et al: Screening and early diagnosis of osteoporosis through X-ray and ultrasound based techniques. World J Radiol. 5(11):398-410, 2013
2. Whitaker M et al: Bisphosphonates for osteoporosis–where do we go from here? N Engl J Med. 366(22):2048-51, 2012
3. Blake GM et al: The role of DXA bone density scans in the diagnosis and treatment of osteoporosis. Postgrad Med J. 83(982):509-17, 2007
4. Kanis JA: Diagnosis of osteoporosis and assessment of fracture risk. Lancet. 359(9321):1929-36, 2002
5. Kanis JA et al: Risk factors in osteoporosis. Maturitas. 30(3):229-33, 1998

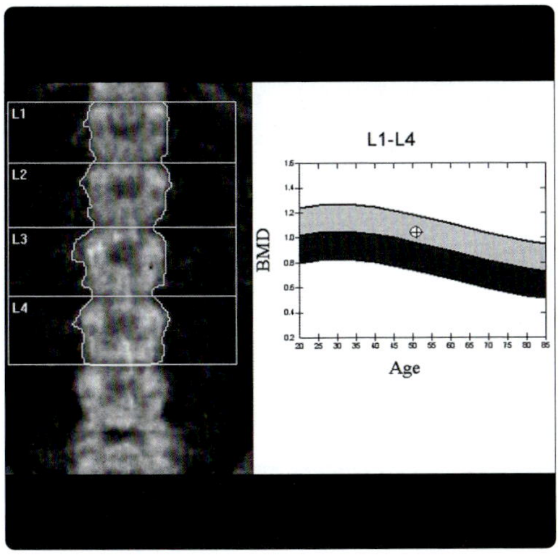

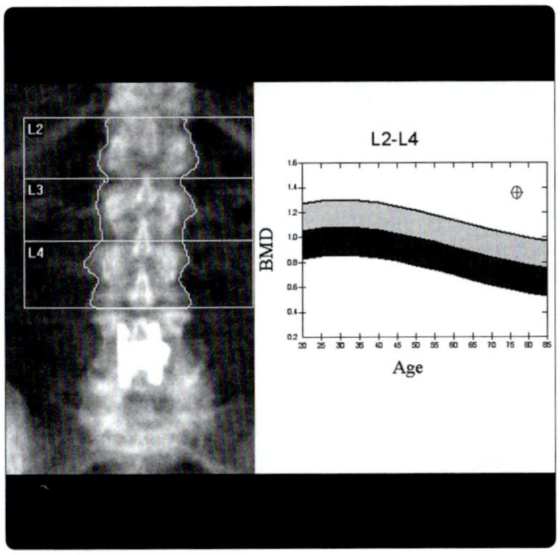

(Left) *Normal DXA of the lumbar spine is shown.* **(Right)** *DXA of the lumbar spine shows a quality control issue: Incorrect numbering of the lumbar spine (should be L1-L3). Metallic hardware overlying the lumbar spine is excluded.*

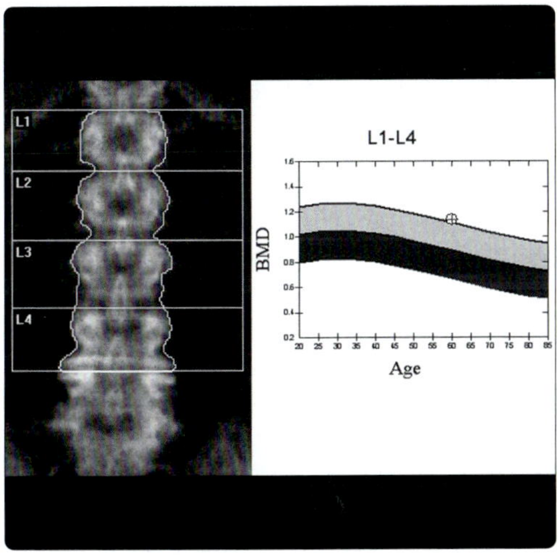

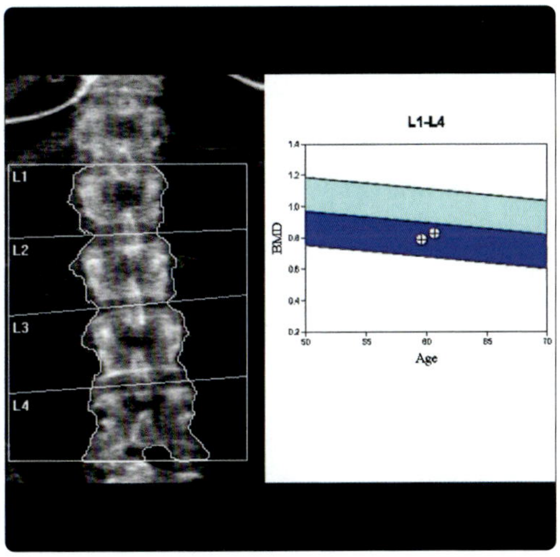

(Left) *DXA of the lumbar spine shows a quality control issue: The L4 vertebral body BMD and T-score are higher than L1-L3. L4 measurements should be excluded secondary to degenerative changes and sclerosis. The result of removing the L4 vertebral will not change the final assessment of normal, but will affect follow-up.* **(Right)** *DXA of the lumbar spine shows T-score of -2.0. The patient is osteopenic by WHO classification.*

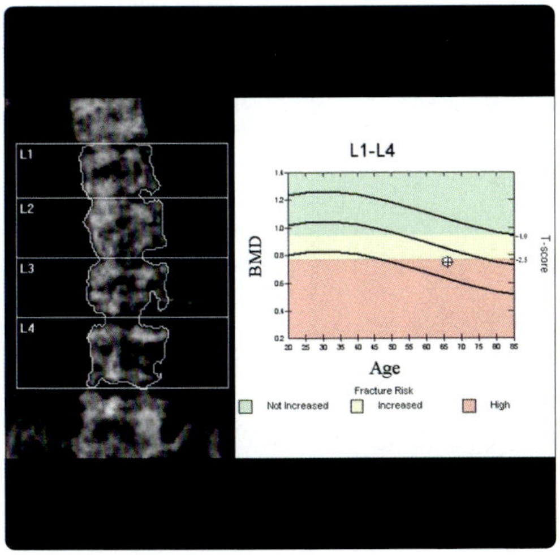

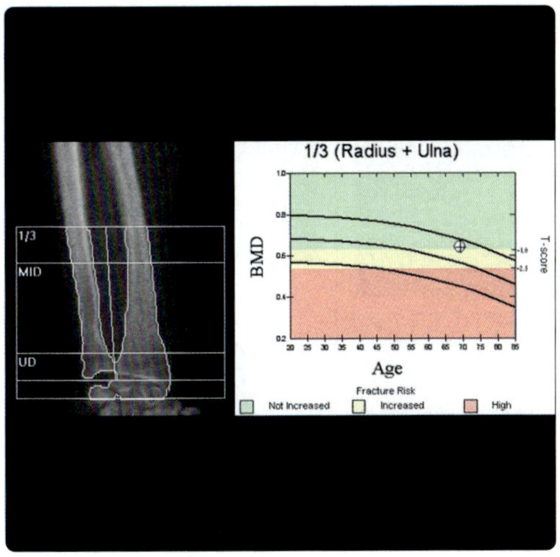

(Left) *DXA of the lumbar spine shows T-score of -2.7. The patient has osteoporosis of the lumbar spine by WHO classification.* **(Right)** *DXA shows the non-dominant wrist in a patient with primary hyperparathyroidism. The T-score of the 1/3 radius and ulna is -0.7, diagnosing the patient as normal.*

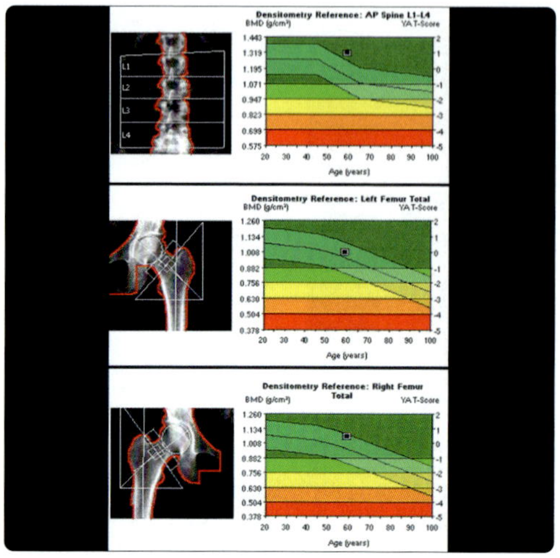

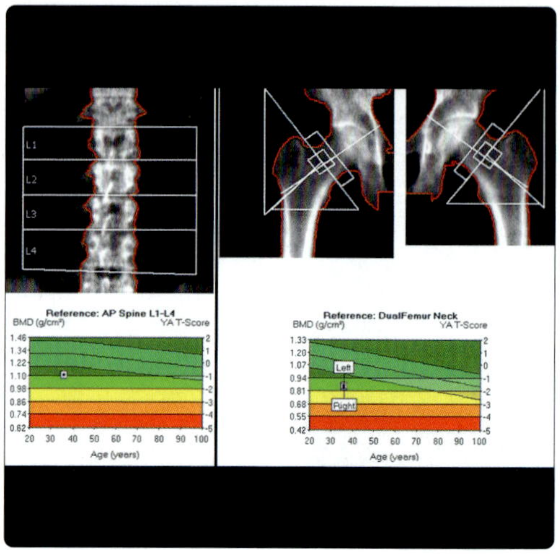

(Left) *A quality control issue in the L4 vertebral body is shown. The T-score is 3.5 compared to negative values for the remainder of the L1-L3 vertebral bodies. L4 shows degenerative changes and sclerosis on the image, and should be excluded. The total hip T-scores are normal and the L1-L3 spine T-scores are in the osteopenia range.* **(Right)** *This male patient under 50 years of age has a Z-score of -1.6 in the lumbar spine and -2.0 for the hips. These Z scores are within the expected range for age.*

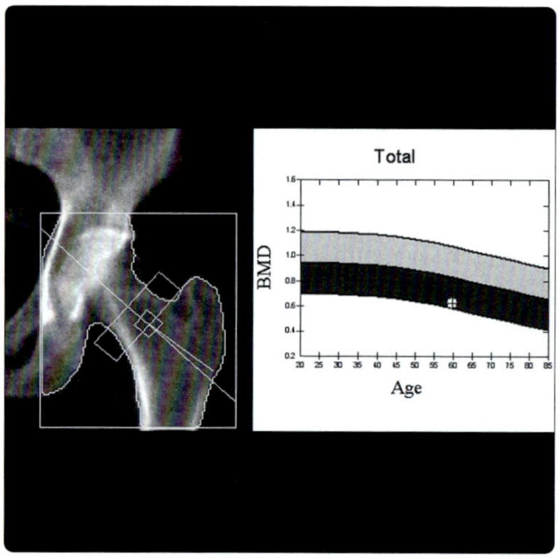

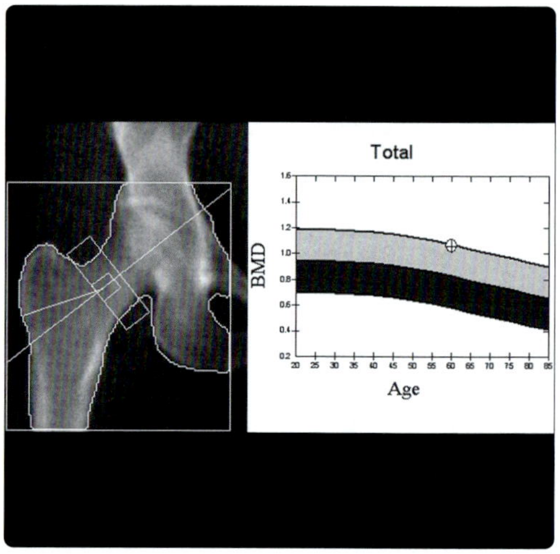

(Left) *DXA scan shows osteoporosis of the left hip with a T-score of -2.6.* **(Right)** *Normal DXA of the right hip shows total hip and femoral neck T-scores of 1.0 and 0.7, respectively.*

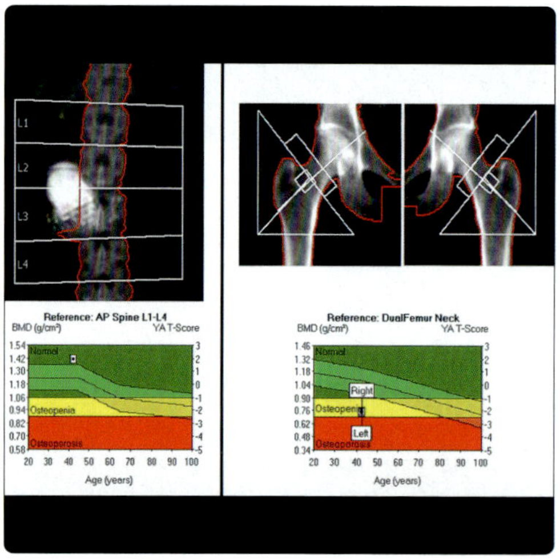

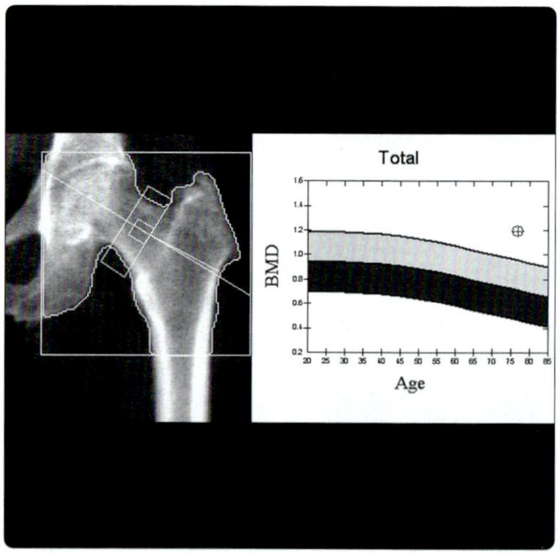

(Left) *A spinal stimulator device overlies the spine. L2-L3 should be excluded from the lumbar BMD measurements. The patient is < 50 years old, therefore Z-scores should be utilized. The Z-score of the lumbar spine is inaccurate secondary to the spinal stimulator device. The Z-score of the hips is -2.4, therefore it is abnormal and outside the expected range for age.* **(Right)** *Normal DXA of the left hip shows total hip T-score of 2.0 (likely due to degenerative changes) and the femoral neck T-score of 1.0.*

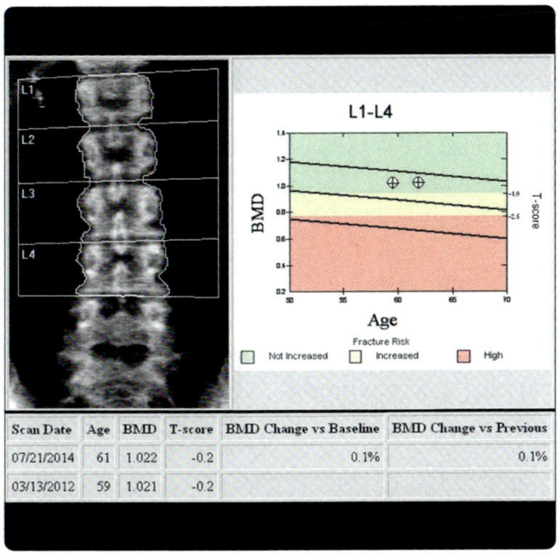

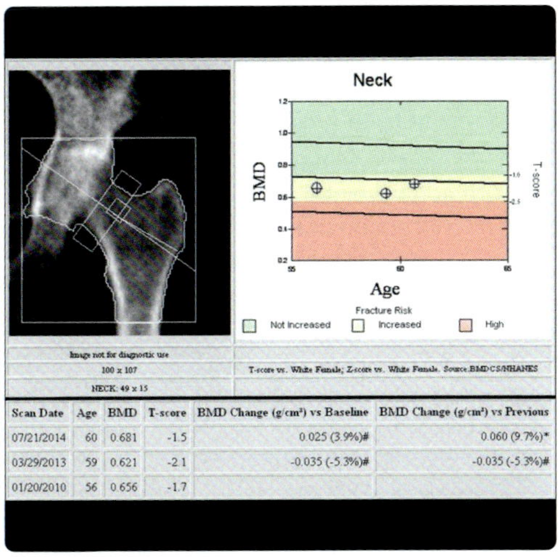

(Left) *DXA scan of the lumbar spine shows no significant change from the prior exam. The patient remains normal by WHO classification.* **(Right)** *Comparison DXA scan of the hip shows a 9.7% increase in BMD from the prior examination, which is considered significant. The patient remains osteopenic by WHO classification.*

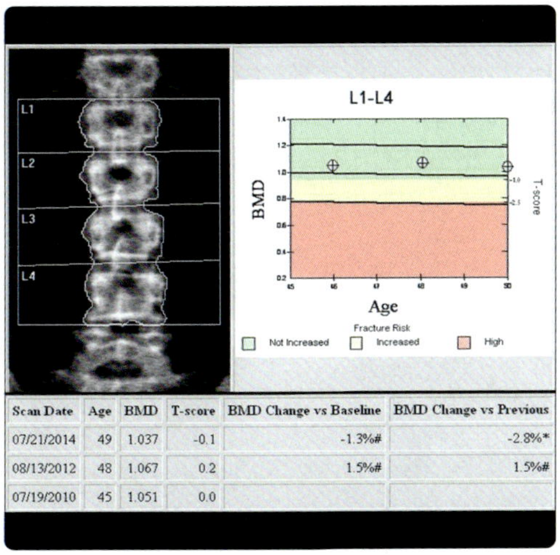

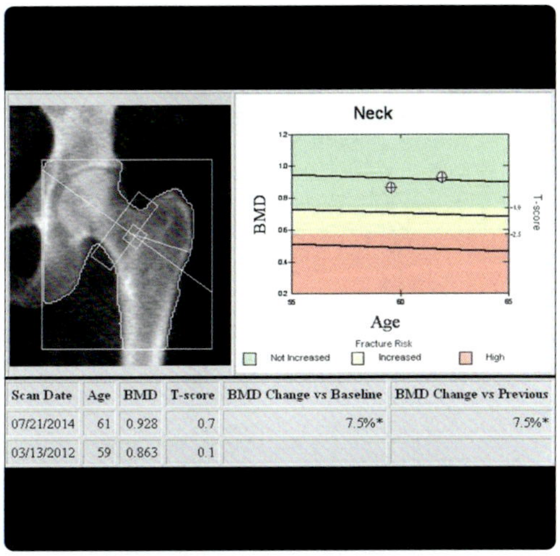

(Left) *Comparison DXA scan of the lumbar spine shows a 2.8% decrease in BMD from the prior examination, which is considered significant. The patient remains normal by WHO classification.* **(Right)** *Comparison DXA scan of the hip shows a 7.5% increase in BMD from the prior examination, which is considered significant. The patient remains normal by WHO classification.*

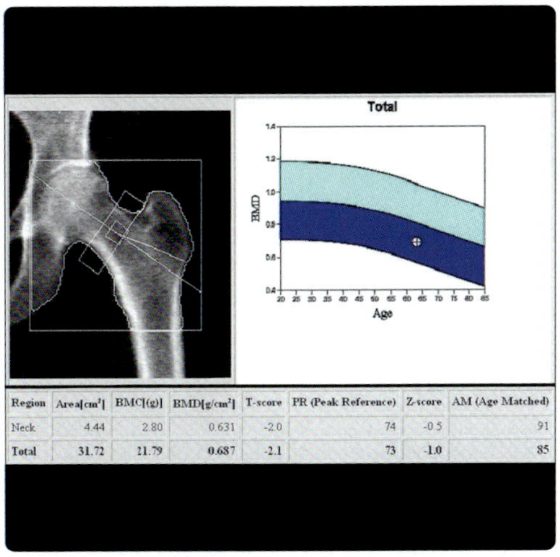

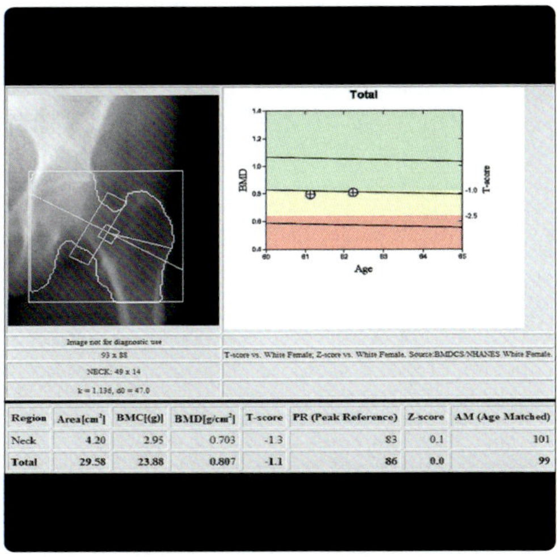

(Left) *DXA scan shows osteopenia with a hip fracture risk of less than 3% and major osteoporotic fracture risk less than 20%.* **(Right)** *DXA scan shows osteopenia with a hip fracture risk of less than 3% and major osteoporotic fracture less than 20%.*

KEY FACTS

IMAGING

- Periprosthetic soft tissue complications
  - Pseudotumor, periprosthetic effusions, synovitis/bursitis, arthrofibrosis, cellulitis
  - Bone scan may be positive in first 2 phases but only mild uptake or absent in 3rd phase
- Diffuse periprosthetic uptake of tracer on skeletal scintigraphy suggests osteolysis from infection or loosening
- 2-3 years after placement, negative study (periprosthetic activity ≤ surrounding nonarticular bone) has very high negative predictive value
- Fractures associated with prosthesis typically present with focally intense fusiform or linear activity along prosthesis
- In-111 leukocyte imaging with Tc-99m sulfur colloid provides most specific and accurate assessment for joint infection and is diagnostic test of choice
- On SPECT, osteomyelitis is likely when uptake of In-111 WBC localizes to bone on 2 or more adjacent tomographic slices
- Labeled leukocytes are mostly neutrophils, which are present in infections and not prevalent in aseptically loosened prosthesis
- False-negative results occur in chronic infections and false-positive results occur in aseptic inflammation
- Newer MR sequences have allowed better evaluation of arthroplasties; advantage of MR would be evaluation of adjacent soft tissue structures for other diagnosis causing painful prosthesis
- F-18 FDG PET/CT is not widely accepted method to evaluate joint prosthesis complications, and sensitivity and specificity are lower than In-111 leukocyte imaging

TOP DIFFERENTIAL DIAGNOSES

- Periprosthetic fracture
- Prosthetic joint loosening
- Prosthetic joint infection

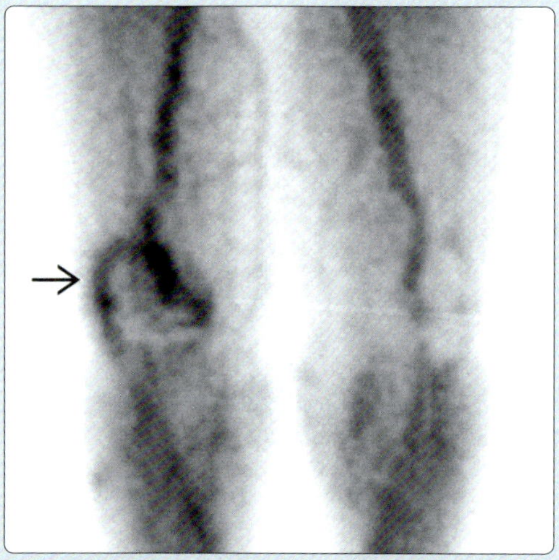

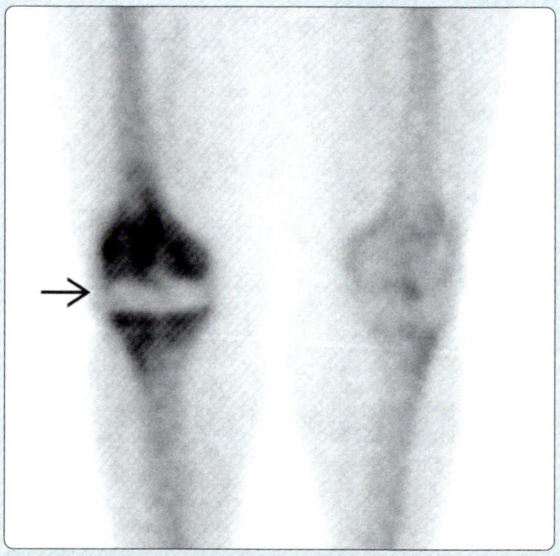

(Left) *Anterior image from the soft tissue phase of a 3-phase bone scan shows periprosthetic hyperemia → to the right knee joint. The perfusion images (not shown) showed hyperperfusion.* **(Right)** *Delayed-phase image from the same patient shows periprosthetic uptake of tracer →. Abnormal 3-phase skeletal scintigraphy could represent aseptic loosening or infection.*

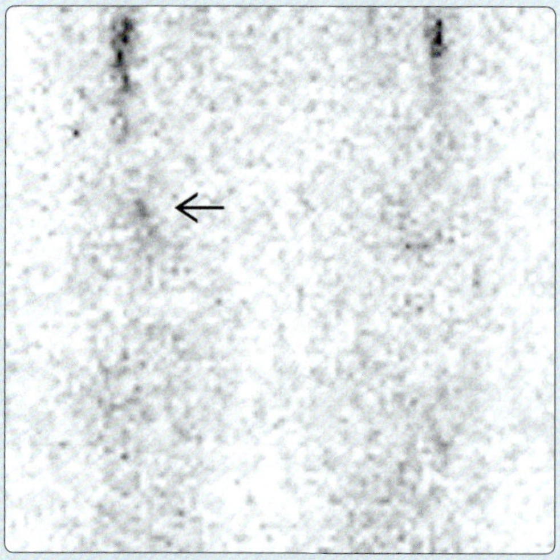

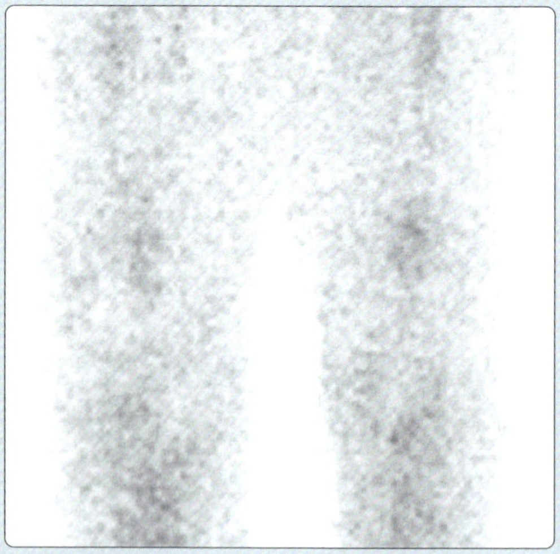

(Left) *In-111 leukocyte imaging in the same patient with abnormal 3-phase skeletal scintigraphy shows a small focus of activity → in the region of the right knee prosthesis.* **(Right)** *Tc-99m sulfur colloid marrow imaging in the same patient shows discordant findings in that no significant uptake is present in the region of the right knee joint. These findings are most compatible with an infected right knee prosthesis.*

TERMINOLOGY

Definitions

- Estimated over 800,000 hip and knee joint arthroplasties performed in USA annually
  - Less frequently shoulder, wrist, and elbow arthroplasty performed
- Prosthesis made of metal (cobalt–chromium or titanium) and ultra high molecular-weight polyethylene material
- Components attached to native bone with surgical cement (polymethylmethacrylate), application of hydroxyapatite compound to their surface, or by constructing prosthetic materials with porous coating to allow bone ingrowth

IMAGING

General Features

- Best diagnostic clue
  - Loosening
    - Activity at tip of prosthesis in cemented hip prosthesis 1 year after placement suggests loosening
    - Diffuse periprosthetic uptake of tracer suggests osteolysis from infection or loosening
  - Infection
    - In-111 leukocyte imaging with Tc-99m sulfur colloid provides most specific and accurate assessment for joint infection and is diagnostic test of choice
    - Diffuse periprosthetic uptake of tracer suggests osteolysis from infection or loosening
  - Fracture
    - 3-phase skeletal scintigraphy typically shows focally intense fusiform or linear activity along prosthesis

Radiographic Findings

- Lucency at bone-prosthesis or bone-cement interface > 2 mm &/or has increased over prior images suggests loosening
- Knee: Thin lucency more common in tibial component
- Periprosthetic fracture
- Tilting of prosthesis suggests loosening and particle disease
- Newer MR sequences have allowed better evaluation of arthroplasties
  - Advantage of MR would be evaluation of adjacent soft tissue structures for other diagnosis causing painful prosthesis

Nuclear Medicine Findings

- Bone scan
  - 10 years after implantation, 50% of prostheses show radiographic evidence of loosening and 30% require revision
    - Accuracy for diagnosing complications of lower extremity joint prostheses is 50-70%
  - Bone scans can serve as screening examination
  - All prosthesis initially show increased activity
    - 2-3 years after placement, negative study (periprosthetic activity ≤ surrounding nonarticular bone) has very high negative predictive value
  - Hip arthroplasty
    - 10% show increased activity at 2 years
    - Periprosthetic activity in porous hip prosthesis 2-3 years after placement
    - Activity at tip of prosthesis in cemented hip prosthesis 1 year after placement
  - Knee arthroplasty
    - Tibial component > femoral component; increased activity frequently persists for years

Imaging Recommendations

- Best imaging tool
  - 3-phase bone scan: Most common screening exam
    - Loosening vs. infection: Delayed phase imaging only or 3-phase imaging cannot reliably differentiate aseptic loosening from infection
    - Fracture: First 2 phases variable/correlate with acuity, focal increased activity at fracture site on delay phase
    - Normal bone scan has high negative predictive value
  - Labeled leukocyte scintigraphy
    - Labeled leukocytes are mostly neutrophils, which are present in infections and not prevalent in aseptically loosened prosthesis
    - Usually matches 3-phase bone scan distribution in infection
    - Compacted marrow from procedure also shows increased activity; therefore, Tc-99m sulfur colloid used in conjunction with accuracy > 90%
    - On SPECT, osteomyelitis is likely when uptake of In-111 WBC localizes to bone on 2 or more adjacent tomographic slices
    - False-negative results occur in chronic infections
    - False-positive results occur in aseptic inflammation
  - Tc-99m sulfur colloid: Used to confirm labeled leukocyte scintigraphy results
    - Localizes to normal marrow, discordant activity to leukocyte scintigraphy indicates infection
  - PET/CT
    - Loosening: Increased activity about majority of or entire component that is confined to bone-prosthesis or bone-cement interface
    - Infection: Increased activity extends to adjacent soft tissues
    - Activity around acetabular component and proximal aspect of femoral component on FDG PET seen frequently, typically not associated with infection
    - Sensitivity and specificity are lower than In-111 leukocyte imaging
    - Not widely accepted method to evaluate joint prosthesis complications
  - Ga-67 scintigraphy
    - Not used commonly
    - Variable sensitivity and specificity reported
    - Negative examination has high negative predictive value
    - In conjunction with bone scan
      - If intensity &/or distribution greater than bone scan, osteomyelitis indicated
      - If intensity and distribution same as bone scan, test equivocal
      - If intensity less than bone scan and distribution same as bone scan, osteomyelitis not indicated
- Protocol advice
  - Triad of imaging studies in violated bone

- Tc-99m MDP/HDP, In-111 WBC, and Tc-99m sulfur colloid
- According to SNMMI, 15% window at 140-keV Tc-99m peak and a 15% window at 247-keV In-111 photopeak are used if Tc-99m dose is injected on day 1 before In-111 leukocyte imaging
- 10% or 15% window at 173-keV In-111 photo peak for delayed In-111 leukocyte images obtained on day 2 (18–30 h) after Tc-99m dose has been injected

- SPECT/CT
  - Differentiates soft tissue from bone uptake
  - Better defines cortical or marrow extent of infection

DIFFERENTIAL DIAGNOSIS

Periprosthetic Fracture

- Risk factors: Poor bone stock (osteoporosis, bone cysts, rheumatoid arthritis, particle disease), male, highly active
- Shoulder: Humerus fracture most common
- Hip: Femur fracture at lateral cortex near stem tip > acetabulum
- Knee: Patella fracture > femur and tibia
- 3-phase bone scan: Focal increased activity at fracture site

Prosthetic Joint Loosening

- Major causes include micromotion over time and osteolysis (e.g., particle disease)
- 3-phase bone scan: Variable activity on first 2 phases, focal activity at bone-prosthesis site of motion on delay phase

Prosthetic Joint Infection

- Infection rate < 1% in primary joint replacement, increased to as high as 15% in revision shoulder arthroplasty
- Vast majority occur < 90 days post operation but may occur > 2 years delay
- 3-phase bone scan: Diffuse increased activity on all phases in early infections; may be more focal in later presentation

Periprosthetic Soft Tissue Complications

- Pseudotumor (e.g., particle disease), periprosthetic effusions, synovitis/bursitis
  - Bone scan may be positive in first 2 phases but weakly increased or absent in 3rd phase; usually diagnosed by CT or MR
- Snapping hip syndrome: Iliopsoas tendon may be evaluated dynamically with fluoroscopic tenography

Heterotopic Ossification

- Bone formation in periprosthetic soft tissues commonly seen post operation due to liberation of primitive bone-forming cells
- 3-phase bone scan: Focal mildly increased activity in soft tissues with corresponding new bone on radiograph

Prosthetic Alignment Abnormality

- Radiographic diagnosis, presentation as recurrent dislocation or limited range of motion

CLINICAL ISSUES

Presentation

- Most common signs/symptoms
  - Painful prosthesis may be due to mechanical hardware failure (e.g., improper alignment, particle disease/metallosis, loosening), infection, or periprosthetic fracture
    - Infection
      - Local: Increased pain or acute decreased range of motion in replaced joint, swelling, erythema, draining wound, fevers
      - Constitutional: Fevers, chills, night sweats, fatigue
    - Loosening
      - Chronic pain that may be exacerbated by weight bearing
    - Fracture
      - Acute pain initially, may become chronic
- Other signs/symptoms
  - C-reactive protein (CRP) or erythrocyte sedimentation rate (ESR) elevated in knee prosthesis infection
  - CRP and ESR elevated in hip prosthesis infection
  - Joint aspiration should be performed in suspected prosthesis infections
    - If nondiagnostic, perform nuclear imaging

Treatment

- In loosening, patient will need single-stage revision arthroplasty
- Treatment of infected hardware is more complex and often requires multiple admissions
  - Surgical debridement of infection may occur followed by IV and oral antibiotics, if infection caught early
  - In most cases, prosthesis is removed and temporary cement spacer treated with antibiotics placed
  - Long course of IV antibiotics
  - Once infection has resolved, revision arthroplasty is performed

DIAGNOSTIC CHECKLIST

Consider

- Identifying timing of prosthesis placement
- Type of prosthesis: Cemented, porous, revision

Image Interpretation Pearls

- Looking for concordant or discordant findings on In-111 leukocyte and Tc-99m sulfur colloid marrow images will differentiate infection from aseptic loosening
- 3-phase skeletal scintigraphy is nonspecific and is most useful when study is normal or identifies fracture or other non prosthesis-related cause of symptoms

SELECTED REFERENCES

1. Palestro CJ: Nuclear medicine and the failed joint replacement: Past, present, and future. World J Radiol. 6(7):446-58, 2014
2. Osmon DR et al: Diagnosis and management of prosthetic joint infection: clinical practice guidelines by the Infectious Diseases Society of America. Clin Infect Dis. 56(1):e1-e25, 2013
3. Palestro CJ: FDG-PET in musculoskeletal infections. Semin Nucl Med. 43(5):367-76, 2013
4. Love C et al: Nuclear medicine and the infected joint replacement. Semin Nucl Med. 39(1):66-78, 2009

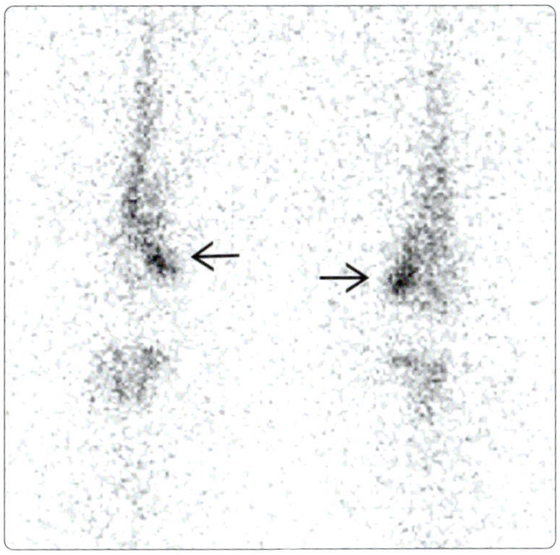
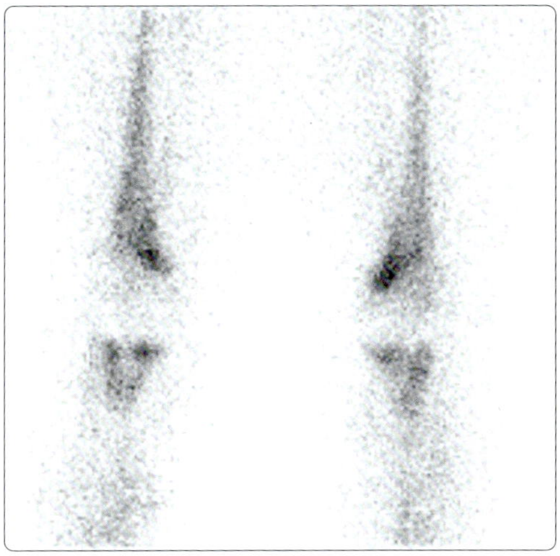

(Left) *Anterior image from an In-111 leukocyte scan shows bilateral knee prosthesis with periprosthetic uptake of tracer most prominent in the medial femoral compartments ➔.* **(Right)** *Anterior image from a Tc-99m sulfur colloid marrow scan in the same patient shows concordant uptake when compared to the In-111 leukocyte scan. There is no scintigraphic evidence of prosthetic infection.*

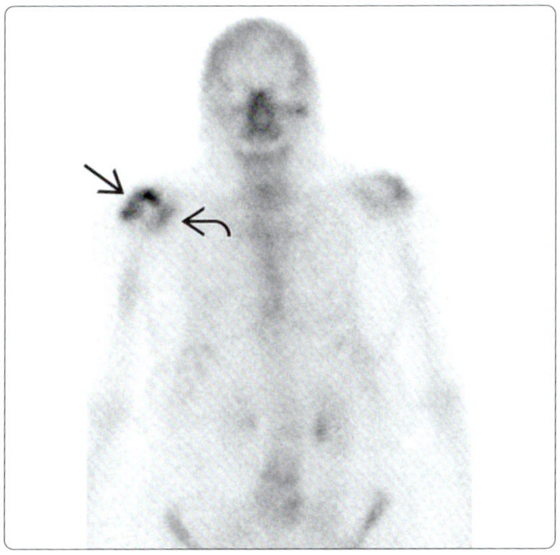
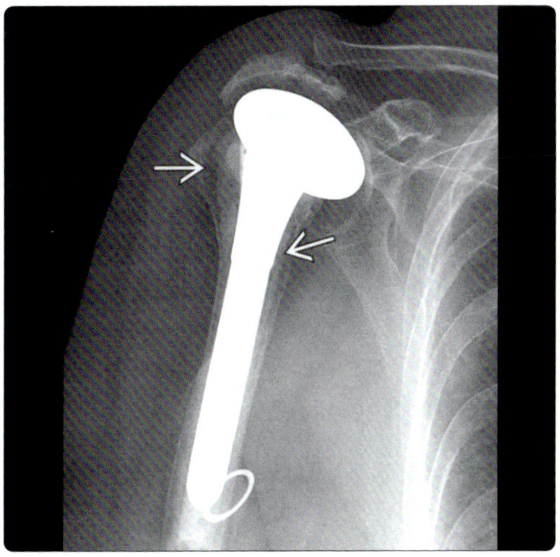

(Left) *Delayed-phase anterior bone scan in a patient with a right shoulder arthroplasty shows moderately increased uptake along the greater tuberosity ➔ and glenoid ➚.* **(Right)** *Corresponding AP radiograph in the same patient shows lucency ➡ at the bone-cement interface. Infection or loosening may show periharware lucency. An In-111 leukocyte scan with Tc-99m sulfur colloid marrow imaging would allow differentiation of aseptic loosening vs. prosthetic infection.*

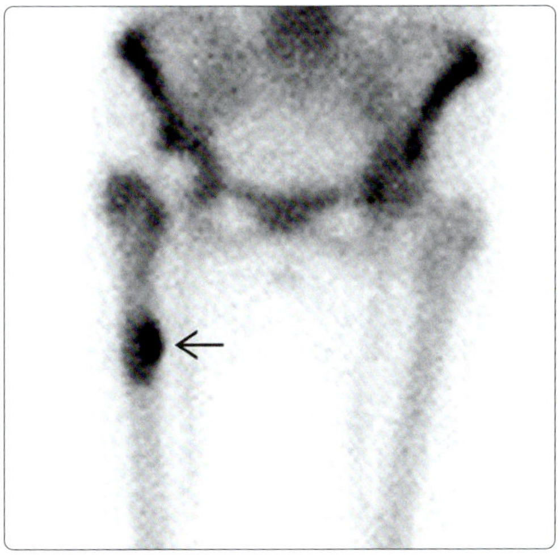
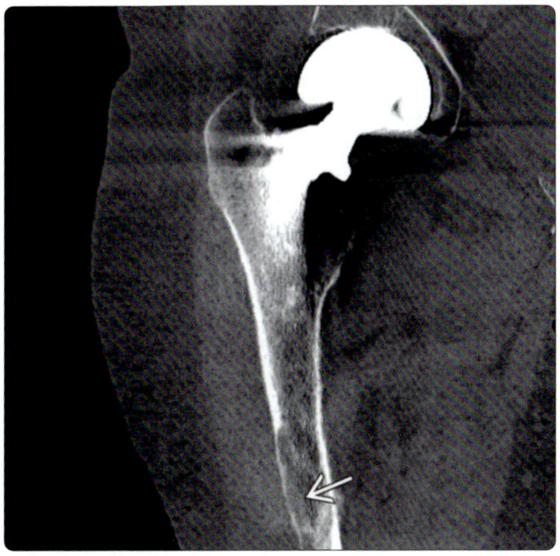

(Left) *Anterior delayed-phase bone scan demonstrates focal fusiform increased activity along the medial margin of the distal femoral component stem ➔. This finding could represent periprosthetic fracture or focal aseptic loosening.* **(Right)** *Sagittal reformatted CT in bone window shows periosteal ➡ new bone formation at a stress fracture site along the posterior, medial margin of the distal femoral component.*

KEY FACTS

IMAGING

- Plain radiography: First-line study in work-up of arthritides
- Bone scans are useful for whole-body evaluation of arthritides, confirmation of diagnosis
- When performing 3-phase bone scan, consider injecting in non-affected extremity or feet to avoid false increased flow
- Longer uptake times from injection to delayed imaging useful in diabetics or patients with poor circulation
- Spot images of both extremities useful for comparison

TOP DIFFERENTIAL DIAGNOSES

- Rarely, pattern of degenerative change may mimic multifocal metastatic disease
- Plain films often indicated for differentiating trauma from arthritis after lesions identified on bone scan
- Septic arthritis more often than OA has periarticular increased activity on all phases of 3-phase bone scan

PATHOLOGY

- Forces exceeding normal stresses on an otherwise healthy joint
- Underlying bony failure because of inherent compromise, vascular disruption, metabolic derangement, inflammation
- Articular cartilaginous degeneration
- Osteophytosis (marginal bone hypertrophy)

DIAGNOSTIC CHECKLIST

- Bone scan to confirm presence of radiographically occult joint disease
- SPECT/CT useful for localizing radiographically occult lesions in spine, postsurgical spine evaluation

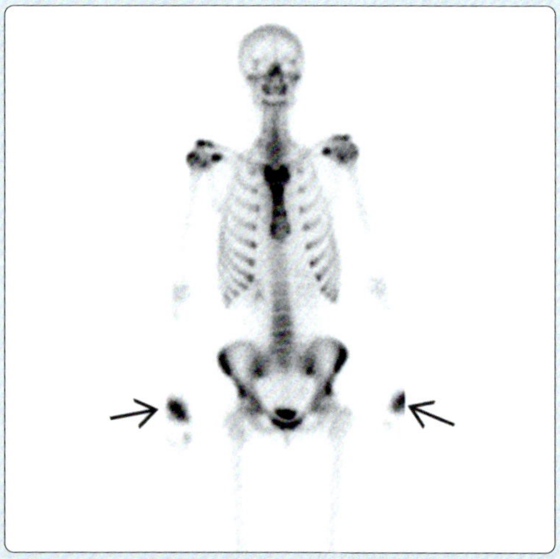

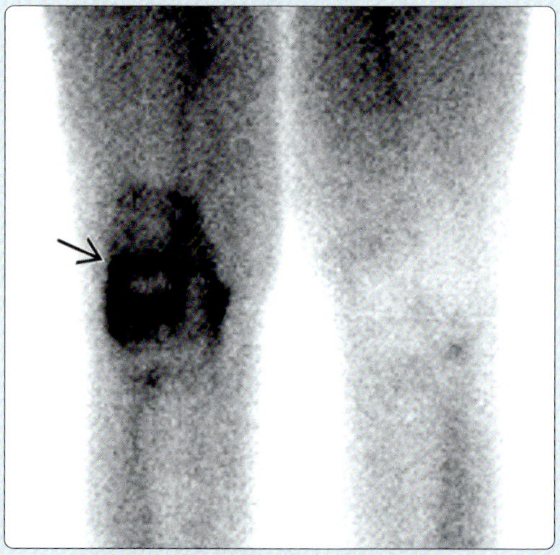

(Left) *Delayed whole-body bone scan in a 19-year old-woman with rheumatoid arthritis (RA) shows increased uptake in the carpal bones of the wrist →, characteristic of RA.* **(Right)** *Anterior flow phase bone scan of the same patient shows a joint-centered hyperperfusion → involving the right knee.*

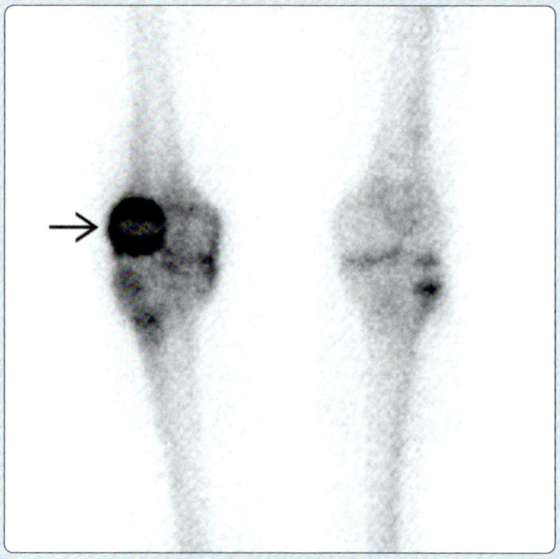

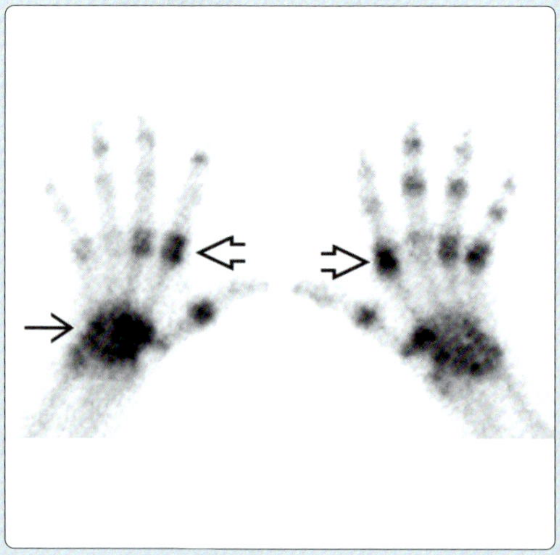

(Left) *Delayed image of the knees shows significantly increased uptake in the right knee, particularly involving the patellofemoral joint →. Findings of active RA in the right knee were confirmed.* **(Right)** *Palmar bone scan of the hands demonstrates distribution of uptake typical of rheumatoid arthritis: Wrists → and MCP ⇨ joints.*

TERMINOLOGY

Definitions

- Osteoarthritis (OA): Deterioration of joints leading to compromise of function with eventual loss of integrity
- Inflammatory arthropathy
  - Rheumatoid
    - Rheumatoid/juvenile rheumatoid arthritis
    - Systemic lupus erythematosus
    - Scleroderma
  - Seronegative spondyloarthropathies
    - Ankylosing spondylitis
    - Psoriatic arthritis
    - Reactive arthritis (Reiter syndrome)
  - Metabolic-induced arthritides
    - Hemochromatosis
    - Calcium pyrophosphate crystal deposition (CPPD) disease/pseudogout
    - Gout

IMAGING

General Features

- Best diagnostic clue
  - Increased joint activity on delayed phase bone scan
- Location
  - OA
    - CMC, DIP and PIP joints
    - MTP joints
    - Hips
    - Knees
    - Spinal facets
  - Inflammatory: Variable, etiology dependent
    - Rheumatoid (e.g., bilateral wrists, feet)
    - Seronegative (e.g., spine, SI joints)
    - Metabolic (e.g., great toe)

Nuclear Medicine Findings

- Bone scan
  - Increased activity about affected joints due to osteoblastic response
  - Can show hyperperfusion, hyperemia, and delayed uptake on 3-phase bone scan
- PET
  - Increased activity on F-18 FDG PET/CT about affected joints due to hypermetabolism in inflammatory response
    - Inflammatory arthritis cannot reliably be distinguished from infectious arthritis
    - Active synovitis considered reason for F-18 FDG accumulation
    - Degree of uptake in RA shows positive correlation with signs and symptoms of disease
  - Most sensitive for spinal osteomyelitis and discitis
    - High negative predictive value

Imaging Recommendations

- Best imaging tool
  - Plain radiography: First-line study in work-up of arthritides
    - Less sensitive than bone scan or MR
  - Bone scan
    - Useful for whole-body evaluation of arthritides, confirmation of diagnosis
    - Confirm radiographically occult joint disease
    - Noninfectious arthritis often incidental finding on whole-body imaging for bone metastases
    - SPECT/CT useful for localizing radiographically occult lesions in spine, postsurgical spine evaluation
    - Active osteoblastic activity of arthritides can be 3-phase bone scan positive
  - MR: Modality of choice for evaluation of localized inflammatory arthritides
    - Best to evaluate for associated fluid collections
- Protocol advice
  - Bone scan
    - 3-phase protocol for extremity joints and proximal appendicular joints (shoulder, hips)
    - Whole-body bone scan for skeletal survey
    - Spot views: Palmar hands, plantar feet
    - SPECT/CT: Preferred for vertebral lesions

Artifacts and Quality Control

- Consider injecting in non-affected extremity or feet to avoid false increased flow
- Spot images of both extremities useful for comparison
- Longer uptake times from injection to delayed imaging useful in diabetics or patients with poor circulation
- Watch for misregistration artifact on SPECT/CT from patient motion or breathing

DIFFERENTIAL DIAGNOSIS

Trauma

- Fracture, subluxation, avulsion
- Plain films often indicated for clarification after lesions identified on bone scan
  - CT may be necessary particularly in spine, pelvis, ribs, sternum

Neoplasm

- Rarely, pattern of degenerative change may mimic multifocal metastatic disease
  - Joints commonly affected by degenerative change
  - Spine metastases can mimic spine OA
    - Metastases more common in vertebral body; OA involves endplates and facets

Osteomyelitis, Septic Arthritis

- Periarticular increased activity on all phases of 3-phase bone scan
- Clinically suggestive picture with symptoms including fever, elevated WBC, constant pain, erythema

Bone Infarction, Avascular Necrosis

- Vascular compromise preceding collapse and subsequent degenerative arthritis
- MR useful in equivocal cases

PATHOLOGY

General Features

- Etiology
  - Forces exceeding normal stresses on an otherwise healthy joint

- Cartilaginous decline with subsequent underlying bony compromise
- Underlying bony failure because of inherent compromise, vascular disruption, metabolic derangement, inflammation
- Autoimmune and metabolic disease

- Genetics
  - OA: Hereditary component
  - Rheumatoid: Associated with HLA-DRB1, 18q21 region of *RNFRSR11A* gene
  - Seronegative spondyloarthropathies: HLA-B27
- Associated abnormalities
  - OA
    - Overweight, prior trauma/sports injuries, developmental anomalies
  - Rheumatoid arthritis
    - Anemia, pulmonary nodules, amyloidosis, inflammatory cardiovascular conditions, ocular, neurological
  - Seronegative spondyloarthropathies
    - Ulcerative colitis, Crohn disease

Gross Pathologic & Surgical Features

- Articular cartilaginous degeneration
- Osteophytosis (marginal bone hypertrophy)
- Synovial hypertrophy and inflammation

CLINICAL ISSUES

Presentation

- Most common signs/symptoms
  - OA
    - Joint pain, swelling, tenderness, stiffness, decreased range of motion, joint effusion
    - Long term: Joint deformity
    - Laboratory: Positive C reactive protein
  - Rheumatoid arthritis
    - Morning stiffness, soft tissue swelling, symmetric arthritis, hands affected
    - Long term: Swan neck deformity
    - Laboratory: Positive rheumatoid factor
  - Seronegative spondyloarthropathies
    - Chronic pain, stiffness
    - Laboratory: Negative rheumatoid factor
    - Reactive: Associated with preceding infection (usually genital, gastrointestinal), uveitis, urethritis

Demographics

- Age
  - OA
    - Incidence increases with age
  - Rheumatoid arthritis
    - Peak 4th to 6th decades
  - Seronegative spondyloarthropathies
    - Younger population (~ 20-40 years)
- Gender
  - OA
    - No predilection
  - Rheumatoid arthritis
    - M:F = 1:2.5
  - Seronegative spondyloarthropathies
    - M > F
- Epidemiology
  - OA
    - Most common joint disorder
    - 33% > 65 years have knee OA on radiograph
  - Rheumatoid arthritis
    - Prevalence up to 1.5%
  - Seronegative spondyloarthropathies
    - Prevalence < 1%

Treatment

- Medical therapy
  - Anti-inflammatory drugs, anti-rheumatoid agents (e.g., methotrexate), antibiotics
- Physical therapy
  - Non-weight-bearing exercise: Swimming, bicycling
  - Weight training, flexibility, stretching exercises
- Surgery
  - Arthroplasty, osteotomy, arthrodesis

DIAGNOSTIC CHECKLIST

Consider

- Bone scan for whole-body evaluation of arthritides, confirmation of diagnosis
- Bone scan to confirm presence of radiographically occult joint disease
- SPECT/CT useful for localizing radiographically occult lesions in spine, postsurgical spine evaluation
- Spot views of palmar hands, plantar feet for best evaluation

Image Interpretation Pearls

- Bone metastases and arthritides can occasionally be confused: Plain film/CT/MR correlation valuable

SELECTED REFERENCES

1. Mosher TJ et al: Osteoarthritis year 2013 in review: imaging. Osteoarthritis Cartilage. Epub ahead of print, 2013
2. van der Laken CJ et al: Nuclear imaging of rheumatic diseases. Best Pract Res Clin Rheumatol. 26(6):787-804, 2012
3. Kubota K et al: FDG PET for rheumatoid arthritis: basic considerations and whole-body PET/CT. Ann N Y Acad Sci. 1228:29-38, 2011
4. Mohan HK et al: SPECT/CT in imaging foot and ankle pathology-the demise of other coregistration techniques. Semin Nucl Med. 40(1):41-51, 2010
5. Costelloe CM et al: Musculoskeletal pitfalls in 18F-FDG PET/CT: pictorial review. AJR Am J Roentgenol. 193(3 Suppl):WS1-WS13, Quiz S26-30, 2009
6. Kubota K et al: Whole-body FDG-PET/CT on rheumatoid arthritis of large joints. Ann Nucl Med. 23(9):783-91, 2009
7. De Leonardis F et al: The role of conventional radiography and scintigraphy in the third millennium. Best Pract Res Clin Rheumatol. 22(6):961-79, 2008
8. Houseni M et al: Facet joint arthropathy demonstrated on FDG-PET. Clin Nucl Med. 31(7):418-9, 2006

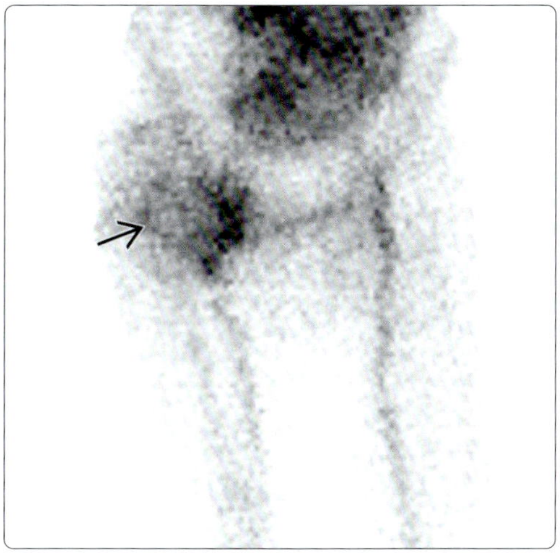

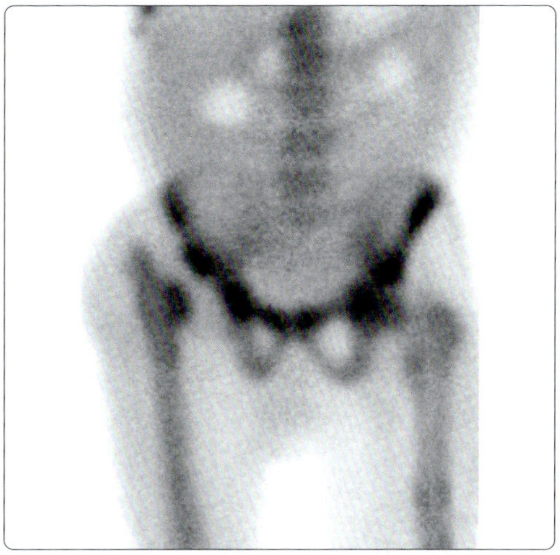

(Left) *Anterior 3-phase bone scan was performed on a 53-year-old man with septic arthritis of the right hip. Angiographic phase shows increased uptake in the region of the right hip and adjacent soft tissues ⇨, concerning for abscess.* **(Right)** *Corresponding delayed image shows normal tracer accumulation within the osseous structures without evidence to suggest osteomyelitis. Note that this patient had undergone right femoral head and neck resection (Girdlestone procedure).*

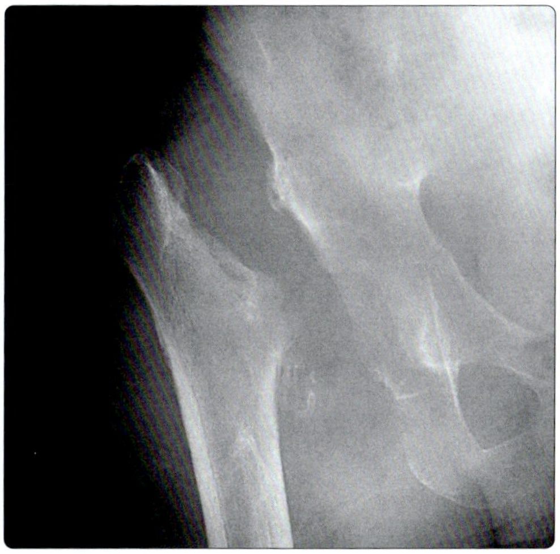

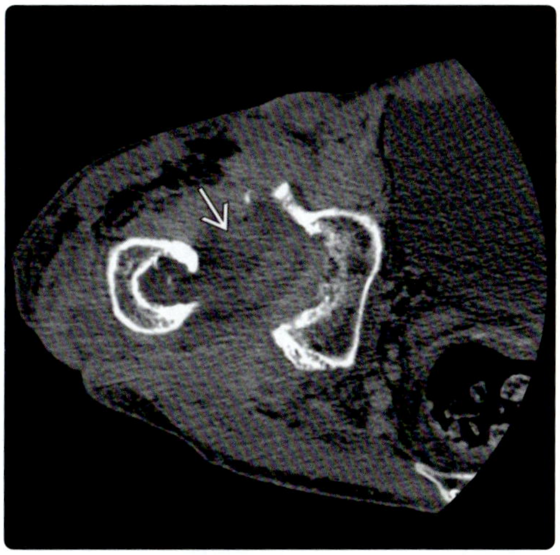

(Left) *AP right hip radiograph shows the altered anatomy after resection arthroplasty due to recurrent septic arthritis in this patient's hip.* **(Right)** *Corresponding noncontrast transaxial CT shows a heterogeneous fluid collection ➡ interposed between the proximal femur and acetabulum, concerning for abscess.*

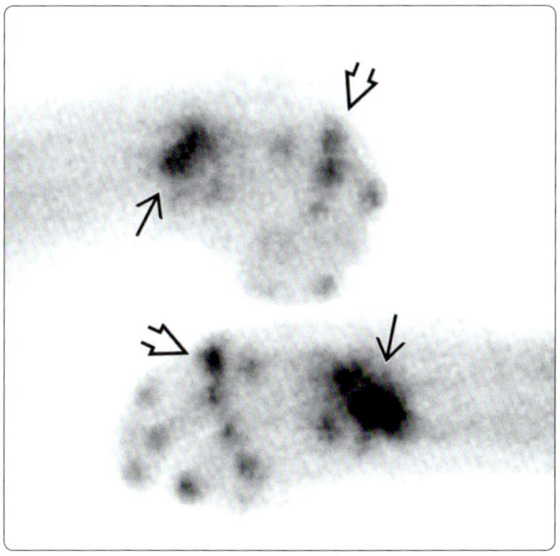

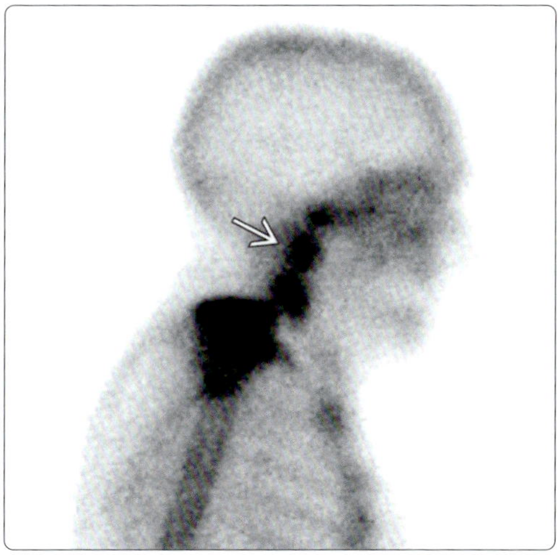

(Left) *Spot images from a bone scan of a 54-year-old woman with inflammatory arthritis demonstrate typical distribution of uptake in wrists ⇨ and MCP ⇨ joints.* **(Right)** *Lateral spot image of the cervical spine from a bone scan of an 81-year-old man with rheumatoid arthritis shows increased activity in the cervical spine ➡, likely a result of RA with superimposed degenerative changes.*

Osteomyelitis and Septic Arthritis

KEY FACTS

TERMINOLOGY

- Local or generalized suppurative process causing progressive destruction of bone

IMAGING

- Classic appearance on 3-phase bone scan: Increased activity on all 3 phases
- Ga-67 preferred over In-111 WBC when evaluating spinal discitis/osteomyelitis
- False-positive WBC scan in recently "violated" bone (e.g., fracture) due to localization in marrow elements
- False-negative WBC scan in chronic infections and spinal discitis/osteomyelitis
- Arthroplasties/prostheses may be 3-phase (+) due to normal hyperemic healing/osteoblastic remodeling ≥ 12 m
- Tc-99m 3-phase bone scan if MR contraindicated: > 95% sensitivity/specificity in patients with pristine bone
- Tc-99m HMPAO WBC scan: Better imaging characteristics; however, requires Tc-99m sulfur colloid marrow map 24-72 hrs later if + (same imaging energy); ↑ blood pool may result in false-positive
- Septic arthritis typically has diffusely increased uptake throughout the joint compared to osteomyelitis that can show focal uptake only on one side of the joint.

PATHOLOGY

- Most common cause: Extension of cellulitis or traumatic direct inoculation in adolescents/adults
- Hematogenous spread (more common in pediatric population)
- Vascular insufficiency (diabetic foot infection)

DIAGNOSTIC CHECKLIST

- Cellulitis, degenerative arthropathy, post-traumatic, postsurgical
- WBC scan with Tc-99m SC discordance is > 90% sensitive, specific for osteomyelitis

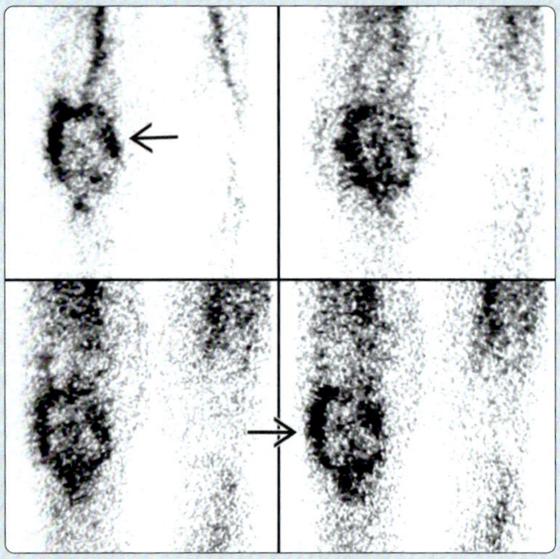

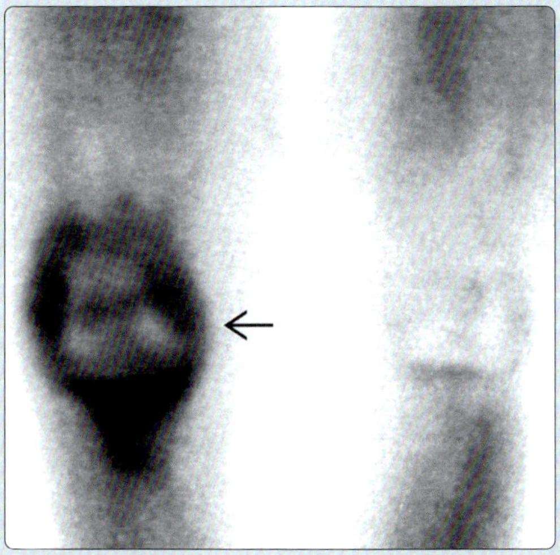

(Left) *Anterior angiographic phase bone scan shows ↑ flow about the right knee ⇨, concerning for postoperative changes, cellulitis, or osteomyelitis.* **(Right)** *Anterior blood pool phase bone scan in the same patient shows hyperemia about the right knee arthroplasty ⇨.*

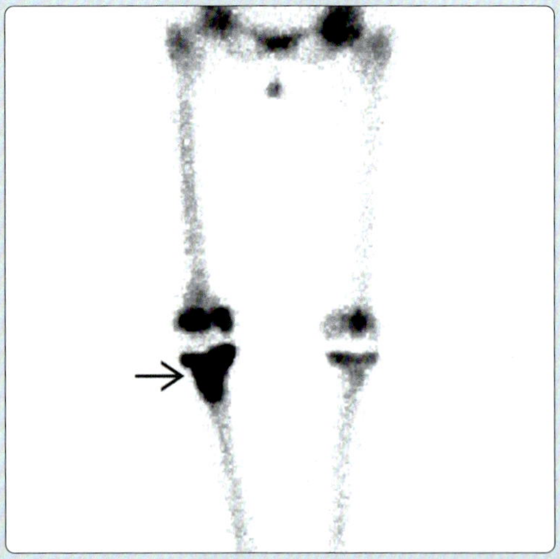

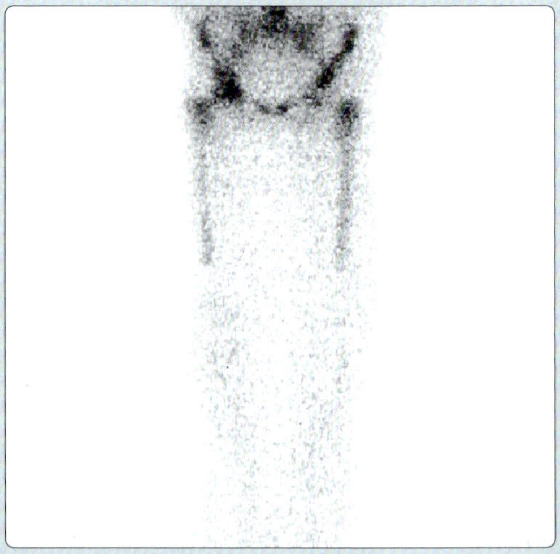

(Left) *Anterior delayed phase bone scan in the same patient shows extensive osteoblastic activity about the right knee arthroplasty ⇨, particularly adjacent to tibial component, prompting In-111 WBC scan.* **(Right)** *Anterior In-111 WBC scan in the same patient shows no abnormal activity, excluding osteomyelitis and indicating cellulitis/postsurgical changes.*

TERMINOLOGY

Definitions

- Local or generalized suppurative process causing progressive destruction of bone
  - Aggressive bone lesion with one or more of the following: Periosteal reaction, soft tissue swelling, subperiosteal abscess, draining sinus
  - Septic arthritis occurs from direct inoculation or hematogenous spread

IMAGING

Nuclear Medicine Findings

- Tc-99m methylene diphosphonate (MDP) and hydroxymethylene diphosphonate (HDP) 3-phase bone scan
  - Classic appearance on 3-phase bone scan: Increased activity on all 3 phases
  - Occasionally photopenic: Marrow thrombosis, ↑ intramedullary pressure (esp. in children)
  - Useful for large region or whole-body imaging or for patients with MR contraindications
  - May be falsely negative in neonates and infants
- Leukocyte imaging and Ga-67 scans
  - Used both in conjunction with bone scans and independent of bone scans for further specificity
  - In-111 or Tc-99m HMPAO WBCs used for leukocyte imaging
  - Both labeled leukocyte imaging and gallium scans show abnormal uptake in osteomyelitis
- F-18 FDG PET/CT
  - Not used widely in clinical practice
  - Most useful in spinal osteomyelitis with high negative predictive value
  - Cannot differentiate aseptic loosening from infection in arthroplasty evaluation
  - Osteomyelitis would show increased activity in affected osseous structure

Imaging Recommendations

- Best imaging tool
  - Tc-99m 3-phase bone scan if MR contraindicated: > 95% sensitivity/specificity in patients with pristine bone
    - Widely available, rarely contraindicated
    - In cases of coexistent bone abnormalities such as arthropathy, trauma, noninfectious process, or surgical change, specificity poor (~ 33%)
    - If nonpristine bone, may require tagged WBC scan for optimal diagnosis
    - Arthroplasties/prostheses may be 3-phase positive due to normal hyperemic healing, osteoblastic remodeling for ≥ 12 months
- Protocol advice
  - 3-phase bone scan
    - Adult dose: 20-25 mCi (740-925 MBq) Tc-99m MDP/HDP IV
    - Angiographic phase: 2-sec planar images for 60 sec in anterior and posterior projections over area of interest
    - Blood pool phase: Static planar image over area of interest, anterior/posterior projections
    - Mineral/delayed phase: Whole-body or spot image in anterior/posterior projections, lateral/oblique projections as needed
    - Delayed: 8 hour and 24 hour images demonstrate progressive uptake; hyperemic delivery of tracer to bone
      - Particularly useful in diabetics, vascular insufficiency, and renal failure patients
    - SPECT/CT is useful for improved anatomic localization
      - Improves contrast resolution, distinguishing soft tissue from bone involvement
- Additional nuclear medicine imaging options
  - Tagged WBC scan
    - In-111 or Tc-99m HMPAO WBCs localize to infection
    - Improves differentiation of aseptic inflammation, cellulitis, osteomyelitis: Estimated accuracy 92%
    - When coexistent arthropathy/trauma/structural deformity present, WBC scan necessary
    - If WBC scan positive, perform Tc-99m sulfur colloid (SC) marrow map to exclude WBC accumulation in activated reticuloendothelial system elements (red marrow, chronic inflammation)
      - Can be performed concurrently if using In-111 labeled WBCs
    - Tc-99m HMPAO WBC scan: Better imaging characteristics; however, requires Tc-99m SC marrow map 24-72 hr later if (+) (same imaging energy); ↑ blood pool may result in false-positive
      - Sensitivity/specificity of Tc-99m HMPAO WBC scans reported > 95% in violated bone
    - Discordant pattern: Areas of WBC activity not concordant on Tc-99m SC are positive for osteomyelitis
    - Concordant pattern: If WBC activity has matching (concordant) Tc-99m SC activity, study is negative for osteomyelitis
      - Concordant activity associated with infiltration of chronic granulomatous cells (e.g., neuropathic arthropathy, surgical changes)
    - WBC scan use to evaluate treatment response
    - False-positive WBC scan in recently violated bone (e.g., fracture, postsurgical) due to localization in marrow elements
    - False-negative WBC scan in chronic infections and spinal discitis/osteomyelitis
  - Tc-99m SC marrow mapping has similar uptake to WBC scan in chronic inflammation or red marrow
  - Ga-67 scintigraphy: Depicts distribution of infection/inflammation (Fe/iron surrogate), may be helpful in chronic osteomyelitis
    - When compared with bone scan, Ga-67 uptake should be greater than bone scan uptake or show uptake of different size (larger or smaller)
    - Preferred over In-111 WBC for spinal discitis/osteomyelitis due to potential false (-) result
  - SPECT and SPECT/CT adds specificity to location of abnormal activity
- Correlative imaging features
  - Plain film: Limited sensitivity and specificity
    - Normal initially; recognition may take 2-3 weeks

– Loss of cortical margins; periosteal reaction, erosions, soft tissue swelling, sequestra, involucra, sclerosis

Artifacts and Quality Control

- Equipment
  - Inadequate imaging technique (missed angiographic phase, not enough delay for delayed images)
  - Equipment failure (failed photomultiplier tube)
  - Wrong collimator or incorrect photopeak
- Radiopharmaceutical
  - Radiochemical impurity with free pertechnetate
  - Too little dose secondary to partial dose extravasation
- Patient
  - Urinary contamination and patient motion
  - Patient clothing and accessories (watch, jewelry) causing photopenic defects
  - Poor hydration or poor renal function

DIFFERENTIAL DIAGNOSIS

Arthropathy

- Neuropathic, osteoarthritic, rheumatoid, gout: Concordant WBC and Tc-99m SC marrow map favors arthropathy

Post-Traumatic

- Clinical history of fracture, surgery, other imaging studies showing post-traumatic changes, focal or linear in pattern

Paget Disease: Osteitis Deformans

- Very intense uptake on bone scan during active phase; involves pelvis, calvarium, and spine; affected bones appear enlarged; can be polyostotic

Osteoid Osteoma

- Typically moderate uptake peripherally and more intense activity centrally in nidus on bones scan; WBC scan can distinguish from osteomyelitis

PATHOLOGY

General Features

- Etiology
  - Usually bacterial, may be polymicrobial
  - Most common cause: Extension of cellulitis or traumatic direct inoculation in adolescents/adults
    - Intraosseous extension via Volkmann (transverse) and haversian (longitudinal) canals
    - Penetrating trauma, decubitus ulcers, wounds
    - Pseudomonas aeruginosa: IV drug users
    - Septic arthritis, prosthesis failure
  - Hematogenous spread
    - Most common in pediatric population with predominantly long bone involvement
    - Less common in adults and typically involves vertebral body
  - Vascular insufficiency
    - Diabetic foot infections
    - Bacteroides fragilosa: Common in diabetics
- Associated abnormalities
  - Cellulitis, infected open wound, sinus tract, frank drainage of pus through skin (advanced cases)
  - Brodie abscess: Cavitary, usually metaphyseal, collection of necrotic debris, WBCs

CLINICAL ISSUES

Presentation

- Most common signs/symptoms
  - Bone pain, erythema, swelling, fluctuance, fever, nausea, malaise, sweats, chills
  - Overlying soft tissue ulcer
  - ↑ WBC count and erythrocyte sedimentation rate
  - Blood cultures: (+) in ~ 50% of patients with osteomyelitis
- Other signs/symptoms
  - Adjacent abscess, local extension into joint, fistula
  - Pathologic fracture

Demographics

- Epidemiology
  - 1/4 of diabetics will suffer severe foot morbidity during their lifetime
    - Especially with ulcerations, wounds, and penetrating injuries of feet
  - In IV drug users, osteomyelitis occurs in unusual locations
  - More common in patients with AIDS, immune suppression, sickle cell anemia
  - Orthopedic procedures and open fractures predispose

Natural History & Prognosis

- Good prognosis if adequate therapy initiated
  - May result in osseous deformity or growth arrest
- Chronic osteomyelitis more likely recalcitrant, especially in diabetics and patients with vascular disease

Treatment

- Eradication through IV antibiotic therapy, wound hygiene, surgical debridement, amputation
  - Chronic osteomyelitis requires surgical intervention

DIAGNOSTIC CHECKLIST

Consider

- Cellulitis, degenerative or inflammatory arthropathy, post-traumatic, postsurgical
- Septic arthritis has increased activity in all phases of 3-phase bone scan
- Septic arthritis typically has diffusely increased uptake throughout joint compared to osteomyelitis that can show focal uptake only on 1 side of joint

Image Interpretation Pearls

- WBC scan (+) with Tc-99m SC (-) discordance is > 90% sensitive, specific for osteomyelitis

Reporting Tips

- Recommend In-111 WBC with Tc-99m SC after abnormal 3-phase bone

SELECTED REFERENCES

1. Love C et al: Radionuclide imaging of inflammation and infection in the acute care setting. Semin Nucl Med. 43(2):102-13, 2013
2. Palestro CJ: FDG-PET in musculoskeletal infections. Semin Nucl Med. 43(5):367-76, 2013
3. van der Bruggen W et al: PET and SPECT in osteomyelitis and prosthetic bone and joint infections: a systematic review. Semin Nucl Med. 40(1):3-15, 2010

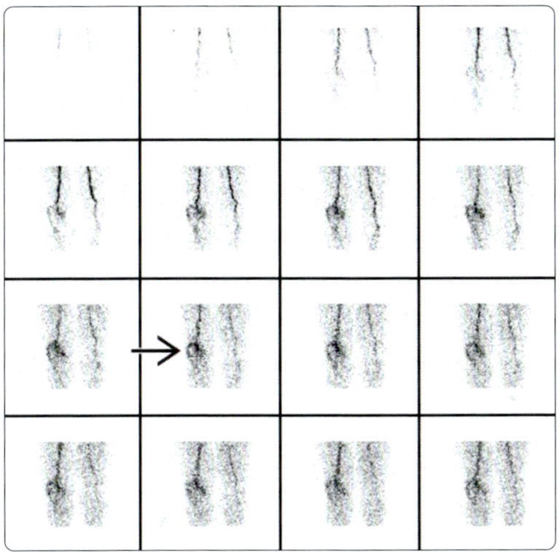

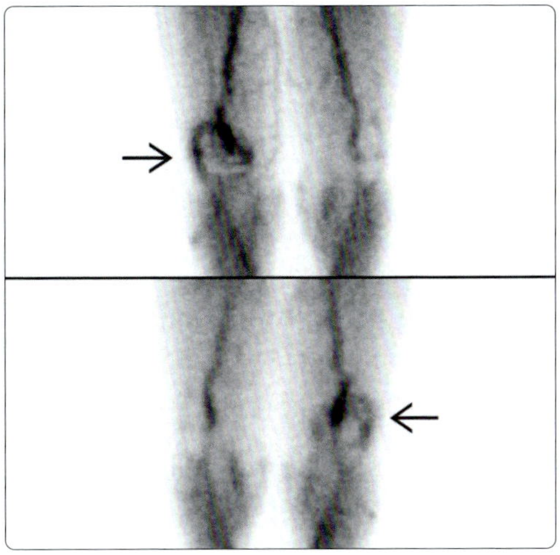

(Left) *Anterior flow images from a 3-phase bone scan show hyperperfusion to a right knee arthroplasty →.* **(Right)** *Anterior (top) and posterior (bottom) immediate static images of the knees show hyperemia to the right knee arthroplasty →.*

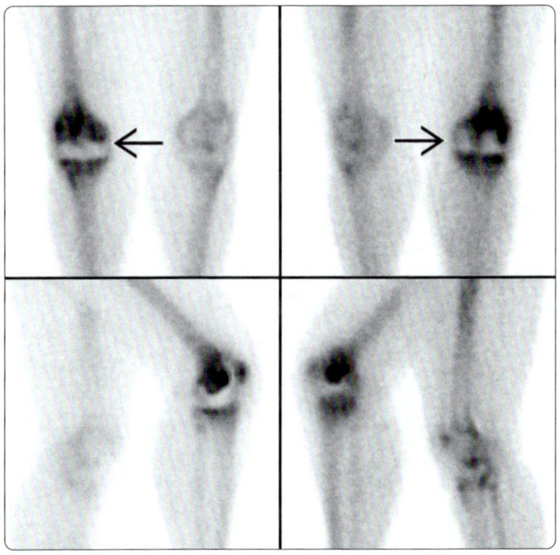

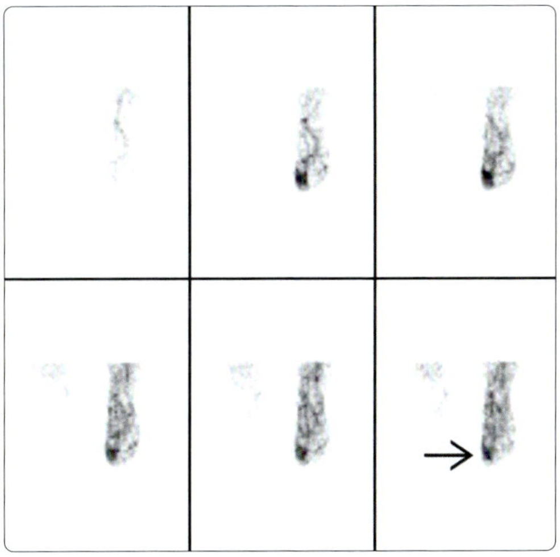

(Left) *Anterior (top left) and posterior (top right) delayed static images and lateral static images (bottom row) show increased tracer localization involving the right knee in a periprosthetic distribution →. Findings are most compatible with infection of the right knee arthroplasty. In-111 WBC scan with same-day bone marrow imaging may be performed to add specificity.* **(Right)** *Plantar flow images from a 3-phase bone scan show hyperperfusion to the foot and more focally to the great toe →.*

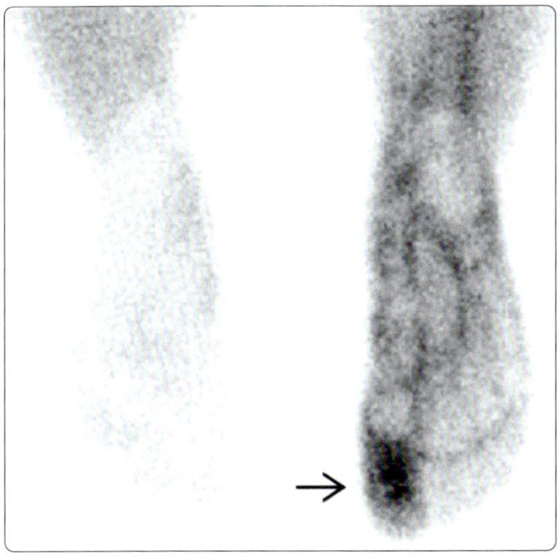

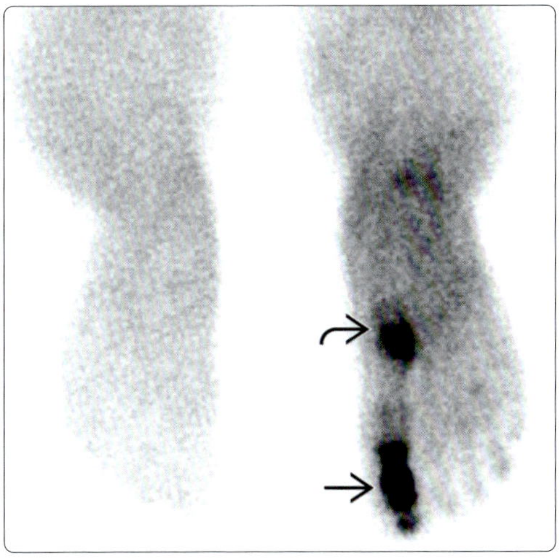

(Left) *Immediate plantar static image shows hyperperfusion to the right great toe →.* **(Right)** *Plantar delayed image shows focal increased tracer localization to the right distal metatarsal and phalanx →. Given the 3-phase positive findings, underlying osteomyelitis is the most likely diagnosis in this patient with a diabetic foot ulcer on his great toe. Additional activity in the base of the 1st metatarsal → was not positive on the 1st 2 phases and is most compatible with osteoarthritis.*

(Left) *Angiographic phase bone scan of a 7-year-old boy with suspected osteomyelitis of the distal left tibia shows increased flow ➔ to the area.* **(Right)** *Blood pool phase image shows hyperemia ➔ of the distal tibia and ankle joint.*

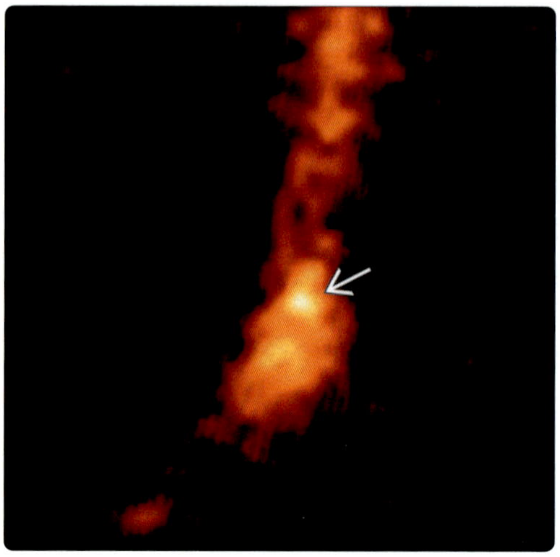

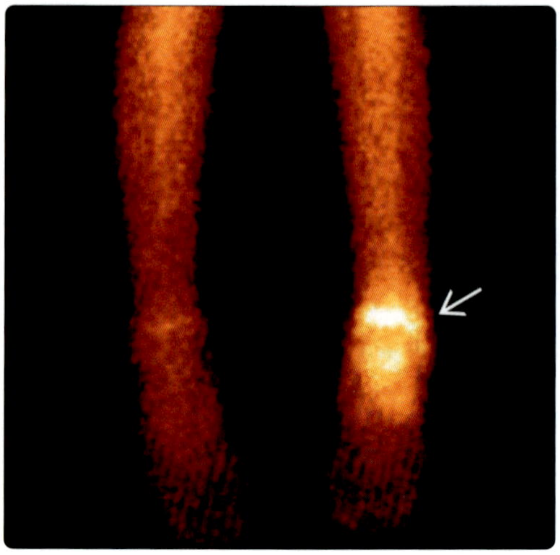

(Left) *Corresponding delayed phase image also shows increased uptake ➔ in the distal tibia. Findings are on both sides of the joint, compatible with septic arthritis and osteomyelitis of the adjacent bone.* **(Right)** *Corresponding lateral radiograph shows no evidence of osteomyelitis. Radiographs are less sensitive than 3-phase skeletal scintigraphy for septic arthritis/osteomyelitis.*

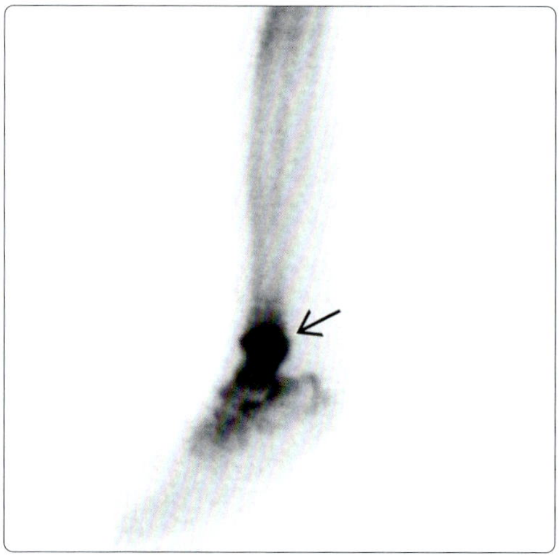

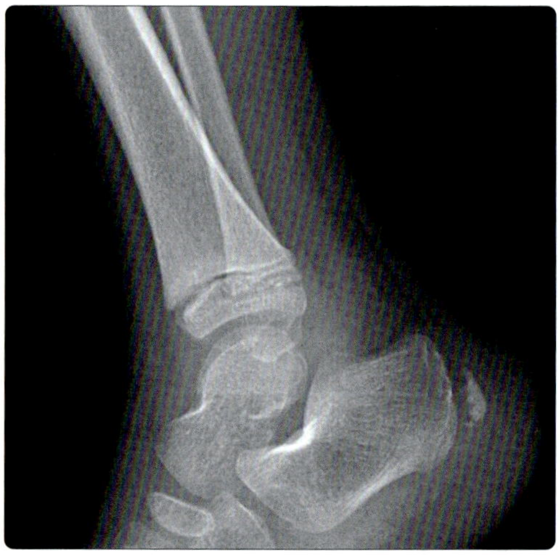

(Left) *Plantar angiographic phase bone scan in a patient with diabetic foot ulcer shows hypervascularity about great toe ➔, suspicious for osteomyelitis.* **(Right)** *Plantar delayed phase bone scan in the same patient shows tracer accumulation in the head of the 3rd metatarsal ➔ and the proximal phalanx of the 3rd digit ➔, indicating osteomyelitis.*

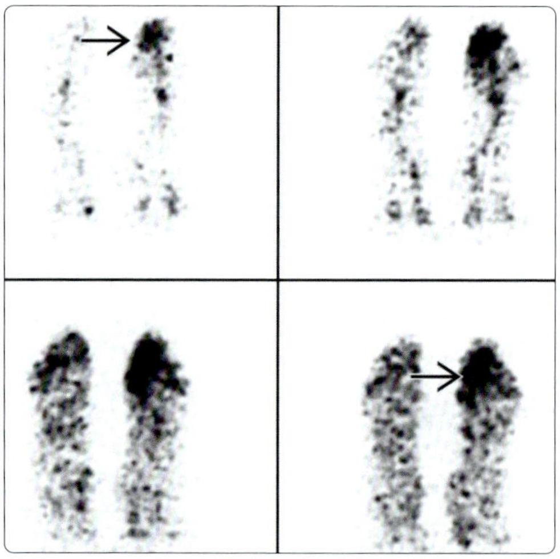

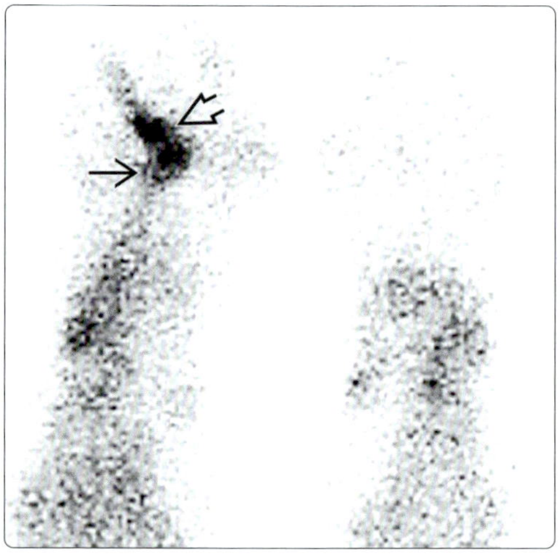

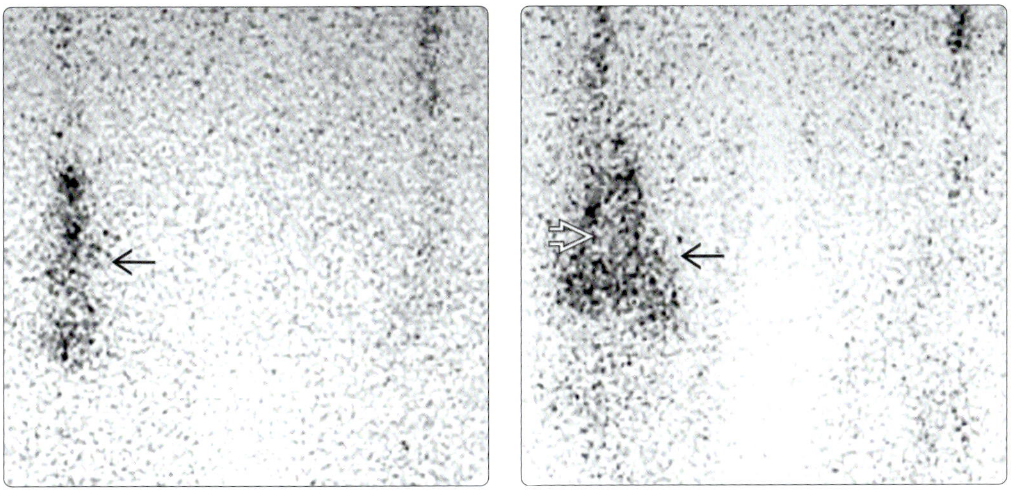

(Left) *Anterior In-111 WBC scan in the same patient shows linear accumulation → in the distal right femur, corresponding to lucent region on plain In-111 WBC scan.* **(Right)** *Anterior Tc-99m SC scan in the same patient shows red marrow distribution →. Focal photopenia ➡ corresponds to WBC accumulation in Brodie abscess. This discordance indicates osteomyelitis.*

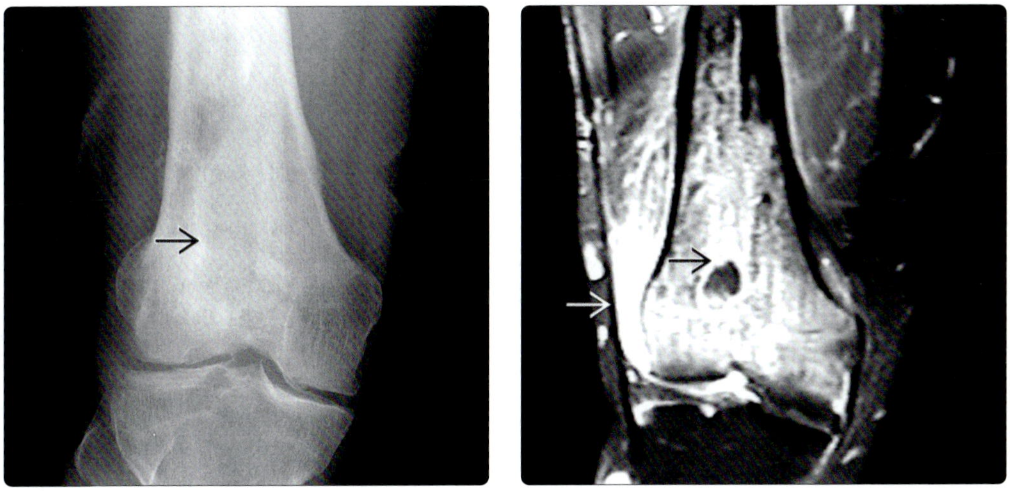

(Left) *Anterior radiograph shows lucent medullary lesion → at site of Brodie abscess.* **(Right)** *Coronal T2-weighted MR in the same patient shows fluid signal lateral to the distal femoral condyle ➡ and at the site of Brodie abscess in the intramedullary region →.*

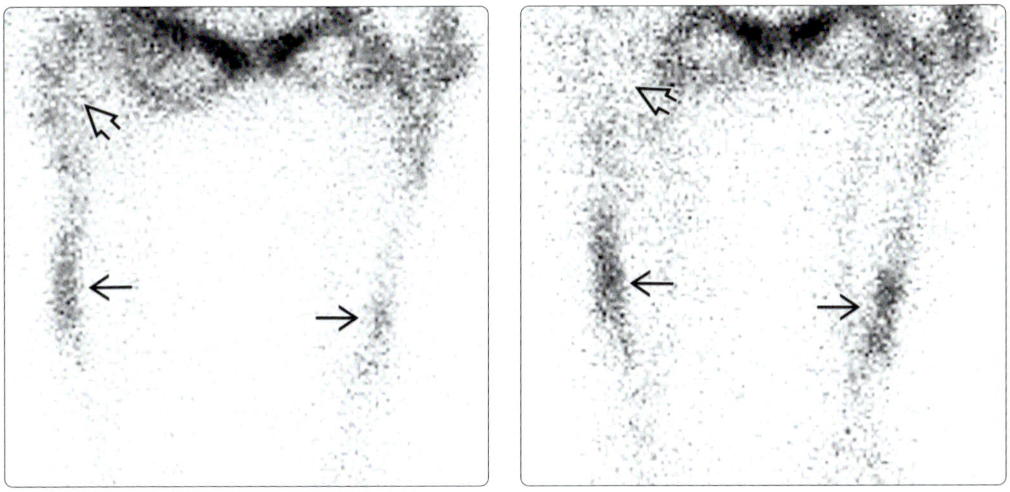

(Left) *Anterior In-111 WBC scan shows leukocyte aggregation in the proximal right → and bilateral mid femurs →, necessitating Tc-99m SC marrow map.* **(Right)** *Anterior Tc-99m SC marrow map in the same patient shows presence of reticuloendothelial system cells (red marrow) in the mid femurs →. Absence of activity in the proximal right femur is consistent with osteomyelitis →.*

KEY FACTS

TERMINOLOGY

- Broad term for diseases that result in bone strength or mineralization abnormalities
- Overlap of bone scan findings of osteomalacia, renal osteodystrophy, and hyperparathyroidism

IMAGING

- **General Findings**
  - Superscan (faint or absent renal activity) presentation
  - Tie sternum: Hot manubrium and increased cortical uptake in sternal body
  - Increased axial and periarticular activity
- **Hyperparathyroidism (HPT)**
  - Extraosseous uptake in lungs, kidneys, and stomach
  - Brown tumors are less common in secondary HPT than in primary HPT
- **Osteomalacia**
  - Costochondral uptake of tracer = beading or rosary bead
  - Pseudofractures (Looser zone or Milkman fractures)
- **Renal osteodystrophy**
  - Can have very high bone:soft tissue ratio
  - More diffuse and symmetric than 2° HPT, which may show focal uptake from cystic changes and brown tumors
- **Paget Disease**
  - Markedly increased uptake in affected regions, but can be normal in sclerotic burned-out areas
  - Bone scan can be used to assess complications of fracture and sarcomatous degeneration, but correlation with conventional imaging suggested to avoid false-negative assessments
- **Osteoporosis**
  - Not specifically associated with abnormal bone scan findings
  - Bone scan useful to diagnose osteoporotic fractures, especially in sacrum and ribs

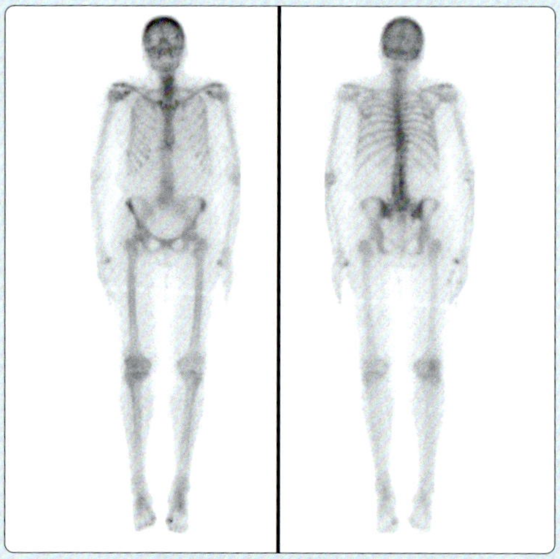

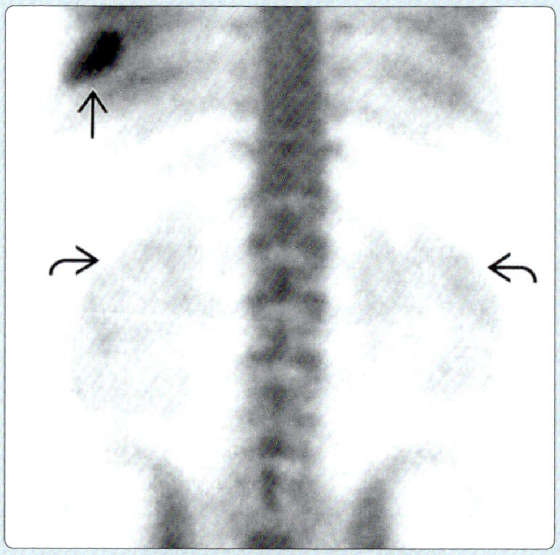

(Left) *Superscan in a patient with renal osteodystrophy is shown. The overall pattern is nonspecific, but there is no focal lesion to suggest pseudofractures or brown tumors.* **(Right)** *Bone scan in a 46-year-old man with secondary hyperparathyroidism (HPT) due to end-stage renal disease shows increased uptake in the brown tumor of a rib ➡, as well as bilateral renal cortical uptake related to HPT ↪.*

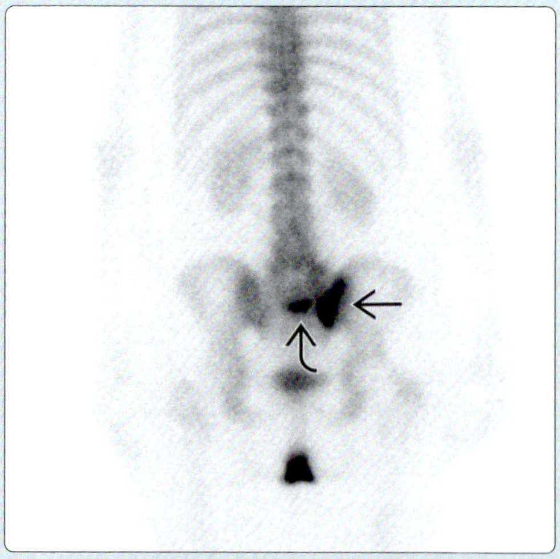

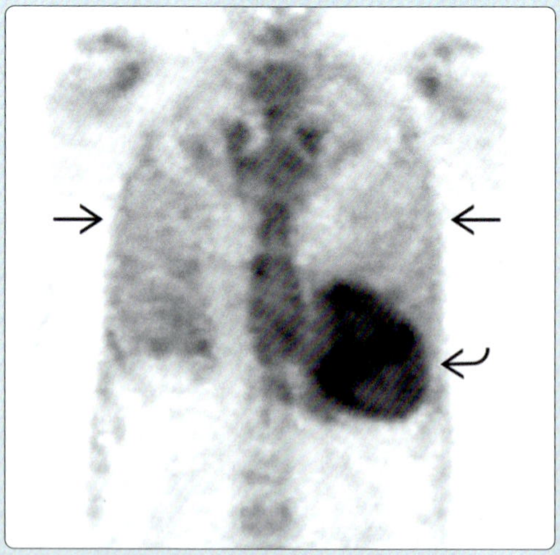

(Left) *A 77-year-old female with osteoporosis presents with pelvic pain. Bone scan shows vertically oriented increased uptake in the right sacrum ➡ and horizontal activity in the mid sacrum ↪, which are most compatible with insufficiency fractures. Osteoporosis does not show increased or decreased uptake.* **(Right)** *Bone scan shows primary HPT with diffuse extraosseous uptake in the lungs ➡ and myocardium ↪, an indication of severe disease.*

TERMINOLOGY

Definitions

- Metabolic bone disease
  - Broad term for diseases that result in bone strength or mineralization abnormalities
  - Common indication for bone scan is increased alkaline phosphatase and bone pain
  - Overlap of bone scan findings of osteomalacia, renal osteodystrophy, and hyperparathyroidism

IMAGING

General Features

- Best diagnostic clue
  - Superscan (faint or absent renal activity) presentation
  - Increased axial and periarticular activity
  - If not superscan, very good bone scan appearance with excellent bone/soft tissue contrast
  - Focal uptake to suggest fracture or pseudofracture in osteomalacia
  - Tie sternum: Hot manubrium and increased cortical uptake in sternal body
  - Prominent uptake in mandible typical for renal osteodystrophy
  - Costochondral uptake of tracer = beading or rosary bead seen in osteomalacia

Nuclear Medicine Findings

- Whole-body bone scan
  - Important to differentiate between metastatic disease and metabolic bone disease
  - Bone scans of hyperparathyroidism (HPT), osteomalacia, and renal osteodystrophy must be differentiated from those of metastatic malignancy
    - Have no role in diagnosis or management of these diseases
- Hyperparathyroidism (HPT)
  - Primary
    - Normal bone scan in 80%
    - Foci of increased uptake: Calvarium, mandible, sternum, acromioclavicular joint, lateral humeral epicondyles, hands
    - Increased uptake in brown tumors
    - Extraskeletal uptake
      - Lungs, kidneys, stomach most common
      - Myocardium, spleen, diaphragm, thyroid, skeletal muscle in severe disease
  - Secondary
    - Superscan
    - Diffuse lung uptake in 60%
    - Brown tumors: Less common than in primary HPT
    - Uptake increased in vertebrae, distal 3rd of long bones, rib
- Osteomalacia
  - Can be normal in early stages of disease
  - Generalized increased uptake in axial skeleton
  - Increased uptake at ends of multiple ribs, with beading appearance along rib cage (rachitic rosary sign)
    - In contrast to linear orientation of metastasis along single rib
    - Can help differentiate metabolic superscan from metastatic disease
  - Increased sternum uptake common
  - Pseudofractures (Looser zone or Milkman fractures) occur in ribs, lateral scapula, clavicles, pubic rami, radius/ulna, and medial femoral cortices
    - Bone scan is more sensitive to diagnose pseudofractures than radiography
    - Often perpendicular to cortex
    - Symmetric in appearance
- Renal osteodystrophy
  - High bone metabolism secondary to chronic kidney disease
  - Can have very high bone:soft tissue ratio, similar to superscan
    - Typically most striking appearance of metabolic bone diseases excluding Paget disease
    - Lack of bladder activity can help differentiate from metastatic superscan
  - Signs of secondary HPT
  - More diffuse and symmetric than secondary HPT, which may show focal uptake from cystic changes and brown tumors
- Paget disease
  - Markedly increased uptake in affected regions
  - Can be normal in sclerotic burned-out areas
  - Pelvis most common site, followed by spine, skull, femur, scapula, tibia, and humerus
  - Bone scan used to determine extent of disease
  - More commonly polyostotic
  - Bone scan can be used to assess complications of fracture and sarcomatous degeneration, but correlation with conventional imaging suggested to avoid false-negative assessments
- Osteoporosis
  - Not specifically associated with abnormal bone scan findings
  - Quantitative evaluation of skeletal uptake at 24 hours cannot differentiate normal vs. osteoporotic bone
  - Bone scan useful to diagnose osteoporotic fractures, especially in sacrum and ribs
  - May take 2 weeks for bone scan to become abnormal in osteoporotic fractures
  - Vertebral fractures normalize on bone scan in 3-18 months (average 9-12 months)

Imaging Recommendations

- Best imaging tool
  - Bone scan offers most information for suspected metabolic disease involving skeleton
- Protocol advice
  - Whole-body imaging allows full skeletal survey
  - 3-phase protocol not typically indicated
  - SPECT/CT useful for improved localization of abnormal uptake in pelvis and improved contrast for more subtle lesions

DIFFERENTIAL DIAGNOSIS

Hyperparathyroidism

- Overproduction of parathyroid hormone
  - Primary: Parathyroid hormone secreting adenoma

- Secondary: Increased production of parathyroid hormone in response to low serum calcium
- Tertiary: Parathyroid tissue unregulated and autonomous after long period of stimulation
- Brown tumor and extraosseous uptake in lungs, stomach, and renal cortex help differentiate from other entities
- Diffuse calvarial and mandibular uptake is typical for HPT

Osteomalacia

- Defective bone mineralization typically caused by vitamin D or calcium deficiency
- Causes rickets in pediatric patients

Renal Osteodystrophy

- Bone demineralization caused by chronic kidney disease
- Renal failure → hyperphosphatemia → hypocalcemia → secondary hyperparathyroidism → bone demineralization
- Can include varying degrees of osteoporosis, osteomalacia, adynamic bone, and secondary HPT

Paget Disease

- Chronic disease of abnormal bone remodeling typically seen in elderly
- Polyostotic involvement
- Increased uptake, except in osteoporosis circumscripta (lytic skull disease) when only margins of lesion show uptake
- Patchy uptake occurs after therapy

Hypertrophic Osteoarthropathy

- Associated with cancer
- Clubbing and periostitis of small joints, especially distal interphalangeal joints (DIPs)
- Uptake along periosteum

Osseous Metastases

- Not uniform and symmetric uptake
- Heterogenous uptake mostly in axial skeleton
- Clinical information useful to distinguish from metabolic disease

Other Causes of Generalized Increased Skeletal Uptake on Bone Scan

- Thyrotoxicosis
- Acromegaly
- Hypervitaminosis D
- Systemic mastocytosis
- Myelofibrosis
- Osteopetrosis

CLINICAL ISSUES

Presentation

- Most common signs/symptoms
  - Increased alkaline phosphatase and bone pain common indication for bone scan
  - Symptoms of hypercalcemia in HPT
    - Bones: Bone pain, osteitis fibrosa cystica, fractures
    - Stones: Kidney stones
    - Groans: Impaired GI motility, constipation, nausea
    - Moans: Psychiatric and neurological symptoms
- Other signs/symptoms
  - Chronic kidney disease
  - Spontaneous tendon rupture
  - Extraskeletal calcifications in skin and vasculature

SELECTED REFERENCES

1. Abdelrazek S et al: Bone scan in metabolic bone diseases. Review. Nucl Med Rev Cent East Eur. 15(2):124-31, 2012
2. Cook GJ et al: Miscellaneous indications in bone scintigraphy: metabolic bone diseases and malignant bone tumors. Semin Nucl Med. 40(1):52-61, 2010
3. Martin KJ et al: Metabolic bone disease in chronic kidney disease. J Am Soc Nephrol. 18(3):875-85, 2007
4. Pour MC et al: Diffuse increased uptake on bone scan: super scan. Semin Nucl Med. 34(2):154-6, 2004
5. Peller PJ et al: Extraosseous Tc-99m MDP uptake: a pathophysiologic approach. Radiographics. 13(4):715-34, 1993
6. Spitz J et al: Scintimetric evaluation of remodeling after bone fractures in man. J Nucl Med. 34(9):1403-9, 1993
7. McAfee JG: Radionuclide imaging in metabolic and systemic skeletal diseases. Semin Nucl Med. 17(4):334-49, 1987

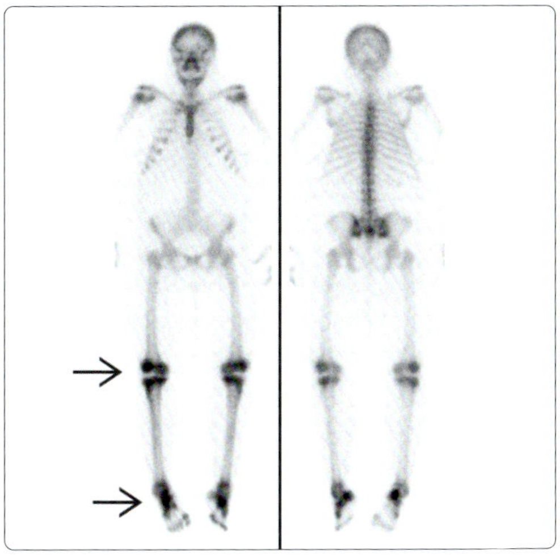

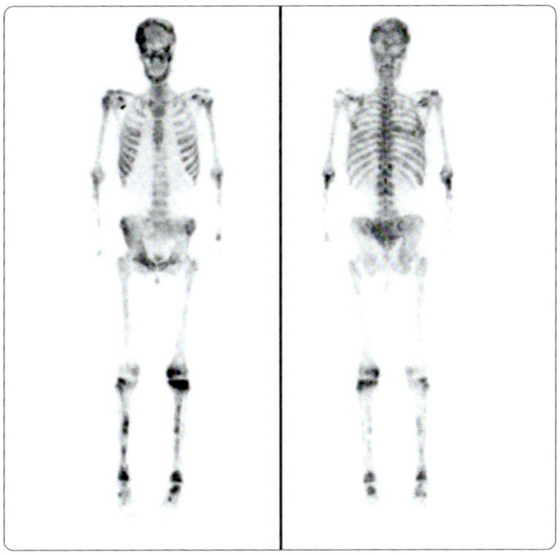

(Left) *Bone scan shows the superscan for metabolic disease due to renal osteodystrophy with increased periarticular uptake →.* **(Right)** *Superscan in a patient with widespread osseous metastasis in the axial and appendicular skeleton is shown. The activity is not uniform, homogenous, or symmetric, as is typical in metabolic disease.*

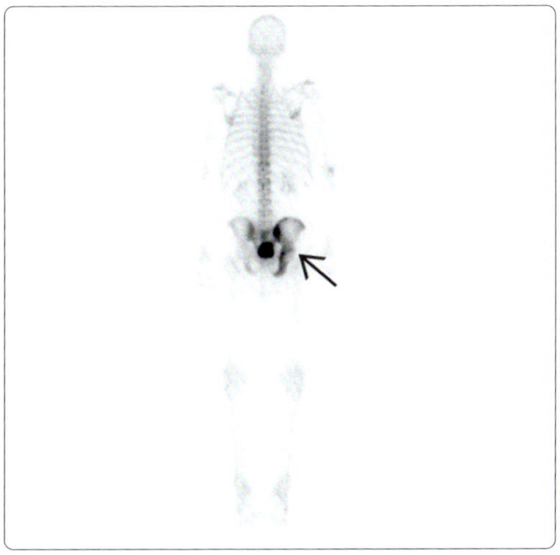

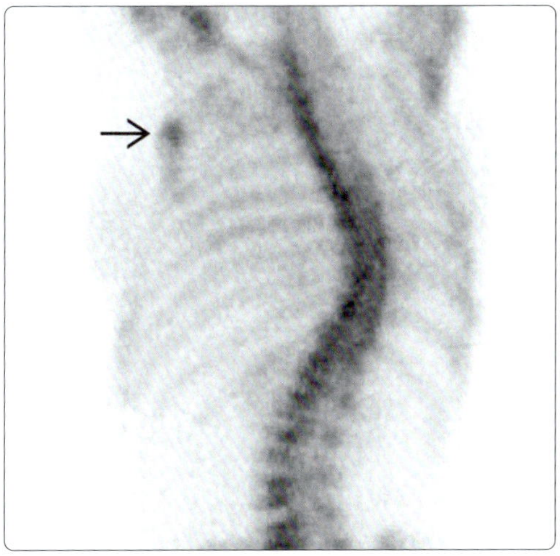

(Left) *Whole-body bone scan in the posterior projection shows homogeneous uptake in an enlarged right hemipelvis → without multifocality. Correlation with radiographs or CT would be useful, if available, but these findings are most compatible with Paget disease.* **(Right)** *Left posterior oblique view of the thorax in a patient with osteomalacia and thoracolumbar scoliosis shows focal increased uptake in the lateral scapula → that is compatible with a pseudofracture (Looser zone).*

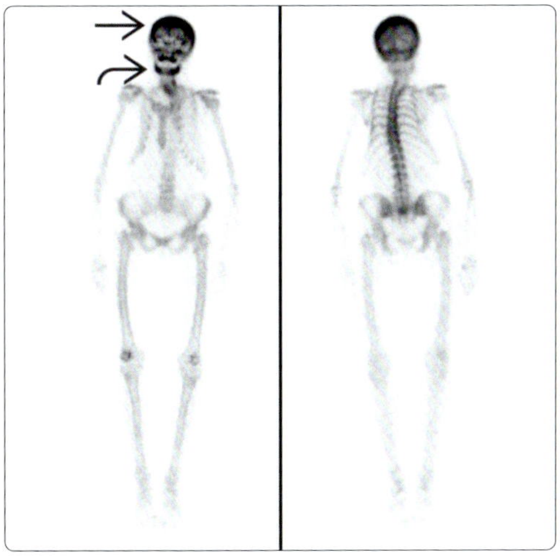

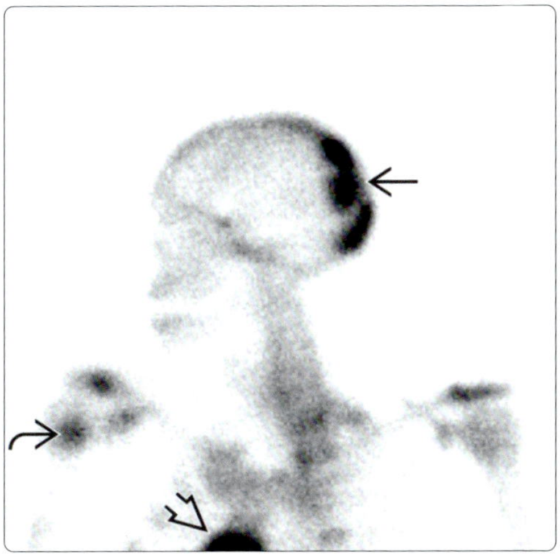

(Left) *Bone scan shows diffuse uptake throughout the axial and appendicular skeleton secondary to hyperparathyroidism (HPT). Marked uniform increased uptake in the skull → and mandible ↗ are more typical in metabolic disease due to HPT.* **(Right)** *Multiple foci of abnormal uptake in the posterior calvarium →, with additional focal uptake in the right humerus ↗ and partially imaged uptake in the sternum, ⇒ is shown on this bone scan. This pattern is typical for metastases, not metabolic bone disease.*

KEY FACTS

TERMINOLOGY

- Extraskeletal osteogenesis
- Acquired: Ectopic ossification, myositis ossificans circumscripta/traumatica
- Hereditary: Atraumatic HO, fibrodysplasia ossificans progressiva (FOP)/ myositis ossificans progressiva (MOP), Münchmeyer disease

IMAGING

- Tc-99m MDP 3-phase and whole-body bone scan more sensitive than other imaging modalities, particularly early in disease
- Bone scan used to follow HO maturation
- Ga-67 scintigraphy: May be incidentally positive on imaging performed for infectious processes
- WBC, Tc-99m sulfur colloid scans: May be positive in mature HO due to red marrow/reticuloendothelial

TOP DIFFERENTIAL DIAGNOSES

- Histology of HO easily mistaken for (osteo)sarcoma; ideally diagnosis established without biopsy
- Osteosarcoma ossifies from center, opposite of HO

DIAGNOSTIC CHECKLIST

- Use 3-phase bone scan to follow maturation course
- Plain film correlation for bone scan findings if HO diagnosis not established
- Vascular (angiographic) and blood pool phases may be more intense than delayed phase images in early HO
- Conventional modalities should demonstrate peripheral to central ossification, central fat in mature lesions

(Left) *Lateral radiograph in a 21-year-old man with persistent pain following ORIF of the right elbow shows extensive heterotopic ossification ➡ anterior and posterior to the elbow joint.* **(Right)** *Corresponding AP radiograph shows extensive ossification ➡ around the joint.*

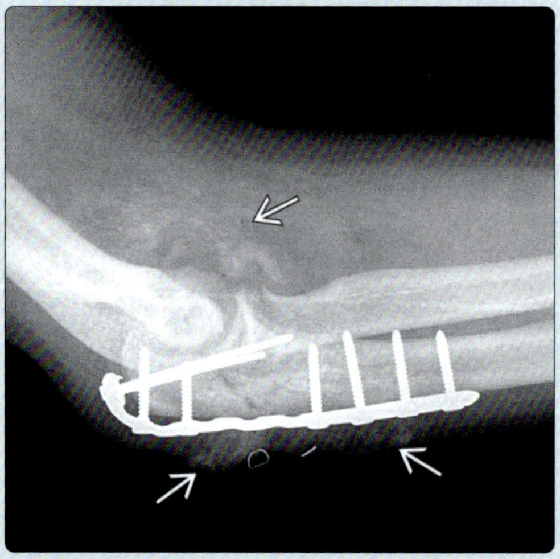

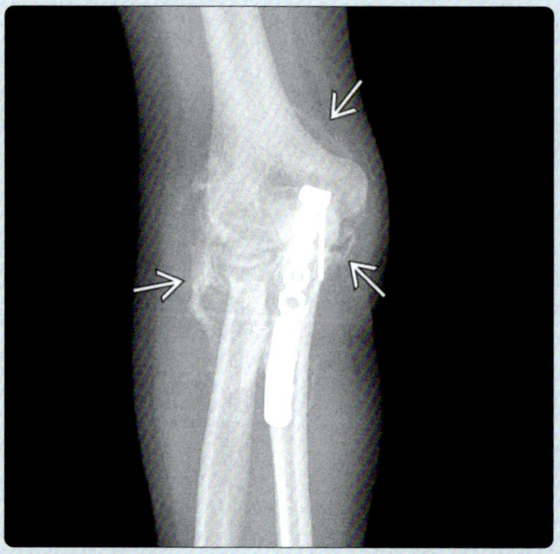

(Left) *Angiographic phase bone scan shows mildly increased flow ➡ at the right elbow. Radiopharmaceutical injection in the right upper extremity was avoided.* **(Right)** *Corresponding delayed phase bone scan shows significantly increased uptake ➡ in the right elbow, consistent with active heterotopic ossification.*

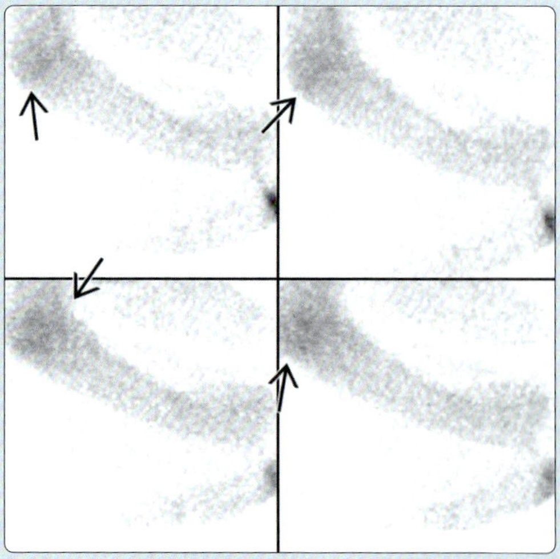

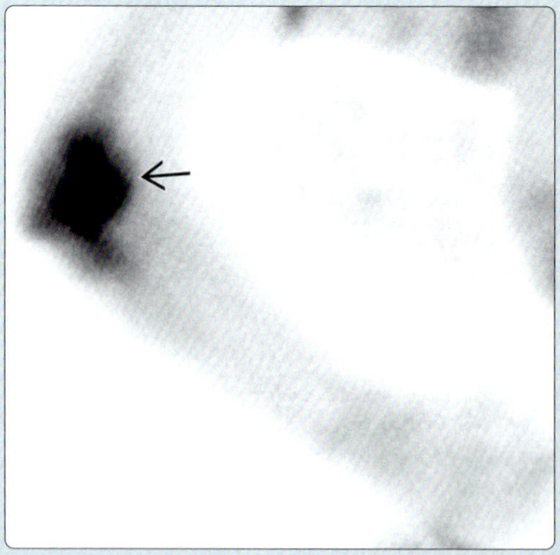

TERMINOLOGY

Abbreviations

- Heterotopic ossification (HO)

Definitions

- Extraskeletal osteogenesis
  - Typically (though not necessarily) in muscle
  - Tendons, fascia (fasciitis ossificans), subcutaneous fat
- Acquired: Ectopic ossification, myositis ossificans circumscripta/traumatica
- Hereditary: Atraumatic HO, fibrodysplasia ossificans progressiva (FOP)/myositis ossificans progressiva (MOP), Münchmeyer disease

IMAGING

General Features

- Best diagnostic clue
  - Amorphous, ill-defined, immature soft tissue bone formation and subsequent ossific maturation
- Location
  - Heterotopic ossification
    - Thighs: Contusion, crush injury
    - Tends to be diaphyseal in thigh (differential Dx: Osteosarcoma, frequently metadiaphyseal)
    - Hips: Arthroplasty, neurologic impairment
    - Most common postsurgically about hip flexors
    - Upper extremities: Elbows, shoulders, brain injury
    - Knees: Spinal cord injury
  - Fibrodysplasia ossificans progressiva (acquired)
    - Spreads from axial to appendicular, proximal to distal, cranial to caudal: Sternocleidomastoid, paraspinous, masticators, shoulder, pelvic muscles
    - Causes progressive limitation of motion
- Morphology
  - Thickened muscle/fascia with edema (CT/MR), amorphous calcification, ossific maturation

Nuclear Medicine Findings

- Tc-99m MDP 3-phase and whole-body bone scan
  - Positive on angiographic, blood pool, delayed bone scan phases during formation, maturation
  - Moderately positive on delayed phase only when lesion becomes stable: Useful to monitor maturation
  - At maturation (6 months to 2 years), lesion matches or is similar to normal bone (i.e., vertebral body) on bone scan
- Ga-67 scintigraphy: May be incidentally positive on imaging performed for infectious processes
- WBC, Tc-99m sulfur colloid scans: May be positive in mature HO due to red marrow

Radiographic Findings

- Plain radiography: May show immature amorphous, ill-defined bone by 2-6 weeks
  - Recommendation is to repeat radiographs in 30 days
  - Subsequent imaging shows progressive ossific maturation/demarcation at ~ 6 weeks
  - 6-12 weeks: Lamellar bone develops at involved boundaries
- Brooker classification for hip HO
  - I: Islands of bone in soft tissue
  - II: Bone spurs with ≥ 1 cm between opposing surfaces
  - III: Spurs with ≤ 1 cm space
  - IV: Ankylosis

CT Findings

- CT/MR: Soft tissue mass with peripheral calcification/bone formation
  - Organization occurs with maturation as above
  - Central fat may be present in mature HO

Ultrasonographic Findings

- Ultrasound: Usually incidental finding (operator dependent) of vascular US for DVT
  - Look for HO concurrently with venous survey
  - Increasingly organized, echogenic margins, central hypoechogenicity: Maturing bone
  - Sheet-like calcification is considered specific

Imaging Recommendations

- Best imaging tool
  - Plain radiographs: First-line imaging modality
    - Inexpensive, widely available, well tolerated
    - Evaluates underlying bony conditions, excludes many other causes
  - Tc-99m MDP 3-phase and whole-body bone scan
    - More sensitive than other imaging modalities, particularly early in disease
      - Blood flow and soft tissue phase abnormal 2-3 weeks post injury
      - Delayed phase abnormalities occurs 3-4 weeks post injury
    - Used to follow HO maturation
      - Most bone scans return to normal 12 months post injury
    - Whole-body survey
    - Can compare region of HO to normal vertebral body uptake to establish maturity
- Protocol advice
  - Tc-99m MDP bone scan
    - Adult dose: 20-25 mCi (740-925 MBq) IV
    - Hydrate patient to improve soft tissue washout
    - Inject in extremity away from site of interest to prevent pooling, venous valvular adherence, subsequent false-positive
    - Angiographic and soft tissue phase: Image over area of interest during and immediately after radiotracer injection
    - Delayed phase: Image at 3-4 hours post injection, Consider longer if renal failure or poor cardiac output
    - SPECT/CT used for improved anatomic localization

DIFFERENTIAL DIAGNOSIS

Deep Venous Thrombosis

- May coexist secondary to local compression
- Pain, erythema, swelling, similar patient population

Extraskeletal (Parosteal) Osteosarcoma, Synovial Sarcoma, Chondrosarcoma

- Histology of HO easily mistaken for (osteo)sarcoma; ideally diagnosis established without biopsy
- HO should have soft tissue plane between adjacent bone

- Osteosarcoma ossifies from center, opposite of HO

Tumoral Calcinosis

- Globular juxtaarticular soft tissue calcifications, encapsulated granulomatous hydroxyapatite

Hematoma

- May be present prior to heterotopic ossification
- Nonenhancing centrally (in contrast to early HO on MR)
- Progressive evolution of blood products on MR, dystrophic calcification may occur
- Spontaneous resorption, persistence/enlargement requiring drainage, or abscess formation may occur

PATHOLOGY

General Features

- Etiology
  - Myositis ossificans traumatica, no significant genetic linkage, most often secondary to trauma
    - Blunt trauma, crush injuries, infection, burns, surgery, immobilization
    - Often hip arthroplasty, ORIF of femur/elbow fractures
    - CNS injury, compromise (25% or more), including poliomyelitis, Guillain-Barré
    - Electrical rhabdomyolysis
    - Common in patients with previous HO
  - FOP, Münchmeyer disease
    - Atraumatic, idiopathic
- Genetics
  - Fibrodysplasia ossificans progressiva, Münchmeyer disease
    - Autosomal dominant, rare, childhood onset
    - Possible link to morphogenic protein receptor gene defect
- Associated abnormalities
  - Post-traumatic form
    - DISH, ankylosing spondylitis, Paget disease
  - Hereditary form, FOP
    - Shortening/segmentation abnormalities of digits (great toe), metatarsals, metacarpals, spine

Gross Pathologic & Surgical Features

- Undifferentiated centrally, mature peripheral bone
  - Progressive from center to periphery
  - Central tissues sufficiently undifferentiated to complicate histologic distinction vs. osteosarcoma
  - Marginal tissues show mature osteoid matrix
  - Biopsy peripheral, central and intermediate regions to establish characteristic zonal maturation
    - If biopsy is performed too early before maturation, it is often too difficult to exclude osteosarcoma

Microscopic Features

- Mesenchymal stem cells develop into spindle cells then osteoblasts
- Osteoblasts produce woven bone with progressive organization forming lamellated bone surrounding trabecular bone
- Microscopic bone formation starts around 1 week, lamellated bone ~ 6 weeks, mature ~ 6-24 months

CLINICAL ISSUES

Presentation

- Most common signs/symptoms
  - Post-traumatic/nonhereditary: Pain, swelling, hard palpable mass, edema, contractures
  - Progressive limitation/restriction of motion

Demographics

- Gender
  - M:F = 2:1 in patients with central cord insult

Natural History & Prognosis

- Lesions may persist permanently, resolution may occur, particularly lesions induced by local damage
  - Neurologically induced lesions unlikely to resolve
- Malignant degeneration to osteosarcoma incidence may be skewed by formidable histologic interpretations

Treatment

- Pharmaceutical prevention: NSAIDs, (indomethacin prophylaxis), diphosphonate therapy (etidronate)
  - Variable success, indomethacin most common
    - Ectopic bone formation decreased, function and pain not significantly different, ↑ complications
  - NSAIDs used as prophylaxis prior to THA
- Physical rehabilitation, range of motion therapy
- External beam radiation
- Surgical intervention
  - After maturation has been established to minimize recurrence and hemorrhage
  - 3-phase bone scans allow maturation surveillance

DIAGNOSTIC CHECKLIST

Consider

- Use 3-phase bone scan to follow maturation course if surgical resection is considered
- Plain film correlation for suspected HO based on bone scan findings if HO diagnosis not established

Image Interpretation Pearls

- Vascular (angiographic) and blood pool phases may be more intense than delayed phase images in early HO
- Conventional modalities should demonstrate peripheral to central ossification, central fat in mature lesions

SELECTED REFERENCES

1. Nauth A et al: Heterotopic ossification in orthopaedic trauma. J Orthop Trauma. 26(12):684-8, 2012
2. Vavken P et al: Economic evaluation of NSAID and radiation to prevent heterotopic ossification after hip surgery. Arch Orthop Trauma Surg. 131(9):1309-15, 2011
3. Crundwell N et al: Non-neoplastic conditions presenting as soft-tissue tumours. Clin Radiol. 62(1):18-27, 2007
4. Shehab D et al: Heterotopic ossification. J Nucl Med. 43(3):346-53, 2002

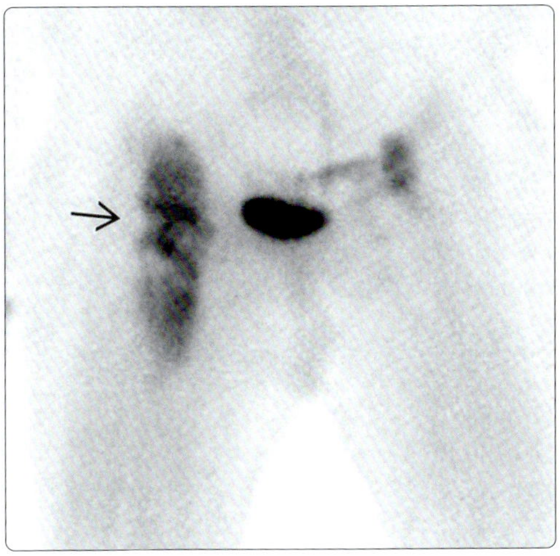

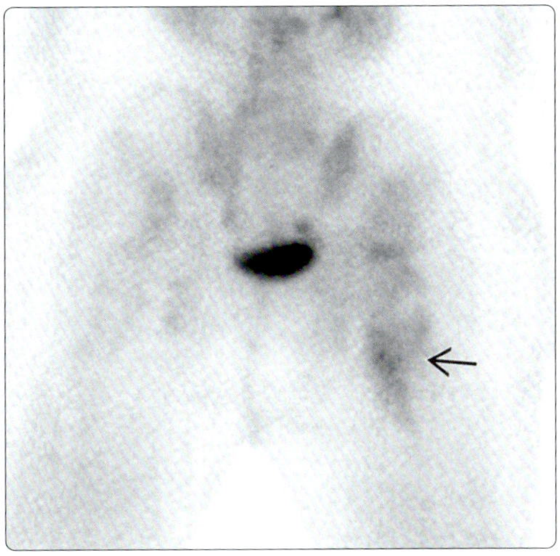

(Left) *Anterior bone scan in a man with right hip pain shows a large area of increased activity overlying the right hip* → *, consistent with heterotopic ossification.* **(Right)** *Corresponding posterior spot image from the bone scan shows heterotopic ossification* → *, which impairs visualization of the right hip joint.*

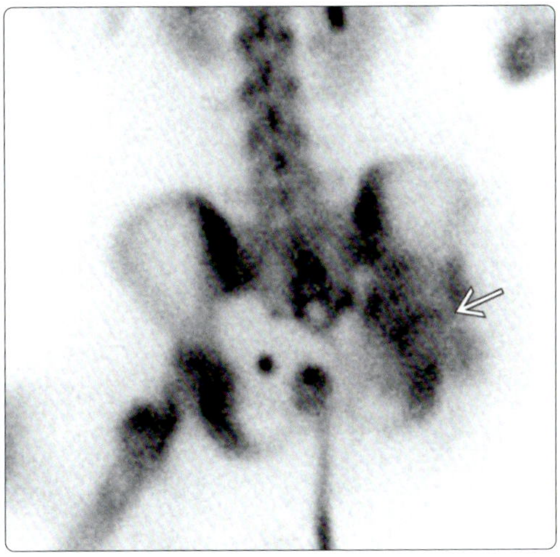

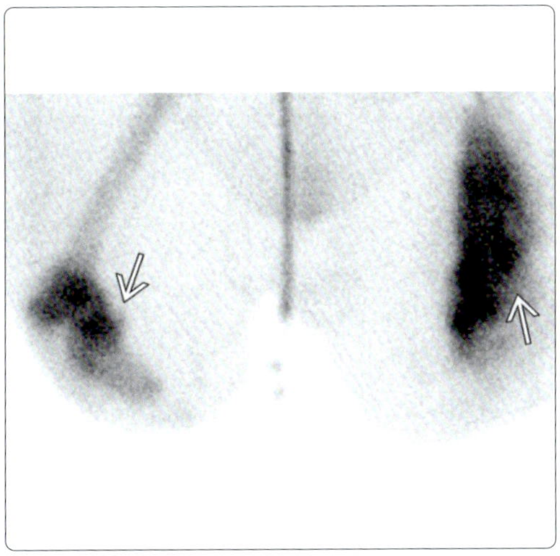

(Left) *Posterior bone scan in a woman post amputation with pelvic pain shows diffuse uptake* ⇨ *in the soft tissues of the right hip, suggestive of early active heterotopic ossification.* **(Right)** *Anterior bone scan in a man with left above the knee amputation and right below the knee amputation shows activity within the soft tissues* ⇨ *surrounding the stumps bilaterally, consistent with heterotopic ossification.*

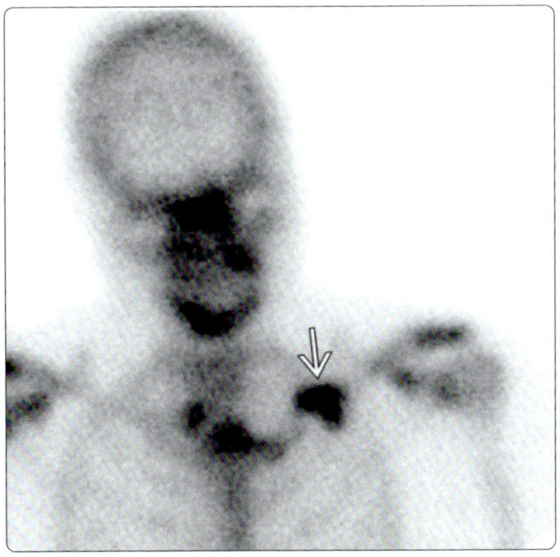

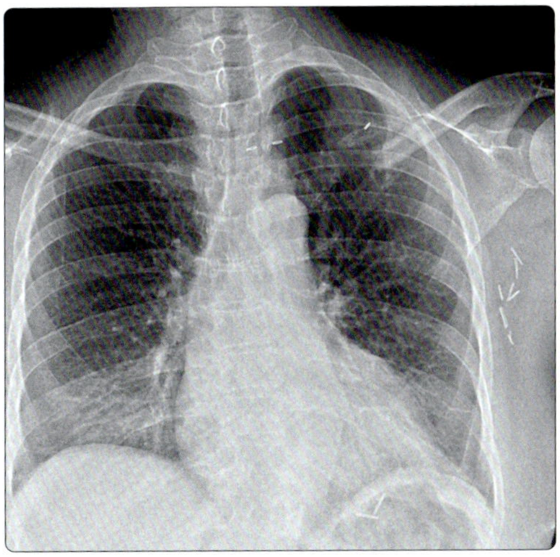

(Left) *Anterior bone scan in a 54-year-old woman s/p left sternoclavicular joint resection shows increased uptake* ⇨ *at the resection site of the clavicle, compatible with heterotopic ossification.* **(Right)** *Corresponding PA radiograph shows the proximal left clavicle resection. Bone scan findings precede significant ossification on this radiograph, showcasing the sensitivity of bone scan over radiography in the detection of early heterotopic ossification.*

Occult Fracture

KEY FACTS

TERMINOLOGY

- Occult fracture (fx): Fracture with no radiographic findings
- Pathologic fracture usually used to describe fx through bone focally weakened by tumor or infection

IMAGING

- 70-85% of fatigue fxs occult on initial radiographs
- Pelvic insufficiency fxs often missed on radiographs unless secondary healing present
- Acute fractures: 80% abnormal on bone scan at 24 hours, 95% at 72 hours, 98% at 1 week (longer in elderly)
- In elderly, uptake poorly localized until ≥ 1 week
- If obtained very early (≤ 2 days) after injury → false-positives due to periosteal reaction, contusion, traumatic synovitis, etc.
- Scintigraphic appearance of fractures depends on time elapsed since injury
  - Acute: Positive on all 3 phases
  - Subacute: ↓ in activity on blood flow and blood pool images with ↑ localization at fracture site
  - Remote: Positive on delayed phase only with gradual decrease in activity as healing occurs
- Negative predictive value (NPV) of bone scan: 98% for scaphoid fx, 94% for femoral neck fx
- Sacrum
  - Vertical component through both ala ± horizontal component through sacrum if bilateral
  - Called H, Honda, or butterfly sign due to characteristic appearance on BS
  - Linear array of lesions in adjacent ribs is typical for fracture with traumatic etiology
  - Single rib lesion in patient with known malignancy: 88-90% due to fx, not malignancy

(Left) *AP radiograph of a 53-year-old woman with right persistent foot pain shows postsurgical changes ➡ of the 1st MTP. No fracture or other abnormality is identified in the 2nd MTP.* **(Right)** *3-phase Tc-99m MDP bone scan (plantar view) of the same patient shows increased uptake in the region of the right 2nd proximal phalanx ➡ in all phases. Differential considerations include occult fracture and infection. On delayed imaging, focal uptake at the right 1st MTP ➡ is likely postsurgical in nature.*

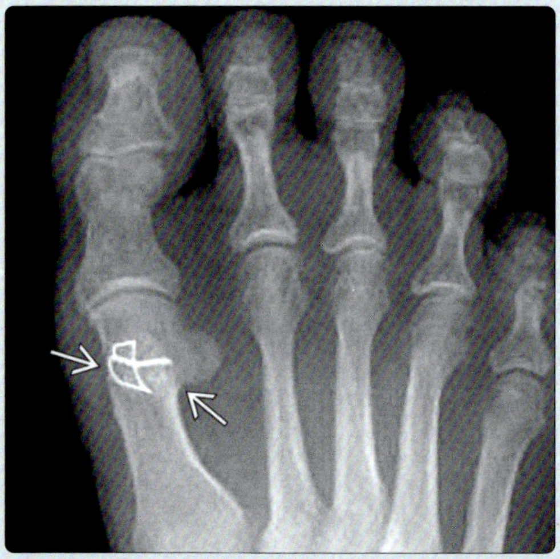

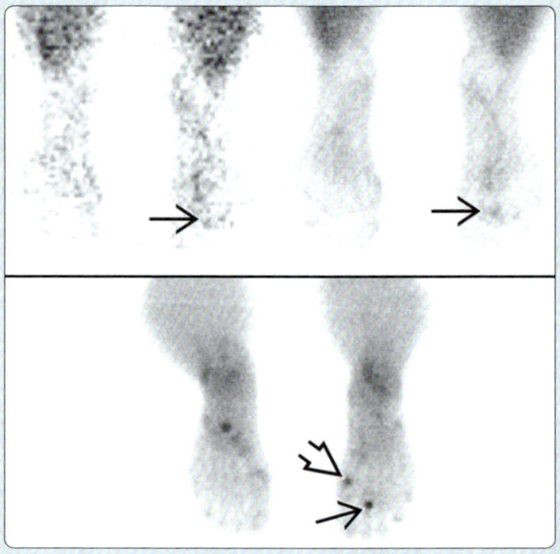

(Left) *LAO Tc-99m MDP bone scan shows uptake ➡ at the anterior portion of the 7th rib. The patient has a remote history of renal cell carcinoma. Given its location and isolated nature, this most likely represents a fracture. Solitary rib metastasis is unlikely and even more so in a patient with RCC, which often presents with a lytic (cold) lesion.* **(Right)** *Axial NECT of the same patient identifies the corresponding skeletal abnormality as a healing anterior rib fracture ➡ due to trauma.*

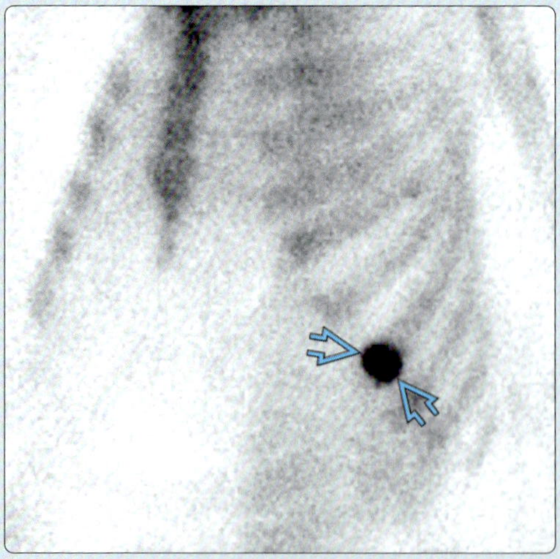

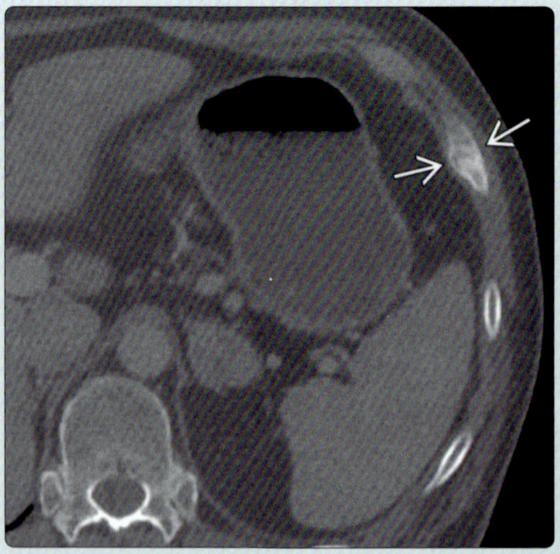

TERMINOLOGY

Definitions

- Occult fracture (fx): Fracture with no radiographic findings
- Pathologic fracture: Used to describe fx through bone focally weakened by tumor or infection

IMAGING

General Features

- Best diagnostic clue
  - Bone scintigraphy (BS): Focally increased uptake on delayed phase
- Location
  - Adults presenting to ED after acute injury
    - Upper extremity: Radial head, carpal bones (scaphoid, triquetrum)
    - Lower extremity: Knee (tibial plateau, Segond, patella), foot (calcaneus, talus)
    - Pelvis/hip: Femoral neck, sacral ala, acetabulum
    - Also: Vertebrae, sternum, and ribs
  - Adults with minor trauma or gradual onset of pain
    - 70-85% of fatigue fxs occult on initial radiographs
    - Pelvic insufficiency fxs often missed on radiographs unless secondary healing present
  - Scaphoid, radial head, femoral neck, calcaneus most common occult fxs overall
- Morphology
  - Sacrum
    - Vertical component through both ala ± horizontal component through sacrum if bilateral
    - Called H, Honda, or butterfly sign due to characteristic appearance on BS
    - More commonly atypical in appearance; often associated with ≥ 1 vertebral fxs
  - Pelvis
    - Common pattern of pubic rami fx + SI joint involvement
  - Ribs
    - Linear array of lesions in adjacent ribs is typical for fracture with traumatic etiology
    - Single rib lesion in patient with known malignancy: 88-90% due to fx, not malignancy
    - Anterior, near costochondral junction more likely benign
  - Sternum
    - Horizontal uptake near manubriosternal junction
      - In patient with breast cancer, sternum may be site of isolated mets
      - Vertical uptake along sternum in patients with sternotomy (sternal split)

Radiographic Findings

- Mandatory to rule out overt fxs, other causes for pain (e.g., osteomyelitis and tumor)
- May be normal early on; subsequent films may show evidence of healing
  - 15-35% sensitivity for stress fractures on initial exam, 30-70% on follow-up
  - Fxs of scaphoid, radial head, and femoral neck initially occult in 10-15% of cases
- Fxs of posterior pelvis and sacrum obscured by overlapping bowel gas

Nuclear Medicine Findings

- Bone scan
  - Tc-99m methylene diphosphonate (MDP) bone scintigraphy: 3 phases
    - Blood flow (or arterial) phase: Assesses vascularity
    - Blood pool (or soft tissue) phase: Assesses presence of tissue hyperemia
    - Delayed (or mineral) phase: Assesses ↑ osteoblastic activity in response to fx
  - Scintigraphic appearance of fractures depends on time elapsed since injury
    - Acute: Positive on all 3 phases
    - Subacute: ↓ in activity on blood flow and blood pool images with ↑ localization at fracture site
    - Remote: Positive on delayed phase only with gradual decrease in activity as healing occurs
  - Acute fractures: 80% abnormal at 24 hours, 95% at 72 hours, 98% at 1 week (longer in elderly)
  - Highly sensitive (95-100%), similar to that of MR; useful to rule out osseous pathology
    - Negative predictive value (NPV): 98% for scaphoid fx, 94% for femoral neck fx
  - **Limitations**
    - In elderly, uptake poorly localized until ≥ 1 week
    - If obtained very early (≤ 2 days) after injury → false-positives due to periosteal reaction, contusion, traumatic synovitis, etc.
    - High bone turnover from osteoporosis may increase background noise → false-negative scan
    - Limited utility for short-term follow-up: Persistent uptake (66% normalize at 1 year, 90% at 2 years)
      - May be longer depending on age, healing status of patient
    - Underlying cause of fracture (benign vs. pathologic) hard to determine
      - May be able to infer cause in some cases based on pattern and distribution of lesions
      - Further correlative imaging often required in indeterminate cases
- PET
  - Increased uptake in acute, subacute fractures
  - Often incidental fractures are noted during oncologic imaging

Imaging Recommendations

- Best imaging tool
  - Bone scintigraphy
    - To rule out occult fx: Sensitivity 95-100%, NPV 95-100% (with SPECT/CT) vs. MR
    - To detect concomitant skeletal injuries without additional radiation
      - Helpful in polytrauma, patient with poorly localized pain
      - Utility in fx of pelvis/sacrum since often multiple, associated with vertebral fx
    - To localize and characterize skeletal injuries in conjunction with SPECT/CT
    - To assess acuity of injury in unclear cases
- Protocol advice

- Tc-99m MDP bone scan
  - Patient preparation
    - Hydrate patient before injection and prior to delayed imaging
    - Should void immediately prior to imaging; may catheterize if visualization of pelvis is essential
  - Radiopharmaceutical
    - Tc-99m MDP: 20-30 mCi (740 MBq to 1.1 GBq) IV
  - Dosimetry
    - Bone receives largest radiation dose
  - Image aquisition
    - 3 phases recommended: Flow, blood pool (tissue), and delayed (mineral) phases
    - Delayed phase: At 2-4 hours, longer (up to 24 hours) if necessary to clear background
    - Use high-resolution collimator, obtain high count images; pinhole collimator when imaging small bones of wrist/ankle; place camera close to patient
    - Whole-body views ± spot images depending on patient history
    - Obtain SPECT/CT
  - Image processing
    - No special processing of planar imaging is required

Artifacts and Quality Control

- Occult fractures often have significant metabolic uptake on F-18 FDG PET/CT, thus creating false-positives for metastatic disease

DIFFERENTIAL DIAGNOSIS

Soft Tissue Conditions

- Hematoma, bone contusions, bursitis, tendinitis
- Usually positive on last 2 phases only

Conditions Associated With Bone Remodeling

- Arthritis (periarticular ± symmetric), gout, Charcot joint, healing osteonecrosis

Pathologic Fracture

- Metastasis (clinical history important; MR definitive)
- Osteomyelitis (hotter with infection than fracture)
- Bone tumor (polyostotic process on BS; may need correlative imaging with MR/CT to exclude)

Other

- Postsurgical change, normal variants (bilateral, usually at points of muscle insertion)

PATHOLOGY

Staging, Grading, & Classification

- Classified by acuity
  - Acute (1-4 weeks)
  - Subacute (6-12 weeks)
  - Remote/chronic (12 weeks to 2 years)

CLINICAL ISSUES

Presentation

- Most common signs/symptoms
  - Persistent localized pain after any form of trauma
    - May only require minor trauma in patients with underlying skeletal disease
  - Swelling, point tenderness typical in acute setting
  - In proximity to joint (radial head, femoral neck): ↓ in both active and passive range of motion

Demographics

- Traumatic: Bimodal age distribution, young adults (accidents, sports) and elderly (falls)
- Fatigue: Active young adults (undernourished female athletes, military recruits, long-distance runners)
- Insufficiency: Risk increases with age; M:F is 1:2 due to osteoporosis

Natural History & Prognosis

- Fractures represent up to 80% of missed diagnoses in emergency departments
- Early detection limits prolonged pain, loss of function, and disability
  - Delayed diagnosis ↑ risk of acute complications: Compartment syndrome, AVN, nonunion
  - Long-term: Chronic pain, deformity, additional fxs, paralysis (vertebral fxs), ↑ mortality

DIAGNOSTIC CHECKLIST

Consider

- Bone scintigraphy
  - Test of choice for radiographically occult fracture if MR not available/contraindicated
  - Best option if multifocal disease is a concern
- MR preferred in elderly hip fx < 72 hours of injury, if ligamentous or articular injury also clinically suspected

Image Interpretation Pearls

- Patient history important
  - Timing of injury if traumatic
  - Reporting of any previous skeletal injuries or surgeries
  - History of malignancy
- Correlation with other anatomic imaging valuable

SELECTED REFERENCES

1. Scheyerer MJ et al: Evaluation of pelvic ring injuries using SPECT/CT. Skeletal Radiol. ePub, 2014
2. Allainmat L et al: Use of hybrid SPECT/CT for diagnosis of radiographic occult fractures of the wrist. Clin Nucl Med. 38(6):e246-51, 2013
3. Querellou S et al: Role of SPECT/CT compared with MRI in the diagnosis and management of patients with wrist trauma occult fractures. Clin Nucl Med. Epub ahead of print, 2013
4. Cannon J et al: Imaging choices in occult hip fracture. J Emerg Med. 37(2):144-52, 2009
5. Bryant LR et al: Comparison of planar scintigraphy alone and with SPECT for the initial evaluation of femoral neck stress fracture. AJR Am J Roentgenol. 191(4):1010-5, 2008

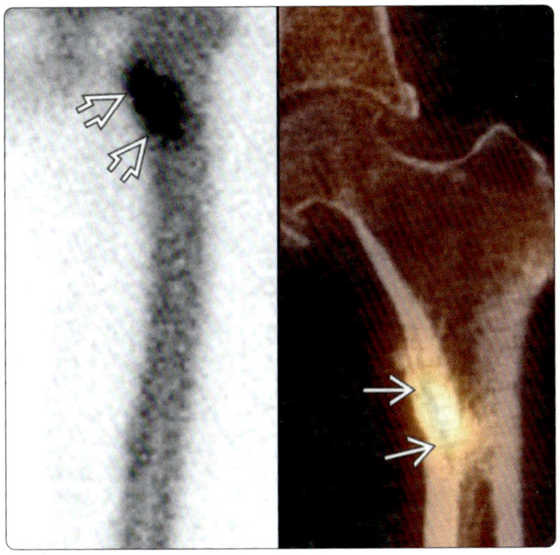

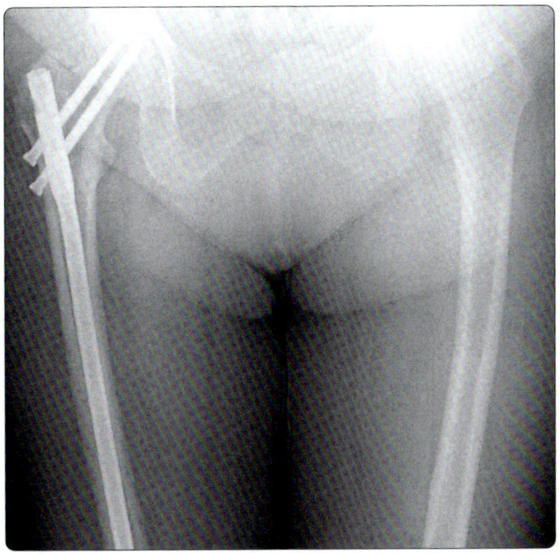

(Left) *Anterior Tc-99m MDP bone scan (left) shows focal increased uptake in the left proximal femur. Coronal fusion image from a SPECT/CT (right) shows a vertical fracture line, which corresponds to the scintigraphic abnormality.* **(Right)** *Hip radiograph of the same patient performed 1 day before the bone scan shows lack of apparent fracture of the left proximal femur.*

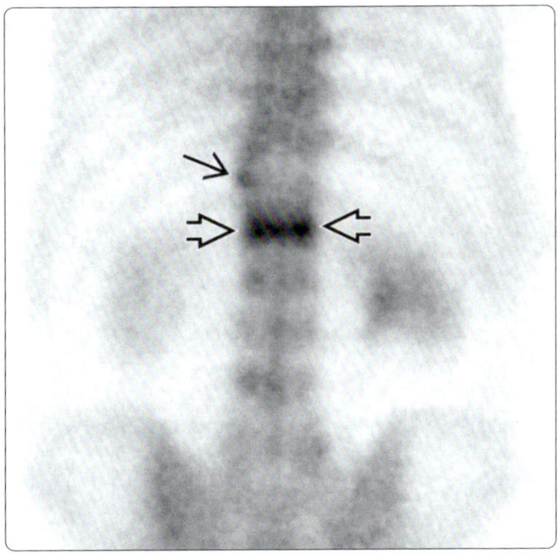

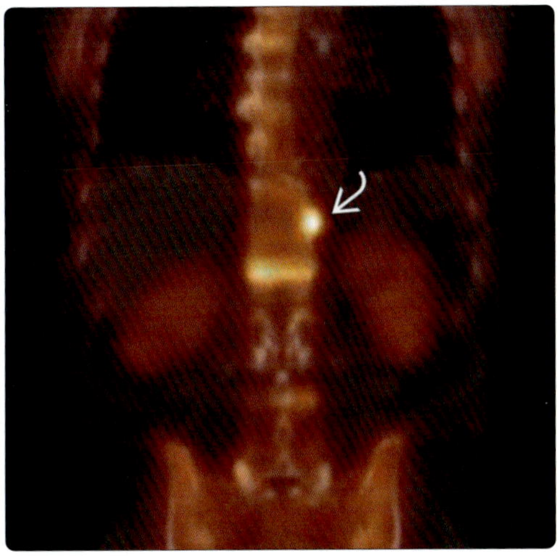

(Left) *Posterior Tc-99m MDP bone scan in a patient with chronic back pain shows intense band-like uptake within the L1 vertebral body consistent with fracture. There is also focal uptake on the left lateral aspect of T11/T12, which is nonspecific but could represent occult fracture.* **(Right)** *Coronal SPECT/CT of the same patient shows that the lateral thoracic uptake corresponds to local osteophyte formation. Arthritis is an important consideration for focal, intense osseous uptake on bone scan.*

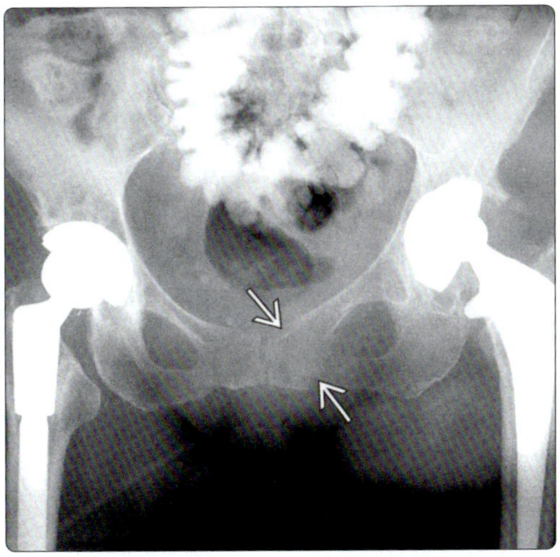

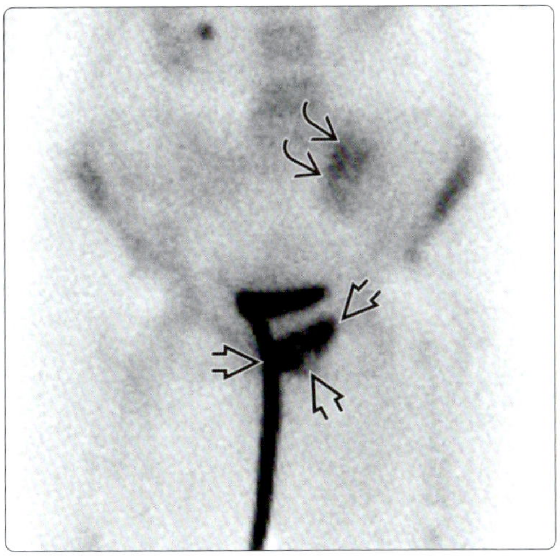

(Left) *Pelvic radiograph of a 75-year-old woman with bilateral hip arthroplasty shows pubic rami fractures immediately adjacent to the symphysis. The sacroiliac joints are obscured by bowel loops filled with enteric contrast.* **(Right)** *Anterior Tc-99m MDP bone scan of the same patient shows expected intense uptake of the left pubic rami near the pubic symphysis. The left sacroiliac joint, which could not be visualized on radiographs, has increased uptake consistent with occult fracture.*

KEY FACTS

TERMINOLOGY

- Stress fracture: Abnormal stress or overuse imposed on otherwise normal bone
- Stress fracture differs from insufficiency fracture: Physiologic stress overwhelming abnormal (insufficient) bone

IMAGING

- Most often lower extremity secondary to stress of weight-bearing, especially in fatigue fractures
- Most common: Tibial shaft (posteromedial cortex of distal 1/3); running, activity requiring rapid decelerations/stops
- Tc-99m MDP 3-phase bone scan: Sensitivity 75-95%, limited specificity
  - Typically positive on all 3 phases
  - Angiographic and blood pool phase positivity may become less conspicuous after 2-4 weeks
- MR: High sensitivity, specificity; advantages include evaluation of adjacent soft tissues, tendons, ligaments; no ionizing radiation

PATHOLOGY

- Wolff law: Bone remodels in response to stress
- Overuse overwhelms accommodative remodeling
- Osteoporosis, eating disorders, amenorrhea may be present in women

CLINICAL ISSUES

- Chronic skeletal pain with weight-bearing or repetitive use in absence of trauma
- Stress fracture may be initial presentation in anorexia nervosa
- Rest, rehabilitation, bracing, surgery in advanced/complicated cases

(Left) *Anterior bone scan of a 72-year-old woman with right hip pain shows a focus of increased uptake over the right midfemoral diaphysis ➜ concerning for stress fracture.* **(Right)** *Corresponding radiograph of this patient's midfemur shows a thin lucency ➜ within a region of cortical thickening consistent with stress fracture.*

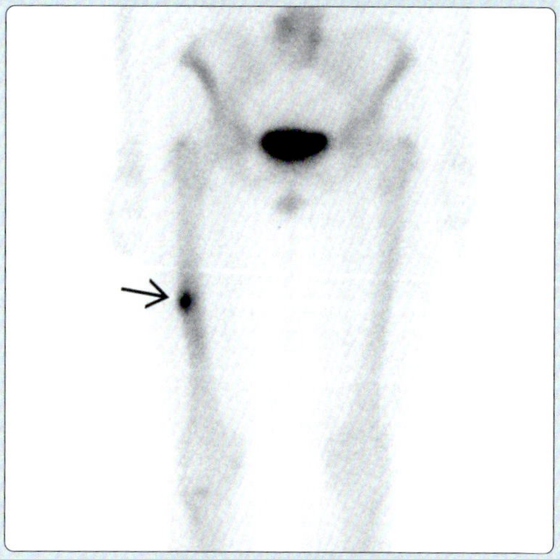

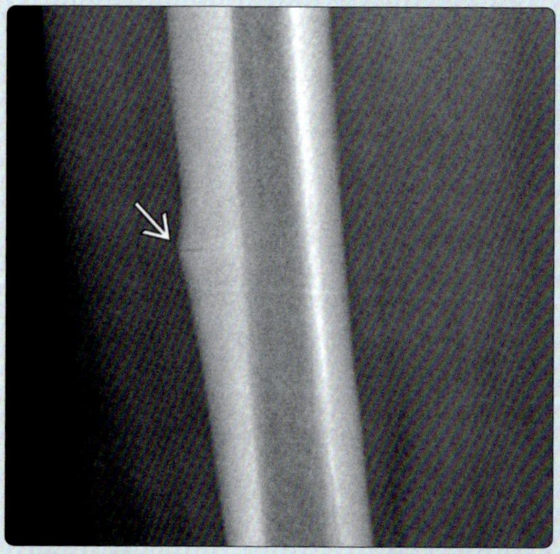

(Left) *Anterior bone scan of a 38-year-old woman with left hip pain following left femoral fixation shows an obliquely oriented region of increase uptake at the left femoral diaphysis ➜.* **(Right)** *Corresponding radiograph shows lucencies ➜ with accompanying periosteal reaction consistent with healing stress fracture.*

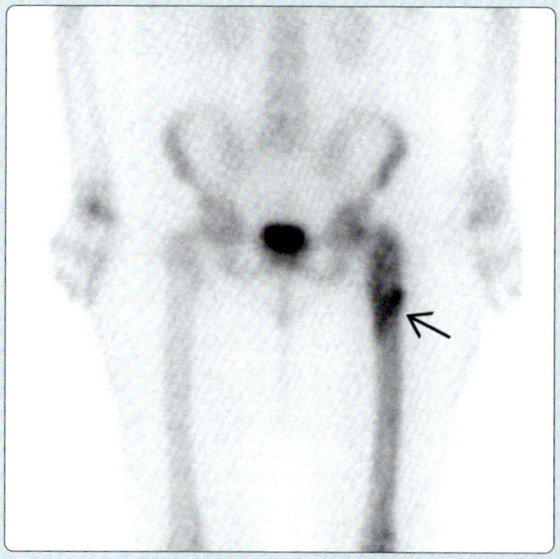

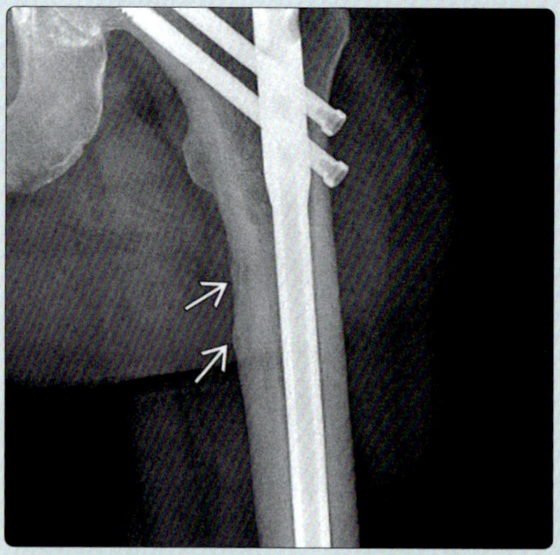

TERMINOLOGY

Definitions

- Stress reaction in bone leading to fracture
- Skeletal trauma secondary to repetitive loading overcoming intrinsic repair rates, resulting in spectrum of progressive bone disruption ranging from micro damage stress reaction to complete fracture
- Stress fracture: Abnormal stress or overuse imposed on otherwise normal bone
- Stress fracture differs from insufficiency fracture: Physiologic stress overwhelming abnormal (insufficient) bone
  - Underlying metabolic or other bony deficiency
- Partial or complete fracture
  - Grade I: < 25% of cortex
  - Grade II: 25-50% cortical involvement
  - Grade III: 50-75% cortical involvement
  - Grade IV: > 75% cortical involvement

IMAGING

General Features

- Best diagnostic clue
  - MR: T1WI hypointensity
  - Tc-99m MDP 3-phase bone scan: Typically focal uptake on all 3 phases
- Location
  - Most often lower extremity secondary to stress of weight-bearing, especially in fatigue fractures
    - Most common: Tibial shaft (posteromedial cortex of distal 1/3); running, activity requiring rapid decelerations/stops
    - Anterior tibial stress fractures uncommon: African American athletes, marching in sand, telemark skiers; mimics direct contusion
    - Tarsal bones: Calcaneus (vertically oriented, parallel to physeal scar), talus, navicular
    - Metatarsals, particularly 2nd and 3rd: Walking, marching, endurance sports, ballet
    - Fibula: Marathon running, jumping, ballet
    - Spine: Pars, pedicles; spondylolysis may occur in young athletes (L5 > L4 > L3); may be incomplete or unilateral; younger patients more likely asymptomatic
    - Sacrum: More common than other pelvic sites; H configuration due to vertical and horizontal fractures implies insufficiency fracture
    - Pelvis: Pubic rami/symphysis pubis, also iliac or supra-acetabular
    - Femur: Most common in medial femoral neck/intertrochanteric region; distal femur most common posteriorly (lateral images helpful)
    - Sesamoids: Running, jumping; DDx: Sesamoiditis
    - Occasionally humerus, radius, ulna, scapula, rib

Nuclear Medicine Findings

- Tc-99m MDP 3-phase bone scan: Sensitivity 75-95%, limited specificity
  - Clinical history important for interpretation
  - Allows whole-body imaging
  - Typically positive on all 3 phases
  - Angiographic and blood pool phase positivity may become less conspicuous after 2-4 weeks
  - Delayed phase abnormality can persist for ≥ 6-12 months
  - Early bone scan limited in patients with osteoporosis (may require 48-72 hours to mount osteoblastic response)
  - Usually focal, fusiform or oval configuration of increased activity
  - Focal activity (e.g., < 1/5 length of tibia)
  - Areas of asymptomatic uptake in athletes: Stress-induced remodeling; may or may not progress to stress fractures

Radiographic Findings

- First-line imaging
- Low sensitivity (10-15%) initially, useful to exclude other pathologies
- Delayed imaging improves accuracy
- Sclerosis, periosteal thickening, callous formation after 2 weeks or more
- Occasionally reveals discrete, visible fracture

CT Findings

- Findings similar to those on radiography, best sensitivity to osteopenia
- High sensitivity 85-95%, high specificity
- Stress fracture may be obscured by coexistent marrow changes in anorexia nervosa

MR Findings

- Increased fat-suppressed T2, PD, or STIR signal: Bone edema suggestive, but nonspecific
- Focal, linear low-density fracture delineation may be revealed on T1WI, corresponding to T2 abnormalities

Imaging Recommendations

- Best imaging tool
  - MR: High sensitivity, specificity; advantages include evaluation of adjacent soft tissues, tendons, ligaments; no ionizing radiation
- Protocol advice
  - Tc-99m MDP 3-phase bone scan
    - Hydrate patient prior to procedure to promote soft tissue washout; improves target to background
    - 20-25 mCi (740-925 MBq) IV
      - □ Inject away from area of interest
    - Angiographic and blood pool phases over area of interest
    - Delayed image at 3-4 hours, 2-3 hours longer in patients with poor cardiac output or renal failure
    - Best target to background ratio at 6-12 hours, can image up to 24 hours in difficult cases
    - Whole-body scan: Evaluate for other abnormalities, no additional radiation
    - SPECT recommended to increase sensitivity, especially when evaluating spine

DIFFERENTIAL DIAGNOSIS

Shin Splints/Tibial Periostitis

- Microavulsion of Sharpey fiber attachments
- Linear, superficial posterior medial tibial cortex, ≥ 1/3 of tibial length

- Angiographic phase hyperemia absent/minimal

Soft Tissue Pathology

- Strains, sprains, contusions, myositis, tendinopathies, neuropathies, compartment syndromes
- Bone may be positive on angiographic and blood pool phases, then negative on mineral phase

Joint Derangement, Trauma, Avulsion

- Suspected on radiography; MR to characterize

Neoplasm: Benign or Malignant

- Radiography often suspicious for diagnosis
- Pathologic fracture
  - Local loss of skeletal integrity secondary to underlying bone lesion
  - More commonly metaphyseal
  - Sclerotic, lytic, or permeative, associated mass, endosteal scalloping by CT
  - Well-defined T1 signal changes in pathologic bone, associated mass, endosteal scalloping, T2 changes nonspecific

PATHOLOGY

General Features

- Etiology
  - Wolff law: Bone remodels in response to stress
  - Overuse overwhelms accommodative remodeling
    - Osteoclastic activity may precede adequate osteoblastic reparative remodeling by weeks
- Associated abnormalities
  - Osteoporosis, eating disorders, amenorrhea may be present in women
  - Spondylolysis, spondylolisthesis

Microscopic Features

- Microdamage with reactive osteoclastic/osteoblastic remodeling

CLINICAL ISSUES

Presentation

- Most common signs/symptoms
  - Chronic skeletal pain with weight-bearing or repetitive use in absence of trauma
  - Symptoms may be vague and mimic other etiologies
  - Stress fracture may be initial presentation in anorexia nervosa

Demographics

- Age
  - ↑ with age (↓ bone density)
- Gender
  - M:F = 1:2
- Epidemiology
  - Up to 10% of sports medicine cases, often overlooked
  - More common in females and nonathletes who undertake new or increased activities
    - In females, high-impact activities (running, cheerleading, gymnastics) have higher correlation with stress fractures
  - Typically occur in situations of normal, healthy patients with overuse activity patterns
  - Insufficiency fractures may result from metabolic bone disorders
    - Senile osteopenia
    - Postmenopausal osteopenia, osteoporosis
    - Previously irradiated bone
    - Vitamin D, phosphate disorders
    - Hyperparathyroidism
    - Chronic renal disease
    - Aluminum, fluoride, heavy metal toxicity

Natural History & Prognosis

- Prognosis generally very good providing early recognition, appropriate therapy, compliance
  - Resolution may take 1-18 months or more
- Insufficiency fractures have compromised bone initially, less inclined to heal
- Complications: Delayed union/nonunion (not uncommon), avascular necrosis, pseudoarthrosis

Treatment

- Rest, rehabilitation, bracing, surgery in complicated cases

DIAGNOSTIC CHECKLIST

Consider

- DDx: Strains, sprains, contusions, derangements, periostitis

Image Interpretation Pearls

- Stress fracture: Positive 3-phase imaging with appropriate history
- Areas of asymptomatic uptake in athletes: Stress-induced remodeling; may or may not progress to stress fractures

SELECTED REFERENCES

1. Bancroft LW: Wrist injuries: a comparison between high- and low-impact sports. Radiol Clin North Am. 51(2):299-311, 2013
2. Liong SY et al: Lower extremity and pelvic stress fractures in athletes. Br J Radiol. 85(1016):1148-56, 2012
3. Murthy NS: Imaging of stress fractures of the spine. Radiol Clin North Am. 50(4):799-821, 2012
4. Bryant LR et al: Comparison of planar scintigraphy alone and with SPECT for the initial evaluation of femoral neck stress fracture. AJR Am J Roentgenol. 191(4):1010-5, 2008
5. Campbell SE et al: Imaging of stress injuries of the pelvis. Semin Musculoskelet Radiol. 12(1):62-71, 2008
6. Lee E et al: Role of radionuclide imaging in the orthopedic patient. Orthop Clin North Am. 37(3):485-501, viii, 2006
7. Gaeta M et al: CT and MR imaging findings in athletes with early tibial stress injuries: comparison with bone scintigraphy findings and emphasis on cortical abnormalities. Radiology. 235(2):553-61, 2005
8. Connolly LP et al: Young athletes with low back pain: skeletal scintigraphy of conditions other than pars interarticularis stress. Clin Nucl Med. 29(11):689-93, 2004
9. Oza UD et al: Multiple insufficiency fractures in a young woman with anorexia nervosa and bulimia. Clin Nucl Med. 28(3):250-1, 2003

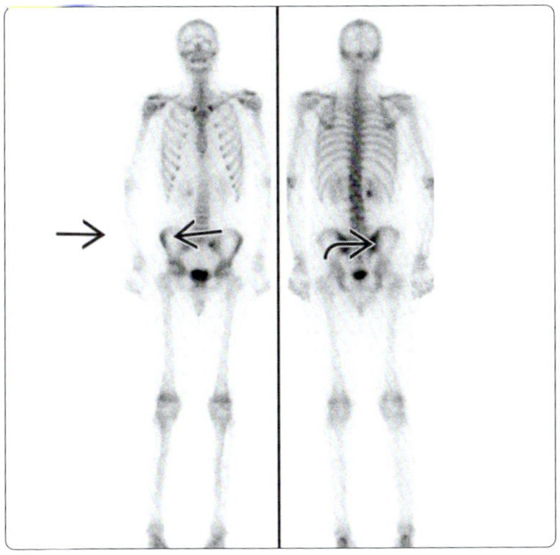
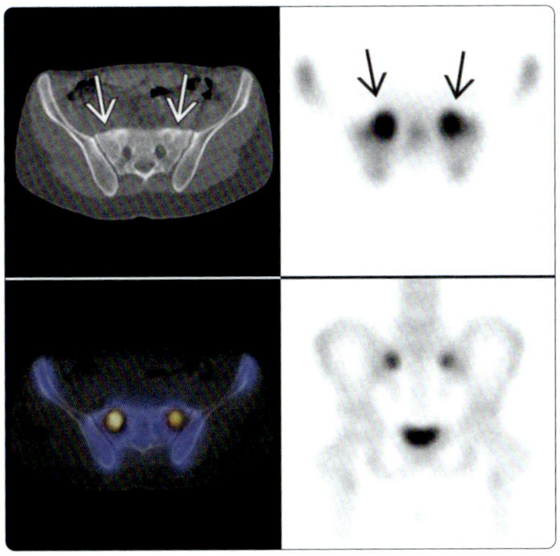

(Left) *Whole-body bone scan in a 16-year-old basketball player with gluteal pain shows bilateral focal uptake of tracer in the sacrum on anterior* → *and posterior* ↪ *views.* **(Right)** *SPECT/CT performed on the same patient confirms uptake of tracer in the bilateral anterior sacrum* → *with corresponding sclerosis on CT images* ➡. *Findings were most compatible with bilateral sacral stress fractures.*

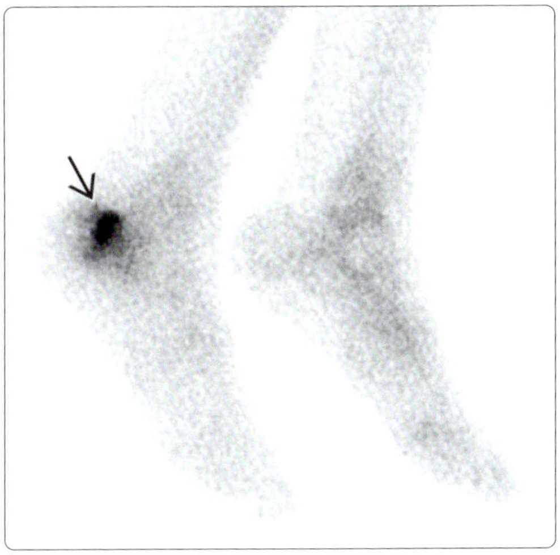
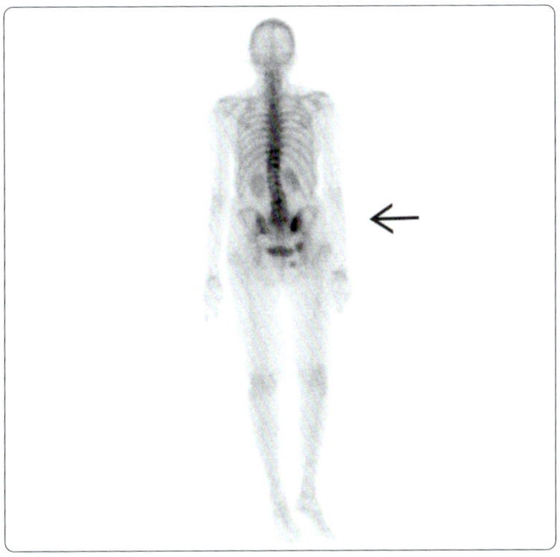

(Left) *Right lateral bone scan shows vertical orientation of uptake in the posterior calcaneus* → *parallel to the physeal scar, most compatible with a stress fracture.* **(Right)** *Posterior whole-body bone scan shows vertically oriented uptake of tracer in the right sacrum* →, *most compatible with a sacral insufficiency fracture.*

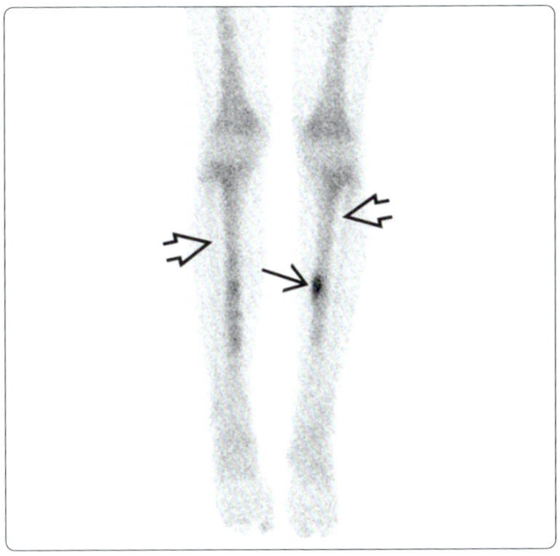
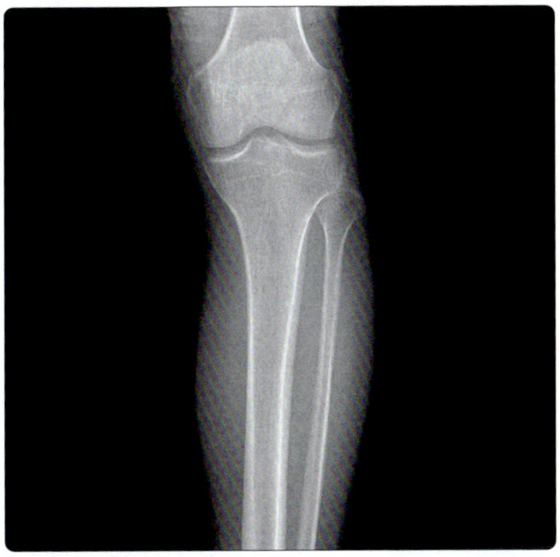

(Left) *Anterior bone scan of a 16-year-old girl with bilateral shin pain shows patchy linear regions of increased activity in both tibias* ⇨ *representing shin splints and an accompanying, more focal oval-shaped region of uptake in the medial left tibia, compatible with a stress fracture* →. **(Right)** *This patient's left lower extremity radiograph shows no acute osseous abnormality. A follow-up radiograph in 2 weeks may show sclerosis and periosteal thickening.*

KEY FACTS

TERMINOLOGY

- Avascular necrosis (AVN): Ischemic death of trabecular bone and marrow

IMAGING

- Bone scan 80-85% sensitive with use of SPECT
- Vascular phase has photopenic defect
- Reparative phase increased activity due to osteoblastic response
- Bone scan more sensitive than plain film
- Useful in identifying multiple sites of involvement
- Femoral head, humeral head most common
- Early subchondral lucency → sclerosis → collapse → secondary degenerative change

CLINICAL ISSUES

- Symptomatic disease may lead to structural failure and severe secondary arthritis
- AVN of hip: Increased risk of involvement of opposite hip
- Male > female (up to 8x in most locations)
- Spontaneous osteonecrosis knee: Elderly females
- Treat underlying disease
- Idiopathic: Treat conservatively and symptomatically
- Decompression: ± bone-grafting
- Joint replacement: For advanced disease
- Osteotomy: Moves area of necrosis away from site of maximum weight bearing

DIAGNOSTIC CHECKLIST

- Use high-resolution/pinhole collimators or SPECT for most sensitive bone scan
- Bone scan less sensitive than MR in most cases
- Bone scan used to identify multiple sites of involvement in patients with risk factors

(Left) *Blood pool phase of a bone scan shows a subtle focus of increased uptake at the distal left radius ⇒. Flow was also increased in this region. When evaluating upper extremity lesions on 3-phase bone scans, avoidance of tracer injection in the arms should be considered.* **(Right)** *Anterior planar static image from a bone scan in the same patient shows increased activity at the distal left radius ⇒ indicative of AVN. This patient had a prior injury, evidenced by increased activity in the ulna ⇒ consistent with internal fixation hardware.*

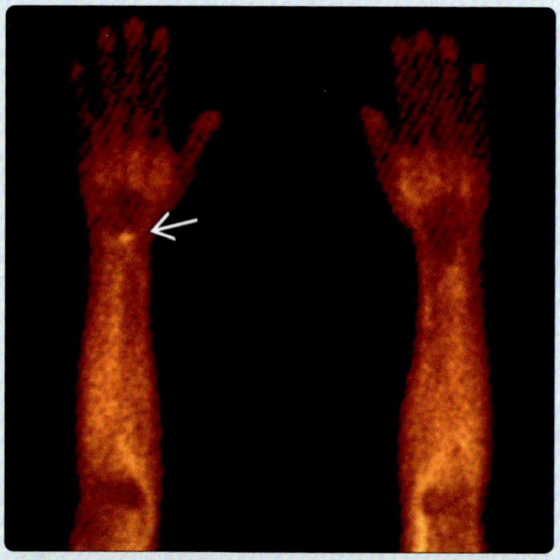

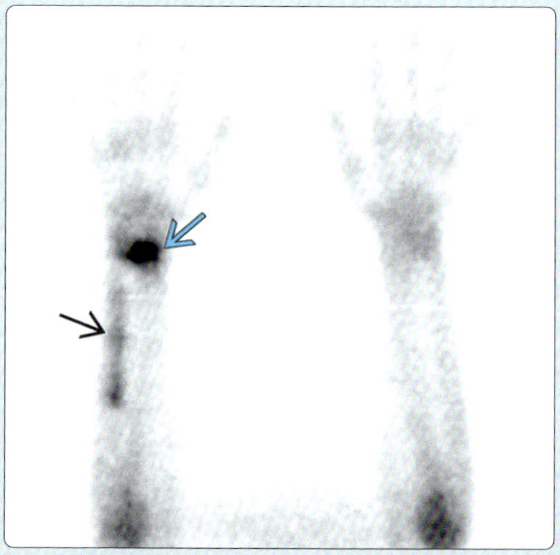

(Left) *Coronal T2-weighted MR of the wrist shows increased marrow signal in the distal radius extending to the cortex ⇒. There is no surrounding soft tissue edema to suggest trauma or infection.* **(Right)** *Axial T1-weighted MR shows an ill-defined region of decreased signal ⇒ in the distal radius characteristic of AVN.*

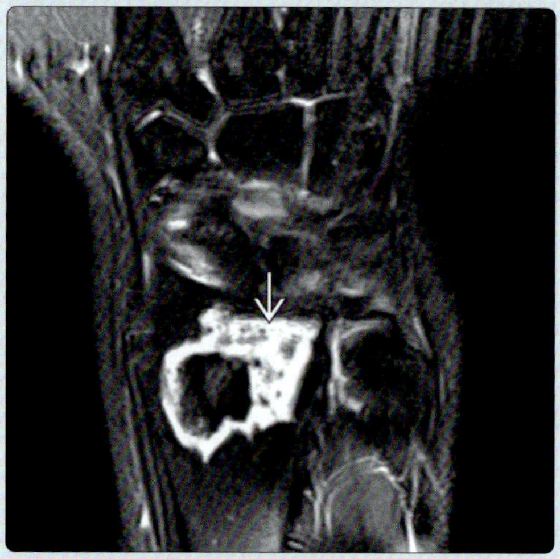

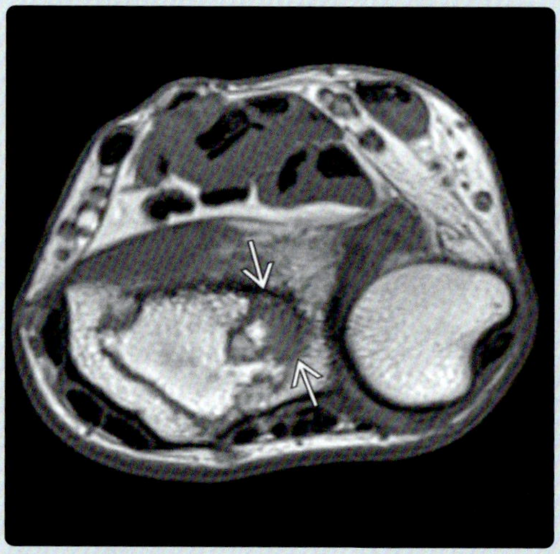

TERMINOLOGY

Abbreviations

- Avascular necrosis (AVN)

Synonyms

- Aseptic necrosis, bone infarct, osteonecrosis, osseous necrosis, ischemic necrosis

Definitions

- Ischemic death of trabecular bone and marrow

IMAGING

General Features

- Location
  - Commonly anterior weight-bearing portion of femoral head, and humeral head
  - Scaphoid
  - Knee: Medial femoral condyle (Blount disease) in pediatrics; idiopathic osteonecrosis (elderly females)
  - Lunate (Kienböck disease)
  - Tarsal navicular (Köhler disease)
  - Talus
  - Proximal tibia
  - Vertebrae (Kummel disease)
  - Small bones of hands and feet
  - Pelvis
  - Metatarsal head (Freiberg disease)
- Morphology
  - Humeral/femoral head: Linear/wedge-shaped photopenia

Nuclear Medicine Findings

- Bone scan
  - 80-85% sensitive with use of SPECT/CT
  - Vascular phase of AVN
    - Photopenic defect
    - May have donut sign due to surrounding hyperemia, adjacent synovitis
    - SPECT/CT imaging helpful in unmasking hyperemia from avascular area
  - Reparative phase of AVN
    - Photopenia diminishes
    - Increased activity due to osteoblastic response
  - May see involvement of multiple joints in patients with underlying disease (e.g., sickle cell disease)
- Tc-99m sulfur colloid
  - Defines distribution of viable red bone marrow (marrow map), reticuloendothelial system
  - Symptomatic sites of AVN: Decreased activity immediately after vaso-occlusive event
  - Asymptomatic sites of AVN: Decreased activity in area of old bone infarct
  - Useful in identifying patients with expanded marrow, such as sickle cell patients
  - Limitations of use of Tc-99m sulfur colloid in AVN
    - Developmental regression of red marrow in extremities (distal to proximal): Adult pattern is axial and proximal appendicular
    - Elderly: May lose red marrow signal in proximal femurs, humeri; may be asymmetrical
    - Loss of red marrow signal with infection, trauma

Radiographic Findings

- Normal → early subchondral lucency → patchy sclerosis → collapse → secondary degenerative change

CT Findings

- Osteopenia → subchondral lucency → sclerosis
- Less sensitive than MR

MR Findings

- T1WI
  - Hypointense peripheral band outlining central region
- T2WI
  - Hyperintense inner border (granulation tissue) parallel to hypointense periphery (sclerosis, fibrosis); known as double-line sign

Imaging Recommendations

- Best imaging tool
  - MR usually most sensitive
    - First-line evaluation
  - Bone scan more sensitive than plain film
    - Useful in identifying multiple sites of involvement
    - Can be used if MR is indeterminate
- Protocol advice
  - Dose: Tc-99m MDP bone scan
    - Adult: 20-30 mCi (740 MBq-1.11 GBq)
    - Inject away from site of interest
  - Angiographic, blood pool static, and delayed planar images
    - AP images with high-resolution or pinhole collimator
    - Symmetric positioning of both affected and unaffected opposite region
    - Beware bladder artifact from high counts in bladder; back projection reconstruction artifact causes loss of counts in adjacent bones, simulates AVN of hip
  - SPECT/CT
    - Increases sensitivity through improved tissue contrast
    - If imaging hip, empty bladder first

DIFFERENTIAL DIAGNOSIS

Fracture

- History of trauma, weakened bone
- Hyperemia and delayed increased uptake

Transient Osteoporosis

- Bone marrow edema syndrome: Femoral head and neck
- Most common in 3rd and 4th decades; may be seen in 3rd trimester of pregnancy
- Hyperemia and diffuse increased uptake of radiotracer
  - Involves femoral head, neck, intertrochanteric region
  - Acetabulum spared
- Resolves over 10-12 month period

Infection

- Acute hematogenous osteomyelitis (pediatric) and chronic post-traumatic osteomyelitis (adult)
- Pain and fever
- Increased uptake of radiotracer on all 3 phases bone scan
- Often involves both sides of joint

Bone Tumor

- Metastasis
  - Most often lung, breast, and prostate
  - Typically increased uptake
  - Extensively lytic or anaplastic lesions may have decreased uptake
- Primary bone tumor: Chondrosarcoma, osteosarcoma
  - Intense increased uptake

Bursitis

- Inflammation of bursa
- Associated with overuse
- Diffuse hyperemia and increased uptake in area of bursa

Osteoarthritis

- Increased uptake in weight-bearing location
- Older population
- Increased uptake in periarticular distribution

PATHOLOGY

General Features

- Etiology
  - Traumatic
    - Disrupted blood supply at time of injury
    - Follows subcapital femoral neck fracture (60-75%), dislocation of hip joint (25%), scaphoid fracture (30-40% in cases with nonunion)
    - Slipped capital femoral epiphysis (15-40%)
    - Anatomic factors may predispose
    - Lunate AVN common with negative ulnar variant wrist
  - Non-traumatic
    - Corticosteroids, alcohol abuse
    - Idiopathic (spontaneous osteonecrosis knees, Legg-Calvé-Perthes, Freiberg disease)
    - Pancreatitis: Fat emboli
    - Organ transplant
    - Sickle cell anemia
    - Antiphospholipid antibodies, coagulopathy
    - Vasculitis: SLE, collagen-vascular disease, XRT
    - Caisson disease: Nitrogen bubbles occlude arterioles
    - Gaucher disease

Gross Pathologic & Surgical Features

- Depends on stage of infarct
- Pale bone marrow with varying degrees of necrosis
- Cystic degeneration in area of infarct
- Secondary osteoarthritis after structural failure and collapse of articular surface

Microscopic Features

- Early
  - Cellular ischemia and death
- Repair
  - Necrotic debris in intertrabecular spaces
  - Ingrowth of mesenchymal cells and capillaries
  - Vascular granulation tissue separates dead/live bone
  - Mesenchymal cells differentiate into osteoblasts
  - Eventual new layers of bone formation

CLINICAL ISSUES

Presentation

- Most common signs/symptoms
  - Clinical features depend on age of disease
    - Pain, initially with sudden onset
    - Warmth, tenderness, erythema with acute infarct
  - May be asymptomatic

Demographics

- Age
  - Depends on underlying disease
    - Sickle cell disease: Presents in 1st decade of life
    - Legg-Calvé-Perthes: Young boys
    - AVN of hip: 20-50 years
- Gender
  - Male > female (up to 8x in most locations)
  - Spontaneous osteonecrosis knee: Elderly females

Natural History & Prognosis

- Symptomatic disease may lead to structural failure and severe secondary arthritis
- Asymptomatic disease may resolve
- AVN of hip: Increased risk of involvement of opposite hip

Treatment

- Treat underlying disease
- Idiopathic: Treat conservatively and symptomatically
  - Hydration, analgesics, limit weight bearing
- Decompression ± bone-grafting
- Osteotomy moves area of necrosis away from site of maximum weight bearing
- Joint replacement for advanced disease
- Diphosphonate therapy

DIAGNOSTIC CHECKLIST

Consider

- Bone scan more sensitive than plain films
  - Use high-resolution/pinhole collimators or SPECT for most sensitive bone scan
  - Bone scan less sensitive than MR in most cases
- Bone scan used to identify multiple sites of involvement in patients with risk factors

SELECTED REFERENCES

1. Joshi JK et al: Role of nuclear medicine imaging in recognizing different causes of osteonecrosis of the jaw. Clin Nucl Med. 38(1):40-3, 2013
2. Buchan CA et al: Imaging of postoperative avascular necrosis of the ankle and foot. Semin Musculoskelet Radiol. 16(3):192-204, 2012
3. Lee GC et al: Are we evaluating osteonecrosis adequately? Int Orthop. 36(12):2433-9, 2012
4. Sohn MH et al: F-18 FDG uptake in osteonecrosis mimicking bone metastasis on PET/CT images. Clin Nucl Med. 32(6):496-7, 2007

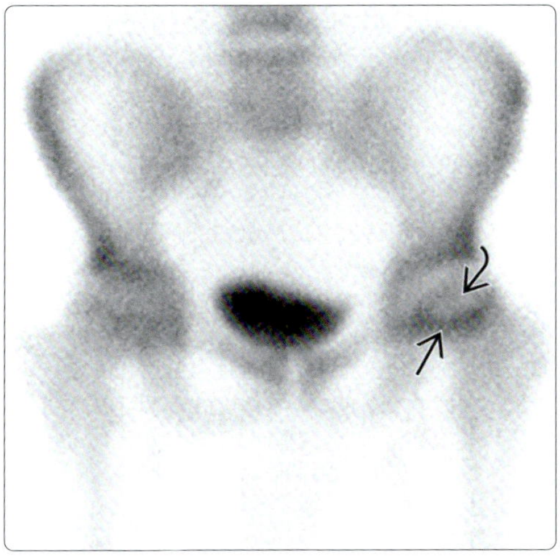

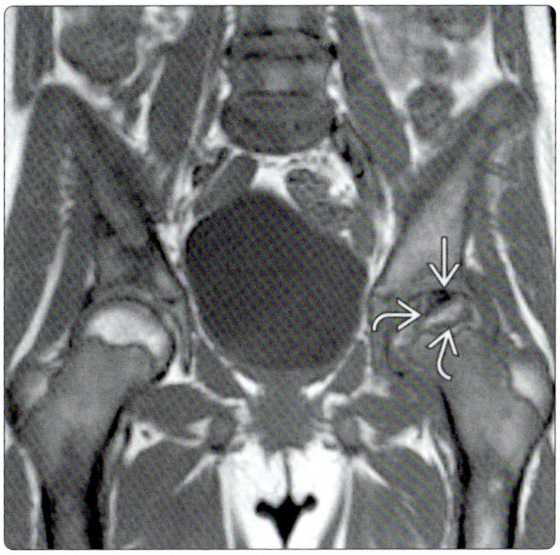

(Left) *Anterior planar bone scan shows central photopenic defect ⇨ with reactive rim of left femoral head ⇨ in a 15-year-old boy with history of steroid use and acute hip pain. This is an early bone scan finding of AVN.* **(Right)** *Coronal T1-weighted MR in the same patient shows a serpiginous line of decreased signal intensity ➡ outlining a geographic focus of AVN in the femoral epiphysis. Subchondral collapse with irregularity of the articular surface ➡ is also present, findings typical of AVN.*

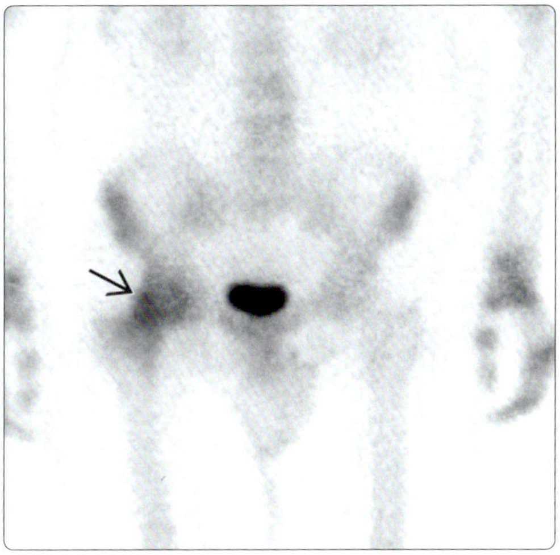

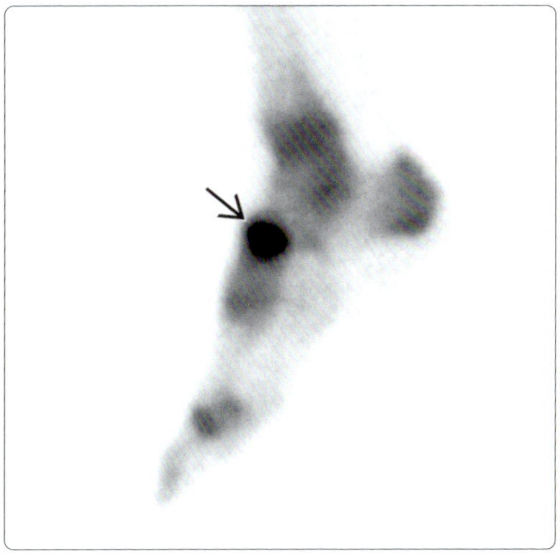

(Left) *Anterior planar bone scan shows increased activity in the right femoral head ⇨ consistent with the reparative phase of AVN.* **(Right)** *Lateral bone scan of the left foot shows increased activity in the region of the navicular bone ⇨ in this patient with Kohler disease (AVN of the navicular bone).*

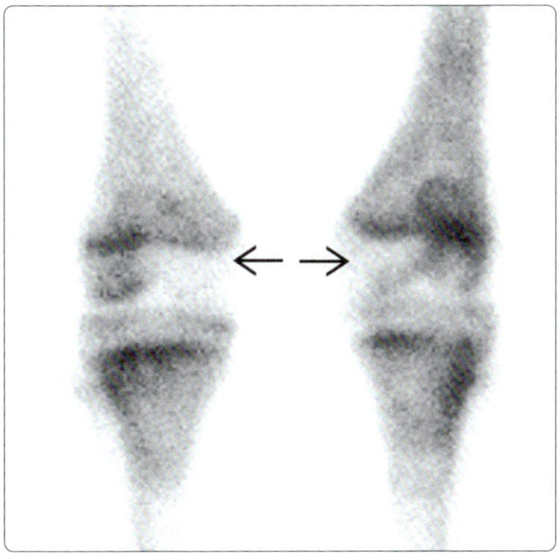

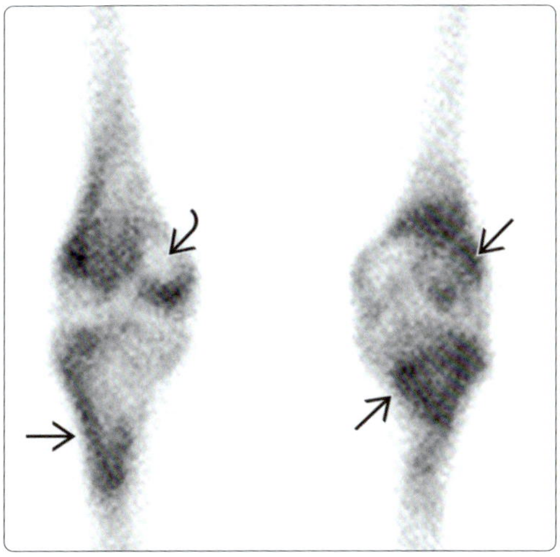

(Left) *Anterior planar bone scan of the knees in a patient with a history of steroid use and acute knee pain shows photopenic defects in the medial femoral condyles ⇨, consistent with early phase AVN.* **(Right)** *Anterior bone scan of the knees in a patient with sickle cell disease shows heterogeneous uptake of radiotracer reflecting multiple evolving bone infarcts in various phases. Note early-phase photopenia ⇨ as well as foci of increased activity ⇨ indicative of reparative phase.*

Complex Regional Pain Syndrome

KEY FACTS

TERMINOLOGY

- Complex regional pain syndrome (CRPS) is painful disorder of extremities
- Cause is likely neurological disorder affecting vascular system, pain receptors
- Usually due to injury, surgery, vascular event
- Usually unilateral; bilateral in ~ 25%
- Two types
  - CRPS type 1 has no detectable nerve lesion
  - CRPS type 2 has detectable nerve lesion
- Staging
  - Stage 1: Extremity pain characterized by aching, throbbing, burning, cold/touch intolerance, swelling
  - Stage 2: Muscle wasting, ↑ soft tissue edema, brawny skin, ↑ pain, vasomotor abnormalities
  - Stage 3: ↓ range of motion, digit/joint contracture, waxy skin, brittle, ridged nails, vasomotor abnormalities, ↓ pain

IMAGING

- Tc-99m MDP bone scan: Classically, increased periarticular activity in affected limb on delayed images
- Classic findings on 3-phase bone scan
  - Angiographic phase: Hyperperfusion to affected limb
  - Blood pool phase: Periarticular hyperemia when compared with unaffected limb
  - Delayed phase: Increased periarticular activity in affected limb; abnormal activity increases distally
- Staging
  - Stage 1: Hyperemia on angiographic phase, increased periarticular activity on blood pool and delayed phase
  - Stage 2: Hyperemia on angiographic phase, increased periarticular activity on blood pool and delayed phase
  - Stage 3: Can present as normal bone scan or just delayed phase periarticular activity
- Pediatric patients may show decreased uptake on all 3 phases

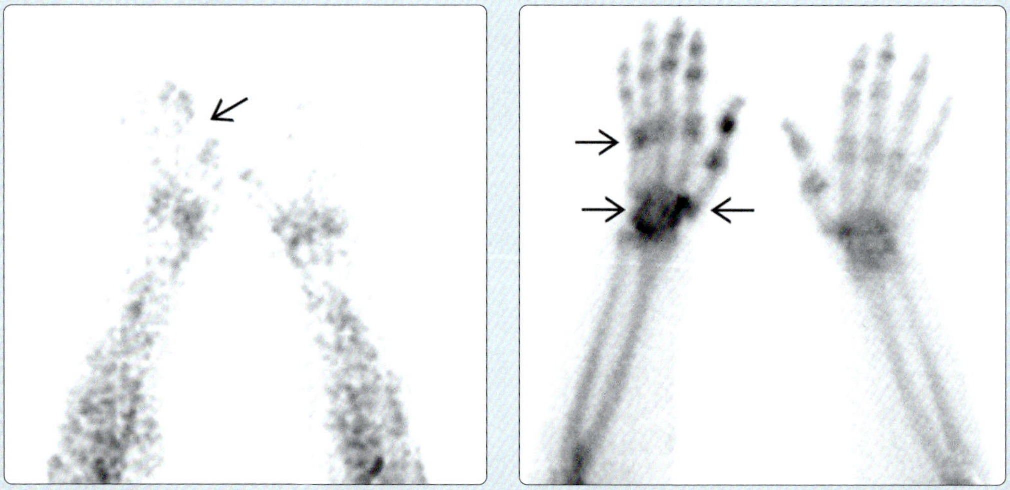

(Left) *Angiographic phase bone scan of a 58-year-old female with suspected complex regional pain syndrome shows mildly increased perfusion to the right hand ➡ compared to the left.* **(Right)** *Delayed bone scan of the same patient shows right-sided increased periarticular uptake ➡ in the wrist and hand.*

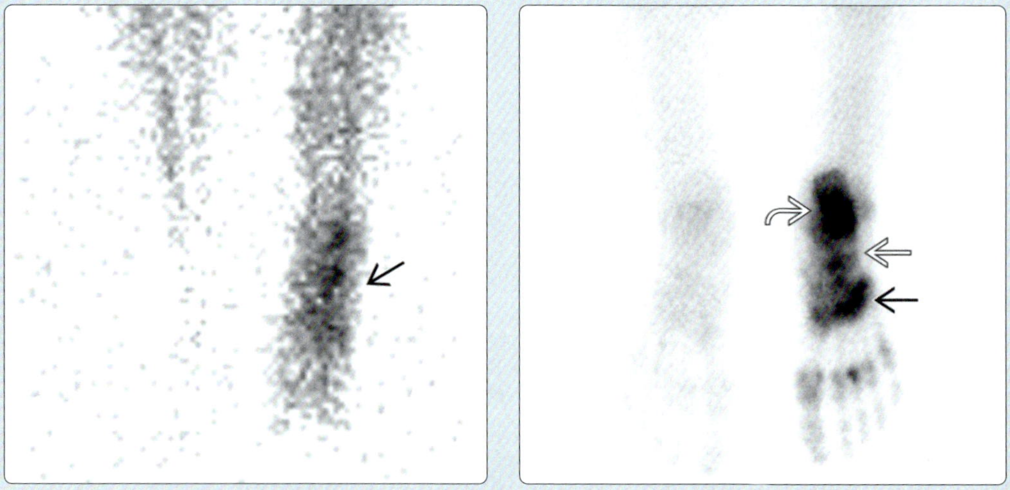

(Left) *Anterior bone scan of 16-year-old female in the angiographic phase demonstrates increased flow to the left foot and ankle ➡, characteristic of stage 1 complex regional pain syndrome.* **(Right)** *Delayed plantar image shows periarticular increase in activity along the left midfoot ➡, metatarsophalangeal ➡, and tibiotalar ➡ joints.*

TERMINOLOGY

Abbreviations

- Complex regional pain syndrome (CRPS)

Definitions

- Painful disorder of extremities
  - Usually due to injury, surgery, vascular event
  - Usually unilateral; bilateral in ~ 25%
- Once thought to be mediated by sympathetic nervous system (not proven)
- Current thought: Likely neurological disorder affecting vascular system, pain receptors
  - CRPS type 1
    - No detectable nerve lesion
    - Reflex sympathetic dystrophy
  - CRPS type 2
    - Detectable nerve lesion
    - Causalgia
- Staging
  - Stage 1: Extremity pain characterized by aching, throbbing, burning, cold/touch intolerance, swelling
    - Early, hyperemic stage
    - Pain, sensory abnormalities predominate
  - Stage 2: Muscle wasting, ↑ soft tissue edema, brawny skin, ↑ pain, vasomotor abnormalities
    - Dystrophic stage
    - 3-6 months after onset of stage 1
    - May last weeks, months
  - Stage 3: ↓ range of motion, digit/joint contracture, waxy skin, brittle, ridged nails, vasomotor abnormalities, ↓ pain
    - Atrophic stage
    - Permanent
    - 6 months to 1 year duration of symptoms

IMAGING

General Features

- Best diagnostic clue
  - Tc-99m MDP bone scan: Classically, increased periarticular activity in affected limb on delayed images
    - Periarticular activity increases distally
- Location
  - Upper, lower extremities most common
  - Face has been reported
  - Usually unilateral; bilateral in ~ 25%

Nuclear Medicine Findings

- Classic findings on 3-phase bone scan
  - Angiographic phase: Hyperperfusion to affected limb
  - Blood pool phase: Periarticular hyperemia when compared with unaffected limb
  - Delayed phase: Increased periarticular activity in affected limb; abnormal activity increases distally
- Pediatric patients may show decreased uptake on all 3 phases
- Findings by stage
  - Stage 1: Hyperemia on angiographic phase, increased periarticular activity on blood pool and delayed phase
  - Stage 2: Hyperemia on angiographic phase, increased periarticular activity on blood pool and delayed phase
    - Decreased blood flow can be seen; suggests vasospasm, more common in children
  - Stage 3: Can present as normal bone scan or just delayed phase periarticular activity

Radiographic Findings

- Most common: Osteopenia, especially subchondral
- Less common: Joint destruction, sclerosis, osteophytosis
- Radiography helpful in stage 2, 3

CT Findings

- Stage 3: Focal areas of osteoporosis

MR Findings

- Stage 2: Soft tissue edema, tissue contrast enhancement, thickened skin, muscle atrophy
- Stage 3: Muscle atrophy, thickened skin

Imaging Recommendations

- Best imaging tool
  - 3-phase bone scan
    - Sensitivity: 75-100%
    - Specificity: 80-100%
- Protocol advice
  - 20-30 mCi (740-1,110 MBq) Tc-99m MDP IV
  - Mechanical issues associated with radiotracer injection (e.g., hyperemia can be caused by tourniquet release) can compromise study
    - If evaluating upper extremity, attempt injection in lower extremity
    - If evaluating lower extremity, inject radiotracer in upper extremity
  - 3-phase bone scan: Always include opposite side for same time (not counts)
    - High-quality planar images of hands (palmar) and feet (plantar) required for optimal periarticular evaluation
    - Angiographic phase: Include distal aspect of affected and unaffected extremity
    - Immediate static (blood pool) phase: Include entire extremity (e.g., shoulders to tips of fingers), affected and unaffected extremity
    - Delayed: Include entire extremity (e.g., shoulders to tips of fingers), affected and unaffected extremity
  - Whole-body scan
    - May be useful for imaging both extremities at once
    - Likely need spot views of most distal extremity nevertheless

DIFFERENTIAL DIAGNOSIS

Disuse

- Post-traumatic, stroke
- Bone scan: Increased periarticular uptake early in disuse is more pronounced proximally, rather than distally; uptake decreased in chronic disuse

Neuropathy

- Nerve impingement, Pancoast syndrome
- Bone scan: Typically normal

Vascular

- Vasculitis, Raynaud syndrome, venous thrombosis, arteriovenous fistula, frostbite
- RSD: Can mimic CRPS with patchy uptake on blood pool; asymmetrical uptake on delayed images

Bone Disorder

- Migratory osteolysis
- Bone scan: Increased uptake in early stages

PATHOLOGY

General Features

- Etiology
  - Peripheral nerve-mediated inflammation and pain
  - Central nervous system likely has role as well
- Genetics
  - *HLA-A3*, *HLA-B7*, *HLA-DR2(15)* implicated
  - *HLA-DR2(15)* associated with poor treatment response
- Associated abnormalities
  - Emotional disturbances
  - Fibromyalgia
  - Sleep disorders

Gross Pathologic & Surgical Features

- Edema
- Muscle atrophy
- Thickened, waxy skin
- Hair loss

Microscopic Features

- Mast cells, neutrophils, macrophages in affected limb
- Inflammatory cytokines in affected limb
- Fibroblasts, macrophages, Schwann cells in affected nerves

CLINICAL ISSUES

Presentation

- Most common signs/symptoms
  - Burning, stinging pain
  - Vasomotor instability
    - Color, temperature, sweating asymmetry
  - Hyperesthesia
- Other signs/symptoms
  - Swelling
  - ↓ range of motion
  - Skin changes (thickened, waxy), hair loss
  - Osteopenia

Demographics

- Age
  - Adults
    - Usually 30-60 years
    - Mean age: 49 years
  - Children < 18 years
    - Lower extremity predominance (5:1 vs. adults)
    - CRPS 1: Girls > boys
    - CRPS 2: Girls = boys
    - Incidence highest ~ puberty
- Gender
  - Females > males
- Ethnicity
  - CRPS 1 may be more common in Caucasians
- Epidemiology
  - Usually precipitating event
    - Soft tissue injury: Cause of 40% of CRPS cases in 1 study
    - Fracture: Cause of 25% of CRPS cases in 1 study
    - Myocardial ischemia: 5-20% patients have CRPS
    - Stroke: 10-20% of patients with hemiplegia
    - Knee: Arthroscopic surgery most common
    - Vascular intervention: AV graft, hemodialysis
  - In ~ 35% of patients with CRPS, no precipitating event

Natural History & Prognosis

- Children
  - Respond well to intensive physical therapy (cure rate of 90% without medications)
  - Recurrence rate: 30-50%
- Adults
  - Recurrence rate: 2% per patient per year
- High intensity uptake on bone scan suggests better prognosis, positive response to therapy
- Early diagnosis and treatment important to prevent permanent sequelae

Treatment

- Physical therapy (particularly with children)
- Medication
  - Tricyclic antidepressants, NSAIDs, steroids, anticonvulsants, bisphosphonates, opioids
- Nerve manipulation
  - Sympathetic blocks, transcutaneous electrical nerve stimulation (TENS), spinal cord stimulation, sympathectomy (not common)

DIAGNOSTIC CHECKLIST

Consider

- Bone scan to look for signs of classic CRPS findings
  - Patient may respond well to course of steroids
- High intensity uptake on bone scan suggests better prognosis, positive response to therapy
- Early bone scan in patient with suspected CRPS to treat early
- Palmar and plantar delayed planar images to best display periarticular activity

SELECTED REFERENCES

1. Moon JY et al: Analysis of patterns of three-phase bone scintigraphy for patients with complex regional pain syndrome diagnosed using the proposed research criteria (the 'Budapest Criteria'). Br J Anaesth. 108(4):655-61, 2012
2. Ringer R et al: Concordance of qualitative bone scintigraphy results with presence of clinical complex regional pain syndrome 1: meta-analysis of test accuracy studies. Eur J Pain. 16(10):1347-56, 2012
3. Lee E et al: Role of radionuclide imaging in the orthopedic patient. Orthop Clin North Am. 37(3):485-501, viii, 2006
4. Wilder RT: Management of pediatric patients with complex regional pain syndrome. Clin J Pain. 22(5):443-8, 2006
5. Intenzo CM et al: The role of nuclear medicine in the evaluation of complex regional pain syndrome type I. Clin Nucl Med. 30(6):400-7, 2005

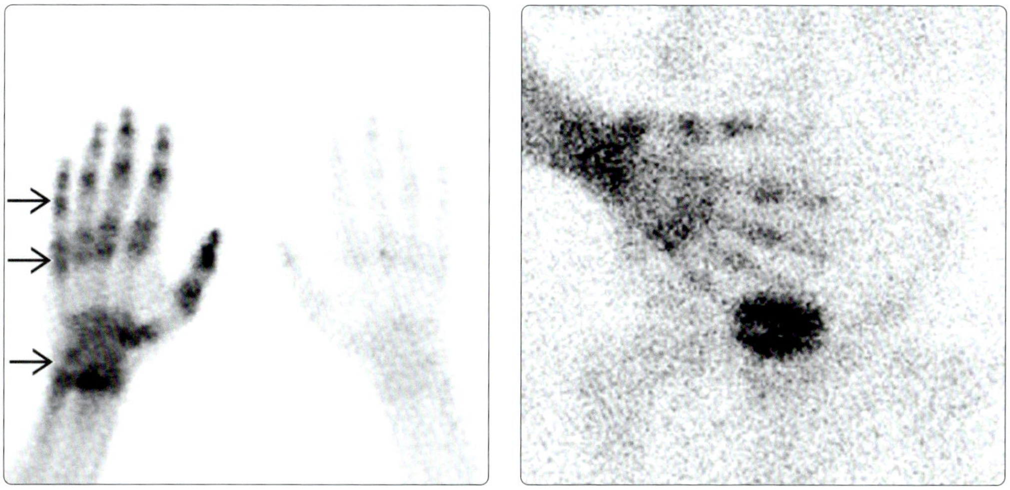

(Left) *Palmar bone scan shows periarticular uptake → in the left hand in a patient with rotator cuff injury. CRPS type 2 was diagnosed. The symptoms were chronic, with hand atrophy compatible with stage 3.* **(Right)** *Bone scan of a 65-year-old man being staged for prostate carcinoma who could not move his right arm shows periarticular uptake. After further questioning, he'd had remote right brachial plexus injury. CRPS type 2 of the right hand was diagnosed.*

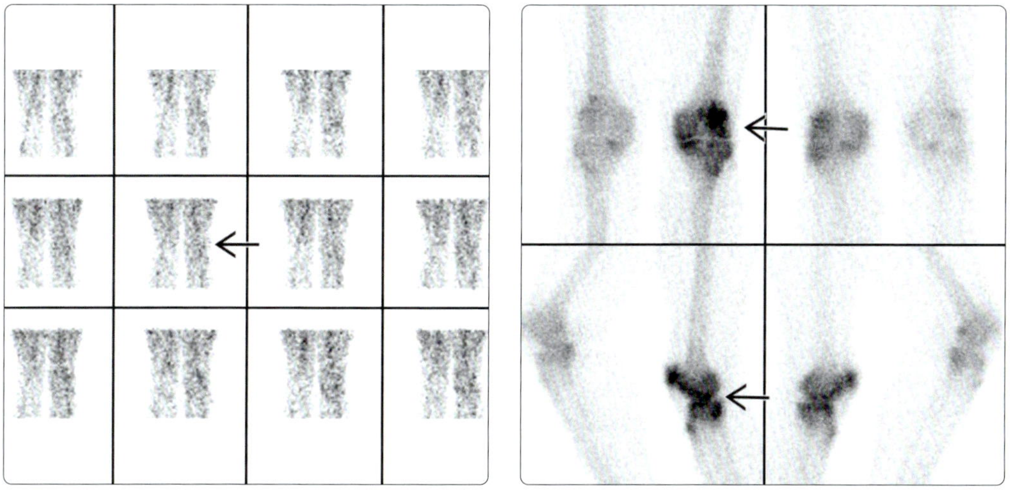

(Left) *Anterior angiographic phase bone scan of the knees shows increased perfusion → to the left knee.* **(Right)** *Delayed phase images of the same patient shows periarticular uptake in the left knee joint →. These findings are nonspecific, but with normal radiographs and appropriate clinical history, CRPS was diagnosed.*

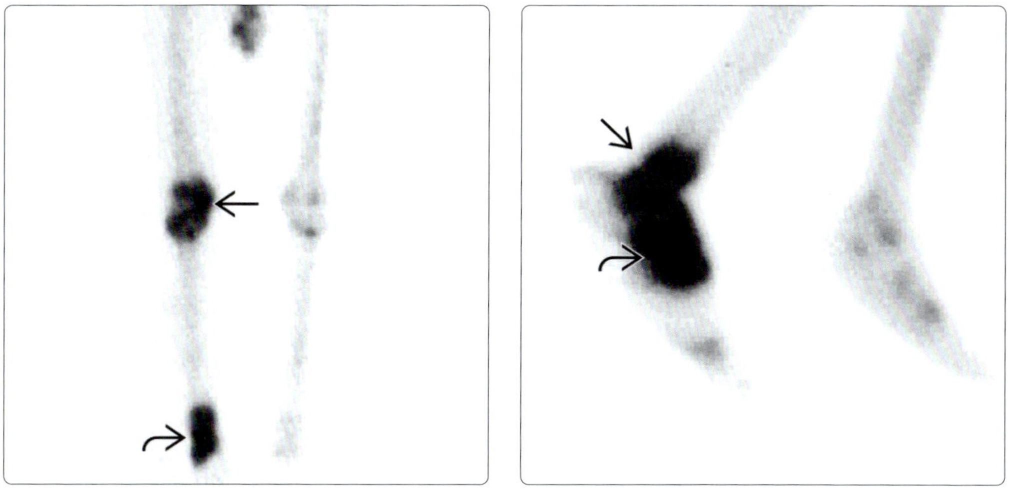

(Left) *Anterior delayed phase bone scan in a patient with right lower extremity pain and no history of injury shows increased periarticular activity involving the right knee → and ankle/foot ↷.* **(Right)** *Lateral view of the feet and ankles in the same patient shows markedly increased periarticular activity in the right ankle → and midfoot ↷. A markedly positive bone scan suggests this patient would have a favorable response to therapy.*

Sickle Cell Disease

KEY FACTS

TERMINOLOGY

- Acute musculoskeletal pain in sickle cell disease (SCD): Primary differential is bone infarction vs. osteomyelitis
- SCD: Genetic disorder of hemoglobin causing deformed (sickled) red blood cells
- Causes wide range of clinical manifestations (e.g., vasoocclusive crisis → bone infarction, autosplenectomy → increased risk of infection)

IMAGING

- Bone infarction: ↓ activity on bone scan if acute; may have no or mild uptake on leukocyte scan
- Osteomyelitis: ↑ activity on 3-phase bone scan and leukocyte scan
- Whole-body scan allows comprehensive skeletal survey for other sites of involvement
- Generalized ↑ uptake in skeleton often seen 2° to chronic anemia → marrow expansion
- Spleen may show extraosseous uptake 2° to infarction, calcification, and fibrosis
- Asymptomatic increased activity: Old infarction, chronic osteomyelitis, bone remodeling/repair (e.g., treated osteomyelitis, trauma)
- Bone infarction: Axial skeleton and long bones most frequently involved (hematopoietic bone marrow)
- Osteomyelitis: Hematogenous spread to vascular bone, usually in long bones (tibia, femur, humerus)

DIAGNOSTIC CHECKLIST

- For problem solving, use both bone scan and marrow map to differentiate osteomyelitis and infarction (increased specificity)
- Osteomyelitis: Usually positive on bone scan but can be negative; normal or increased uptake on marrow map; usually increased on In-111 WBC, Ga-67

(Left) *Anterior In-111 WBC scan of a 45-year-old male with SCD shows relative photopenia ⇨ at the left femoral head. Note the absence of splenic activity in this patient with a history of SCD and autosplenectomy.* **(Right)** *Corresponding radiograph of the left hip shows avascular necrosis of the left femoral head with subchondral collapse ➡ and fragmentation.*

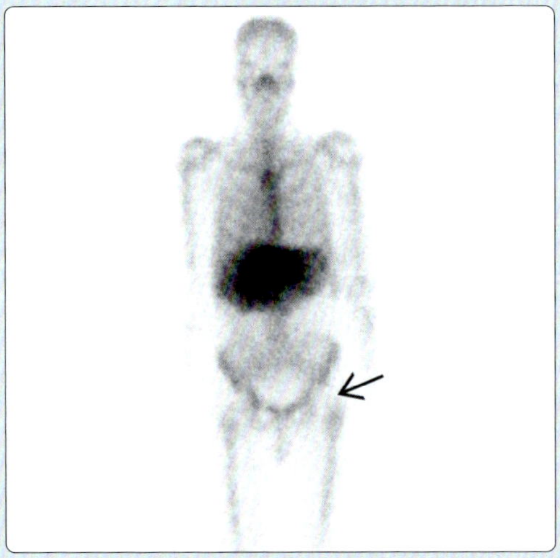

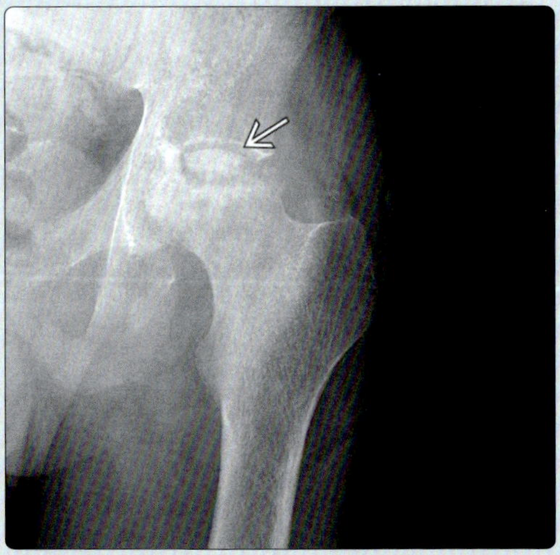

(Left) *Anterior planar image from a bone scan of a 20-year-old woman with SCD and leg pain shows increased uptake at the distal left tibia ⇨ with differential considerations, including infarction and osteomyelitis.* **(Right)** *Corresponding bone marrow imaging with Tc-99m shows increased uptake ⇨ concordant with the prior bone scan and an In-111 WBC scan (not shown). These findings suggest reparative phase of bone infarction.*

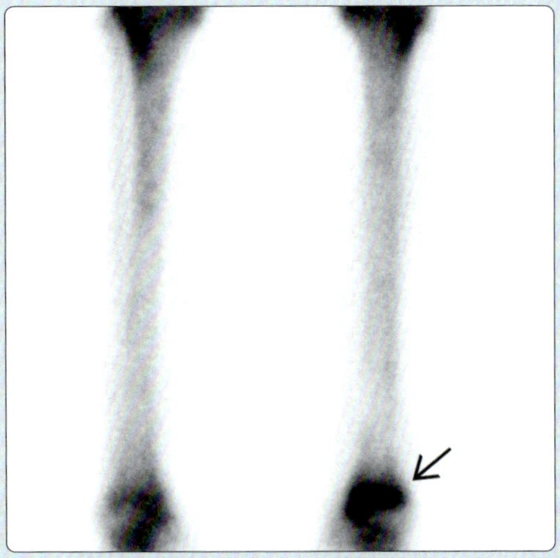

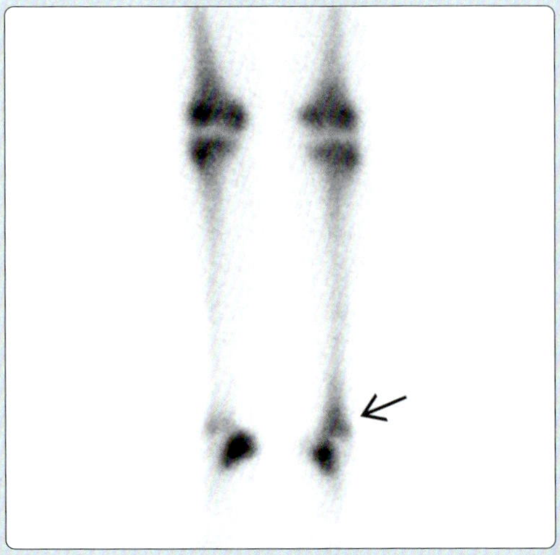

TERMINOLOGY

Abbreviations

- Sickle cell disease (SCD)

Definitions

- Genetic disorder of hemoglobin
  - Single base substitution in gene encoding beta-globin subunit
  - Deformed (sickled) RBCs
  - Causes wide range of clinical manifestations (e.g., vasoocclusive crisis → bone infarction, autosplenectomy → increased risk of infection)
- Acute musculoskeletal pain in SCD: Primary differential = bone infarction vs. osteomyelitis
  - Both present with pain, swelling, fever
  - Blood cultures can be negative in up to 50% of cases of acute osteomyelitis
  - Treatments vastly different
    - Bone infarction: Analgesics, hydration
    - Osteomyelitis: Long-term antibiotics
  - Early diagnosis important
  - Bone infarction more common than osteomyelitis

IMAGING

General Features

- Best diagnostic clue
  - First-line modality: MR
    - T1WI C+: Hypointense in acute bone infarction, may have enhancing rim with healing
    - T1WI C+: Osteomyelitis enhances
  - Nuclear medicine: Findings on most modalities nonspecific, reserved for problem solving
    - Bone infarction: ↓ activity on bone scan if acute; may have no or mild uptake on leukocyte scan
    - Osteomyelitis: ↑ activity on 3-phase bone scan and leukocyte scan
- Location
  - Bone infarction
    - Axial skeleton and long bones most frequently involved (hematopoietic bone marrow)
    - Most common long bone site: Proximal femur/humerus/tibia, distal femur
  - Osteomyelitis
    - Hematogenous spread to vascular bone
    - Usually in long bones: Tibia, femur, humerus
- Morphology
  - Bone infarction: Highly variable; does not extend beyond bone or involve soft tissues
  - Osteomyelitis: Can extend beyond bone into soft tissues (cellulitis, edema)

Nuclear Medicine Findings

- Tc-99m MDP bone scan
  - Tracer localizes to regions of osteoblastic activity, hyperemia
  - Bone infarction
    - Acute (days): ↓ uptake
    - Subacute (1 week): ↑ uptake
    - Remote (years): Old infarcts can show ↑ activity due to continued bone remodeling
  - Acute osteomyelitis
    - ↑ activity on all phases of 3-phase bone scan
    - Occasionally cold on 3rd phase of bone scan (especially vertebral osteomyelitis)
  - Whole-body scan allows comprehensive skeletal survey for other sites of involvement
    - Generalized ↑ uptake in skeleton often seen 2° to chronic anemia → marrow expansion
    - Spleen may show extraosseous uptake 2° to infarction, calcification, and fibrosis
    - Asymptomatic increased activity: Old infarction, chronic osteomyelitis, bone remodeling/repair (e.g., treated osteomyelitis, trauma)
- Tc-99m sulfur colloid scan bone marrow map
  - Decreased uptake in either bone infarct or infection
  - Symptomatic sites: ↓ activity in marrow space immediately following vasoocclusive event due to bone marrow edema
  - Asymptomatic regions of ↓ activity = old bone infarction (more commonly seen in older children, adults)
  - Whole-body scan allows comprehensive skeletal survey for other sites of involvement
  - Absence of splenic activity often due to autoinfarction, functional asplenia
- Image interpretation: Nuclear medicine findings frequently not specific
  - Osteomyelitis: ↑ activity on bone scan and WBC scan, ↓ on bone marrow scan
  - Bone infarction: Variable activity on bone scan, ↓ on bone marrow scan, ↓ or mild ↑ on WBC scan
- WBC scan: Absence of activity suggests infarction; increased uptake may signify either infection or infarction with secondary inflammation

Radiographic Findings

- Radiograph: Normal in early bone infarction and osteomyelitis
  - May show periosteal changes (can be seen with bone infarction and osteomyelitis)

MR Findings

- Bone infarction: Marrow edema ± thin rim of enhancement around nonenhancing marrow
- Osteomyelitis: Geographic, irregular marrow enhancement with contrast
- High signal intensity of hematopoietic bone in children can → false-positives
- Diagnosis of acute osteomyelitis: 92% sens, 96% spec
- Can be difficult to distinguish osteomyelitis from bone infarction in some cases

Ultrasonographic Findings

- Osteomyelitis: Subperiosteal fluid collection
- Allows for concurrent aspiration, cultures

Imaging Recommendations

- Best imaging tool
  - MR: Focal examination of symptomatic site(s)
- Additional nuclear medicine imaging options
  - In-111 WBC scintigraphy

- Helpful to differentiate acute osteomyelitis and infarction in equivocal cases
- Look for areas of ↑ activity discordant to bone or bone marrow scan findings
- If negative, can exclude infection
  - Ga-67 scintigraphy
    - May show ↓ activity in acute bone infarction
    - Normal activity in healing infarcts
    - Best for spinal and chronic osteomyelitis
    - If negative, can exclude osteomyelitis
  - F-18 PET/CT
    - Possible role in distinguishing infection vs. infarction, not yet validated

DIFFERENTIAL DIAGNOSIS

Sclerotic Bone Tumor

- Increased uptake on bone scan
- Decreased uptake on bone marrow and WBC scan

Lytic Bone Tumor

- Bone typically photopenic with possible rim of activity
- Photopenic on bone marrow scan (marrow replacement)

Septic Arthritis

- Positive 3-phase bone scan and ↑ periarticular uptake
- Positive In-111 WBC scan

Gout

- Positive periarticular activity on bone scan
- May have positive WBC scan (intense inflammation)

Chronic Inflammation (not Infected)

- Increased uptake on bone scan
- Increased uptake on WBC and bone marrow scan (mononuclear cell infiltration)

PATHOLOGY

General Features

- Genetics
  - Autosomal recessive → instability in RBC morphology in deoxygenated state
  - Amino acid substitution (valine ↔ glutamate), at 6th position of β-chain in hemoglobin molecule
- Associated abnormalities
  - Coexisting thalassemia: Includes disorders affecting α hemoglobin as well as β hemoglobin genes

Gross Pathologic & Surgical Features

- Bone infarction: Elongated pale region of bone marrow with hyperemic border sharply demarcated from cortex
- Osteomyelitis: Inflammatory changes, edema, necrosis

Microscopic Features

- Infarction: Cystic spaces due to fat necrosis, focal calcifications, dead trabeculae
  - Late stages: Ingrowth of granulation tissue
- Osteomyelitis: In SCD, usually hematogenous spread of infection, infiltration of WBCs into bone elements, thrombosis, necrosis

CLINICAL ISSUES

Presentation

- Most common signs/symptoms
  - Acute pain, fever
- Other signs/symptoms
  - Acute chest syndrome, jaundice, anemia, infection, stroke, pulmonary hypertension, stunted growth, priapism

Demographics

- Epidemiology
  - Most common: Sub-Saharan Africans and descendants
  - 1 in 12 African Americans have SC trait (Hb AS)
  - Also found in people of Mediterranean, Indian, and Middle Eastern heritage

Natural History & Prognosis

- Life expectancy for homozygotes: ~ 45 years
- Multiorgan damage from chronic vasoocclusions and hemolysis
- Heterozygotes have more indolent course and near normal life expectancy

Treatment

- Bone infarction: Hydration, pain control
  - Symptoms usually improve < 1 week
- Osteomyelitis: Long-term IV antibiotics

DIAGNOSTIC CHECKLIST

Consider

- For problem-solving, use both bone scan and marrow map to differentiate osteomyelitis and infarction (increased specificity)
- Osteomyelitis: Usually positive on bone scan but can be negative; normal or increased uptake on marrow map; usually increased on In-111 WBC, Ga-67
- Bone infarction: Variable activity on bone scan; ↓ activity on marrow map; variable activity on Ga-67, In-111 WBC

Image Interpretation Pearls

- History, clinical presentation, time course of symptoms important for diagnosis
- Dynamic changes in bone scan appear over time

SELECTED REFERENCES

1. Pratesi A et al: Sickle cell-related bone marrow complications: the utility of diffusion-weighted magnetic resonance imaging. J Pediatr Hematol Oncol. 35(4):329-30, 2013
2. Saito N et al: Clinical and radiologic manifestations of sickle cell disease in the head and neck. Radiographics. 30(4):1021-34, 2010
3. Ziakas PD et al: Bone marrow necrosis in sickle cell anaemia. Blood Transfus. 8(3):211, 2010
4. Cerci SS et al: Different findings in Tc-99m MDP bone scintigraphy of patients with sickle cell disease: report of three cases. Ann Nucl Med. 21(5):311-4, 2007
5. Ejindu VC et al: Musculoskeletal manifestations of sickle cell disease. Radiographics. 27(4):1005-21, 2007
6. Kim SK et al: Natural history and distribution of bone and bone marrow infarction in sickle hemoglobinopathies. J Nucl Med. 43(7):896-900, 2002
7. Skaggs DL et al: Differentiation between bone infarction and acute osteomyelitis in children with sickle-cell disease with use of sequential radionuclide bone-marrow and bone scans. J Bone Joint Surg Am. 83-A(12):1810-3, 2001

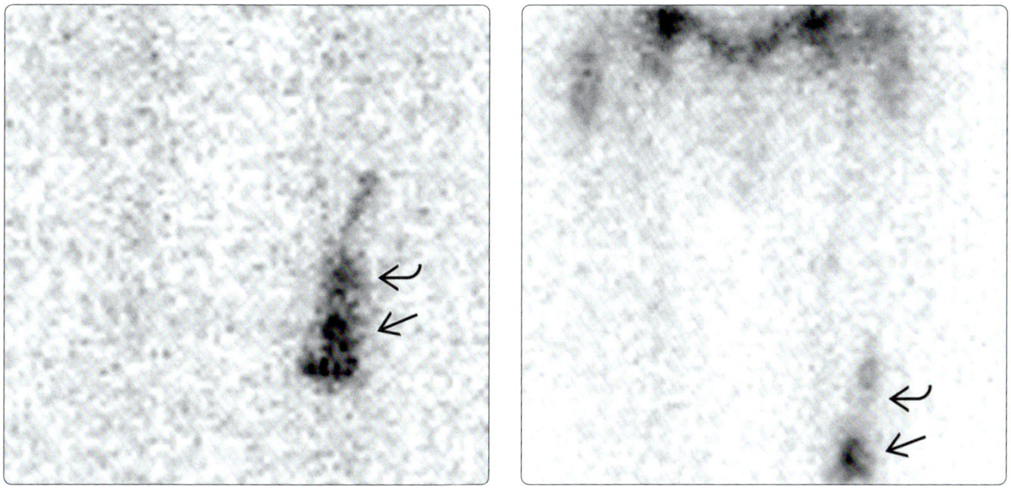

(Left) *Anterior In-111 WBC scan of the bilateral femurs shows moderately intense activity in the distal diaphysis* → *and metadiaphysis* ↪. **(Right)** *Subsequent anterior Tc-99m sulfur colloid scan of the femur shows more mild uptake of tracer in the metadiaphysis* → *and a smaller region of activity involving the distal diaphysis* ↪. *These discordant findings are most compatible with underlying osteomyelitis.*

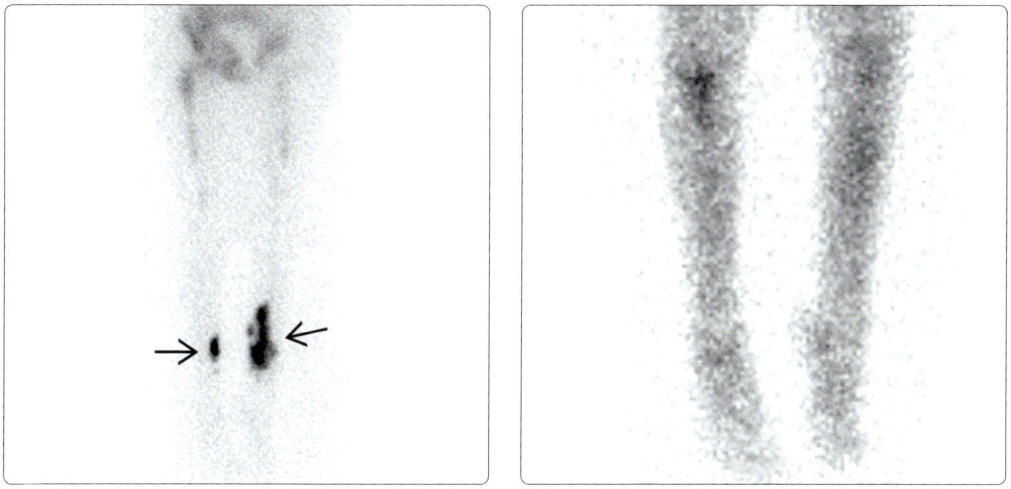

(Left) *Anterior In-111 WBC scan shows multifocal uptake* → *in the bilateral distal tibias.* **(Right)** *Subsequent Tc-99m sulfur colloid scan shows discordant findings of absent activity in the distal tibias. These findings are most compatible with osteomyelitis and probable adjacent soft tissue infection of the bilateral tibias.*

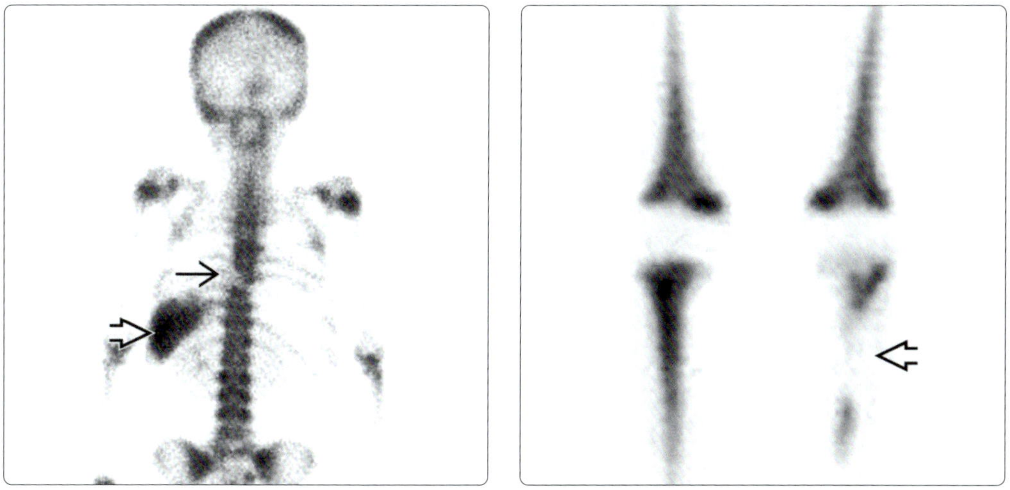

(Left) *Posterior bone scan of a patient with SCD shows photopenic defect in the thoracic vertebra* →, *suggesting an acute bone infarction. Uptake in the spleen* ⇨ *can be due to acute sickle crisis or autoinfarction with calcification.* **(Right)** *Tc-99m sulfur colloid bone scan shows photopenic defect in the proximal left tibia* ⇨ *in a patient with SCD and acute leg pain, most suggestive of a bone infarction.*

SECTION 6

Thyroid and Parathyroid

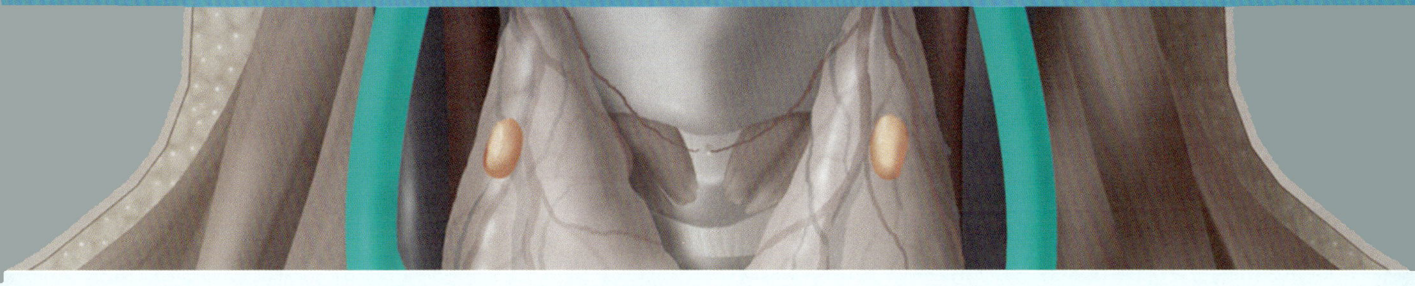

Introduction

Thyroid

Parathyroid

Introduction

Thyroid imaging scans and quantitative thyroid uptake determinations remain a high proportion of the clinical nuclear medicine practice, particularly to characterize nodular thyroid disease and diagnose and treat patients with hyperthyroidism. With the advent of minimally invasive parathyroidectomy techniques in the 1990s, the Tc-99m sestamibi parathyroid scan was developed to localize parathyroid adenomas and direct surgical approach. In recent years, SPECT/CT has been added to parathyroid scan protocols to provide valuable 3-dimensional localization.

Thyroid Scan

Thyroid scan with I-123 is indicated for patients with indeterminate thyroid nodules on ultrasound &/or biopsy. In the case of indeterminate biopsy results, if the nodule is hot on thyroid scan, a hyperfunctioning nodule is confirmed and malignancy is unlikely. In addition, Tc-99m pertechnetate or I-123 thyroid scans are useful to confirm the etiology of hyperthyroidism and help to guide therapy.

Traditionally, planar images with anterior and anterior oblique images over the thyroid were obtained. However, SPECT or SPECT/CT images are now common, as they have better resolution, can be more easily compared to ultrasound, and generally take less time than traditional planar imaging (20 minutes vs. 40-60 minutes).

- Toxic adenoma: On thyroid scan, toxic adenoma appears as solitary hot nodule with relative suppressed uptake of radiotracer in remainder of thyroid gland
- Toxic multinodular goiter: On thyroid scan, toxic multinodular goiter appears as multiple hot and cold nodules in normal-sized or enlarged thyroid gland
- Graves disease: On thyroid scan, Graves disease appears as homogeneous, intense uptake in diffusely enlarged thyroid gland; physiologic salivary gland uptake is decreased

Thyroid Uptake

Thyroid uptake determinations show how much radioactive iodine is absorbed by the thyroid gland. Four or 24 hours after administration of a small amount of I-131 or I-123, a gamma probe over the patient's neck counts gamma rays emitted for 1 minute. This is compared to counts from a standard dose of radioactive iodine counted in a neck phantom (100% uptake). Physiological background uptake in the patient (gamma probe counts over the thigh) is subtracted. Although normal iodine uptake values can vary depending on regional iodine ingestion, the typical normal value at 24 hours ranges from 15-30%.

In patients with hyperthyroidism, uptake percentages help clinicians determine the etiology of hyperthyroidism and the appropriate dose of I-131 for therapy.

- Toxic adenoma: Thyroid uptake determination is often low-normal or normal, as most of uptake occurs in toxic adenoma
- Toxic multinodular goiter: Thyroid uptake determination is often normal or mildly elevated (< 50%)
- Graves disease: Thyroid uptake value is usually >50% and often 80-90%

Parathyroid Imaging

In the 1980s, the standard of care for patients with hypercalcemia due to primary hyperparathyroidism was a bilateral neck dissection and exploration. The surgeon would locate all parathyroid glands at surgery, biopsy normal and abnormal glands, and remove any adenomatous parathyroid glands after confirmation from pathological intraoperative frozen section. The cure rate was > 95%. However, the morbidity associated with a bilateral neck dissection included risks of anesthesia, bleeding, nerve damage, and a large neck scar. In an effort to reduce morbidity, surgeons developed a minimally invasive parathyroidectomy in the 1990s, which at its best could be done under local anesthesia with a 1 cm incision.

Parathyroid scans with Tc-99m sestamibi, a traditional cardiac radiopharmaceutical, came into use as the standard preoperative localization study. Immediate planar images 20 minutes after radiopharmaceutical injection show the thyroid gland and parathyroid adenoma in relation to each other. Delayed images after washout of the thyroid gland show just the parathyroid adenoma. The benefits of parathyroid scans included localization of ectopic parathyroid adenomas in addition to those located posterior to the thyroid gland. SPECT and SPECT/CT are valuable adjuncts to planar imaging, particularly in the case of ectopic adenomas and those that descend into the tracheoesophageal groove.

Local surgical practice significantly affects how the reading physician interprets the parathyroid scan. For example, some surgeons place an incision based on whether the origin of the parathyroid adenoma is superior or inferior. Other surgeons base their incision on where the parathyroid adenoma sits anatomically, depending heavily on the SPECT/CT images. Some surgeons only require left or right localization because they perform a hemi-neck exploration. Communication between the surgeon and the reading physician helps to tailor the parathyroid scan interpretation for the type of surgery planned.

More recently, surgeons perform office-based ultrasound to detect parathyroid adenomas prior to parathyroidectomy. Therefore, Tc-99m sestamibi parathyroid scans are now usually reserved for more complicated cases, such as

- No parathyroid adenoma detected on clinical ultrasound
- Indeterminate findings on clinical ultrasound
- Recurrent hypercalcemia after parathyroidectomy for parathyroid adenoma or hyperplasia
- Coexisting thyroid nodules

Any ectopic parathyroid adenomas detected on parathyroid scan are usually followed by contrast-enhanced CT or MR for optimal anatomic characterization of findings and surgical planning. Given these clinical scenarios, SPECT/CT, thyroid scans as well as anatomic imaging with MR and CECT have all become useful adjuncts to the planar parathyroid scan.

Selected References

1. Hoang JK et al: Imaging thyroid disease: updates, imaging approach, and management pearls. Radiol Clin North Am. 53(1):145-61, 2015
2. Hindié E et al: The role of radionuclide imaging in the surgical management of primary hyperparathyroidism. J Nucl Med. 56(5):737-744, 2015

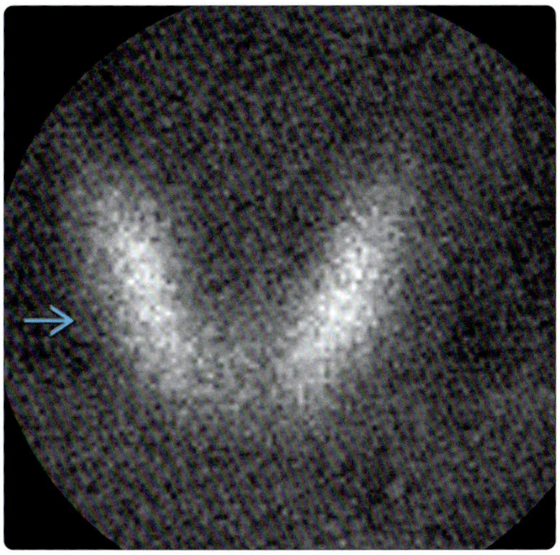

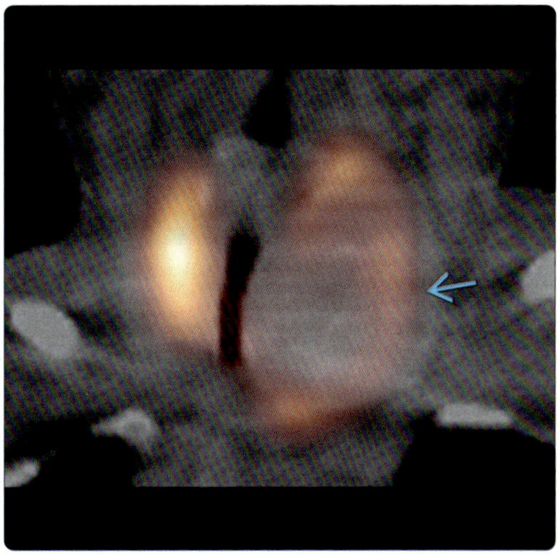

(Left) *Anterior thyroid scan shows homogeneous uptake* ➡ *throughout a normal thyroid gland.* **(Right)** *Anterior Tc-99m pertechnetate SPECT/CT of the thyroid shows an enlarged left thyroid lobe with a dominant cold nodule* ➡ *compressing the trachea.*

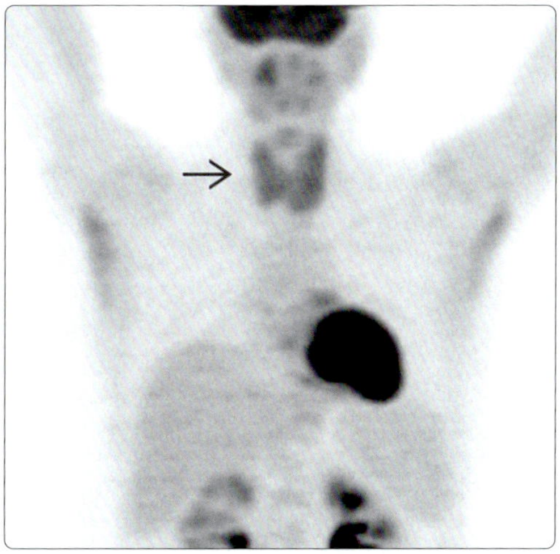

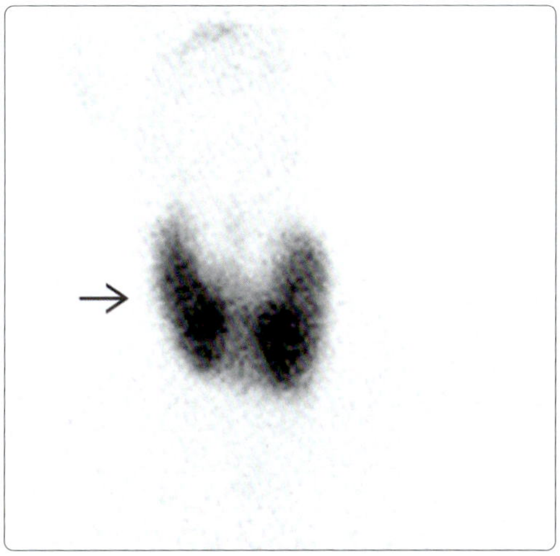

(Left) *Anterior F-18 FDG PET shows diffusely increased uptake in an enlarged thyroid gland* ➡*, suggestive of Graves disease or other diffuse thyroid process such as thyroiditis.* **(Right)** *Anterior thyroid scan shows diffuse, homogeneous uptake in an enlarged thyroid gland* ➡*, consistent with Graves disease. Note absent salivary gland uptake.*

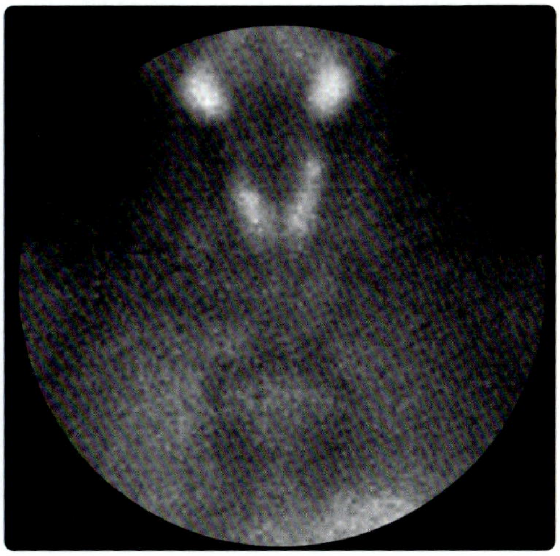

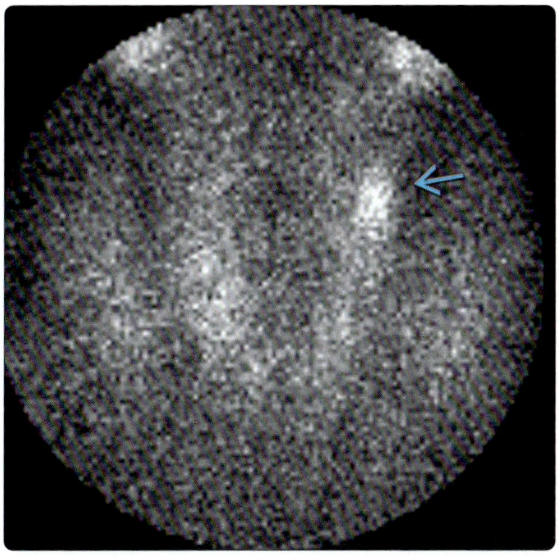

(Left) *On this anterior Tc-99m sestamibi parathyroid scan, images were obtained from the angle of the mandible to the heart border to survey for ectopic adenomas.* **(Right)** *Anterior parathyroid scan in the same patient shows retention of radiotracer in a left superior parathyroid adenoma* ➡*.*

KEY FACTS

TERMINOLOGY

- Graves disease: Autoimmune thyrotoxicosis induced by thyroid-stimulating antibodies (TSAs)

IMAGING

- Tc-99m pertechnetate or I-123 thyroid scan
  - Homogeneously enlarged thyroid with markedly increased radiotracer uptake
  - Decreased uptake in salivary glands
  - Superimposed nodules occur in 5-10%
- Radioactive iodine uptake
  - Usually > 50%, often 80-90%

TOP DIFFERENTIAL DIAGNOSES

- Subacute thyroiditis
- Multinodular goiter, toxic adenoma
- Hyperthyroid autoimmune thyroiditis
- Medication/contrast effects
- Non-thyroid endogenous sources

CLINICAL ISSUES

- Presentation
  - Anxiety
  - Appetite stimulation (weight loss or gain, depending on calories consumed)
  - Heat intolerance
  - Palpitations/arrhythmia
  - Tremor
  - Ophthalmopathy
- Demographics
  - Most common: 3rd-5th decade
  - M < F (1:7-8)
  - Most common etiology of hyperthyroidism in pediatric population
- Radioactive iodine (I-131) therapy
  - Empiric standard dose or calculated dose: Typically 15-20 mCi (555-740 MBq) I-131 p.o.
  - Hypothyroidism is goal of therapy

(Left) *Anterior thyroid scan in a patient with Graves disease shows homogeneous uptake in an enlarged thyroid gland and pyramidal lobe. Note lack of salivary gland uptake, a common finding in thyroid scans of Graves disease.* **(Right)** *Anterior thyroid scan shows a cold nodule in the interpolar right thyroid lobe. Prior to treatment with radioactive iodine, ultrasound is indicated to evaluate for malignant characteristics.*

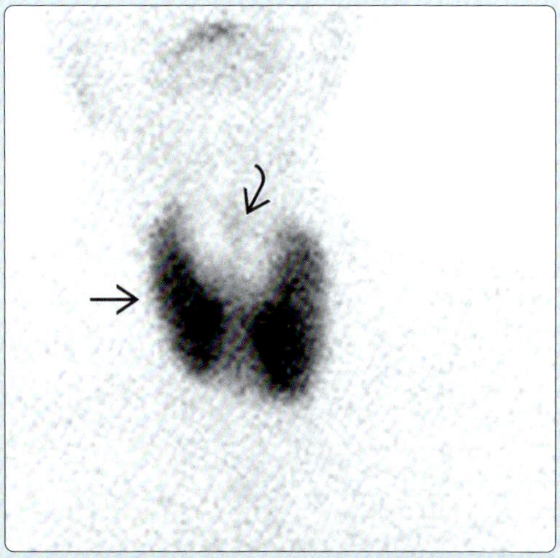

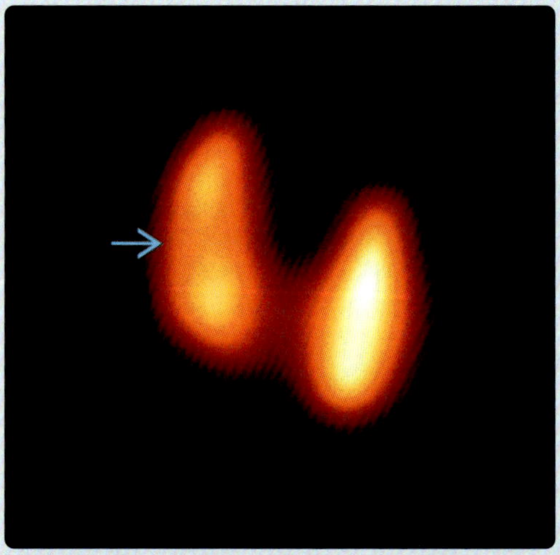

(Left) *Anterior thyroid scan in a patient with Graves disease shows an enlarged, heterogeneous, nodular pattern with a dominant cold nodule. This nodule showed benign characteristics at ultrasound. Note that 5-10% of patients with Graves disease have superimposed thyroid nodules.* **(Right)** *Anterior thyroid scan shows a diminutive left thyroid lobe in a patient with prior left hemithyroidectomy and subsequent development of Graves disease.*

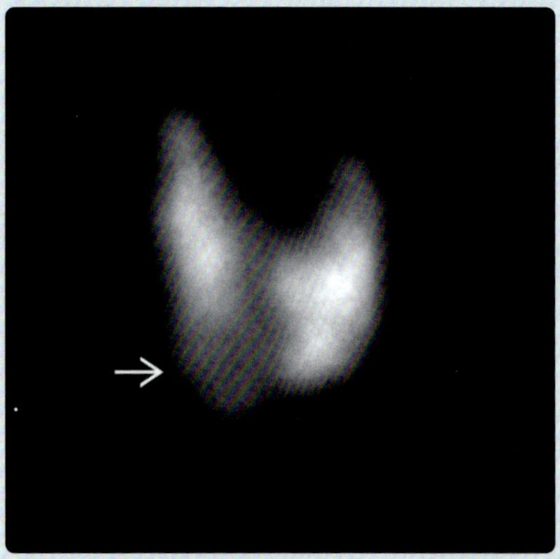

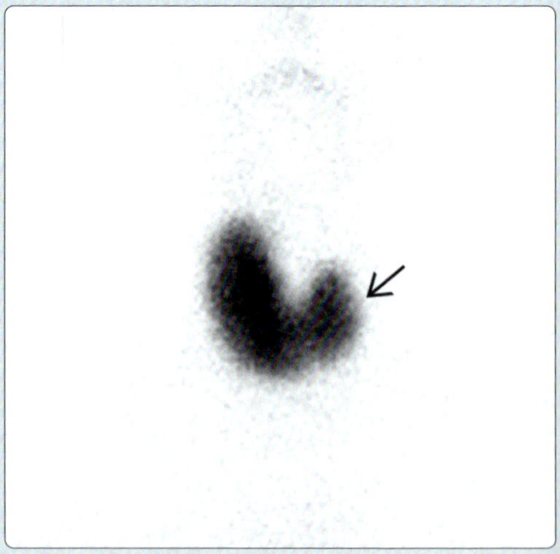

TERMINOLOGY

Definitions

- Graves disease
  - Autoimmune thyrotoxicosis induced by thyroid-stimulating antibodies (TSAs)
  - Thyroid functions autonomously, independent of pituitary thyrotropin-stimulating hormone (TSH)

IMAGING

Nuclear Medicine Findings

- Tc-99m pertechnetate or I-123 thyroid scan
  - Homogeneously enlarged thyroid with markedly increased radiotracer uptake
  - Decreased uptake in salivary glands
  - High target to background levels
  - Superimposed nodules occur in 5-10%
    - Consider Marine-Lenhart syndrome
      - Graves plus multinodular goiter or autonomous nodule(s)
- Radioactive iodine uptake: Usually > 50%, often 80-90%

Imaging Recommendations

- Best imaging tool
  - Thyroid scan
    - Tc-99m pertechnetate
      - Lower radiation exposure compared to I-123
      - Discordant nodules possible, although rare: Nodules hot on Tc-99m pertechnetate may be cold on I-123
    - I-123
      - I-123 trapped and organified by thyroid nodules
      - No discordant nodules
  - Thyroid uptake
    - High turnover in high uptakes; not all trapped iodine organified, so lower 24-hr measurement more indicative of true uptake
    - Patients with high iodine turnover may require higher dose radioactive iodine therapy
- Protocol advice
  - Thyroid scan
    - Patient preparation
      - Review history of medications, diet, history
      - Kelp, cough medicines, vitamins, thyroid hormone, amiodarone can decrease thyroid uptake of radiopharmaceuticals
      - Antithyroid medications (methimazole, propylthiouracil): Discontinue 3-5 days prior to scan
      - IV contrast agents can reduce thyroid uptake for 1-2 months
      - Amiodarone can decrease thyroid uptake for 3-6 months
    - Radiopharmaceutical: I-123 (200-400 μCi [7.4-14.8 MBq] p.o., absorbed by intestine) or Tc-99m pertechnetate (2-10 mCi [74-370 MBq] IV)
      - Tc-99m pertechnetate: Lower radiation dose to thyroid compared with I-123
      - Tc-99m pertechnetate: Trapped but not organified by thyroid gland
      - I-131: Not used for imaging in benign disease due to beta emissions/high radiation dose to thyroid
    - Normal thyroid scan biodistribution: Radioactive iodine and Tc-99m pertechnetate taken up by thyroid, salivary glands, gastric mucosa, choroid plexus
  - Dosimetry
    - I-123: Thyroid receives largest radiation dose followed by urinary bladder
    - Tc-99m pertechnetate: Thyroid receives largest radiation dose
  - Image acquisition
    - I-123: 3-24 hr after p.o. dose
    - Tc-99m pertechnetate: 5-30 min after IV injection
    - SPECT/CT imaging (~ 20 min): Patient positioned supine, head immobilized
    - Pinhole collimator imaging (~ 45-60 min): Patient positioned supine or at 45°, neck extended, head immobilized
      - Anterior, LAO, RAO static images, 10-15 mins each
  - I-123 or I-131 uptake measurement at 4/24 hr
    - Patient preparation
      - Similar to preparation for thyroid scan
    - Radiopharmaceutical
      - I-131: Can use 5-10 μCi (0.2-0.4 MBq) I-131 for uptake if planning Tc-99m pertechnetate scan
      - I-123: I-123 allows uptake and scan with single radiopharmaceutical
      - Tc-99m pertechnetate: Commonly used for scan; can be used for uptake (not common)
  - Uptake acquisition
    - 24 hr most common, may add 4 hr uptake to evaluate for rapid turnover
    - Sitting or supine, head extended
    - Counts using open-faced collimated detector probe, 20-30 cm away from neck
  - Uptake measurement and calculation
    - Counts per 1 min over thyroid
    - Counts per 1 min over mid thigh (background) at same distance used for thyroid counts
      - Urinary bladder excluded from detector field
    - Counts per 1 min over identical-activity I-131 as that given patient in standardized Lucite neck phantom at same distance used for thyroid counts
      - Can use dose given to patient, then correct for decay
    - Counts per 1 min of room background
    - Radioactive iodine uptake (RAIU) = (neck counts - thigh counts) / (phantom counts - background counts) x 100%
  - Normal RAIU values (vary by institution)
    - 4 hr: ~ 5-15%
    - 24 hr: ~ 10-35%

DIFFERENTIAL DIAGNOSIS

Subacute Thyroiditis

- Self-limiting postviral autoimmune thyrotoxicosis
  - Autoimmune thyroid stimulation → hormone release, suppressing TSH
  - Clinical diagnosis difficult in prolonged cases or when prior upper respiratory illness not apparent

- Very low or absent radioactive iodine uptake (< 5%)
- Medical symptom management; not treated with radioactive iodine

Multinodular Goiter, Toxic Adenoma

- Normal to elevated radioactive iodine uptake; nodularity on scan
- Generally requires higher levels of I-131 (≥ 20-30 mCi [740-1,110 MBq]) for therapy

Hyperthyroid Autoimmune Thyroiditis

- Hashimoto disease with hashitoxicosis
  - Chronic thyroiditis characterized by anti-thyroid antibodies: Anti-thyroperoxidase, anti-thyroglobulin, and anti-mitochondrial antibodies
  - 3-5% develop transient thyrotoxicosis
- Silent thyroiditis, postpartum thyroiditis
  - Painless, self-limited autoimmune thyrotoxicosis characterized by lymphocytic infiltration
- Not treated with radioactive iodine

Medication/Contrast Effects

- Thyroiditis factitia: Exogenous thyroid hormone ingestion
- Amiodarone-induced thyroiditis: Effects may last weeks to months
- Jod-Basedow phenomenon: Iodine-induced thyrotoxicosis in endemic (iodine-deficient)/nonendemic goiter, other diseases, normal thyroid

Non-Thyroid Endogenous Sources

- Pheochromocytoma, trophoblastic tumors, metastatic thyroid cancer

PATHOLOGY

General Features

- Etiology
  - Susceptibility increased by combined genetic and environmental factors; history of triggering event such as surgery may be elicited
  - Frequent familial history of autoimmune thyroiditis: Graves, Hashimoto, postpartum thyroiditis
- Associated abnormalities
  - Thyroid function laboratory findings
    - ↓ TSH most sensitive
    - Elevated T4, T3 despite ↓ TSH typical
  - Anti-thyroid antibodies: Anti-TSH receptor in serum
    - Anti-thyrotropin receptor antibodies ↑ thyroid hormone production
    - Antibodies to thyroglobulin, thyroid peroxidase, and sodium-iodide symporter frequently detected

CLINICAL ISSUES

Presentation

- Most common signs/symptoms
  - Anxiety, weight loss, heat intolerance, tremor, palpitations/arrhythmia
  - Graves ophthalmopathy
    - Exophthalmos, diplopia: Seen in 25-30% patients
    - Treat with high-dose glucocorticoids
    - Effects of I-131 therapy controversial; rare cases of ↑ ophthalmopathy with radioiodine therapy reported, may be coincidental

Demographics

- Age
  - Most common: 3rd to 5th decade
  - Most common etiology of hyperthyroidism in pediatric population
- Gender
  - M < F (1:7-8)

Natural History & Prognosis

- Presents with moderate/severe hyperthyroidism
  - Cardiac complications: Heart failure, arrhythmia (atrial fibrillation)
  - Thyrotoxic crisis/storm: Rare but potentially life-threatening acute thyroid hormone discharge
  - Osteoporosis

Treatment

- Antithyroid medication: Propylthiouracil (PTU) or methimazole (Tapazole)
  - Often used temporarily (side effects or relapse in > 50%)
    - Rare agranulocytosis (0.2-0.5%), hepatic dysfunction
- Radioactive iodine (I-131)
  - Empiric standard dose or calculated dose: Typically 15-20 mCi (555-740 MBq) I-131 p.o.
  - Calculated dose based on uptake measurement and thyroid size
    - 8-10 mCi (296-370 MBq) into thyroid gland (# mCi desired divided by 4/24-hr uptake)
    - Higher doses for large goiter, low uptake value, repeat therapy
  - Hypothyroidism is goal of therapy
    - Difficult to achieve euthyroidism, may undertreat hyperthyroidism if attempted
    - Lifelong thyroid hormone replacement required
  - Post-therapy side effects rare but include
    - Radiation thyroiditis: Locally inflamed thyroid (treat with acetaminophen, corticosteroid taper)
    - Thyroid storm: Treat with β-blockers
  - ~ 5% require retreatment after 6-12 months
- Thyroidectomy
  - Patients with large, compressive goiters
  - Risks: Laryngeal nerve trauma, bleeding, infection, scar, death
  - As with radioactive iodine therapy, total thyroidectomy requires lifelong thyroid hormone replacement
  - Used in patients with contraindications to other therapy
    - Medical: Hepatic disease, medically refractive hyperthyroidism
    - Radioactive iodine: Unable to follow radiation safety precautions, patient bias against radiation treatment

SELECTED REFERENCES

1. Society of Nuclear Medicine and Molecular Imaging. ACR–SNM–SPR Practice Guideline for the Performance of Thyroid Scintigraphy and Uptake Measurements. http://snmmi.files.cms-plus.com/docs/Thyroid_Scintigraphy_1382732120053_10.pdf. Created October 1, 2009. Accessed July 31, 2015

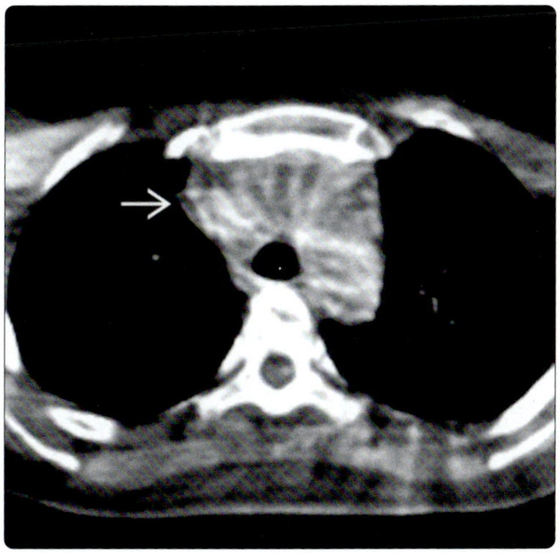

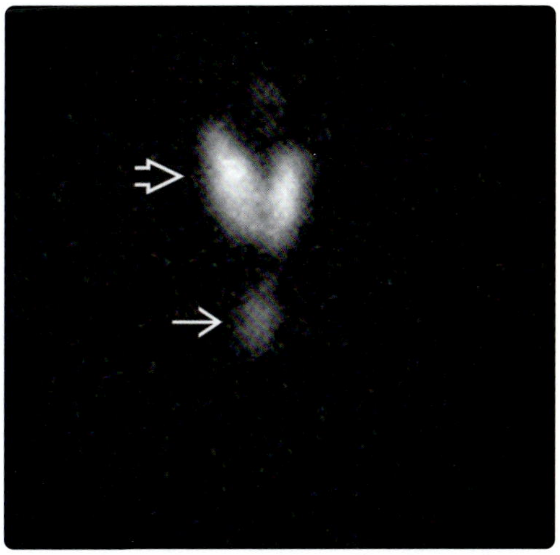

(Left) *Axial CT in a patient with Graves disease shows anterior mediastinal mass →. Thymic hyperplasia is common in Graves disease and often resolves after successful treatment.* **(Right)** *Anterior thyroid scan in a patient with Graves disease shows an enlarged, homogeneous thyroid gland → with substernal uptake →. This could be low-level radiotracer uptake in thymic hyperplasia or a focus of ectopic thyroid tissue.*

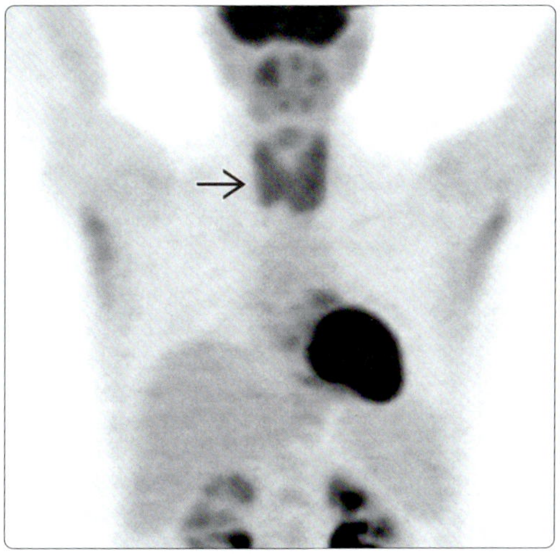

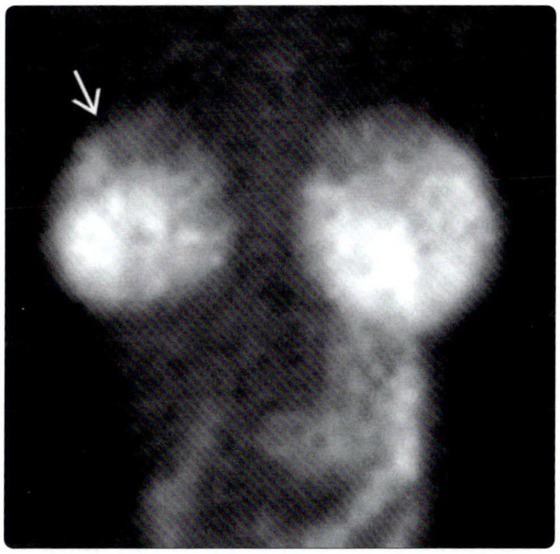

(Left) *F-18 FDG PET shows incidental imaging of diffusely enlarged, hypermetabolic thyroid gland → in a patient with Graves disease.* **(Right)** *Anterior thyroid scan with I-123 in a currently lactating patient shows bilateral breast uptake →. Lactating breasts take up and excrete iodine, therefore breast milk should be discarded after thyroid scans, depending on the half-life of the radiotracer used. Therapy with I-131 should be delayed until 1-3 months after lactation has ceased to avoid unacceptable breast irradiation.*

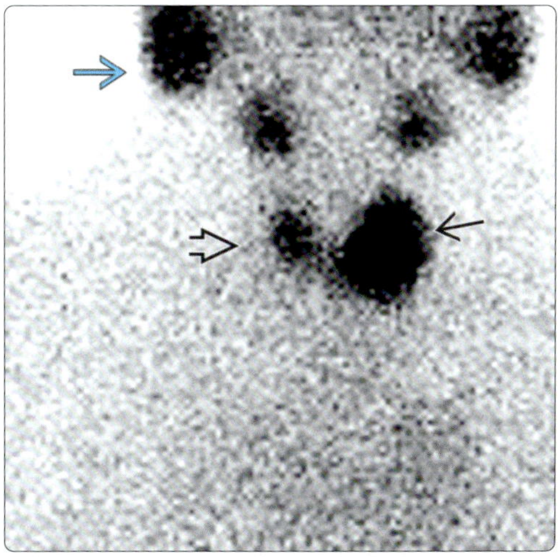

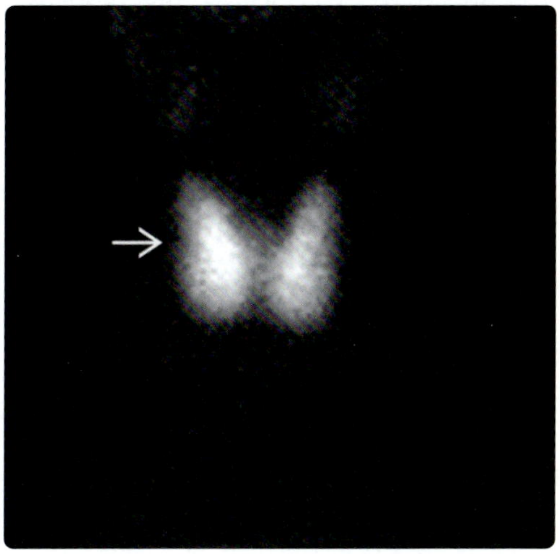

(Left) *Anterior thyroid scan in a patient presumed to have Graves disease shows left thyroid nodule → and relative suppression of the right thyroid lobe →, consistent with toxic nodular etiology for hyperthyroidism. Note salivary gland uptake →, uncommon in Graves disease.* **(Right)** *Anterior thyroid scan in a 13 year old with Graves disease shows an enlarged thyroid →. A therapy dose of at least 15 mCi I-131 is recommended for pediatric patients, as a sublethal dose of I-131 could theoretically induce thyroid cancer later in life.*

KEY FACTS

IMAGING

- Variable uptake of thyroid nodules on scintigraphy
    - Hyperfunctioning (hot)
        - Increased uptake compared with surrounding thyroid
        - < 1% chance of malignancy
    - Isofunctioning (warm)
        - Similar uptake to surrounding thyroid
        - 10-15% chance of malignancy
    - Nonfunctioning (cold)
        - Uptake less than surrounding thyroid
        - 10-15% chance of malignancy in solitary cold nodule
- Multinodular goiter (MNG) on thyroid scintigraphy
    - Heterogeneous uptake in enlarged thyroid gland with multiple variable-intensity nodules
    - Dominant cold nodule in MNG: 5% chance of malignancy
- Hypermetabolic nodule on F-18 FDG PET
    - ~ 33% risk of malignancy in hypermetabolic thyroid nodules

CLINICAL ISSUES

- I-123
    - I-123 trapped by thyroid and incorporated into thyroglobulin for thyroid hormone production (organification)
    - No discordant nodules
- Tc-99m pertechnetate
    - Tc-99m pertechnetate trapped, but not organified
    - Discordant nodules possible, although rare: Nodules hot on Tc-99m pertechnetate may be cold on I-123 scan
- Radioactive iodine uptake
    - Can get thyroid uptake values using I-131 or I-123 (Tc-99m pertechnetate less common)
    - Can be low, normal, or mildly elevated (often < 50%) in thyroid nodular disease
    - Obtained in patients with hyperthyroidism
    - Useful for diagnosis and radioactive iodine therapy planning

(Left) *Anterior thyroid scan shows normal thyroid. Note the right lobe is most often bigger than the left lobe.* **(Right)** *Anterior thyroid scan shows a very large multinodular goiter with substernal extension.*

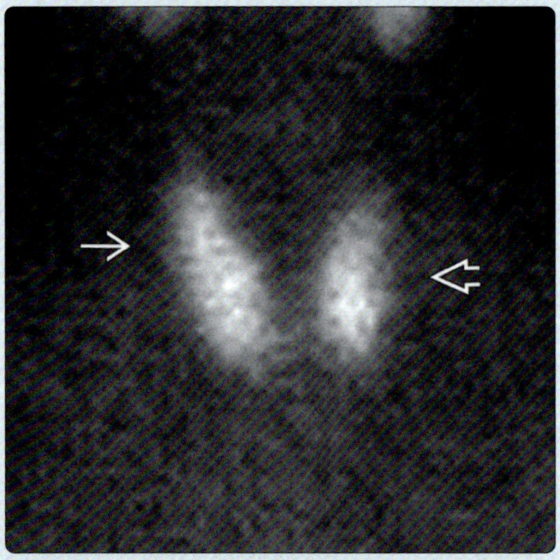

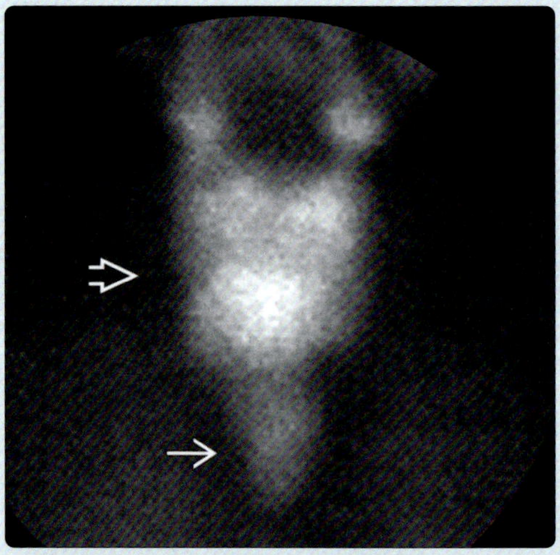

(Left) *Anterior F-18 FDG PET shows focal increased activity in the left thyroid lobe. Because of increased risk of malignancy, incidental hypermetabolic thyroid nodules should undergo ultrasound and fine-needle aspiration if indicated by ultrasound.* **(Right)** *Anterior thyroid scan shows a large cold nodule encompassing the majority of the left thyroid lobe. Cold nodules should undergo ultrasound evaluation due to an increased risk of malignancy.*

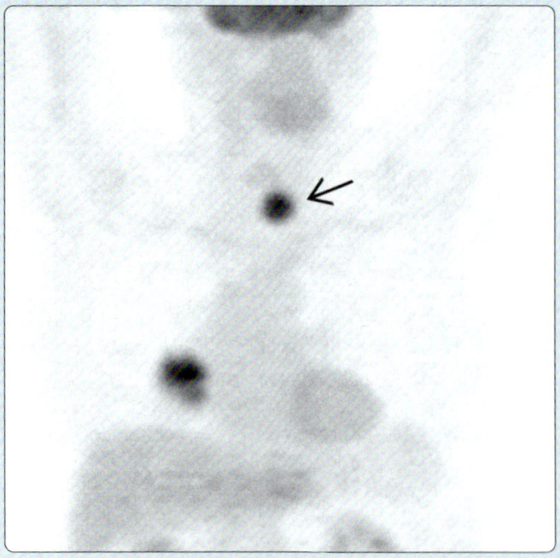

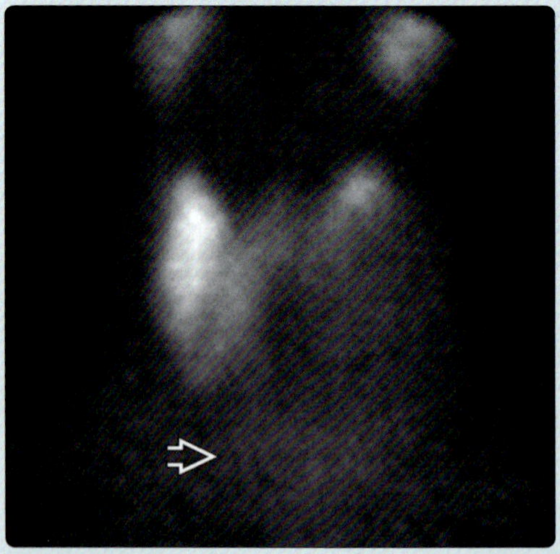

IMAGING

Nuclear Medicine Findings

- Thyroid nodules have variable uptake on thyroid scan
  - Hyperfunctioning (hot): Increased uptake compared with surrounding thyroid
    - < 1% risk of malignancy
  - Isofunctioning (warm): Similar uptake to surrounding thyroid
    - 10-15% risk of malignancy
    - Also called indeterminate nodules, as many are nonfunctioning
  - Nonfunctioning (cold): Uptake less than surrounding thyroid
    - 10-15% risk of malignancy in solitary cold nodule
- Multinodular goiter (MNG) on thyroid scintigraphy
  - Heterogeneous uptake in enlarged thyroid with multiple variable-intensity nodules
  - May extend substernally
  - Evaluate for dominant cold nodule (large, cold nodule when compared with other nodules)
  - Dominant cold nodule: 5% risk of malignancy
- Thyroid nodule on F-18 FDG PET/CT
  - Incidental hypermetabolic thyroid nodules detected in 1-2% of patients undergoing PET/CT
  - ~ 33% risk of malignancy in hypermetabolic thyroid nodules
  - Requires ultrasound and fine-needle aspiration as indicated
  - TSH level recommended (may represent toxic adenoma)

Imaging Recommendations

- Best imaging tool
  - Thyroid scintigraphy
    - I-123
      - I-123 trapped by thyroid follicular cells and incorporated into thyroglobulin for thyroid hormone production (organification)
      - No discordant nodules
    - Tc-99m pertechnetate
      - Discordant nodules rare: Nodules hot on Tc-99m pertechnetate may be cold on I-123 scan
      - Tc-99m pertechnetate trapped, but not organified
  - Radioactive iodine uptake
    - Can be low, normal, or mildly elevated (often < 50%) in thyroid nodular disease
    - Obtained in patients with hyperthyroidism
    - Used for diagnosis and radioactive iodine therapy planning
- Protocol advice
  - Thyroid scintigraphy
    - Patient preparation
      - Antithyroid medications (methimazole, propylthiouracil): Discontinue 3-5 days prior to scan
      - Amiodarone decreases thyroid uptake (3-6 months)
      - IV contrast agents reduce thyroid uptake (1-2 months)
      - Kelp, cough medicines, vitamins, thyroid hormone decrease thyroid uptake
      - Lactating patient: Since lactating breasts take up radiotracer, use Tc-99m pertechnetate; breast milk pumped/discarded for 24 hours
    - Radiopharmaceutical
      - Tc-99m pertechnetate: 2-10 mCi (74-370 MBq) IV
      - I-123: 200-400 µCi (7.4-14.8 MBq) p.o.
      - I-131: Not used for imaging in benign disease due to beta emissions/high radiation dose to thyroid (1 rad/µCi)
    - Dosimetry
      - Tc-99m pertechnetate: Thyroid receives largest radiation dose; lower radiation dose to thyroid compared with I-123
      - I-123: Thyroid receives largest radiation dose followed by urinary bladder (urinary excretion)
      - Normal biodistribution: I-123 and Tc-99m pertechnetate taken up by salivary glands, thyroid, gastric mucosa, choroid plexus
      - Radioactive iodine concentrated by lactating breast tissue; often precludes imaging with RAI; treatment with I-131 absolutely contraindicated
    - Image acquisition
      - Tc-99m pertechnetate: 5-30 min after IV injection
      - I-123: 3-24 hours after p.o. dose
      - SPECT/CT (~ 20 min imaging time): Patient supine, head immobilized
      - Pinhole collimator imaging (~ 1 hour imaging time): Supine or at 45°, neck extended, head immobilized; anterior, LAO, RAO
      - Pinhole collimator imaging: Each image acquired for ~ 100K counts
  - I-123 or I-131 RAI uptake measurement at 4/24 hours
    - Patient preparation
      - Similar to preparation for thyroid scan
      - Note renal failure patients can have lower uptake due to impaired iodine clearance
    - Radiopharmaceutical
      - I-131: Can use 5-10 µCi (0.19-0.37 MBq) I-131 for uptake if planning Tc-99m pertechnetate scan
      - I-123: Allows uptake and scan with single radiopharmaceutical
      - Tc-99m pertechnetate commonly used for scan; can be used for uptake, but not common
  - Uptake measurement and calculation
    - Counts per 1 min over thyroid
    - Counts per 1 min over midthigh at same distance used for thyroid counts
      - Urinary bladder excluded from detector field
    - Counts per 1 min over identical-activity I-131 as that given patient in standardized Lucite neck phantom at same distance used for thyroid counts
      - Can use I-131 dose given to patient, then correct for decay
    - Counts per 1 minute of room background
    - % radioactive iodine uptake (RAIU) = [neck counts - thigh counts] / (phantom counts - background counts) x 100
  - Normal RAIU values (vary by institution)
    - 4-6 hours: ~ 5-15%
    - 24 hours: ~ 10-35%

Differential Diagnosis: Thyroid Nodules

Cold/Warm	Hot
Cyst: Simple, hemorrhagic, colloid	Adenoma, functioning
Adenoma, nonfunctioning/involuted	Thyroiditis, focal
Thyroiditis, focal	Discordant nodule (hot on Tc-99m pertechnetate, cold on I-123)
Carcinoma: Thyroid, lymphoma, metastases	
Hematoma	
Granuloma	
Abscess	
Infiltrative disorders (e.g., amyloid)	
Parathyroid adenoma/cyst	

A cold/warm thyroid nodule has a 10-15% risk of malignancy. Hot nodules have < 1% risk of malignancy. Discordant nodules are rare.

Artifacts and Quality Control

- Thyroid scintigraphy
  - Poor uptake of radiopharmaceutical may be due to medication/IV contrast/diet/renal failure
  - Radiotracer in esophagus may mimic thyroid tissue (reimage after administering water to patient)
- I-123 or I-131 RAI uptake
  - 4-6 hour values useful for Graves patients, as rapid-turnover Graves may show high uptake at 4-6 hours and only normal or mildly elevated values at 24 hours

DIFFERENTIAL DIAGNOSIS

Toxic or Autonomous Nodule (Plummer Disease)

- Single or multiple toxic nodules causing hyperthyroidism
- Often suppresses uptake in balance of thyroid

Multinodular Goiter

- Enlarged thyroid with multiple hot, warm, cold nodules
- If associated with hyperthyroidism, called toxic multinodular goiter

Nodular Graves Disease

- Heterogeneous, enlarged thyroid: High radioactive iodine uptake, signs/symptoms of Graves disease
- Solitary cold nodule in Graves needs ultrasound ± fine-needle aspiration

Hashimoto Disease

- Autoimmune chronic thyroiditis; + antithyroid antibodies
- Hashimoto typically hypofunctional goiter; often similar appearance to MNG
- Can have transient hyperthyroidism (Hashitoxicosis)

CLINICAL ISSUES

Presentation

- Most common signs/symptoms
  - Neck mass with palpable nodules
  - If thyroid nodular disease and hyperthyroid, symptoms may be subtle
    - Weight loss, anxiety, palpitations, menstrual irregularity, atrial fibrillation, congestive heart failure
    - Subclinical hyperthyroidism (normal T4/T3 but suppressed TSH)

Treatment

- Surgery often required for large MNG, or MNG with compressive symptoms
- Toxic MNG or toxic adenoma
  - Medication
    - Propylthiouracil (PTU) and methimazole
      - Thyroid organification blockers
      - Bone marrow, hepatic toxicity may limit use
    - β blockers
      - Cardioprotective, symptomatic relief
  - Radioactive iodine (I-131) therapy
    - Effective treatment for toxic adenoma and MNG
    - Note transient swelling in MNG after I-131 if compressive symptoms
    - Often bulk of MNG does not decrease significantly after I-131
    - Larger I-131 doses (> 20 mCi (740 MBq), sometimes 30-40 mCi [1.1-1.4 GBq]) required compared to Graves disease therapy
    - May require multiple doses
  - Surgery
    - Often required for large toxic MNG or MNG with compressive symptoms

Malignant Potential of Thyroid Nodules

- Ultrasound has replaced thyroid scan for evaluation of thyroid nodules for malignant potential
- When fine-needle aspiration of suspicious nodule shows follicular neoplasm or indeterminate cytology, I-123 scintigraphy may be considered
  - Concordant autonomously functioning nodule on I-123 scintigraphy is reassuring and thyroid lobectomy/thyroidectomy may be avoided

SELECTED REFERENCES

1. Hoang JK et al: Imaging thyroid disease: updates, imaging approach, and management pearls. Radiol Clin North Am. 53(1):145-61, 2015
2. American Thyroid Association (ATA) Guidelines Taskforce on Thyroid Nodules and Differentiated Thyroid Cancer et al: Revised American Thyroid Association management guidelines for patients with thyroid nodules and differentiated thyroid cancer. Thyroid. 19(11):1167-214, 2009

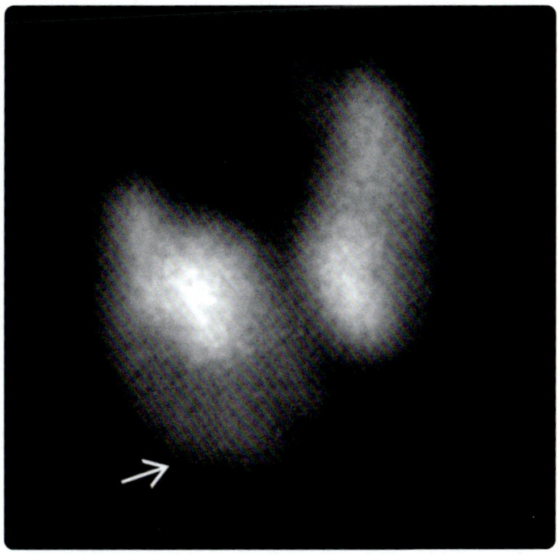
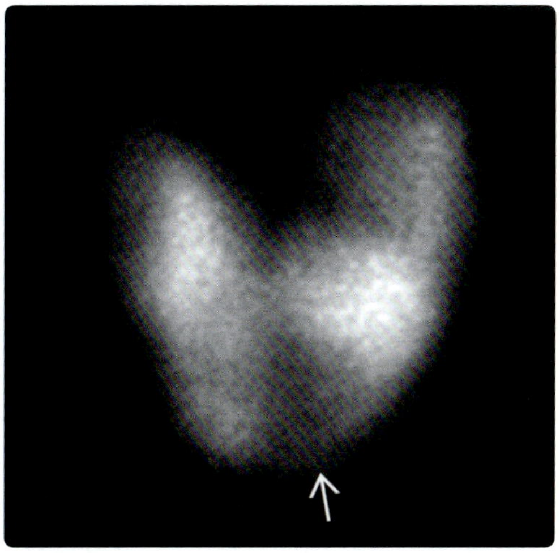

(Left) *Anterior thyroid scan shows a warm nodule* → *in the inferior pole of the right thyroid lobe.* **(Right)** *Right anterior oblique thyroid scan in same patient shows that the nodule* → *is more photopenic than evident on anterior image.*

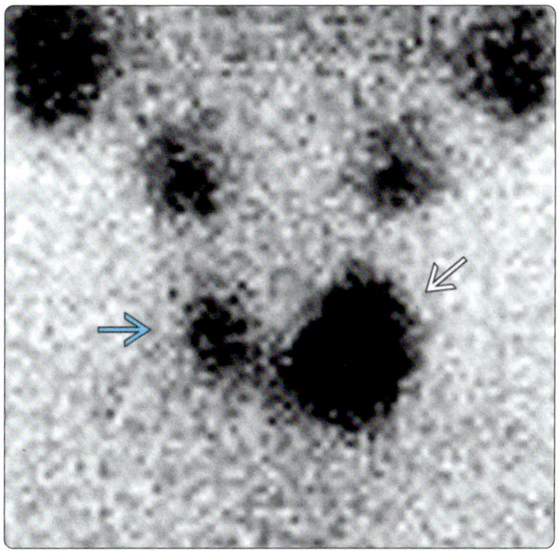
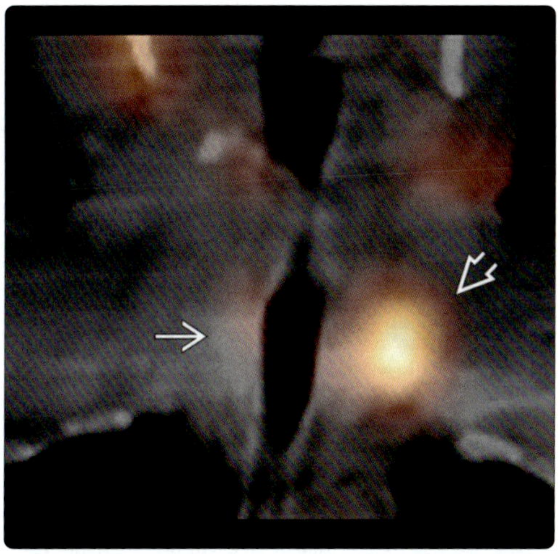

(Left) *Anterior thyroid scan in a hyperthyroid patient shows a hot nodule in the left thyroid lobe* → *that is suppressing uptake in the normal right thyroid lobe* →*, also called a toxic adenoma.* **(Right)** *Coronal SPECT/CT thyroid scan shows increased uptake in a left toxic adenoma* → *with complete suppression of the right thyroid lobe* →.

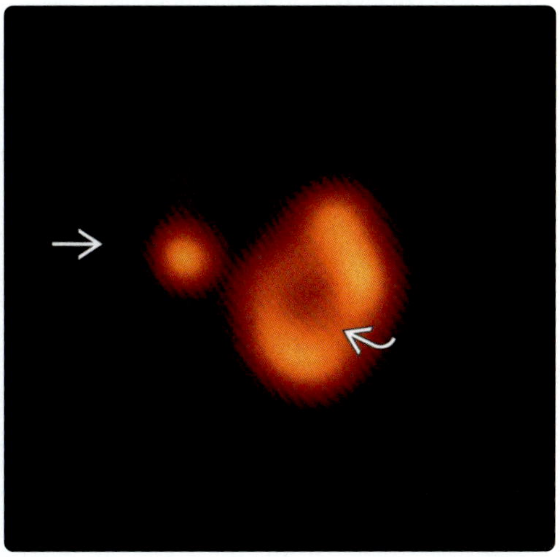
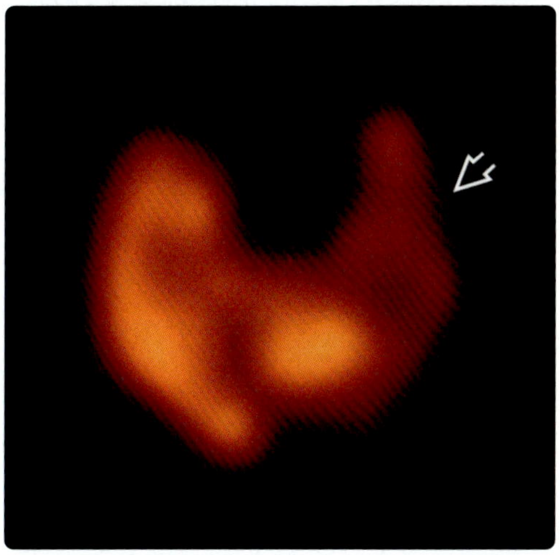

(Left) *Anterior thyroid scan in a hyperthyroid patient shows a degenerating toxic adenoma, an enlarged hot nodule with a photopenic center* → *that suppresses the right thyroid lobe* →. **(Right)** *Anterior thyroid scan shows multinodular goiter with a dominant cold nodule* → *that should undergo ultrasound to evaluate for malignant features.*

Parathyroid Adenoma

KEY FACTS

TERMINOLOGY

- Parathyroid adenoma
  - Enlarged parathyroid gland with normal cellular structure
  - May be posterior to thyroid gland or ectopic
  - Causes primary hyperparathyroidism (symptomatic or asymptomatic hypercalcemia)

PATHOLOGY

- Perithyroidal (90-95%)
  - Posterior or inferior to thyroid (most common)
  - Subcapsular (3-8%): Under fibrous capsule surrounding thyroid
  - Intrathyroidal (2%): Within thyroid parenchyma
- Ectopic (5-10%)
  - Parathyroid glands also found in carotid sheath, mediastinum, great vessels, cardiac border due to embryological dysgenesis
  - Inferior parathyroid glands more likely to be ectopic
- Supranumerary glands
  - 25% may have 5 or more glands
- Multiple adenomas
  - 4-5% have multiple adenomas
  - Consider parathyroid hyperplasia

DIAGNOSTIC CHECKLIST

- False-negatives
  - Radiotracer may wash out of adenoma before delayed images; however, early planar images may be adequate for localization
  - SPECT/CT images obtained after washout from parathyroid adenoma
  - Photopenic nodule posterior to or inferior to thyroid suggests cystic degeneration or necrosis
  - Limited field of view: Image from carotid sheath to inferior cardiac border to search for ectopic adenomas
  - Avoid satisfaction of search: Multiple adenomas may be present

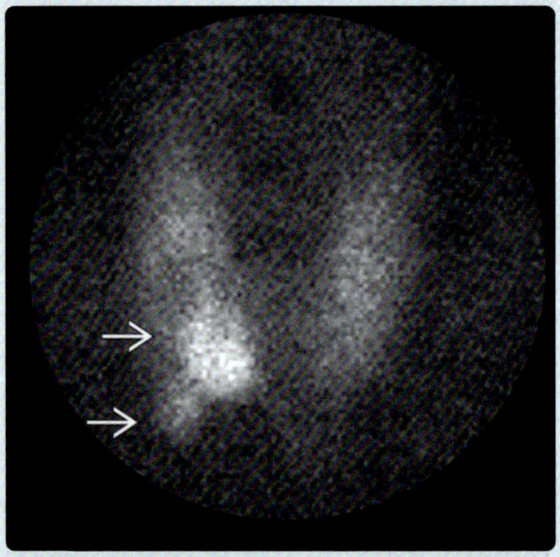
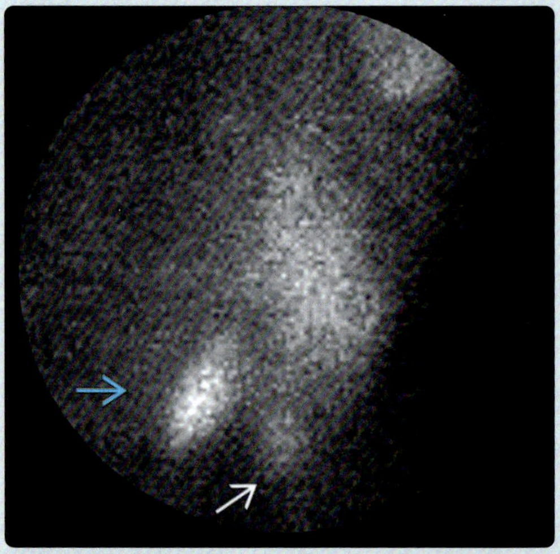

(Left) *Anterior parathyroid scan shows 2 foci of increased activity ➔ adjacent to the inferior pole of the right thyroid lobe.* **(Right)** *Right lateral parathyroid scan in same patient shows 2 parathyroid adenomas, 1 posterior to ➔ and 1 inferior to ➔ the inferior pole of the right thyroid lobe. Double parathyroid adenomas can be seen in up to 5% of patients with primary hyperparathyroidism.*

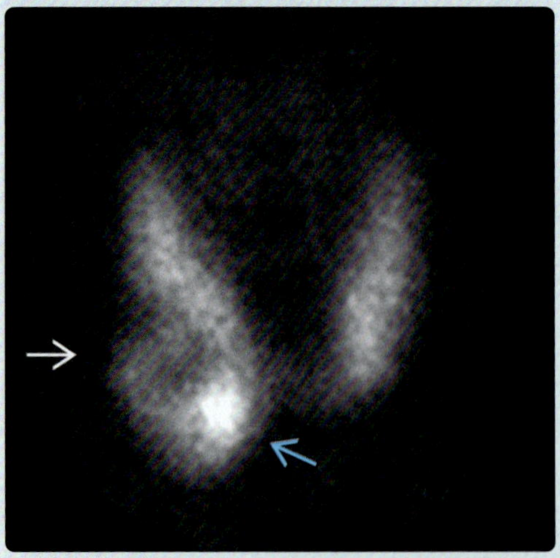
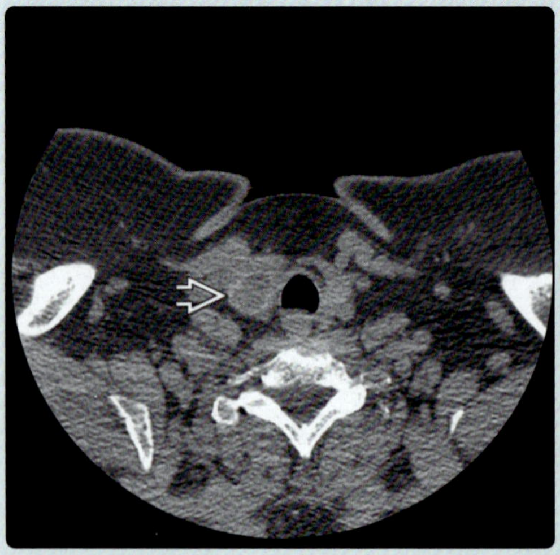

(Left) *Anterior parathyroid scan shows a focus of abnormally increased activity ➔ with central photopenia ➔. This suggests a cystic parathyroid adenoma.* **(Right)** *Axial CT in same patient shows the hypointense, cystic parathyroid adenoma ➔.*

TERMINOLOGY

Definitions

- Parathyroid adenoma
  - Most common cause of primary hyperparathyroidism
    - Hypercalcemia due to increased production of parathyroid hormone (PTH) by parathyroid gland(s)
  - Enlarged parathyroid gland with normal cellular structure
  - May be posterior to thyroid gland or ectopic

IMAGING

Nuclear Medicine Findings

- Dual-phase Tc-99m sestamibi parathyroid scintigraphy
  - Early images
    - 10-20 min post injection
    - Activity in thyroid and parathyroid adenoma
  - Delayed images
    - 90 min post injection
    - Activity in thyroid washes out, activity in adenoma persists
      - ~ 60% of adenomas retain radiotracer longer than thyroid
  - SPECT/CT
    - SPECT/CT at 90 min (after thyroid washes out)
    - Better to localize activity posterior to thyroid, in tracheoesophageal groove, or to ectopic site
- Dual radiotracer protocol
  - Tc-99m sestamibi parathyroid scintigraphy to localize thyroid and parathyroid adenoma
  - Thyroid-only radiotracer to distinguish borders of thyroid gland: Tc-99m pertechnetate or I-123
  - Often used when Tc-99m sestamibi parathyroid scintigraphy indeterminate

Imaging Recommendations

- Best imaging tool
  - Ultrasound localizes adenoma in 80% (usually performed in office by surgeon)
  - Dual-phase Tc-99m sestamibi parathyroid scintigraphy for adenoma not localized by ultrasound
- Protocol advice
  - Radiopharmaceutical for localizing parathyroid tissue
    - 20-30 mCi (740 MBq to 1.1 GBq) Tc-99m sestamibi, tetrofosmin
  - Radiopharmaceutical for localizing thyroid-only tissue
    - 10-20 mCi (370-740 MBq) Tc-99m pertechnetate, 200-400 μCi (7.4-14.8 MBq) I-123
  - Dosimetry
    - Largest dose to bladder
  - Image acquisition: Single vs. dual radiopharmaceutical
    - Single radiopharmaceutical
      - Anterior planar images of chest and neck obtained at 10-30 min and again at 90-180 min
    - Dual radiopharmaceutical
      - Radiopharmaceutical that accumulates only in thyroid tissue
      - Planar images obtained of thyroid, then subtracted from parathyroid scintigraphy
  - SPECT/CT
    - Increases contrast in adenoma
    - May show smaller adenoma
    - Confirms tracheoesophageal groove location
    - Identify ectopic parathyroid adenomas
- Parathyroid adenoma on correlative imaging
  - Ultrasound
    - Homogeneous, hypoechoic, hypervascular mass ± cystic regions
    - Surrounded by thin echogenic rim (fat) if intrathyroidal
  - MR
    - T1 low intensity; T2 ≥ fat intensity
  - CECT
    - Homogeneous, enhancing mass

DIFFERENTIAL DIAGNOSIS

Benign Thyroid Pathology

- Thyroid adenoma
- Multinodular goiter
- Ectopic thyroid

Parathyroid Carcinoma

- Scintigraphic appearance identical to parathyroid adenoma, unless lymphadenopathy evident on images
- Regional lymph node metastases at presentation as high as 17%
- Heterogeneous, often calcified nodules

Other Malignancy

- Thyroid, lung, lymphoma, head and neck cancer

Infection/Inflammation

- Benign lymphadenopathy
- Abscess

PATHOLOGY

General Features

- Etiology
  - Primary hyperparathyroidism
    - Parathyroid adenoma: Cause of 75-85% of primary hyperparathyroidism cases
    - Parathyroid hyperplasia: 10-15%
    - Parathyroid carcinoma: 0.5-5.0%
      - Enlarged parathyroid gland with cellularity consistent with carcinoma
      - Lymphadenopathy may be present
- Genetics
  - 95% of cases are sporadic
  - 5% of cases due to multiple endocrine neoplasia syndromes (MEN1, MEN2a), familial hypocalciuric hypercalcemia
- Associated abnormalities
  - Increased PTH production causes mobilization of calcium from bones and renal conservation of calcium
    - Osteitis fibrosa cystica: Resorption of bone, especially distal phalanges; increased alkaline phosphatase
    - Brown tumors: Fibrous lytic lesions of bone
    - Metastatic calcification of organs
    - Nephrolithiasis
    - Peptic ulcer disease (usually with MEN1)

- Weakness
- Mental confusion
- Arrhythmia

Gross Pathologic & Surgical Features

- Well-circumscribed, soft, tan nodule
- May show cystic degeneration
- 0.5-5.0 g

Microscopic Features

- Fibrous capsule
- Predominately chief cells
- Nests of oxyphil cells
- Rarely, oxyphil or water-clear cells predominate

Anatomic Location of Parathyroid Glands

- Perithyroidal (90-95%)
  - Posterior or inferior to thyroid (most common)
  - Subcapsular (3-8%): Under fibrous capsule surrounding thyroid
  - Intrathyroidal (2%): Within thyroid parenchyma
- Ectopic (5-10%)
  - Parathyroid glands also found in carotid sheath, mediastinum, great vessels, cardiac border due to embryological dysgenesis
  - Inferior parathyroid glands more likely to be ectopic
- Supranumerary
  - 25% may have 5 or more glands
- Multiple adenomas
  - 4-5% have multiple adenomas
  - Consider parathyroid hyperplasia

CLINICAL ISSUES

Presentation

- Most common signs/symptoms
  - Asymptomatic hypercalcemia most common; found on routine lab work
  - Mental confusion, sleep disorders
  - Bone pain: Compression fractures
  - Renal colic: Nephrolithiasis

Demographics

- Age
  - Peak incidence > 50 years
- Gender
  - M:F = 1:3

Treatment

- Minimally invasive parathyroidectomy
  - Very small incision (0.5 inch)
  - Distinction between superior or inferior origin important, so dissection does not extend over recurrent laryngeal nerve and fascial planes
  - First localize parathyroid adenoma in right or left neck
  - Then localize parathyroid adenoma in anteroposterior plane compared with thyroid
    - Posteriorly displaced adenomas: Superior in origin
    - Inferiorly displaced adenomas: Inferior in origin
    - Closely apposed to thyroid: Mid to superior pole of thyroid lobe = superior in origin; inferior pole of thyroid lobe = inferior in origin
- Unilateral cervical exploration
  - Incision from midline neck laterally (1-2 inches)
  - Important to localize parathyroid adenoma in right or left neck
- Bilateral cervical exploration
  - Historically popular treatment
  - Still used in cases of hyperparathyroidism with
    - Concurrent multinodular goiter, thyroid adenomas
    - Recurrent hyperparathyroidism
    - Negative parathyroid scan (adenoma with no uptake, hyperplasia)

DIAGNOSTIC CHECKLIST

Image Interpretation Pearls

- False-negatives
  - Radiotracer may wash out of adenoma before delayed images; however, early planar images may be adequate for localization
  - SPECT/CT images obtained after washout from parathyroid adenoma
  - Photopenic nodule posterior to or inferior to thyroid suggests cystic degeneration or necrosis
  - Limited field of view: Image from carotid sheath to inferior cardiac border to search for ectopic adenomas
  - Avoid satisfaction of search: Multiple adenomas may be present
- False-positives
  - Thyroid adenomas
  - Multinodular goiter
  - Asymmetric activity in salivary glands can resemble ectopic parathyroid adenoma in carotid sheath
  - Single or multiple foci in lateral neck suggest lymphadenopathy and malignant etiology (parathyroid carcinoma, thyroid cancer)

SELECTED REFERENCES

1. Schenk WG 3rd et al: Surgeon-performed ultrasound for primary hyperparathyroidism. Am Surg. 79(7):681-5, 2013
2. Greenspan BS et al: SNM practice guideline for parathyroid scintigraphy 4.0. J Nucl Med Technol. 40(2):111-8, 2012
3. Mohebati A et al: Imaging techniques in parathyroid surgery for primary hyperparathyroidism. Am J Otolaryngol. 33(4):457-68, 2012
4. Carlson D: Parathyroid pathology: hyperparathyroidism and parathyroid tumors. Arch Pathol Lab Med. 134(11):1639-44, 2010
5. Baliski CR et al: Selective unilateral parathyroid exploration: an effective treatment for primary hyperparathyroidism. Am J Surg. 189(5):596-600; discussion 600, 2005
6. Cohen MS et al: Outpatient minimally invasive parathyroidectomy using local/regional anesthesia: a safe and effective operative approach for selected patients. Surgery. 138(4):681-7; discussion 687-9, 2005
7. Gilat H et al: Minimally invasive procedure for resection of a parathyroid adenoma: the role of preoperative high-resolution ultrasonography. J Clin Ultrasound. 33(6):283-7, 2005
8. Clark P et al: Providing optimal preoperative localization for recurrent parathyroid carcinoma: a combined parathyroid scintigraphy and computed tomography approach. Clin Nucl Med. 29(11):681-4, 2004
9. Clark PB et al: Enhanced scintigraphic protocol required for optimal preoperative localization before targeted minimally invasive parathyroidectomy. Clin Nucl Med. 28(12):955-60, 2003

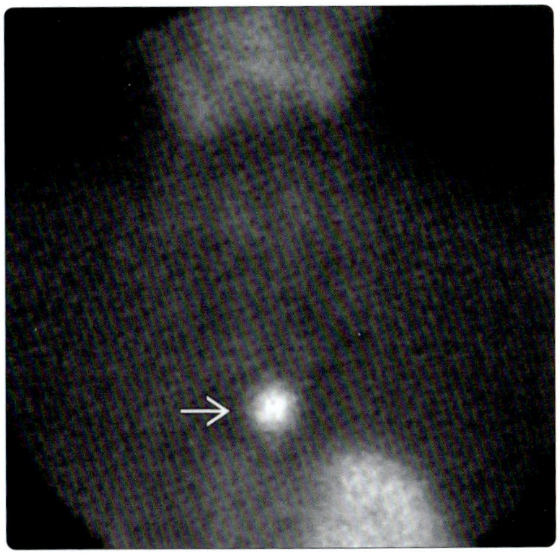

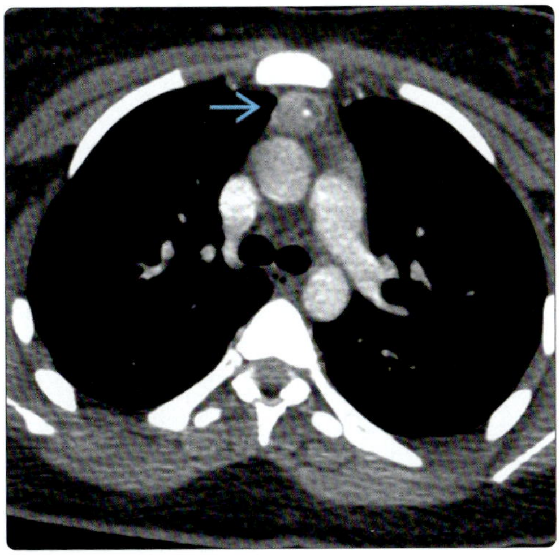

(Left) *Anterior parathyroid scan shows a focus of abnormal activity in the thorax, likely an ectopic parathyroid adenoma. This needs to be confirmed on anatomic imaging.* **(Right)** *Axial CECT in the same patient shows an enhancing ectopic parathyroid adenoma.*

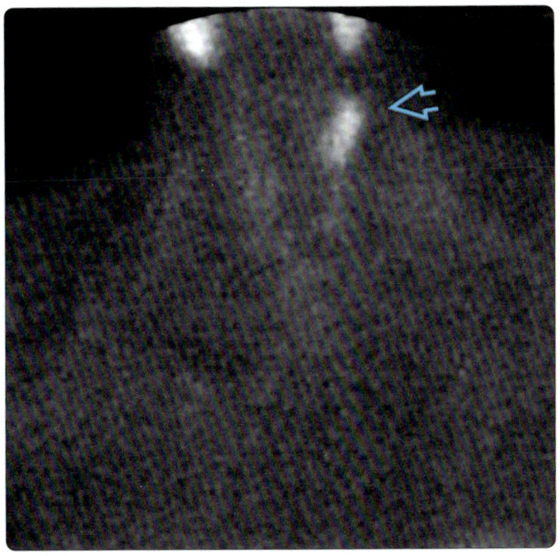

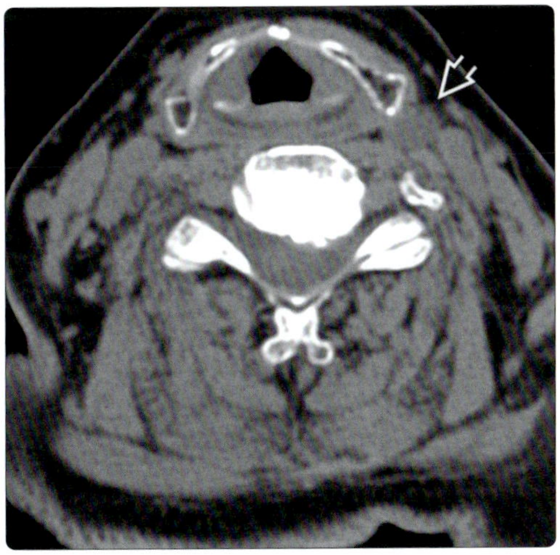

(Left) *Anterior parathyroid scan shows increased activity superolateral to the left thyroid bed.* **(Right)** *Axial CT in same patient performed for neck pain shows an ectopic parathyroid adenoma adjacent to the carotid artery.*

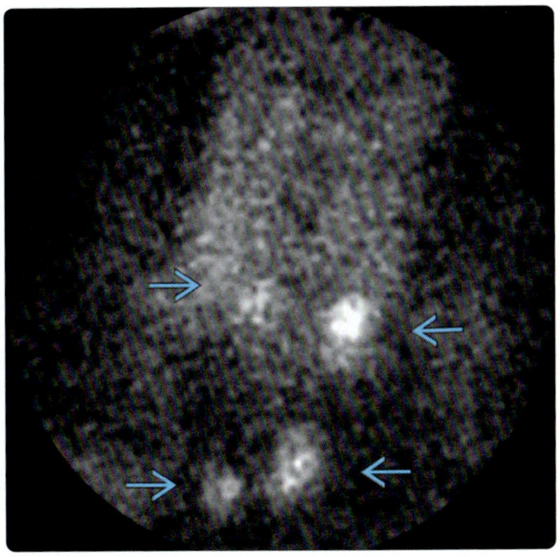

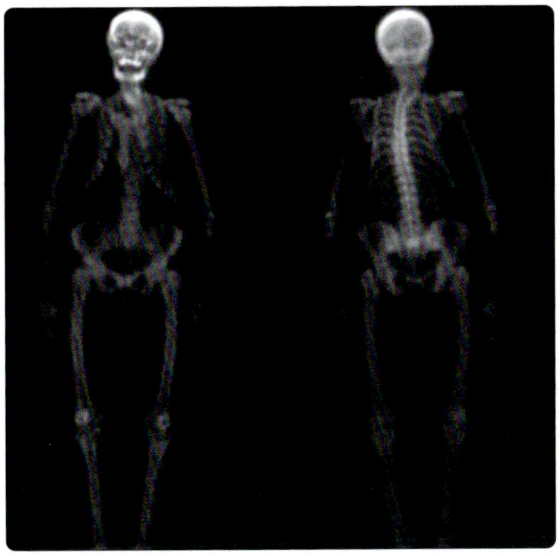

(Left) *Anterior parathyroid scan shows 4 foci of abnormal activity after washout of the thyroid gland, consistent with 4-gland hyperplasia. If hyperplastic glands get large enough, they can be seen on parathyroid scan.* **(Right)** *Anterior and posterior bone scan in a patient with parathyroid carcinoma shows a superscan due to metabolic bone disease (hyperparathyroidism).*

SECTION 7

Thoracic

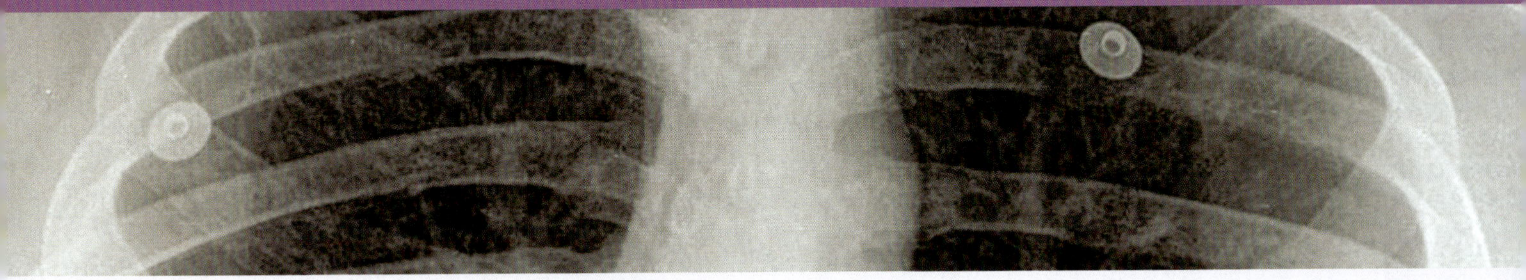

Introduction

Infection and Inflammation

Lung Perfusion and Ventilation

Introduction

Functional imaging of lung perfusion and ventilation (VQ) has been performed for over 40 years, its advent a medical breakthrough in that it replaced invasive pulmonary angiography for the diagnosis of pulmonary embolism. VQ scans remain an important part of the clinical nuclear medicine practice despite the advent of CT angiography, particularly in efforts to reduce radiation dose. Evolving interpretation algorithms have made it easier for readers to interpret exams and for clinicians to understand the interpretation for their clinical practice. Thoracic surgeons rely on quantitative lung perfusion analysis for patients with borderline lung function who may undergo lobectomy or pneumonectomy, ensuring that patients will have sufficient postsurgical lung capacity.

Once a robust indication, the characterization of atypical, opportunistic, and neoplastic pulmonary diseases in immunocompromised hosts using Ga-67 and Th-201 scans has largely been replaced with high-resolution CT and bronchoscopy. However, characterization of active versus inactive granulomatous disease using nuclear medicine continues to support clinical therapeutic decision-making.

Ventilation-Perfusion Scans for Diagnosis of Pulmonary Embolism

When first introduced in the 1970s, the VQ scan replaced invasive pulmonary angiography for the diagnosis of pulmonary embolism. By the 1990s, a large, prospective clinical trial of mostly inpatients, called the Prospective Investigation of Pulmonary Embolism Diagnosis (PIOPED), was published, giving physicians an interpretation algorithm fraught with confusing terms and indeterminate findings. It is understandable that with the advent of CT angiogram (CTA) in the 1990s, VQ scans for the diagnosis of pulmonary embolism fell out of favor as CTA was more readily available and VQ scan interpretations could be difficult to apply clinically.

Over the years, reanalysis of the valuable PIOPED data and further studies have refined VQ interpretation algorithms, making interpretation easier. As the data have been reexamined, CTA and VQ scan have been shown to have similar diagnostic accuracy. In one study, emergency department patients with suspected pulmonary embolism were triaged based on chest x-ray: If normal, the patient underwent VQ instead of CTA. The number of positive VQ scans was ~ 4%, and the number of positive CTAs was 13%. The false-negative rates on these studies were the same at 1%.

The clinical value of VQ scans becomes apparent in light of radiation dose received for a study with similar diagnostic accuracy as CTA. The American College of Radiology recently studied this problem, finding the estimated dose to the breast using a 4-slice CTA somewhere between 20 and 60 mSv. In contrast, a complete VQ scan is estimated to deliver < 1 mSv to the breast. Even lower radiation doses can be achieved using perfusion-only scans and doses as low as 1 mCi (370 MBq) Tc-99m MAA for the perfusion scan, a method of particular importance for pregnant patients. In one center, it was estimated that over 95% of pregnant patients undergoing perfusion-only scan for suspected pulmonary embolism had a normal perfusion-only scan.

A simplified trinary interpretation algorithm for VQ scans is now being advocated, in which conclusions are reported as pulmonary embolism likely, unlikely, or nondiagnostic. Training readers in this interpretation algorithm may also improve ordering clinician confidence in VQ interpretations.

- PE likely/present: High probability scan, with inclusion of a single-segmental VQ mismatch in the high probability category
- PE unlikely/absent: Normal and very low probability scans
- Nondiagnostic for PE: All others

A single-segmental mismatch in a patient with no underlying cardiopulmonary disease has a positive predictive value of 86%.

Quantitative Lung Perfusion Analysis

Quantitative analysis of relative regional lung perfusion remains valuable in patients undergoing lung reduction surgery (e.g., lung cancer or bullectomy). Prior to lobectomy or pneumonectomy, pulmonary function tests are performed. Typically, if the forced expiratory volume in 1 second is below expected values, a lung perfusion analysis can quantify the relative functioning lung mass. Normally, with region of interest analysis, the right lung encompasses 55% of the entire lung perfusion capacity and the left lung, 45%. Each lung can be further subdivided into 3 regions. The portion planned for resection can be factored in with preoperative lung function values, giving an estimate of postoperative lung function. Often, tumor in 1 region is already compromising pulmonary blood flow and this analysis can reassure surgeons that patients will not be harmed by a lobectomy or pneumonectomy.

Atypical Pulmonary Infection and Granulomatous Disease

Historically, the indication for nuclear medicine evaluation of pulmonary diseases was strong. Particularly in patients with HIV, Ga-67 and Th-201 narrowed the differential diagnosis in atypical and opportunistic infections such as PJP, MAC, and CMV pneumonia as well as diagnosis of Kaposi sarcoma and lymphoma. This gave clinicians valuable information for treating these unusual diseases. However, diagnosis with high-resolution CT &/or bronchoscopy has largely replaced this indication.

Characterization of granulomatous disease (such as sarcoidosis) with Ga-67 and F-18 FDG- PET/CT remains a robust clinical indication. These scans can determine disease activity, enhancing therapeutic decision-making. Additionally, an accurate assessment of pulmonary and extrapulmonary organ involvement can be challenging for clinicians. Diagnosis of granulomatous disease in the heart, skin, eyes, and lymphatic system can be made using nuclear medicine scans, allowing for the use of immunomodulating drugs as indicated.

Selected References

1. Kim NH et al: Chronic thromboembolic pulmonary hypertension. J Am Coll Cardiol. 62(25 Suppl):D92-9, 2013
2. Glaser JE et al: Successful and safe implementation of a trinary interpretation and reporting strategy for V/Q lung scintigraphy. J Nucl Med. 52(10):1508-12, 2011

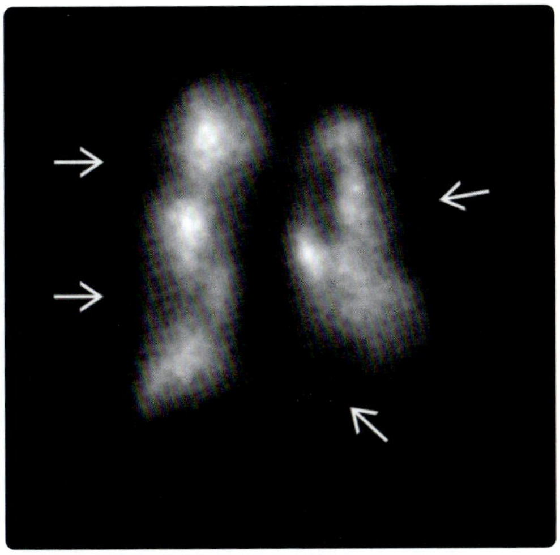

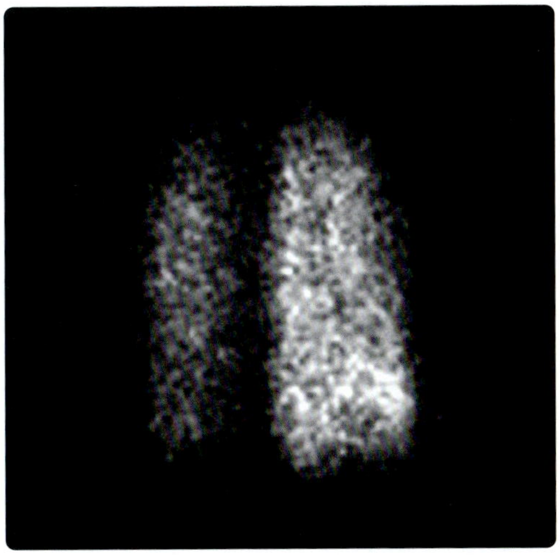

(Left) *RPO Tc-99m MAA pulmonary perfusion scan shows multiple peripheral, wedge-shaped perfusion defects.* **(Right)** *RPO Xe-133 pulmonary ventilation scan in the same patient shows virtually normal ventilation, confirming pulmonary embolism in a hypercoagulable patient.*

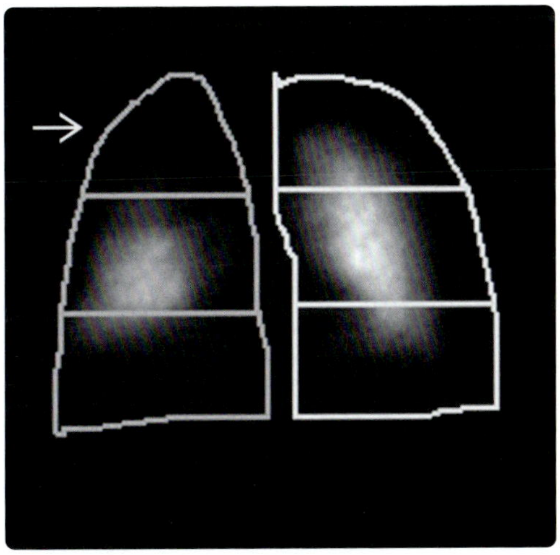

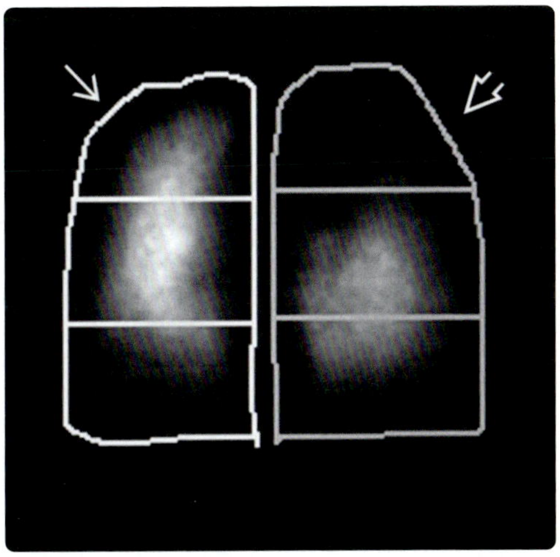

(Left) *Anterior Tc-99m MAA quantitative lung perfusion scan in a patient with lung cancer shows decreased perfusion in the right apex due to tumor involvement.* **(Right)** *Posterior Tc-99m MAA quantitative lung perfusion scan in the same patient shows region of interest analysis around the left and right lungs, further subdivided into 3 zones per lung. Right upper lobectomy should have little impact on current lung function, given absent perfusion in this area.*

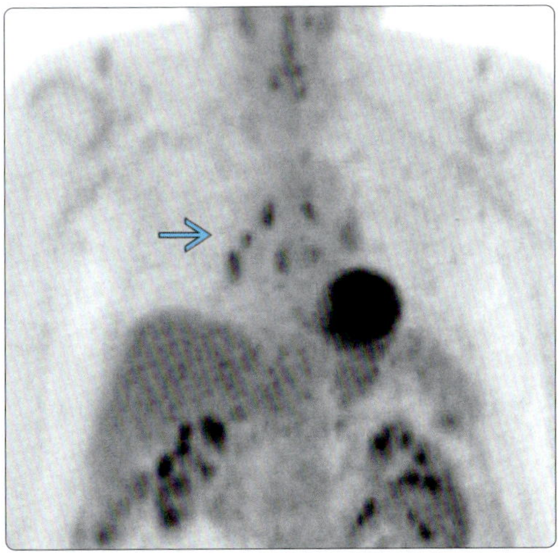

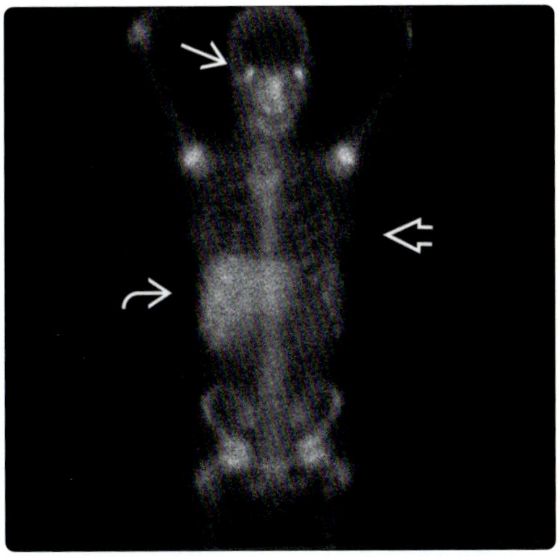

(Left) *Anterior F-18 FDG PET in a patient with sarcoidosis shows increased uptake in mediastinal and bihilar lymph nodes, consistent with active disease.* **(Right)** *Anterior Ga-67 scintigraphy in a patient with inactive sarcoidosis shows normal Ga-67 biodistribution, including lacrimal glands, bone, and liver.*

KEY FACTS

TERMINOLOGY

- Atypical pneumonias and opportunistic infections
  - Affect patients with HIV, cancer, or those on immunosuppressive therapy

IMAGING

- HRCT most often sufficient to diagnose atypical/opportunistic infection
- Ga-67 scintigraphy and F-18 FDG PET/CT sensitive for active cellular infiltration, but nonspecific
- Combined Tl-201 and Ga-67 imaging can help narrow DDx
- Pattern important for diagnosis of atypical/opportunistic infection

TOP DIFFERENTIAL DIAGNOSES

- Characteristic patterns on Ga-67 scintigraphy
  - (PJP): Intense diffuse pulmonary uptake
  - Tuberculosis (TB): Patchy/lobar pulmonary plus hilar nodal uptake
  - *Mycobacterium avium* complex: Patchy/lobar pulmonary plus hilar/extrahilar nodal uptake
  - Cytomegalovirus (CMV): Diffuse low-grade pulmonary uptake with perihilar prominence; concomitant eye, adrenal, or colonic uptake
  - Bacterial pneumonia: Lobar uptake
  - Kaposi sarcoma: No uptake
- Characteristic patterns on combined thallium/gallium imaging
  - PJP: Diffuse pulmonary thallium negative/gallium positive
  - Mycobacterial infection: Mediastinal thallium negative/gallium positive
  - Bacterial pneumonia: Focal pulmonary thallium negative/gallium positive
  - Kaposi sarcoma: Pulmonary and mediastinal thallium positive/gallium negative
  - Lymphoma: Pulmonary and mediastinal thallium positive/gallium positive

(Left) *Frontal chest radiograph in a 54-year-old man with HIV presenting with fever and shortness of breath demonstrates diffuse interstitial opacities and small bilateral effusions. The differential included infection and pulmonary edema.* **(Right)** *Anterior Ga-67 scintigram in the same patient demonstrates diffuse, intense uptake throughout both lungs ➡, consistent with infection/inflammation. This patient was found to have Pneumocystis jiroveci infection.*

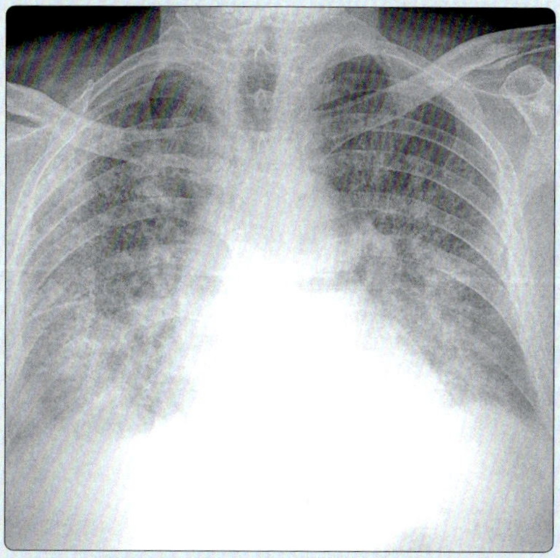

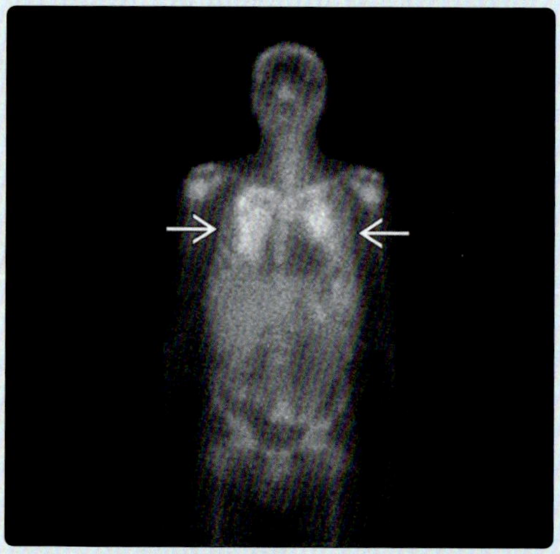

(Left) *Axial chest CT in a 75-year-old woman with a history of MAC infection and breast cancer demonstrates multiple nodular opacities ➡ in the left lung as well as scattered tree-in-bud nodularity.* **(Right)** *Axial PET in the same patient demonstrates hypermetabolic activity in the 2 more posterior left-sided opacities ➡, most consistent with active MAC infection. These improved following therapy for MAC. The more anterior nodule is only mildly hypermetabolic ➡, suggesting it is more chronic.*

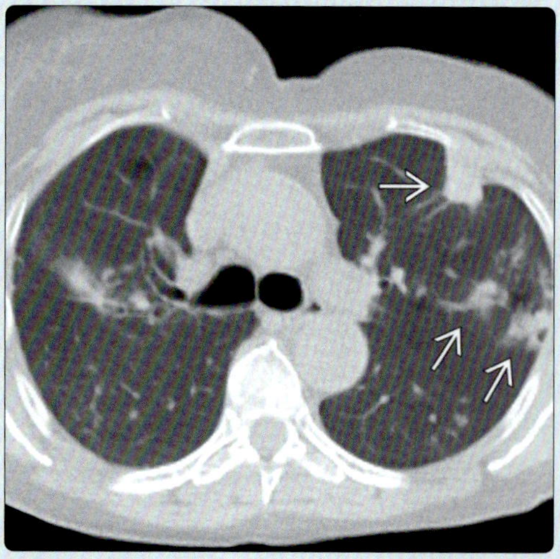

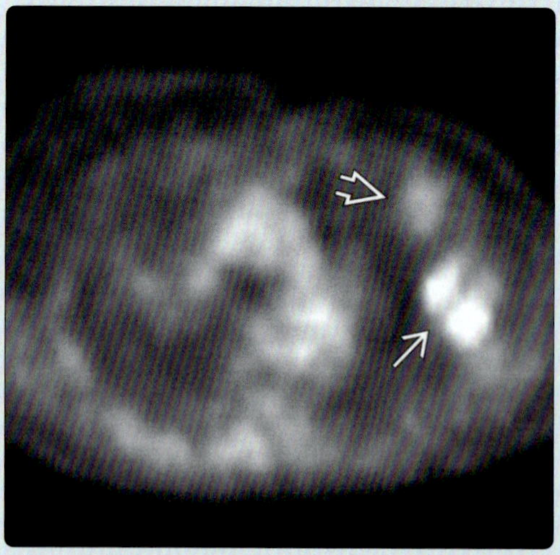

TERMINOLOGY

Definitions

- Atypical pneumonias and opportunistic infections
  - Affect patients with HIV, cancer, or those on immunosuppressive therapy (for collagen vascular disease, asthma, rheumatoid arthritis, inflammatory bowel disease, post transplant)

IMAGING

Nuclear Medicine Findings

- Ga-67 scintigraphy
  - *Pneumocystis jiroveci* pneumonia (PJP)
    - Early infection: Intense diffuse pulmonary uptake of Ga-67; no nodal uptake; may precede radiographic and physiologic abnormalities
    - Partial treatment with aerosolized pentamidine: May show uptake in only lower/upper lung zones
    - Prophylactic therapy: Very mild uptake, confined to upper lungs
    - Preterminal AIDS: Ga-67 uptake may be absent
    - Grading system
      - Grade 0 (normal): Uptake ≤ adjacent soft tissue; high negative predictive value with normal CXR
      - Grade 1: Uptake > soft tissue, but less than rib
      - Grade 2: Uptake > rib, but less than liver
      - Grade 3: Uptake = hepatic uptake, photopenic cardiac silhouette
      - Grade 4 (strongly positive): Uptake > liver
  - Tuberculosis (TB): Patchy/lobar pulmonary plus hilar nodal Ga-67 uptake
  - *Mycobacterium avium* complex (MAC): Patchy/lobar pulmonary plus hilar/extrahilar nodal Ga-67 uptake
  - Cytomegalovirus (CMV) pneumonia
    - Diffuse low-grade Ga-67 uptake with perihilar prominence; no nodal uptake
    - Look for eye (retinitis), adrenal (adrenalitis), renal, and persistent colonic (diarrhea) uptake
  - Kaposi sarcoma: No Ga-67 uptake
  - Bacterial pneumonia: Lobar Ga-67 uptake
  - Lymphoid interstitial pneumonia: Diffuse low-grade Ga-67 uptake; no nodal uptake
  - Lymphoma: Bulky nodal Ga-67 uptake, typically abdominal
- F-18 FDG PET/CT
  - Sensitive for infection, but cannot differentiate from malignancy
  - Increased F-18 FDG uptake implies active infection/inflammation
  - HIV viremia causes mildly F-18 FDG-avid lymphadenopathy
- Tl-201 and Ga-67 combined imaging
  - PJP: Thallium negative/gallium positive; diffuse pulmonary uptake
  - Mycobacterial infection: Thallium negative/gallium positive; mediastinal uptake
  - Bacterial pneumonia: Thallium negative/gallium positive; focal pulmonary uptake
  - Kaposi sarcoma: Thallium positive/gallium negative; pulmonary and mediastinal uptake
  - Lymphoma: Thallium positive/gallium positive; pulmonary and mediastinal uptake
  - No disease: Thallium negative/gallium negative

Imaging Recommendations

- Best imaging tool
  - HRCT may be sufficient in majority of cases to diagnose atypical/opportunistic infection
  - Ga-67 scintigraphy sensitive for active cellular infiltration, but is nonspecific
    - 1-3 day delay between injection and imaging
  - F-18 FDG PET/CT also sensitive for active infection/inflammation
    - Better resolution, higher target to background ratio, faster imaging time, lower radiation dose when compared to Ga-67 scintigraphy
  - Consider Tl-201 scan with immediate &/or 3 hour imaging followed by Ga-67 injection with imaging at 24-48 hours to help narrow differential
- Protocol advice
  - Ga-67 scintigraphy
    - Radiopharmaceutical: Ga-67 citrate
      - Physical t1/2: 78 hours
      - Principal photopeaks: 93 keV (40%), 184 keV (24%), 296 keV (22%), and 388 keV (7%)
      - Excretion: 10-25% by kidneys in first 24 hours, followed by gastrointestinal tract
    - Dose: 4-6 mCi (150-220 MBq) IV
    - Dosimetry
      - Effective dose equivalent: 0.44 rem/mCi
      - Lower large intestine receives largest dose
    - Image acquisition
      - Large field-of-view multipeak gamma camera with medium-energy parallel hole collimator
      - Anterior and posterior scintigrams obtained 24-72 hours after injection
      - 250k-1 mil total counts for chest
      - 1.5-2 mil total counts for whole body
  - F-18 FDG PET/CT
    - Standard oncologic protocol
  - Tl-201 scintigraphy
    - Radiopharmaceutical: Tl-201 chloride
      - Physical t1/2: 73 hours
      - Principal photopeaks: 68-80 keV (abundant), 170 keV (10%), 135 keV (3%)
      - Excreted slowly in both urine and feces
    - Dose: 3-5 mCi (111-185 MBq) IV
    - Dosimetry: Blood clearance primarily by myocardium, kidneys (largest dose), thyroid, liver, and stomach
    - Image acquisition: Scintigrams obtained 20-60 min after injection; delayed (3-hour) images in lymphoma and sarcoma

DIFFERENTIAL DIAGNOSIS

Pneumocystis jiroveci Pneumonia

- Ga-67 scintigraphy mostly used when chest radiograph, sputum/BAL sampling, and HRCT are nondiagnostic; this should not delay empiric therapy
- HRCT: Diffuse, bilateral ground-glass opacities

Tuberculosis

- F-18 FDG PET/CT useful in monitoring response to therapy
- Less pronounced apical predominance and cavitary disease in immunocompromised patients, with more frequent extrapulmonary disease

Non-Tuberculosis Mycobacteria

- Most commonly MAC
- HRCT
  - Non-HIV MAC infection: Upper lobe involvement ± cavitation in men; right middle lobe &/or lingular involvement in elderly women
  - HIV MAC infection: Multifocal bronchiectasis
  - Non MAC infection: Bilateral interstitial infiltrates

Cytomegalovirus Pneumonia

- Less intense pulmonary uptake than PJP
- Accompanying eye, adrenal, or colonic activity
- HRCT: Patchy or diffuse ground-glass opacities, small pulmonary nodules, and airspace consolidation
- CMV pneumonia more common in transplant recipients
- CMV retinitis more common in HIV-infected patients

Fungal Pneumonia

- Pulmonary aspergillosis
  - Cavitary upper lobe lesions most characteristic
  - Risk factors: Neutropenia, steroids, and CD4 count < 50
- Cryptococcosis
  - Diffuse interstitial infiltrates with pulmonary disease
  - Typically disseminated infection with meningitis
- Histoplasmosis, blastomycosis, coccidioidomycosis

Kaposi Sarcoma

- Negative gallium scan with abnormal chest radiograph &/or increased thallium activity highly suggestive
- Most common AIDS-defining tumor
- Multifocal and aggressive; affecting skin, nodes, GI tract, oral cavity, lung, liver, spleen
- Skin lesions diagnosed by biopsy

Bacterial Pneumonia

- Typical pneumonia, most common infection in HIV patients
  - Lobar Ga-67 uptake, infiltrate on chest radiograph
- Actinomycosis and nocardiosis
  - HRCT: Pulmonary consolidation with cavitation &/or mediastinal adenopathy
  - Hematogenous spread to CNS and subcutaneous tissues, leading to abscess formation
  - Increased skeletal uptake with extension to bone

Toxoplasmosis

- Parasitic infection most commonly causing encephalitis
  - Nonspecific diffuse interstitial or reticulonodular infiltrates
  - CNS lesions: Decreased F-18 FDG uptake relative to CNS lymphoma

Lymphoma

- Non-Hodgkin lymphoma: 2nd most common AIDS-related malignancy; usually high grade, aggressive, and widely disseminated
- Bulky lymphadenopathy with intense F-18 FDG uptake, also affecting liver and spleen
- Intense F-18 FDG uptake helps to differentiate primary CNS lymphoma from cerebral toxoplasmosis
- F-18 FDG PET/CT useful in monitoring treatment response

Lymphoid Interstitial Pneumonia

- Diffuse low-grade pulmonary gallium uptake
- Parotid uptake helps to differentiate from PJP, although this is also seen with sarcoidosis

Esophageal Candidiasis

- Nonspecific, diffusely increased esophageal F-18 FDG uptake
- Can usually be diagnosed with endoscopy, upper GI series

CLINICAL ISSUES

Natural History & Prognosis

- Antiretroviral therapy has led to longer lives, meaning more patients will eventually have opportunistic infections

DIAGNOSTIC CHECKLIST

Consider

- Nuclear medicine imaging mostly used when chest radiograph, sputum/BAL sampling, and HRCT are nondiagnostic
- Nuclear medicine imaging may be useful to evaluate response to therapy

SELECTED REFERENCES

1. Zanoni BC et al: Update on opportunistic infections in the era of effective antiretroviral therapy. Infect Dis Clin North Am. 28(3):501-518, 2014
2. Pupaibool J et al: Other HIV-associated pneumonias. Clin Chest Med. 34(2):243-54, 2013
3. Sathekge M et al: FDG-PET imaging in HIV infection and tuberculosis. Semin Nucl Med. 43(5):349-66, 2013
4. Sathekge M et al: Nuclear medicine imaging in tuberculosis using commercially available radiopharmaceuticals. Nucl Med Commun. 33(6):581-90, 2012
5. Liu Y: Demonstrations of AIDS-associated malignancies and infections at FDG PET-CT. Ann Nucl Med. 25(8):536-46, 2011
6. Nakazato T et al: Pneumocystis jiroveci pneumonia detected by FDG-PET. Ann Hematol. 89(8):839-40, 2010
7. Palestro J et al. Society of Nuclear Medicine Procedure Guideline for Gallium Scintigraphy in Inflammation. http://snmmi.files.cms-plus.com/docs/Gallium_Scintigraphy_in_Inflammation_v3.pdf. Created June 2, 2004. Accessed July 31, 2015
8. Raoof S et al: Imaging of unusual diffuse lung diseases. Curr Opin Pulm Med. 10(5):383-9, 2004
9. Schuster DM et al: Gallium and other agents in diseases of the lung. Semin Nucl Med. 32(3):193-211, 2002
10. Turoglu HT et al: Tumor and infection localization in AIDS patients: Ga-67 and Tl-201 findings. Clin Nucl Med. 23(7):446-59, 1998
11. Thallous chloride Tl 201 Injection. http://www.nuclearonline.org/PI/Nycomed%20Tl-201%20Tl%20Chloride.pdf. Arlington Heights, IL: Amersham, 1995
12. Vanarthos WJ et al: Diagnostic uses of nuclear medicine in AIDS. Radiographics. 12(4):731-49; discussion 749-52, 1992
13. Reiss TF et al: Abnormal lung gallium-67 uptake preceding pulmonary physiologic impairment in an asymptomatic patient with Pneumocystis carinii pneumonia. Chest. 97(5):1261-3, 1990
14. Kramer EL et al: Gallium-67 scans of the chest in patients with acquired immunodeficiency syndrome. J Nucl Med. 28(7):1107-14, 1987
15. Barron TF et al: Pneumocystis carinii pneumonia studied by gallium-67 scanning. Radiology. 154(3):791-3, 1985

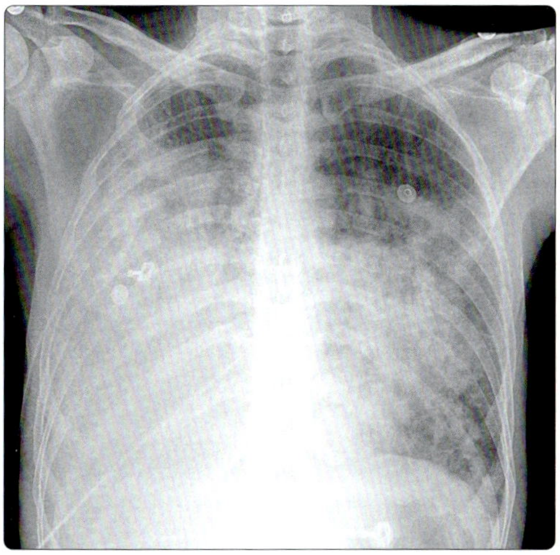

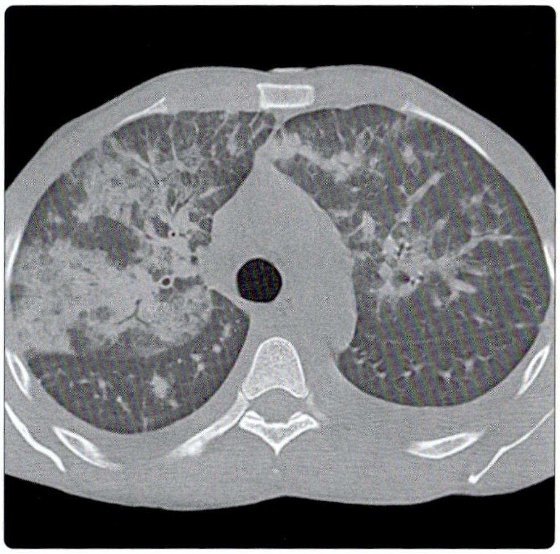

(Left) *Frontal chest radiograph in a 39-year-old man with AIDS demonstrates extensive airspace consolidation in the right lung and more patchy airspace opacities in the left lung.* **(Right)** *Axial chest CT in the same patient demonstrates extensive interstitial and airspace opacities bilaterally in a peribronchovascular distribution, most pronounced in the right upper lobe.*

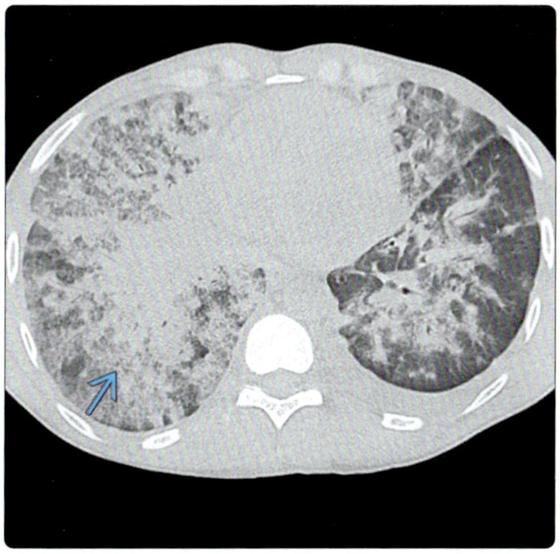

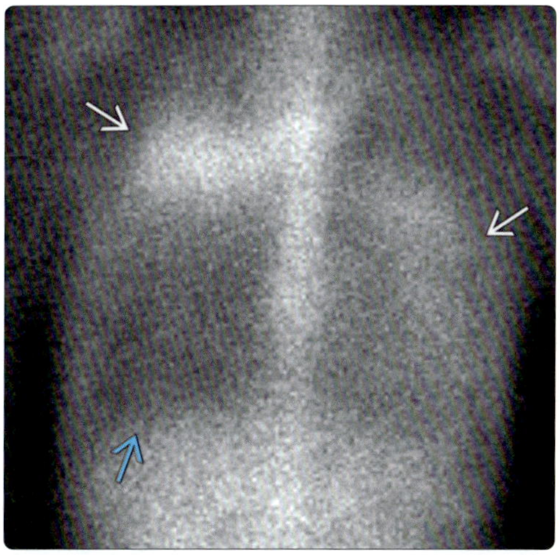

(Left) *Axial chest CT at a lower level in the same patient demonstrates more pronounced consolidation in the right lung base* ⇨*. The CT was consistent with extensive pneumonia, likely due to PJP &/or other infectious etiologies.* **(Right)** *Subsequent anterior Ga-67 scintigraphy demonstrates patchy uptake in the right upper and left lungs* ➡*, consistent with active infection. There is a relative paucity of uptake in the area of extensive consolidation in the right lower lung* ⇨*, secondary to superimposed Kaposi sarcoma.*

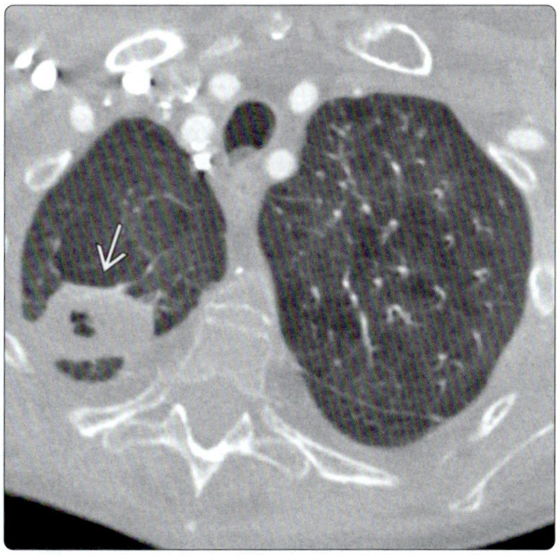

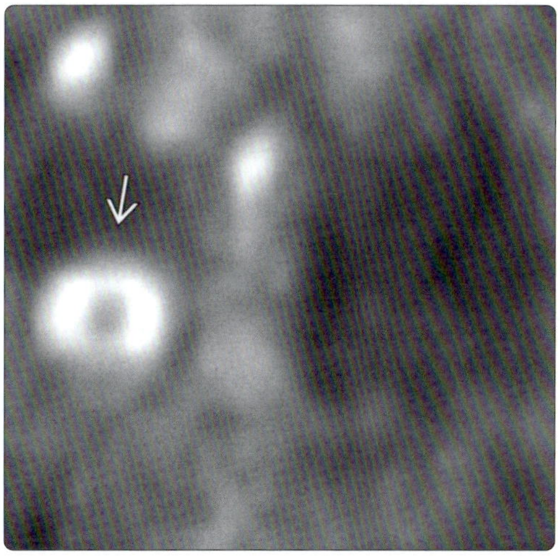

(Left) *Axial chest CT in a 77-year-old woman with emphysema demonstrates a thick-walled cavitary lesion in the right upper lung* ➡*, which was concerning for malignancy.* **(Right)** *Axial F-18 FDG PET demonstrates hypermetabolic activity associated with the cavity* ➡*. Although infection was within the differential, malignancy remained the primary concern. Fine-needle aspiration was negative for malignancy, but did show evidence of fungal infection (Aspergillus).*

Granulomatous Disease

KEY FACTS

IMAGING

- Increased Ga-67 and F-18 FDG uptake indicates active disease
- Uptake inversely proportional to degree of fibrosis
- F-18 FDG PET/CT cannot differentiate granulomatous disease from malignancy
- Ga-67 and F-18 FDG PET/CT signs suggestive of sarcoidosis
  - Lambda sign
    - Result of bilateral hilar and right paratracheal activity
    - Highly suggestive
  - Panda sign
    - Result of lacrimal and parotid gland activity
- HRCT helpful in differentiating granulomatous diseases

TOP DIFFERENTIAL DIAGNOSES

- Sarcoidosis
  - Increased bilateral hilar and right paratracheal activity
  - Radiographic stages from 0 (normal) to 4 (pulmonary fibrosis)
  - HRCT: Upper lobe predominant perilymphatic micronodularity, which may progress to pulmonary fibrosis
- Mycobacterial infection
  - Pulmonary tuberculosis (TB)
    - Primary TB is lower lobe predominant
    - Post primary TB has upper lung predilection
    - F-18 FDG PET/CT useful in evaluating treatment response
  - Nontuberculosis mycobacterial pulmonary disease
- Hypersensitivity pneumonitis
- Langerhans cell histiocytosis
- Chronic granulomatous disease: Recurrent bacterial and fungal infections
- ANCA-associated vasculitis
  - Granulomatosis with polyangiitis: Involves upper airways, lower respiratory tract, and kidneys
  - Churg-Strauss syndrome: Asthma, hypereosinophilia, and necrotizing vasculitis

(Left) *Coronal Ga-67 scintigraphy in a 35-year-old man with sarcoidosis demonstrates increased bilateral hilar and less pronounced right paratracheal activity.* **(Right)** *A frontal chest radiograph in the same patient was read as normal (stage 0).*

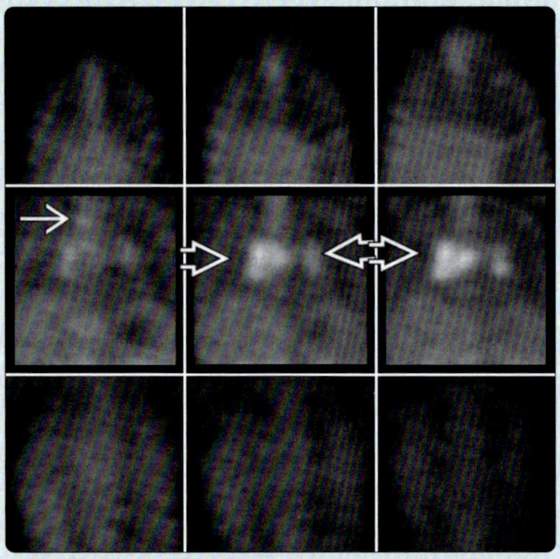

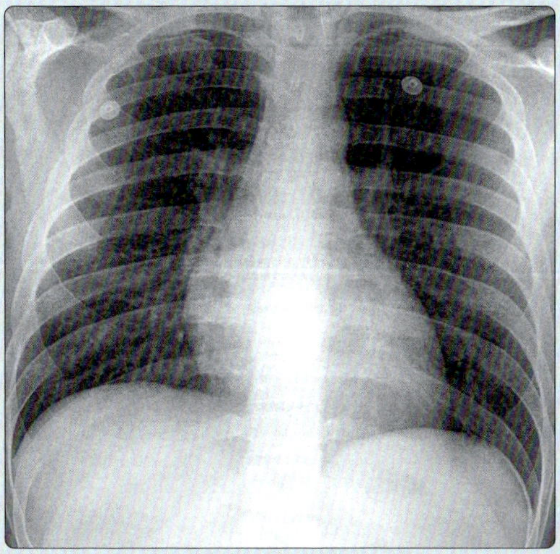

(Left) *Anterior F-18 FDG PET in a patient with pancreatic adenocarcinoma shows malignant abdominal adenopathy. There is also F-18 FDG uptake in the bilateral parotid glands (panda sign) and mild uptake in hilar adenopathy in this patient with sarcoidosis.* **(Right)** *Axial CT in the same patient demonstrates partially calcified hilar adenopathy, consistent with sarcoidosis.*

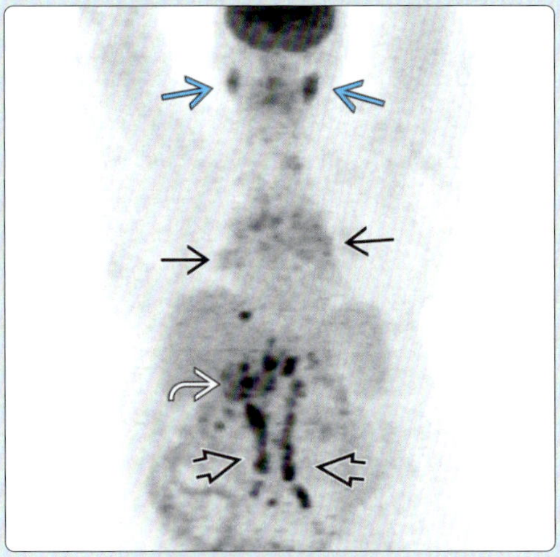

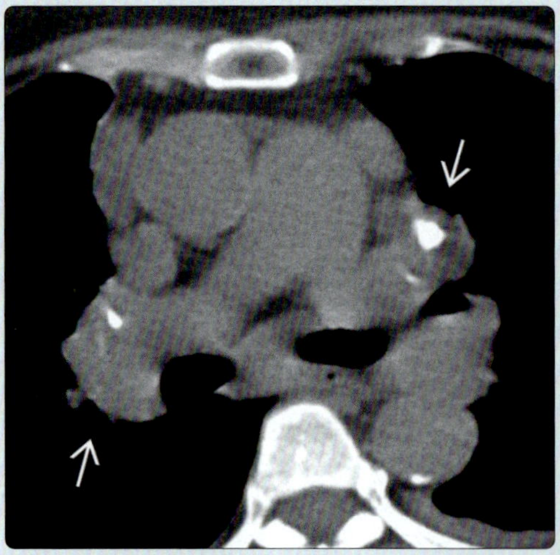

TERMINOLOGY

Definitions

- Disease characterized by formation of granulomas, either infectious or noninfectious
  - Sarcoidosis, mycobacterial infections, hypersensitivity pneumonitis, Langerhans cell histiocytosis, granulomatosis with polyangiitis, chronic granulomatous disease

IMAGING

General Features

- Best diagnostic clue
  - Increased Ga-67 and F-18 FDG uptake indicates active disease
    - Lambda sign: Increased bilateral hilar and right paratracheal activity in sarcoidosis
    - Panda sign: Increased lacrimal and parotid gland activity in sarcoidosis

Nuclear Medicine Findings

- Ga-67 scintigraphy
  - Uptake proportional to degree of inflammation
  - Uptake inversely proportional to degree of fibrosis
- F-18 FDG PET/CT
  - Similar distribution as Ga-67, may be more sensitive
  - Accurate assessment of disease activity
  - Cannot distinguish from malignancy

Radiographic Findings

- Sarcoidosis has radiographic stages
  - Stage 0: Normal
  - Stage 1: Lymphadenopathy, typically bilateral and symmetric
  - Stage 2: Lymphadenopathy and parenchymal lung disease
  - Stage 3: Parenchymal lung disease only
  - Stage 4: Pulmonary fibrosis

Imaging Recommendations

- Best imaging tool
  - Radiography or HRCT often sufficient for diagnosis and follow-up
  - Ga-67 is useful for initial diagnosis of sarcoidosis
  - Ga-67 and F-18 FDG PET/CT can differentiate active and inactive disease
- Protocol advice
  - Gallium-67 scintigraphy
    - Radiopharmaceutical: Gallium-67 citrate
      - Physical t1/2 of 78 hours
      - Principal photopeaks: 93 keV (40%), 184 keV (24%), 296 keV (22%), and 388 keV (7%)
      - Excretion: 10-25% excreted by kidneys in 1st 24 hours, then principally excreted by gastrointestinal tract
    - Dose
      - Adults: 4-6 mCi (150-220 MBq)
      - Children: 0.04-0.07 mCi/kg (1.5-2.6 MBq/kg); minimum dose of 0.25-0.5 mCi
    - Dosimetry (effective dose equivalent)
      - Adults: 0.44 rem/mCi
      - Children: 1.5 rem/mCi
      - Lower colon receives largest dose
    - Image acquisition
      - Large FOV multipeak gamma camera with a medium-energy parallel hole collimator
      - Anterior and posterior scintigrams obtained 24-72 hours after injection
      - 250,000 to 1 million total counts (5-20 min) for chest scintigraphy
      - 1.5-2 million total counts (25-35 min) for whole-body scintigraphy
  - F-18 FDG PET/CT
    - Standard oncologic protocol

CT Findings

- Typical sarcoid features and anatomic distribution
  - Bilateral hilar and right paratracheal lymph node enlargement
  - Upper lobe predominant perilymphatic micronodularity
- Findings of reversible parenchymal inflammation
  - Nodularity, airspace consolidation, ground-glass opacities
- Findings of irreversible pulmonary fibrosis
  - Honeycombing, architectural distortion, traction bronchiectasis, upper lobe volume loss, and hilar retraction
- Broader differential in patients with unilateral disease, cavitary lung lesions, &/or pleural fluid

DIFFERENTIAL DIAGNOSIS

Sarcoidosis

- Symmetric hilar and right paratracheal activity
- Upper lobe predilection for pulmonary disease
- Lambda sign on Ga-67 or F-18 FDG PET/CT results from symmetric hilar and right paratracheal activity; highly suggestive of sarcoidosis
- Panda sign on Ga-67 or F-18 FDG PET/CT results from symmetric lacrimal and parotid gland activity; supportive of diagnosis, especially in combination with lambda sign &/or characteristic radiographic/HRCT findings

Mycobacterial Infection

- Pulmonary tuberculosis
  - Primary: F-18 FGD-avid middle and lower lobe predominant parenchymal disease, pleural effusions, lymphadenopathy, &/or miliary disease
  - Post primary: Patchy consolidation involving apical and posterior segments of upper lobes and superior segments of lower lobes ± cavitation
  - F-18 FDG PET/CT can evaluate treatment response
- Nontuberculosis mycobacterial pulmonary disease
  - Radiography: Infiltrates, multiple nodules, &/or cavitation
  - HRCT: Multiple small nodules or multifocal bronchiectasis

Hypersensitivity Pneumonitis

- Acute or insidious onset without fibrosis: Diffuse &/or centrilobular ground-glass opacities, air-trapping, &/or head cheese sign

- Insidious onset with fibrosis: Reticulation with relative sparing of extreme apices and bases, traction bronchiectasis, and honeycombing

Langerhans Cell Histiocytosis

- Radiography: Ill-defined nodules and reticular opacities with mid to upper lung predominance; may present with pneumothorax
- HRCT: Centrilobular micronodularity progressing to confluent cystic changes and honeycombing

Chronic Granulomatous Disease

- Recurrent bacterial and fungal infections
- Radiography: Consolidation, reticulonodular opacities, and scarring
- HRCT: Nonspecific pulmonary findings; can form mycetomas; infection may spread to pleura or chest wall, potentially leading to osteomyelitis

ANCA-Associated Vasculitis

- Granulomatosis with polyangiitis (formerly Wegener granulomatosis)
  - Involves upper and lower respiratory tract and kidneys
  - HRCT: Nodules and cavitating masses, consolidation, and bronchial wall thickening
- Churg-Strauss syndrome
  - Asthma, hypereosinophilia, and necrotizing vasculitis
  - HRCT: Patchy consolidation

Fungal Infection

- Coccidioidomycosis, histoplasmosis, blastomycosis, aspergillosis, cryptococcosis, sporotrichosis
- Lymphadenopathy more likely asymmetric

Bacterial Infection

- Brucellosis, granuloma inguinale, melioidosis, cat-scratch disease, Whipple disease

Protozoa and Trematodes

- Leishmaniasis, toxoplasmosis, schistosomiasis

Nongranulomatous Disease

- Silicosis and coal worker's pneumoconiosis
- Metastatic malignancy, lung cancer
- Lymphoma

PATHOLOGY

Microscopic Features

- Sarcoidosis: Noncaseating, perilymphatic granulomas surrounded by lymphocytes, plasma cells, and fibroblasts
- Infectious granulomas may be necrotic; caseating granulomas in tuberculosis

CLINICAL ISSUES

Presentation

- Most common signs/symptoms
  - Sarcoidosis may present with respiratory symptoms, fatigue, weight loss; as many as 50% are asymptomatic
  - Increased ACE level, hypercalcemia, restrictive ventilatory defect

Demographics

- Age
  - Peak incidence of sarcoidosis in 3rd decade of life
- Gender
  - Slightly higher incidence in females
- Ethnicity
  - Most prevalent in African Americans, Swedes, and Danes
  - More likely attributable to tuberculosis, leprosy, and fungal infections in less developed countries and immunocompromised patients

Natural History & Prognosis

- Most patients stable or in remission at 10 years
- ~ 20% develop chronic lung disease and pulmonary fibrosis
- < 5% die from disease, usually from respiratory failure or cardiac/neurologic involvement
- Poor prognostic factors: Stage 2-3 at diagnosis, onset after age 40, black race, hypercalcemia
- Favorable prognostic factors: Fever, polyarthritis, erythema nodosum, bilateral hilar lymphadenopathy

Treatment

- Systemic &/or inhaled corticosteroids, cytotoxic drugs, &/or anti-TNF agents
- Infectious etiologies treated with specific antimicrobials

DIAGNOSTIC CHECKLIST

Image Interpretation Pearls

- Degree of uptake on Ga-67 or F-18 FDG PET/CT is proportional to disease activity
- Lambda &/or panda signs are highly suggestive of sarcoidosis

SELECTED REFERENCES

1. Skoura E et al: Imaging in tuberculosis. Int J Infect Dis. 32:87-93, 2015
2. Society of Nuclear Medicine. Procedure Guideline for Gallium Scintigraphy in Inflammation, Version 3.0. http://snmmi.files.cms-plus.com/docs/Gallium_Scintigraphy_in_Inflammation_v3.pdf. Approved June 2, 2004. Accessed August 3, 2015
3. Baughman RP et al: Medical therapy of sarcoidosis. Semin Respir Crit Care Med. 35(3):391-406, 2014
4. Castañer E et al: Imaging findings in pulmonary vasculitis. Semin Ultrasound CT MR. 33(6):567-79, 2012
5. Mukhopadhyay S et al: Causes of pulmonary granulomas: a retrospective study of 500 cases from seven countries. J Clin Pathol. 65(1):51-7, 2012
6. Oksüz MO et al: 18F-FDG PET/CT for the diagnosis of sarcoidosis in a patient with bilateral inflammatory involvement of the parotid and lacrimal glands (panda sign) and bilateral hilar and mediastinal lymphadenopathy (lambda sign). Eur J Nucl Med Mol Imaging. 38(3):603, 2011
7. Criado E et al: Pulmonary sarcoidosis: typical and atypical manifestations at high-resolution CT with pathologic correlation. Radiographics. 30(6):1567-86, 2010
8. Towbin AJ et al: Chronic granulomatous disease. Pediatr Radiol. 40(5):657-68; quiz 792-3, 2010
9. Basu S et al: Functional imaging of inflammatory diseases using nuclear medicine techniques. Semin Nucl Med. 39(2):124-45, 2009
10. Hirschmann JV et al: Hypersensitivity pneumonitis: a historical, clinical, and radiologic review. Radiographics. 29(7):1921-38, 2009
11. Sundar KM et al: Pulmonary Langerhans cell histiocytosis: emerging concepts in pathobiology, radiology, and clinical evolution of disease. Chest. 123(5):1673-83, 2003
12. Koh WJ et al: Nontuberculous mycobacterial pulmonary diseases in immunocompetent patients. Korean J Radiol. 3(3):145-57, 2002
13. Sy WM et al: The evolutional stage changes in sarcoidosis on gallium-67 scintigraphy. Ann Nucl Med. 12(2):77-82, 1998
14. Sulavik SB et al: Specificity and sensitivity of distinctive chest radiographic and/or 67Ga images in the noninvasive diagnosis of sarcoidosis. Chest. 103(2):403-9, 1993

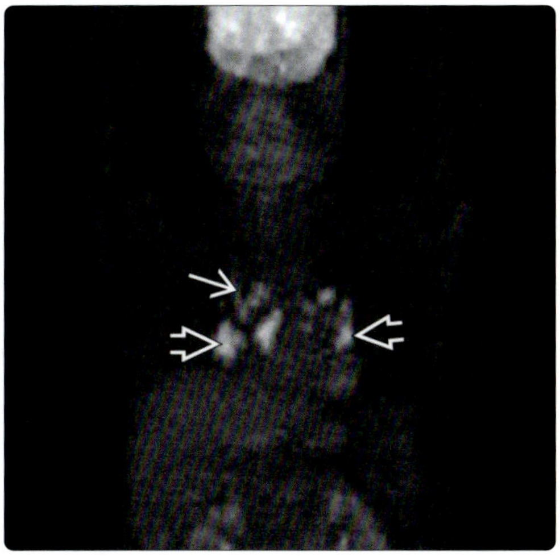

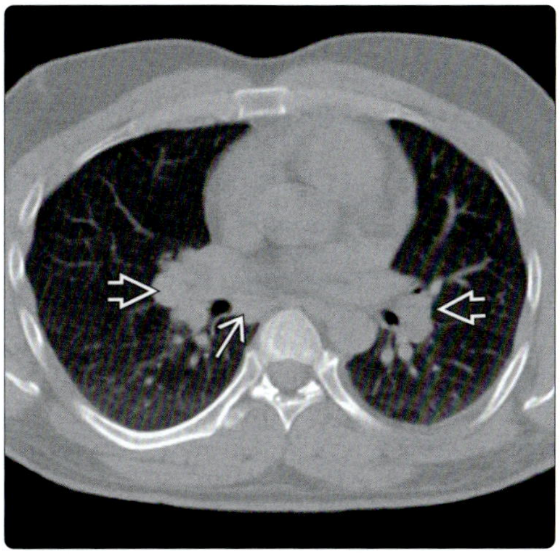

(Left) *Anterior F-18 FDG PET in a 42-year-old man with sarcoidosis shows active disease in hilar ➡ and mediastinal lymph nodes, including the right paratracheal ➡ region.* **(Right)** *Axial CT of the same patient demonstrates bilateral hilar ➡ and subcarinal ➡ lymph node enlargement.*

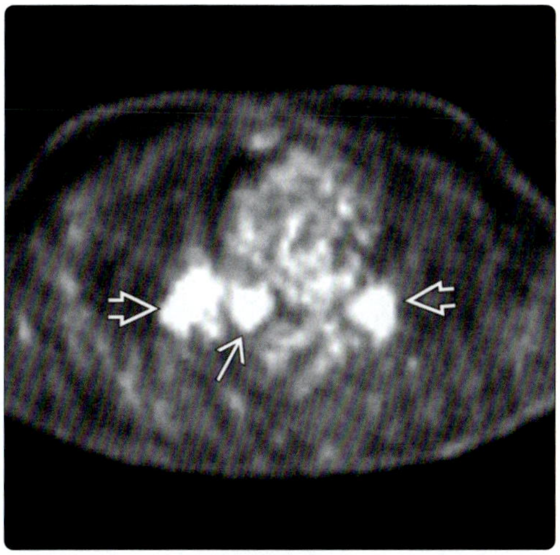

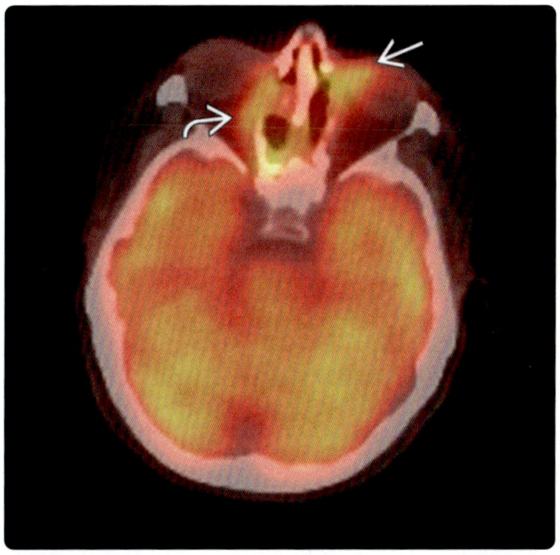

(Left) *Axial F-18 FDG PET shows increased uptake in the enlarged hilar ➡ and subcarinal ➡ lymph nodes, consistent with active sarcoidosis.* **(Right)** *Axial fused F-18 FDG PET/CT in a patient with granulomatosis with polyangiitis shows hypermetabolic soft tissue in the nasal cavity with bony destruction ➡. There is also hypermetabolic soft tissue in the medial left orbit ➡ due to associated nasolacrimal duct obstruction.*

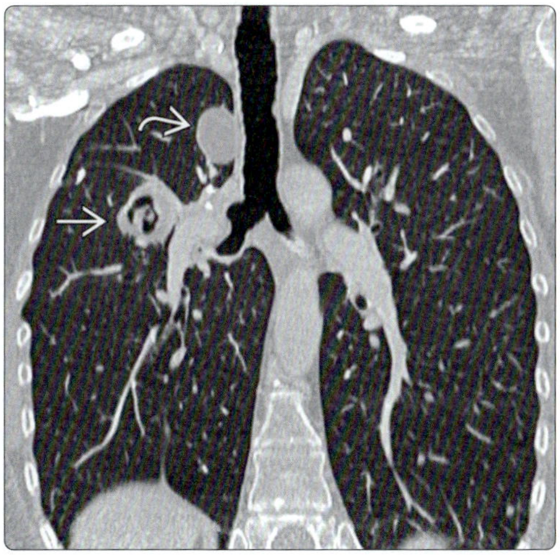

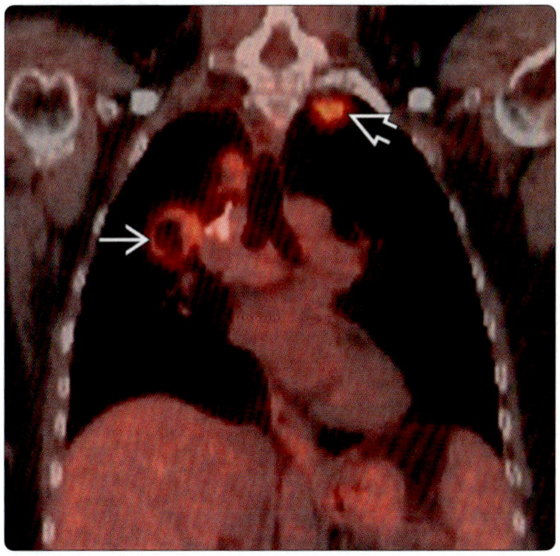

(Left) *Coronal CT in a 51-year-old patient with a history of granulomatosis with polyangiitis demonstrates enlarging pulmonary nodules ➡ bilaterally, one of which is cavitary ➡.* **(Right)** *Coronal fused F-18 FDG PET/CT in the same patient demonstrates uptake within the bilateral cavitary ➡ and noncavitary ➡ nodules. Following immunosuppressive therapy, these nodules resolved.*

Pulmonary Embolism

KEY FACTS

IMAGING

- Pulmonary embolism (PE)
  - Segmental or subsegmental lung perfusion defects with normal ventilation on ventilation/perfusion (V/Q) scan are highly specific for PE
    - Lower lobes >> upper lobes
    - Bilateral in majority of cases
    - Pleural-based, wedge-shaped with apex of wedge directed toward pulmonary hilum
  - Defect size
    - Large: > 75% of segment
    - Moderate: 26-74% of segment
    - Small: < 25% of segment
  - CXR should be used as adjunct to interpretation of V/Q scan, useful to exclude clinical mimics of PE
  - V/Q scan is 95% sensitive for emboli that completely occlude pulmonary arterioles > 2 mm
- Airway disease (obstruction, mucous plugging, pneumonia)
  - Ventilation larger than perfusion abnormality
- Parenchymal lung disease (tumor, infection, COPD, asthma)
  - Ventilation = perfusion abnormality (matched defect)

DIAGNOSTIC CHECKLIST

- Normal V/Q scan
  - Excludes clinically significant PE
- Low-probability V/Q and low clinical likelihood
  - Does not require further study or treatment
- Low-probability V/Q scan with intermediate/high clinical likelihood
  - Further evaluation with lower extremity venous Dopplers, CTA
- High-probability V/Q with low clinical likelihood
  - Requires further study (CTA)
- High-probability V/Q with high clinical likelihood
  - Requires treatment; no further test necessary

(Left) *Normal Tc-99m MAA lung perfusion scan shows anterior, posterior, right lateral, and left lateral views. This photopenic* ➡ *defect is caused by the heart.* **(Right)** *Normal Tc-99m MAA lung perfusion scan shows right anterior oblique, left anterior oblique, right posterior oblique, and left posterior oblique views. This photopenic* ➡ *defect is caused by the heart.*

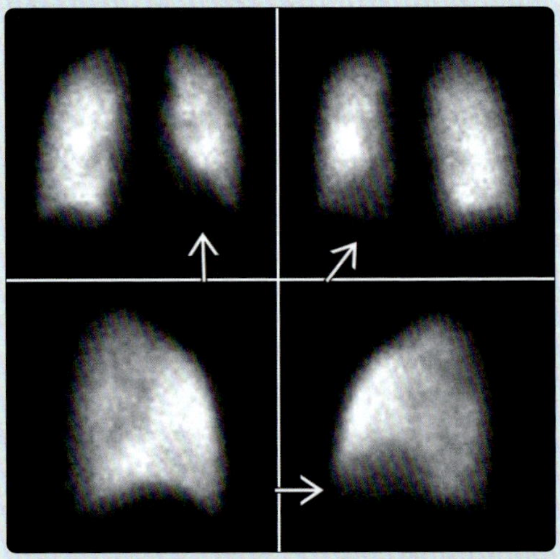

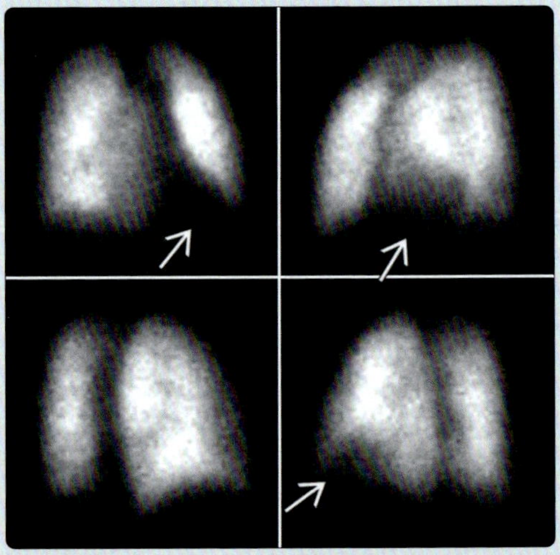

(Left) *Graphic shows the pulmonary segments in the anterior, posterior, right lateral, and left lateral views.* **(Right)** *Normal lung ventilation scan shows right posterior oblique* ➡ *and left posterior oblique* ➡ *views with corresponding normal washout.*

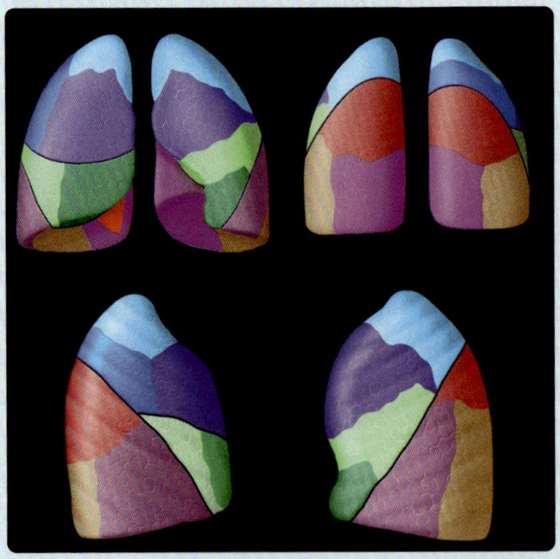

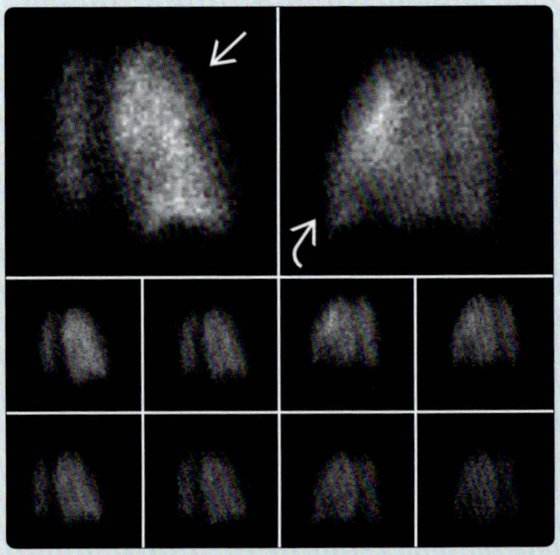

IMAGING

General Features

- Best diagnostic clue
  - Pulmonary embolism (PE) on ventilation/perfusion (V/Q) scan
    - Peripheral, wedge-shaped segmental or subsegmental lung perfusion defects with normal ventilation
  - Overall, V/Q scan has 85% sensitivity, 93% specificity for PE
  - False-negatives
    - Partially occluded vessel
    - Low clot burden
    - Subacute clot (retracted)
- Location
  - Lower lobes >> upper lobes
  - Bilateral in majority of cases
- Size
  - Defect size on V/Q scan
    - Large: > 75% of segment
    - Moderate: 26-74% of segment
    - Small: < 25% of segment
  - Embolus size
    - V/Q scan is 95% sensitive for emboli that completely occlude pulmonary arterioles > 2 mm
- Morphology
  - Wedge-shaped with apex of wedge directed toward pulmonary hilum
  - Pleural-based, includes fissures

CT Findings

- CTA
  - Direct visualization of thromboembolism in pulmonary arteries
    - Partial or complete intraluminal filling defect(s) in pulmonary arteries
    - Abrupt pulmonary artery vessel cutoff
  - Technical/clinical Issues
    - CTA is most common first-line PE exam in clinical practice today
      - 83% sensitivity, 96% specificity for PE
      - Negative predictive value ~ 100%
      - May provide etiology of alternate diagnosis if PE excluded
      - Higher interobserver agreement than V/Q
    - Technically inadequate studies occur in 2-4% of patients

Nuclear Medicine Findings

- V/Q scan
  - Perfusion (Q) defect
    - Highly sensitive alone for PE when in segmental distribution
    - Parenchymal lung disease can also cause decreased perfusion, reducing specificity for PE
  - Ventilation (V) defect
    - V > Q abnormality
      - Airway disease (obstruction, mucous plugging, pneumonia)
    - V = Q abnormality (matched)
      - Parenchymal lung disease (tumor, infection, COPD, asthma)
  - V/Q mismatch
    - Perfusion abnormality with normal ventilation and clear radiograph in that region is specific for PE
  - Interpretive criteria
    - PIOPED study (1990)
      - Established sensitivity/specificity of V/Q scan for PE by prospectively comparing V/Q scan to pulmonary angiography
    - Original PIOPED criteria
      - Categorizations: High, intermediate, low, very low probability, and indeterminate
      - Complex to apply and resulted in many indeterminate studies
    - Modified PIOPED II criteria (2008)
      - Derived from analysis of PIOPED II data (2006) and modified by reanalysis of data
      - Reduced number of indeterminate studies
    - PISAPED criteria (1996) and perfusion-only modified PIOPED II criteria (2008)
      - Accurately diagnose PE without ventilation

Radiographic Findings

- CXR should be used as adjunct to interpretation of V/Q scan, useful to exclude clinical mimics of PE
- Most patients with acute PE have radiographically normal chest
- Atelectasis or opacity in affected segment is most common positive finding in patients ± PE

Imaging Recommendations

- Protocol advice
  - Patient preparation
    - Obtain CXR in posteroanterior and lateral projections (preferred) or portable anteroposterior CXR (acceptable); CXR within a few days may be adequate in patients with no changes in signs or symptoms
    - Chest CT can substitute for CXR
  - Radiopharmaceuticals
    - Doses of radiopharmaceuticals vary depending on perfusion-first or ventilation-first protocol
    - Ventilation imaging
      - 5-20 mCi (185-740 MBq) Xe-133; 0.3 mCi/kg (10-12 MBq/kg) for pediatric patients
      - Aerosols: 25-35 mCi (925-1,300 MBq) Tc-99m diethylenetriaminepentaacetic acid or Tc-99m sulfur colloid
    - Perfusion imaging
      - 1-4 mCi (37-148 MBq) Tc-99m macroaggregated albumin
  - Image acquisition
    - Low-energy all-purpose parallel hole collimator
    - Perfusion images
      - 8 views of lungs (anterior, posterior, right and left lateral, left anterior oblique, right anterior oblique, left posterior oblique, right posterior oblique)
      - 100k counts each
    - Ventilation images

Diagnostic Criteria for Pulmonary Embolism

Modified PIOPED II Criteria	Perfusion-Only Modified PIOPED II Criteria	Perfusion-Only PISAPED Criteria
PE Present/High Probability	**PE Present**	**PE Present**
≥ 2 large mismatched V/Q segmental defects*	≥ 2 large mismatched Q/CXR segmental defects*	≥ 1 wedge-shaped Q defect(s)
Nondiagnostic	**Nondiagnostic**	**Nondiagnostic**
All other findings	All other findings	Cannot classify as PE present or PE absent
Very Low Probability	**PE Absent**	**PE Absent**
Nonsegmental defect(s)	Nonsegmental defect(s)	Normal or near-normal Q scan
Up to 3 small segmental defects*	Up to 3 small segmental defects *	Non-wedge-shaped Q defect(s)
Solitary matched V/Q defect with corresponding CXR lesion in mid or upper lung occupying no more than 1 segment	Solitary Q defect with corresponding CXR match in mid or upper lung occupying no more than 1 segment	Contour defect caused by enlarged heart, mediastinum, or diaphragm
Q defect smaller than corresponding CXR lesion	Q defect smaller than corresponding CXR lesion	
Stripe sign (linear perfused region between nonperfused region and pleural surface)	Stripe sign (linear perfused region between nonperfused region and pleural surface)	
Solitary large pleural effusion (≥ 1/3 of lung field)	Solitary large pleural effusion (≥ 1/3 of lung field)	
2 or more matched V/Q defects without corresponding CXR lesions	No Q defect(s)	
Normal		
No Q defect(s)		

**Or arithmetic equivalent. V/Q = ventilation/perfusion scan.*

Adapted with permission from Parker JA et al: SNM practice guideline for lung scintigraphy 4.0. J Nucl Med Technol. 40(1):57-65, 2012

- ▫ If using Xe-133, left posterior oblique and right posterior oblique projections, or posterior projection only
- ▫ If using aerosol, 8 views of lungs to match perfusion images
- – Perfusion-first protocol
  - ▫ May omit ventilation if perfusion study is normal or matches CXR findings
- – Ventilation-first protocol
  - ▫ Perfusion imaging contributes background activity to ventilation image; thus it is common to perform ventilation before perfusion imaging

DIFFERENTIAL DIAGNOSIS

Chronic or Unresolved PE

- Often indistinguishable from acute PE without prior scan
- Other patterns include heterogeneous perfusion
- CT: Vascular pruning, mosaic attenuation

Nonthromboembolic Intraluminal Occlusions

- Tumor
- Foreign body
- Septic emboli

Pulmonary Vascular Abnormalities

- Unilateral decrease/absent perfusion in pulmonary artery
  - Extrinsic compression: Tumor, adenopathy
  - Intrinsic vascular obliteration: Vasculitis, pulmonary artery tumor
- Congenital
  - Pulmonary artery agenesis, hypoplasia

CLINICAL ISSUES

Treatment

- Anticoagulation with heparin, warfarin: Prevents further thromboembolism
- Thrombolytic therapy: Decreases clot burden in lungs
- Venous filters: When thromboembolism occurs despite medical management or if contraindication to anticoagulation

DIAGNOSTIC CHECKLIST

Image Interpretation Pearls

- Normal V/Q scan
  - Excludes clinically significant PE
- Low-probability V/Q and low clinical likelihood
  - Does not require further study or treatment
- Low-probability V/Q scan with intermediate/high clinical likelihood
  - Further evaluation with lower extremity venous Dopplers, CTA
- High-probability V/Q with low clinical likelihood
  - Requires further study (CTA)
- High-probability V/Q with high clinical likelihood
  - Requires treatment; no further test necessary

SELECTED REFERENCES

1. Parker JA et al: SNM practice guideline for lung scintigraphy 4.0. J Nucl Med Technol. 40(1):57-65, 2012

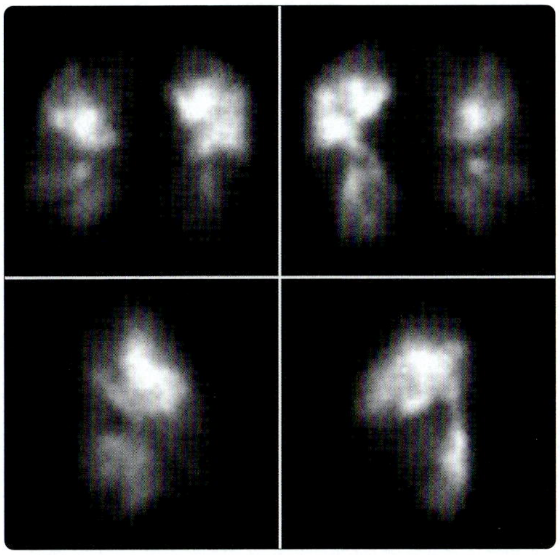

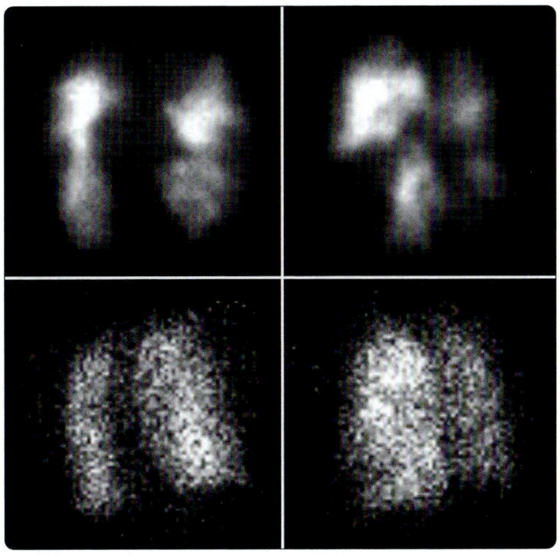

(Left) *Anterior, posterior, right lateral, and left lateral Tc-99m MAA lung perfusion images show multiple large segmental perfusion defects.* **(Right)** *Left posterior oblique and right posterior oblique perfusion (top) and ventilation (bottom) images show multiple large mismatched perfusion defects, a high-probability ventilation/perfusion (V/Q) scan by modified PIOPED II criteria.*

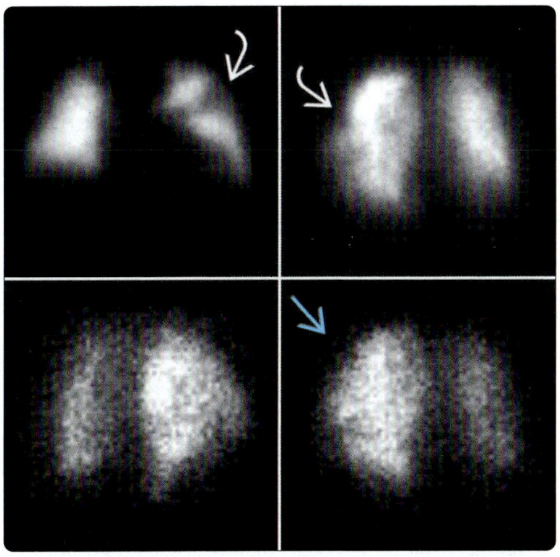

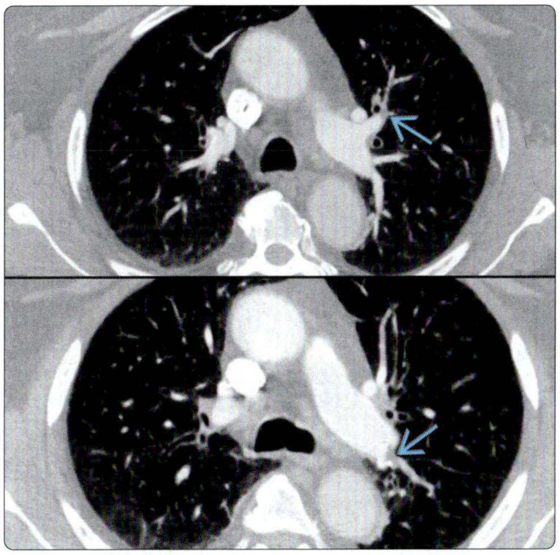

(Left) *Anterior and left posterior oblique perfusion images (top) show a large segmental defect ➔ without a corresponding ventilation defect ➔ on posterior oblique images. This is a nondiagnostic scan by modified PIOPED II criteria and warranted further study by CTA.* **(Right)** *Axial CTA in the same patient shows arterial filling defects ➔ consistent with PE.*

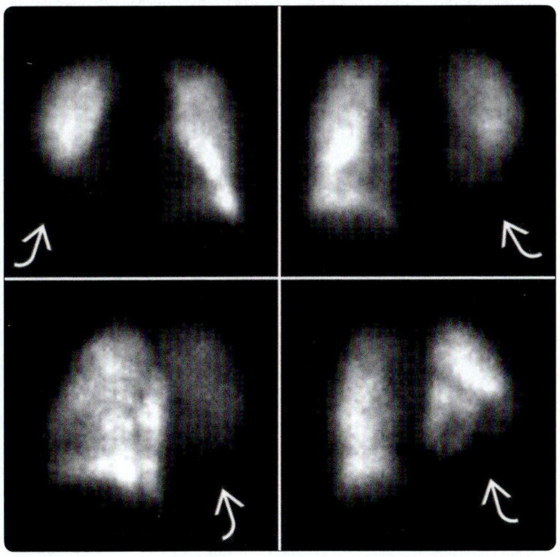

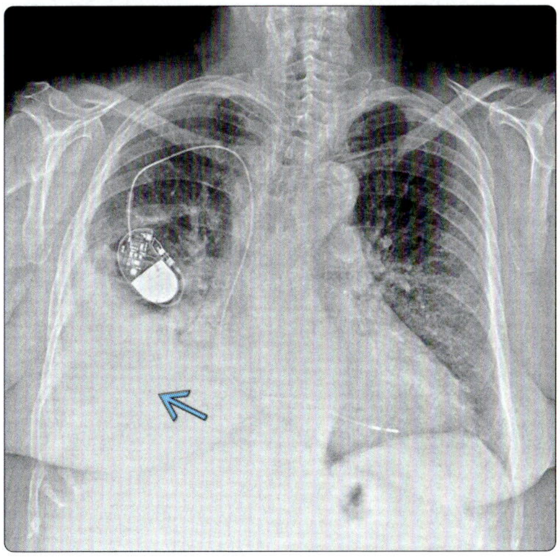

(Left) *Anterior, posterior, left posterior oblique, and right posterior oblique views of a perfusion-only lung scan show a prominent defect in the right base ➔.* **(Right)** *Plain film of chest in the same patient shows a prominent right effusion ➔, which corresponds to perfusion scan findings. As this effusion is approximately 1/3 of the lung field, this is interpreted as very low probability for PE (or PE absent).*

KEY FACTS

TERMINOLOGY

- Quantitative analysis of pulmonary perfusion, often used as presurgical or postprocedure evaluation

IMAGING

- Tc-99m MAA pulmonary perfusion study
  - Perfusion defects correspond to regions of vascular compromise
  - Preoperative planning for pulmonary resection
    - Pneumonectomy: Predicted postoperative FEV_1 = preoperative FEV_1 x (1-fraction of total perfusion for resected lung)
    - Lobectomy: Perfusion of upper, mid, and lower regions of interest can give an estimate of relative contribution to FEV_1
  - Congenital heart anomalies and pulmonary right-to-left shunts
    - Asymmetry of lung perfusion, assess treatment response (e.g., pulmonary artery stent or dilatation)
  - Pre- and postoperative lung transplant evaluation
    - Can assess vascular anastomosis with baseline post-transplant study
    - In single-lung transplants VQ scans can be helpful for diagnosing obliterative bronchiolitis
- Anterior and posterior images over the lungs using low-energy all purpose parallel hole collimator
  - Regions of interest drawn around both lungs
  - Each lung divided into 3 regions of interest
  - Geometric mean analysis of anterior and posterior planar data
  - Geometric mean: Square root of the product of anterior and posterior counts

DIAGNOSTIC CHECKLIST

- Normal lung perfusion is relatively symmetrical
  - 55% right, 45% left
- Review correlative imaging, if available, prior to interpretation

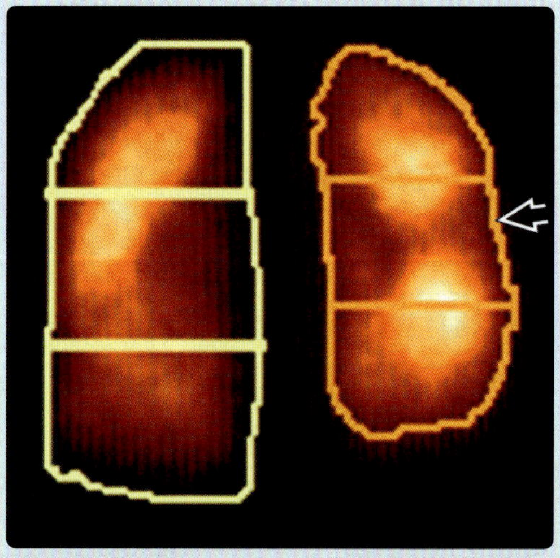
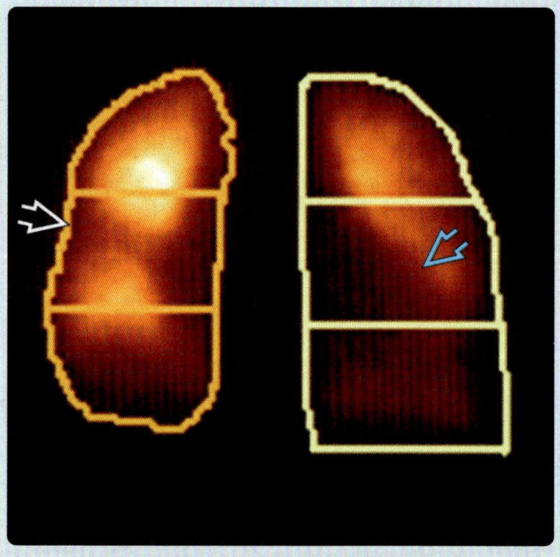

(Left) *Posterior pulmonary perfusion scan in a patient with sarcoidosis and concern for pulmonary arterial compromise shows diminished perfusion in the right midlung* ➡. **(Right)** *Anterior pulmonary perfusion scan in the same patient shows the right midlung* ➡ *perfusion defect and cardiomegaly* ➡*. Overall, quantitative relative lung perfusion was symmetrical, with the right lung providing 56% of relative lung function.*

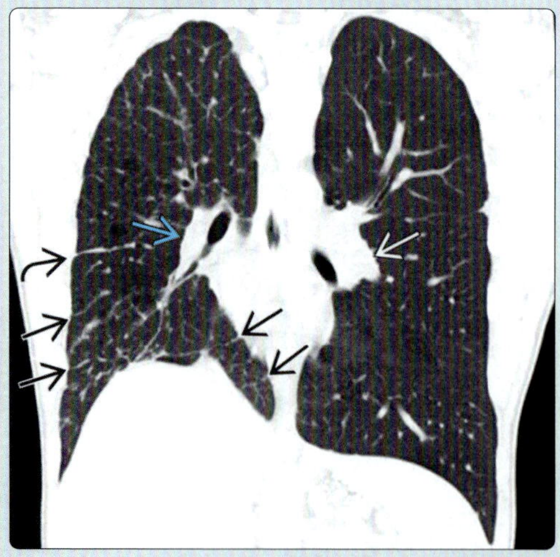
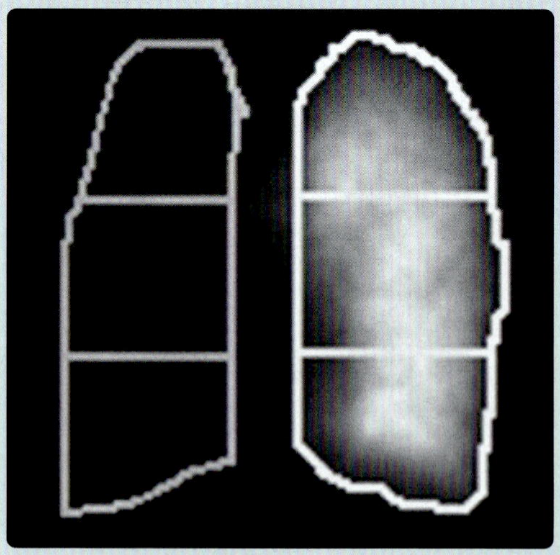

(Left) *Coronal CT in a patient with a history of total anomalous pulmonary venous drainage repaired in infancy shows that total occlusion of right pulmonary veins occurred postoperatively. The right interlobar pulmonary artery* ➡ *is small compared to the left* ➡*. Interlobular septal edema signifies venous obstruction* ➡*. Edema thickens the minor fissure* ➡*.* **(Right)** *Anterior quantitative relative lung perfusion scan in the same patient shows that the left lung receives 98% of the total lung perfusion.*

TERMINOLOGY

Definitions

- Quantitative analysis of pulmonary perfusion, often used as presurgical or postprocedure evaluation

IMAGING

Nuclear Medicine Findings

- Tc-99m macroaggregated albumin (MAA) pulmonary perfusion study
  - Perfusion defects correspond to regions of vascular compromise
  - Preoperative planning for pulmonary resection
    - Lower postoperative FEV_1 or DLCO is associated with worse postoperative morbidity and mortality
    - Pneumonectomy: Predicted postoperative FEV_1 = preoperative FEV_1 x (1-fraction of total perfusion for resected lung)
    - Operative risk is considered reasonable if predicted postoperative FEV_1 and DLCO are > 40%
    - Lobectomy: Perfusion of upper, mid, and lower regions of interest can give an estimate of relative contribution to FEV_1
    - Lobectomy alternate anatomic method: Predicted postoperative FEV_1 = preoperative FEV_1 x (1- y/z), whereby the number of functional segments to be removed is y and the total number of functional segments is z
  - Congenital heart anomalies and pulmonary right-to-left shunts
    - Asymmetry of lung perfusion, assess treatment response (e.g., pulmonary artery stent or dilatation)
    - Note: Brain and kidney uptake of Tc-99m MAA with right-to-left shunt
  - Pre- and postoperative lung transplant evaluation
    - Ventilation and perfusion (VQ) studies performed
    - Prelung transplant
      - VQ scan identifies lung with worse function for single lung transplantation
    - Postlung transplant
      - Can assess vascular anastomosis with baseline post-transplant study
      - In single-lung transplants VQ scans can be helpful for diagnosing obliterative bronchiolitis
      - Diminished early perfusion may be a risk factor for development of chronic rejection
      - Serial scans can detect subtle compromise (e.g., rejection, infection)

Imaging Recommendations

- Best imaging tool
  - Planar Tc-99m MAA pulmonary perfusion imaging data are a reasonable representation of regional lung function
    - SPECT imaging improves regional assessment but increases scanner time and is not necessary
  - CT and PET/CT: Essential for preoperative planning for lung cancer and other pulmonary parenchymal disease resection
  - MR and ultrasound: Often valuable in interpretation of perfusion imaging in congenital heart disease
- Protocol advice
  - Quantitative lung perfusion scan
    - Patient preparation
      - Have patient cough and take deep breaths prior to injection
      - Patients with asthma can use bronchodilators prior to injection
    - Radiopharmaceutical
      - Tc-99m MAA
    - Dose
      - Adults:1-4 mCi (40-150 MBq) IV
      - Children: 0.03 mCi/kg (1.11 MBq/kg) IV
      - Do not inject in a line with a filter; direct intravenous injection is best
    - Dosimetry
      - Lungs receive highest dose
    - Image acquisition
      - Low-energy all-purpose parallel hole collimator
      - Anterior and posterior images over both lungs
      - 100K counts each image
    - Image processing
      - Regions of interest drawn around both lungs
      - Each lung divided into 3 regions of interest
      - Geometric mean analysis of anterior and posterior planar data
      - Geometric mean: Square root of the product of anterior and posterior counts

DIFFERENTIAL DIAGNOSIS

Diminished Lung Perfusion

- Pulmonary embolism
- Vasculitis
- Mass obstructing or encasing the pulmonary artery
- Asthma
- Other pulmonary parenchymal disease inducing redistribution of blood flow

DIAGNOSTIC CHECKLIST

Image Interpretation Pearls

- Review chest radiographs, CT &/or PET/CT, and angiography, if available, prior to interpretation
- Normal lung perfusion is relatively symmetrical
  - 55% right, 45% left
- Focal increased activity in lungs can be caused by blood clotting in syringe or line

SELECTED REFERENCES

1. ACR–SPR–STR practice parameter for the performance of pulmonary scintigraphy. American College of Radiology website. http://acr.org/~/media/860d4274393a477daa0d6acf663c9ed8.pdf. Updated September 3, 2014. Accessed June 9, 2015
2. Brunelli A et al: Physiologic evaluation of the patient with lung cancer being considered for resectional surgery: Diagnosis and management of lung cancer, 3rd ed: American College of Chest Physicians evidence-based clinical practice guidelines. Chest. 143(5 Suppl):e166S-90S, 2013
3. Parker JA et al: SNM practice guideline for lung scintigraphy 4.0. J Nucl Med Technol. 40(1):57-65, 2012
4. Mazzone PJ: Preoperative evaluation of the lung cancer resection candidate. Expert Rev Respir Med. 4(1):97-113, 2010
5. MacDonald A et al: Infrequently performed studies in nuclear medicine: part 2. J Nucl Med Technol. 37(1):1-13, 2009

SECTION 8
Urinary Tract

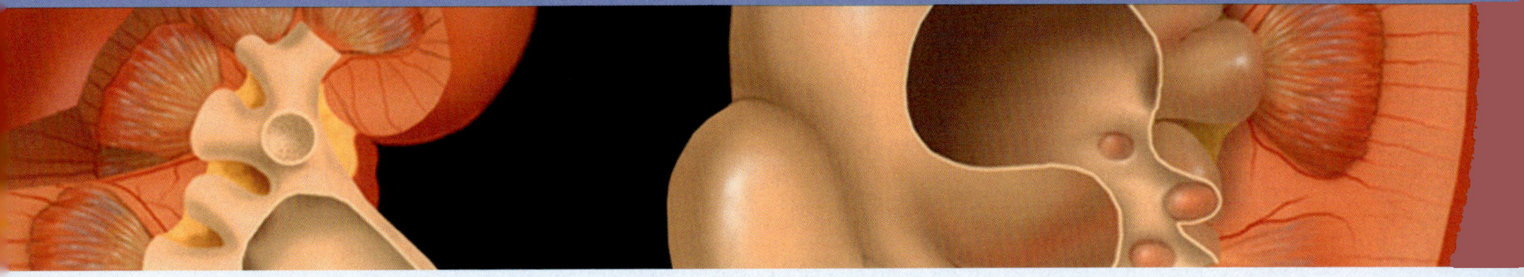

Introduction

Infection and Inflammation

Renal Function

Introduction

The majority of nuclear imaging of the urinary tract focuses on the kidney, designed to assess 1 or more elements of renal blood flow, structure, function, and collecting system drainage. Commonly used radiopharmaceuticals designed to achieve this include

- Radiopharmaceuticals that are cortically bound: Tc-99m dimercaptosuccinic acid (DMSA), Tc-99m glucoheptonate
- Radiopharmaceuticals that are secreted by the tubules: Tc-99m mercaptoacetyltriglycine (MAG3)
- Radiopharmaceuticals that are filtered: Tc-99m diethylene triamine pentaacetic acid (DTPA), I-131 hippuran

The other commonly performed nuclear imaging study of the urinary tract is radionuclide cystography. Nuclear cystograms are generally performed in children and are designed to evaluate for vesicoureteral reflux (VUR) that might predispose to pyelonephritis and renal scarring.

Renal Cortex

Renal cortical scanning detects parenchymal defects related to scarring or acute pyelonephritis. Radiopharmaceuticals employed for renal cortical scanning (Tc-99m DMSA, glucoheptonate) concentrate in the renal cortex by binding the proximal convoluted tubules. Pinhole and SPECT imaging are commonly employed to obtain high-resolution images of the kidney to allow detection of small parenchymal defects. Both acute pyelonephritis and renal scarring can appear as focal or multifocal, wedge-shaped defects. It is primarily the time course that distinguishes the 2, with defects visible after more than 6 months reflective of scarring. More established or extensive scarring may appear as a global decrease in renal size.

Previously, renal cortical scanning was largely used as a secondary assessment in the work-up of suspected VUR, which was generally evaluated with a "bottom up" approach aimed at identifying the presence of VUR. More recently, some have been advocating for a "top down" approach in which DMSA is the primary study, arguing that prevention of renal parenchymal injury is the primary aim of VUR therapy.

Renal Obstruction

The assessment of renal obstruction focuses on distinguishing the dilated, nonobstructed collecting system from the obstructed collecting system. This can be a question in both the native kidney (commonly ureteropelvic junction obstruction) and the transplant kidney (anastomotic obstruction). Tc-99m MAG3 is the primary radiopharmaceutical used for assessment of renal collecting system drainage. Most examinations aimed at assessing collecting system drainage consist of a set of baseline images in which the radiopharmaceutical is administered and serial images are obtained as it is extracted from the blood pool, passes through the renal parenchyma, and appears in the collecting system. Split renal function (based on differential perfusion) can also be derived from this baseline set of images. Subsequently, a diuretic is administered and further serial images are obtained as the collecting system progressively fills and drains. Creation and evaluation of clearance curves are critical to the interpretation of both phases of the exam with clearance T 1/2 derived from the postdiuretic curves used to quantify the efficacy of renal collecting system drainage.

Renal Transplant

Following renal transplantation, there are multiple processes that can compromise function of the transplant, including but not limited to acute tubular necrosis (ATN), rejection, drug toxicity, collecting system obstruction, and vascular anastomotic narrowing. Renal scintigraphy allows noninvasive assessment of renal transplant function and can be used to assess perfusion, parenchymal function, and collecting system drainage. Renal scintigraphy also has value in determining the etiology of peritransplant fluid collections.

Tc-99m MAG3 is the most commonly employed radiopharmaceutical in the evaluation of renal transplants though DMSA may be employed when assessment of renal parenchyma is needed. As with native collecting system obstruction, diuretics are often used when collecting system obstruction is suspected.

Generally, planar imaging is sufficient for the evaluation of a renal transplant. Unlike imaging of the native kidneys, the camera head should be positioned anteriorly or dual-head imaging should be performed when evaluating a heterotopic renal transplant. SPECT and SPECT/CT may add value when renal cortical imaging is performed or in the assessment of peritransplant fluid collections.

Renovascular Hypertension

Renovascular abnormalities can result in hypertension that is difficult to control medically. Scintigraphy plays an important role in the work-up of renovascular hypertension as not all cases have macroscopic vascular abnormalities (e.g., main renal artery stenosis) that can be identified on anatomic imaging.

Imaging of renovascular hypertension is generally performed with Tc-99m MAG3 ± angiotensin-converting enzyme inhibitor (ACEI) administration.

Vesicoureteral Reflux

Nuclear cystography is a "bottom up" approach to identifying VUR as a cause of recurrent urinary tract infections, pyelonephritis, and renal parenchymal injury. Nuclear cystography entails obtaining dynamic or serial images while the bladder is filled 1 or more times after a bolus of radiopharmaceutical, commonly Tc-99m DTPA. Any radiopharmaceutical seen extending into the ureters or to the level of the kidney is reflective of VUR.

Nuclear cystography is more sensitive than fluoroscopic voiding cystourethrography (VCUG) but cannot identify grade I VUR and gives less anatomic detail. As such, some practitioners will use VCUG as the first test in a child with suspected VUR, following with nuclear cystography.

Calculation of Glomerular Filtration Rate

Renal function as measured by glomerular filtration rate (GFR) can be calculated by obtaining serial blood samples or serial images following injection of a small amount of a radiopharmaceutical that is cleared by glomerular filtration. Scintigraphically determined GFRs are more accurate than GFRs calculated from serum creatinine or other serum markers of renal function.

Selected References

1. Taylor AT: Radionuclides in nephrourology, part 1: radiopharmaceuticals, quality control, and quantitative indices. J Nucl Med. 55(4):608-15, 2014
2. Taylor AT: Radionuclides in nephrourology, Part 2: pitfalls and diagnostic applications. J Nucl Med. 55(5):786-98, 2014

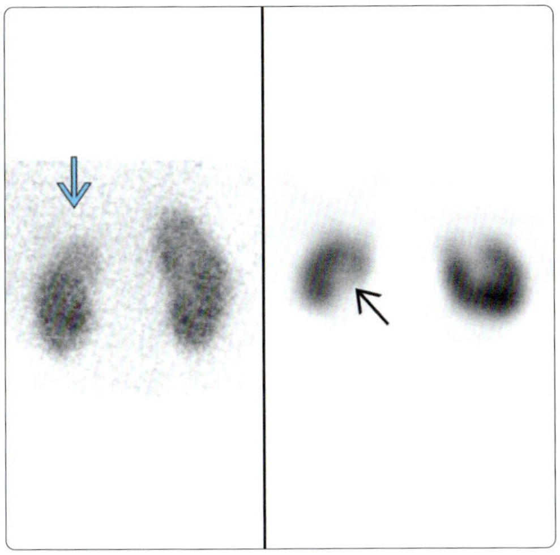

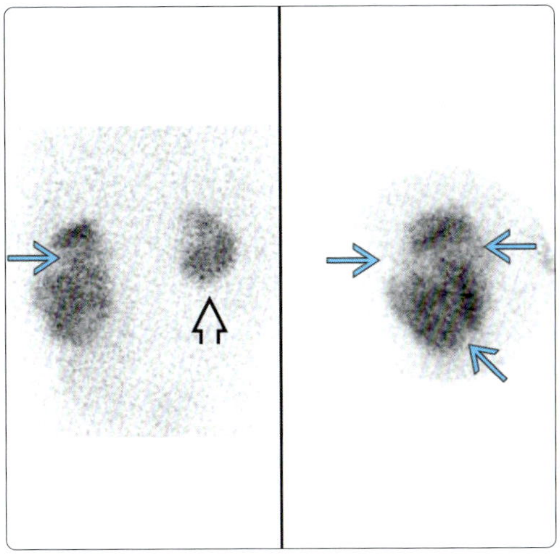

(Left) *Posterior planar (left) and axial SPECT (right) images from a Tc-99m DMSA scan in an 8 year old with hypertension show a small right kidney with a moderate-sized parenchymal defect in the upper pole, reflective of scarring.* **(Right)** *Posterior planar (left) and LPO pinhole (right) images from a Tc-99m DMSA scan in an 8 month old with recurrent pyelonephritis show a globally scarred, small right kidney and multifocal defects in the left kidney, compatible with a combination of scar and acute pyelonephritis.*

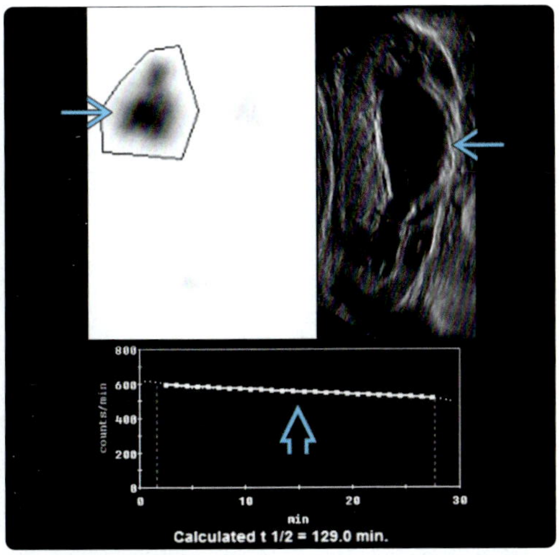

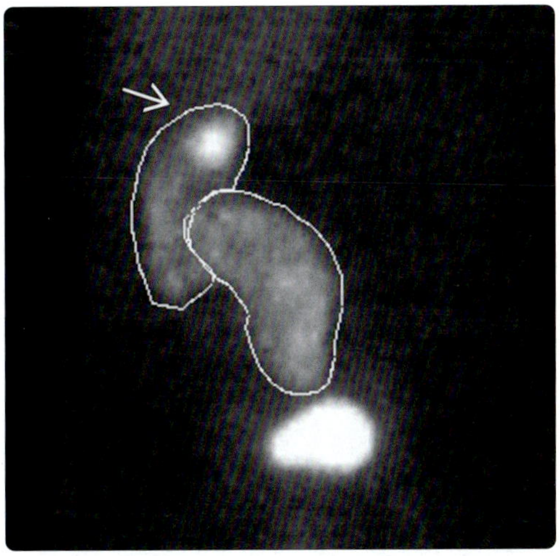

(Left) *Tc-99m MAG3 diuretic renal scan and corresponding ultrasound in a 15 month old show moderate to marked left hydronephrosis with no clearance following diuretic administration, compatible with UPJ obstruction.* **(Right)** *Anterior Tc-99m MAG3 renogram in a patient with 2 transplanted kidneys shows focal calyceal retention in the upper pole of 1 kidney, without global obstruction.*

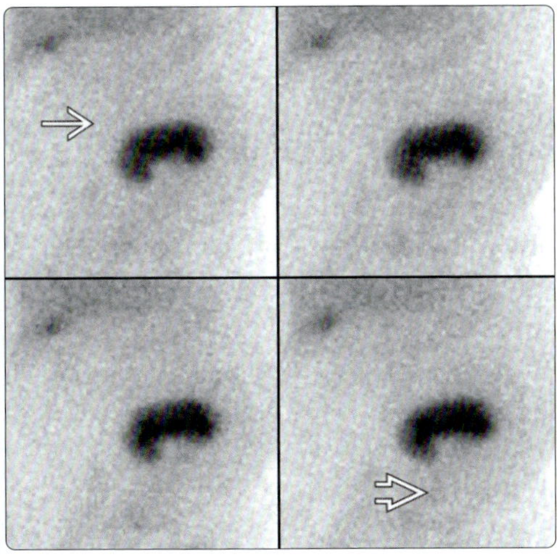

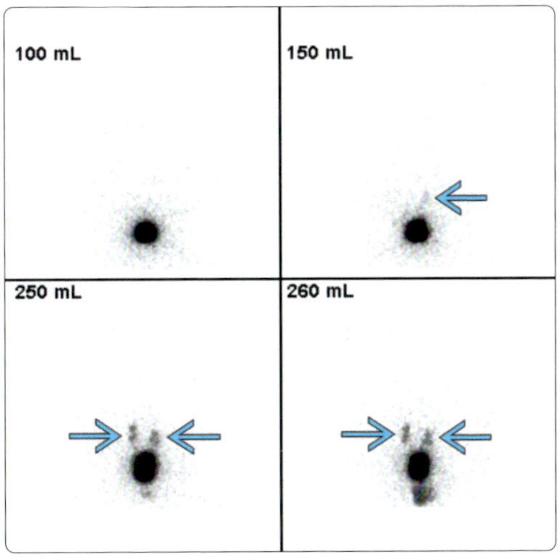

(Left) *Anterior Tc-99m MAG3 renogram of a transplant kidney shows progressive parenchymal accumulation of radiotracer without excretion into the urinary bladder, consistent with acute tubular necrosis.* **(Right)** *Selected posterior projection images from Tc-99m DTPA cystogram in a 1 year old with recurrent UTIs shows bilateral vesicoureteral reflux to the level of the renal pelves, which is comparable to radiographic grade II VUR.*

Renal Scar and Pyelonephritis

KEY FACTS

IMAGING

- Cortical defect on Tc-99m dimercaptosuccinic acid (DMSA) renal cortical imaging
  - Due to acute pyelonephritis or scar
    - Pyelonephritis: Photopenic defects extend to hilum
    - Cortical scar: Photopenic defects more superficial
  - Upper > lower > mid pole for pyelonephritis, vesicoureteral reflux-induced scar
  - Defect not due to other cause, such as mass or fetal lobulation
  - Renal cortical scintigraphy detects 2x as many defects as ultrasound, 4x as many as intravenous urography
- In-111 WBC scan
  - Uptake sensitive and specific for pyelonephritis
  - No normal uptake in kidneys
- Ga-67 citrate scan
  - Sensitive but not specific for acute pyelonephritis
  - Bilateral renal Ga-67 uptake > 48 hr post injection: Renal insufficiency and interstitial nephritis; mimics diffuse acute pyelonephritis
  - Focal increased Ga-67 uptake: Acute pyelonephritis, lymphoma, leukemia, metastases

CLINICAL ISSUES

- Pyelonephritis and reflux-induced renal scarring
  - Major predisposing factor for proteinuria, hypertension, ultimate renal failure
- Treatment
  - Acute pyelonephritis
    - ~ 2-week course of antibiotics; may start IV and switch to oral (prophylactic with documented vesicoureteral reflux)
  - Vesicoureteral reflux
    - Watchful waiting in low-grade reflux (80% resolve spontaneously)
    - Surgical/endoscopic correction in high grade/scar

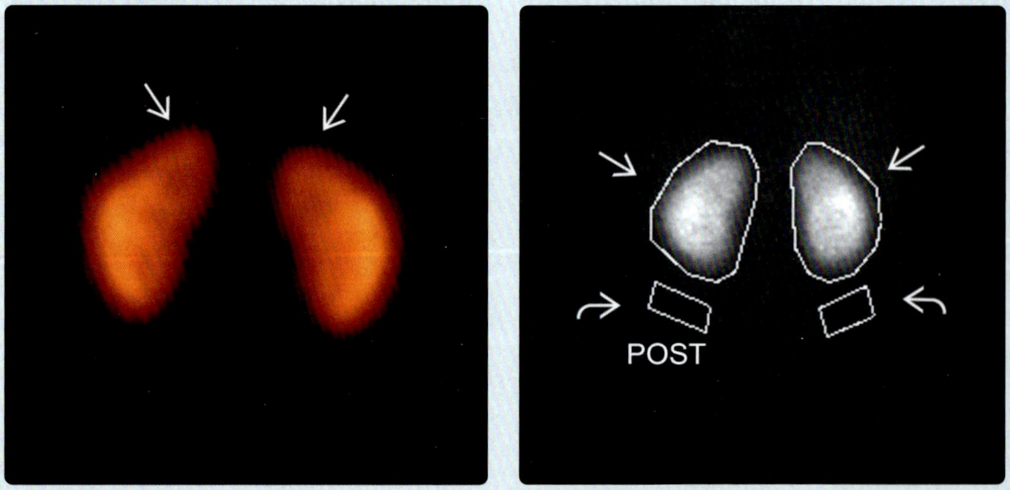

(Left) *Tc-99m dimercaptosuccinic acid (DMSA) renal cortical scan shows normal uptake in both kidneys. Note the relatively decreased activity in upper poles* ➔. **(Right)** *Posterior Tc-99m DMSA renal cortical scan shows region-of-interest analysis of bilateral kidneys* ➔ *and background activity* ➔, *which allows for calculation of relative functioning renal mass.*

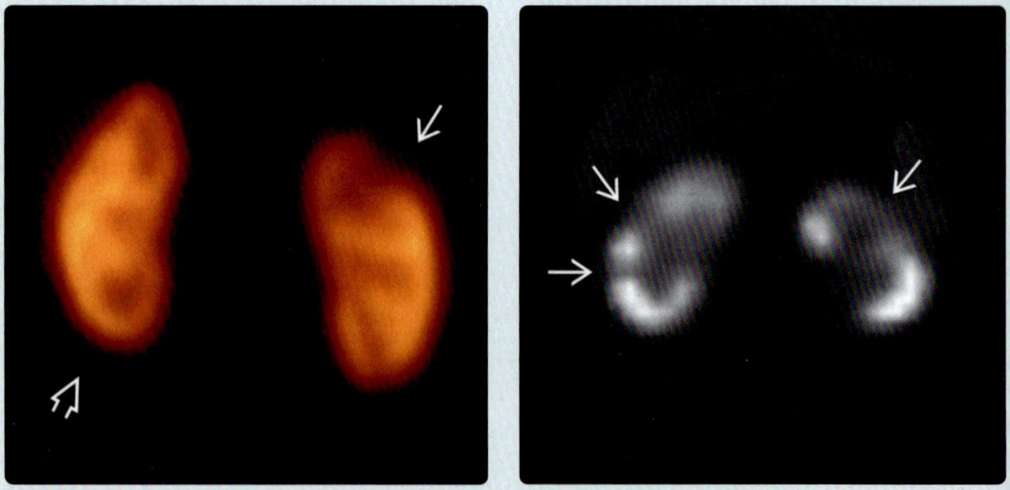

(Left) *Tc-99m DMSA renal cortical scan shows normal left renal cortical uptake* ➔ *and a focal photopenic defect in the upper pole of the right kidney* ➔, *consistent with a scar.* **(Right)** *Tc-99m DMSA renal cortical scan shows multiple foci of cortical scar* ➔ *in a patient with vesicoureteral reflux.*

IMAGING

General Features

- Best diagnostic clue
  - Cortical defect on Tc-99m dimercaptosuccinic acid (DMSA) renal cortical imaging
    - Due to acute pyelonephritis or scar
      - Upper > lower > mid pole for pyelonephritis, vesicoureteral reflux (VUR)-induced scar
    - Defect not due to other cause, such as mass or fetal lobulation

Nuclear Medicine Findings

- Tc-99m DMSA renal cortical scan
  - Gold standard for renal cortical scar/infarct
    - Cortical scintigraphy detects 2x as many defects as ultrasound, 4x as many as intravenous urography
  - Typical cause of renal scar: Pyelonephritis, VUR
  - Pyelonephritis-induced renal scar
    - Acute pyelonephritis: Striated uptake appearance on Tc-99m DMSA
      - Pattern usually extends toward hilum (scar tends to be more superficial)
    - Acute 1st time pyelonephritis (< 1 week): Renal cortical scan demonstrates cortical abnormalities in 50-79% (US misses 61% of these)
      - Acute pyelonephritis-related cortical defects can resolve by 6 weeks
    - Late post-pyelonephritis (12-24 months): Resolution of 50% of cortical defects apparent at ≤ 6 months
    - Persistent scars after acute pyelonephritis necessitates evaluation for correction of underlying structural causes of infection
      - Pyelonephritis-induced renal scar in absence of VUR can be from abnormal bladder dynamics
  - VUR-induced renal scarring
    - VUR found in > 58% of children with 1st time acute pyelonephritis and scars on renal cortical scan
    - Male patients with high-grade reflux presenting with 1st UTI: Nearly 1/2 have renal parenchymal damage on renal cortical scan
    - Scars on renal cortical scan correlate with ↑ grade VUR: Indication for surgical correction rather than watchful waiting, prophylactic antibiotics
    - New renal cortical scars with UTI despite antibiotic prophylaxis: Indication for surgical correction
    - High-grade VUR without UTI: Renal cortical scars in 65%
    - Recommendations for renal cortical scan in VUR: ↑ grade reflux (grade ≥ 3); reflux with recurrent UTI
  - Vascular insult, embolization, trauma, renal transplant: Renal cortical scan useful in assessing extent of damage, residual functioning renal mass
- Labeled WBC scan: Identification of acute pyelonephritis in complicated cases
  - In-111 WBC scan: No normal uptake in kidneys; ↑ uptake sensitive and specific for pyelonephritis
  - Tc-99m HMPAO WBC scan: Normal uptake in kidneys and bladder; ↓ sensitivity, specificity for pyelonephritis
- Ga-67 citrate scan: Incidental identification of renal infection when patient scanned for other reasons
  - Sensitive but not specific for acute pyelonephritis
  - Normal symmetrical Ga-67 renal uptake up to 48 hr post injection
  - Bilateral renal Ga-67 uptake > 48 hr post injection: Renal insufficiency and interstitial nephritis; mimics diffuse acute pyelonephritis
  - Focal increased Ga-67 uptake: Acute pyelonephritis, lymphoma, leukemia, metastases

Imaging Recommendations

- Best imaging tool
  - Tc-99m DMSA renal cortical scan with SPECT
    - Identifying renal parenchymal lesions following acute pyelonephritis, scar in chronic pyelonephritis
    - Identifies scar related to VUR, especially of "breakthrough UTI" while on prophylactic antibiotics
    - Evaluation of renal function post VUR surgical correction: Differential renal Tc-99m DMSA uptake, scar assessment
    - Identify cortical infarction following trauma, embolic event, vascular injury
- Protocol advice
  - Tc-99m DMSA renal cortical scan
    - Children: 40-50 μCi (1.48-1.85 MBq)/kg, minimum activity 350 μCi (13 MBq) IV
    - Adults: 5 mCi (185 MBq) IV
    - Tc-99m DMSA: 40-65% injected dose bound to cortical proximal convoluted tubules 2 hr post injection
    - Preferred tracer in small infants (permits best cortical resolution)
    - Patients with renal tubular acidosis have decreased concentration of Tc-99m DMSA tracer in tubules, causes increased urinary excretion
    - Renal failure: ↑ hepatic clearance
  - Tc-99m glucoheptonate scan
    - Children: 80-120 μCi (3-4.5 MBq)/kg (minimum activity 0.5 mCi [18.5 MBq]) IV
    - Adults: 8 mCi (300 MBq) IV
    - Glucoheptonate: 10-20% bound to proximal convoluted tubule at 2 hr, remainder excreted glomerular filtration
    - Partial glomerular filtration permits dynamic and static imaging within 20-30 min of injection
    - Initial renal scan to evaluation flow, function
    - Delayed planar/SPECT at 2-4 hr post injection
- Patient preparation
  - No prep needed if no planned conscious sedation
  - If child not able to cooperate, consider conscious sedation with pediatric anesthesia, including informed consent
  - Obtain history of prior GU surgery, congenital anomalies, urinary obstruction, possible renal masses
- Dosimetry
  - Renal cortical exposure similar with both Tc-99m DMSA and Tc-99m glucoheptonate, but Tc-99m DMSA provides lower gonadal/bladder wall exposure
  - Tc-99m DMSA: Administered activity 0.04-0.05 mCi (1.5-1.85 MBq)/kg
    - Critical organ: Kidneys (0.45 mGy/MBq)
    - Effective dose of 0.039 mSv/MBq

- Tc-99m GH: Administered activity 0.08-0.12 mCi (3-4.5 MBq)/kg
  - Critical organ: Bladder wall (0.15 mGy/MBq)
  - Effective dose of 0.024 mSv/MBq
- Image acquisition
  - Posterior and anterior supine planar images with low-energy, all-purpose parallel hole collimator at 2 hr post injection
    - Differential renal function calculated using geometric mean method
      - Geometric mean: Square root of product of anterior and posterior counts
    - Place regions of interest over each kidney and background areas on posterior imaging
  - If poor renal function, delayed images can be performed to permit longer uptake time
  - SPECT for best 3D cortical evaluation
    - If SPECT not available, anterior, posterior, and bilateral posterior oblique images
    - High- or ultra-high-resolution collimator; 300-500 K/image
    - If known or suspected horseshoe kidney, image from anterior to discern connecting bridge of renal tissue between lower pole moieties ventral to spine

Artifacts and Quality Control

- If distended or neurogenic bladder, place bladder catheter and allow continuous drainage
  - Prevents back-pressure effect and interference from retained collecting system activity
- If patulous or obstructed collecting system, can use furosemide before delayed images or patient can return for delays 24 hr after tracer injection
- Too much air within tracer reaction vial causes degradation of Tc-99m DMSA complex → increased renal uptake, increased hepatic background activity

DIFFERENTIAL DIAGNOSIS

Pyelonephritis

- Cortical scar: Photopenic defects more superficial
- Pyelonephritis: Photopenic defects extend to hilum

Renal Masses

- Focal region of absent Tc-99m DMSA uptake ± mass effect

Renal Cyst

- Discrete, sharp, rounded focus of absent Tc-99m DMSA

Polyarteritis Nodosa

- Striated appearance: Mimics acute pyelonephritis
- Correlate with history, CTA findings, and available histopathology

Fetal Lobulation

- Normal variant: Focal indentation between lobules may mimic scar

Interstitial Nephritis

- May mimic diffuse bilateral pyelonephritis on Ga-67

Splenic Impression

- Normal variant: Smooth indentation/flattening along anterior aspect of left renal upper pole may mimic scar

PATHOLOGY

General Features

- Etiology
  - Pyelonephritis
    - Underlying VUR evident in 1/3 of pediatric patients
    - *Escherichia coli* > *Klebsiella*

CLINICAL ISSUES

Presentation

- Most common signs/symptoms
  - Acute pyelonephritis: Fever, abdominal pain, irritability (infants), frequency, strong-smelling urine

Demographics

- Gender
  - Pyelonephritis and VUR: M:F = 1:2

Natural History & Prognosis

- Pyelonephritis and reflux-induced renal scarring: Major predisposing factor for proteinuria, hypertension, ultimate renal failure
- Risk factors for renal parenchymal damage with VUR: History of UTIs, reflux grade, age at diagnosis

Treatment

- Acute pyelonephritis
  - ~ 2-week course of antibiotics; may start IV and switch to oral (prophylactic with documented VUR)
- Vesicoureteral reflux
  - Watchful waiting in low-grade reflux (80% resolve spontaneously)
  - Surgical/endoscopic correction in high grade

DIAGNOSTIC CHECKLIST

Consider

- Renal cortical scintigraphy detects 2x as many defects as ultrasound, 4x as many as intravenous urography

Image Interpretation Pearls

- Tc-99m DMSA renal cortical scan
  - Pyelonephritis: Photopenic defects extend to hilum
  - Cortical scar: Photopenic defects more superficial
  - Fetal lobulation, normal variant causing focal indentation between lobules on renal cortical scan, may mimic scar
  - Spleen can cause smooth indentation/flattening along anterior aspect of left renal upper pole, which can mimic scar

SELECTED REFERENCES

1. American College of Radiology. ACR-SPR Practice Parameter for the Performance of Renal Scintigraphy. 2014
2. Agras K et al: Resolution of cortical lesions on serial renal scans in children with acute pyelonephritis. Pediatr Radiol. 37(2):153-8, 2007
3. Temiz Y et al: The efficacy of Tc99m dimercaptosuccinic acid (Tc-DMSA) scintigraphy and ultrasonography in detecting renal scars in children with primary vesicoureteral reflux (VUR). Int Urol Nephrol. 38(1):149-52, 2006
4. Ataei N et al: Evaluation of acute pyelonephritis with DMSA scans in children presenting after the age of 5 years. Pediatr Nephrol. 20(10):1439-44, 2005
5. Lin KY et al: Acute pyelonephritis and sequelae of renal scar in pediatric first febrile urinary tract infection. Pediatr Nephrol. 18(4):362-5, 2003
6. Mandell et al. Society of Nuclear Medicine Procedure Guideline for Renal Cortical Scintigraphy in Children version 3.0. 195-8, 2003

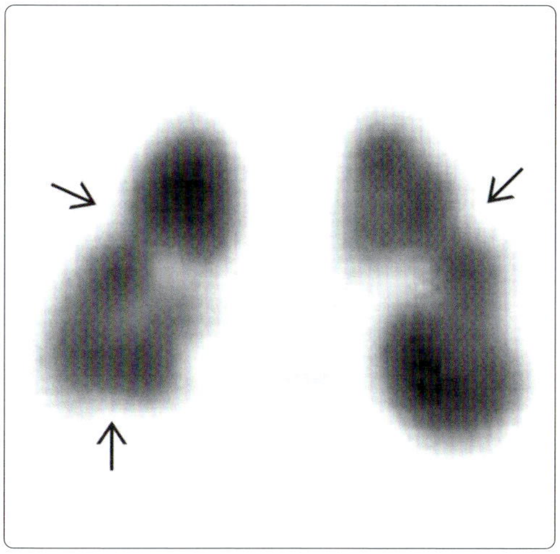

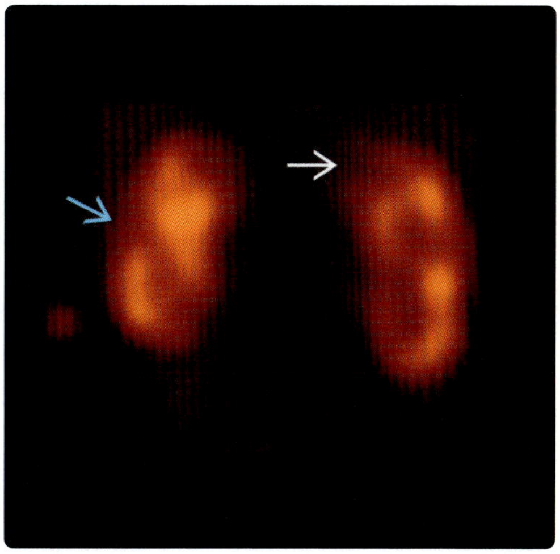

(Left) *Tc-99m DMSA renal SPECT shows multiple bilateral cortical defects* ➔ *in a patient with bilateral high-grade reflux and multiple previous urinary tract infections. Fetal lobulation could also have this appearance.* **(Right)** *Tc-99m DMSA renal cortical scan in a patient with fever, UTI, and vesicoureteral reflux shows multiple photopenic defects that likely represent pyelonephritis* ➔ *and scar* ➔*.*

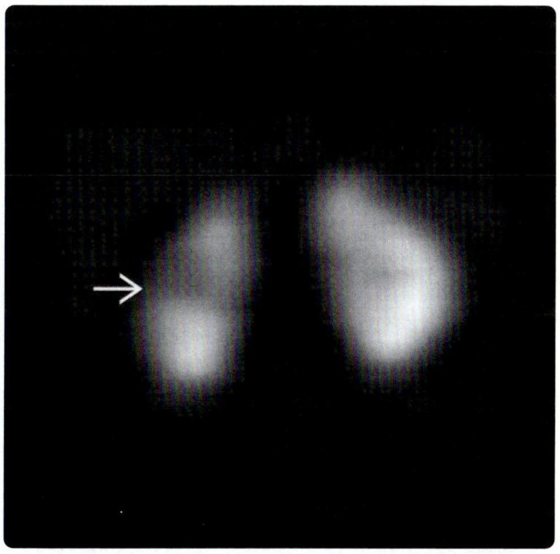

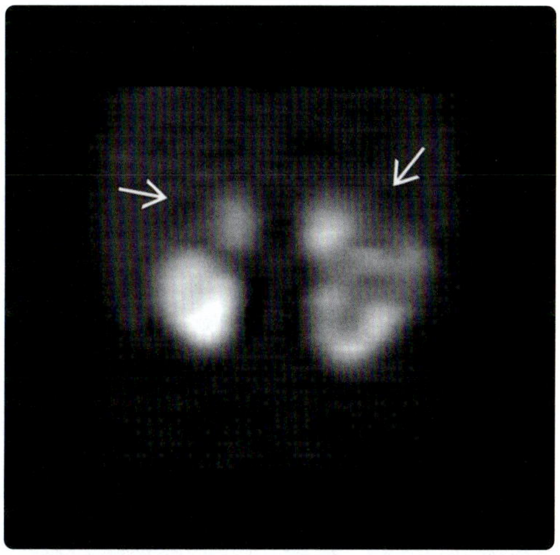

(Left) *Tc-99m DMSA renal cortical scan shows a rounded lesion in interpolar left kidney* ➔*, a cyst on ultrasound.* **(Right)** *Tc-99m DMSA renal cortical SPECT shows multiple cortical defects* ➔ *in a patient with acute pyelonephritis.*

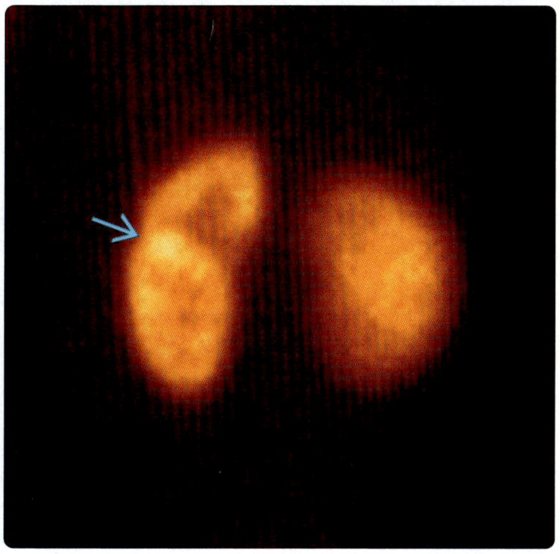

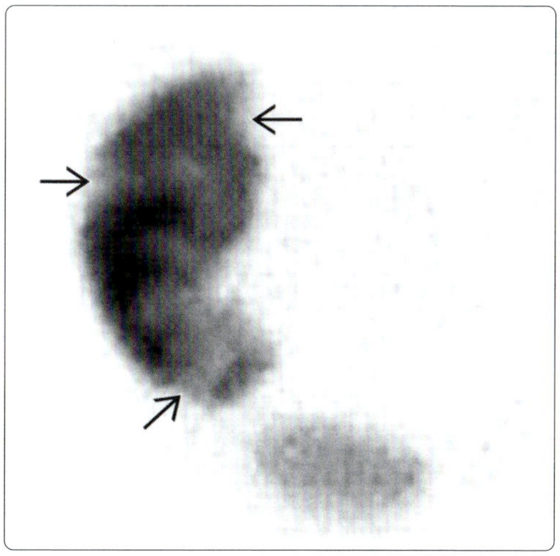

(Left) *Posterior Tc-99m DMSA scan shows focally increased activity* ➔*, suggesting a hypertrophied column of Bertin.* **(Right)** *Anterior Tc-99m glucoheptonate renal cortical scan in a transplant kidney shows multiple cortical defects* ➔*. It is postulated that acute rejection episodes and renal infarcts cause these defects.*

Hydronephrosis

KEY FACTS

IMAGING

- Renal scintigraphy: Anatomic and functional imaging using Tc-99m MAG3 with furosemide (Lasix) to evaluation patency of collecting system
- Normal renogram curve
  - Spontaneous washout of activity from collecting system prior to furosemide administration (washout t1/2 < 10 min)
- High-grade obstruction curve
  - Progressive rise in activity in collecting system, even after furosemide
- Partial obstruction curve
  - Activity continues to rise until furosemide; thereafter decreases but washout t1/2 > 10 min
- Functional obstruction curve
  - Activity continues to rise until furosemide given, then washes out normally (washout t1/2 ≤ 10 min)
- False-positive or indeterminate furosemide washout
  - ↓ renal function, ↓ response to furosemide, severely dilated nonobstructed collecting system, immature kidney, dehydration

TOP DIFFERENTIAL DIAGNOSES

- Intrinsic vs. extrinsic urinary tract obstruction
- Dilated, nonobstructed collecting system
- Vesicoureteral reflux
- Acute tubular necrosis
- Renal artery stenosis
- Renal vein thrombosis
- Medical renal disease

DIAGNOSTIC CHECKLIST

- Immature kidneys may produce false-positive or indeterminate results: Wait until 6-8 weeks of age before furosemide renography
- Postural drainage maneuver increases specificity of furosemide renography

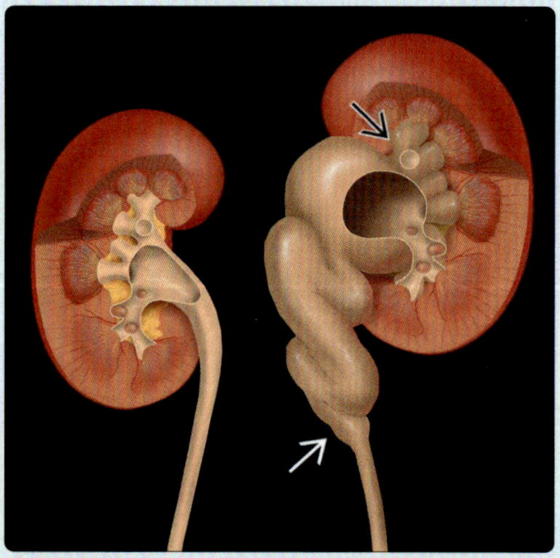
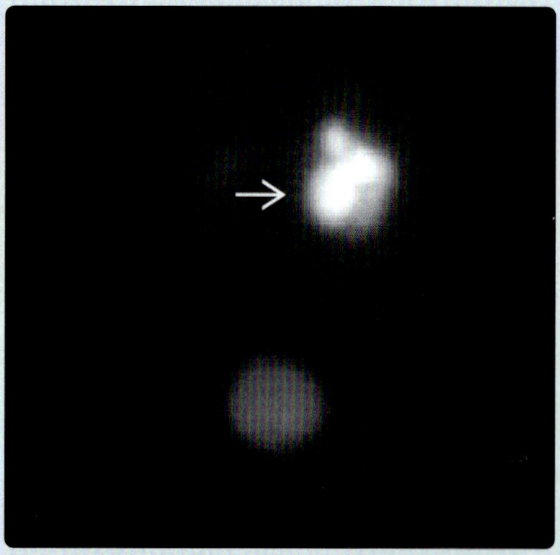

(Left) *Graphic shows unilateral dilated calyces ⇨ and dilated, corkscrew renal pelvis ➡ to the level of the ureteropelvic junction, consistent with UPJ obstruction.* **(Right)** *Renogram shows the UPJ obstruction with a dilated right renal pelvis ➡ and calyces to the level of the ureteropelvic junction.*

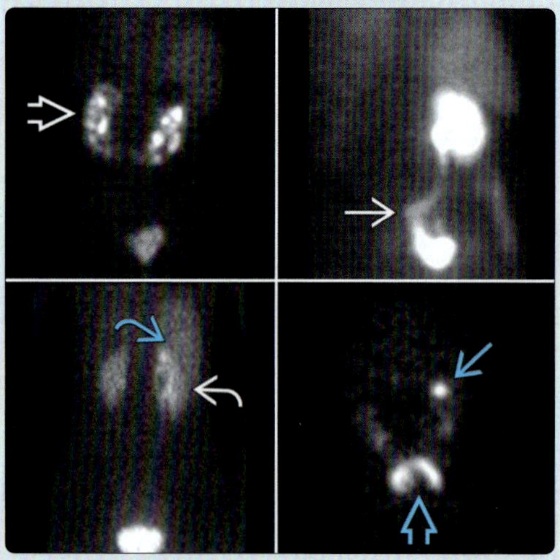
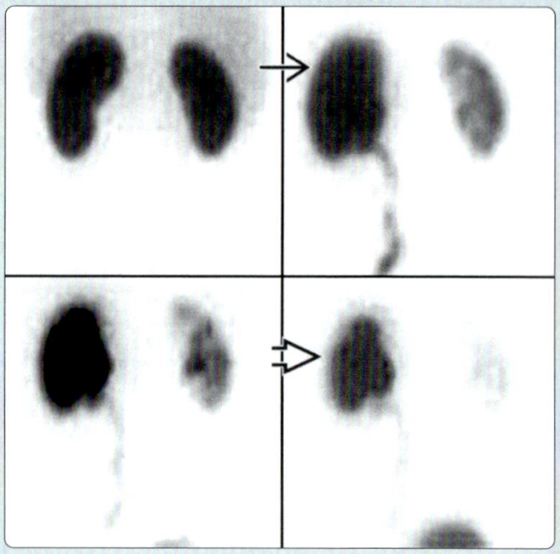

(Left) *Renogram shows a horseshoe kidney ➡, a right ileal conduit with tracer in bowel ➡, a right duplicated system (upper ⇨ & lower ➡ moiety), and a duplicated right system with upper pole retention due to obstruction ⇨. Note photopenic ureterocele ⇨ in bladder.* **(Right)** *Tc-99m MAG3 renogram in a 6 week old with left hydronephrosis ⇨ shows retention of radiotracer despite furosemide administration. This study is positive for left UPJ obstruction ⇨.*

TERMINOLOGY

Definitions

- Hydronephrosis
  - Dilation of collecting system, which can be caused by obstruction of urinary outflow
  - Hydroureter/hydronephrosis may persist after obstruction has resolved

IMAGING

General Features

- Renal scintigraphy
  - Anatomic and functional imaging using Tc-99m mercaptoacetyltriglycine (MAG3) with furosemide (Lasix) to evaluate patency of collecting system
    - Characterize hydronephrosis
    - Estimate relative renal function

Nuclear Medicine Findings

- Relative renal mass
  - Differential or split renal function
  - ROI drawn around each kidney
  - 1-3 min after injection, values are selected and reported as percentage
    - Normal: 45-55%
- Angiographic phase
  - Flow to kidneys is seen quickly after aorta
  - Cortex should accumulate radiotracer over 1-3 min
    - Should be homogeneous
    - Cortical defects may indicate scar
  - If decreased renal function, uptake will be delayed
- Clearance phase
  - Calyceal activity within 5 min
  - Bladder activity within 10-15 min
- Renogram curve
  - Graphic representation of uptake and excretion of Tc-99m MAG3 by kidneys plotted on time-activity curve
  - t1/2
    - Amount of time it takes for 1/2 of maximum cortical activity to clear
      - Normal: < 10 min
  - Must be read with images

Imaging Recommendations

- Best imaging tool
  - Acute obstruction: IVP or NECT
  - Chronic obstruction: Tc-99m MAG3 renography with furosemide
- Protocol advice
  - Patient preparation
    - Patient hydration with oral or IV fluids
    - No furosemide day of exam (±)
    - Void prior to study
      - Full bladder, incomplete voiding, bladder outlet obstruction, or vesicoureteral reflux will greatly complicate results
      - Consider Foley catheter placement if necessary
  - Radiopharmaceutical
    - Tc-99m MAG3
      - Cleared nearly entirely by tubular secretion
      - Uptake decreased by poor renal function
      - Adults: Up to 10 mCi (370 MBq) Tc-99m MAG3 IV
      - Pediatrics: 0.05-0.1 mCi/kg Tc-99m MAG3 IV (min: 0.5 mCi [18.5 MBq]; max: 5 mCi [185 MBq])
    - Tc-99m diethylenetriamine pentaacetic acid (DTPA)
      - Cleared through glomerular filtration
      - Convenient, inexpensive
      - Usually reserved for GFR calculations
  - Dosimetry
    - Urinary bladder receives largest radiation dose
  - Image acquisition
    - Patient supine, gamma camera posterior
    - Angiographic sequence
      - 1-2 sec images for 1-2 min
    - Dynamic sequence
      - 15-60 sec images for 20-30 min
    - Diuresis sequence
      - Patient given furosemide and additional 15-60 sec images for 20-30 min
    - Postvoid images
      - At conclusion of exam, obtain supine posterior planar image x 1 min (prevoid)
      - Postural drainage maneuver: Patient upright x 10 min (void during interval)
      - 10 min after prevoid image: Repeat supine posterior image x 1 min (postvoid)
  - Pharmacologic intervention
    - Furosemide
      - Differentiates between dilated without obstruction vs. dilated with urodynamically significant obstruction
      - Administer IV when collecting system well visualized on side of obstruction (typically @ 15 min)
      - Administer slowly over 1 min
      - Adults: 0.5 mg/kg (max: 40 mg)
      - Pediatrics: 1 mg/kg (max: 40 mg)
      - Azotemia (↑ Cr, ↓ GFR) may require higher dose (80-150 mg)
  - Imaging processing
    - Quantitative analysis
      - Angiographic phase: Region of interest around whole kidney, differential renal function (1-2 min post injection for MAG3)
      - Furosemide washout curves: Region of interest around whole kidney plus dilated portions of collecting system

DIFFERENTIAL DIAGNOSIS

Mechanical Obstruction

- Intrinsic
  - Upper tract obstruction
    - Congenital, stricture, stone, or urothelial mass
  - Lower tract obstruction
    - Tumor, stricture, prostate pathology, or posterior urethral valve
- Extrinsic
  - Mass, retroperitoneal fibrosis

Renogram

	Relative Renal Mass	Angiographic Phase	Clearance Phase	Renogram Curve
Normal	45-55%	Renal cortex seen within 1-3 sec after aorta; symmetric; no cortical defects	Calyceal activity: < 5 min; bladder activity: Within 10-15 min	Spontaneous washout of activity from collecting system
High-grade or complete obstruction	Cannot predict functional potential in face of high-grade obstruction	Normal to delayed	Calyceal activity usually normal, unless renal function is impaired secondary to obstruction; no bladder activity if obstruction is upper tract and bilateral	Progressive rise in activity, even after furosemide; delayed time to cortical peak; washout t1/2 > 20 min
Partial obstruction	Normal to low	Normal	Normal calyceal activity time, bladder activity may be delayed if bilateral	Washout delayed until furosemide or postvoid procedure, then will decrease but still delayed; low-grade (questionable clinical significance): t1/2 10-15 min; partial obstruction, clinically significant: t1/2 15-20 min +
Functional obstruction	Normal (unless prior high-grade obstruction caused residual decreased renal function)	Normal	Calyceal activity < 5 min; may have delayed bladder activity	Washout delayed until furosemide or postvoid procedure; then washes out normally (t1/2 < 10 min)
Renal artery stenosis	Asymmetric, with decreased relative renal mass on affected side	Delayed	Delayed calyceal activity time	Normal time-activity curve appearance, but peak is delayed

Functional Obstruction

- Dilated, nonobstructed collecting system
- May show persistent hydronephrosis in absence of, or after relief of, obstruction

Vesicoureteral Reflux

- May mimic obstruction if bladder not catheterized during furosemide renography; obstruction and reflux may coexist

Acute Tubular Necrosis

- Renal blood flow normal to slightly ↓; rising (delayed) nephrogram

Renal Artery Stenosis

- Small kidney; ± ↓ renal blood flow; delayed nephrogram; ↓ excretion; esp. with ACE inhibitors

Renal Vein Thrombosis

- Similar findings to complete obstruction: ↓ renal blood flow/function, rising nephrogram, ↓ collecting system visualization

CLINICAL ISSUES

Presentation

- Renal colic
- Impaired renal function
- Infectious symptoms
- Hydronephrosis on prenatal ultrasound

Natural History & Prognosis

- High-grade obstruction: Renal functional impairment, infection
- Low-grade obstruction: Variable outcome, careful observation if no treatment

Treatment

- Mechanical relief of obstruction: Stent, nephrostomy, pyeloplasty, urinary diversion, lithotripsy

DIAGNOSTIC CHECKLIST

Consider

- Immature kidneys may produce false-positive or indeterminate results: Wait until 6-8 weeks of age before furosemide renography

Image Interpretation Pearls

- Postural drainage maneuver: Increases specificity of furosemide renography
  - Many causes of false-positive or indeterminate scans show normal emptying in upright position
    - Severely dilated, nonobstructed kidney
    - Poor furosemide response: Poor renal function; already on furosemide
    - Atonic collecting system

SELECTED REFERENCES

1. Roudakova K et al: The evolving epidemiology of stone disease. Indian J Urol. 30(1):44-8, 2014
2. Estrada CR Jr: Prenatal hydronephrosis: early evaluation. Curr Opin Urol. 18(4):401-3, 2008
3. Karam M et al: Diuretic renogram clearance half-times in the diagnosis of obstructive uropathy: effect of age and previous surgery. Nucl Med Commun. 24(7):797-807, 2003
4. Itoh K: 99mTc-MAG3: review of pharmacokinetics, clinical application to renal diseases and quantification of renal function. Ann Nucl Med. 15(3):179-90, 2001

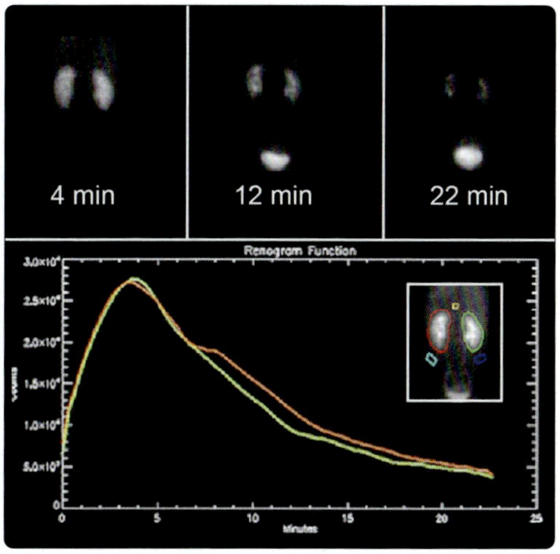

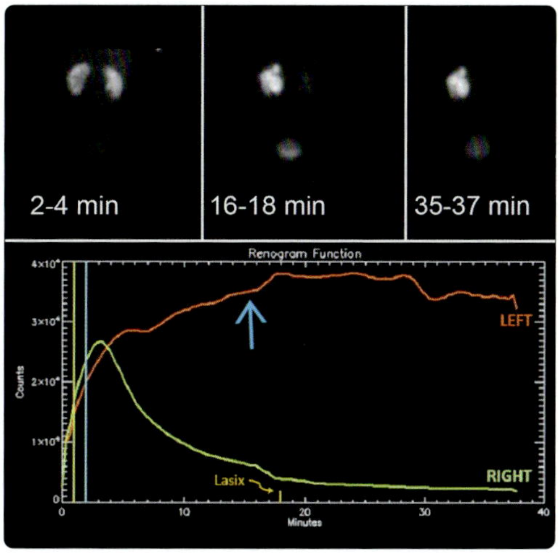

(Left) *Normal, symmetric bilateral renal function, flow, and excretion are shown without evidence of obstruction.* **(Right)** *Normal renogram of right kidney shows no obstruction. Left kidney shows complete obstruction with progressive rise in activity → in collecting system, even after furosemide.*

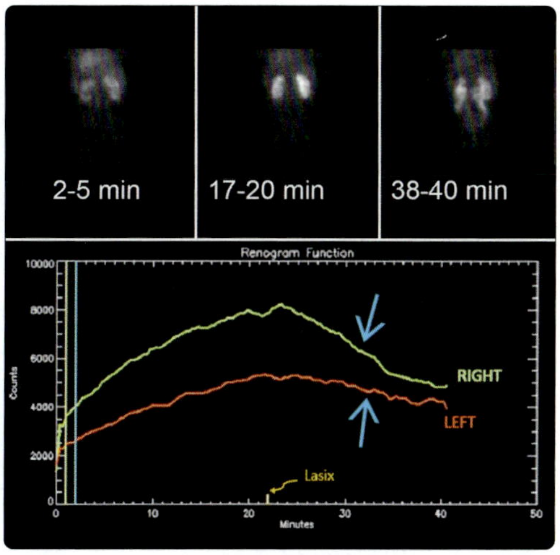

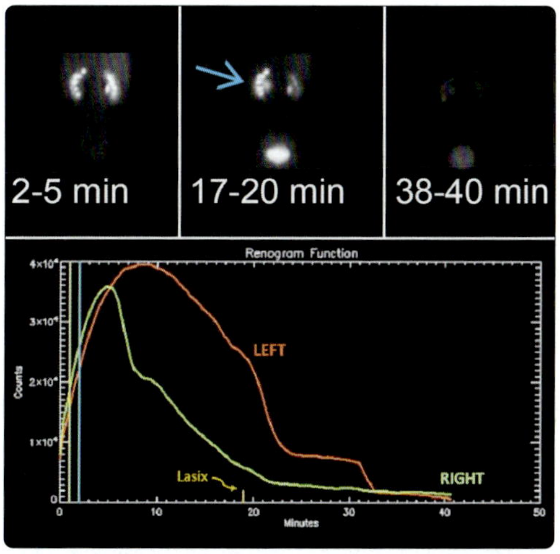

(Left) *Bilateral partial obstruction is shown. Time to calyceal activity is > 5 min and activity continues to rise until furosemide; thereafter decreases → but washout t1/2 > 10 min. Additionally, the relative functional renal mass is greater on the right. There is minimal bladder activity.* **(Right)** *Left kidney shows patulous renal collecting system → with delayed spontaneous excretion, which normalizes after furosemide. Right kidney shows normal renal function.*

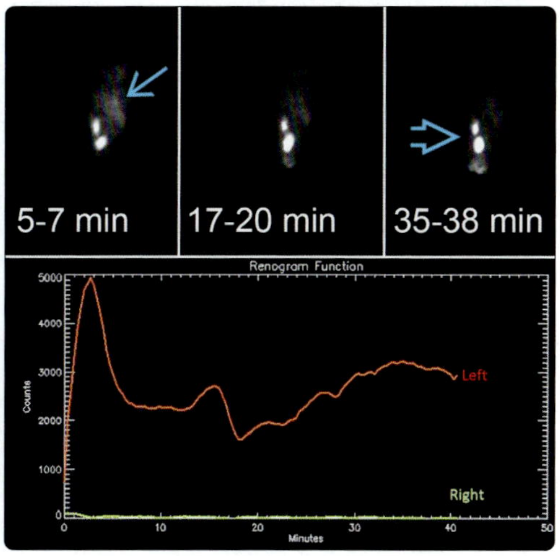

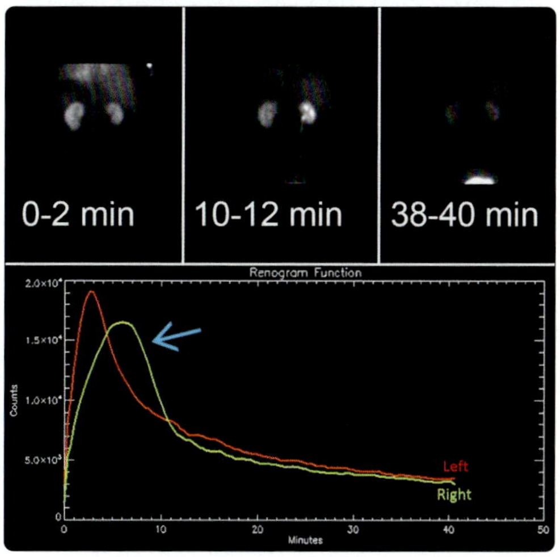

(Left) *Nonfunctioning right kidney is shown with no appreciable blood flow or uptake →. Left kidney is nonobstructed, but fluctuant activity in the pelvis and ureter ⇒ is consistent with vesicoureteral reflux. Relative renal mass is 100% on the left.* **(Right)** *Right renal artery stenosis is shown. Relative functioning renal mass is 62% on left, 38% on right. The right kidney is smaller than the left with delayed time to peak with normal washout →. There is a normal left renogram curve.*

KEY FACTS

IMAGING

- Tc-99m pertechnetate nuclear cystogram: Reflux of radiotracer from bladder into ureter, intrarenal collecting system
  - 0.5-1 mCi (18.5-37 MBq) Tc-99m pertechnetate instilled as bolus into bladder through catheter
- Sedation of young patients during study common
  - Image acquisition: Filling, voiding, post void

PATHOLOGY

- 80% of patients outgrow reflux, usually by puberty; presumably due to changes at ureterovesical junction
  - Low-grade vesicoureteric reflux (VUR) more likely to resolve
- Associated abnormalities
  - Multicystic dysplastic kidney
  - Ectopic kidneys
  - Repaired bladder exstrophy
  - Neurogenic bladder
  - Voiding dysfunction
- May also result from periureteral diverticulum, ureterocele, bladder outlet obstruction

CLINICAL ISSUES

- Serial follow-up
  - Low-grade VUR may resolve spontaneously
- Medical management
  - Prophylactic antibiotics to prevent pyelonephritis
- Surgical management
  - Ureteral reimplantation
- Minimally invasive
  - Endoscopic periureteral injections of bulking agents

DIAGNOSTIC CHECKLIST

- Tc-99m pertechnetate nuclear cystogram: More sensitive than VCUG for VUR, but gives less anatomic detail
- Tc-99m DMSA renal scan most accurate method to identify scar

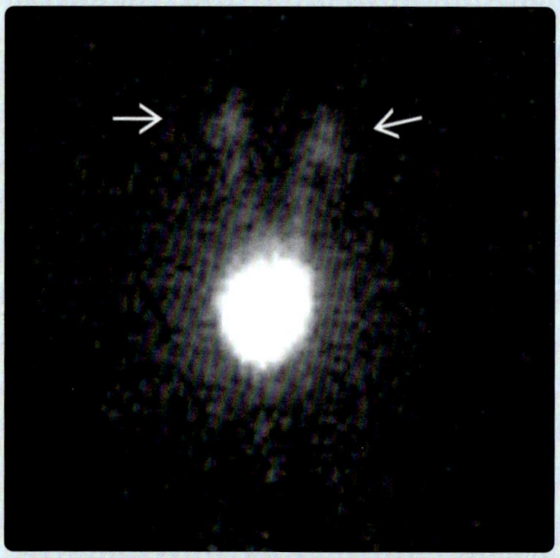

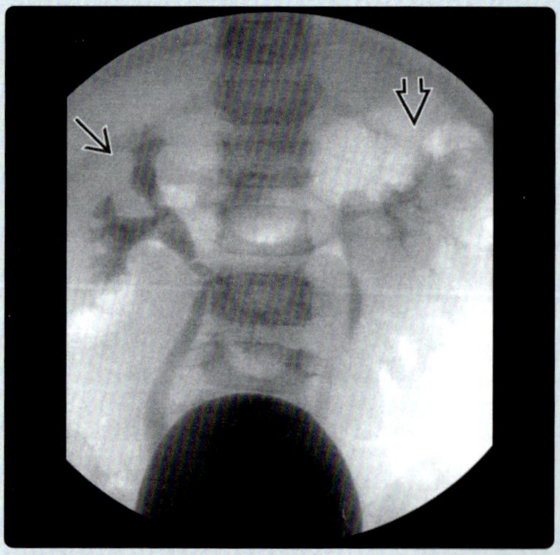

(Left) *Posterior Tc-99m pertechnetate nuclear cystogram shows bilateral vesicoureteral reflux* ➡ *to the level of the collecting systems. The right collecting system may be dilated.* **(Right)** *Voiding cystourethrogram in the same patient shows contrast in a dilated collecting system on the right* ➡ *and contrast to the level of the collecting system on the left* ⇨*.*

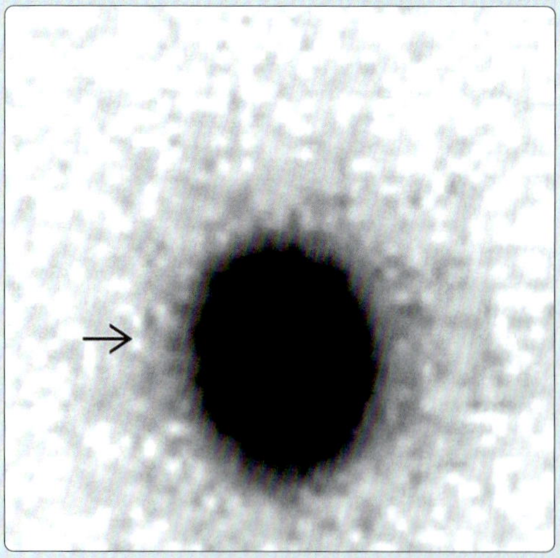

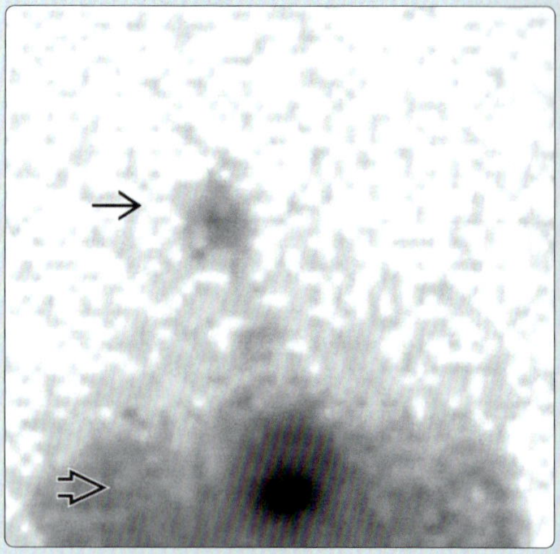

(Left) *Posterior Tc-99m pertechnetate nuclear cystogram shows radiotracer in the bladder* ➡ *and no vesicoureteric reflux on prevoid images.* **(Right)** *Posterior Tc-99m pertechnetate nuclear cystogram in the same patient after voiding shows left vesicoureteric reflux with a dilated collecting system* ➡ *and activity in the bladder and diaper* ⇨*.*

TERMINOLOGY

Abbreviations

- Vesicoureteric reflux (VUR)

Definitions

- Retrograde flow of urine from bladder into ureter &/or renal pelvis

IMAGING

Nuclear Medicine Findings

- Nuclear cystogram
  - Reflux of Tc-99m pertechnetate from bladder into ureter &/or renal collecting system on filling or voiding
  - Dynamic images during filling and voiding increases detection of VUR, including transient reflux
  - Difficult to grade VUR on nuclear cystogram due to lack of anatomic resolution
    - Qualitatively reported as mild, moderate, or severe

Fluoroscopic Findings

- Voiding cystourethrogram
  - VCUG: Anatomic information in addition to reflux evaluation
  - Early filling image of bladder best shows intraluminal abnormalities: Ureterocele, polyp, mass
  - Iodinated contrast in ureter, renal collecting system on filling or voiding = VUR
  - Oblique views of distended bladder help show periureteral diverticula and ureteric insertion into bladder in cases of VUR
  - Voiding images of urethra to exclude distal pathology: Contribute to back pressure, bladder outlet obstruction
  - Grading of VUR

Ultrasonographic Findings

- Normal US
- Pelvicalyceal, ureteral, collecting system dilatation
- US not sensitive or specific for VUR

Imaging Recommendations

- Best imaging tool
  - Nuclear cystogram
    - Serial evaluation in patients with VUR to assess for spontaneous resolution
    - Follow-up after antireflux procedure or after antibiotic therapy
    - Initial evaluation of females with UTI
    - Screening of patients who have a sibling with VUR
    - Used in patients with neurogenic bladder to diagnose VUR
    - Used to quantify postvoid residual volume in urinary bladder
    - Voiding cystourethrography is usually initial study if high clinical suspicion for VUR or if anatomic detail needed
      - Preferred for anatomic detail of upper tracts and evaluation of urethral anatomy
      - More radiation than nuclear cystogram
  - Tc-99m dimercaptosuccinic acid (DMSA) renal scan
    - Best method to identify scarring secondary to reflux or infection
    - Planar or SPECT images may be obtained
  - Tc-99m diethylenetriamine pentaacetic acid (DTPA) or MAG3 renogram
    - Can diagnose VUR indirectly using renogram
      - Perform conventional dynamic renogram prior to voiding phase
      - After activity clears from kidneys and ureters, record dynamic images during voiding
      - Avoids bladder catheterization
      - Less sensitive than direct radionuclide cystography
      - Not recommended in non-toilet-trained children
- Protocol advice
  - Patient voids prior to procedure
  - Sedation of patient during study may be performed
  - Bladder catheterization using sterile technique
  - Patient position
    - Filling phase
      - Supine
      - Camera posterior
    - Voiding phase
      - Infants, toddlers, and uncooperative children are supine
      - Cooperative children sit upright
      - Camera posterior
  - Radiopharmaceutical instilled as bolus into bladder through catheter
    - Tc-99m pertechnetate
      - Activity of 0.25-0.5 mCi (9.25-18.5 MBq) for infants and toddlers
      - Administered activity 0.5-1 mCi (18.5-37 MBq) for adults
    - Tc-99m sulfur colloid or Tc-99m DTPA can also be used
    - Bolus administration ensures entire amount of radiotracer delivered to bladder
  - Instillation of fluid volume after radiotracer bolus
    - Bladder volume goal: [Age in years + 2] x 30 cc
    - Normal saline, water
    - Gravity instill fluid 70-100 cm above patient via catheter
    - Record volume at which VUR occurs
    - Record volume of voided urine
  - Image acquisition
    - Protect camera from urine contamination
    - Low-energy, all-purpose collimator or high-resolution collimator
    - 64 x 64 acquisition matrix
    - Posterior images of pelvis and abdomen, unless calculation of residual bladder volume is planned
      - Anterior and posterior images required for residual bladder volume calculation
    - Filling and voiding dynamic images at 5-10 sec/frame, posterior
    - Once bladder goal volume is reached, instruct patient to void
    - Prevoid and postvoid static images, 3-5 minutes each
  - Image processing
    - Residual volume quantification

- Prevoid and postvoid anterior and posterior images
- Regions of interest (ROI) drawn over bladder
- Residual volume (mL) = (voided volume in mL x postvoid bladder ROI count) / (initial bladder ROI count - postvoid bladder ROI count)

DIFFERENTIAL DIAGNOSIS

Radiotracer Contamination

- Contamination may occur with urination, radiotracer activity on skin or in diaper
- May mimic VUR on nuclear cystography

Bladder Diverticulum

- Primary (congenital defect, protrusion through bladder wall) or secondary (obstruction, neurogenic dysfunction)
- May mimic VUR on nuclear cystography

PATHOLOGY

General Features

- Associated abnormalities
  - Vesicoureteral reflux has clear association with acute pyelonephritis, renal scarring
  - Multicystic dysplastic kidney
  - Ectopic kidneys
    - Note that VUR most commonly involves contralateral orthotopic kidney
  - Repaired bladder exstrophy
  - Neurogenic bladder
  - Voiding dysfunction
- May also result from periureteral diverticulum, ureterocele, bladder outlet obstruction

Staging, Grading, & Classification

- Nuclear cystogram grading
  - Mild: Reflux in ureter
  - Moderate: Reflux to nondilated ureter and renal pelvis
  - Severe: Reflux to dilated collecting system
- Scale used for VCUG is not used in nuclear cystography; best to be descriptive

Gross Pathologic & Surgical Features

- Deficiency or immaturity of longitudinal muscle in submucosal ureter
- Distortion of ureteral insertion by adjacent bladder anomaly
- Abnormal angle of ureteral insertion through bladder wall (tends to correct as ureter grows and elongates)

CLINICAL ISSUES

Presentation

- Most common signs/symptoms
  - Most often discovered during work-up of UTI
  - Higher grades of reflux may be suspected on prenatal ultrasound
  - ~ 50% of patients with UTIs have reflux
  - Prevalence of UTIs in infants, young children: 5%

Demographics

- Age
  - VUR most common in children < 2 years
- Gender
  - F:M = 2:1
- Ethnicity
  - More common in Caucasians than African Americans (reports of 3:1 to 20:1)
- Epidemiology
  - Incidence varies; reported as low as < 1% and as high as 1-2% of general population
  - VUR in 25-40% of children with acute pyelonephritis
  - VUR seen in 5-50% of asymptomatic siblings of children with documented VUR

Natural History & Prognosis

- 80% outgrow VUR before puberty
  - Low-grade VUR more likely to resolve
- Can lead to renal scar, renal insufficiency, hypertension, end-stage renal disease
- Prognosis is dependent upon degree and duration of VUR, presence of UTIs, scarring

Treatment

- Treat infection before performing VCUG, nuclear cystogram
- Medical management
  - Prophylactic antibiotics to prevent pyelonephritis
- Surgical management
  - Ureteral reimplantation
  - Minimally invasive endoscopic periureteral injections of bulking agents
- Definitive treatment indicated with repeated infections despite antibiotic prophylaxis; evidence of renal scarring by Tc-99m DMSA renal scan

DIAGNOSTIC CHECKLIST

Consider

- Tc-99m pertechnetate nuclear cystogram: More sensitive than VCUG for VUR but gives less anatomic detail
- Tc-99m DMSA most accurate method for identifying scarring

Image Interpretation Pearls

- Reporting of nuclear cystogram
  - Number of attempted bladder fills
  - Total volume instilled into bladder
  - Bladder volume at reflux
  - Assessment of VUR magnitude
  - Whether VUR occurred at filling or voiding
  - Qualitative/quantitative residual bladder volume

SELECTED REFERENCES

1. American College of Radiology. ACR–SPR–SNM Practice Guideline for the Performance of Adult and Pediatric Radionuclide Cystography. 2010
2. Boubaker A et al: Radionuclide investigations of the urinary tract in the era of multimodality imaging. J Nucl Med. 47(11):1819-36, 2006
3. Piepsz A et al: Pediatric applications of renal nuclear medicine. Semin Nucl Med. 36(1):16-35, 2006
4. Unver T et al: Comparison of direct radionuclide cystography and voiding cystourethrography in detecting vesicoureteral reflux. Pediatr Int. 48(3):287-91, 2006

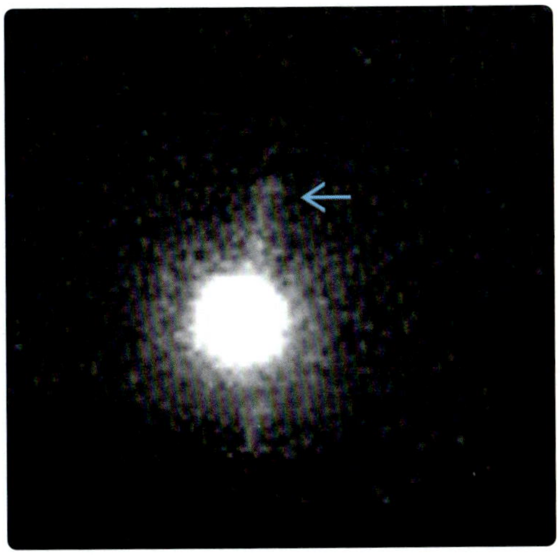

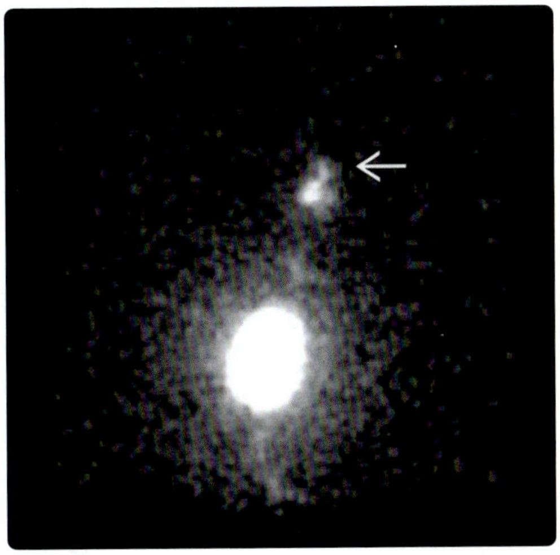

(Left) *Posterior Tc-99m pertechnetate nuclear cystogram shows vesicoureteral reflux to the mid right ureter* ⇨*, which is not dilated.* **(Right)** *Posterior Tc-99m pertechnetate nuclear cystogram shows vesicoureteral reflux into the right renal pelvis* ➡*, which is dilated.*

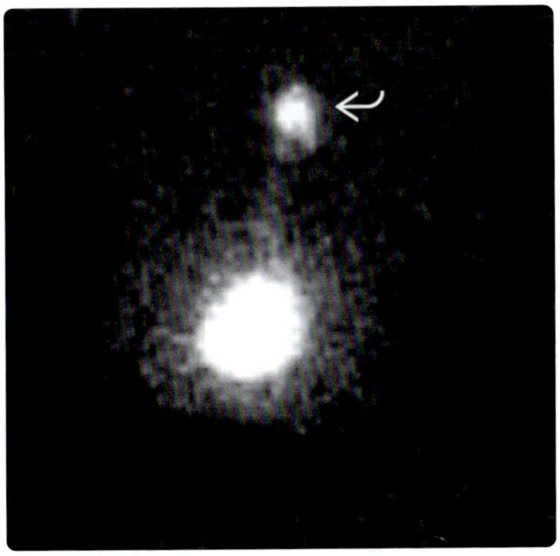

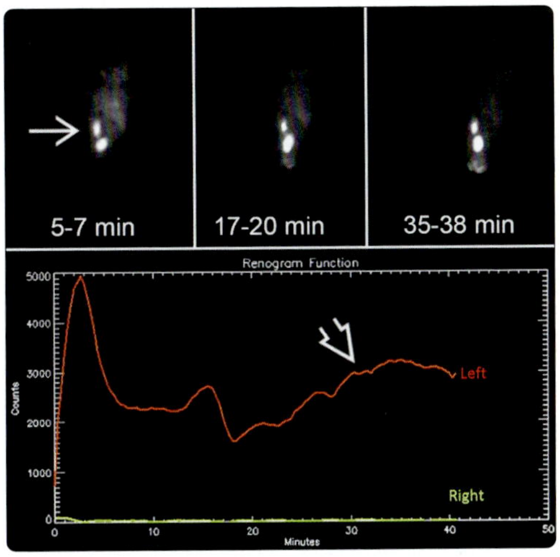

(Left) *Posterior Tc-99m pertechnetate nuclear cystogram shows vesicoureteral reflux into a dilated right renal pelvis* ➡*.* **(Right)** *Posterior indirect cystogram using Tc-99m MAG3 renogram shows radiotracer in the left renal collecting system* ➡ *that increases over time due to vesicoureteric reflux* ➡*.*

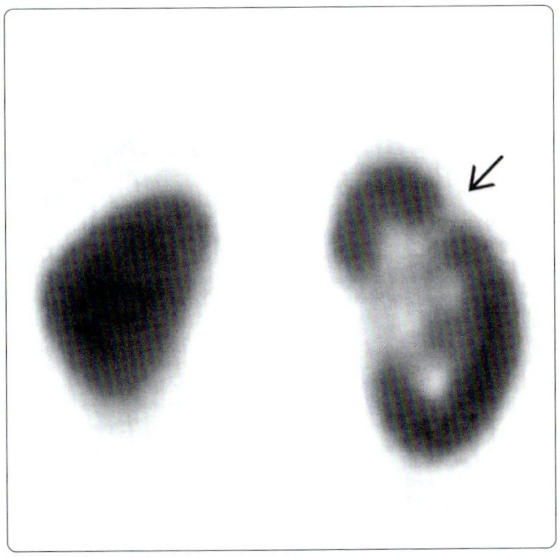

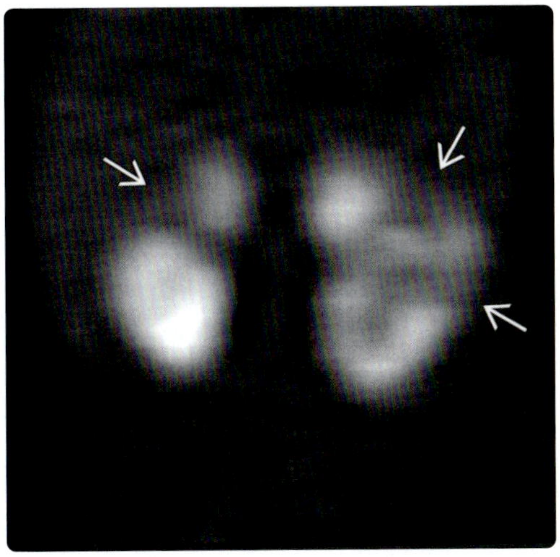

(Left) *Coronal Tc-99m DMSA renal scan SPECT shows cortical scarring in superolateral upper pole of the left kidney* ⇨*, a typical pattern resulting from high-grade reflux.* **(Right)** *Coronal Tc-99m DMSA renal scan SPECT shows multifocal cortical scars* ➡ *in a patient with vesicoureteric reflux and chronic urinary tract infections.*

KEY FACTS

TERMINOLOGY

- Renal scintigraphy can assist in setting of renal transplant to evaluate and potentially differentiate cause of early or late allograft dysfunction
- Acute tubular necrosis (ATN): Poor function immediately post transplant from preoperative ischemic/reperfusion injury to allograft
- Acute rejection (AR): Cellular or humoral antibody-mediated rejection
- AR occurs any time: Most common ~ 5-7 days to 1st few months
- Chronic rejection (CR): Untreatable delayed humoral process of fibrosis, cortical loss

IMAGING

- Cortical retention seen in AR and ATN
- Time course of events highly important: ATN typically presents earlier and improves
- Perfusion in AR generally worse than function: Often technically difficult to visualize
- Drug toxicity can appear very similar to ATN
- Sensitivity and specificity lower for late AR: May be superimposed on CR (biopsy required)
- Urinoma/urine leak: Days to weeks postoperatively; ↑ creatine due to reabsorbed urine
- Lymphocele: Typically 2-4 months postoperatively

DIAGNOSTIC CHECKLIST

- Activity in bladder from native kidneys may mask obstruction
- Full bladder or reflux may mimic obstruction: Empty bladder critical for renal scan
- Small IV site, poor bolus, or extravasation of dose: Mimic decreased blood flow to transplant
- Hypotension can mimic decreased flow and excretion from transplant

(Left) *Whole-body scan from a Tc-99m methylene diphosphonate bone scan in a patient with chronic back pain demonstrates normal uptake of radiotracer in a transplant kidney in the right lower quadrant.* **(Right)** *Transplant renogram in the left lower quadrant demonstrates normal flow during the angiographic phase of imaging.*

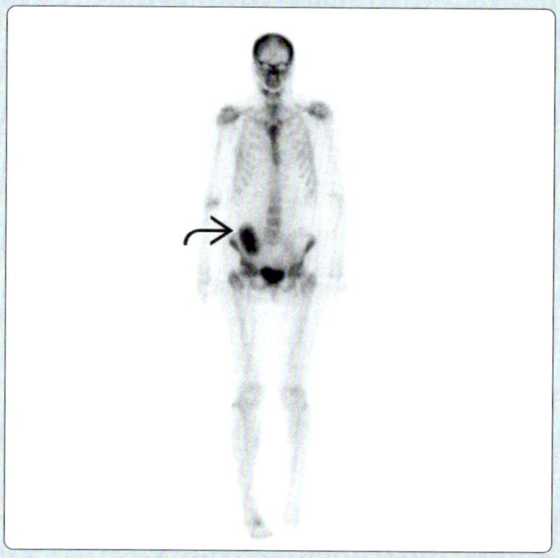

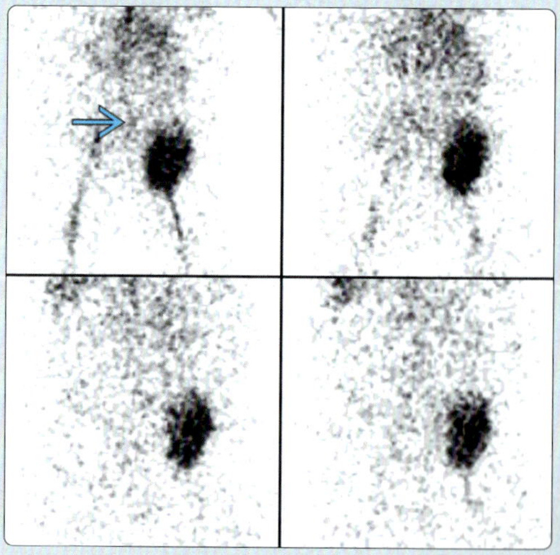

(Left) *Excretion images from a Tc-99m mercaptoacetyltriglycine (MAG3) transplant renogram demonstrate normal excretion from the transplant kidney with expected accumulation of radiotracer in the bladder.* **(Right)** *Normal time-activity curve in the same patient shows rapid peak uptake and washout of radiotracer in a baseline exam of a living related donor allograft.*

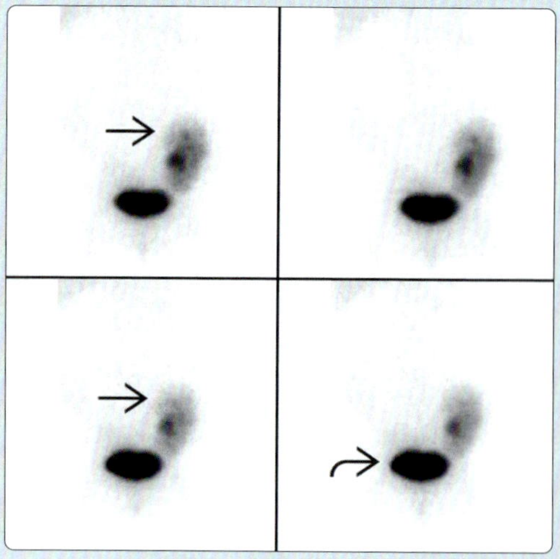

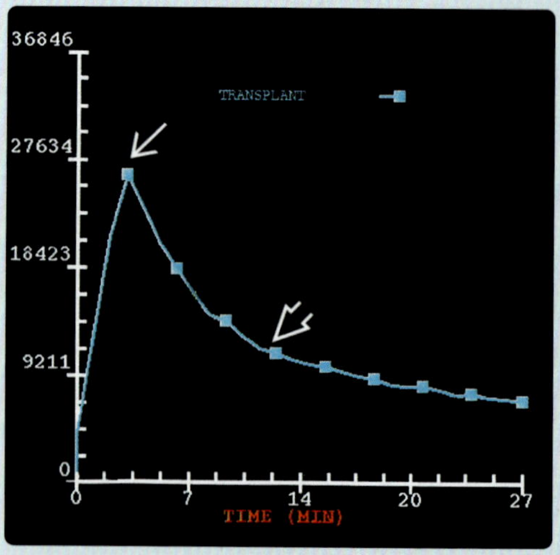

TERMINOLOGY

Definitions

- Renal transplant evaluation with Tc-99m mercaptoacetyltriglycine (MAG3) and diethylene-triamine-pentaacetate (DTPA) renography
  - Assists in setting of renal transplant to evaluate and potentially differentiate cause of early or late allograft dysfunction
    - Vascular complications
    - Acute rejection (AR) and chronic rejection (CR)
    - Acute tubular necrosis (ATN)
    - Obstruction
    - Urinoma and lymphocele formation

IMAGING

Nuclear Medicine Findings

- Renal scintigraphy
  - Tc-99m MAG3
    - Renal tubular agent, preferred for renal transplant evaluation
  - Tc-99m DTPA
    - Slower clearance than MAG3, limited utility in cases of poor renal function with extraction fraction << MAG3 (cleared by glomerular filtration)
    - Renogram curves in ATN and AR are different with DTPA, reflecting different mechanisms (filtered instead of excreted)
  - Tc-99m dimercaptosuccinic acid (DMSA)
    - Incorporated into tubular cells
    - For parenchymal imaging in pyelonephritis and cortical scarring

Imaging Recommendations

- Protocol advice
  - Baseline renogram at 24-48 hr to assess function and allow better differentiation of ATN and AR
    - Knowing baseline uptake slope and degree of cortical retention critical in identification of developing/worsening AR
  - Patient preparation: 300-500 mL water p.o. or IV hydration (7 mL/kg)
  - Patient voids immediately before exam or bladder catheterized in those with incomplete emptying
  - Patient position: Supine with camera anterior, centered over side of pelvis containing transplant
  - Camera: Low-energy, all-purpose collimator
  - Computer: Acquire study in 2 phases, angiogram and functional
    - Angiogram: Dynamic 1-2 sec/frame for 60 sec
    - Functional: 15-60-sec frames for 20-30 min followed by prevoid and postvoid images
  - Radiotracer
    - Tc-99m MAG3: Up to 10 mCi (370 MBq) IV in adults; 0.05-0.1 mCi (1.85-3.7 MBq)/kg in pediatrics, max 5 mCi (185 MBq)
    - 2nd line: Tc-99m DTPA, up to 15 mCi (555 MBq) IV in adults; 0.1-0.2 mCi (3.7-7.4 MBq)/kg in pediatrics, max 5 mCi (185 MBq)
    - Tc-99m DMSA: Up to 5 mCi (185 MBq) in adults; 0.05-0.1 mCi (1.85-3.7 MBq)/kg in pediatrics, max 3 mCi (111 mBq)
    - Positioning arm at 90° angle to body will minimize axillary retention of tracer
  - Diuretic: Furosemide (0.5 mg/kg, max 40 mg in adults, 1 mg/kg in pediatrics) if obstruction suspected; administer 20-30 min after radiotracer injection if good function
  - Processing
    - Region of interest (ROI) around kidney, background next to kidney (can be cortical or whole-kidney ROI)
    - Background ROI preferences vary: Crescent or encircle allograft
    - Time-activity curve (TAC) processing: For blood flow and dynamic function phases
    - Measures of excretion: Seen in 3rd phase of TAC and ratios of late counts to peak counts (e.g., 20/max ratio)
  - Calculate measures of excretion/cortical retention
    - Perfusion index: Kidney to aorta (iliac artery for transplant) ratio
    - t1/2: Time required to go from maximal counts to 1/2-maximal counts (normal 6.6 ± 2.8 min)
    - 20/max count ratio: Ratio of counts at 20 min to peak counts; > 0.35 is abnormal for cortical ROIs
  - Calculate glomerular filtration rate or effective renal plasma flow (ERPF): May allow earliest identification of chronic allograft nephropathy
  - Dosimetry
    - Critical organ is bladder
    - Hydration lowers dose, no safety precautions required after study completion
    - Effective dose ~ 3 mSv
- Interpretation
  - Perfusion to allograft: Normally within 4 sec of radiotracer bolus passing through iliac artery
  - Normal peak cortical activity 3-5 min post injection
  - Normal renal transit: Tracer in collecting system, bladder by 6 min
  - By end of exam, cortex should clear or be significantly less than early in exam if no cortical retention
  - Cortical retention seen in ATN, AR, CR
  - Cortical loss and dilated pelvis helpful identifiers in CR
- Additional nuclear medicine imaging options
  - Labeled leukocyte scintigraphy: Patchy or focal uptake may indicate pyelonephritis (low sensitivity)
    - In-111 preferred over Tc-99m HMPAO WBCs: Tc-99m HMPAO metabolites excreted by kidneys
    - In-111 WBCs typically show diffuse uptake even in healthy transplants due to mononuclear cell residence from previous rejection

DIFFERENTIAL DIAGNOSIS

Vascular Complications

- Fairly rare: Occlusions seen < 1% and renal artery stenosis (RAS) up to 10%
  - Renal vein thrombosis (RVT): Different pattern in transplant vs. native kidney RVT
    - Transplant RVT: Lack of draining collaterals, overall perfusion ↓ causing absent or photopenic transplant

- Imaging appearance therefore similar to arterial thrombosis
  - Native kidney RVT: Large, hot kidney as activity accumulates in but does not clear
- Renal artery thrombosis: Also shows absent function; can be patchy if distal; Tc-99m DMSA renal scan can be useful
- RAS: Typically late complication (> 1 year post transplant)
  - Imaging pattern similar to that for native kidney captopril renography

Acute Tubular Necrosis

- Classically presents with relatively preserved perfusion and delayed uptake/excretion (tubular agents)
- Abnormal baseline renal scan at 24 hr (AR typically occurs later)
- In severe cases, diminished flow may also be present, making distinction from rejection and other entities difficult
- Bladder activity classically absent; background activity increases over time (e.g., gallbladder with MAG3)

Acute Rejection

- Perfusion in AR generally worse than function: Often technically difficult to visualize
- ↑ cortical retention compared with baseline from 1 week to < 1 year: Sensitive, fairly specific for AR
- Specificity of cortical retention low without baseline as scar; incomplete resolution of ATN may be present
- Late-developing AR and immunosuppressive drug toxicity appear similar
- Sensitivity and specificity lower for late AR: May be superimposed on CR (biopsy required)

Chronic Rejection

- Rare in transplant < 1 year unless prior episodes of severely compromised function
- 1st sign: ↓ blood flow, ERPF with relatively spared function
- Over time, cortical thinning with worsening uptake and clearance develop, along with ↑ cortical dilation
- Furosemide may help differentiate from obstruction

Drug Toxicity

- Calcineurin inhibitors (cyclosporine and tacrolimus) cause nephrotoxicity through arteriolar vasoconstriction and tubulointerstitial injury
- Imaging appearance is similar to and difficult to distinguish from ATN (preserved perfusion and poor tubular function)
  - Typically presents later than ATN (time course very important)

Surgical Complications

- Obstruction: May occur from days to years postoperatively
  - Activity in bladder from native kidneys may mask obstruction
  - Full bladder or reflux may mimic obstruction: Empty bladder critical for renal scan
- Urinoma/urine leak: Days to weeks postoperatively; ↑ creatinine due to reabsorbed urine
- Lymphocele: Typically 2-4 months postoperatively

Pyelonephritis

- More common in allografts than general population, ↑ with vesicoureteral reflux

PATHOLOGY

General Features

- Delayed graft function: Definition varies but generally refers to oliguria or need for dialysis within 1st week post transplant
  - Most commonly due to ATN: Ischemic injury- and reperfusion-related free radical damage
  - More common in cadaveric allografts (up to 50%); only 5% in live donors
  - Usually resolves/improves spontaneously, severe cases that do not resolve indicate poor prognosis
- Rejection: Autoimmune response mounted against transplanted allograft, usually T-cell mediated
  - Hyperacute: Rejection of graft immediately after release of vascular cross clamp; caused by deposition of preformed antibodies; now largely eliminated by better screening
  - Accelerated: Specific form of AR occurring in previously sensitized patients with anti-HLA antibodies; usually presents 3-5 days post transplant
  - AR: Cellular or humoral antibody-mediated rejection
    - AR occurs any time: Most common ~ 5-7 days-1st few months
    - AR is rare > 1st year
    - Tubulitis and arteritis are principle lesions indicative of AR on pathology per Banff classification
  - CR: Untreatable delayed humoral process of fibrosis, cortical loss
    - Progressive decline in renal function due to failure to maintain immunosuppression of antigraft lymphocytes or antibodies
    - CR is currently most common cause of graft loss due to advances in AR therapy

DIAGNOSTIC CHECKLIST

Image Interpretation Pearls

- Bladder emptying critical to accurate interpretation
- Tc-99m DTPA has different renogram curves for ATN and AR, potential for more diagnostic utility
- False-positives
  - Small IV site, poor bolus, or extravasation of dose: Mimic decreased blood flow to transplant
  - Hypotension can mimic decreased flow and excretion from transplant
  - Full bladder can mimic obstruction and obscure visualization of urinoma (use Foley catheter if urinoma suspected)

SELECTED REFERENCES

1. Taylor AT: Radionuclides in nephrourology, part 1: radiopharmaceuticals, quality control, and quantitative indices. J Nucl Med. 55(4):608-15, 2014
2. Taylor AT: Radionuclides in nephrourology, part 2: pitfalls and diagnostic applications. J Nucl Med. 55(5):786-98, 2014
3. Nankivell BJ et al: Rejection of the kidney allograft. N Engl J Med. 363(15):1451-62, 2010
4. Russell CD et al: Prediction of renal transplant survival from early postoperative radioisotope studies. J Nucl Med. 41(8):1332-6, 2000
5. Dubovsky EV et al: Report of the Radionuclides in Nephrourology Committee for evaluation of transplanted kidney (review of techniques). Semin Nucl Med. 29(2):175-88, 1999

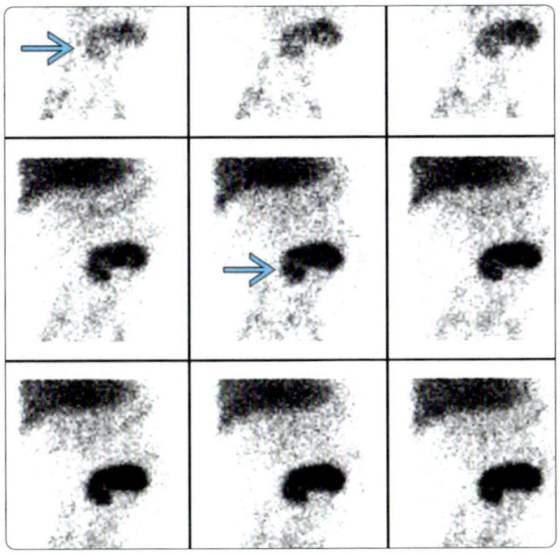
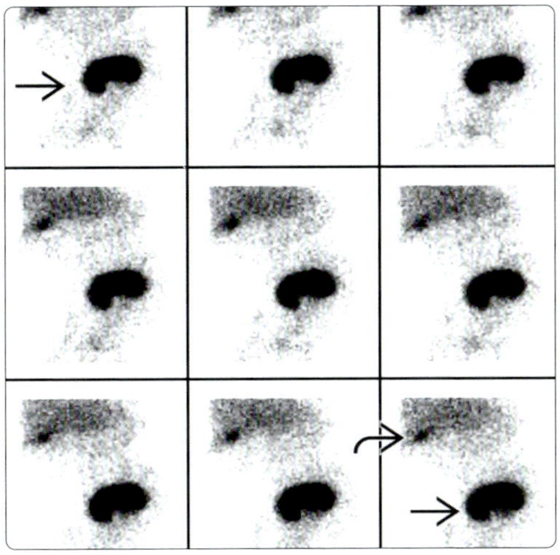

(Left) *Anterior MAG3 renogram shows left pelvic transplant kidney ➔ with normal perfusion. Radiopharmaceutical should be evident in transplant within 4 sec of iliac vessel visualization.* **(Right)** *Excretion images from a transplant Tc-99m MAG3 renogram demonstrate progressive cortical accumulation of the radiotracer and no significant excretion ➔. Also note the accumulation of background activity, including the gallbladder ↪, a pattern typical of acute tubular necrosis.*

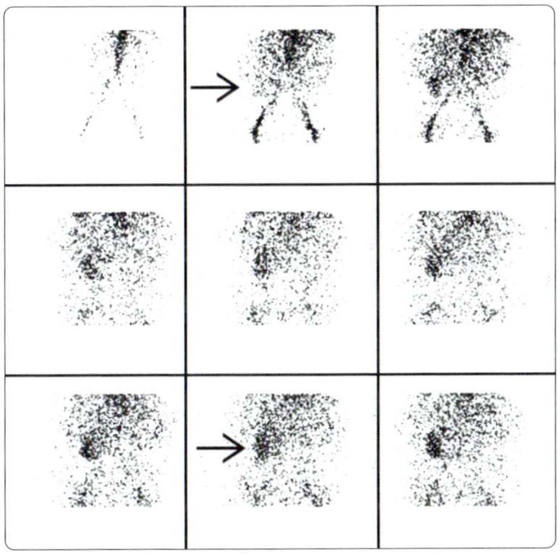
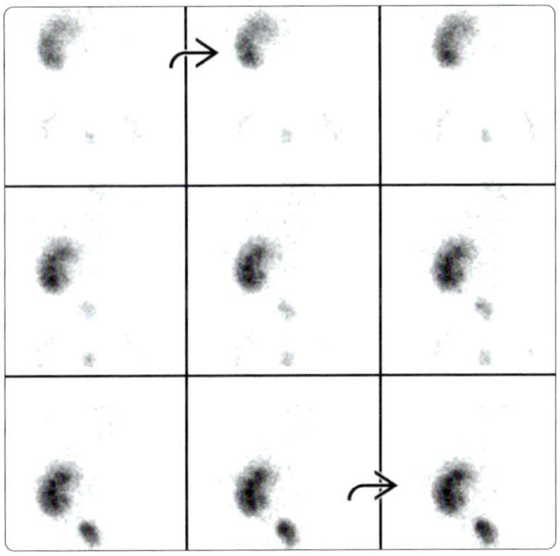

(Left) *Perfusion images from a Tc-99m MAG3 renogram demonstrate decreased perfusion to a right lower quadrant renal transplant ➔.* **(Right)** *Excretion images from a Tc-99m MAG3 renogram demonstrate decreased excretion and mild cortical retention from a right lower quadrant renal transplant ↪. This patient had chronic rejection.*

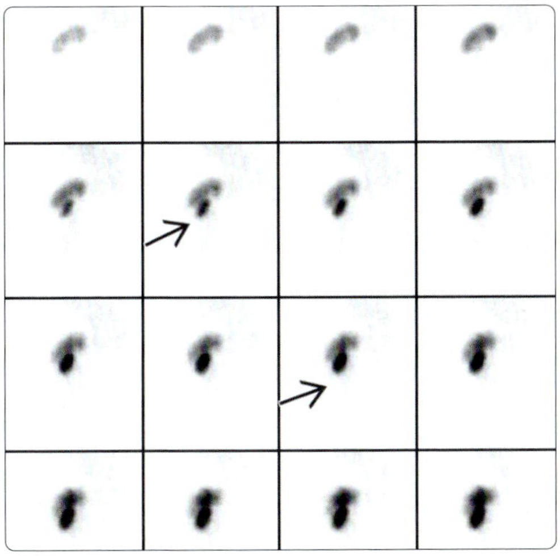
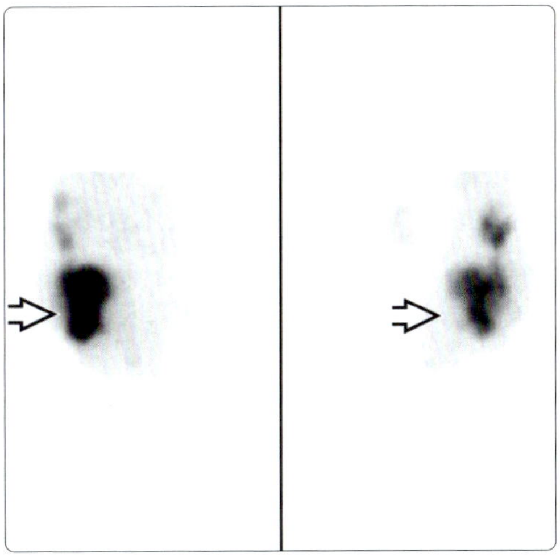

(Left) *Excretion images from a Tc-99m MAG3 renogram demonstrate accumulation of tracer inferior to the right lower quadrant renal transplant ➔.* **(Right)** *Delayed postvoid images demonstrate accumulation of radiotracer in the right flank ⇨, confirming the suspected diagnosis of urinoma. Utilizing different projections is often useful and necessary to distinguish urinomas from anatomy.*

KEY FACTS

IMAGING

- ACE-inhibited (ACEI) renography is excellent way to detect clinically significant renal artery stenosis (RAS)
- Unilateral parenchymal retention following ACEI administration is most important diagnostic criterion
- Bilateral abnormalities are often nonspecific, chronic, or procedure related
- In patients with normal or minimally reduced renal function (creatinine < 1.7 mg/dL); sensitivity and specificity are ~ 90%
- Sensitivity and specificity of study are improved when gold standard is response to revascularization, rather than anatomic presence of RAS
- Probability of renovascular hypertension (RVHT) is graded as low, intermediate, or high
    - High-probability scan with Tc-99m MAG3: Increased peak time by 2-3 min or 40%

CLINICAL ISSUES

- RAS is most common cause of secondary hypertension (HTN)
- Untreated RVHT leads to irreversible renal damage, may cause chronic renal failure
- ACEI renography can be more cost effective 1st test than CTA or MRA in appropriately selected population
- ACEI renography is far more useful in non-azotemic patients (up to 50% of azotemic patients have intermediate probability study)
- RAS can be detected with conventional imaging
    - Not all patients with RAS have RVHT
- RVHT is related to but distinct from RAS and can be detected with ACEI renography uniquely
- ACEI-induced renographic changes indicate high probability that HTN will be cured or improved after revascularization

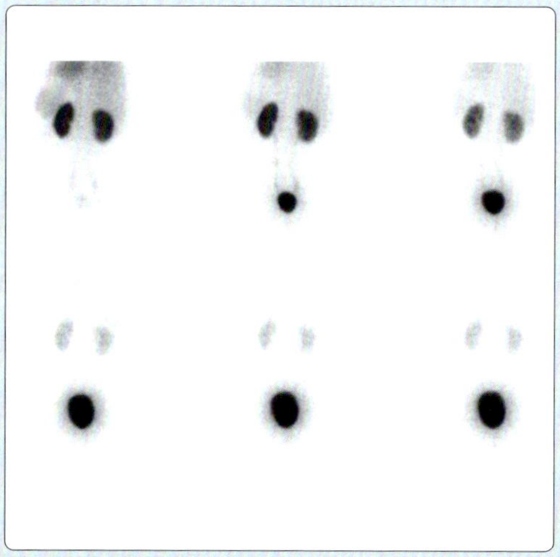

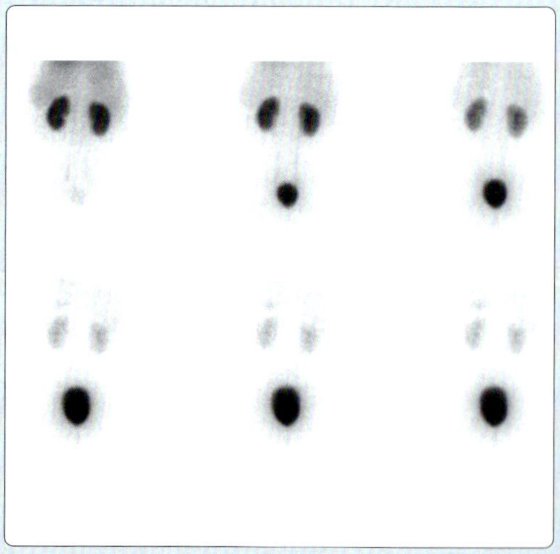

(Left) *Pre-captopril posterior ACE-inhibited renography demonstrates normal symmetric excretion bilaterally.* **(Right)** *Post-captopril posterior ACE-inhibited renography demonstrates normal symmetric excretion bilaterally.*

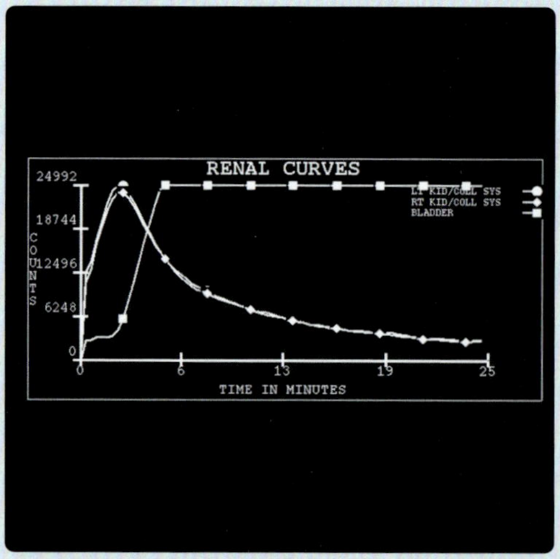

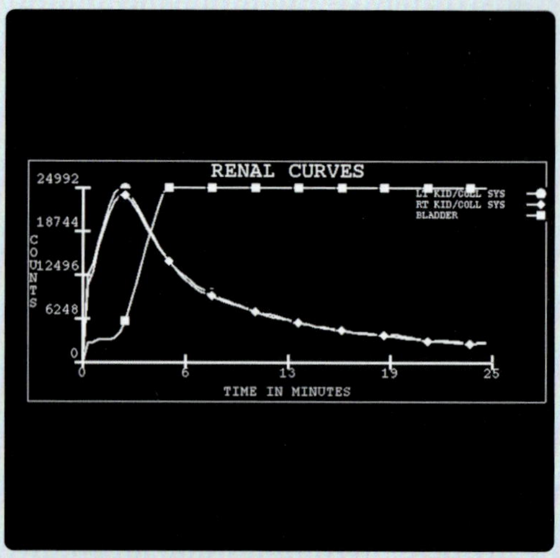

(Left) *Chart shows pre-captopril posterior ACE-inhibited renography, demonstrating normal symmetric excretion bilaterally.* **(Right)** *Chart shows post-captopril posterior ACE-inhibited renography, demonstrating normal symmetric excretion bilaterally.*

TERMINOLOGY

Abbreviations

- Renovascular hypertension (RVHT)

Definitions

- Hypertension (HTN) caused by hemodynamically significant renal artery stenosis (RAS) activating renin-angiotensin system

IMAGING

General Features

- Best diagnostic clue
  - ACE inhibitor (ACEI) renogram showing functional deterioration after ACEI administration compared with baseline renogram

Nuclear Medicine Findings

- Baseline Tc-99m mercaptoacetyltriglycine (MAG3) renogram (without ACEI)
  - Blood flow usually not perceptibly altered; nonspecific small kidney or ↓ function could be seen but scan often normal
  - Nonspecific: Any abnormality could be caused by numerous etiologies (e.g., obstruction)
- ACEI renogram: Excellent detection of clinically significant RAS; sensitivity > 90% and specificity 95% in those with good renal function
  - Patients without RVHT show no significant change from baseline
  - Functional deterioration after ACEI compared with baseline identifies patients with reversible RVHT with high accuracy
  - Angiographic phase unreliable: Technically difficult to perform, flow often normal or ↓ due to low tissue volume in small kidneys
- Time-activity curves and renal-function images will vary depending on radiopharmaceutical
- Renogram using Tc-99m DTPA: Shows overall decrease in uptake and function of kidney with RAS after ACEI
  - Renal excretion of DTPA exclusively by glomerular filtration and directly reflects glomerular filtration rate (GFR)
- Renogram using Tc-99m MAG-3: Shows significant cortical retention of radiotracer in kidney with RAS after ACEI
  - MAG-3 excreted by tubular secretion, so drop in GFR does not affect uptake

Imaging Recommendations

- Protocol advice
  - Patient preparation
    - Stop ACEI 3-7 days prior to exam; if not, sensitivity decreases (~ 15-17%)
      - Stop short-acting ACEI (e.g., captopril) 3 days before; 5-7 days for long-acting ACEI
      - Also stop angiotensin II receptor blockers, e.g., losartan
    - Stop diuretics and calcium channel blockers, if safe
    - Hydrate p.o.; 7 mL/kg 30-60 min before study
    - Place IV for radiopharmaceutical injection and IV fluids in case of hypotension post ACEI, or if receiving IV enalapril
    - Empty bladder immediately before exam
    - Position patient supine with camera posterior for native kidneys and anterior for renal transplant
  - Radiotracer: MAG3 adult 1-10 mCi/kg (37-370 MBq/kg), child 0.1 mCi/kg (3.7 MBq/kg); DTPA adult 1-10 mCi/kg (37-370 MBq/kg), child 0.1 mCi/kg (3.7 MBq/kg)
  - Choose 1-day or 2-day protocol depending on clinical suspicion or patient population
    - 2-day protocol (low probability of disease): ACEI scan 1st; if abnormal, baseline scan 1-2 days later; routine radiotracer dose used for each exam
    - 1-day protocol (high probability of disease): 1 mCi (37 MBq) low-dose baseline followed by 5-10 mCi (200-400 MBq) high-dose ACEI scan
      - Time required between 2 depends on dose; if 1 mCi is used, begin 2nd part as soon as 1st study has concluded
  - ACEI
    - Captopril: 25-50 mg p.o. (may crush tablets), monitor blood pressure every 5-15 min for 1 hr; patient should be n.p.o. 4-6 hr for best absorption
      - Wait 60 min to administer radiopharmaceutical
    - Enalapril: 40 μg/kg IV up to 2.5 mg given over 3-5 min
      - Wait 15 min to administer radiopharmaceutical
      - Advantages include shorter study time, no interference with absorption; disadvantages include higher risk of procedural hypotension
  - Diuretic: Furosemide (20 mg) during imaging may improve accuracy of exam
    - Increases washout of tubular agents, improves sensitivity of cortical retention
    - Can be used at beginning of both studies; higher risk of hypotension
  - Acquisition
    - Camera: Low-energy, parallel hole collimator; 15-20% photopeak centered at 140 keV; large field of view
    - Computer: Blood flow 1-2-sec frames/60 sec and dynamic 30-sec frames for 25-30 min; prevoid, postvoid static images
  - Processing: Regions of interest (ROIs) over closest adjacent vessel (iliac artery) and around kidney with background area near/around kidney
    - ROIs typically done as whole kidney; addition of cortical ROIs can be helpful if there is retention of tracer in pelvocalyceal system
  - Dosimetry
    - Critical organ is bladder wall
    - Effective dose ~ 4 mSv
- Interpretation: Probability of RVHT caused by RAS graded as low, intermediate, or high
  - Low probability (< 10%): Pre and post renograms normal or improvement after ACEI
  - Intermediate (indeterminate) probability: Abnormal baseline findings that are unchanged after ACEI
    - Small, poorly functioning kidney (< 30%) may not respond appropriately
    - Symmetric bilateral abnormalities most often due to factors such as dehydration
    - Cortical retention, ratio counts at 20 to 3 minutes (20/3 ratio) ~ 0.1-0.5
    - Reduced uptake of DTPA of 5-9%

- High probability (> 90%)
  - MAG-3: ↑ peak time (by 2-3 min or at least 40%)
  - DTPA: ↓ peak and ↓ relative uptake or GFR > 10%
  - MAG-3: Increase in 20- or 30-min/peak ratio of ≥ 0.15 from baseline study
  - Decrease in MAG-3 uptake > 10%
  - Marked unilateral parenchymal retention of DTPA after ACEI compared with baseline study

DIFFERENTIAL DIAGNOSIS

Primary (Essential) HTN

- HTN of unknown cause

Secondary HTN

- HTN due to underlying, potentially correctable cause
  - RVHT
  - Medications
  - Endocrine disorders
  - Rare: Pheochromocytoma, coarctation of aorta (children)

PATHOLOGY

General Features

- Renin-angiotensin system increases renal blood flow when renal hypoperfusion detected
  - Diminished renal blood flow causes ↑ renin secretion by renal juxtaglomerular cells
  - Renin from kidneys converts angiotensinogen from liver into angiotensin I, which is then converted by ACE into angiotensin II
  - Angiotensin II causes preferential vasoconstriction of efferent arteriole of glomerulus
    - ↑ blood pressure maintains renal perfusion and GFR
- ACEI drugs prevent formation of angiotensin II, causing renal function to fall in patients with RVHT
  - Renovascular disease left untreated can result in RVHT, renal failure, end-stage renal disease
    - Not all RAS leads to RVHT, and treating RAS does not always reverse HTN
  - ACEI antihypertensive medications (e.g., captopril and enalapril) are used to identify RVHT on renogram

CLINICAL ISSUES

Presentation

- Most common signs/symptoms
  - Presentation of RVHT typically nonspecific, difficult to distinguish clinically from other causes of HTN
  - Per SNMMI guidelines, cost effectiveness and utility higher when appropriate patients are selected
    - Abrupt onset or severe HTN
    - HTN resistant to 3-drug therapy in compliant patient
    - Abdominal or flank bruits
    - Unexplained azotemia in elderly hypertensive patient
    - Worsening renal function during antihypertensive therapy, especially with ACEIs or angiotensin II receptor blockers
    - Grade 3 or 4 hypertensive retinopathy
    - Occlusive disease in other vascular beds
    - Onset of HTN in patients < 30 or > 55 years
    - HTN in children

Demographics

- RAS is most common cause of secondary HTN
  - 60-90% of cases related to atherosclerotic disease; 10% due to fibromuscular dysplasia
- 30-50% of normotensive patients may have moderate to severe RAS
- 7% of population > 65 years have RAS
- RAS is present in 1-5% of patients with HTN

Natural History & Prognosis

- Untreated RVHT leads to irreversible renal damage, may cause chronic renal failure
- Rapid identification and therapy required to prevent irreversible damage

Treatment

- Treatment options include medical therapy vs. angioplasty &/or stenting
  - Recent studies have significantly impacted views toward invasive therapy for RAS
  - STAR, ASTRAL, and most recently CORAL studies have failed to demonstrate significant improvement in outcomes for angioplasty/stenting over optimal medical therapy in patients with RAS
  - Identification and targeted therapy for these patients remains important (whether invasive or optimized medical management)

DIAGNOSTIC CHECKLIST

Consider

- False-negatives
  - RAS > 90 % (insufficient compensation at baseline to allow detectable change with ACEI)
  - Patients on chronic ACEI therapy
  - Baseline renal insufficiency (when unilateral, lack of captopril response could be due to RAS or unilateral parenchymal disease)
  - Poor p.o. absorption of ACEI
- False-positives
  - Bilateral hydronephrosis or patulous collecting system (furosemide can help)
  - Hypotension related to ACEI administration
  - Poor hydration

SELECTED REFERENCES

1. Cooper CJ et al: Stenting and medical therapy for atherosclerotic renal-artery stenosis. N Engl J Med. 370(1):13-22, 2014
2. Taylor AT: Radionuclides in nephrourology, Part 2: pitfalls and diagnostic applications. J Nucl Med. 55(5):786-98, 2014
3. Cooper CJ et al: Stent revascularization for the prevention of cardiovascular and renal events among patients with renal artery stenosis and systolic hypertension: rationale and design of the CORAL trial. Am Heart J. 152(1):59-66, 2006
4. Taylor AT Jr et al: Procedure guideline for diagnosis of renovascular hypertension. Society of Nuclear Medicine. J Nucl Med. 39(7):1297-302, 1998
5. Taylor A et al: Consensus report on ACE inhibitor renography for detecting renovascular hypertension. Radionuclides in Nephrourology Group. Consensus Group on ACEI Renography. J Nucl Med. 37(11):1876-82, 1996

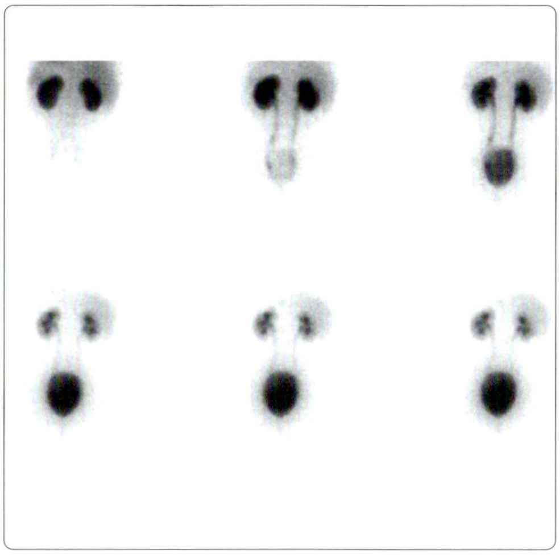

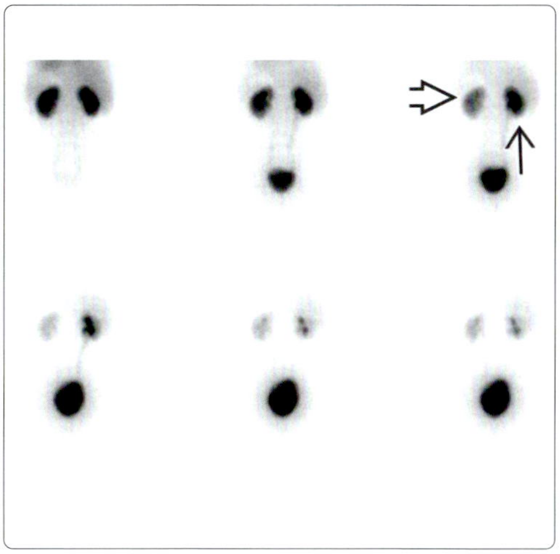

(Left) *Pre-captopril posterior ACE inhibited (ACEI) renography demonstrates normal symmetric excretion bilaterally.* **(Right)** *Post-captopril renogram demonstrates decreased excretion from the right ⇨ kidney relative to the left ⇨.*

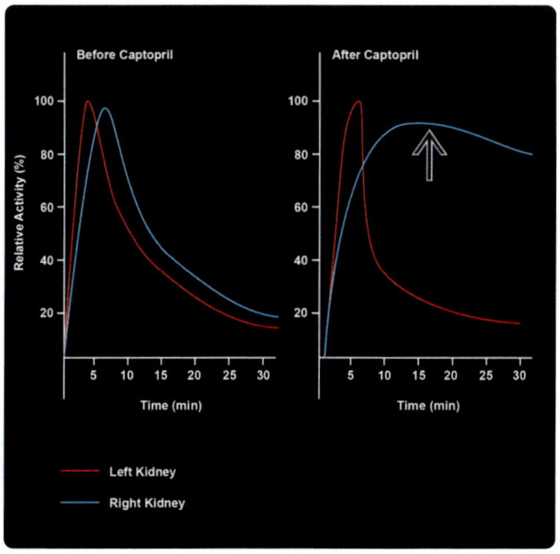

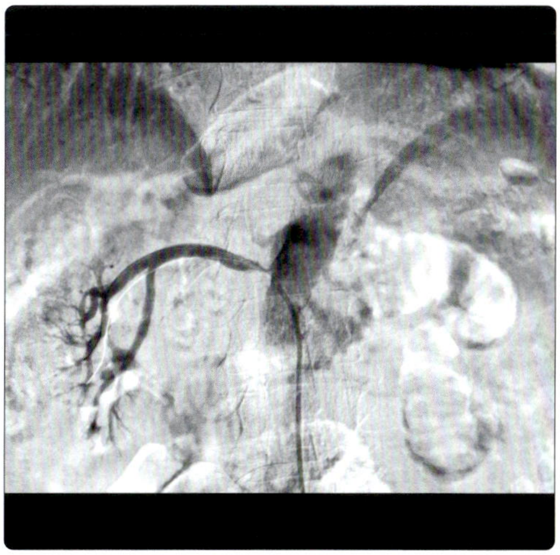

(Left) *Tc-99m MAG3 time-activity curves show typical cortical retention ⇨ seen after ACEI administration in a patient with renovascular hypertension from right renal artery stenosis.* **(Right)** *Angiographic image demonstrates high-grade stenosis at the ostium of the right renal artery.*

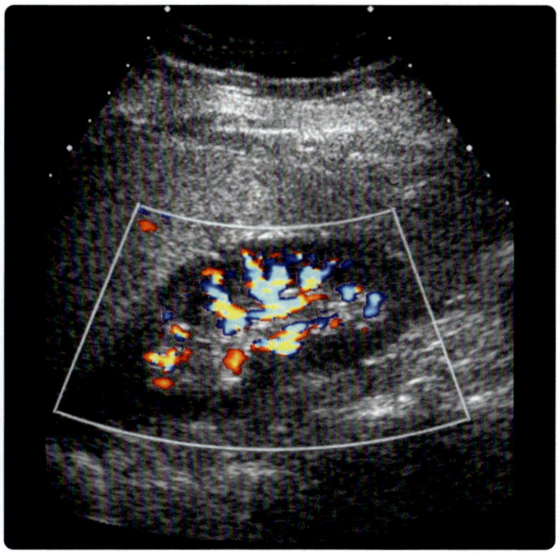

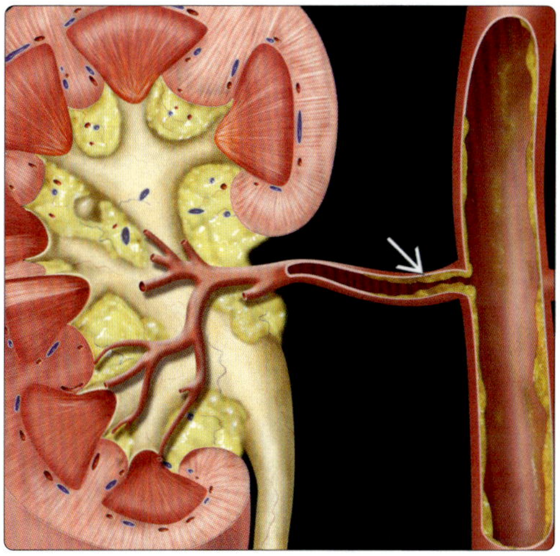

(Left) *Color Doppler ultrasound of the right kidney demonstrates normal flow. No evidence of hydronephrosis is seen.* **(Right)** *Graphic shows luminal renal artery narrowing → from atherosclerosis, the most common cause of renal artery stenosis, a condition that may result in renovascular hypertension.*

SECTION 9

Pediatrics

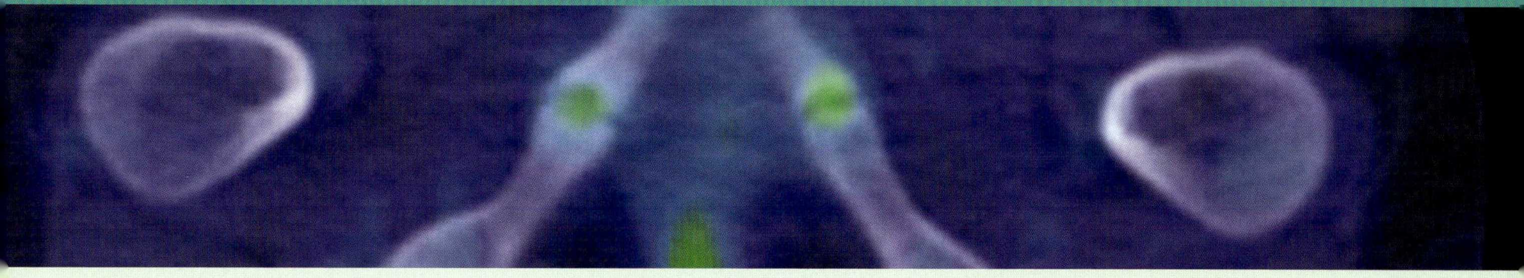

Introduction

Central Nervous System

Thyroid

Gastrointestinal

Hepatobiliary

Infection and Inflammation

Musculoskeletal

Introduction

Pediatric imaging in nuclear medicine encompasses imaging of a broad spectrum of developmental and pathologic entities. Some of these entities are unique to children and young adults while others impact both adults and young patients. Independent of differences in pathologic entities, there are several unique considerations when imaging a child or young adult.

ALARA

The concept of "as low as is reasonably achievable" (ALARA) applies to all medical imaging that involves ionizing radiation, but it has received particular attention in the pediatric and young adult population predicated on the understanding that the risk of radiation-induced malignancy is higher in this population than in the adult population. In nuclear medicine, there are 3 ways to adhere to ALARA.

- Avoiding unnecessary exams
- Appropriate radiopharmaceutical dosing
- Appropriate application of correlative imaging

Radiopharmaceutical Dosing

Unlike with adult patients in whom a fixed dose of radiopharmaceutical is more commonly used, pediatric radiopharmaceutical dosing is typically weight-based. The longstanding approach to determine pediatric dosing was to divide the child's weight in kilograms by an idealized adult weight of 70 kg and multiply that by the standard radiopharmaceutical dose administered to an adult patient (child's weight in kg/70)*(adult dose). More recently, consensus guidelines have been developed and published by both North American and European groups to standardize administered activity based on not only weight but experience using the radiopharmaceuticals in pediatric patients. Differences exist between the North American Consensus Guidelines and the European Association of Nuclear Medicine dosage card, but efforts to harmonize those guidelines are underway. In the interim, dosing according to either guideline as well as altering administered activities based on the clinical indication is considered acceptable.

Appropriate Application of Correlative Imaging

Other than the administered radiopharmaceutical, the other source of medical radiation exposure in nuclear medicine is correlative imaging, chiefly CT. In general, it is appropriate to limit the use of CT and the CT exposure parameters in pediatric patients to maintain dose from the CT component at ALARA while still obtaining the necessary diagnostic information.

For PET/CT, CT optimization means tailoring the CT parameters to the clinical question, which can range from attenuation correction only (lowest dose), to bone detail CT, localization CT, or diagnostic CT. CT parameters in each of these categories should also be adjusted to patient size.

For SPECT/CT, CT parameters should similarly be tailored to the clinical question. More importantly, it may be that CT is not needed for every SPECT examination. In some settings, a negative SPECT is sufficient to rule out abnormality, and in other settings, correlation to anatomic imaging can be achieved through review of previously performed diagnostic imaging or post-hoc fusion.

Need for Distraction or Sedation/Anesthesia

In general, pediatric patients have more difficulty holding still for imaging procedures than adult patients do. This can be particularly problematic in nuclear medicine in which both static and tomographic images may require several minutes to obtain. Many examinations can be achieved in pediatric patients without sedation or anesthesia through the application of coaching, distraction techniques (video goggles, etc.), and careful imaging technique (posterior positioning of the camera head). Sedation or general anesthesia may be required for some patients undergoing some examinations to obtain good quality images and answer the clinical questions (e.g., very young patients undergoing F-18 FDG PET/CT or I-123 MIBG exams). Sedation and anesthesia can be administered for most nuclear medicine studies without compromising the study itself. F-18 FDG PET/CT is one exception where sedation can impact the distribution of radiotracer, particularly in the brain. As such, for F-18 FDG PET/CT exams, sedation/anesthetic induction should be held until 30-45 minutes into the uptake period.

Anatomy-Based Imaging Issues

Knowledge of the normal distribution of radiotracer in pediatric and young adult patients is critically important for the appropriate interpretation of nuclear medicine examinations. Sources of variant radiotracer in young patients include growth centers and physiologic uptake that is more common than in adult patients.

- Physes, apophyses, and synchondroses can all be sources of normal radiotracer uptake on bone scan and PET/CT
- Lymphoid tissue is a more prominent source of F-18 FDG uptake in pediatric and young adult patients
- Thymic tissue, which can be present in widely varying amounts, takes up both F-18 FDG and I-123 MIBG
- Brown fat is more common in pediatric and young adult patients and takes up both F-18 FDG and I-123 MIBG

Selected References

1. Davidson AJ et al: Anesthesia and the developing brain: a way forward for clinical research. Paediatr Anaesth. 25(5):447-52, 2015
2. Fahey FH et al: Standardization of administered activities in pediatric nuclear medicine: a report of the first nuclear medicine global initiative project, part 1-statement of the issue and a review of available resources. J Nucl Med. 56(4):646-51, 2015
3. Grant FD et al: Radiation doses for pediatric nuclear medicine studies: comparing the North American consensus guidelines and the pediatric dosage card of the European Association of Nuclear Medicine. Pediatr Radiol. ePub, 2014
4. Lassmann M et al: Paediatric radiopharmaceutical administration: harmonization of the 2007 EANM paediatric dosage card (version 1.5.2008) and the 2010 North American consensus guidelines. Eur J Nucl Med Mol Imaging. 41(5):1036-41, 2014
5. Zacharias C et al: Pediatric CT: strategies to lower radiation dose. AJR Am J Roentgenol. 200(5):950-6, 2013
6. DiMaggio C et al: Early childhood exposure to anesthesia and risk of developmental and behavioral disorders in a sibling birth cohort. Anesth Analg. 113(5):1143-51, 2011
7. Gelfand MJ et al: Pediatric radiopharmaceutical administered doses: 2010 North American consensus guidelines. J Nucl Med. 52(2):318-22, 2011
8. Alessio AM et al: Weight-based, low-dose pediatric whole-body PET/CT protocols. J Nucl Med. 50(10):1570-7, 2009
9. Lassmann M et al: The new EANM paediatric dosage card: additional notes with respect to F-18. Eur J Nucl Med Mol Imaging. 35(9):1666-8, 2008
10. Lassmann M et al: The new EANM paediatric dosage card. Eur J Nucl Med Mol Imaging. 35(9):1748, 2008

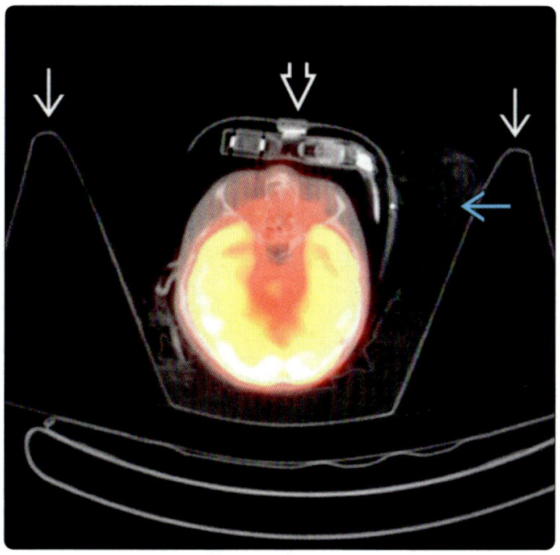

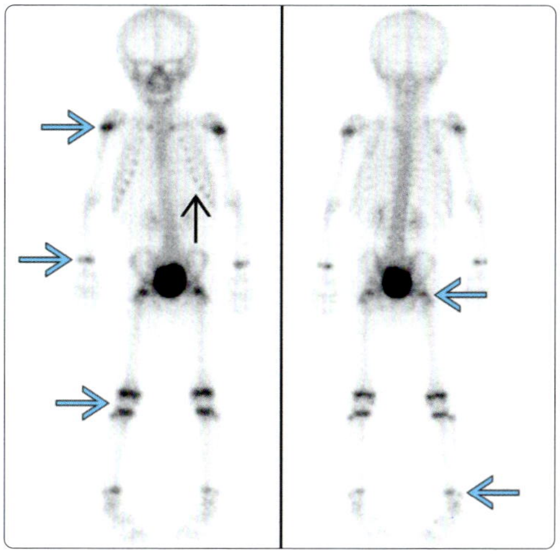

(Left) *Axial fused F-18 FDG PET/CT in a 7-year-old child undergoing whole-body scan shows multiple methods to maintain patient positioning in this awake child, including video goggles* ➡, *passive head holder* ➡, *and linen to support the head and limit motion* ➡. **(Right)** *Anterior and posterior whole-body Tc-99m MDP bone scan in a 3-year-old child shows normal increased uptake at the physes* ➡ *and at the costochondral junctions* ➡.

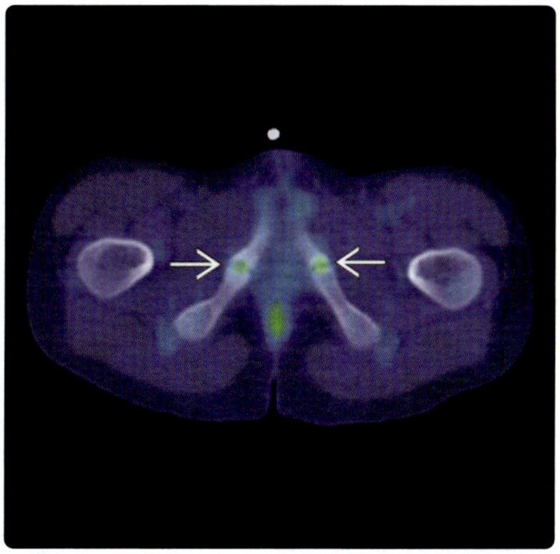

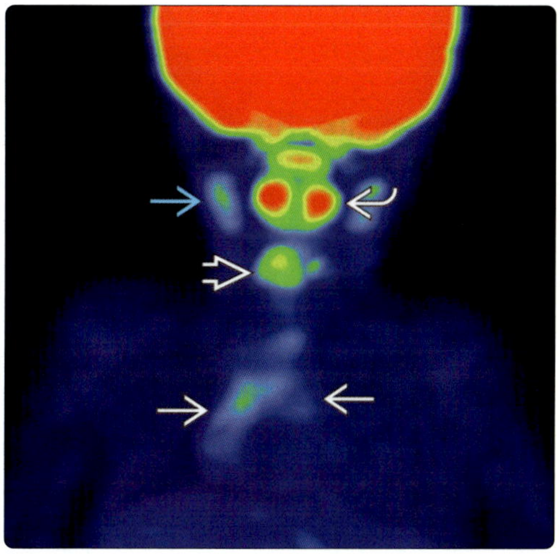

(Left) *Fused axial F-18 FDG PET/CT in a 10 year old shows normal uptake at the ischiopubic synchondroses* ➡. *The synchondroses can appear asymmetrically irregular and uptake can be variably asymmetric.* **(Right)** *Coronal MIP F-18 FDG PET in a 3-year-old child shows normal uptake in lymphoid tissue of Waldeyer ring* ➡, *salivary glands* ➡, *tongue and sublingual muscles* ➡, *and the thymus* ➡. *Thymic uptake should be uniform and in the shape of an inverted "V", or chevron, as seen in this case.*

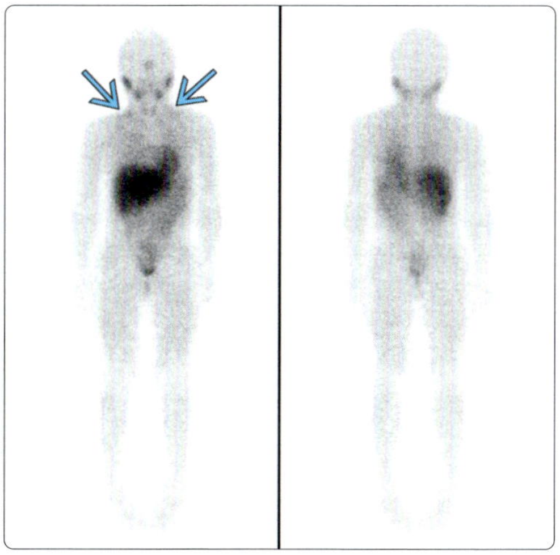

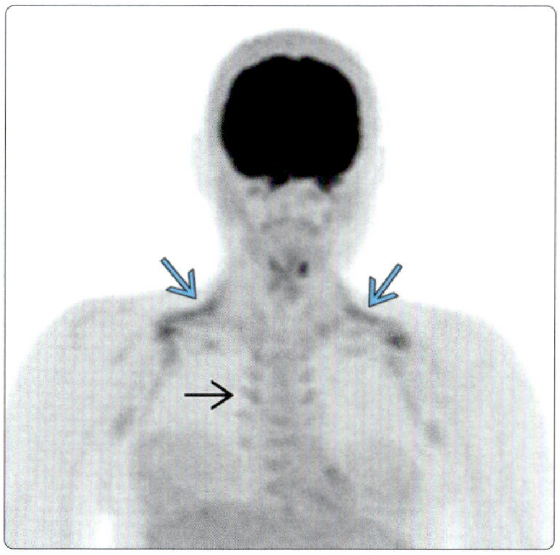

(Left) *Anterior and posterior MIBG scan in a 6 year old shows physiologic distribution of the radiotracer (salivary glands, nasal mucosa, thyroid, heart, liver, and GI and GU tracts) with normal variant uptake in supraclavicular brown fat* ➡. **(Right)** *Coronal MIP F-18 FDG PET in a 16 year old shows uptake in supraclavicular* ➡ *and costovertebral* ➡ *brown fat. Uptake in brown fat can be mitigated by warming the patient or administering pharmacologic blocking agents.*

KEY FACTS

IMAGING

- Nuclear imaging not part of routine evaluation of isolated seizures
  - Plays important role in multidisciplinary/multimodality work-up of intractable epilepsy
- Nuclear imaging may identify structurally inconspicuous epileptogenic foci
- SPECT: Radiotracer deposition reflects regional cerebral blood flow
  - Interictal: Epileptogenic focus appears as area of decreased radiotracer deposition (hypoperfusion)
  - Ictal: Epileptogenic focus appears as area of increased radiotracer deposition (hyperperfusion)
  - SISCOM may identify epileptogenic foci that are inconspicuous on visual assessment of ictal and interictal SPECT images
- F-18 FDG PET: Epileptogenic focus appears as area of hypometabolism (larger than epileptogenic focus)
  - Statistical parametric mapping (SPM) can help detect and confirm foci of hypometabolism
- MR is ideal modality to identify structural causes of seizure/epilepsy
  - Mesial temporal sclerosis: Decreased volume, increased T2 signal in hippocampus
  - Focal cortical dysplasia (FCD): Focal cortical thickening and increased T2 signal, blurring of gray-white junction

CLINICAL ISSUES

- Most common cause of epilepsy
  - Young: FCD
  - Adolescent/young adult: Mesial temporal sclerosis
- Antiepileptic drugs are first line of therapy
- Surgical resection: Reserved for patients with intractable, focal epilepsy

(Left) *FLAIR MR in a 16-year-old male with intractable epilepsy shows an area of gliosis in the left parietal lobe related to remote trauma →.* **(Right)** *Interictal Tc-99m ECD SPECT in the same patient shows hypoperfusion corresponding to the left parietal gliosis ➔ and involving the adjacent parietal lobe →.*

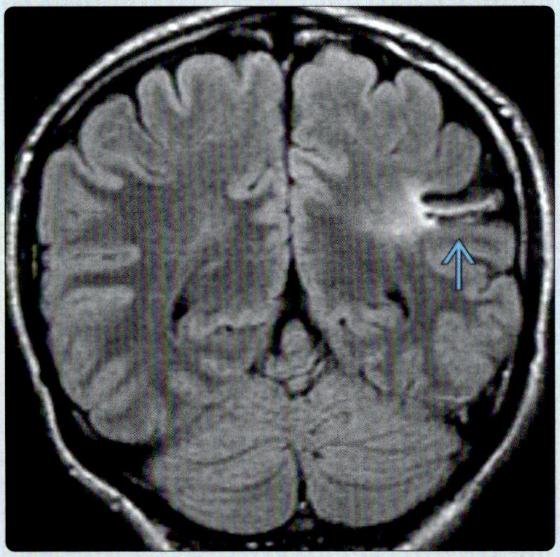

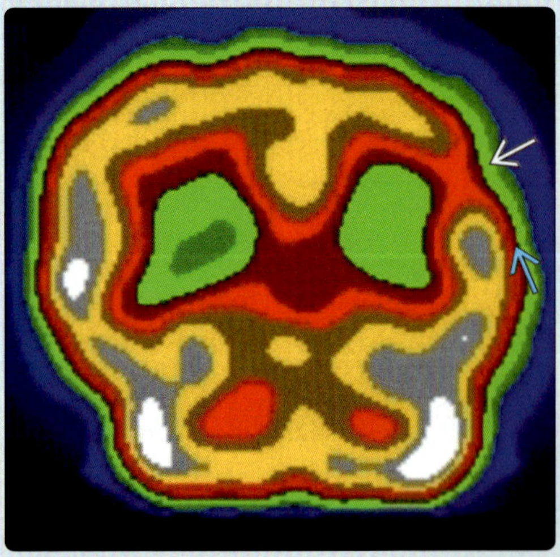

(Left) *Ictal Tc-99m ECD SPECT in the same patient shows hypoperfusion corresponding to the left parietal gliosis ➔. The adjacent parietal lobe, however, is hyperperfused (relative to the right) reflecting seizure activity.* **(Right)** *F-18 FDG PET in the same patient shows hypometabolism corresponding to the left parietal gliosis ➔, as well as hypometabolism (relative to the right) of adjacent parietal lobe →. This corroborates the SPECT findings and suggests a seizure focus.*

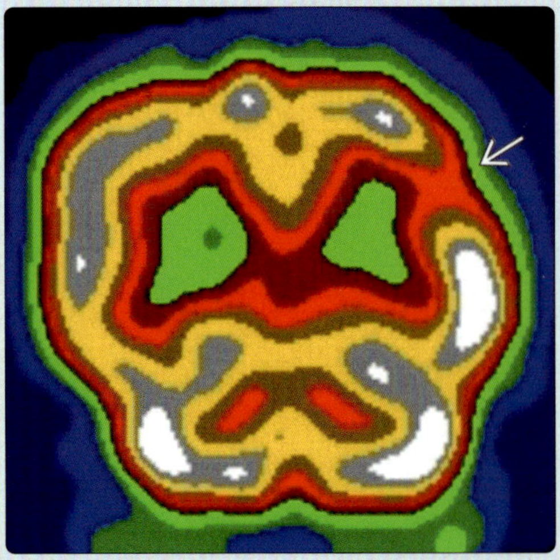

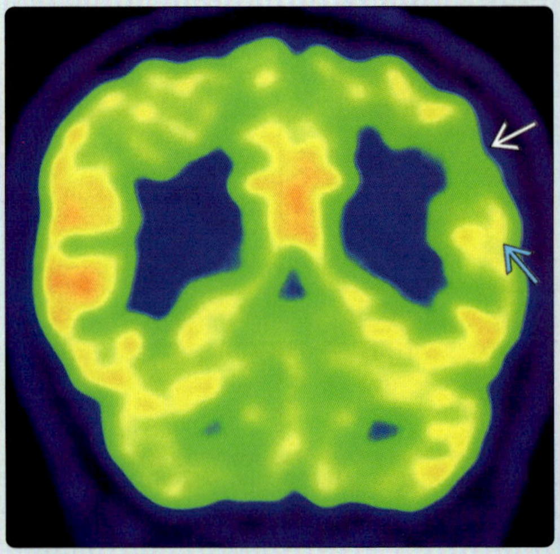

TERMINOLOGY

Definitions

- Seizure: Clinical manifestation of aberrant neuronal electrical discharge(s) in brain
- Epilepsy: 2 or more unprovoked, afebrile seizures

IMAGING

General Features

- Imaging of isolated/acute seizures is generally structural (CT/MR) and reserved for patients with focal or complex seizures or focal neurologic signs
- Imaging is an important component in management of epilepsy
  - Structural imaging (CT/MR) often performed at diagnosis to exclude structural cause
  - Multimodality imaging (including nuclear) plays substantial role in work-up of intractable epilepsy
- Work-up of intractable epilepsy is multidisciplinary/multimodality process
  - Clinical assessment: History, seizure semiology
  - Electroencephalography (EEG): Scalp and intracranial
  - MR: Structural, ± functional
  - Perfusion (SPECT) imaging
  - Metabolic (F-18 FDG PET) imaging
  - Magnetoencephalography

Nuclear Medicine Findings

- Nuclear imaging not part of routine evaluation of isolated seizures
- May identify structurally inconspicuous epileptogenic foci
- **SPECT perfusion**
  - Radiotracer deposition reflects regional cerebral blood flow
    - Tc-99m hexamethylpropyleneamine oxime (HMPAO) and Tc-99m ethyl cysteinate dimer (ECD) most commonly used tracers
      - Lipophilic, small molecules diffuse across blood-brain barrier
      - ECD clears more rapidly from blood pool, has more linear extraction at high blood flow rates; less nonspecific scalp and soft tissue uptake than HMPAO
    - High first-pass extraction, peak accumulation in ~ 2 min, no substantial redistribution
      - Can image for at least 2 hrs after injection without substantial loss of fidelity
  - Interictal SPECT
    - Epileptogenic focus appears as area of decreased radiotracer deposition (hypoperfusion)
  - Ictal SPECT
    - Epileptogenic focus appears as area of increased radiotracer deposition (hyperperfusion)
      - Correspondence to epileptogenic focus depends on interval between seizure onset and injection; longer intervals allow more propagation to surrounding tissue
      - Beware of pseudonormalization where hyperperfusion during ictus makes a baseline hypoperfused focus appear symmetric to normal side
    - Higher sensitivity than interictal SPECT for epileptogenic focus
  - Subtraction ictal SPECT coregistered to MR (SISCOM)
    - Means to compare ictal and interictal SPECT imaging and localize abnormalities to MR
    - Foci of ictal hyperperfusion that correspond with interictal hypoperfusion appear as foci of activity on SISCOM
    - May identify epileptogenic foci that are inconspicuous on visual assessment of ictal and interictal SPECT images
- **F-18 FDG PET**
  - Interictal exam due to prolonged (~ 30 min) uptake of F-18 FDG
    - If seizure occurs during uptake phase, may see hypermetabolism at epileptogenic focus
  - Indirect marker of neuronal activity
  - Epileptogenic focus appears as area of hypometabolism
    - Area of hypometabolism is generally larger than epileptogenic focus
  - Highest accuracy in temporal lobe epilepsy (TLE), less likely to identify epileptogenic focus in extratemporal epilepsy
  - Adds most value in cases of structurally inconspicuous TLE
  - Higher sensitivity than interictal SPECT
  - Post-processing with statistical parametric mapping (SPM) can help detect and confirm foci of hypometabolism
    - SPM compares, on pixel by pixel basis, F-18 FDG uptake in patient to normal database to identify foci of abnormally decreased uptake
- With both SPECT and PET imaging, may see corresponding downstream abnormality in cerebellar hemisphere opposite involved cerebral hemisphere
  - Decreased radiotracer uptake on interictal SPECT and F-18 FDG PET
  - Increased radiotracer uptake on ictal SPECT
- **Other tracers**
  - C-11 flumazenil: Binds CNS gamma-aminobutyric acid (GABA) receptors; GABA receptors are decreased in epileptogenic foci

MR Findings

- Mesial temporal sclerosis: Decreased volume and increased T2 signal in mesial temporal structures including hippocampal formation
  - Resultant asymmetry in size of temporal horn of lateral ventricle
- Focal cortical dysplasia (FCD): Cortical thickening and increased T2 signal, extension of T2 signal to ventricle, blurring of gray-white junction

DIFFERENTIAL DIAGNOSIS

CNS Tumor

- May or may not be cause of seizures
- May appear as focus of hypo- or hyperperfusion on SPECT
- May appear as a focus of hypometabolism on F-18 FDG PET if low grade

Congenital Anomalies

- Structural abnormalities: Heterotopic gray matter, abnormal sulcation, schizencephaly
- May appear as focus of hypometabolism on FDG PET even if not epileptogenic

Tuberous Sclerosis

- Can be difficult to identify epileptogenic focus as majority of tubers are hypoperfused and hypometabolic
- Epileptogenic tubers generally show perfusion/metabolic abnormalities larger than area of structural abnormality

Rasmussen Encephalitis

- Progressive inflammatory process involving unilateral cerebral hemisphere, generally with progressive cerebral atrophy
- Appears as large areas (lobar or hemispheric) of perfusion or metabolic abnormality

PATHOLOGY

Gross Pathologic & Surgical Features

- Mesial temporal sclerosis: Hard, shrunken hippocampus
- Focal cortical dysplasia (FCD): Firm, rubbery cortical focus

Microscopic Features

- Mesial temporal sclerosis
  - Variable distribution of pyramidal neuronal loss
  - Gliosis
- FCD: Abnormalities in neuronal migration resulting in cortical dyslamination
  - Type I: Abnormal cortical layering
  - Type II: Abnormal cortical layering **and** cytologic abnormalities
  - Type III: Abnormal cortical layering associated with primary brain lesion (adjacent or in same lobe)

CLINICAL ISSUES

Demographics

- Epidemiology
  - Seizure
    - Most common causes of acute seizures: Fever, infection, head injury
    - Febrile seizures
      - Usually occur between 6 months and 5 years of age
      - Occur in 3-8% of children < 5 years
      - 60% risk of recurrence
  - Epilepsy
    - Highest incidence in first year of life (~ 90-200 per 100,000)
    - Prevalence higher in rural areas
    - Risk factors
      - Family history
      - Prior febrile seizure: 2-7% develop epilepsy
    - Most common causes
      - Young: FCD
      - Adolescent/young adult: Mesial temporal sclerosis
    - Intractable epilepsy occurs in 20-30%

Natural History & Prognosis

- Epilepsy subtypes: Current terminology
  - Genetic: Genetic abnormality without discrete structural abnormality
  - Structural or metabolic
    - Discrete structural epileptogenic lesion
      - Many of these are genetic in etiology
    - Metabolic condition leading to propensity for seizures
  - Unknown cause
- FCD: Malformation of cortical development
  - Secondary to insult (genetic, infectious, ischemic) during development
- Mesial temporal sclerosis
  - Often secondary to insult (infection, trauma, febrile seizures) early in life

Treatment

- Antiepileptic drugs
  - First line of therapy
  - Managing clinician will often try multiple agents and combinations of agents to achieve seizure reduction (or freedom) with minimum of side effects
- Ketogenic diet
- Vagal nerve stimulator
  - Often used in patients with intractable epilepsy
- Surgical resection: Reserved for patients with intractable, focal epilepsy
  - Outcomes better if resection includes sites identified on SISCOM
  - Outcome of surgery for FCD is better if lesion is visible by MR

SELECTED REFERENCES

1. Wilmshurst JM et al: The challenges and innovations for therapy in children with epilepsy. Nat Rev Neurol. 10(5):249-60, 2014
2. Miyata H et al: Surgical pathology of epilepsy-associated non-neoplastic cerebral lesions: a brief introduction with special reference to hippocampal sclerosis and focal cortical dysplasia. Neuropathology. 33(4):442-58, 2013
3. Sidhu R et al: Pediatric seizures. Pediatr Rev. 34(8):333-41; 342, 2013
4. Blümcke I et al: The clinicopathologic spectrum of focal cortical dysplasias: a consensus classification proposed by an ad hoc Task Force of the ILAE Diagnostic Methods Commission. Epilepsia. 52(1):158-74. 2011
5. Kim S et al: SPECT Imaging of Epilepsy: An Overview and Comparison with F-18 FDG PET. Int J Mol Imaging. 2011:813028, 2011
6. la Fougère C et al: PET and SPECT in epilepsy: a critical review. Epilepsy Behav. 15(1):50-5, 2009
7. Rastogi S et al: Neuroimaging in pediatric epilepsy: a multimodality approach. Radiographics. 28(4):1079-95, 2008
8. O'Brien TJ et al: Subtraction peri-ictal SPECT is predictive of extratemporal epilepsy surgery outcome. Neurology. 55(11):1668-77, 2000
9. Won HJ et al: Comparison of MR imaging with PET and ictal SPECT in 118 patients with intractable epilepsy. AJNR Am J Neuroradiol. 20(4):593-9, 1999
10. Devous MD Sr et al: SPECT brain imaging in epilepsy: a meta-analysis. J Nucl Med. 39(2):285-93, 1998
11. Spencer SS: The relative contributions of MRI, SPECT, and PET imaging in epilepsy. Epilepsia. 35 Suppl 6:S72-89, 1994
12. Friston KJ et al: Comparing functional (PET) images: the assessment of significant change. J Cereb Blood Flow Metab. 11(4):690-9, 1991

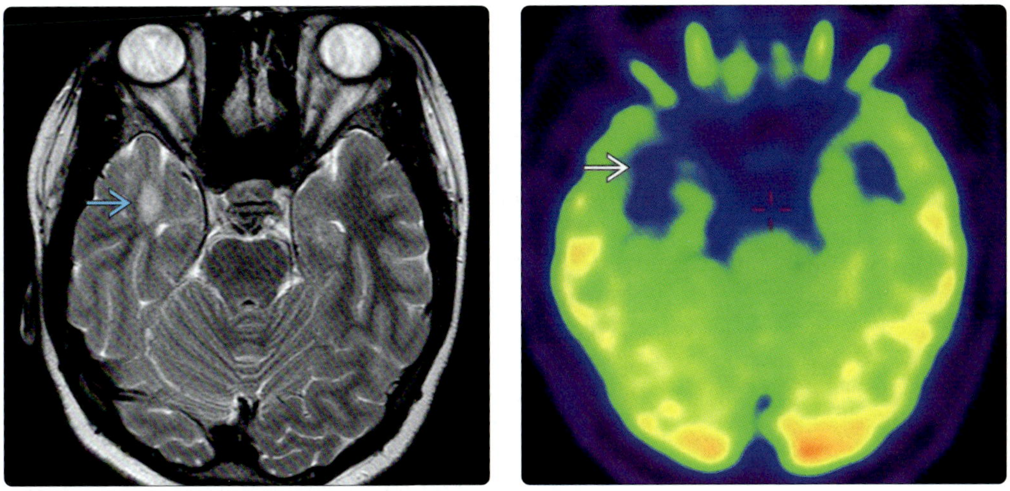

(Left) *Axial T2-weighted MR in a 12-year-old female with epilepsy shows a right temporal focal cortical dysplasia (FCD), apparent as cortical and subcortical increased signal* →. **(Right)** *Axial F-18 FDG PET in the same patient shows hypometabolism associated with the FCD* ➔*, supporting the epileptogenic nature of this lesion.*

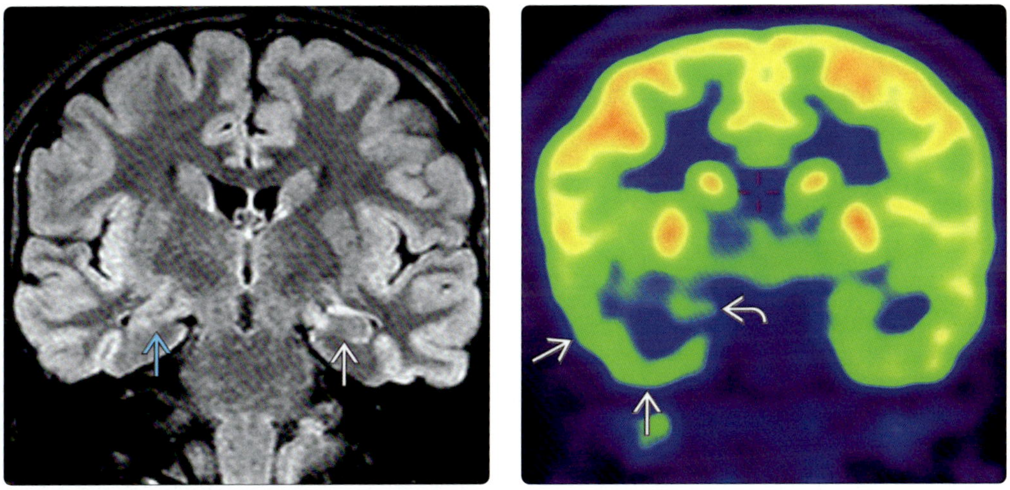

(Left) *Coronal FLAIR MR in the same patient shows right mesial temporal sclerosis associated with the FCD. The right hippocampus is decreased in volume and small* → *compared to the left* ➔*. The combination of an FCD and MTS is considered a type IIIa lesion.* **(Right)** *Coronal F-18 FDG PET in the same patient shows global hypometabolism of the right temporal lobe* ➔ *with more conspicuous hypometabolism of the hippocampus* ↪*. These findings support a right temporal localization of the epileptogenic focus.*

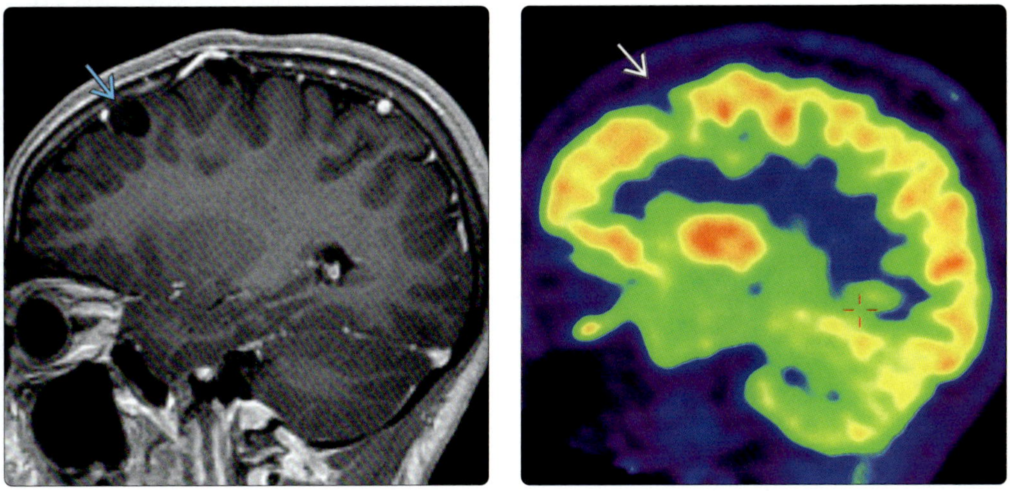

(Left) *Sagittal T1 C+ MR in a 17-year-old female shows a frontal dysembryoplastic neuroepithelial tumor (DNET) as a nonenhancing, low-signal lesion* →. **(Right)** *Sagittal F-18 FDG PET in the same patient shows focal hypometabolism associated with the DNET* ➔*. In this case, the hypometabolism is reflective of both the low grade of this tumor and its epileptogenicity.*

Congenital Hypothyroidism

KEY FACTS

TERMINOLOGY

- Primary congenital hypothyroidism (CH): Developmental defects in thyroid, can be permanent or transient (due to maternal effects, iodine exposure or deficiency)
  - Dysgenesis (70%)
    - Ectopia, hypogenesis, agenesis
    - Usually sporadic
- Dyshormonogenesis (20%)
  - Usually a defect in thyroid hormone synthesis
    - TSH receptor insensitivity, iodide transporter and organification defects, iodine recycling defects, thyroglobulin synthesis defects
  - TSH usually very high on newborn screening
  - Usually transmitted as autosomal recessive trait
  - Genetic counseling indicated for future pregnancies

IMAGING

- Infant screening programs allow early identification of CH
- Imaging performed once CH confirmed with serum TSH, T3 and T4 testing
- I-123 thyroid scan or Tc-99m pertechnetate scan are scintigraphic tests of choice
  - I-123 may be more sensitive and allow assessment of organification defects with perchlorate
  - Tc-99m pertechnetate allows earlier imaging
- Ultrasound useful to confirm structural abnormalities of thyroid: Athyroisis, hypoplasia, goiter
  - Less sensitive than scintigraphy for ectopic thyroid

CLINICAL ISSUES

- Untreated CH can have dramatic effects on growth, intellectual and motor development
- Developmental and IQ prognosis is excellent if CH identified early and treatment initiated
- If CH due to dyshormonogenesis or maternal autoimmune thyroiditis, counseling warranted for future pregnancy risk

(Left) *Tc-99m pertechnetate scan in a 4-week-old boy with congenital hypothyroidism and thyroid agenesis shows absence of uptake in the expected location of the thyroid. There are no foci of uptake outside of the thyroid bed to suggest ectopic tissue. Expected uptake is visible in the stomach.* **(Right)** *Transverse grayscale ultrasound of the thyroid bed in a 2-year-old girl with treated congenital hypothyroidism due to agenesis shows no normal thyroid tissue. Note trachea and carotid arteries.*

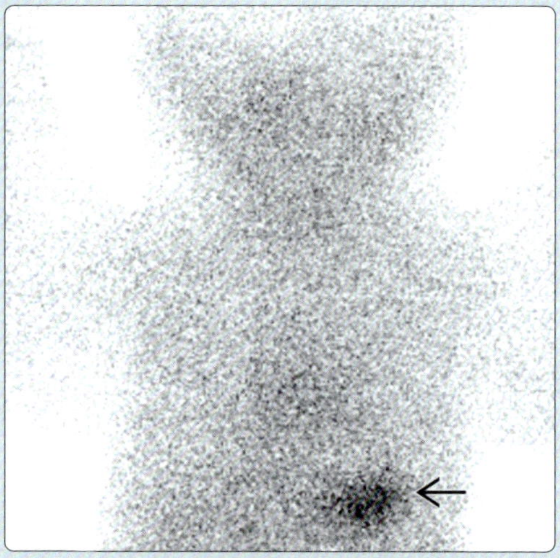

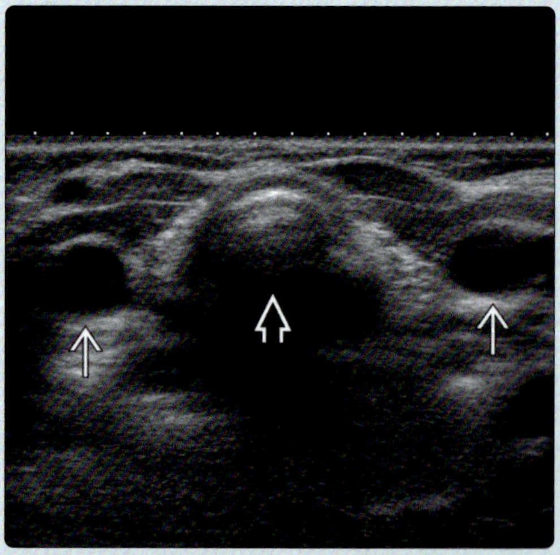

(Left) *Anterior I-123 thyroid scan shows unilateral uptake in a patient with hemiagenesis of the thyroid. Note how the single lobe is enlarged.* **(Right)** *Lateral Tc-99m pertechnetate scan in a 2-year-old boy with congenital hypothyroidism shows no uptake of tracer in the expected location of the thyroid gland. Focal uptake in the tongue base is compatible with ectopic (lingual) thyroid. Note normal lower level uptake in the salivary glands and uptake in the stomach.*

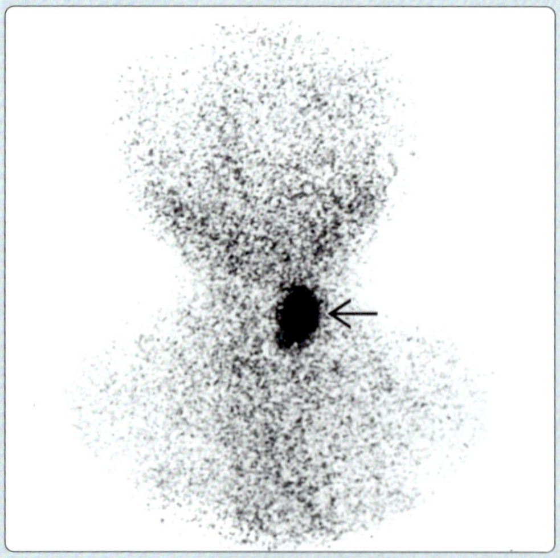

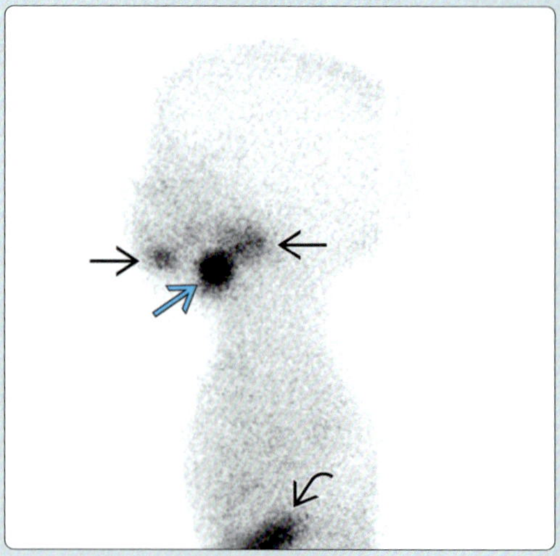

TERMINOLOGY

Definitions

- Congenital hypothyroidism (CH): Inadequate thyroid hormone production or insensitivity to thyroid hormone, manifested in infancy
  - Primary CH: Developmental defects in thyroid, can be permanent or transient (due to maternal effects, iodine exposure or deficiency)
    - Dysgenesis (70%)
      - Ectopia, hypogenesis, agenesis
      - Usually sporadic
    - Dyshormonogenesis (20%)
      - Usually a defect in thyroid hormone synthesis (e.g., TSH receptor insensitivity, iodide transporter and organification defects, iodine recycling defects, thyroglobulin synthesis defects)
      - TSH usually very high on newborn screening
      - Usually transmitted as autosomal recessive trait
      - Genetic counseling indicated for future pregnancies
  - Secondary CH: Developmental defects (anatomic or functional) in pituitary or hypothalamus

IMAGING

General Features

- Infant screening programs detect hypothyroidism for early identification of CH
  - Heel prick between 2-5 days of age, TSH measured in blood sample
- Imaging performed once CH confirmed with TSH, T3 and T4 testing

Nuclear Medicine Findings

- **Tc-99m pertechnetate or I-123 thyroid scan**
  - Athyrosis/agenesis
    - No focal radiotracer uptake between base of tongue and upper chest
  - Hypoplasia/partial agenesis
    - Decreased (or normal) uptake in small, abnormally shaped eutopic gland
  - Ectopy
    - Focal/multifocal radiotracer uptake in neck
    - Along course of normal thyroid from foramen cecum in tongue to thyroid bed
  - Dyshormonogenesis
    - High uptake in ± enlarged, eutopic gland
    - Partial organification defect: Perchlorate test washout 10-50%
    - Complete organification defect: Perchlorate test washout > 90%
  - TSH receptor abnormality
    - Faint or absent uptake in eutopic gland
  - Sodium iodine symporter (NIS) defect
    - Faint or absent uptake in eutopic gland
  - Maternal antithyroid antibodies
    - Faint or absent uptake in eutopic gland

Ultrasonographic Findings

- Grayscale ultrasound
  - Useful to confirm absence, partial agenesis or hypoplasia of thyroid
  - Ectopic thyroid: Soft tissue nodule with echotexture of thyroid gland outside of thyroid bed
    - Less sensitive than scintigraphy for identification of ectopic thyroid
- Color Doppler
  - Ectopic thyroid is hypervascular

Imaging Recommendations

- Best imaging tool
  - I-123 thyroid scan or Tc-99m pertechnetate scan
    - I-123 thyroid scan may be more sensitive for small or hypofunctioning foci of thyroid tissue
    - I-123 thyroid scan may allow assessment of organification defects through perchlorate washout testing
    - Tc-99m pertechnetate scan allows earlier imaging
- Protocol advice
  - Patient preparation
    - If imaging in neonatal period, no need to stop thyroid replacement as TSH levels remain elevated for several days after initiation of therapy
    - If imaging older child with treated CH, need to hold thyroid replacement to allow optimal detection of thyroid tissue
  - I-123 thyroid scan
    - Radiopharmaceutical
      - No consensus guidelines; suggested administered activity: 3-10 μCi/kg (0.111-0.37 MBq/kg) (max 200 μCi [7.4 MBq])
    - Dosimetry
      - Effective dose = 0.81 rad/mCi (depends on thyroid uptake)
      - Critical organ = thyroid (16.6 rad/mCi, depends on thyroid uptake)
    - Image acquisition
      - Image at 3-6 hours, delayed image as needed at 24 hours for low-level uptake
    - Perchlorate washout test: Uncommonly performed but can identify organification defects
      - After imaging of radiotracer uptake, potassium perchlorate administered orally and repeat imaging obtained at 60-90 minutes
      - Dosing: 10 mg/kg in infant, 400 mg in child, 1,000 mg in adult
      - Normal = washout < 10%
      - Partial organification defect = washout 10-50%
      - Complete organification defect = washout > 90%
  - Tc-99m pertechnetate thyroid scan
    - Radiopharmaceutical
      - No consensus guidelines; suggested administered activity: 66 μCi/kg (2.4 MBq/kg) (max 3 mCi [111 MBq])
    - Dosimetry
      - Effective dose = 0.05 rad/mCi
      - Critical organ = thyroid (~ 0.1-0.2 rad/mCi)
    - Image acquisition
      - Image at 10-20 min

- Typically acquire anterior and posterior planar images with parallel hole collimator to look for thyroid tissue
- Pinhole collimator for more detailed assessment of tissue in thyroid bed
- Salivary gland uptake can mask subtle thyroid uptake, delayed imaging may allow washout of salivary glands
- Can also stimulate washout of salivary glands through administration of lemon juice

DIFFERENTIAL DIAGNOSIS

Thyroid Dysgenesis

- Ectopy, athyrosis, hypoplasia
  - Ectopy: 2/3 of dysgenesis
  - Athyrosis: Complete absence of thyroid tissue
  - Hypoplasia

Dyshormonogenesis

- Defects can occur anywhere along uptake, synthesis, secretion, and utilization pathways

Central Hypothyroidism

- Pituitary dysgenesis
- Pituitary dysfunction
- Hypothalamic dysfunction

Maternal Factors

- Autoimmune thyroiditis
  - TSH-R blocking antibodies (e.g., Hashimoto disease) cross placenta
  - Antibodies clear from infant circulation by 6 months; thyroid function normalizes
- Anti-thyroid medication: Propylthiouracil, methimazole
- Maternal iodine overload: Amiodarone, iodinated contrast, iodine cleansing agents
- Maternal I-131 therapy for hyperthyroidism or cancer

Congenital Hepatic Hemangiomas

- Consumptive hypothyroidism due to production of type 3 iodothyronine deiodinase

PATHOLOGY

General Features

- Etiology
  - Majority sporadic
  - Rare hereditary forms
- Genetics
  - Genetic abnormalities uncommonly identified (~ 2%)
  - Dyshormonogenesis: Autosomal recessive

CLINICAL ISSUES

Presentation

- Most common signs/symptoms
  - Majority asymptomatic, identified by newborn screening
- Other signs/symptoms
  - Gestation > 42 weeks (seen in ~ 20%)
  - Birth weight > 90th percentile (seen in ~ 33%)
  - Prolonged jaundice (> 3 weeks)
  - Feeding difficulty
  - Lethargy
  - Hoarse cry
  - Constipation
  - Macroglossia
  - Hypothermia
  - Edema
  - Cold or mottled skin
  - Wide posterior fontanelle (> 5 mm)
  - Umbilical hernia
- **10% of patients with primary CH have associated congenital anomalies**
  - 50% congenital cardiac defects
  - Others: Spiky hair, cleft palate, neurologic abnormalities, genitourinary malformations
- **Secondary CH**
  - Generally associated with deficiencies in other pituitary hormones

Demographics

- Age
  - CH present at birth, most diagnosed < 2-3 weeks
- Gender
  - F:M = 2:1
- Epidemiology
  - Incidence: 1:3,000-4,000 live births
    - Increased incidence in Hispanics (1:2,000)
    - Decreased incidence in African Americans (1:10,000)
  - Higher frequency in areas with iodine deficient diet

Natural History & Prognosis

- Treated CH
  - Excellent developmental and IQ prognosis if identified early and treatment initiated
- Untreated CH
  - Mental retardation: IQ highly dependent on timing of initiation of therapy
    - Before 3 months: Generally normal development
  - Growth retardation
  - Delayed motor development
- Counseling important in documented cases of CH due to dyshormonogenesis or maternal autoimmune thyroiditis
  - Dyshormonogenesis: 25% occurrence rate in future pregnancies
  - Maternal autoimmune thyroiditis: High rate of occurrence in future pregnancies

Treatment

- Thyroid hormone replacement

SELECTED REFERENCES

1. Grüters A et al: Detection and treatment of congenital hypothyroidism. Nat Rev Endocrinol. 8(2):104-13, 2011
2. Rastogi MV et al: Congenital hypothyroidism. Orphanet J Rare Dis. 5:17, 2010
3. Clerc J et al: Scintigraphic imaging of paediatric thyroid dysfunction. Horm Res. 70(1):1-13, 2008
4. Schoen EJ et al: The key role of newborn thyroid scintigraphy with isotopic iodide (123I) in defining and managing congenital hypothyroidism. Pediatrics. 114(6):e683-8, 2004
5. el-Desouki M et al: Thyroid scintigraphy and perchlorate discharge test in the diagnosis of congenital hypothyroidism. Eur J Nucl Med. 22(9):1005-8, 1995

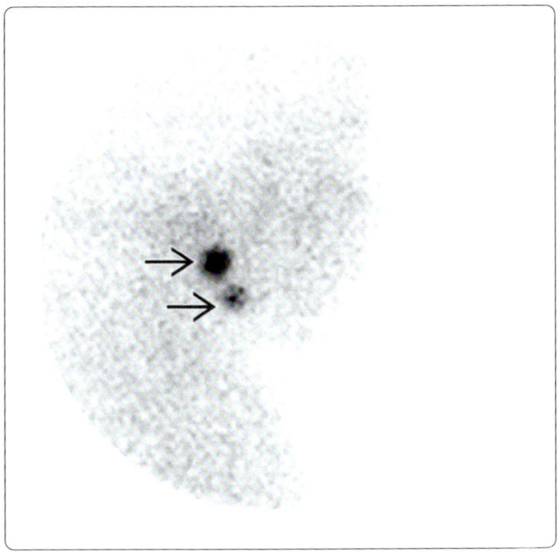

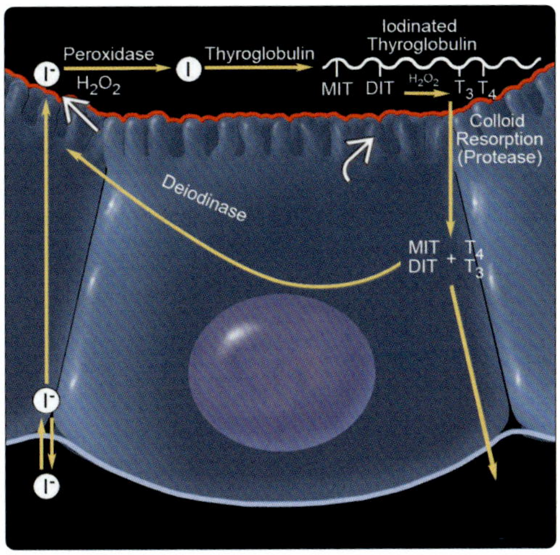

(Left) *Lateral I-123 thyroid scan in a 2-week-old girl with congenital hypothyroidism shows no normal uptake of iodine in the thyroid bed. 2 foci of uptake are present in the upper neck reflective of ectopic thyroid tissue.* **(Right)** *Graphic shows thyroid hormone production by thyroid follicles. Note iodide is trapped by the thyroid and organified, playing an essential role in thyroid hormone production.*

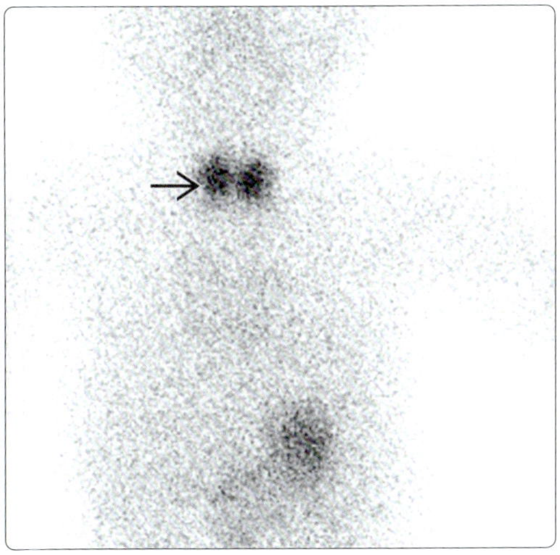

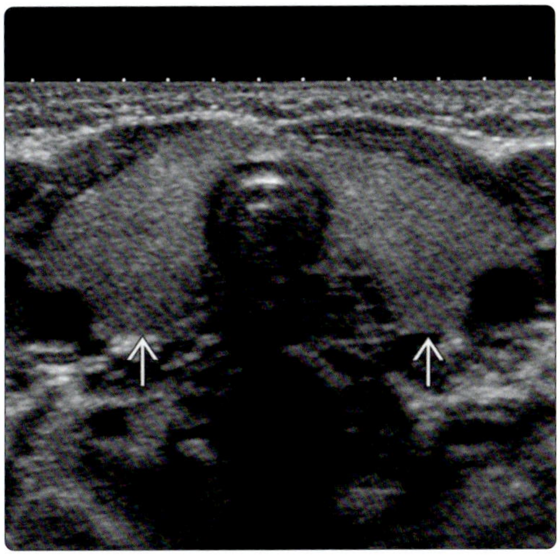

(Left) *Anterior Tc-99m pertechnetate scan in a 3-month-old girl with congenital hypothyroidism shows increased uptake in an enlarged, bilobed, eutopic thyroid. These findings suggest the presence of dyshormonogenesis (an organification defect).* **(Right)** *Transverse ultrasound of the neck in the same patient shows an enlarged, homogeneous bilobed thyroid in its normal location.*

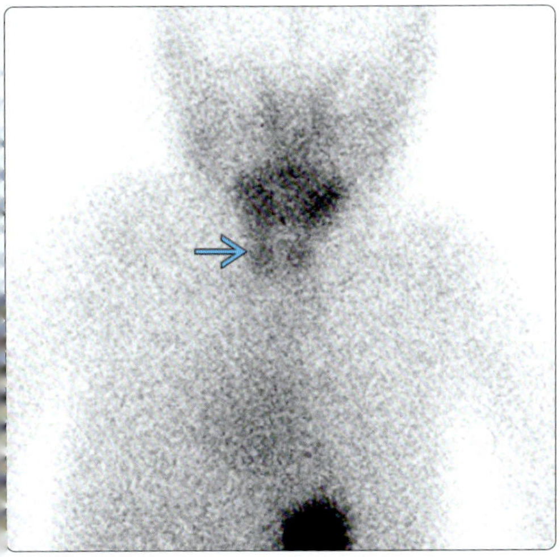

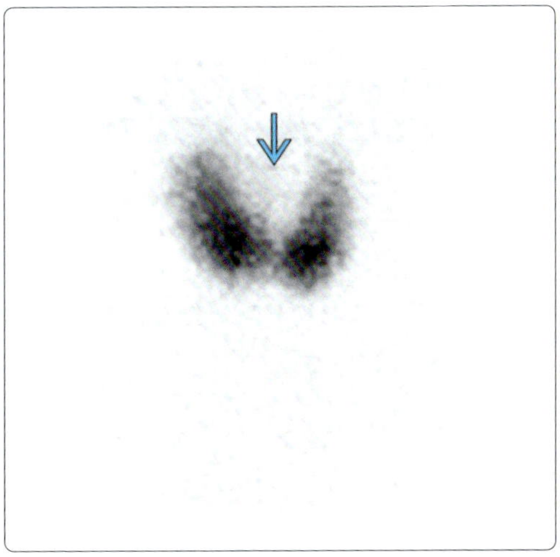

(Left) *Anterior Tc-99m pertechnetate scan in a 3-year-old girl with congenital hypothyroidism shows a bilobed, eutopic thyroid with diffusely decreased uptake. This reflects hypofunctioning of the gland with the exact etiology in this case undetermined.* **(Right)** *Pinhole image from a Tc-99m pertechnetate scan in an 11 day old with Pendred syndrome (sensorineural deafness, CH with goiter) shows an enlarged gland with increased radiotracer uptake and a prominent pyramidal lobe.*

KEY FACTS

TERMINOLOGY

- Gastroparesis = delayed gastric emptying in absence of mechanical obstruction

IMAGING

- Solid gastric emptying is diagnostic test of choice for gastroparesis
- Milk study allows assessment of both reflux and gastric emptying in infants
- Normative data for infant and pediatric gastric emptying is sparse and variable
- Liquid and solid emptying are not equivalent; one may be normal when other is not
- For young (< 8 years) and small (< 30 kg) patients, can image with single head
- In young adults and larger patients, need dual head imaging with calculation of gastric emptying based on geometric mean

CLINICAL ISSUES

- Gastroparesis more common in patients with diabetes mellitus or muscular dystrophy

DIAGNOSTIC CHECKLIST

- Regions of interest are key for accurate assessment of emptying
- Comparison to previously performed fluoroscopic upper GI exams or cross-sectional imaging (CT or MR) helpful to identify location and shape of stomach and course of adjacent bowel
- In patients with rapid emptying, some emptying may have occurred prior to "time zero" image; may need to calculate emptying relative to total abdominal counts (stomach and bowel)
- In general, geometric mean is most appropriate method to calculate retained activity/emptying

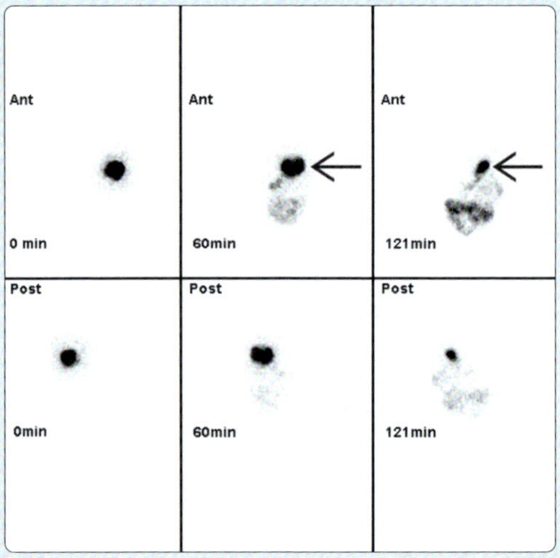

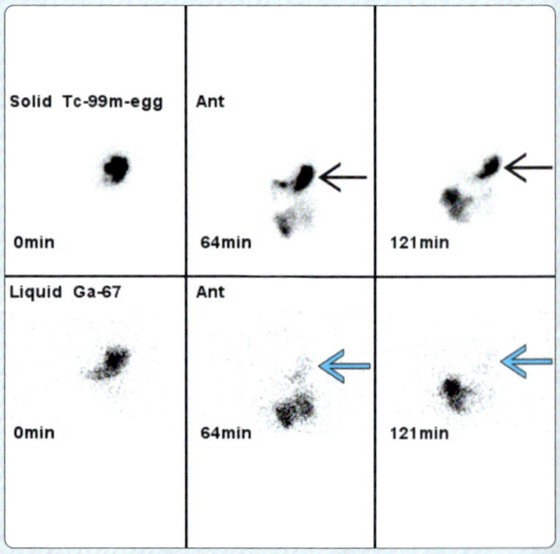

(Left) *Anterior and posterior solid phase gastric emptying study in a 12 year old with history of fundoplication shows normal emptying (decreased activity in the stomach, 70% at 2 hrs ➡).* **(Right)** *Anterior dual phase gastric emptying scan shows normal partial gastric emptying of the solid phase (57% at 2 hrs) ➡ and gastric emptying of most of the liquid phase (89% at 2 hrs) ➡.*

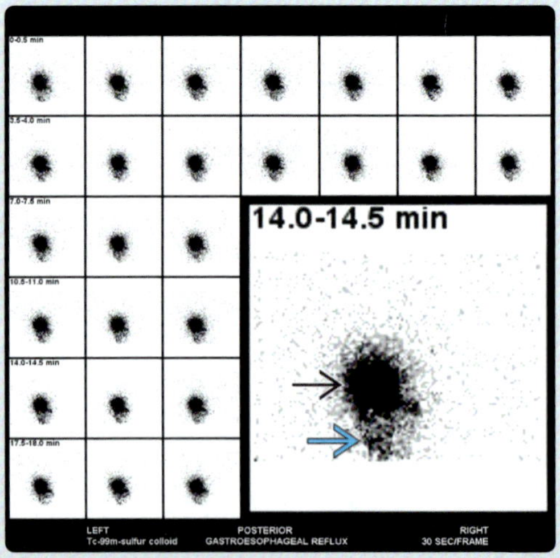

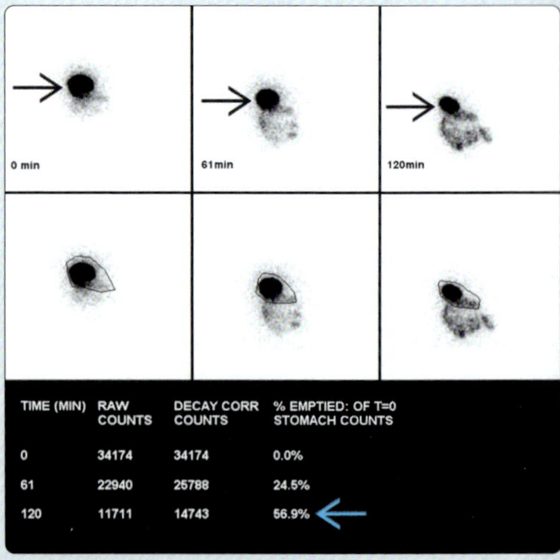

(Left) *Serial 30 second posterior images from dynamic portion of a normal milk scan are shown with a single image magnified for detail. Activity is visible in the stomach ➡ and intestine ➡ without any observed episodes of gastroesophageal reflux.* **(Right)** *Posterior projection images from a normal milk study show progressive emptying of the stomach ➡ over 2 hrs (57% emptying at 2 hrs ➡).*

TERMINOLOGY

Definitions

- Gastroparesis = delayed gastric emptying in absence of mechanical obstruction

IMAGING

General Features

- Best diagnostic clue
  - Delayed gastric emptying of scintigraphic solid meal

Nuclear Medicine Findings

- **Milk (reflux) study**
  - Used in infants with symptoms of gastroesophageal reflux (GER)
  - Allows assessment of frequency and severity of reflux and of gastric emptying
  - Milk and formula behave more like solid than liquid in acidic environment of stomach
  - Variable norms for gastric emptying (limited data)
    - Signer, 1975: 48-70% emptying at 60 min, 24-48% emptying at 2 hrs
    - Knatten et al, 2013: 43-79% emptying at 60 min
  - 1 hr emptying is poor predictor of 2 hr emptying; need to image for full 2 hrs
- **Routine gastric emptying study**
  - Older (non-infant) patients, used to assess gastric motility
  - Criteria for delayed emptying are highly variable and not well established in children
    - Chogle et al, 2013: Retention > 90% at 1 hr, > 60% at 2 hrs, > 30% at 4 hrs
    - Rodriguez et al, 2012: ≤ 40% emptying at 1 hr
    - Waseem et al, 2012: Half-time of > 90 min for solids, > 60 min for liquids
  - Liquid and solid emptying are not equivalent
    - Liquid emptying may remain normal even in setting of severe gastroparesis
    - Considered by some to be an end-stage indicator of gastroparesis

Imaging Recommendations

- Best imaging tool
  - Solid gastric emptying study
- Protocol advice
  - Preparation
    - Fast 4-6 hrs prior to study
    - Promotility medications should be held for 48-72 hrs prior to study (unless referring MD wants to see effect of medication)
  - Solid meal used for gastric emptying scintigraphy is carefully standardized in adults but less so in children
    - Typical meal of egg (or egg substitute), bread with butter and water commonly used
    - Some centers use oatmeal or cheese based on pediatric preferences
  - Radiopharmaceutical
    - Milk (or formula) for reflux study generally labeled with Tc-99m DTPA or Tc-99m sulfur colloid
      - Consensus guidelines suggest 0.25-1 mCi (9-37 MBq)
      - Formula volume titrated based on patient age
    - Solid emptying
      - Generally labeled with Tc-99m DTPA or Tc-99m sulfur colloid
      - Consensus guidelines suggest 0.25-0.5 mCi (9-18.5 MBq) in children
    - Liquid emptying (combined scan with solid emptying)
      - Generally labeled with either I-111 or Ga-67 when performed as dual phase study
      - In-111: 125 µCi (adult dosing)
      - Ga-67: 0.0015 mCi/kg
  - Dosimetry
    - Tc-99m sulfur colloid
      - Effective dose = 0.44-1.3 mSv depending on weight if above dosing used
      - Critical organ = colon (2-6 mGy)
  - Image acquisition
    - Milk study
      - Anterior or posterior single head images, every 5-30 sec for 1 hr
        - Assess for number and severity (proximal extent) of reflux events
      - Anterior or posterior single head images at time zero, 1 hr, and 2 hrs, corrected for decay
        - Assess gastric emptying
    - Routine gastric emptying
      - Can use single head, posterior camera for young (< 8 years) and small (< 30 kg) patients
      - In young adults and larger patients, need dual head imaging with calculation of gastric emptying based on geometric mean
      - Low-energy collimator for solid emptying studies
      - Medium-energy collimator for liquid/solid dual label studies
      - Duration of imaging in pediatric patients highly variable; many centers moving to adult standard of 4 hrs
      - Images acquired at time zero, 1 hr, 2 hrs, ± 4 hrs, corrected for decay

DIFFERENTIAL DIAGNOSIS

Gastroesophageal Reflux

- Caused by increased duration and frequency of relaxation of lower esophageal sphincter &/or by compromised esophageal clearance, sphincter hypotonia, increased gastric acidity or delayed gastric emptying

Peptic Ulcer Disease

- Ulceration of stomach/proximal duodenum, sometimes associated with *Helicobacter pylori* infection

Functional Dyspepsia

- Upper abdominal pain, nausea, and early satiety without structural cause

Dumping Syndrome

- Abnormal rapid emptying of stomach causes abdominal discomfort, nausea, diarrhea

PATHOLOGY

General Features

- Normal elements of gastric emptying
  - Fundal accommodation/receptive relaxation
  - Tonic contraction of fundus: Necessary for emptying of liquids
  - Antral peristalsis: Necessary for emptying of solids
  - Gastric trituration
  - Restricted emptying by pylorus: Allows only 1 mm and smaller particles to leave stomach
- Most common causes in children are
  - Idiopathic
  - Post viral
  - Medication effect
  - Postsurgical

CLINICAL ISSUES

Presentation

- Most common signs/symptoms
  - Nausea
  - Vomiting
  - Early satiety
  - Bloating
  - Abdominal pain
  - Weight loss
- Other signs/symptoms
  - Infants: Failure to thrive, irritability

Demographics

- Age
  - All ages
- Gender
  - Overall relatively even M:F, though becomes more common in females as age increases
- Epidemiology
  - More common in patients with diabetes mellitus
  - More common in patients with muscular dystrophy

Natural History & Prognosis

- Most cases improve with time, though can take years
- Complications include
  - Gastroesophageal reflux
  - Esophagitis
  - Gastritis

Treatment

- Medications
  - Proton pump inhibitors
  - Promotility medications: Tegaserod, erythromycin, metoclopramide, domperidone
- Diet modification: Small frequent meals, decreased fat, lactose-free diet
- Surgery
  - Gastrostomy/gastrojejunostomy tubes: Generally used in cases with severe weight loss/failure to thrive to provide nutritional support
  - Pyloroplasty
  - Fundoplication

DIAGNOSTIC CHECKLIST

Image Interpretation Pearls

- Regions of interest are key
  - Poorly placed regions of interest limit accuracy of results
  - Comparison to previously performed fluoroscopic upper GI exams or cross-sectional imaging (CT or MR) helpful to identify location and shape of stomach and course of adjacent bowel
  - In patients with rapid emptying, some emptying may have occurred prior to "time zero" image; may need to calculate emptying relative to total abdominal counts (stomach and bowel)
- In general, geometric mean is most appropriate method to calculate retained activity/emptying
- Gastric and liquid emptying do not necessarily correspond; possible to have abnormality of just 1 of 2 phases

SELECTED REFERENCES

1. Grant FD et al: Radiation doses for pediatric nuclear medicine studies: comparing the North American consensus guidelines and the pediatric dosage card of the European Association of Nuclear Medicine. Pediatr Radiol. ePub, 2014
2. Chogle A et al: Gastroparesis in children: the benefit of conducting 4-hour scintigraphic gastric-emptying studies. J Pediatr Gastroenterol Nutr. 56(4):439-42, 2013
3. Drubach LA et al: Gastric emptying in children: what is the best acquisition method? J Pediatr Gastroenterol Nutr. 55(2):191-3, 2012
4. Rodriguez L et al: Clinical presentation, response to therapy, and outcome of gastroparesis in children. J Pediatr Gastroenterol Nutr. 55(2):185-90, 2012
5. Waseem S et al: Spectrum of gastroparesis in children. J Pediatr Gastroenterol Nutr. 55(2):166-72, 2012
6. Gelfand MJ et al: Pediatric radiopharmaceutical administered doses: 2010 North American consensus guidelines. J Nucl Med. 52(2):318-22, 2011
7. Warrington JC et al: Pediatric gastrointestinal nuclear medicine. Semin Nucl Med. 37(4):269-85, 2007
8. Gelfand MJ et al: Gastric emptying in infants and children: limited utility of 1-hour measurement. Radiology. 178(2):379-81, 1991
9. Signer E: Gastric emptying in newborns and young infants. Measurement of the rate of emptying using indium-113m-microcolloid. Acta Paediatr Scand. 64(3):525-30, 1975

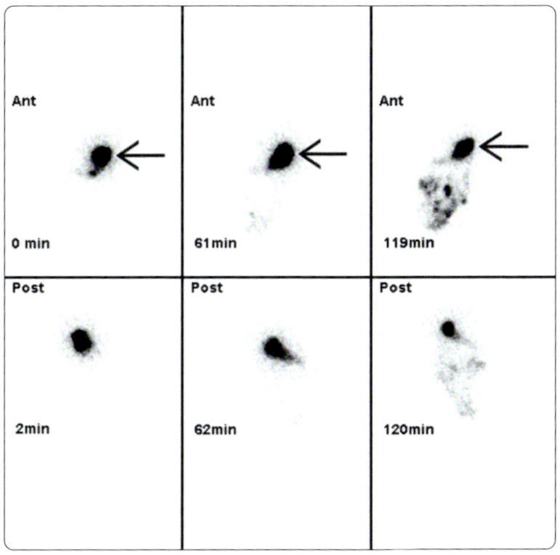

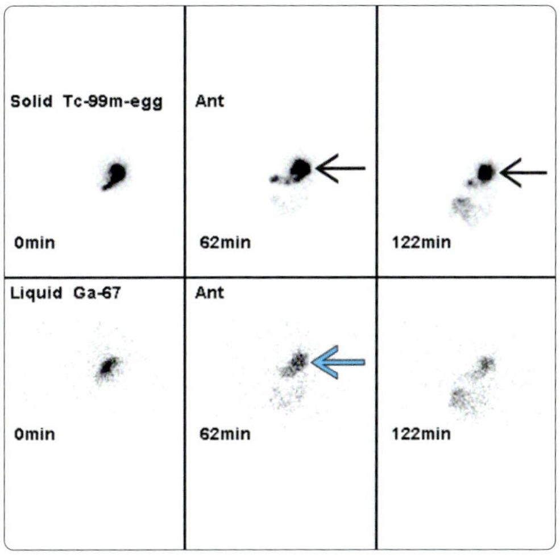

(Left) *Anterior and posterior solid phase gastric emptying scan shows delayed gastric emptying* → *(25% at 2 hrs).* **(Right)** *Anterior dual phase gastric emptying scan in a 10 year old with reflux and vomiting shows retention of radiotracer in the stomach, reflecting delayed gastric emptying of both the solid* → *(27% at 2 hrs) and liquid* → *(38% at 2 hrs) phases.*

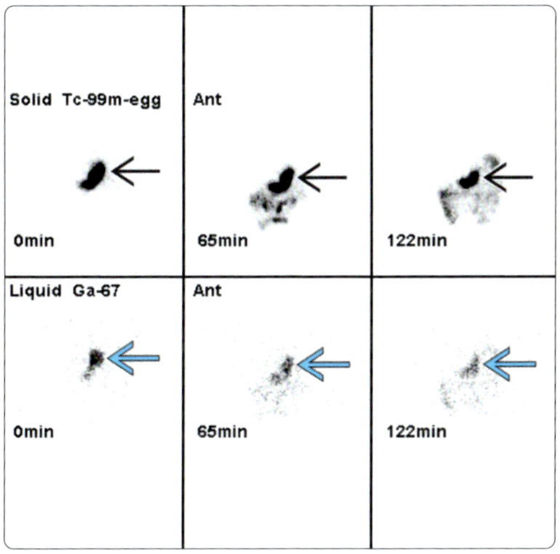

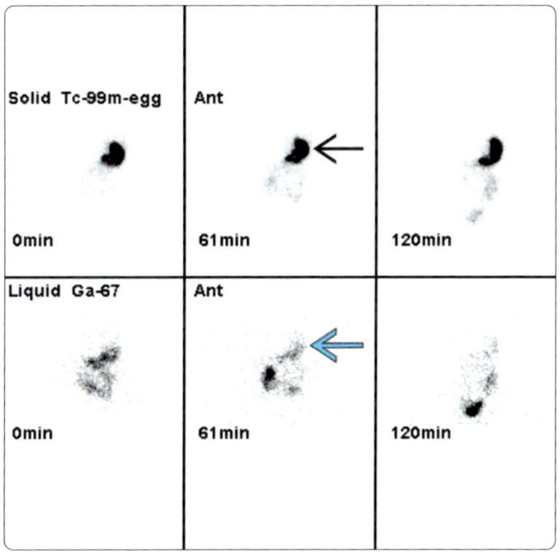

(Left) *Anterior dual phase gastric emptying scan in a 13 year old with nausea and Nissen fundoplication shows normal gastric emptying of solid phase (60% at 2 hrs)* → *but delayed gastric emptying of liquid phase (56% at 2 hrs)* →*.* **(Right)** *Anterior gastric emptying scan in a 12 year old with known gastroparesis shows retention of Tc-99m sulfur colloid in stomach* → *with partial clearance of Ga-67* →*, reflective of delayed solid emptying (3% at 2 hrs) with borderline liquid emptying (65% at 2 hrs).*

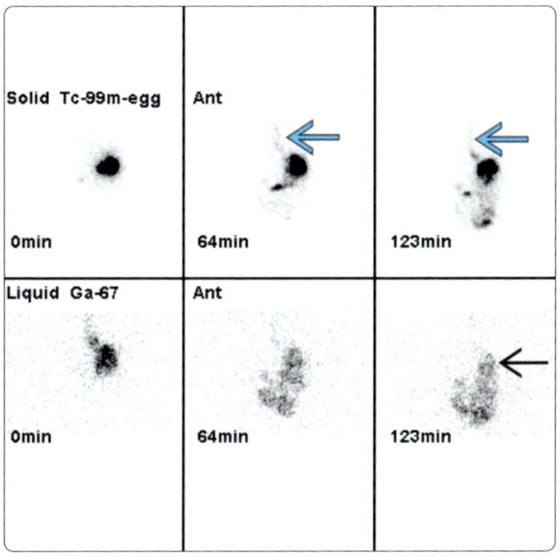

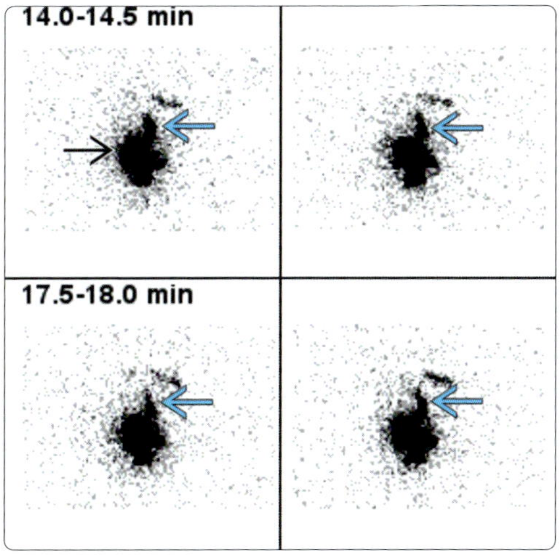

(Left) *Anterior dual phase gastric emptying scan shows retention of radiotracer in the stomach* → *on both phases, reflective of delayed emptying (59% liquid, 27% solid emptying at 2 hrs). Radiotracer is also seen in the esophagus due to gastroesophageal reflux* →*.* **(Right)** *Posterior images from dynamic portion of milk scan show activity extending from the stomach* → *into the lower esophagus* → *and persisting for more than 4 min, reflective of gastroesophageal reflux.*

KEY FACTS

TERMINOLOGY

- Meckel diverticulum: True diverticulum related to incomplete closure of omphalomesenteric duct
  - Most common congenital GI tract anomaly

IMAGING

- **Tc-99m pertechnetate scintigraphy**
  - Imaging test of choice in suspected Meckel diverticulum with GI bleeding
  - Taken up and secreted by tubular glands of gastric mucosa
  - Will only be positive if diverticulum contains heterotopic gastric mucosa
  - Focus of radiotracer accumulation (generally in right lower quadrant) that typically appears coincident with gastric mucosa
- Premedication with histamine (H2) blocker before imaging improves detection
- Activity should not migrate/disperse (vs. activity from GI bleed)
- Position of diverticula can vary and change during exam
- SPECT or SPECT/CT may be helpful to better localize foci of activity, particularly in subtle or confusing cases

CLINICAL ISSUES

- Most commonly presents with painless GI bleeding
- May present with abdominal pain due to obstruction, diverticulitis

DIAGNOSTIC CHECKLIST

- Key finding is **focal** uptake that appears coincident with gastric activity
- Important to differentiate activity in Meckel from excreted activity in urinary tract and activity cleared from stomach
- Negative Meckel scan does not mean absence of Meckel diverticulum; just means no Meckel diverticulum containing gastric mucosa

(Left) *Anterior Meckel scan in a 6-year-old boy with anemia and bloody stools shows the classic scintigraphic appearance of Meckel diverticulum. Focal radiotracer uptake similar to gastric uptake is present in the right lower quadrant* →. **(Right)** *Normal Meckel scan in a 5-year-old girl with bloody stools shows accumulation of activity in the stomach* → *with excreted activity in the bladder* ⇨. *Postvoid and lateral imaging shows no obscured focus of activity to suggest a Meckel diverticulum.*

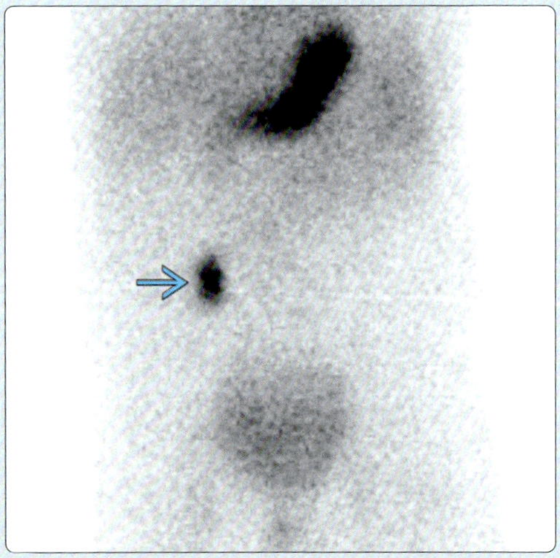

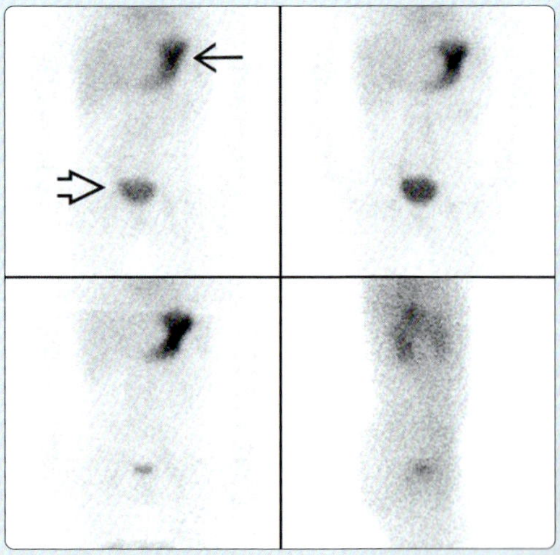

(Left) *Meckel scan in an 11-month-old girl with a Meckel diverticulum in the left abdomen shows an elongated focus of radiotracer uptake in the left mid abdomen* → *that persists through 40 min of imaging.* **(Right)** *Upright abdominal radiograph in a 7-year-old boy shows air-fluid levels* → *in dilated small bowel loops reflective of a small bowel obstruction found to be due to a Meckel diverticulum with adhesive bands.*

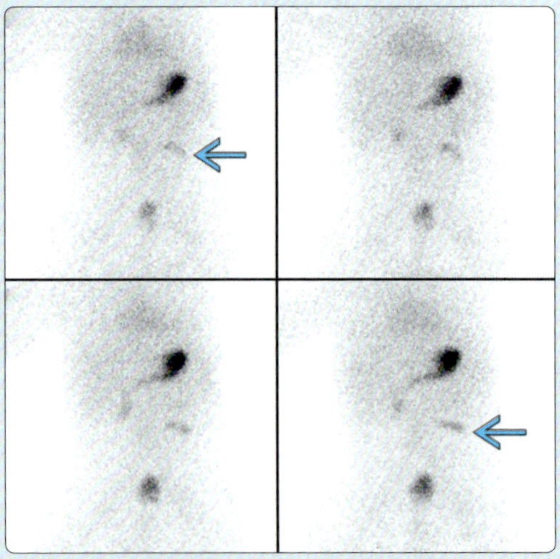

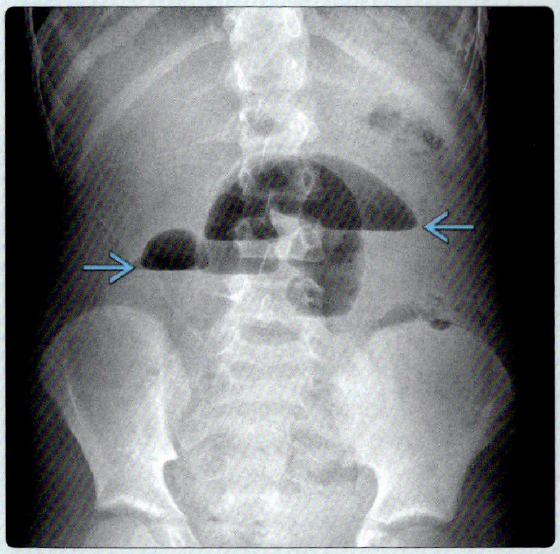

TERMINOLOGY

Definitions

- True diverticulum related to incomplete closure of omphalomesenteric duct

IMAGING

General Features

- Location
  - 50-100 cm from ileocecal valve
  - Usually located in right lower quadrant of abdomen
    - May be periumbilical or in the left abdomen
    - Can be mobile within abdomen
- Size
  - Variable; up to 15 cm in length
  - Considered giant if > 5-6 cm in diameter

Nuclear Medicine Findings

- **Tc-99m pertechnetate scintigraphy**
  - Taken up and secreted by tubular glands of gastric mucosa
  - Should be reserved for symptomatic cases with documented substantial GI bleeding (generally resulting in hematocrit drop)
  - Focus of radiotracer accumulation (generally in right lower quadrant) that (typically) appears coincident with gastric mucosa
    - Generally discrete focus
    - May appear ill defined if infected
    - May have delayed uptake
  - Will only be positive if diverticulum contains heterotopic gastric mucosa
    - Will miss diverticula lined by small bowel mucosa
    - May miss diverticula with small amounts of gastric mucosa
  - Activity should not migrate/disperse (vs. activity from GI bleed)
    - Activity persists throughout imaging
    - Diverticula may move in abdomen (e.g., left lower quadrant to right lower quadrant)
      - Focus of activity moves but maintains shape and does not disperse
  - False-positives
    - Duplication cysts with heterotopic gastric mucosa
    - Ulcerative or inflammatory processes
    - Active GI bleeding
    - Intussusception
    - GU activity
- **Tc-99m red blood cell or sulfur colloid scintigraphy**
  - Not test of choice for Meckel diverticulum but may be performed due to GI bleeding
  - Will only be positive in cases with active bleeding
  - Radiotracer accumulation in right lower quadrant with intraluminal migration

Imaging Recommendations

- Protocol advice
  - **Tc-99m pertechnetate scintigraphy**
  - Patient preparation
    - NPO 3-6 hr prior to imaging
    - Premedication with histamine (H2) blocker
      - Ranitidine 2-3 mg/kg (max dose 150 mg) commonly used
      - Recommended duration of premedication variable: SNMMI recommends 2 days for oral cimetidine, no specific recommendation for ranitidine; in practice 1 hr is sufficient for oral ranitidine (peak plasma half-life achieved ~ 90 min)
      - Slows secretion of pertechnetate allowing improved visualization of ectopic mucosa in diverticulum
      - If patient chronically on H2 blocker or proton pump inhibitor (PPI), no need to premedicate
    - Use of glucagon (to slow/stop peristalsis) has been described; not routinely used
      - Goal is to prevent gastric secretions from traveling downstream and causing false-positive or obscuring diverticulum
    - Can give super saturated potassium iodide (SSKI) after completion of study to protect thyroid
  - Radiopharmaceutical
    - Tc-99m sodium pertechnetate
      - 0.05 mCi (1.85 MBq)/kg IV (minimum 0.25 mCi)
  - Dosimetry
    - Effective dose = 0.86-1.04 mSv depending on patient weight
    - Critical organ = colon (~ 3 mGy)
  - Image acquisition
    - Single head anterior gamma camera with low-energy all-purpose or high-resolution collimator
    - Dynamic imaging for 35-45 min
    - Right lateral view can confirm anterior position of focal right lower quadrant activity and can separate Meckel from GU activity
    - Post-void imaging may be helpful to clear GU activity
    - SPECT or SPECT/CT may be helpful to better localize focal activity, particularly in subtle cases

Radiographic Findings

- Useful for identification of secondary findings including obstruction, perforation
- May identify enterolith (laminated calculus in right lower quadrant)

CT Findings

- Uncomplicated diverticula can be identified by CT, but CT more useful for assessment of complications (obstruction, diverticulitis, etc.)
  - Diverticulitis: Thick-walled, irregular diverticulum with surrounding inflammation, ± perforation
- May identify enteroliths

DIFFERENTIAL DIAGNOSIS

Spectrum of Omphalomesenteric Duct Remnants

- Umbilico-ileal fistula: Tubular connection between umbilicus and ileum
- Umbilical sinus: Blind-ending tract from umbilicus extending into abdomen
- Umbilical cyst: Cyst within fibrous remnant of omphalomesenteric duct without patent connection to either umbilicus or ileum

- Persistent fibrous cord: Connects umbilicus to ileum

Enteric Duplication Cyst

- May be indistinguishable on scintigraphy from Meckel diverticulum
- Located on mesenteric side of bowel

Gastrointestinal Bleeding From Other Causes

- Activity moves intraluminally in abdomen
- Timing of appearance of activity often different from that of stomach

Renal Excretion

- Can cause false-positive results

Gastrointestinal Excretion

- Stomach may excrete radiotracer despite administration of H2 blockers
- Left lateral decubitus positioning may limit this
- Administration of water by mouth and reimaging may help dilute excreted activity

PATHOLOGY

General Features

- Etiology
  - Incomplete closure/atrophy of omphalomesenteric (vitelline) duct
    - Omphalomesenteric duct is embryonic communication between yolk sac and midgut
  - Meckel diverticulum is most common (98%) of spectrum of omphalomesenteric duct remnants

Gross Pathologic & Surgical Features

- Blind-ending outpouching from antimesenteric side of distal ileum
- May have have fibrous connection to umbilicus
- May have fibrous connections/adhesions to adjacent ileum (mesodiverticular bands)
- Blood supply via remnant of omphalomesenteric artery

Microscopic Features

- True diverticulum containing all layers of bowel wall
- Lined by small bowel mucosa
- 50% contain heterotopic tissue
  - Gastric mucosa most common (23-50%)
  - Pancreatic tissue in 5-16%
  - Colonic or biliary mucosa more rare
- Ulceration may occur within diverticulum or in adjacent ileum
- May harbor small foci of carcinoid tumor

CLINICAL ISSUES

Presentation

- Most common signs/symptoms
  - Painless GI bleeding
- Other signs/symptoms
  - Abdominal pain
    - Due to obstruction
    - Due to Meckel diverticulitis
      - Generally also have fever and vomiting
      - May mimic acute appendicitis
    - Due to enterolith formation
    - Due to volvulus or torsion of diverticulum
  - Obstruction
    - Due to intussusception or inversion of diverticulum
    - Due to adhesions/mesodiverticular bands
  - Littre hernia: Inguinal hernia containing Meckel diverticulum

Demographics

- Age
  - Of symptomatic cases, 60% before age 10
- Epidemiology
  - Most common congenital GI tract anomaly
  - 2-3% of population

Natural History & Prognosis

- 4% lifetime risk of developing complications

Treatment

- Surgery
  - Reserved for symptomatic cases

DIAGNOSTIC CHECKLIST

Image Interpretation Pearls

- Tc-99m pertechnetate is test of choice for Meckel diverticulum-containing heterotopic gastric mucosa
- Key finding is **focal** uptake that appears coincident with gastric activity
- Important to differentiate activity in Meckel from excreted activity in urinary tract and activity cleared from stomach
- Negative Meckel scan does not mean absence of Meckel diverticulum; just means no Meckel diverticulum-containing gastric mucosa

SELECTED REFERENCES

1. Grant FD et al: Radiation doses for pediatric nuclear medicine studies: comparing the North American consensus guidelines and the pediatric dosage card of the European Association of Nuclear Medicine. Pediatr Radiol. ePub, 2014
2. Sinha CK et al: Meckel's scan in children: a review of 183 cases referred to two paediatric surgery specialist centres over 18 years. Pediatr Surg Int. 29(5):511-7, 2013
3. Gelfand MJ et al: Pediatric radiopharmaceutical administered doses: 2010 North American consensus guidelines. J Nucl Med. 52(2):318-22, 2011
4. Dillman JR et al: Utility of SPECT/CT with Meckel's scintigraphy. Ann Nucl Med. 23(9):813-5, 2009
5. Kiratli PO et al: Detection of ectopic gastric mucosa using 99mTc pertechnetate: review of the literature. Ann Nucl Med. 23(2):97-105, 2009
6. Levy AD et al: From the archives of the AFIP. Meckel diverticulum: radiologic features with pathologic Correlation. Radiographics. 24(2):565-87, 2004
7. Richards DA: Comparative pharmacodynamics and pharmacokinetics of cimetidine and ranitidine. J Clin Gastroenterol. 5 Suppl 1:81-90, 1983
8. Gelfand MJ et al: Radionuclide imaging of Meckel's diverticulum in children. Clin Nucl Med. 3(1):4-8, 1978

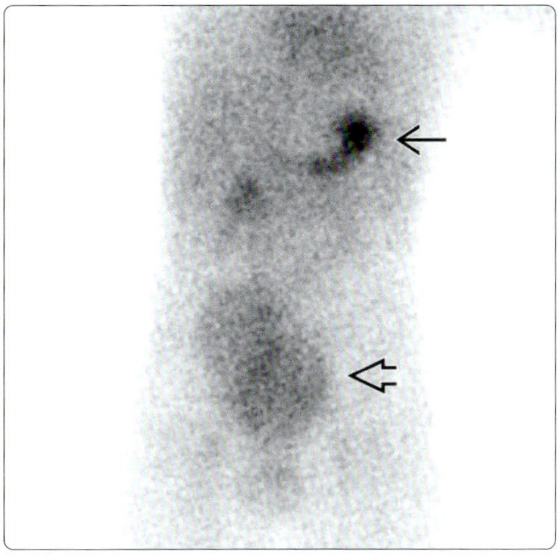
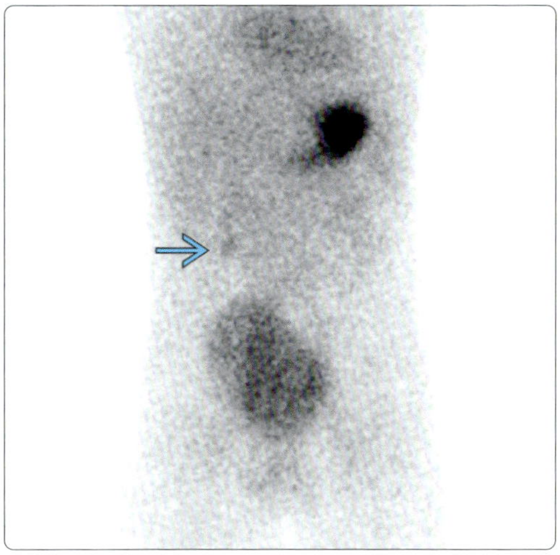

(Left) *Meckel scan in a 5 year old with rectal bleeding and anemia shows accumulation of activity in the stomach → and bladder ⇨, but no focal uptake to suggest a Meckel diverticulum.* **(Right)** *Subsequent image in the same patient shows a focus of activity in the left mid abdomen → that first appeared at 40 min and persisted through 90 min. This case illustrates the occasional delayed appearance of uptake in ectopic gastric mucosa in a Meckel diverticulum.*

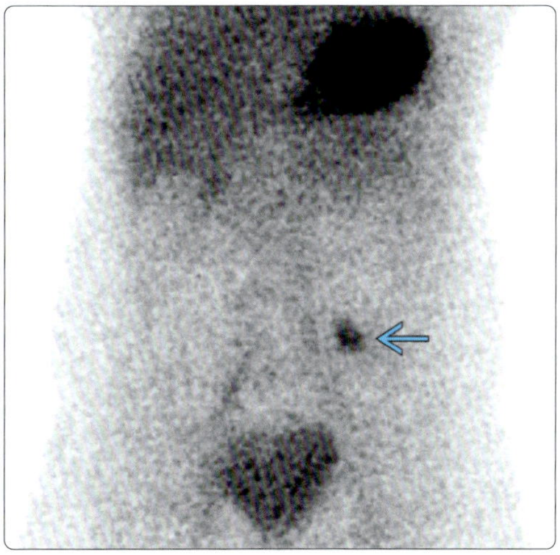
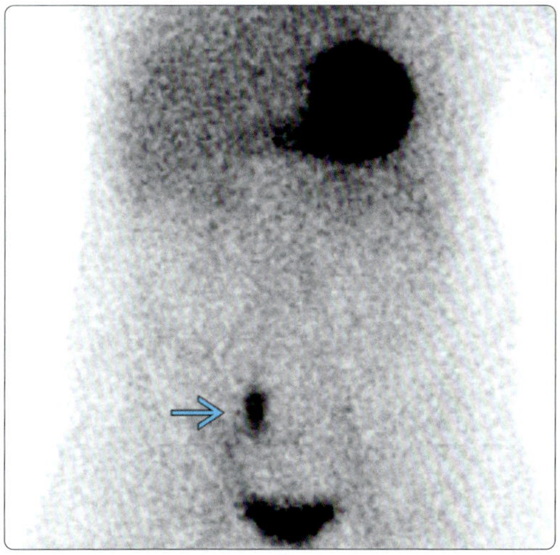

(Left) *Meckel scan in a 10-year-old girl with bloody stool shows a focus of radiotracer accumulation in the left mid abdomen →.* **(Right)** *Subsequent image in the same patient shows that the focus of radiotracer maintains its shape and intensity of radiotracer uptake but migrates to the right lower quadrant →. Some Meckel diverticula (like this case) can move within the abdomen.*

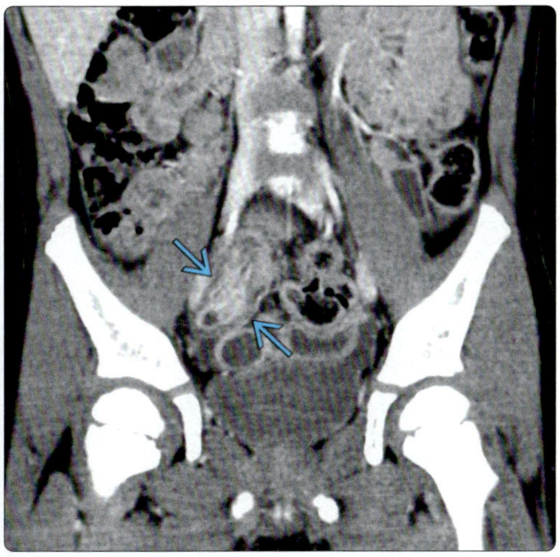
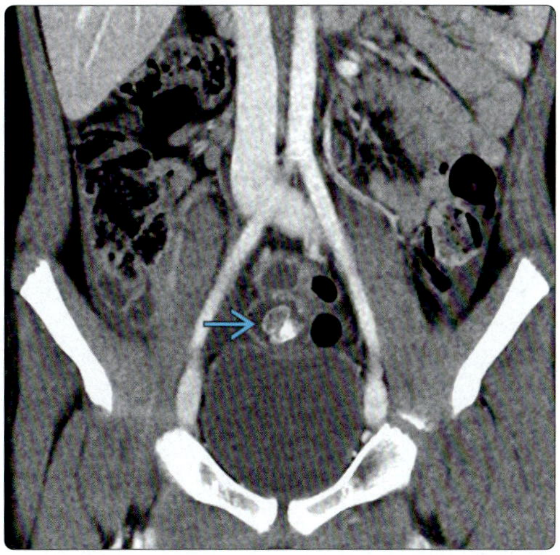

(Left) *Coronal CECT in a 5-year-old boy with abdominal pain shows a hyperenhancing, blind-ending loop of bowel in the right lower quadrant with surrounding inflammatory change →. Not shown is free intraperitoneal air in this patient with perforated Meckel diverticulitis.* **(Right)** *Coronal CT in a 10-year-old boy shows coarse calcifications → within a loop of bowl above the dome of the bladder reflecting enteroliths in a Meckel diverticulum.*

Biliary Atresia

KEY FACTS

TERMINOLOGY

- Obliterative cholangiopathy of neonates involving intrahepatic and extrahepatic ducts to varying degrees
- Resulting cholestasis leads to cirrhosis and death if untreated

IMAGING

- Hepatobiliary scintigraphy with Tc-99m iminodiacetic acid (IDA) derivative
  - Extremely sensitive; clear demonstration of biliary-to-bowel transit excludes biliary atresia
  - Specificity lower; many other causes of cholestasis can mimic biliary atresia
- Premedication essential to increase hepatic transport of radiotracer and improve specificity
  - Most common agent: Phenobarbital 5 mg/kg/day in 2 divided doses for at least 3 and preferably 5 days prior to scan
- Nonvisualization of bowel on delayed imaging at 24 hrs raises possibility of biliary atresia

TOP DIFFERENTIAL DIAGNOSES

- Neonatal hepatitis
- Choledochal cyst
- Choledocholithiasis
- Paucity of intrahepatic ducts

DIAGNOSTIC CHECKLIST

- Facilitate prompt scheduling of hepatobiliary scan when ordered; delay in surgical treatment may significantly increase risk of poor outcome
- Presence of gallbladder does not exclude biliary atresia
- Even if hepatobiliary scan strongly suggests neonatal hepatitis, cannot exclude biliary atresia unless bowel activity evident

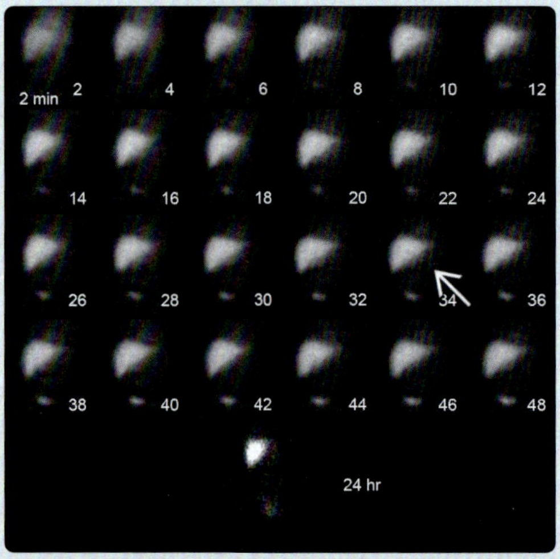

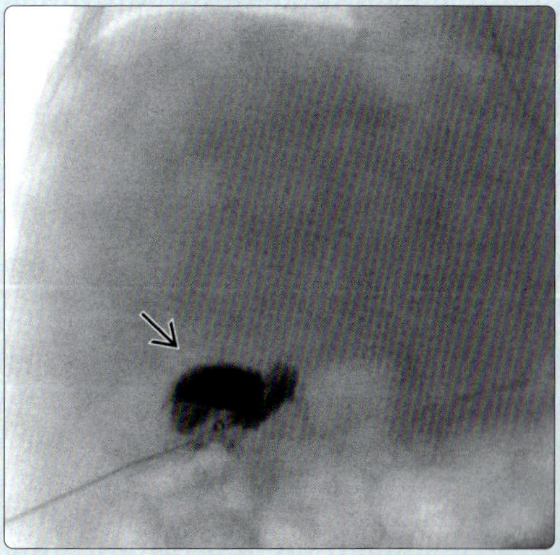

(Left) *Anterior Tc-99m HIDA scan shows uniform intense uptake in the liver and prompt clearance from the blood pool in this neonate with biliary atresia. There is no gallbladder activity and no intestinal activity, even at 24 hours. Faint nonmotile activity in the left upper quadrant* ➔ *represents renal excretion of radiotracer.* **(Right)** *Intraoperative cholangiogram in the same patient shows that contrast fills the gallbladder* ➔ *but does not enter the common bile duct, confirming biliary atresia.*

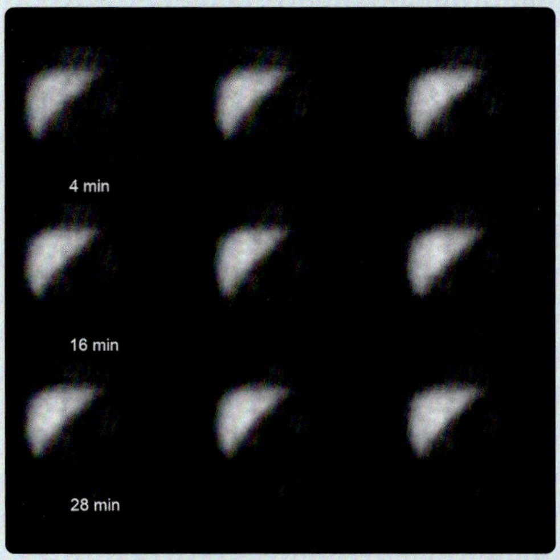

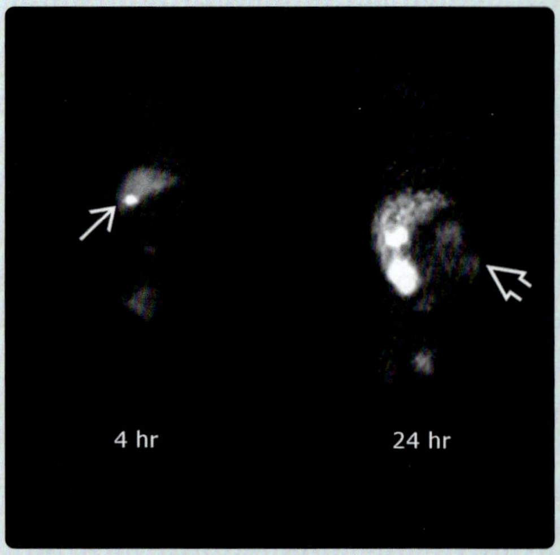

(Left) *Initial segment of a hepatobiliary scan in this jaundiced infant without biliary atresia shows uptake in the liver and clearance of tracer from blood pool without gallbladder or bowel activity. At this point, biliary atresia cannot be excluded.* **(Right)** *Delayed image at 4 hours shows gallbladder activity* ➔*; however, a minority of patients with biliary atresia can show this finding. Activity in the bowel throughout the abdomen* ➔ *is seen at 24 hours, excluding biliary atresia.*

TERMINOLOGY

Definitions

- Obliterative cholangiopathy of neonates involving intrahepatic and extrahepatic ducts to varying degrees
  - Resulting cholestasis leads to cirrhosis and death if untreated

IMAGING

Nuclear Medicine Findings

- Hepatobiliary scintigraphy
  - Normal
    - Prompt clearance of radiotracer from blood pool
    - Uniform hepatic uptake
      - Gallbladder (GB) and bile ducts may not be seen in neonates
    - Bowel activity within 60 min
  - Biliary atresia
    - Prompt clearance of radiotracer from blood pool
    - Uniform hepatic uptake
    - Nonvisualization of bowel on delayed imaging (24 hrs)
    - Patients who have developed hepatic impairment can show delayed clearance from blood pool and decreased hepatic uptake
  - Neonatal hepatitis
    - Delayed clearance from blood pool
    - Poor hepatic uptake
    - Bowel activity often present
      - May be minimal or absent depending on degree of hepatic dysfunction

Imaging Recommendations

- Best imaging tool
  - Hepatobiliary scintigraphy with Tc-99m iminodiacetic acid (IDA) derivative
    - Extremely sensitive; clear demonstration of biliary-to-bowel transit excludes biliary atresia
    - Specificity lower; many other causes of cholestasis can mimic biliary atresia
- Protocol advice
  - Patient preparation
    - Premedication essential to increase hepatic transport of radiotracer and improve specificity
      - Most common agent: Phenobarbital 5 mg/kg/day in 2 divided doses for at least 3 and preferably 5 days prior to scan
      - Alternative agent: Ursodeoxycholic acid 20 mg/kg/day in 2 divided doses for 2-3 days prior to scan; continue use until scan complete
    - Fasting 2 hours prior
      - Clear liquids can be given in this time period if necessary
  - Radiopharmaceutical
    - 0.05 mCi (1.85 MBq)/kg Tc-99m mebrofenin administered intravenously
      - Mebrofenin preferred over disofenin due to better hepatic extraction
    - Minimum dose 1 mCi (37 MBq)
      - Note minimum dose 0.5 mCi (18.5 MBq) for other indications where delayed imaging typically not necessary
  - Dosimetry
    - Effective dose: 0.37 rem/mCi to gallbladder, 0.17 rem/mCi to colon
  - Image acquisition
    - Large field-of-view gamma camera
    - 128 x 128 matrix with electronic acquisition zoom
    - Low-energy all-purpose or low-energy high-resolution collimator
    - Dynamic anterior planar images
      - 1 min/frame x 60 min
      - Displaying in cine mode may increase sensitivity for subtle bowel activity
      - Can compress data as needed to increase counts per frame
    - Static anterior planar images at delayed time points until bowel visualized or until 24 hours after injection
    - Lateral or oblique planar images or SPECT to evaluate questionable bowel activity
      - For SPECT, consider omitting attenuation correction CT to reduce radiation exposure

Artifacts and Quality Control

- Potential false-negative test: Urinary tract activity and urine contamination can simulate bowel activity
  - Lateral planar images or SPECT can distinguish
  - Change diaper and clean skin
- Potential false-positive test: Insufficient phenobarbital level decreases hepatic transit
  - Goal serum level 14-15 μg/mL; typically achieved by empiric dosing
  - Level can be measured prior to exam, or afterward if exam is positive

Ultrasonographic Findings

- Usually 1st imaging test in work-up
  - Can show signs of many different hepatobiliary conditions
- Biliary atresia
  - Triangular cord sign
    - Triangular echogenic structure ≥ 4 mm thick adjacent to portal vein
    - Fibrosed remnant of extrahepatic biliary system
    - Highly specific for biliary atresia
    - Wide range of sensitivity reported
  - Absent or small, irregular gallbladder
  - Lack of gallbladder contraction after feeding
  - Hepatosplenomegaly (nonspecific)

Other Modality Findings

- Intraoperative cholangiography
  - Definitive test to evaluate biliary anatomy
  - Some centers use percutaneous GB cholangiogram (if GB present on US or hepatobiliary scintigraphy) or ERCP

DIFFERENTIAL DIAGNOSIS

Neonatal Hepatitis

- Term applied when underlying etiology of cholestasis is not discovered

- Incidence decreasing due to improved diagnosis of other causes of cholestasis
  - Viral or bacterial infection
  - α-1-antitrypsin deficiency
  - Inborn errors of metabolism
  - Shock
  - Total parenteral nutrition-associated cholestasis
- Similar findings on hepatobiliary scan regardless of underlying etiology
- Clinical presentation often indistinguishable from biliary atresia

Choledochal Cyst

- May see photopenic defect centrally on early images, which slowly accumulates tracer over time
- Large cysts can obstruct common bile duct and mimic biliary atresia

Choledocholithiasis

- Rare in this age group, look for associated bile duct anomalies

Paucity of Intrahepatic Ducts

- Can be isolated or syndromic (Alagille syndrome)
- Slow washout from liver periphery with prompt clearance of central liver and bowel arrival may be seen but can also mimic biliary atresia pattern

PATHOLOGY

General Features

- Etiology
  - Unknown; inflammation, viral infection, genetic factors, and vascular insult have been proposed
- Associated abnormalities
  - Biliary atresia isolated in 80-90% of cases
  - Most common syndromic presentation is biliary atresia splenic malformation syndrome
    - Splenic malformations include polysplenia, asplenia, double spleen
    - Other associations in this condition include small bowel malrotation, cardiac defects, interrupted IVC, preduodenal portal vein, and situs inversus

Staging, Grading, & Classification

- Japanese Association of Pediatric Surgeons classification; based on location of proximal most atretic segment
  - Type I: Common bile duct
  - Type II: Common hepatic duct
  - Type III: Porta hepatis (~ 85%)

CLINICAL ISSUES

Presentation

- Most common signs/symptoms
  - Persistent jaundice beyond 2 weeks of age in term infants or 3 weeks of age in preterm infants
- Other signs/symptoms
  - Conjugated hyperbilirubinemia
  - Elevated serum γ-glutamyltransferase
  - Acholic stools
  - Dark urine
  - Failure to thrive
  - Coagulopathy

Natural History & Prognosis

- Untreated biliary atresia fatal by 2 years
- Progressive biliary cirrhosis with hepatic failure

Treatment

- Kasai portoenterostomy
  - Excision of extrahepatic bile ducts to level of porta hepatis and anastomosis of a jejunal loop to cut liver surface with exposed intrahepatic ductules
  - Palliative procedure; inflammation and fibrosis of intrahepatic ducts continues after portoenterostomy
  - Durability dependent on age at surgery, extent of liver damage, and surgical expertise
    - Goal is surgery by 60 days of age
    - Some centers will not perform Kasai after 100 days of age
- Liver transplantation
  - Majority of patients eventually require transplant
    - Kasai allows time for growth of patient and planning transplant
  - Long-term survival after transplant very good (i.e., 10-year survival > 85%)
  - Biliary atresia does not recur after transplant

DIAGNOSTIC CHECKLIST

Consider

- Facilitate prompt scheduling of hepatobiliary scan when ordered; delay in surgical treatment may significantly increase risk of poor outcome

Image Interpretation Pearls

- Presence of GB does not exclude biliary atresia
  - Type I biliary atresia (~ 5-10%) is patent to level of common bile duct; gallbladder can be seen on hepatobiliary scan
  - ~ 20% of type III cases have mucus-filled gallbladder that can appear normal on ultrasound
- Even if hepatobiliary scan strongly suggests neonatal hepatitis, cannot exclude biliary atresia unless bowel activity evident

SELECTED REFERENCES

1. Moreira RK et al: Biliary atresia: a multidisciplinary approach to diagnosis and management. Arch Pathol Lab Med. 136(7):746-60, 2012
2. Tulchinsky M et al: SNM practice guideline for hepatobiliary scintigraphy 4.0. J Nucl Med Technol. 2010 Dec;38(4):210-8. Epub 2010 Nov 15. Erratum in: J Nucl Med Technol. 40(3):17A, 2012
3. De Bruyne R et al: Clinical practice: neonatal cholestasis. Eur J Pediatr. 170(3):279-84, 2011
4. Mittal V et al: Role of abdominal sonography in the preoperative diagnosis of extrahepatic biliary atresia in infants younger than 90 days. AJR Am J Roentgenol. 196(4):W438-45, 2011
5. Rozel C et al: Imaging of biliary disorders in children. Pediatr Radiol. 41(2):208-20, 2011

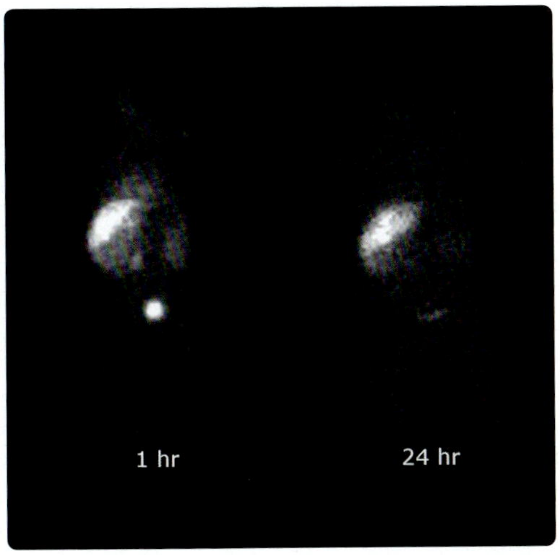

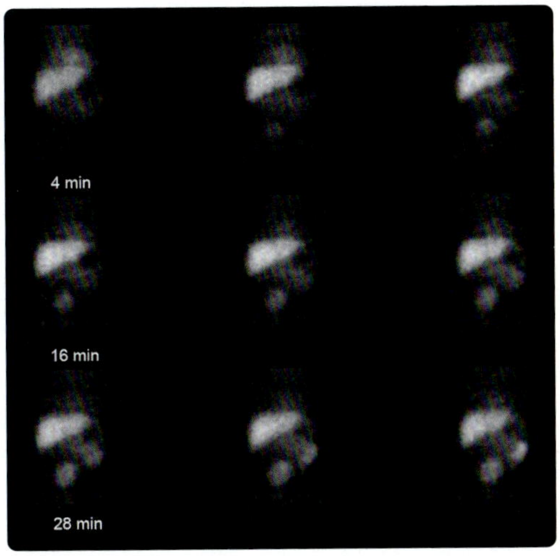

(Left) *Infant with biliary atresia is shown. Despite normal hepatic uptake of tracer, no biliary-to-bowel transit is seen over 24 hours. Note the relatively extensive urinary tract activity, which can be distinguished from bowel using cine images, lateral views, or SPECT if necessary.* **(Right)** *Prompt biliary-to-bowel transit is shown in this jaundiced infant without biliary atresia. Delayed images need not be obtained in this situation.*

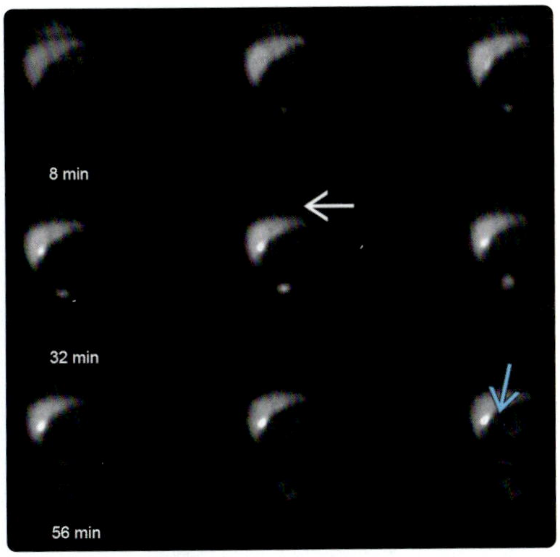

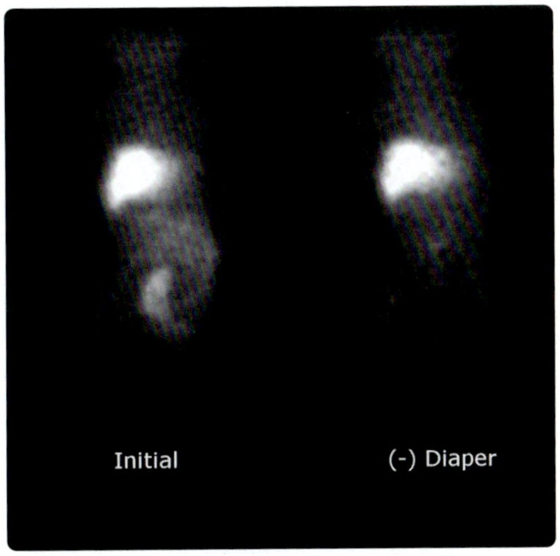

(Left) *This infant with neonatal hepatitis has prolonged activity in the cardiac blood pool* ➡*. Note the intensity is higher relative to hepatic uptake than on some of the other images. Despite this, biliary-to-bowel* ⇨ *transit is clearly seen.* **(Right)** *Delayed static images from a hepatobiliary scan appear to show activity throughout the abdomen, which could be interpreted as bowel. After the diaper was removed and patient cleaned, this activity was no longer seen.*

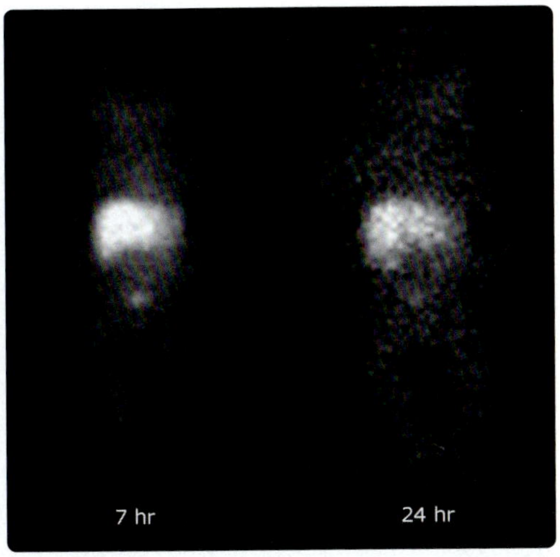

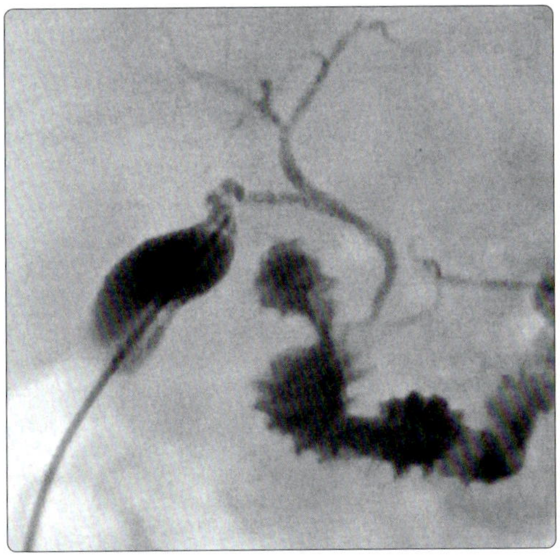

(Left) *Hepatobiliary scan in an infant shows no biliary-to-bowel transit over 24 hours. Biliary atresia cannot be excluded.* **(Right)** *Intraoperative cholangiogram in the same patient shows filling of the gallbladder, cystic duct, common bile duct, and central intrahepatic ducts. The hepatobiliary scan was falsely positive for biliary atresia.*

Fever of Unknown Origin

KEY FACTS

IMAGING

- Small case series have shown diagnostic value of F-18 FDG PET/CT for children with occult infection
  - F-18 FDG PET/CT contributed to final diagnosis in 45%
- In 5-year study published in 1991, bone scan led to diagnosis in 2% of 109 cases
  - 1 case showed uptake in bone related to osteomyelitis, 1 case showed decreased uptake in femoral head of unknown etiology
- 1993 study of Ga-67 scintigraphy in 30 children with FUO found little benefit in absence of focal symptoms
  - 4 positive scans: Pyelonephritis, chronic osteomyelitis, sinusitis, sarcoidosis
- In-111 white blood cell (WBC) scintigraphy
  - In 1991 study, WBC scintigraphy led to diagnosis in 5% of 109 cases
  - 4 of 5 cases showed cardiac uptake: Toxoplasmosis with pericardial effusion, autoimmune disease, presumed Kawasaki, 1 case undiagnosed

TOP DIFFERENTIAL DIAGNOSES

- Pneumonia
- Inflammatory bowel disease
- Kawasaki disease
- Collagen vascular disease
- Malignancy

CLINICAL ISSUES

- Definition of FUO is very specific: Fever > 38°C for ≥ 14 consecutive days
- Approach to FUO in children is very clinical with little role for imaging
  - Series of histories and clinical exams, laboratory tests (trended over time)
  - Imaging only applied if there are localizing signs or concern for malignancy
  - Majority of febrile children have viral illness
- In order, infectious, inflammatory, and neoplastic causes dominate ultimately identified causes of FUO

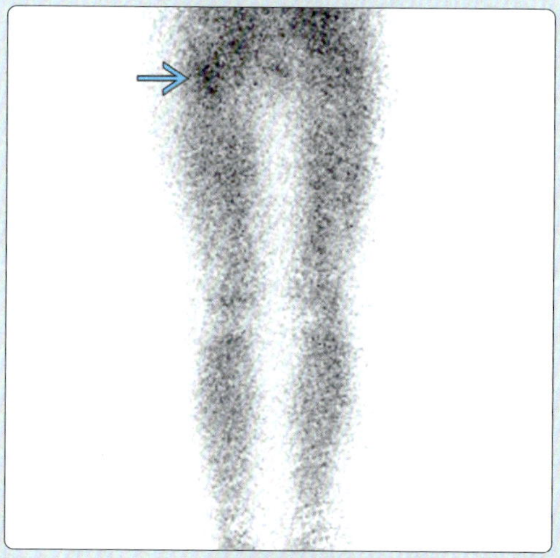

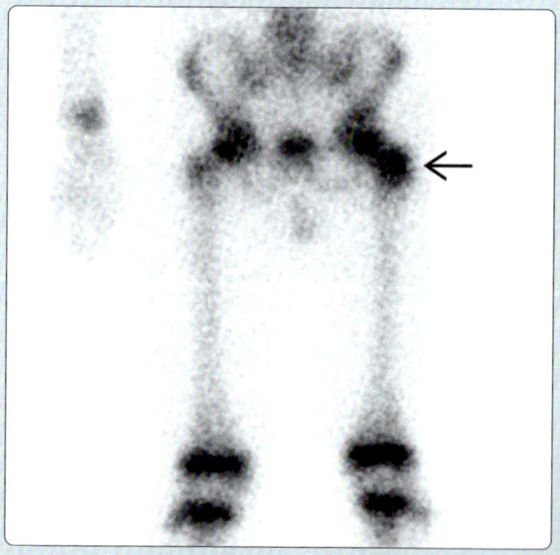

(Left) *Posterior blood pool image from a Tc-99m MDP bone scan in a 5 year old with fever of unknown origin shows increased blood pool activity at the level of the left proximal femur* ➡. **(Right)** *Anterior delayed image in the same patient shows abnormal uptake in the left proximal femur* ➡. *The combination of the blood pool and delayed imaging findings are consistent with osteomyelitis.*

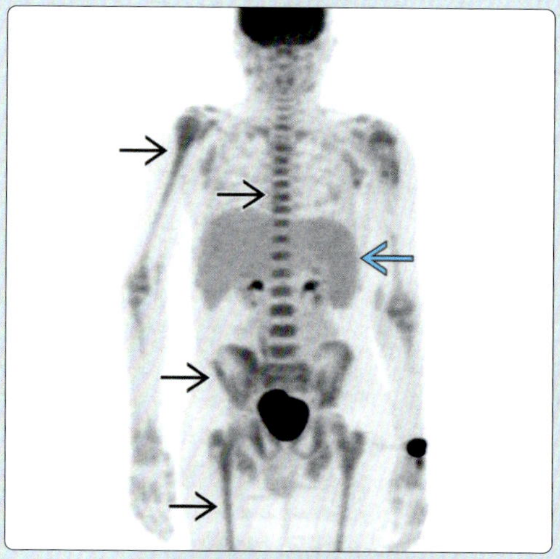

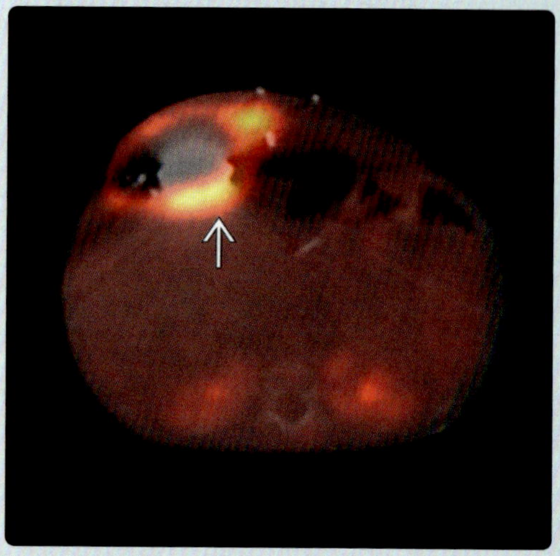

(Left) *Anterior MIP F-18 FDG PET in a 15 year old with fever of unknown origin shows diffusely increased marrow uptake of F-18 FDG* ➡ *and splenomegaly with diffusely increased splenic uptake* ➡ *reflecting involvement by disease in this patient ultimately diagnosed with ALL.* **(Right)** *Fused axial F-18 FDG PET/CT in a 2 year old with fever of unknown origin shows abnormal uptake surrounding an implanted pacer/defibrillator generator in the abdominal wall* ➡ *reflecting device infection as the source of fever.*

IMAGING

Nuclear Medicine Findings

- Bone scan
  - In 5-year study published in 1991, bone scan led to diagnosis in 2% of 109 cases of fever of unknown origin (FOV)
    - 1 case showed uptake in bone related to osteomyelitis, 1 case showed decreased uptake in femoral head of unknown etiology
- PET/CT
  - Advantage of F-18 FDG PET/CT is ability to screen whole body
  - Small case series have shown diagnostic value for children with occult infection
  - Largest study to date of mix of patients with FUO and unexplained inflammation (n=77)
    - F-18 FDG PET/CT contributed to final diagnosis in 45%
    - In other 55%, F-18 FDG PET/CT resulted in unnecessary testing
- Ga-67 scintigraphy
  - In 1991 study, Ga-67 scintigraphy led to diagnosis in 1% of 109 cases
    - Single positive case showed abnormal osseous uptake related to osteomyelitis
  - 1993 study of Ga-67 scintigraphy in 30 children with FUO found little benefit in absence of focal symptoms
    - 4 positive scans: Pyelonephritis, chronic osteomyelitis, sinusitis, sarcoidosis
- In-111 white blood cell (WBC) scintigraphy
  - In 1991 study, WBC scintigraphy led to diagnosis in 5% of 109 cases
    - 4 of 5 cases showed cardiac uptake: 1 case of toxoplasmosis with pericardial effusion, 1 case of autoimmune disease, 1 case of presumed Kawasaki, 1 undiagnosed
    - 1 case showed uptake around heart and in abdominal nodes related to *Bartonella* infection

DIFFERENTIAL DIAGNOSIS

Pneumonia

- Appears as focal accumulation of labeled WBCs or of F-18 FDG with associated parenchymal consolidation on CT

Inflammatory Bowel Disease

- Appears as segmental/multisegmental accumulation of labeled WBCs or F-18 FDG

Kawasaki Disease

- Appears as F-18 FDG avidity associated with wall thickening of involved large vessels, commonly aorta

Collagen Vascular Disease

- Clinical diagnosis without specific scintigraphic findings

Malignancy

- Most commonly leukemia, neuroblastoma

Parasitic Infection

- No typical imaging features, ultimately clinical/laboratory diagnosis

CLINICAL ISSUES

Natural History & Prognosis

- In order, infectious, inflammatory, and neoplastic causes dominate ultimately identified causes of FUO
  - Fair number of cases are never diagnosed
- 2010 systematic review of ultimate diagnoses of pediatric patients with FUO
  - 51% infection
    - 59% bacterial infection
    - 23% pneumonia
    - 10% parasitic infection (generally developing world)
    - 7% viral infection
  - 11% other diagnoses (e.g., inflammatory bowel disease, Kawasaki disease, etc.)
  - 9% collagen vascular disease (e.g., juvenile idiopathic arthritis, etc.)
  - 6% malignancy (e.g., leukemia, lymphoma, neuroblastoma, etc.)
  - 23% no diagnosis
    - 49% of undiagnosed fevers resolved

Treatment

- Some argue for empiric antibiotics until diagnosis is made, then directed therapy; others advocate avoidance of non-targeted antimicrobials

Background

- Fever = elevated core body temperature ≥ 38°C
- Fever is common occurrence in children
  - Fever accounts for 10-25% of emergency department visits, up to 70% of all acute pediatric primary care visits
  - Majority of febrile children have viral illness
- Definition of FUO is very specific
  - Prolonged fever, longer than typical for self-limited infectious process (> 7 days)
    - Original definition specifically defined FUO as fever ≥ 3 weeks, without source after 1 week of investigation
    - Definition used in published series highly variable
    - Current reasonable definition of FUO is fever > 38°C for ≥ 14 consecutive days

General Approach

- Approach is very clinical with little role for imaging
- Series of histories and clinical exams, laboratory tests (trended over time)
- Imaging only applied if there are localizing signs or concern for malignancy

SELECTED REFERENCES

1. Marshall GS: Prolonged and recurrent fevers in children. J Infect. 68 Suppl 1:S83-93, 2014
2. Arora R et al: Evaluation of child with fever without source: review of literature and update. Pediatr Clin North Am. 60(5):1049-62, 2013
3. del Rosal T et al: ^{18}F-FDG PET/CT in the diagnosis of occult bacterial infections in children. Eur J Pediatr. 172(8):1111-5, 2013
4. Chow A et al: Fever of unknown origin in children: a systematic review. World J Pediatr. 7(1):5-10, 2011
5. Jasper N et al: Diagnostic value of [(18)F]-FDG PET/CT in children with fever of unknown origin or unexplained signs of inflammation. Eur J Nucl Med Mol Imaging. 37(1):136-45, 2010
6. Buonomo C et al: Gallium scanning in children with fever of unknown origin. Pediatr Radiol. 23(4):307-10, 1993

Osteomyelitis and Septic Joint

KEY FACTS

IMAGING

- Radiograph useful as 1st test to exclude other causes of symptoms (e.g., fracture, tumor)
- Tc-99m MDP bone scan
  - **Osteomyelitis**
  - Classic scintigraphic findings of osteomyelitis: Increased uptake on all 3 phases of bone scan
  - Cold osteomyelitis: Variant with decreased uptake on delayed phase
  - Metaphyseal osteomyelitis can be subtle, appearing as blurring of physeal uptake or uptake extending beyond normal boundary of physis on bone scan
  - In patients with septic arthritis, adjacent focal uptake on delayed phase bone scan suggests osteomyelitis
  - **Septic arthritis**
  - Uptake on both sides of joint during any/all phases of 2-3 phase scan
  - In patients with septic arthritis of hip, decreased uptake in proximal femoral epiphysis suggests tamponade

TOP DIFFERENTIAL DIAGNOSES

- Trauma, fracture, joint derangement
- Transient/toxic synovitis
- Cellulitis/soft tissue infection
- Legg-Calvé-Perthes disease
- Chronic recurrent multifocal osteomyelitis

CLINICAL ISSUES

- Osteomyelitis
  - Localized, constant pain
  - Limp, guarding, refusal to bear weight or move extremity
  - Septic arthritis
  - Fever
  - Ill appearing
  - Refusal to bear weight

(Left) *Medial blood pool image in a 13 year old with left ankle pain shows diffusely increased soft tissue activity ➔ with more focal increased activity at the level of the distal tibia ➔.* **(Right)** *Medial delayed phase image in the same patient shows abnormal uptake in the distal tibial metaphysis ➔ reflective of osteomyelitis. Note how this obscures the normal physeal uptake. Increased uptake in the bones of the foot ➔ reflects reactive hyperemia.*

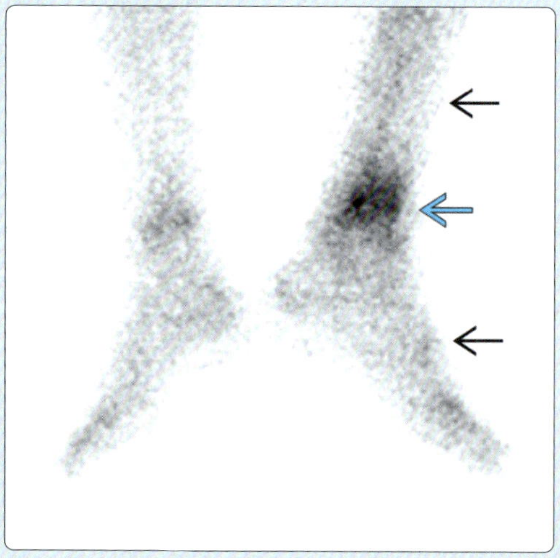

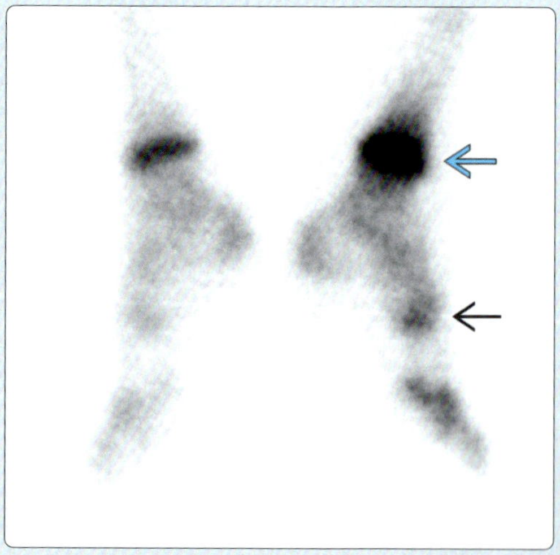

(Left) *Anterior delayed phase bone scan in a 15 year old with left wrist pain shows uptake on both sides of the wrist joint ➔, with more focal uptake in the distal radius ➔. Findings are consistent with osteomyelitis of the radius with associated septic arthritis.* **(Right)** *Anterior and posterior whole-body delayed phase bone scan in an 8 year old with chronic recurrent multifocal osteomyelitis shows multifocal radiotracer uptake ➔ at sites of disease.*

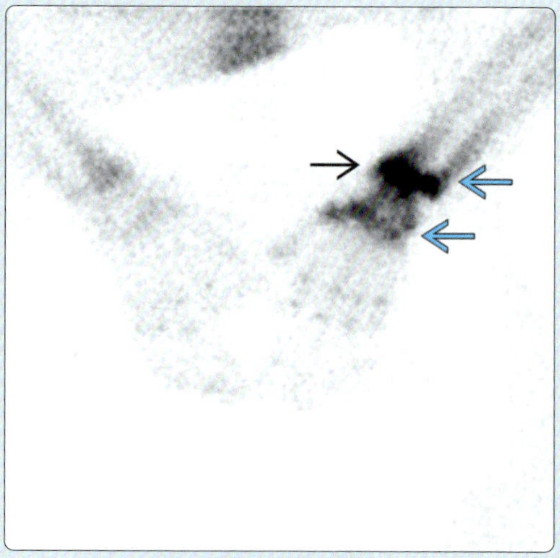

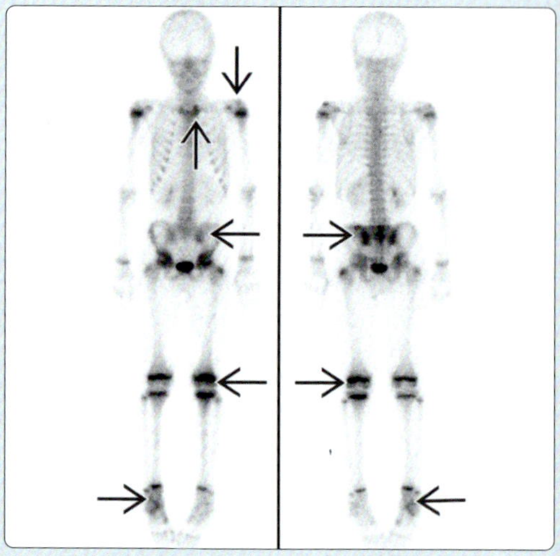

TERMINOLOGY

Definitions

- Osteomyelitis: Infection of bone
  - Usually in lower extremity long bones or pelvis
  - Epiphysis/metaphysis in infants, metaphysis in young children
- Septic arthritis: Infection of joint
  - Generally lower limb

IMAGING

Nuclear Medicine Findings

- Bone scan
  - Osteomyelitis
    - Historically considered highly sensitive (95%), more recent studies show less sensitive (53%)
    - Positive within days of symptom onset
    - Allows whole-body evaluation for multifocal disease
    - Classic findings: Increased uptake on all phases
      - Metaphyseal disease may appear as blurring of normal physeal uptake or as uptake extending beyond normal boundaries of physis
    - Cold osteomyelitis: Variant with decreased uptake on delayed phase
  - Septic arthritis
    - Uptake on both sides of joint during any/all phases of 2-3 phase bone scan
    - May see decreased uptake in proximal femoral epiphysis due to tamponade
- PET/CT
  - Not 1st-line imaging modality for pediatric osteomyelitis
  - 2011 meta-analysis (based largely on adult data) found F-18 FDG PET performed better than Tc-99m MDP scintigraphy
  - Osteomyelitis appears as focal uptake in bone
- Ga-67 scintigraphy
  - Not used in children and young adults due to dosimetry
  - Will show uptake in bone and surrounding soft tissues at sites of infection
- Leukocyte scintigraphy
  - Generally only done in older patients (required volume of blood too much for infants/small children)
  - 2011 meta-analysis (based largely on adult data) found leukocyte scintigraphy statistically performed as well as F-18 FDG PET

Radiographic Findings

- Useful as 1st test to exclude other causes of symptoms (e.g., fracture, tumor)
- Osteomyelitis
  - Radiographic findings apparent only at ≥ 2 weeks include: Demineralization, frank destruction, periosteal new bone formation
- Septic joint
  - During acute phase may be normal, may see displacement of fat planes due to effusion

MR Findings

- Osteomyelitis
  - Positive within days of symptom onset
  - Provides anatomic and soft tissue information that is not well seen by scintigraphy
  - Edema-like increased fluid signal (T2, STIR), decreased T1 signal in marrow
  - Abnormal increased or decreased enhancement of marrow
  - Decreased enhancement of articular cartilage in young patients
  - Subperiosteal fluid collection(s)
- Septic arthritis
  - Joint effusion
  - Synovial enhancement
  - In advanced disease will see cartilage destruction

Ultrasonographic Findings

- Osteomyelitis
  - Soft tissue inflammation (thickening, increased echogenicity), soft tissue hyperemia, soft tissue fluid collection, periosteal elevation, cortical disruption
- Septic joint
  - Joint effusion, most conspicuous along femoral neck

Imaging Recommendations

- Protocol advice
  - **Tc-99m MDP bone scan**
  - Patient preparation
    - Empty bladder prior to imaging
  - Radiopharmaceutical
    - Tc-99m methylene diphosphonate (MDP)
    - 0.25 mCi (9 MBq)/kg IV (North American Consensus Guidelines)
    - Minimum 1 mCi (37 MBq)
    - Inject in extremity away from sites of interest to prevent false-positives from endovascular pooling, venous valvular adherence
  - Dosimetry
    - 2.5-3.7 mSv depending on patient weight if North American Consensus Guideline dosing used
    - Critical organ = bone (39-48 mGy)
  - Image acquisition
    - Low-energy, all-purpose parallel hole collimator or high-resolution collimator
    - Obtain 2-phase (pool + delayed) or 3-phase (flow, pool, delayed) bone scans
      - Flow images should be targeted to area of symptoms but rarely add value
      - Immediate static images can either be targeted to area of symptoms or can be done for whole body
      - Delayed images obtained at 1.5-2 hr, ~ 3 min each (5-600 k counts)
    - Pinhole images improve assessment of joints and tissue immediately adjacent to physes
    - Companion view of asymptomatic side may be helpful
    - For older patients, sit-on-detector views may be helpful if bladder activity cannot be cleared around pelvis
    - SPECT improves sensitivity, can help better define anatomical complex areas (i.e., midfoot)
    - SPECT/CT can improve localization of uptake and can add anatomic information

DIFFERENTIAL DIAGNOSIS

Trauma, Fracture, Joint Derangement

- Including nonaccidental trauma

Transient/Toxic Synovitis

- Self-limited synovitis of hip

Cellulitis/Soft Tissue Infection

- Positive on flow &/or blood pool phase, negative on delayed phase

Legg-Calvé-Perthes Disease

- Idiopathic avascular necrosis of hip

Chronic Recurrent Multifocal Osteomyelitis

- Autoinflammatory disorder with nonspecific inflammation
- Classically involves long bones, pelvis, clavicles, spine

Neoplasm

- Neuroblastoma, osteosarcoma, Ewing sarcoma, leukemia, primary lymphoma of bone

Rheumatologic Disease

- Joint space narrowing, periarticular osteopenia, erosions

Avascular Necrosis

- Sickle cell disease, bone infarct, vaso-occlusive crises

PATHOLOGY

General Features

- Etiology
  - Osteomyelitis
    - Usually hematogenous spread, may also occur due to penetrating trauma, local wound extension
    - *Staphylococcus aureus* most common
  - Septic arthritis
    - Hematogenous spread, direct inoculation (trauma, iatrogenic), contiguous spread from adjacent osteomyelitis

CLINICAL ISSUES

Presentation

- Most common signs/symptoms
  - Osteomyelitis
    - Localized, constant pain
    - Fever
    - Limp, guarding, refusal to bear weight or move extremity
  - Septic arthritis
    - Fever
    - Ill-appearing
    - Refusal to bear weight

Demographics

- Age
  - Osteomyelitis
    - 50% < 5 years
  - Septic arthritis
    - Most common in infants and toddlers
- Epidemiology
  - France (2008-2009)
    - 7.1 per 100,000 incidence of bone/joint infection
      - 50% septic arthritis
      - 41% osteomyelitis
      - 7% spondylodiscitis
    - 80% involved lower limb

Natural History & Prognosis

- Osteomyelitis
  - Involvement of articular cartilage = high risk of growth deformity
  - Up to 10% recur, may develop chronic osteomyelitis
- Septic arthritis
  - Orthopedic emergency

Treatment

- Osteomyelitis
  - Cultures important for optimizing treatment
  - Abscesses require drainage
  - Antibiotic therapy, usually 4-8 weeks, initially IV
  - Surgical debridement as necessary
- Septic arthritis
  - Urgent surgical drainage and joint lavage

DIAGNOSTIC CHECKLIST

Image Interpretation Pearls

- Osteomyelitis
  - Metaphyseal osteomyelitis can be subtle, appearing as blurring of physeal uptake or uptake extending beyond normal boundary of physis on bone scan
  - Evaluate bone scan for decreased bone uptake, signifying cold osteomyelitis
- Septic arthritis
  - No definitive features distinguish reactive from infected effusion by MR or US
  - In patients with septic arthritis, adjacent focal uptake on delayed phase bone scan suggests osteomyelitis
  - In patients with septic arthritis, decreased uptake in proximal femoral epiphysis suggests tamponade

SELECTED REFERENCES

1. Mitha A et al: Community-acquired bone and joint infections in children: a 1-year prospective epidemiological study. Arch Dis Child. 100(2):126-9, 2015
2. Guillerman RP: Osteomyelitis and beyond. Pediatr Radiol. 43 Suppl 1:S193-203, 2013
3. DiPoce J et al: Pediatric osteomyelitis: a scintigraphic case-based review. Radiographics. 32(3):865-78, 2012
4. Hatzenbuehler J et al: Diagnosis and management of osteomyelitis. Am Fam Physician. 84(9):1027-33, 2011
5. Wang GL et al: A meta-analysis of fluorodeoxyglucose-positron emission tomography versus scintigraphy in the evaluation of suspected osteomyelitis. Nucl Med Commun. 32(12):1134-42, 2011
6. Browne LP et al: Optimal imaging strategy for community-acquired Staphylococcus aureus musculoskeletal infections in children. Pediatr Radiol. 38(8):841-7, 2008
7. Mellado Santos JM: Diagnostic imaging of pediatric hematogenous osteomyelitis: lessons learned from a multi-modality approach. Eur Radiol. 16(9):2109-19, 2006
8. Connolly LP et al: Assessing the limping child with skeletal scintigraphy. J Nucl Med. 39(6):1056-61, 1998

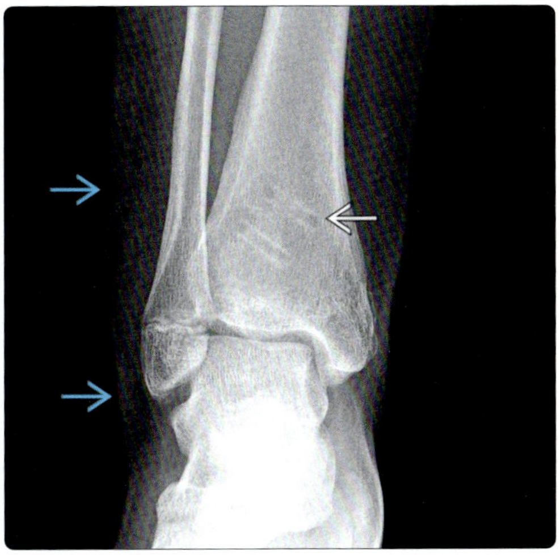

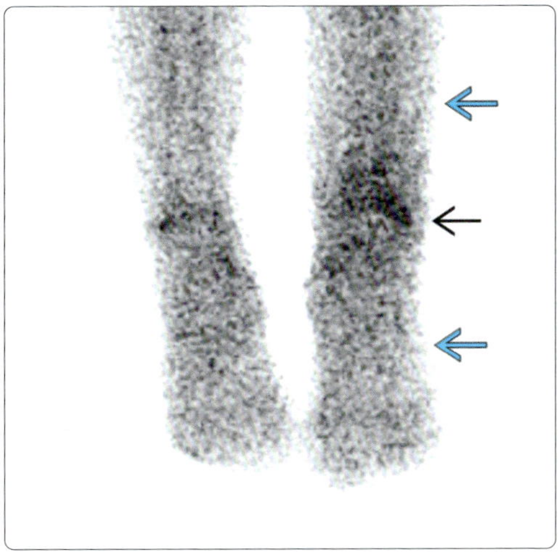

(Left) *Frontal radiograph in a 13 year old with swelling and pain following distal tibial screw removal 2 weeks ago shows screw tracts and soft tissue swelling.* **(Right)** *Posterior blood pool image in the same patient shows diffusely increased soft tissue activity (cellulitis and hyperemia) with focally increased uptake at the level of the distal tibia.*

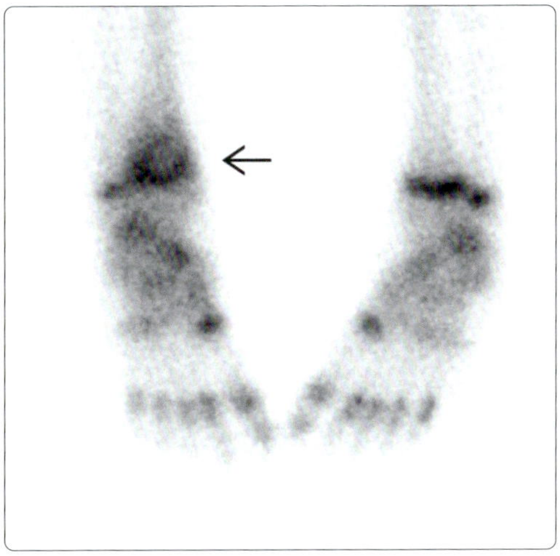

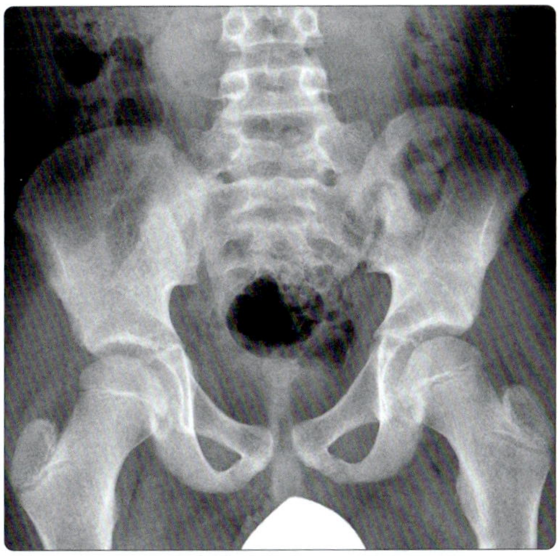

(Left) *Delayed anterior projection image in the same patient shows focally increased uptake in the distal tibial metaphysis reflective of osteomyelitis.* **(Right)** *Frontal radiograph of the pelvis in an 8 year old with left hip pain shows no abnormality, demonstrating the insensitivity of radiographs, especially early in the course of osteomyelitis.*

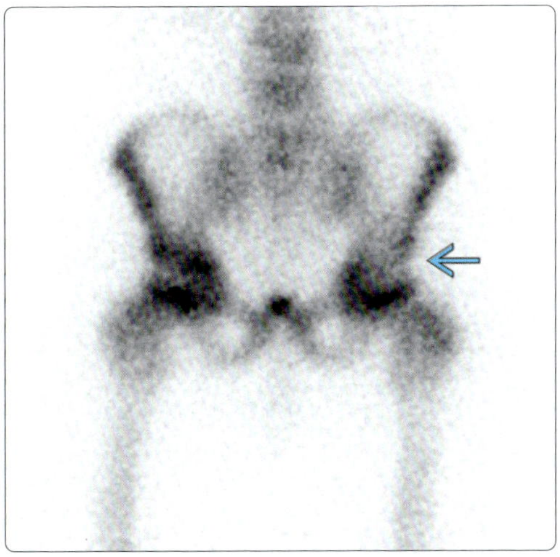

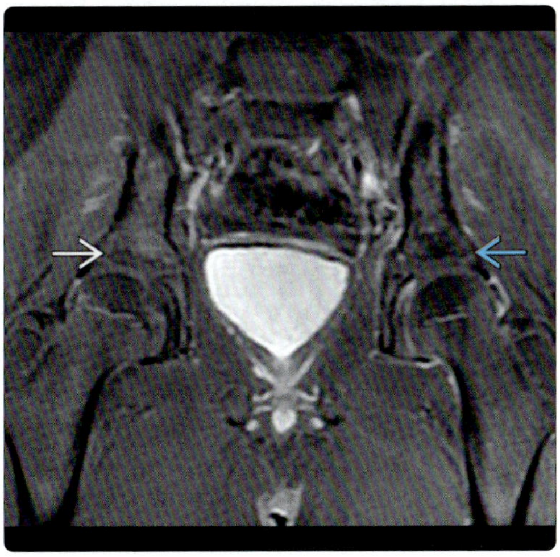

(Left) *Delayed phase bone scan in the same patient shows focally decreased uptake at the level of the acetabular roof on the left reflective of cold osteomyelitis.* **(Right)** *Coronal T1 C+ FS MR in the same patient shows decreased enhancement of the left acetabular roof compared to the normal right side. This may reflect purulent material or ischemia related to the infection.*

KEY FACTS

IMAGING

- Bone scan: Photopenic defect in acute phase, increasing uptake during reparative phase, which begins peripherally
- Pinhole imaging very helpful in assessment of joints, especially hip
  - Provide high-resolution images and better separate physeal, epiphyseal, and acetabular activity
- Classic appearance on MR: Serpentine low signal line on T1, serpentine double line on T2 (high signal inner line, low signal outer line)
- Dynamic gadolinium-enhanced MR can be used to assess revascularization/neovascularization in manner similar to scintigraphy
- Classic appearance on CT: Serpentine or geographic areas of peripheral sclerosis, generally in metaphyses or epiphyses
- Avascular necrosis (AVN) can occur anywhere but is most commonly metaphyseal or epiphyseal
- Radiographs recommended as initial study when avascular necrosis suspected; however, radiographs insensitive to early osteonecrosis
- MR or bone scan both acceptable 2nd tests; MR may be more sensitive but bone scan allows screening for polyostotic involvement

TOP DIFFERENTIAL DIAGNOSES

- Dysplasia epiphysealis capitis femoris (Meyer dysplasia)
- Septic arthritis

PATHOLOGY

- Wide variety of causes with final common pathway of ischemia

CLINICAL ISSUES

- Outcomes relate to shape and surface contour of healed femoral head

(Left) *AP radiograph in 9 year old with right hip pain shows no abnormality highlighting the insensitivity of radiographs for early changes of avascular necrosis.* **(Right)** *Anterior delayed phase bone scan of the pelvis in the same patient shows photopenia in the right proximal femoral epiphysis → compared with the normal left proximal femoral epiphysis →. This is consistent with LCP disease.*

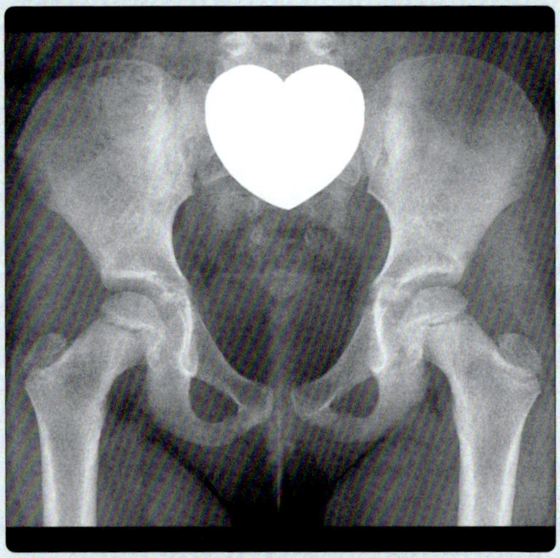

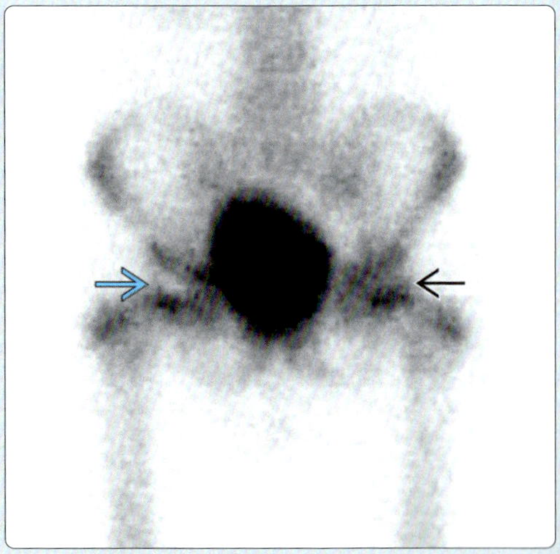

(Left) *Pinhole bone scan of the hips in the same patient provides a higher resolution view of photopenia in the right proximal femoral epiphysis →.* **(Right)** *Six-month follow-up radiograph in the same patient shows radiographic findings of LCP disease with collapse, irregularity, and sclerosis of the right proximal femoral epiphysis →.*

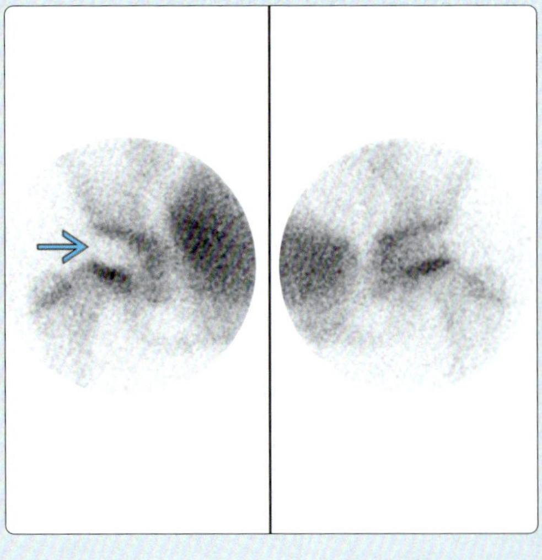

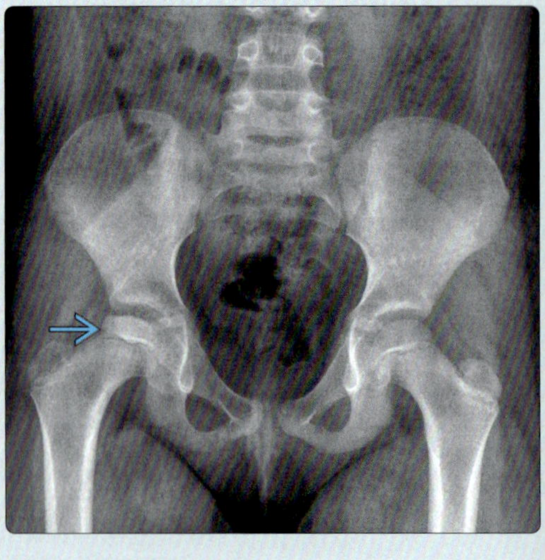

TERMINOLOGY

Abbreviations

- Avascular necrosis (AVN)

Definitions

- Osseous necrosis involving marrow and trabecular bone related to ischemia
  - Also called osteonecrosis, bone infarct, medullary infarct, osseous necrosis
  - Predisposing history: Sickle cell disease, corticosteroids, chemotherapy

IMAGING

General Features

- Best diagnostic clue
  - Bone scan: Photopenic defect in acute phase, increasing uptake during reparative phase, which begins peripherally
  - Classic appearance on MR: Serpentine low signal line on T1, serpentine double line on T2 (high signal inner line, low signal outer line)
  - Classic appearance on CT: Serpentine or geographic areas of peripheral sclerosis, generally in metaphyses or epiphyses
- Location
  - AVN can occur anywhere but is most commonly metaphyseal or epiphyseal

Nuclear Medicine Findings

- Bone scan
  - Osteonecrosis
    - Acute phase: Photopenic defect with possible peripheral uptake related to hyperemia
      - If involves articular surface, may see reactive synovitis
    - Revascularization phase (1-3 weeks): Osteoblastic repair results in increasing radiotracer uptake, generally beginning peripherally
  - Legg-Calvé-Perthes (LCP) disease
    - Appears initially as photopenia in proximal femoral epiphysis, characteristic pattern of revascularization/neovascularization (reappearance of uptake)
    - Staging scheme defined by Conway based on revascularization (A) versus neovascularization (B)
      - Stage 1A: Complete photopenia of proximal femoral epiphysis
      - Stage 2A: Uptake in lateral column, medial photopenia
      - Stage 3A: Anterior and medial extension of uptake
      - Stage 4A: Complete revascularization
      - Stage 1B: Complete photopenia of proximal femoral epiphysis
      - Stage 2B: Base filling: Widening of physeal activity (no lateral column filling)
      - Stage 3B: Mushrooming: Progressive cranial extension of activity from physis into epiphysis
      - Stage 4B: Complete revascularization: Proximal femoral epiphysis poorly defined and irregular
    - Conway staging has prognostic value for development of long-term sequelae
      - A pathway: Associated with good final outcome
      - B pathway: Poorer prognosis
- Tc-99m sulfur colloid
  - Accumulates in areas of normal bone marrow, areas of infarction appear photopenic
  - Limited by inherent heterogeneity of red marrow distribution in the aging population

Imaging Recommendations

- Best imaging tool
  - Radiographs recommended as initial study when AVN suspected
  - Bone scan and MR both acceptable 2nd tests; MR may be more sensitive but bone scan allows screening for polyostotic involvement
- Protocol advice
  - **Tc-99m MDP bone scan**
  - Patient preparation
    - Patient should empty bladder immediately prior to delayed imaging
  - Radiopharmaceutical
    - Tc-99m methylene diphosphonate (MDP)
    - 0.25 mCi (9 MBq)/kg, 1 mCi (37 MBq) minimum activity administered (North American Consensus Guidelines)
  - Dosimetry
    - 2.5-3.7 mSv depending on patient weight (if North American Consensus Guidelines dosing is used)
    - Critical organ = bone (39-48 mGy)
  - Image acquisition
    - Single-head or dual-head gamma camera equipped with a low-energy, high-resolution parallel hole collimator
    - Delayed imaging with pinhole collimator helpful in assessment of joints, especially hip
      - Provides high-resolution images and better separates physeal, epiphyseal, and acetabular activity
      - Pinhole FOV should be centered on epiphysis with collimator aperture as close to patient as possible
    - 3-phase protocol
      - Angiographic phase imaging can be used to dynamically assess perfusion in LCP (30 frames in 64 x 64 or greater matrix at 1-3 per frame)
      - Blood pool images add little value in assessment of AVN
      - Delayed images: Planar statics or SPECT acquired 2-5 hrs after tracer injection
      - SPECT/CT may better define disease and allows correlation with CT findings

Radiographic Findings

- Insensitive to early osteonecrosis
- LCP
  - Established LCP: Irregularity, fragmentation, mixed lysis and sclerosis, height loss of proximal femoral epiphysis
  - Delayed LCP: May regain some height, may develop metaphyseal and epiphyseal broadening
  - Multiple radiographic classification schemes exist (Catterall, Herring, Salter-Thompson)

- Osteonecrosis
  - Established osteonecrosis: Serpentine sclerotic lines, generally in metaphysis and epiphyses
  - Ficat classification scheme for osteonecrosis of hip

MR Findings

- Dynamic gadolinium-enhanced MR can be used to assess revascularization/neovascularization in manner similar to scintigraphy

DIFFERENTIAL DIAGNOSIS

Toxic Synovitis

- Increased uptake of Tc-99m MDP on both sides of joint due to hyperemia

Septic Arthritis

- Increased uptake of Tc-99m MDP on both sides of joint, may see secondary epiphyseal ischemia due to tamponade

Slipped Capital Femoral Epiphysis

- Poorly defined physis on Tc-99m MDP bone scan, ± epiphyseal photopenia, clearly distinguishable by radiographs due to shift of proximal femoral epiphysis relative to metaphysis

Juvenile Idiopathic Arthritis

- Increased uptake of Tc-99m MDP on both sides of joint due to hyperemia

Osteomyelitis

- Cold osteomyelitis may mimic early findings of bone ischemia (photopenia)
- Hot osteomyelitis may mimic healing changes of bone infarct

Dysplasia Epiphysealis Capitis Femoris (Meyer Dysplasia)

- Delayed, irregular ossification of proximal femoral epiphysis without necrosis
- Resolves spontaneously, generally by 6 years of age

PATHOLOGY

General Features

- Etiology
  - Wide variety of causes with final common pathway of ischemia
    - Trauma, steroid use, HIV, sickle cell anemia, vasculitis, Gaucher disease, Caisson disease

CLINICAL ISSUES

Presentation

- Most common signs/symptoms
  - LCP
    - Asymptomatic early
    - Pain and limited range of motion develop after weeks to months
  - Osteonecrosis
    - Variable depending on cause: Asymptomatic to severe pain

Demographics

- LCP
  - 2-12 years of age
  - More common in Caucasians
  - More common in males
  - Increased risk with obesity
  - 0.2-19.1 per 100,000

Natural History & Prognosis

- LCP
  - Outcomes relate to shape and surface contour of healed femoral head
  - Poor contour/lateral extrusion can result in lifelong abnormal biomechanics and development of degenerative changes
  - Outcomes generally better in children < 6 years of age

Treatment

- LCP
  - Goal is to achieve good conformity of femoral head/acetabulum at maturity
  - Majority of cases treated conservatively
  - Some cases require proximal femoral osteotomy &/or acetabular shelf osteotomy to regain contiguity between femoral head and acetabulum
- Osteonecrosis
  - Physical therapy
  - Bisphosphonates may be considered for Ficat stages 0-2
  - Core decompression ± placement of vascularized graft
- Total hip replacement indicated for advanced femoral head collapse

DIAGNOSTIC CHECKLIST

Image Interpretation Pearls

- Radiographs insensitive for early osteonecrosis
- Pinhole images are key in the assessment of proximal femoral osteonecrosis
- Attention to stages of revascularization/neovascularization in LCP

SELECTED REFERENCES

1. Grant FD et al: Radiation doses for pediatric nuclear medicine studies: comparing the North American consensus guidelines and the pediatric dosage card of the European Association of Nuclear Medicine. Pediatr Radiol. ePub, 2014
2. Mazloumi SM et al: Evolution in diagnosis and treatment of Legg-Calve-Perthes disease. Arch Bone Jt Surg. 2(2):86-92, 2014
3. Roca I et al: Evaluation of bone viability. Pediatr Radiol. 43(4):393-405, 2013
4. Gelfand MJ et al: Pediatric radiopharmaceutical administered doses: 2010 North American consensus guidelines. J Nucl Med. 52(2):318-22, 2011
5. Segall G et al: SNM practice guideline for sodium 18F-fluoride PET/CT bone scans 1.0. J Nucl Med. 51(11):1813-20, 2010
6. Stauss J et al: Guidelines for paediatric bone scanning with 99mTc-labelled radiopharmaceuticals and 18F-fluoride. Eur J Nucl Med Mol Imaging. 37(8):1621-8, 2010
7. Dasa V et al: F-18 fluoride positron emission tomography of the hip for osteonecrosis. Clin Orthop Relat Res. 466(5):1081-6, 2008
8. Comte F et al: Confirmation of the early prognostic value of bone scanning and pinhole imaging of the hip in Legg-Calve-Perthes disease. J Nucl Med. 44(11):1761-6, 2003
9. Lamer S et al: Femoral head vascularisation in Legg-Calvé-Perthes disease: comparison of dynamic gadolinium-enhanced subtraction MRI with bone scintigraphy. Pediatr Radiol. 32(8):580-5, 2002
10. Harel L et al: Meyer dysplasia in the differential diagnosis of hip disease in young children. Arch Pediatr Adolesc Med. 153(9):942-5, 1999
11. Smith SW et al: Interobserver reliability and intraobserver reproducibility of the modified Ficat classification system of osteonecrosis of the femoral head. J Bone Joint Surg Am. 78(11):1702-6, 1996

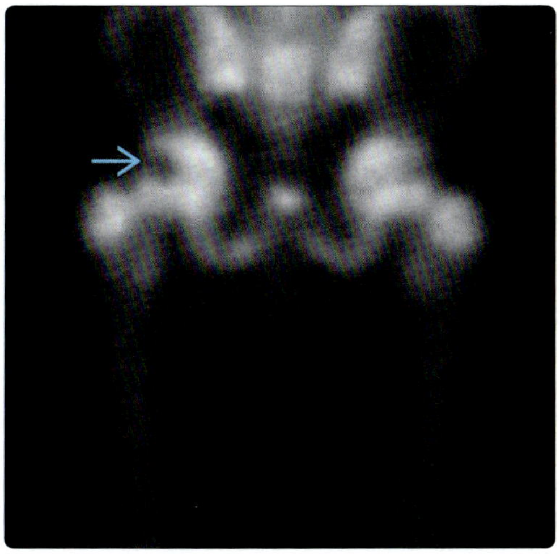

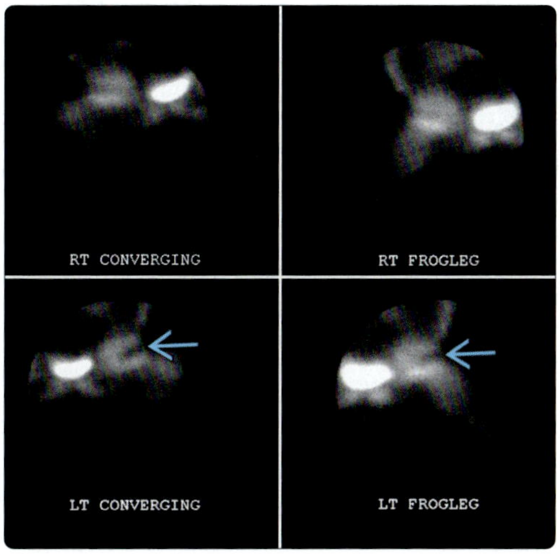

(Left) *Posterior delayed-phase bone scan demonstrates photopenia* ⇒ *in the left proximal femoral epiphysis compatible with avascular necrosis (LCP disease).* **(Right)** *Anterior pinhole scans of both hips confirm the lack of uptake in the proximal femoral epiphysis* ⇒ *in this patient with LCP disease.*

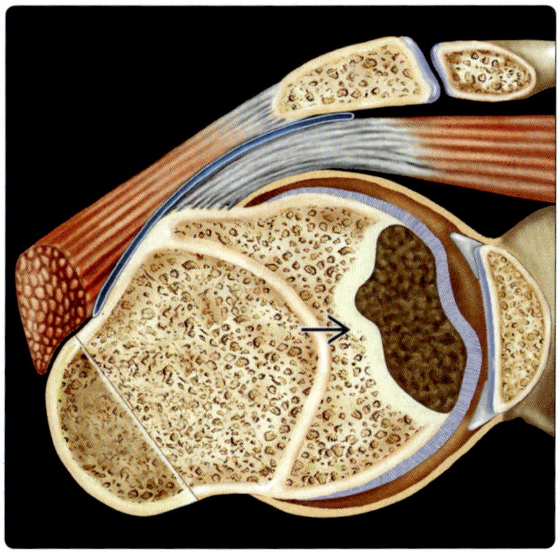

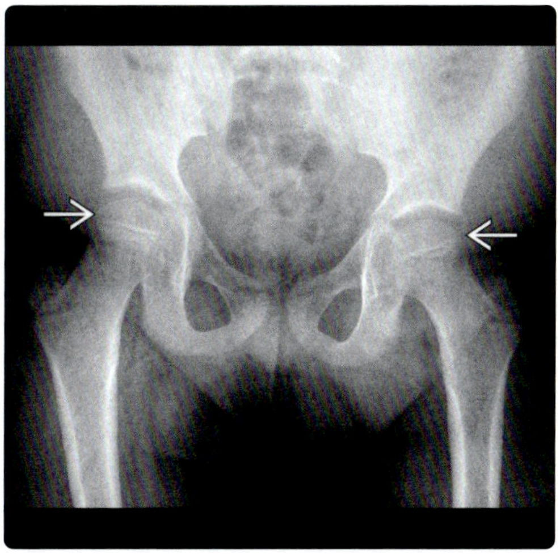

(Left) *Graphic of the glenohumeral joint shows avascular necrosis of the humeral head* ⇒*. The humeral and femoral heads are most common sites of AVN.* **(Right)** *Normal AP radiograph of the pelvis is shown in a 7 year old with hip pain. The femoral heads* ⇒ *are symmetric and smooth without sclerosis or collapse.*

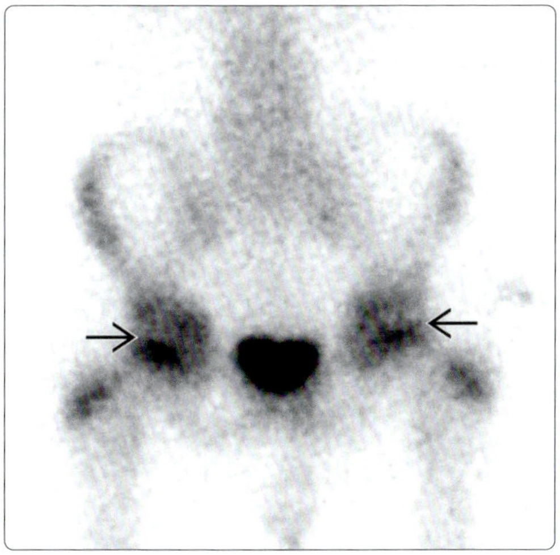

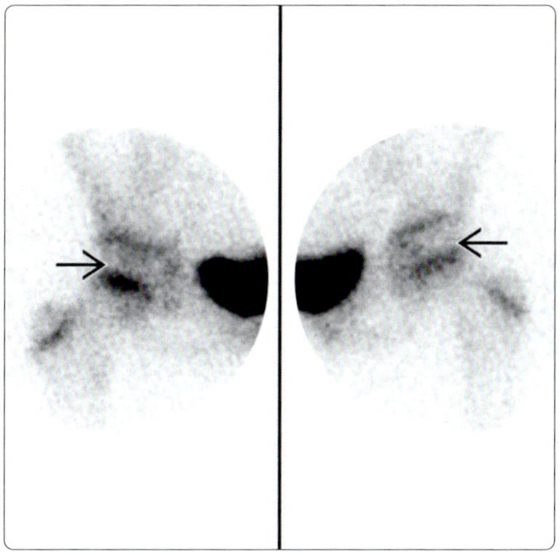

(Left) *Normal anterior delayed-phase bone scan in the same patient shows symmetric, normal uptake of radiotracer in the proximal femoral epiphyses* ⇒*.* **(Right)** *Normal anterior pinhole images of the hips in the same patient show symmetric uptake in the proximal femoral epiphyses* ⇒*. Contrast this with the other cases with various stages of avascular necrosis.*

(Left) *AP radiograph of the pelvis in a 3 year old with known LCP shows fragmentation, height loss, and sclerosis of the right proximal femoral epiphysis → with sclerosis and irregularity of the proximal metaphysis and some lateral extrusion of the right hip.* **(Right)** *Anterior pinhole images of the hips in the same patient show findings of early revascularization. Photopenia in the right proximal femoral epiphysis → is surrounded by a rim of uptake and uptake is present in the medial aspect of the epiphysis →.*

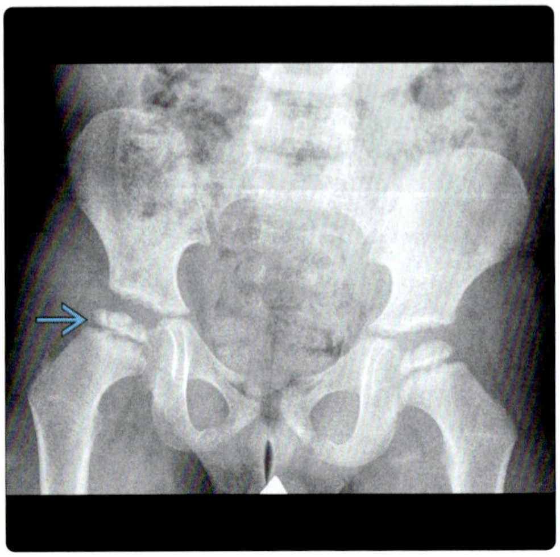

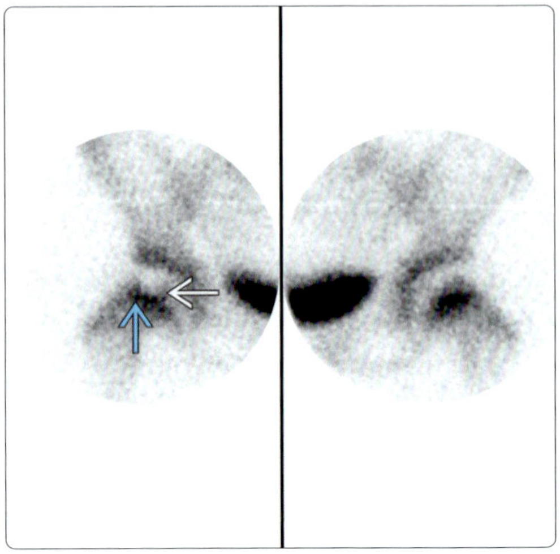

(Left) *Frog leg radiograph of the pelvis in an 8 year old with hip pain shows changes of LCP disease in the left hip with irregularity, mixed lysis and sclerosis, and height loss of the proximal femoral epiphysis →.* **(Right)** *Pinhole images of the hips in the same patient show a normal right hip →. On the left, the physis is poorly defined → but there is uptake in the abnormal proximal femoral epiphysis → reflecting revascularization in the healing phases of LCP disease.*

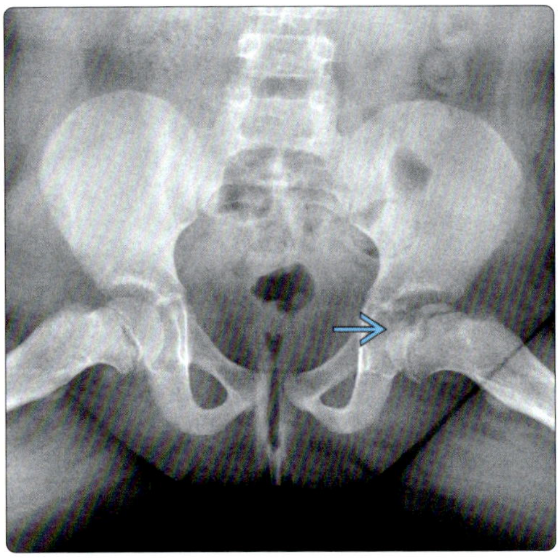

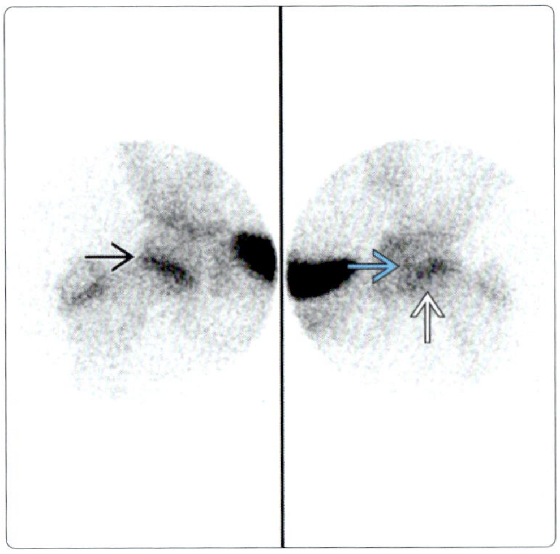

(Left) *AP radiograph of the pelvis is a 5 year old with bilateral leg pain shows irregularity and decreased height of the right proximal femoral epiphysis →. The differential diagnosis for this finding is Meyer dysplasia vs. LCP disease.* **(Right)** *Anterior pinhole images in the same patient show preserved uptake in the right proximal femoral epiphysis → and a normal configuration of the proximal femoral physis → in this patient with Meyer dysplasia.*

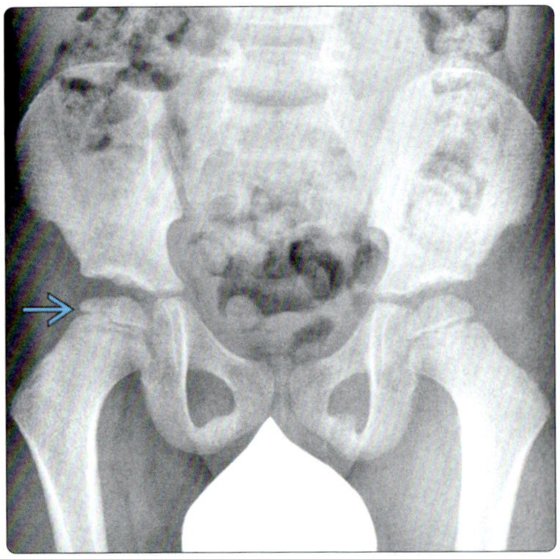

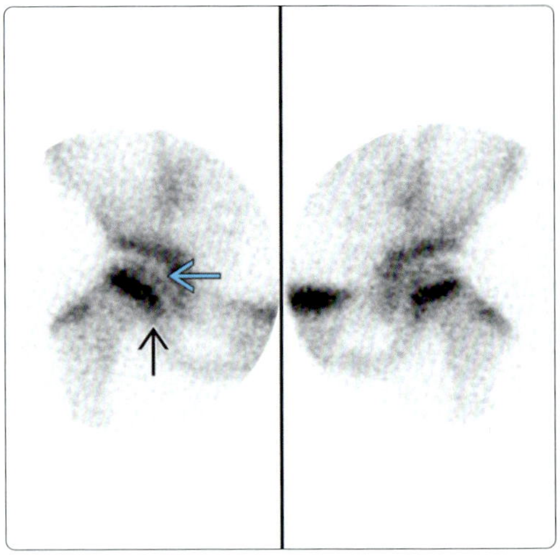

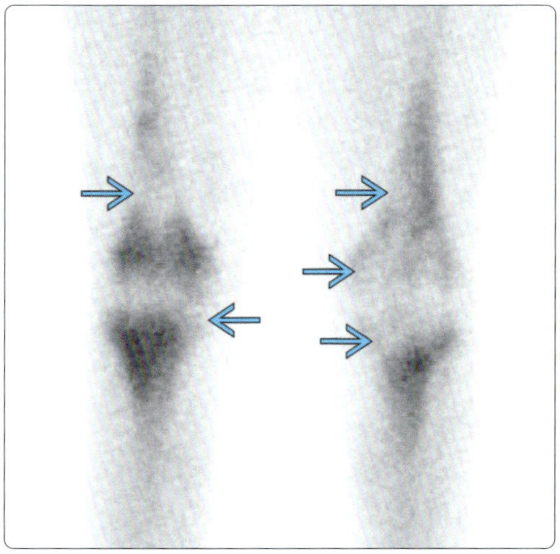

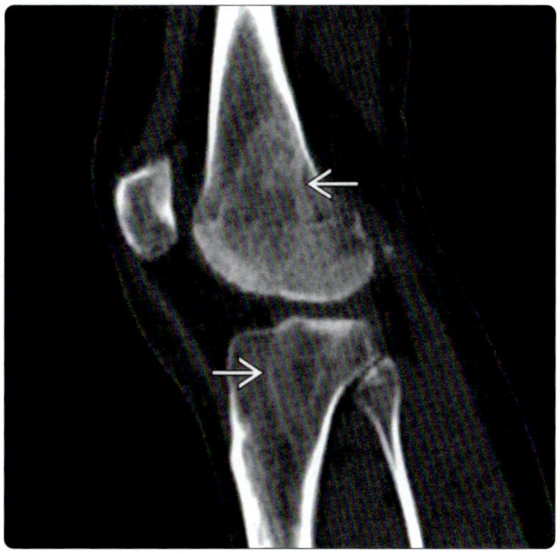

(Left) *Anterior delayed bone scan of the knees in a 19 year old with acute lymphoblastic leukemia (ALL) undergoing treatment shows geographic areas of photopenia on both sides of both knee joints in a background of increased physeal activity.* **(Right)** *Sagittal CT of the right knee in the same patient shows typical findings of osteonecrosis with serpentine sclerosis marginating geographic areas of infarct in the distal femoral and proximal tibial metaphyses.*

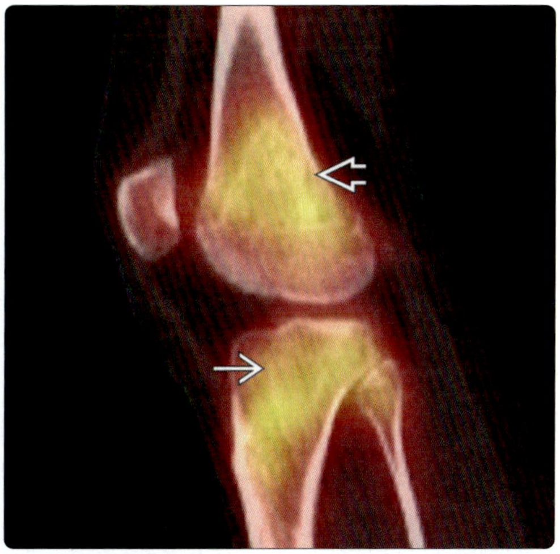

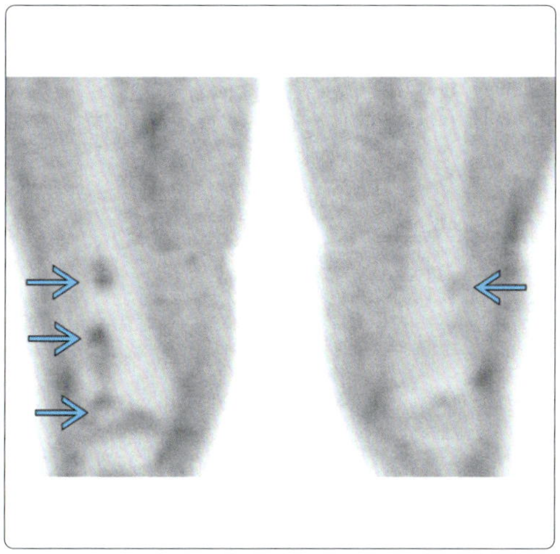

(Left) *Sagittal fused SPECT/CT bone scan of the right knee in the same patient shows uptake surrounding the serpentine areas of sclerosis in the metaphyses of both the distal femur and proximal tibia compatible with bone infarcts.* **(Right)** *Coronal F-18 FDG PET in a 19 year old undergoing therapy for stage IV Hodgkin lymphoma shows patchy and geographic areas of uptake in the distal metadiaphyses and epiphyses of both femurs.*

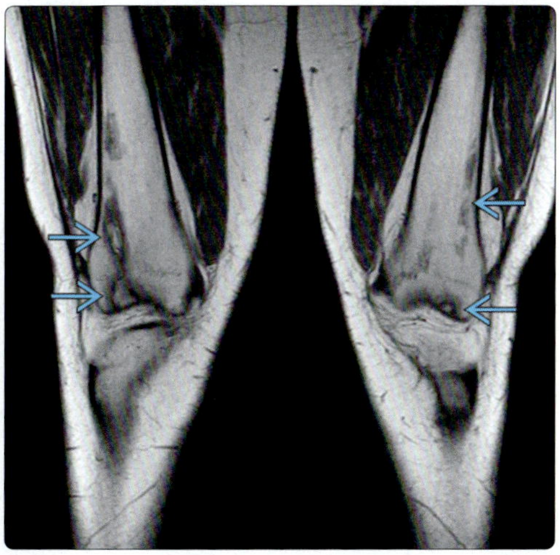

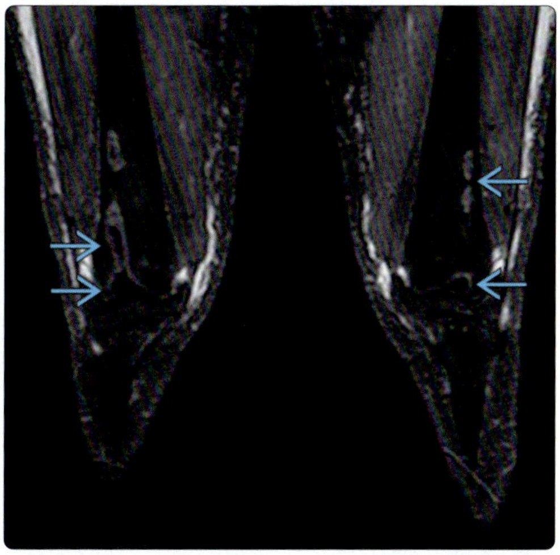

(Left) *Coronal T1-weighted MR in the same patient shows irregular and geographic areas in the medullary space and along the articular surface of both distal femurs marginated by low signal lines consistent with bone infarcts.* **(Right)** *Coronal STIR MR in the same patient shows irregular high signal marginating geographic areas of decreased signal in both distal femurs consistent with bone infarcts. Note how signal in the areas of infarction is lower than the low signal of suppressed normal marrow fat.*

Pediatric Lower Back Pain

KEY FACTS

IMAGING

- Radiograph recommended as initial study
- MR for neurologic red flags and assessment of soft tissues
- Bone scan allows assessment of whole spine and is more sensitive than radiographs
  - SPECT ± CT adds substantial value in localization of uptake and definition of abnormality
  - CT should be targeted at areas of abnormality on SPECT or correlative imaging and does not need to include entire SPECT field of view
- Pars injury is most common structural cause of low back pain in children and young adults
  - Spectrum of injury from stress (uptake + sclerosis, no fracture) to spondylolysis (uptake + pars fracture) to nonunion (no uptake + pars fracture, often with sclerotic margins)
  - Injury may be unilateral or bilateral and may have different grade of injury on each side
- Transitional vertebra is additional common cause of low back pain
  - Symptomatic forms show uptake at abnormal articulation between transitional vertebra (enlarged transverse processes) with sacrum
- Abnormalities in all components of lumbosacral spine and surrounding tissues can result in lower back pain

CLINICAL ISSUES

- Low back pain not related to acute trauma occurs in ~ 40% of pediatric population
  - Structural cause identified in only 12-26%
- Red flag symptoms warrant more urgent work-up
  - Fever
  - Weight loss
  - Acute trauma
  - Neurologic symptoms

(Left) *Delayed planar whole-body images demonstrate subtle increased activity in the posterior elements at the L5 level ⇨.* **(Right)** *SPECT of the same patient substantially increases the conspicuity of bilateral L5 pars uptake ⇨.*

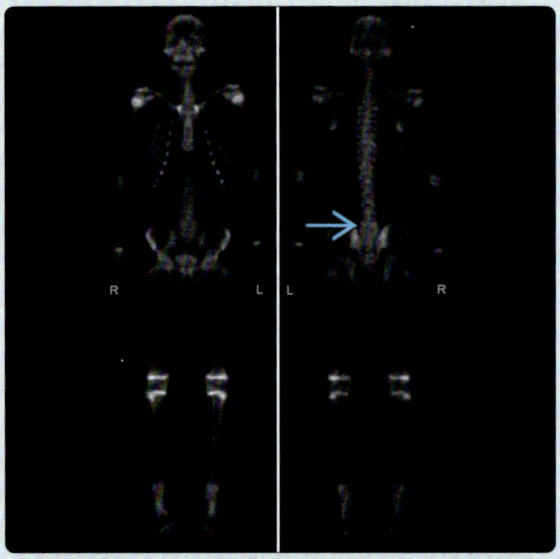

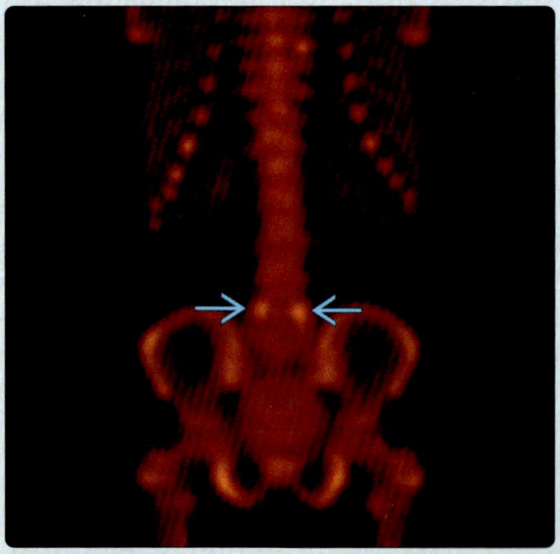

(Left) *Coronal reformatted SPECT/CT of the thoracolumbar spine demonstrates symmetric increased uptake at the L5 pars interarticularis ➡, compatible with bilateral pars injuries.* **(Right)** *Sagittal reformatted CT of the lumbar spine in the same patient confirms a left L5 spondylolysis ⇨. Right spondylolysis was also present (not shown).*

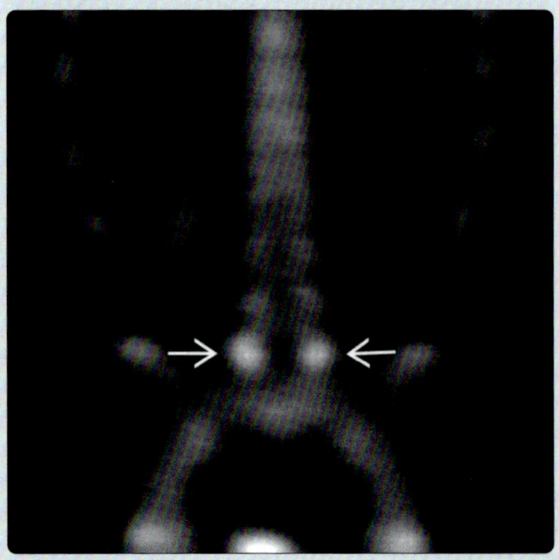

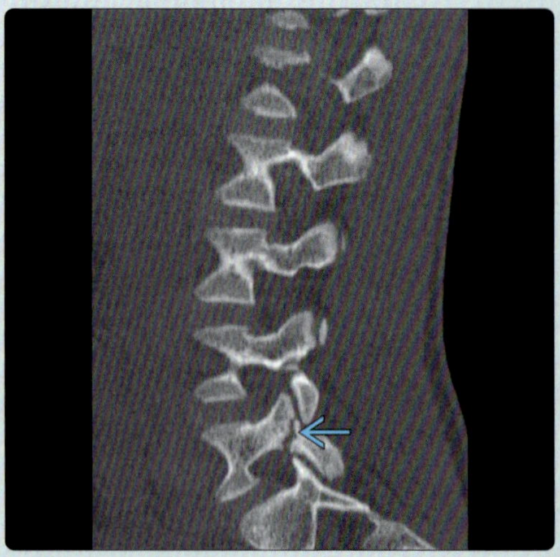

IMAGING

General Features

- Location
  - Abnormalities in all components of lumbosacral spine and surrounding tissues can result in lower back pain

Nuclear Medicine Findings

- Bone scan
  - Bone scan findings depend on etiology of low back pain
  - SPECT ± CT adds substantial value in localization of uptake and definition of abnormality
  - Posterior element uptake
    - Pars injury: Uptake at level of pars interarticularis (unilateral or bilateral)
      - Spectrum of injury from stress (uptake with sclerosis, no fracture) to spondylolysis (uptake with pars fracture) to nonunion (no uptake with pars fracture, often with sclerotic margins)
      - Injury may be unilateral or bilateral and may have different grade of injury on each side
    - Facet hypertrophy/arthropathy: Uptake localized to facet with joint space narrowing, irregularity, sclerosis, hypertrophy on CT
    - Pedicle fracture: Unilateral or bilateral focal radiotracer uptake in pedicles with fracture on CT
      - Distinguished from pars injury based on location
    - Lumbar interspinous bursitis (Baastrup disease): Focal radiotracer uptake in adjacent spinous processes in close approximation on CT
      - May see reactive changes in impinging spinous processes
    - Spinous process avulsion: Focal radiotracer uptake associated with bone fragment separated from tip of spinous process
      - Can be difficult to distinguish from accessory ossification center: Look for fragmentation, disproportionate displacement, healing changes
  - Lateral element uptake
    - Transitional vertebra: Uptake at abnormal articulation between transitional vertebra (enlarged transverse processes) with sacrum
    - Fracture vs. unfused ossification center: Asymmetric radiotracer uptake associated with transverse process
      - CT can be helpful to distinguish fracture and unfused ossification center based on irregularity, symmetry to contralateral side, and healing changes
  - Vertebral body uptake
    - Endplate-apophyseal injury: Radiotracer uptake in region of endplates on planar images
      - Schmorl node: Central uptake and focal endplate depression/irregularity/sclerosis on CT
      - Limbus vertebra: Uptake at anterior corner of vertebra with displaced, often triangular, bone fragment on CT
    - Compression fracture
      - < 4 weeks: Diffuse uptake along depressed vertebral endplate
      - 4 weeks-2 months: Linear uptake at healing fracture
      - > 2 months: Gradually decreasing uptake
    - Degenerative disc: Uptake along endplate with accompanying disc height loss, sclerosis, and osteophytosis on CT
    - Discitis/osteomyelitis: Radiotracer uptake in opposing endplates with disc height loss, endplate irregularity, often sclerosis and surrounding soft tissue inflammation
  - Sacral uptake
    - Stress fracture: Linear uptake ± linear sclerosis on CT
  - Tumoral uptake
    - Benign tumors: Typically in posterior elements
      - Osteoid osteoma: Focal intense uptake in nidus with surrounding halo of less intense uptake, central radiolucency on CT with surrounding sclerosis
      - Osteoblastoma: Large region of uptake with expansile mixed sclerotic/lytic lesion on CT
      - Aneurysmal bone cyst: Diffuse or peripheral uptake with expansile lytic lesion (± thin septations) on CT
    - Malignant tumors: More likely to represent metastatic disease with multifocal uptake
      - Metastatic disease: Most common malignant tumor, generally multifocal uptake
      - Osteosarcoma: Reactive bone formation with amorphous radiotracer uptake
      - Ewing sarcoma: Less reactive bone/uptake than osteosarcoma
- PET/CT
  - Should not be used as 1st test in pediatric/adolescent low back pain
  - Valuable in setting of primary or metastatic malignancy
  - Has role in vertebral osteomyelitis (less dose than Ga-67)
- Ga-67 scintigraphy
  - Performs better than labeled white blood cell scan for vertebral osteomyelitis
  - Rarely performed in children due to dosimetry

Imaging Recommendations

- Best imaging tool
  - Radiograph recommended as initial study
  - MR for neurologic red flags and assessment of soft tissues
  - Bone scan allows assessment of whole spine and is more sensitive than radiographs
    - SPECT has higher sensitivity and specificity than planar imaging
  - CT to identify/assess intraabdominal causes of back pain
  - F-18 FDG PET/CT for suspected disseminated malignancy
- Protocol advice
  - Patient preparation
    - Patient should empty bladder immediately prior to delayed imaging
  - Radiopharmaceutical
    - Tc-99m methylene diphosphonate (MDP)
    - 0.25 mCi (9 MBq)/kg, 1 mCi (37 MBq) minimum activity administered (North American Consensus Guidelines)
  - Dosimetry
    - 2.5-3.7 mSv depending on patient weight if North American Consensus Guideline dosing is used
    - Critical organ = bone (39-48 mGy)

- Imaging
  - Images obtained 1.5-2 hr after radiopharmaceutical administration
  - Anterior and posterior planar whole-body or sequential spot images obtained with large field-of-view camera and low-energy, high-resolution collimator
  - SPECT imaging focused on clinical area of concern and abnormalities identified on planar imaging
    - Correlative CT targeted only at SPECT abnormalities or abnormalities on other imaging (e.g., prior radiographs)

Radiographic Findings

- Initial imaging test for episode of back pain
- Primary function is to exclude traumatic abnormality and gross malalignment
- Can be used to assess dynamic stability

MR Findings

- Test of choice for assessment of low back pain with neurologic red flags
- Valuable for assessment of soft tissues and intraspinal extension of paraspinal soft tissue abnormalities
- Adds value in assessment and characterization of benign and malignant spinal, paraspinal, and intraspinal tumors

CT Findings

- Useful for assessment of acute trauma
- Useful for assessment of intraabdominal and referred causes of low back pain
- Valuable adjunct to SPECT to better characterize and localize scintigraphic abnormalities

DIFFERENTIAL DIAGNOSIS

Chronic Recurrent Multifocal Osteomyelitis

- Imaging findings similar to multifocal osteomyelitis best identified as uptake on blood pool and delayed whole-body imaging

Paraspinal Muscle Abscess

- Rim-enhancing complex collection best identified on CECT or MR

Epidural Abscess

- Rim-enhancing epidural fluid collection with local mass effect
- Best evaluated/identified by MR

Referred Symptoms

- Multiple intrathoracic and intraabdominal pathologies can present as back pain

Metastatic Disease

- Neuroblastoma, rhabdomyosarcoma, Wilms tumor, primary bone sarcomas, etc.

Hematologic Malignancy

- Diffuse or multifocal marrow involvement

CLINICAL ISSUES

Presentation

- Most common signs/symptoms
  - Most commonly present following trauma
  - Sport or activity related pain
- Other signs/symptoms
  - Red flag symptoms warrant more urgent work-up
    - Fever
    - Weight loss
    - Severe, constant, nocturnal, &/or progressive pain
    - Acute trauma
    - History of malignancy or tuberculosis
    - Neurologic dysfunction

Demographics

- Low back pain not related to acute trauma occurs in ~ 40% of pediatric population
- Structural cause identified in only 12-26%

Treatment

- In absence of red flags, generally initially treated conservatively
- Further evaluation including imaging if symptoms do not resolve with conservative management
- Further treatment depends on identified cause

DIAGNOSTIC CHECKLIST

Consider

- SPECT should be considered in all cases regardless of planar imaging findings
- CT may not be needed if planar, SPECT, and previously performed correlative imaging all negative
- CT should be targeted at areas of abnormality on SPECT or correlative imaging and does not need to include entire SPECT field of view

Image Interpretation Pearls

- Pars injury is spectrum progressing from pars stress (uptake with sclerosis but no fracture) to spondylolysis (uptake with pars fracture) to nonunion (no uptake with pars fracture, often with marginal sclerosis)
  - With unilateral spondylolysis, be attentive for associated contralateral pars stress
- SPECT or SPECT/CT invaluable for improved localization of abnormal uptake and identification of etiology
- Be alert for sometimes subtle findings of hematologic malignancy: Increased uptake in medullary space, most conspicuous in long bones

Reporting Tips

- Important to report involved vertebral level and degree of injury if pars injury identified

SELECTED REFERENCES

1. Trout AT et al: Spondylolysis and Beyond: Value of SPECT/CT in Evaluation of Low Back Pain in Children and Young Adults. Radiographics. 35(3):819-34, 2015
2. Nigrovic PA. Evaluation of the child with back pain. UpToDate. http://www.uptodate.com/contents/evaluation-of-the-child-with-back-pain. Accessed on May 16, 2015
3. Calvo-Muñoz I et al: Prevalence of low back pain in children and adolescents: a meta-analysis. BMC Pediatr. 13:14, 2013
4. Standaert CJ: Low back pain in the adolescent athlete. Phys Med Rehabil Clin N Am. 19(2):287-304, ix, 2008
5. Connolly LP et al: Young athletes with low back pain: skeletal scintigraphy of conditions other than pars interarticularis stress. Clin Nucl Med. 29(11):689-93, 2004

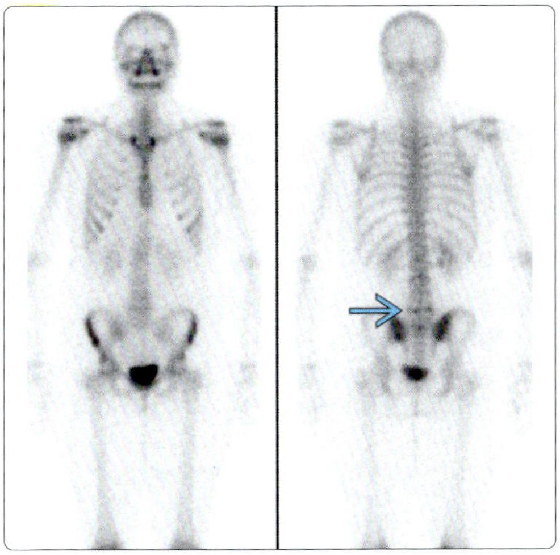

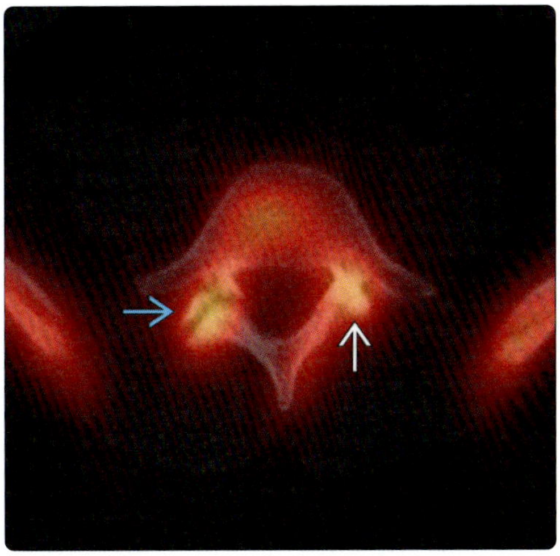

(Left) *Anterior and posterior whole-body bone scan in a 15 year old with low back pain shows increased uptake in the posterior elements at the L5 level.* **(Right)** *Axial fused SPECT/CT in the same patient localizes the increased uptake to a right L5 spondylolysis and left L5 pars stress without lysis.*

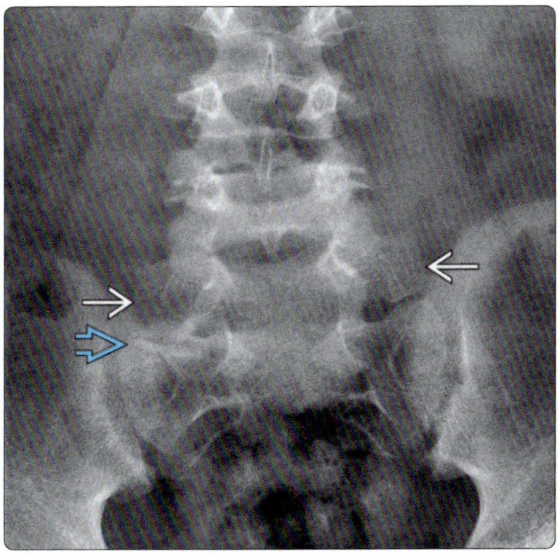

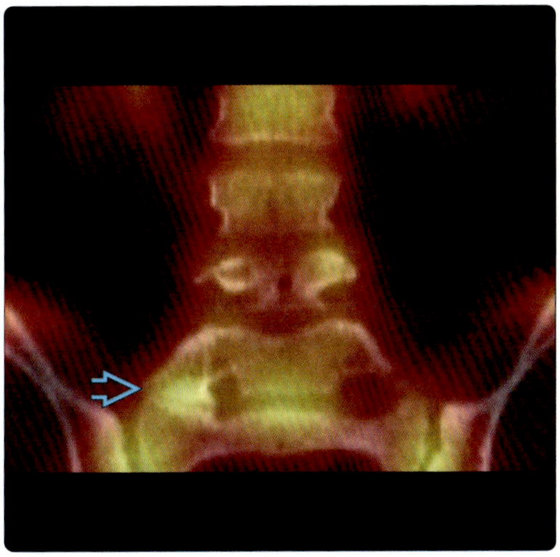

(Left) *AP radiograph of the lumbar spine shows transitional vertebral anatomy at the lumbosacral junction with pseudoarthrosis on the right.* **(Right)** *Coronal fused SPECT/CT from a bone scan in the same patient shows abnormally increased uptake at the pseudoarthrosis between the transitional vertebral body and the sacrum.*

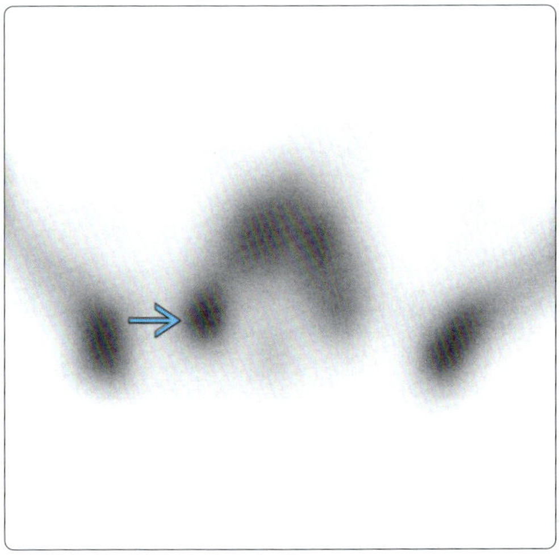

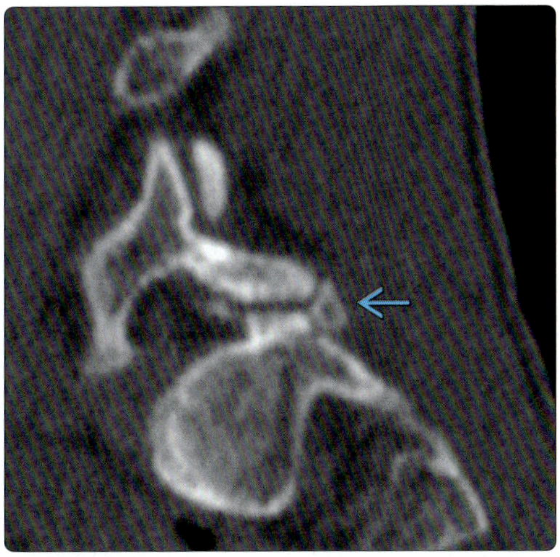

(Left) *Axial reformatted SPECT of the lumbar spine in a 14 year old with low back pain shows focally increased uptake in the right posterior elements.* **(Right)** *Sagittal CT focused at the area of abnormal uptake shows joint space narrowing, irregularity, sclerosis, and hypertrophy of the right L5/S1 facet joint reflective of facet arthropathy.*

Nonaccidental Trauma

KEY FACTS

TERMINOLOGY

- Nonaccidental skeletal injuries are suspected in injury of nonambulatory child, incompatible injury and explanation, delay in seeking medical attention, multiple fractures, and fall as explained etiology for fracture

IMAGING

- Imaging features suggestive of abuse: Multiple fractures of varying age with inconsistent history &/or high-specificity fractures
- Fractures with high specificity for abuse: Rib fractures (especially posterior), classic metaphyseal lesions (CMLs), spinous process fracture, scapular fracture, sternal fracture
- Radiographic skeletal survey is initial imaging exam of choice
    - Repeat skeletal survey (at ~ 2 weeks) increases sensitivity and specificity
- Scintigraphy is complementary to (but cannot replace) skeletal survey
    - Higher diagnostic yield than skeletal survey in anatomically complex sites (pelvis, feet)
    - Lower sensitivity than skeletal survey for CMLs and skull fractures

TOP DIFFERENTIAL DIAGNOSES

- Trauma
- Nutritional rickets

CLINICAL ISSUES

- Fractures 2nd most common finding in cases of abuse
- Substantiated maltreatment (of any form) in 1 in 8 children by age 18
    - ~ 30% of infants have sentinel injury prior to diagnosis of abuse
- 37% of siblings of abused children also abused

DIAGNOSTIC CHECKLIST

- Ethical duty to report suspected abuse in most states

(Left) *Posterior Tc-99m MDP bone scan in a 25 day old with suspected abuse shows multiple posterior rib fractures ➩.* **(Right)** *AP radiograph of the chest in the same patient shows posterior rib fractures in various stages of healing ➩.*

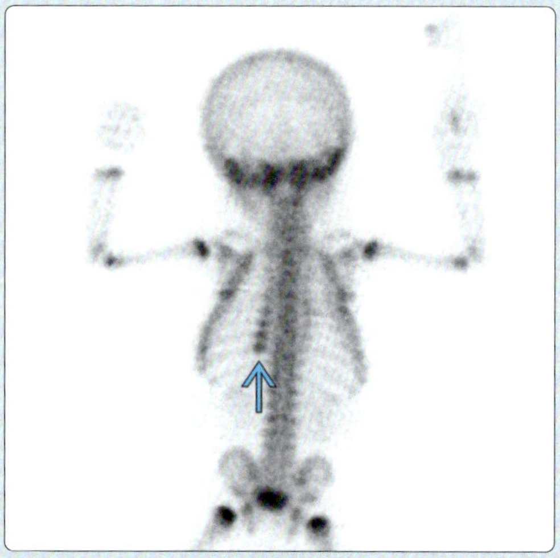

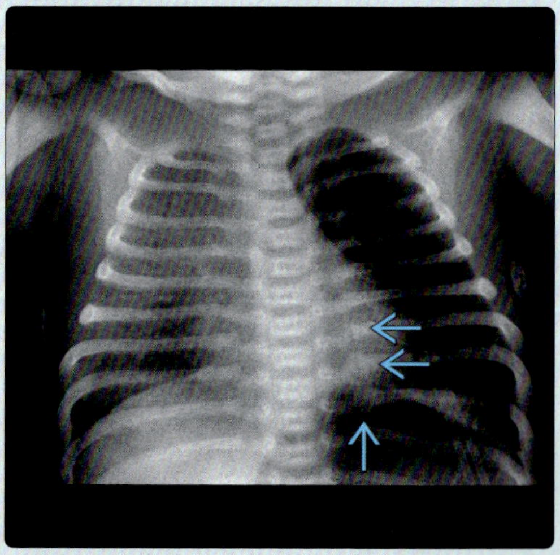

(Left) *Frontal radiograph of the chest demonstrates a healing left clavicle fracture ➩ and multiple healing posterior left rib fractures ➡ suspicious for nonaccidental trauma.* **(Right)** *LPO Tc-99m MDP bone scan shows varying degrees of uptake in the healing left clavicle ➩ and multiple left rib ➡ fractures confirming fractures in varying states of healing suspicious for nonaccidental trauma.*

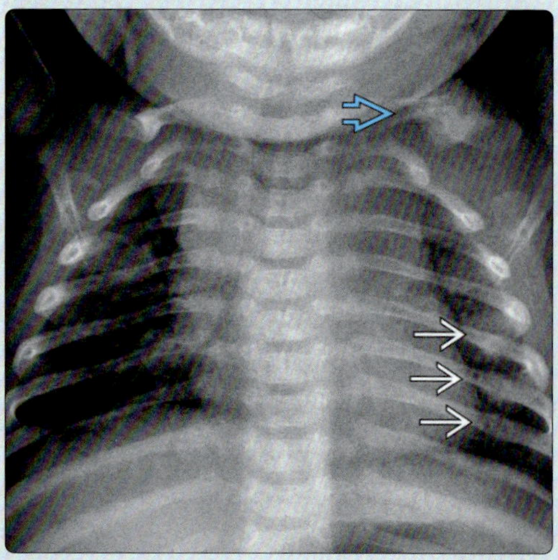

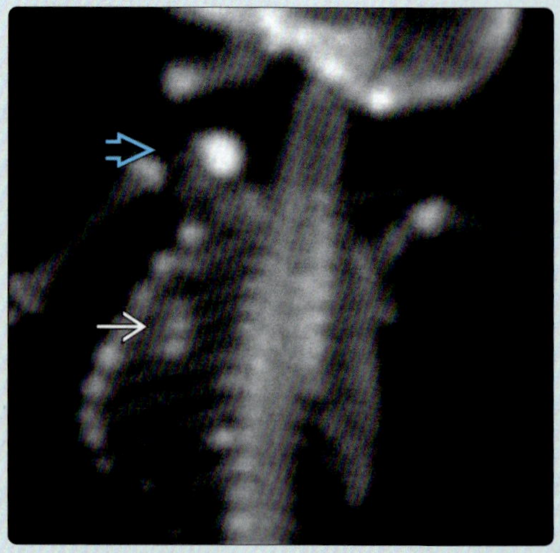

TERMINOLOGY

Definitions

- Nonaccidental skeletal injuries are suspected in injury of nonambulatory child, incompatible injury and explanation, delay in seeking medical attention, multiple fractures, and fall as explained etiology for fracture
- Child maltreatment is broad term encompassing abuse (physical, emotional, sexual) and neglect (physical, emotional, medical, educational, supervisional)
- Physical abuse is inflicted injury to child

IMAGING

General Features

- Best diagnostic clue
  - Diagnosis of child abuse can never be solely based on imaging and requires combination of clinical, investigative, and social findings
  - Imaging features suggestive of abuse: Multiple fractures of varying age with inconsistent clinical history &/or high-specificity fractures
- Location
  - No individual fracture is pathognomonic for abuse
  - Fractures with high specificity for abuse
    - Rib fractures (especially posterior)
    - Classic metaphyseal lesions (CMLs): Corner fractures, bucket handle fractures
    - Spinous process fracture
    - Scapular fracture
    - Sternal fracture

Nuclear Medicine Findings

- Bone scan
  - Focal/multifocal radiotracer uptake at fracture sites
    - Will show uptake prior to healing changes being visible on radiographs
      - Can be seen as early as 24 hr after acute trauma and typically normalizes within 6 months
    - Higher diagnostic yield than skeletal survey in anatomically complex sites (pelvis, feet)
    - Lower sensitivity than skeletal survey for CMLs and skull fractures
    - May identify abuse cases that are occult on initial skeletal survey (complimentary modalities)
    - Typical findings
      - Uptake in multiple adjacent ribs
      - CMLs appear as blurring of physeal uptake or eccentrically increased metaphyseal uptake
      - Soft tissue uptake in the setting of associated soft tissue injury
- F-18 sodium fluoride PET
  - Focal/multifocal radiotracer uptake at fracture sites
    - Higher sensitivity than radiographic skeletal survey for detection of fractures related to abuse
      - Reflects increased sensitivity for rib and other thoracic fractures
    - Lower sensitivity than radiographic skeletal survey for detection of CMLs
  - CMLs appear as blurring of physeal uptake or eccentrically increased metaphyseal uptake

Imaging Recommendations

- Best imaging tool
  - Radiographic skeletal survey is initial imaging exam of choice
  - Bone scintigraphy or F-18 sodium fluoride PET can complement skeletal survey
    - Cannot replace radiographic skeletal survey due to poor sensitivity for CMLs
- Protocol advice
  - **Tc-99m MDP bone scan**
    - Patient preparation: Patient should empty bladder immediately prior to delayed imaging
    - Radiopharmaceutical
      - Tc-99m methylene diphosphonate (MDP)
      - 0.25 mCi/kg (9 MBq), 1 mCi (37 MBq) minimum activity administered (North American Consensus Guidelines)
    - Dosimetry
      - 2.5-3.7 mSv depending on patient weight if North American Consensus Guideline dosing is used
      - Critical organ = bone (39-48 mGy)
    - Image acquisition
      - Single-head or dual-head gamma camera equipped with low-energy, high-resolution parallel hole collimator
      - Images obtained 1.5-2 hr after radiopharmaceutical administration
      - Planar whole-body images or spot images of skeletal segments
      - Pinhole images provide increased resolution of metaphyses
  - **F-18 NaF PET**
    - Patient preparation: Patient should empty bladder immediately prior to imaging
    - Images obtained 15-30 min after administration of the radiopharmaceutical
    - Radiopharmaceutical
      - F-18 NaF (sodium fluoride)
      - 60 μCi (2.2 MBq)/kg, max dose 4 mCi (148 MBq)
    - Dosimetry
      - Reported to be similar to that of Tc-99m MDP imaging

Radiographic Findings

- Classic findings: Multiple fractures in various stages of healing
- Performed as skeletal survey with prescribed series of radiographs focused on each skeletal segment
- Repeat skeletal survey (at ~ 2 weeks) increases sensitivity and specificity

DIFFERENTIAL DIAGNOSIS

Trauma

- Fractures are common in children
  - 42% of boys will have fracture before age 16
  - 27% of girls will have fracture before age 16
- Pattern of injury generally different in abuse than trauma

Osteogenesis Imperfecta

- Diffusely decreased bone mineral density

- Pathologic fractures, often multiple and in various stages of healing

Menkes Syndrome

- X-linked recessive syndrome with disordered copper metabolism
- Constellation of brain parenchymal volume loss, hemorrhage, and metaphyseal lesions

Copper Deficiency

- Nutritional, occasionally seen in long-term total parenteral nutrition use when copper supplementation omitted

Nutritional Rickets

- Osteopenia, cupped and frayed metaphyses
- May have pathologic fractures due to poor mineralization

Osteopetrosis

- Diffusely dense/sclerotic appearing bones
- Pathologic fractures due to abnormal bone

Birth Injuries

- Timing relative to delivery important
- Common fractures: Clavicle, humerus
- May have small amount of subdural bleeding

CLINICAL ISSUES

Presentation

- Most common signs/symptoms
  - Cutaneous findings (bruises, contusions) most common findings in abuse
    - Bruising in child < 9 months, not yet cruising should raise concern
  - Fractures 2nd most common finding
    - Often multiple and in various stages of healing
- Other signs/symptoms
  - Varying degrees of trauma: Mild to severe including death
  - Failure to thrive
  - Seizure

Demographics

- Epidemiology
  - Substantiated maltreatment (of any form) in 1 in 8 children by age 18
    - Neglect most common (70-80%)
  - 5-8% of pediatric emergency room visits related to child abuse or neglect
  - 37% of siblings of abused children also abused
  - Risk factors (child)
    - Age < 4 years of age
    - Child with special needs
  - Risk factors (caregiver)
    - Maternal depression
    - Parental history of abuse
    - Nonbiologic male caregiver in home
    - Parental substance abuse
    - Income inequality
  - Risk factors (social)
    - Community violence

Natural History & Prognosis

- Many patients ultimately diagnosed as abused have previously presented for injury
  - ~ 30% of infants have sentinel injury prior to diagnosis of abuse
    - 80% of sentinel injuries are bruises
  - 2002 study of children who died from abuse found 55% had been seen for traumatic injury within prior month

Treatment

- Larger institutions often have child abuse teams who coordinate multidisciplinary process of diagnosis, work to protect children, and interface with social and criminal justice systems

DIAGNOSTIC CHECKLIST

Consider

- Multiple fractures in various stages of healing, particularly in child with limited mobility or with inconsistent clinical history should raise concern for abuse

Image Interpretation Pearls

- Attention to physeal and metaphyseal uptake on scintigraphy (subtle abnormalities can herald CMLs)
- Scintigraphic studies may miss skull fractures and CMLs
  - Cannot substitute for radiographic skeletal survey
- Multiplicity of injury and fractures specific for abuse should raise concern
  - Fractures with high specificity: Posterior rib fractures, CMLs, scapular fracture, spinous process fracture, sternal fracture
- No fracture is pathognomonic for abuse

Reporting Tips

- Ethical duty to report suspected abuse in most states
- Careful documentation of identified injuries and appropriate reporting is paramount

SELECTED REFERENCES

1. Jackson AM et al: Aspects of abuse: recognizing and responding to child maltreatment. Curr Probl Pediatr Adolesc Health Care. 45(3):58-70, 2015
2. Sheybani EF et al: Pediatric nonaccidental abdominal trauma: what the radiologist should know. Radiographics. 34(1):139-53, 2014
3. Kleinman PK et al: Yield of radiographic skeletal surveys for detection of hand, foot, and spine fractures in suspected child abuse. AJR Am J Roentgenol. 200(3):641-4, 2013
4. van Rijn RR et al: Educational paper: imaging child abuse: the bare bones. Eur J Pediatr. 171(2):215-24, 2012
5. Meyer JS et al: ACR Appropriateness Criteria on suspected physical abuse-child. J Am Coll Radiol. 8(2):87-94, 2011
6. Drubach LA et al: Skeletal trauma in child abuse: detection with 18F-NaF PET. Radiology. 255(1):173-81, 2010
7. Stauss J et al: Guidelines for paediatric bone scanning with 99mTc-labelled radiopharmaceuticals and 18F-fluoride. Eur J Nucl Med Mol Imaging. 37(8):1621-8, 2010
8. Offiah A et al: Skeletal imaging of child abuse (non-accidental injury). Pediatr Radiol. 39(5):461-70, 2009
9. Section on Radiology; American Academy of Pediatrics: Diagnostic imaging of child abuse. Pediatrics. 123(5):1430-5, 2009

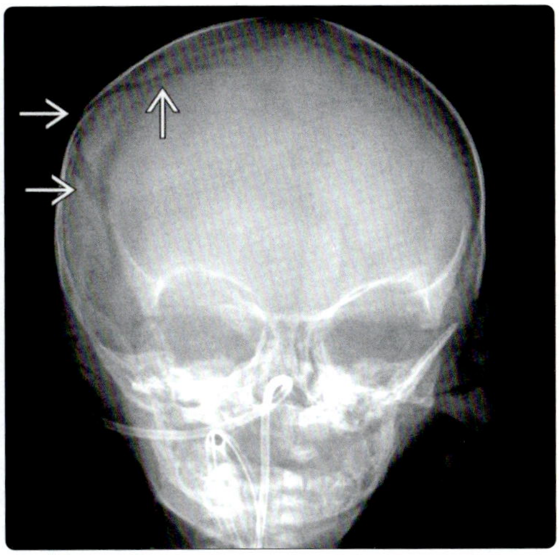

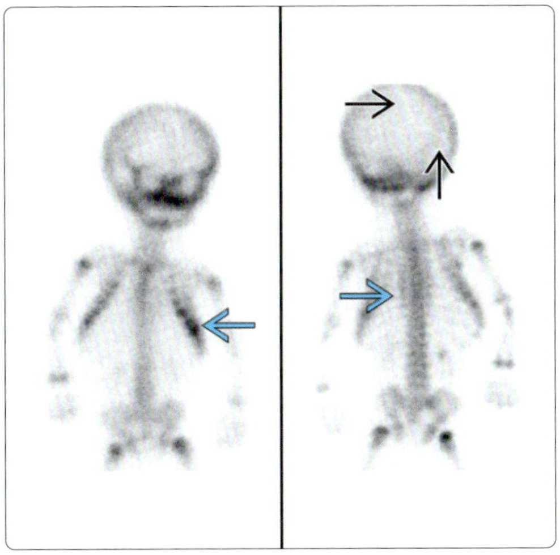

(Left) *AP radiograph of the skull in a 1 month old with suspected abuse shows a right parietal skull fracture* ➡. **(Right)** *Anterior and posterior whole-body bone scan in the same patient shows anterior and posterior rib fractures* ➡. *The known skull fracture is only subtly visible as a linear area of photopenia* ➡.

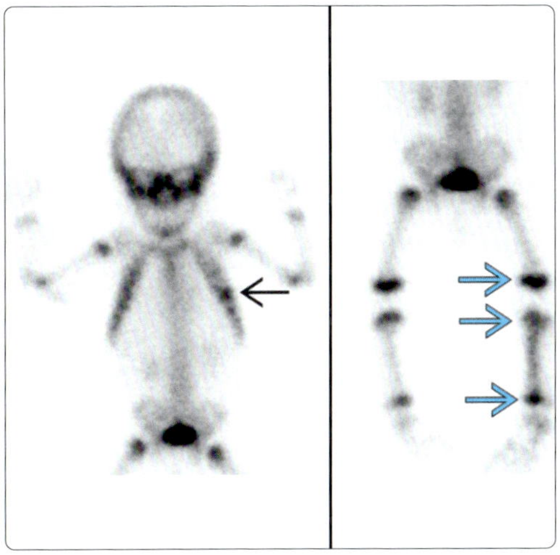

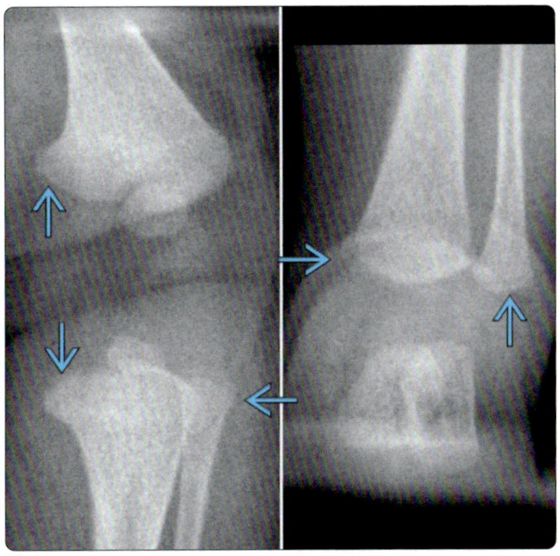

(Left) *Anterior whole-body bone scan in a 6 week old with suspected abuse shows anterior rib fractures* ➡ *and diffusely increased uptake throughout the left tibia, with more focally increased uptake at the proximal and distal tibial metaphyses and at the distal femoral metaphysis* ➡ *reflective of metaphyseal fractures of abuse.* **(Right)** *AP radiographs of the left knee (left) and ankle (right) in the same patient show classic metaphyseal lesions* ➡, *manifest as bucket handle fractures in this projection.*

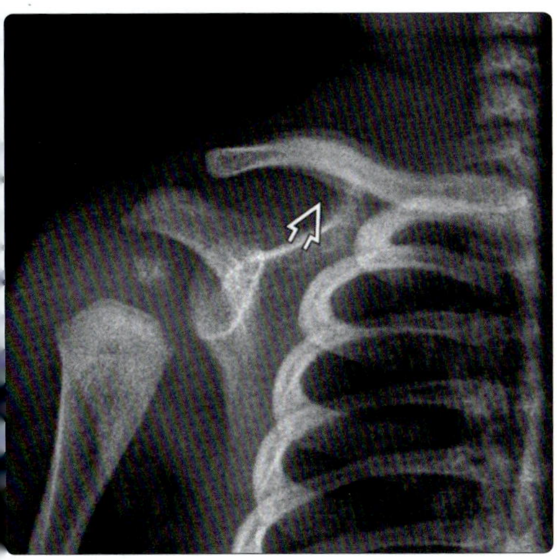

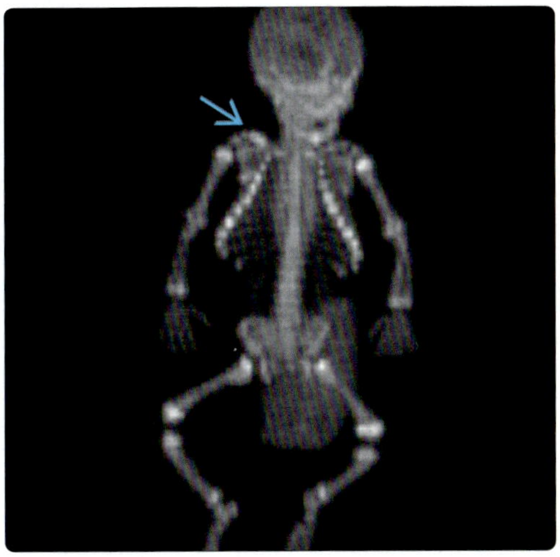

(Left) *Frontal radiograph of the chest demonstrates a healing right clavicle fracture* ➡. **(Right)** *Whole-body F-18 NaF PET to evaluate for additional fractures in the setting of suspected nonaccidental trauma confirms uptake in the healing right clavicle fracture* ➡ *without evidence of additional fractures.*

SECTION 10
Miscellaneous

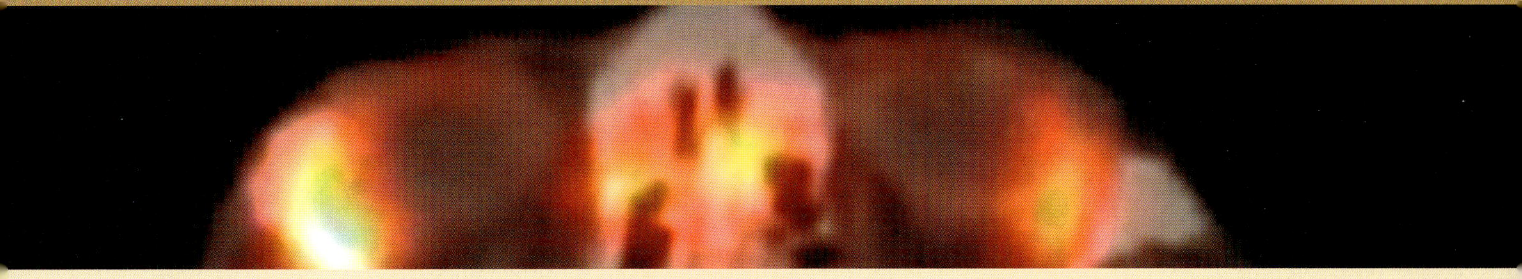

Lacrimal Complex Dysfunction

KEY FACTS

TERMINOLOGY

- Epiphora: Tear overflow, often as result of irritation of the eye or obstruction of the lacrimal system
- Complete obstruction: Obstruction of lacrimal system resulting in radiotracer pooling at site of obstruction and no passage of radiotracer distal to obstruction
- Partial obstruction: Stenosis of lacrimal system resulting in radiotracer pooling at site of obstruction and delayed passage of radiotracer distal to obstruction
- Functional obstruction: Abnormal lacrimal pump function

IMAGING

- Dacryoscintigraphy provides functional information in a manner that mimics physiologic lacrimal flow
  - Tc-99m pertechnetate: 0.1 mCi/mL normal saline
    - 1-2 drops per eye
- Site of obstruction marked by pooling of radiotracer
  - No passage of radiotracer distal to pooling = complete obstruction
  - Passage of radiotracer distal to pooling = partial obstruction
- Compare both sides to qualitatively assess function of lacrimal system

CLINICAL ISSUES

- Most common signs/symptoms
  - Epiphora, watery/mucoid discharge
- Treatment
  - Massage, probing, balloon dacryoplasty, dacryocystorhinostomy; manage underlying cause

DIAGNOSTIC CHECKLIST

- Dacryoscintigraphy recommended over CT/MR dacryocystography
  - Forced injection of contrast with CT/MR dacryocystography can overcome partial obstructions, potentially leading to false-negatives

(Left) *The left lacrimal complex consists of the 1) inner canthus; 2) ampulla; 3) superior, inferior, and common canaliculi. Obstruction can occur anywhere from inner canthus to valve of Hasner (mucosal fold partially covering the opening of the nasolacrimal duct into the nasal cavity).* **(Right)** *Anterior dacryoscintigraphy of left eye shows activity throughout nasolacrimal system, including medial canthus, nasolacrimal sac, nasolacrimal duct, valve of Hasner, and nasal cavity.*

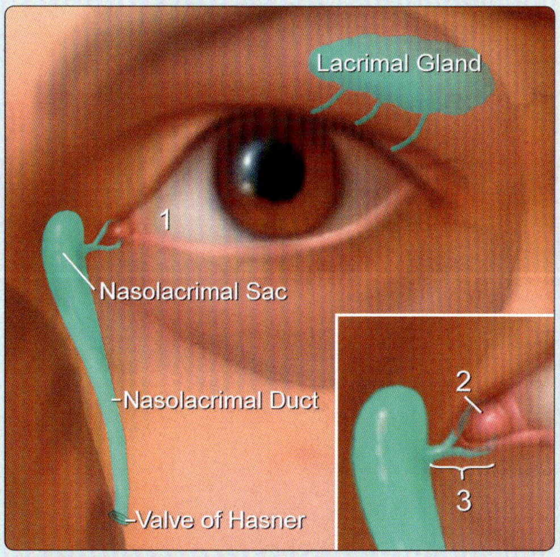

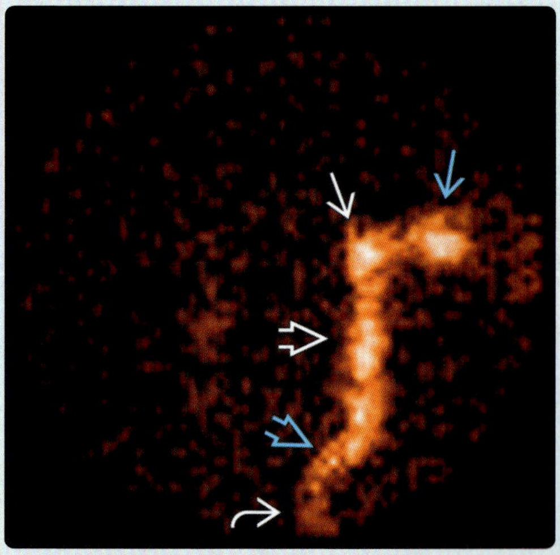

(Left) *Anterior dacryoscintigraphy shows no radiotracer activity in left nasolacrimal duct, consistent with obstruction at nasolacrimal sac.* **(Right)** *Anterior dacryoscintigraphy of left eye shows activity pooling in nasolacrimal sac and nasolacrimal duct with minimal flow into the nasal cavity, suggesting sites of partial obstruction.*

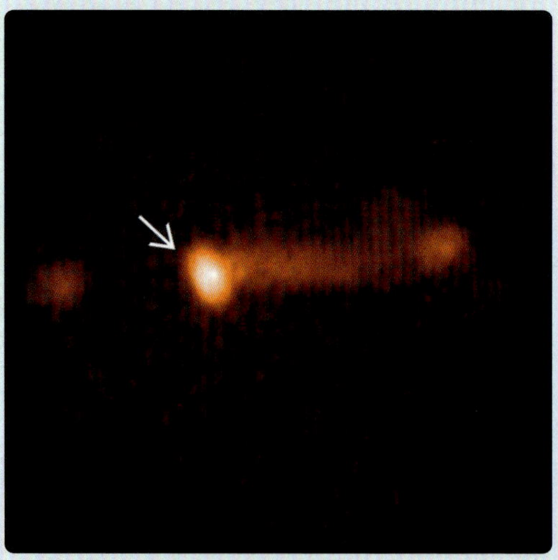

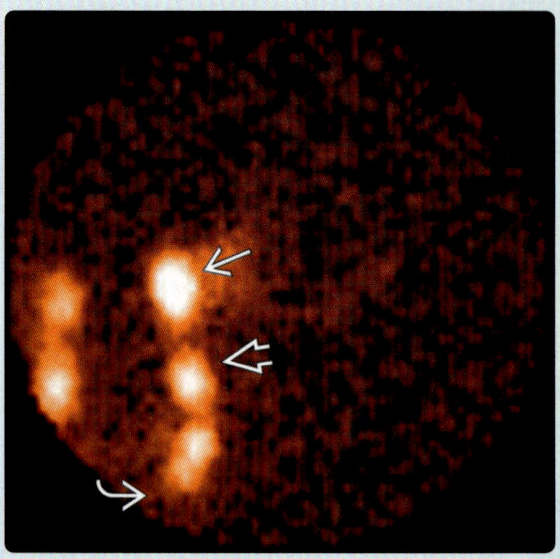

TERMINOLOGY

Definitions

- Dacryoscintigraphy is used to evaluate etiology of obstruction in patients with epiphora (tear overflow, often as a result of eye irritation or obstruction of lacrimal system)
  - Mechanical obstruction
    - Complete obstruction: Obstruction of lacrimal system resulting in radiotracer pooling at site of obstruction and no passage of radiotracer distal to obstruction
    - Partial obstruction: Stenosis of lacrimal system resulting in radiotracer pooling at site of obstruction and delayed passage of radiotracer distal to obstruction;
  - Functional obstruction
    - Defined as epiphora in setting of lacrimal system that is patent to syringing
      - Secondary to abnormal lacrimal pump function
- Dacryoscintigraphy replaces dacryocystography (imaging of lacrimal system using radiopaque dye injected into lacrimal complex)

IMAGING

General Features

- Best diagnostic clue
  - Dacryoscintigraphy: Scintigraphy of lacrimal system using Tc-99m pertechnetate
    - Used to assess patency of lacrimal system
    - Highly underutilized, sensitive, noninvasive imaging modality
  - Images are qualitatively evaluated by comparing both sides
  - Quantitative methods exist for determining conjunctival lacrimal clearance rates
    - Comparison of initial and final counts over conjunctival and nasolacrimal areas through time (e.g., 0 min, 2 min, 5 min, 10 min)
      - Helps quantify radioactive material overflow/loss (i.e., cheek overflow)
- Location
  - Site of obstruction marked by pooling of radiotracer
    - Can be anywhere from medial canthus to valve of Hasner (mucosal fold partially covering opening of nasolacrimal duct into nasal cavity)
      - Valve of Hasner is most common site

Nuclear Medicine Findings

- Tc-99m pertechnetate dacryoscintigraphy
  - Normal
    - Symmetrical passage of radiotracer through lacrimal sac, lacrimal duct, valve of Hasner, into nasal cavity
  - Abnormal
    - Passage of radiotracer distal to pooling = partial obstruction
    - No passage of radiotracer distal to pooling = complete obstruction

Imaging Recommendations

- Best imaging tool
  - Dacryoscintigraphy recommended over CT/MR dacryocystography in evaluation of lacrimal system function
    - Positive-pressure, forced injection of contrast medium with CT/MR dacryocystography can overcome partial obstructions, potentially leading to false-negatives
    - Dacryoscintigraphy mimics physiologic lacrimal system flow, enabling more sensitive study of partial and functional obstructions
- Protocol advice
  - Patient preparation
    - Eyewear, including contact lenses, must be removed
  - Radiopharmaceutical
    - Tc-99m pertechnetate: 0.1 mCi/mL normal saline
      - 1-2 drops per eye
    - Examine less symptomatic eye first
    - Capture radioactive tears with tissue paper to decrease contamination of skin over lacrimal complex
  - Dosimetry
    - Eye receives most radiation
  - Image acquisition
    - Pinhole collimator over eye and nose for 15 min
  - Image processing
    - One image set showing right eye and one showing left eye
    - Another image set showing both eyes
    - Snapshot

DIFFERENTIAL DIAGNOSIS

Anatomic Abnormality

- Ectropion = outward folding of eyelid (usually lower)
- Entropion = inward folding of eyelid (usually lower)
- Trichiasis = abnormally positioned eyelashes, often resulting in corneal &/or conjunctival irritation
- Congenital
  - Most commonly a membranous obstruction at valve of Hasner
  - Facial abnormalities (e.g., Down syndrome and other midline facial anomalies)
- Trauma

Mass Effect

- Basal cell carcinoma, squamous cell carcinoma, metastatic disease (rare, but usually from breast or prostate), congenital, dacroliths

Tear Overproduction

- Conjunctivitis, corneal irritation, drug-induced, psychogenic

Environmental

- Allergies, workplace exposures

Exogenous

- Eye drops, radiation, systemic chemotherapy, bone marrow transplantation

Postsurgical

- Orbital decompression, nasal, paranasal, and other craniofacial procedures

PATHOLOGY

General Features

- Etiology
  - Congenital
    - Most commonly a membranous obstruction at valve of Hasner at distal nasolacrimal duct
    - Stenosis of lacrimal duct is 2nd most common cause of obstruction
    - Lacrimal pump dysfunction
  - Acquired
    - Age-related change
    - Infection (dacryocystitis)
    - Inflammatory disease (e.g., granulomatous)
    - Neoplasm
    - Surgical complication
    - Trauma

Gross Pathologic & Surgical Features

- Nasolacrimal duct stenosis
- Aberrant or blocked lacrimal punctum
- Lacrimal excretion pump dysfunction
- Dacryocystocele

Microscopic Features

- Fibrosis
- Scarring

CLINICAL ISSUES

Presentation

- Most common signs/symptoms
  - Epiphora
  - Watery &/or mucoid discharge
  - Painful medial canthus &/or lacrimal sac
- Clinical profile
  - Past ocular history
    - Previous eye or lid surgery
    - Glaucoma
    - Chronic use of eye drops
    - Previous or current eye infections
  - Physical exam findings
    - Tender, fluctuant mass over medial canthus or lacrimal sac
    - Debris on lashes
    - Visual acuity changes
    - Erythematous, swollen lids

Demographics

- Nasolacrimal obstruction is most common cause of epiphora and ocular discharge in children
  - Present in up to 20% of newborns and symptomatic in up to 6% during 1st year of life
- No sex predilection
- Increased risk in Down syndrome, craniosynostosis, and any other midline facial anomalies

Natural History & Prognosis

- Spontaneous resolution in up to 90% of congenital cases during 1st year of life
- In unresolved cases, probing is approximately 80% successful
- Craniofacial abnormalities reduce probing success rate

Treatment

- Massage is typically first-line treatment
  - Moderate pressure over lacrimal sac in downward motion; perform 2-3x daily
- Probe through lower canaliculus into lacrimal complex
  - Performed by ophthalmologist with small blunt probe or irrigation canula
- Balloon dacryoplasty to dilate incomplete obstruction
- Dacryocystorhinostomy
  - Creation of epithelialized tract between lacrimal sac and nose
- Treat underlying cause

DIAGNOSTIC CHECKLIST

Consider

- Dacryoscintigraphy recommended over CT/MR dacryocystography in assessment of obstructions because dacryoscintigraphy mimics physiologic lacrimal system flow

Image Interpretation Pearls

- Literature does not define normal transit time for nasolacrimal system
- Compare both sides to qualitatively assess function
- Site of obstruction marked by pooling of radiotracer
  - Distal passage of tracer = partial obstruction
  - No passage of tracer = complete obstruction

Reporting Tips

- Mention sites of pooling because these could represent partial obstruction
- Mention most distal site of radiotracer activity
  - Lack of radiotracer transit distal to site indicates complete obstruction
- Mention medial or lateral external radiotracer leakage (on skin) that could be misinterpreted as normal transit
- Mention patient motion and whether this limits interpretation
  - Repeat study if patient motion severely limits interpretation

SELECTED REFERENCES

1. Detorakis ET et al: Lacrimal outflow mechanisms and the role of scintigraphy: current trends. World J Nucl Med. 13(1):16-21, 2014
2. Kemeny-Beke A et al: Simultaneous dacryocystography and dacryoscintigraphy using SPECT/CT in the diagnosis of nasolacrimal duct obstruction. Clin Nucl Med. 37(6):609-10, 2012
3. Palaniswamy SS et al: Dacryoscintigraphy: an effective tool in the evaluation of postoperative epiphora. Nucl Med Commun. 33(3):262-7, 2012
4. Chung YA et al: The clinical value of dacryoscintigraphy in the selection of surgical approach for patients with functional lacrimal duct obstruction. Ann Nucl Med. 19(6):479-83, 2005

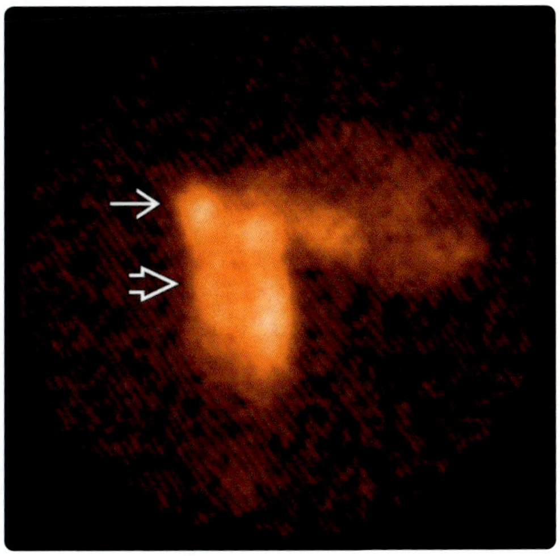

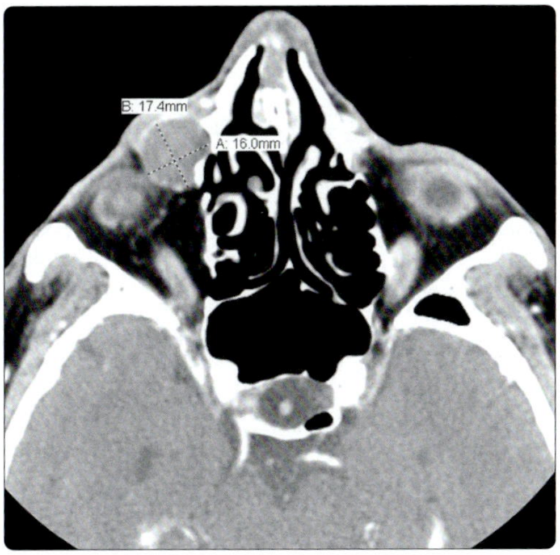

(Left) *Anterior dacryoscintigraphy shows effect of lateral patient movement during exam, with "widened" nasolacrimal sac and nasolacrimal duct.* **(Right)** *Axial CECT shows a dacryocystocele at the right medial canthal fold, one cause of lacrimal complex dysfunction.*

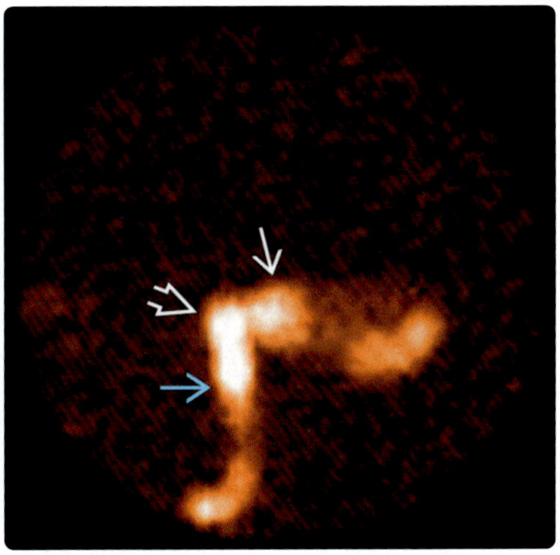

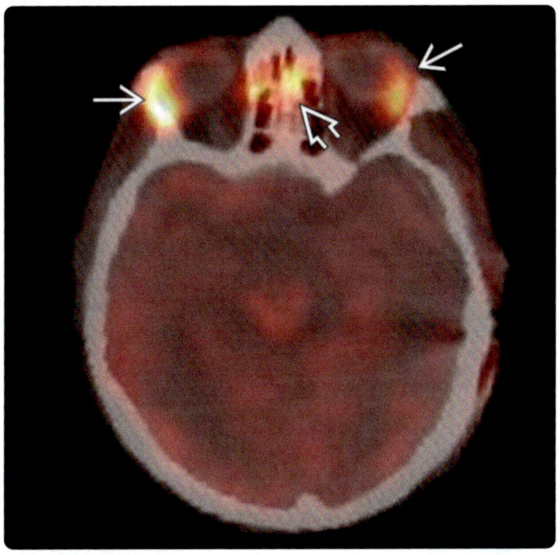

(Left) *Anterior dacryoscintigraphy shows partial obstruction at midportion of left nasolacrimal duct, evidenced by differential activity throughout nasolacrimal duct. Note medial canthus and nasolacrimal sac.* **(Right)** *Axial F-18 FDG PET/CT shows lymphomatous involvement of bilateral lacrimal glands and ethmoid sinus, one cause of lacrimal complex dysfunction.*

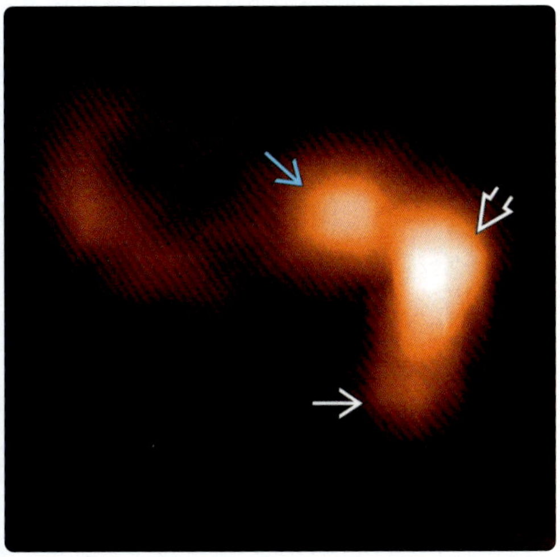

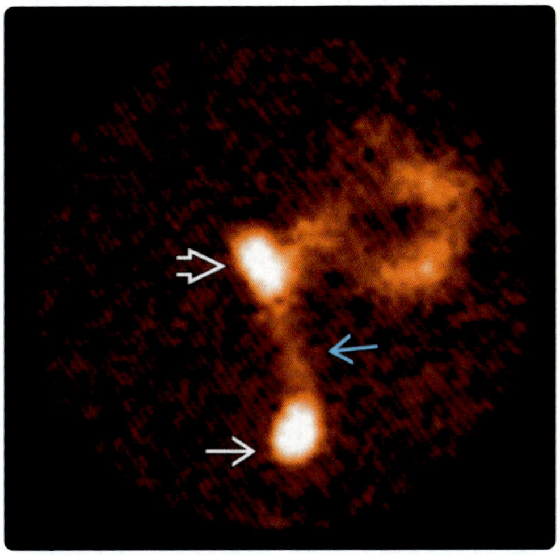

(Left) *Anterior dacryoscintigraphy of right eye shows obstruction at right nasolacrimal duct, evidenced by visualization of nasolacrimal sac and no activity distal to nasolacrimal duct. Note medial canthus.* **(Right)** *Anterior dacryoscintigraphy of left eye shows obstruction at valve of Hasner with no distal flow of radiotracer. Note nasolacrimal sac and nasolacrimal duct.*

Salivary Gland Scintigraphy

KEY FACTS

IMAGING

- Tc-99m pertechnetate salivary gland scintigraphy
  - Demonstrates function of parotid and submandibular glands, including blood flow and excretion
- Normal scan
  - Radiotracer uptake should occur within 1 min of injection, peak activity within 10-21 min
  - After administration of lemon juice, radiotracer excretion should occur immediately, with radiotracer evident in oral cavity

TOP DIFFERENTIAL DIAGNOSES

- Acute sialadenitis
  - Increased blood flow with marked uptake and retention of radiotracer
- Chronic sialadenitis
  - Variable radiotracer uptake, depending on stage
  - Late stage: Little to no uptake in salivary glands
- Sjögren syndrome
  - Decreased uptake and excretion of radiotracer
- Obstruction
  - Prior to lemon juice: Uptake may be increased (acute inflammation), normal, or decreased (functional deterioration due to obstruction)
  - After lemon juice: Poor or absent radiotracer excretion; dilated ducts may be seen
- Warthin tumor
  - Warthin tumor: Takes up Tc-99m pertechnetate and retains it after lemon juice administration

DIAGNOSTIC CHECKLIST

- In addition to images, region of interest analysis is valuable to show uptake and excretion graphically
- Dynamic imaging protocol requires thoughtful preparation and execution for proper timing, patient positioning, imaging, and lemon juice administration

(Left) *Anterior Tc-99m pertechnetate salivary gland scan shows normal blood flow to the parotid glands, submandibular glands, and the thyroid gland.* **(Right)** *Anterior salivary gland scintigraphy in the same patient shows mildly asymmetric uptake in bilateral parotid glands, left greater than right. Peak activity normally occurs within 10-20 min.*

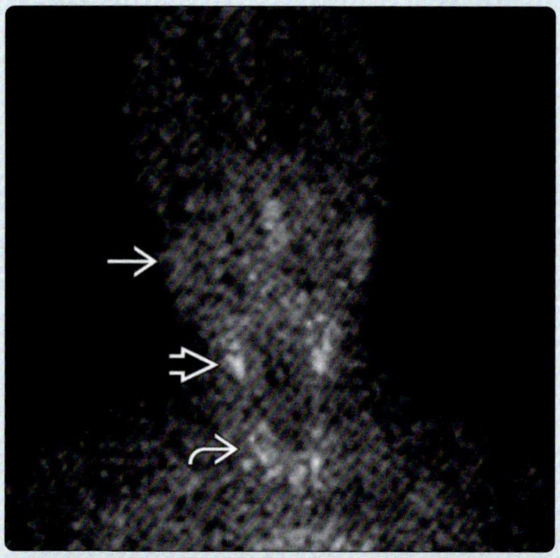

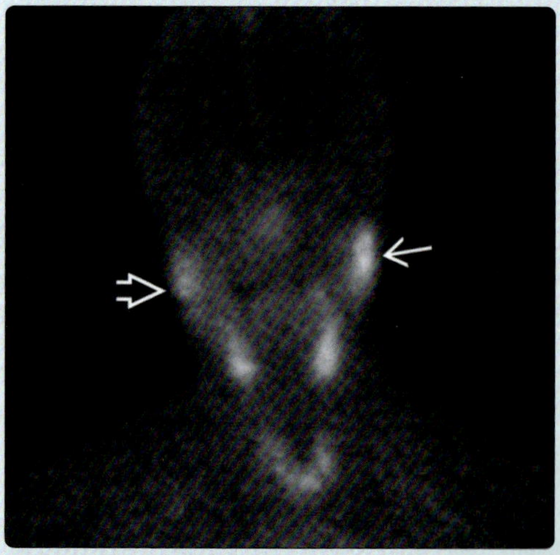

(Left) *Anterior salivary gland scintigraphy after lemon juice shows excretion of radiotracer from the salivary glands, evidenced by decreased salivary gland activity and secretion into the oropharynx.* **(Right)** *Graph of region of interest analysis of salivary gland scintigraphy in the same patient shows immediate salivary gland excretion after lemon juice administration, a normal finding.*

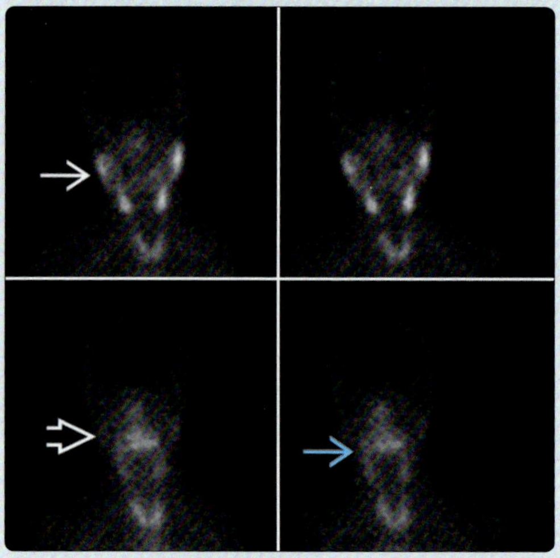

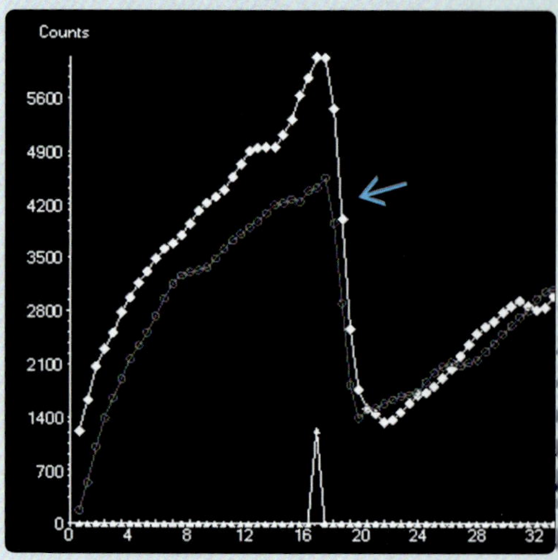

TERMINOLOGY

Definitions

- 3 major pairs of exocrine salivary glands secrete saliva into mouth through salivary ducts
  - Parotid glands: Anterior and inferior to ears
  - Submandibular glands: Under mandible in floor of mouth
  - Sublingual glands: In floor of mouth, lateral to tongue
- Dysfunction can occur due to autoimmune disease, external beam radiation or I-131 therapy, infection, stones, and benign and malignant neoplasms

IMAGING

Imaging Recommendations

- Best imaging tool
  - Tc-99m pertechnetate salivary gland scintigraphy
    - Demonstrates function of parotid and submandibular glands, including blood flow and excretion
    - Detects obstruction
    - Helps to characterize tumors
  - Normal scan
    - Radiotracer uptake should occur within 1 min of injection, peak activity within 10-21 min
    - After administration of lemon juice, radiotracer excretion should occur immediately, with radiotracer evident in oral cavity
- Protocol advice
  - Patient preparation
    - No thyroid-blocking agents prior to scan
    - Ask if patient has any food allergies (do not specify lemon juice, as physiologic stimulation of salivary glands can occur)
  - Radiopharmaceutical and dose
    - 15 mCi (555 MBq) Tc-99m pertechnetate
  - Dosimetry
    - Upper large intestine receives largest dose
  - Image acquisition
    - Patient lies supine with chin and nose touching low energy, all purpose parallel hole collimator
    - Radiotracer administered IV, while dynamic images are obtained for 3-5 seconds per frame for 1-2 min
    - 20 additional min of dynamic imaging at 2-3 min per frame
    - Continue imaging while patient sips mouthful of lemon juice via straw
    - Ask patient to hold lemon juice in mouth for 3-5 seconds before swallowing
    - Coach patient to move as little as possible during the maneuver
    - Continue with 20 additional min of dynamic imaging at 2-3 min per frame
    - Intermittent lateral images of parotids as desired
  - Image processing
    - Region of interest (ROI) analysis with regions drawn over parotid and submandibular glands can graph blood flow and excretion to aid interpretation

DIFFERENTIAL DIAGNOSIS

Acute Sialadenitis

- Acute bacterial infection of salivary glands
- Increased blood flow with marked uptake and retention of radiotracer
- May affect single or multiple glands

Chronic Sialadenitis

- Low-grade, chronic salivary gland infection
- Variable radiotracer uptake, depending on stage
- Late stage: Little to no uptake in salivary glands
- May affect single or multiple glands

Sjögren Syndrome

- Decreased uptake and excretion of radiotracer
- Most commonly affects all salivary glands
- Autoimmune disease with diminished salivary and lacrimal gland excretion

Obstruction

- Prior to lemon juice: Uptake may be increased (acute inflammation), normal, or decreased (functional deterioration due to obstruction)
- After lemon juice: Poor or absent radiotracer excretion; dilated ducts may be seen

Warthin Tumor

- Warthin tumor: Takes up Tc-99m pertechnetate and retains it after lemon juice administration
- Many salivary gland masses take up Tc-99m pertechnetate nonspecifically

CLINICAL ISSUES

Presentation

- Most common signs/symptoms
  - Sialadenitis: Swelling, pain, redness, tenderness
  - Sialolithiasis: Pain and swelling, may be intermittent
  - Xerostomia: Due to decreased saliva production/excretion after fibrosis of salivary ducts
  - Radiation sialadenitis: Pain, swelling, tenderness; dry, burning mouth; decreased sense of taste

Treatment

- Conservative management includes oral hydration, gland massage/"milking," moist heat compresses, sialogogues (e.g., lemon drops), NSAIDs, antibiotics

DIAGNOSTIC CHECKLIST

Consider

- In addition to images, region of interest analysis is valuable to show uptake and excretion graphically
- Dynamic imaging protocol requires thoughtful preparation and execution for proper timing, patient positioning, imaging, and lemon juice administration

SELECTED REFERENCES

1. MacDonald A et al: Infrequently performed studies in nuclear medicine: part 2. J Nucl Med Technol. 37(1):1-13, 2009

SECTION 11

Oncology

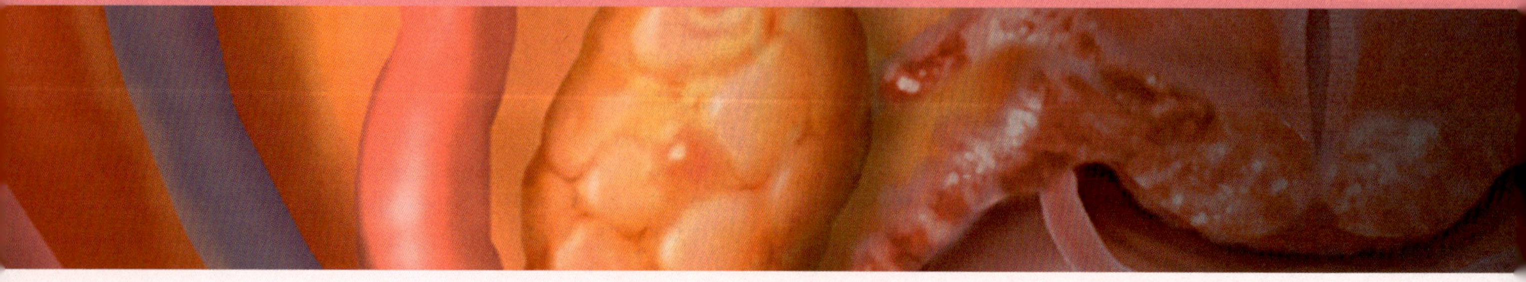

Introduction

Breast

Central Nervous System

Cutaneous

Gastrointestinal Tract

Head and Neck

Hepatobiliary

Lymphoma

Musculoskeletal

Neuroendocrine

Pancreas

Reproductive Organs

Thoracic

Thyroid

Urinary Tract

Pediatrics

Oncologic Imaging in Nuclear Medicine

In oncology, nuclear medicine provides whole-body analysis using various radiotracers that are utilized by tumors in such molecular pathways as glucose utilization, neurotransmitter function, and receptor uptake. The most commonly used oncology studies are F-18 FDG PET/CT and Tc-99m MDP bone scan.

F-18 FDG PET/CT: A glucose analog, F-18-labeled fluorodeoxyglucose is taken up by many types of tumor cells in the glycolysis pathway and is trapped after phosphorylation by hexokinase. Three-dimensional images are obtained with a circular array of detectors and a CT scanner in the PET/CT bore.

MIBG scintigraphy: An analog of norepinephrine, metaiodobenzylguanidine, localizes in benign and malignant neural crest tissue, where it is stored in neurosecretory granules. Imaging with I-123 MIBG is most common; therapy with I-131 MIBG is also available at some centers.

Gallium-67 scintigraphy: Rapidly dividing tumor cells utilize Ga-67 similarly to ferric ion and thus show higher uptake compared to surrounding tissue. Historically used to stage and follow therapy in lymphoma patients, it has been largely replaced by F-18 FDG PET/CT.

In-111 octreotide scintigraphy: A somatostatin analog, In-111 octreotide localizes to neuroendocrine and carcinoid tumors that have somatostatin receptors with a detection sensitivity of ~ 80%. As F-18 FDG has low or variable avidity for these types of tumors, somatostatin receptor scintigraphy remains common in oncologic imaging.

Tc-99m MDP and F-18 Na-F bone scan: Both Tc-99m MDP and F-18 NaF localize to regions of increased bone perfusion and osteoblastic response. Both types of bone scans can be used in oncologic imaging, although Tc-99m MDP bone scans are performed more commonly.

I-123 and I-131 thyroid cancer scintigraphy: Radioactive iodine is incorporated into normal and cancerous thyroid tissue through the sodium-iodide symporter. Dedifferentiated tumors may lose this symporter and thus their radioactive iodine avidity.

F-18 FDG PET/CT

F-18 FDG PET/CT provides whole-body analysis of functional and anatomic data and is commonly utilized in melanoma, head and neck cancers, breast, lung, and colon cancers, and lymphoma. Clinical oncologic applications include

- Staging and restaging
- Response to therapy
- Detection of unknown primary tumor
- Detection of incidental malignancy

MIBG Scintigraphy

Most commonly used to detect primary pheochromocytoma and paragangliomas and metastatic neuroblastoma, scintigraphy with the norepinephrine analog MIBG remains common. The sensitivity of MIBG for neuroblastoma is ~ 90%. The sensitivity of MIBG for pheochromocytoma and paraganglioma is 80-90%, with reports of non-MIBG-avid pheochromocytomas. F-18 FDG PET/CT is sensitive for these tumors as well, however, and provides a higher resolution scan in a shorter time.

Ga-67 Scintigraphy

The oncologic utility of Ga-67 in staging and follow-up of patients with lymphoma has largely been replaced by F-18 FDG PET/CT. It remains valuable as an infection/inflammation imaging agent.

In-111 Octreotide Scintigraphy

In-111 octreotide scintigraphy remains valuable for detection of primary and metastatic carcinoid and neuroendocrine tumors, medullary thyroid cancer, and gastrinomas, improving detection compared with anatomic imaging alone. Sensitivity is reported for these tumors as follows

- Carcinoid: 80-100%
- Pheochromocytoma: 87%
- Neuroblastoma: 89%
- Gastrinoma: 60-90%
- Medullary thyroid cancer: 40-90%

Tc-99m MDP and F-18 Na-F Bone Scan

Most often sufficient for diagnosis and staging of osteoblastic bone metastases, Tc-99m MDP whole-body bone scan continues to be used first-line as a readily available overview of tumor burden in the entire skeleton. F-18 NaF PET shows uptake in osteolytic and osteoblastic lesions and provides improved resolution when compared to planar and SPECT or SPECT/CT bone scans. In general, F-18 NaF PET provides greater sensitivity for the number of bone lesions and is most often a second-line modality after nondiagnostic Tc-99m bone scans.

I-123 or I-131 Thyroid Cancer Scintigraphy

Whole-body radioactive iodine scans in patients post-thyroidectomy for thyroid cancer show the location of residual thyroid tissue and quantitate the amount of tissue that needs to be ablated with radioactive iodine therapy. These scans detect occult lymph node metastasis and metastatic disease to the lungs or bones, which affects the dose of radioactive iodine administered as well as directing future follow-up of the patient. In patients with nonradioactive iodine-avid disease or negative whole-body radioactive iodine scans with rising tumor markers, F-18 FDG PET/CT detects disease, allowing for further treatment, including empiric I-131 therapy, surgery, or external beam radiotherapy.

Clinical Implications

The value of nuclear medicine in oncologic imaging is unequivocal. Nuclear medicine studies help characterize indeterminate lesions on anatomic imaging and add sensitivity for the number of malignant lesions detected when compared with anatomic imaging alone. In addition to the specialized staging applications of scans using I-123 MIBG, radioactive iodine, and In-111 octreotide, F-18 FDG PET/CT provides standard-of-care staging for the majority of cancers today.

Selected References

1. Uslu L et al: Value of 18F-FDG PET and PET/CT for evaluation of pediatric malignancies. J Nucl Med. 56(2):274-86, 2015
2. Turkington TG et al: Clinical oncologic positron emission tomography: an introduction. Semin Roentgenol. 37(2):102-9, 2002

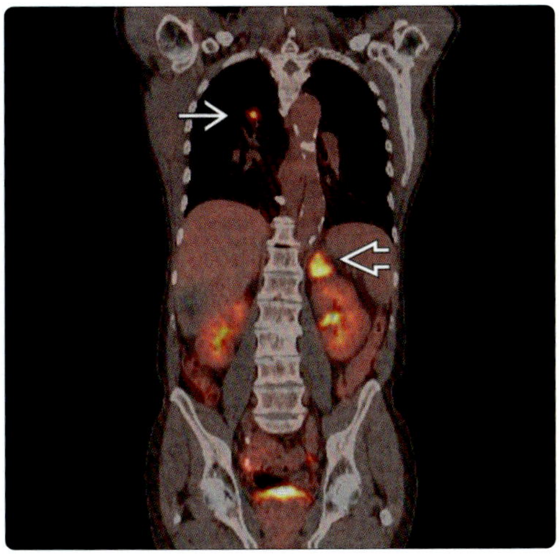
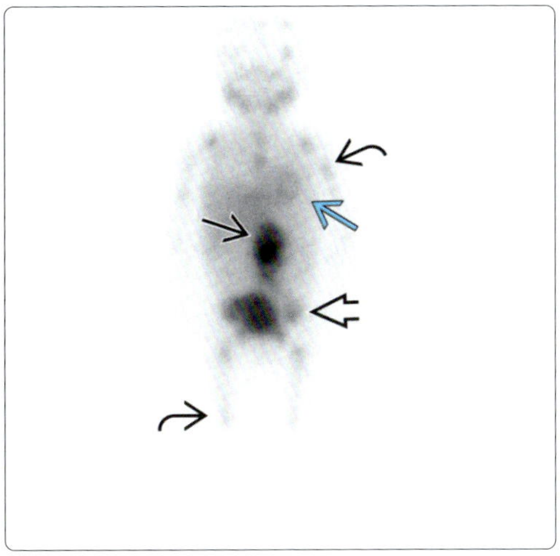

(Left) *Coronal fused F-18 FDG PET/CT shows a patient with primary lung adenocarcinoma of the right lung and a left adrenal metastasis.* **(Right)** *Anterior MIBG in a child with neuroblastoma shows the primary tumor as well as axial and appendicular bone metastases. Note physiologic cardiac uptake.*

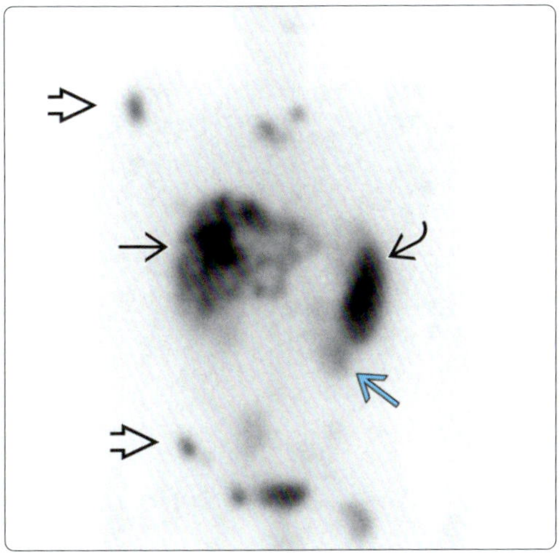
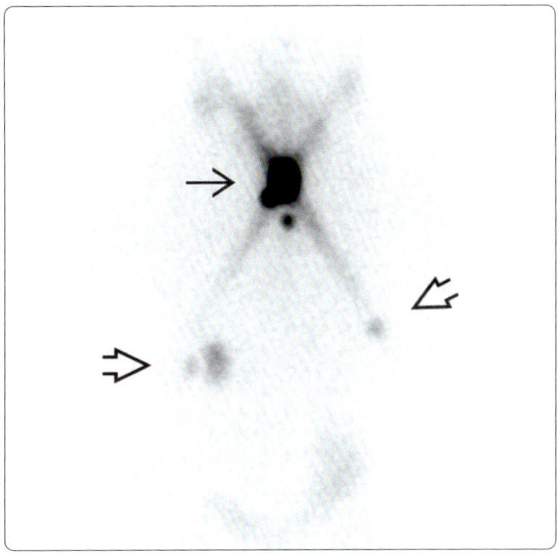

(Left) *Anterior octreotide scan in a patient with carcinoid syndrome shows hepatic and bone metastases. Note physiologic spleen and renal uptake.* **(Right)** *Anterior post I-131 therapy whole-body scan in a patient with recurrent thyroid cancer shows uptake in residual thyroid tissue in the neck and pulmonary metastases.*

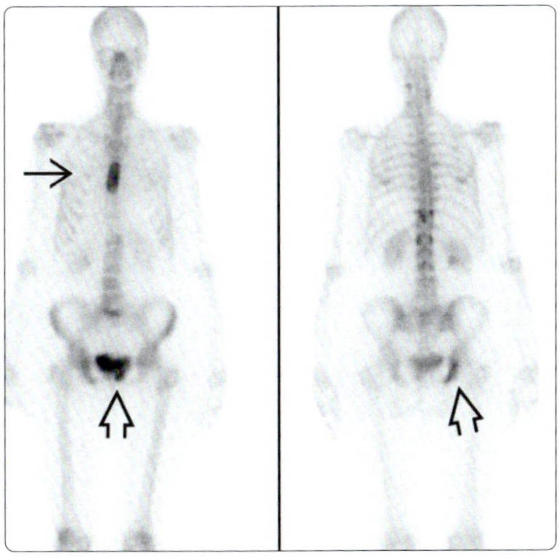
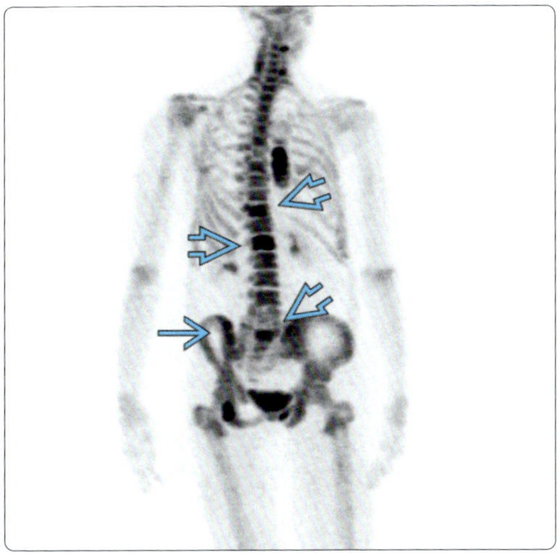

(Left) *Anterior and posterior Tc-99m MDP bone scan in a patient with breast cancer shows metastatic lesions in the sternum and pelvis.* **(Right)** *Maximum-intensity projection F-18 NaF PET bone scan in the same patient shows additional lesions in the spine and pelvis.*

Benign Breast Disease

KEY FACTS

TERMINOLOGY

- Benign conditions in breast may mimic breast carcinoma on PET/CT
- Inflammatory lesions are most common cause for benign FDG uptake in breast

IMAGING

- PET/CT is used in conjunction with other imaging modalities, such as mammography, sonography, and breast MR to make diagnosis
- Common benign causes for FDG uptake on PET include dense breast tissue, fat necrosis, lactation, silicone rupture/granulomas, infection, trauma, recent interventional procedures, and benign breast conditions such as fibroadenomas and fibrocystic change
- Benign breast conditions without significant FDG uptake include cystic lesions, cystic tumors, intramammary nodes, and some benign breast tumors

TOP DIFFERENTIAL DIAGNOSES

- Top differential considerations for benign FDG uptake in breast include poorly FDG-avid tumors such as DCIS, lobular carcinoma, and small tumors (< 2.5 cm)

CLINICAL ISSUES

- Correlation with patient history and symptomatology are keys to correct diagnosis

DIAGNOSTIC CHECKLIST

- Benign disease may be FDG-avid (although typically demonstrates milder uptake compared to breast malignancy)
- False-negatives may arise with small, slow-growing, or noninvasive tumors

(Left) *MIP image from FDG PET demonstrates moderately intense uptake within the regions of the bilateral breasts, gluteal regions, and thighs, compatible with history of free silicone injections.* **(Right)** *Axial FDG PET/CT fusion image shows scattered, moderately intense FDG uptake secondary to free silicone injections. The uptake of FDG is related to foreign body granulomatous reactions.*

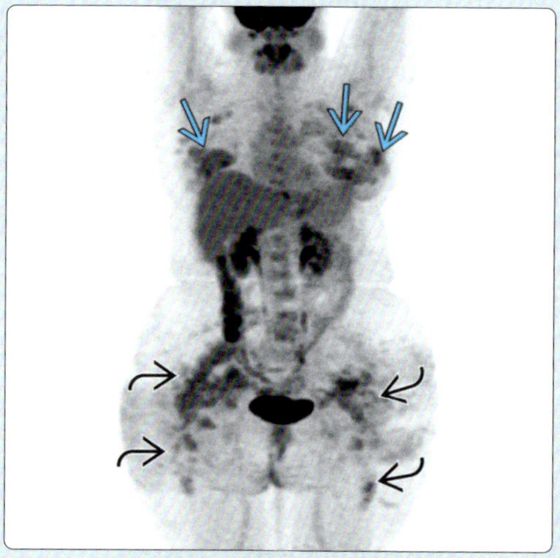

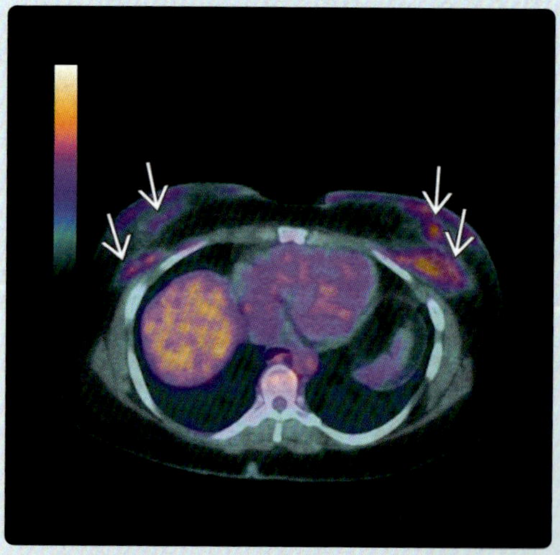

(Left) *Axial FDG PET/CT fusion image shows mild bilateral FDG activity associated with dense breast tissue seen bilaterally. This is a typical finding in premenopausal patients.* **(Right)** *Axial FDG PET/CT fusion image shows minimal FDG activity within fatty breast tissue bilaterally. This minimal activity is centered at the nipples.*

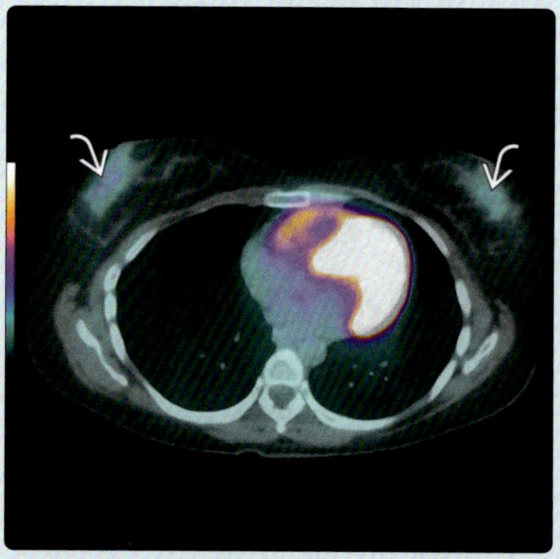

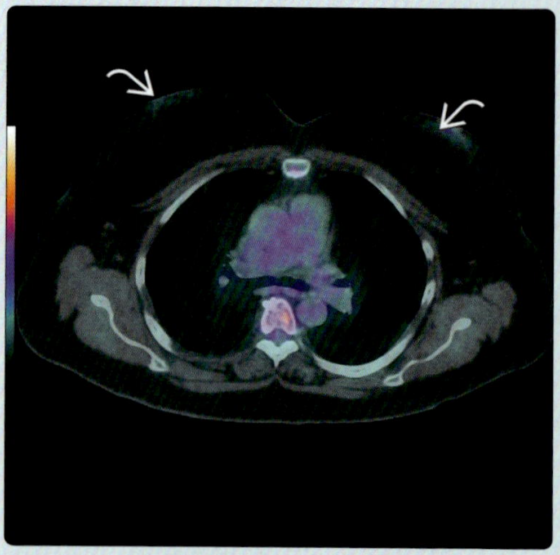

TERMINOLOGY

Definitions

- Benign conditions of breast that may mimic carcinoma
  - Benign lesions with ↑ FDG uptake common
    - Found in 1/4 of all PET/CT scans
  - Although a sensitive imaging technique for malignant tumors, not tumor-specific
  - Underlying inflammatory processes most common cause

IMAGING

General Features

- Best diagnostic clue
  - Mammogram, ultrasound, and MR features of benign breast disease used in conjunction with PET/CT
  - Clinical/surgical history important in identifying benign causes of ↑ FDG uptake
  - Whole-body PET/CT not currently indicated for 1° breast cancer detection 2° to high number false-positives
    - Low sensitivity for small, nonpalpable, and low-grade malignancies
- Location
  - Location for various benign breast tumors variable
    - Correlate with mammography/sonography results for greatest accuracy
    - Patient and clinical history key for ↑ FDG uptake from possible trauma, post intervention, fat necrosis
    - Low-grade malignancies, like high-grade malignancies, are most prevalent in upper outer quadrant of breast
    - Benign tumors without quadrant preference
    - Silicone rupture: ↑ FDG uptake along implant margins
      - □ Variable axillary and internal mammary lymph node uptake
- Size
  - Variable, depending on condition of interest
    - Lactational changes: Increased size of breasts due to proliferation of ductal structures/mammary tissue, typically fairly symmetric distribution
    - Excisional/surgical defects usually minimal in size, but depends on surgical technique
    - Trauma: Size of bruising/hematoma dependent upon severity/force of impact
    - Fat necrosis: Size dependent upon extent of prior trauma/surgery
- Morphology
  - Size, shape, and appearance of benign breast conditions may be similar to that for malignancies
    - Multimodality approach (correlation with prior mammography, sonography, MR) and clinical/personal patient history keys for correct diagnosis
    - Silicone rupture may mimic DCIS on mammography; can exhibit extensive FDG uptake and mimic widespread malignancy in extreme cases
    - Fat necrosis can demonstrate spiculated appearance on mammography; sonography not helpful for differentiation from malignancy
      - □ Usually minimal if any uptake on FDG PET

Nuclear Medicine Findings

- Benign conditions with increased uptake on FDG PET
  - Normal breast tissue
    - FDG uptake is proportional to tissue density and hormonal/menopausal status
      - □ Dense breasts have significantly ↑ FDG uptake compared to fatty breasts
      - □ Breasts in premenopausal patients demonstrate ↑ FDG uptake compared to postmenopausal patients
      - □ ↑ SUV in central breast as opposed to peripheral breast (more fatty tissue in peripheral breast)
    - Breast density typically decreases with increasing age; however, no significant correlation between age and normal breast tissue FDG uptake
  - Fat necrosis
    - May exhibit ↑ FDG uptake from various traumatic events/interventions
      - □ Most common etiologies: Breast trauma, diagnostic interventions & surgical procedures
    - Sterile inflammatory process 2° to previous breast trauma, diagnostic procedure, or surgery
      - □ TRAM reconstruction: Typically ↑ FDG uptake along incisional margins 2° to fat necrosis
    - ↑ FDG uptake 2° to metabolically active inflammatory cells
    - Variable appearance on mammography, dependent upon age
      - □ May present as coarse calcifications, microcalcifications, lipid cysts, focal asymmetry or spiculated masses
    - Sonography may confuse clinical picture (may appear as suspicious hypoechoic, shadowing mass)
    - MR shows ↓ signal intensity on T1-/T2-weighted images with variable enhancement
  - Lactation
    - Lactating glandular tissue: Intense, nearly symmetric FDG uptake
      - □ Slight asymmetry between breasts normal
    - Breast tissue proliferates with lactation and involutes with breastfeeding cessation
    - Increased FDG uptake physiologically related to infant suckling
      - □ Intracellular trapping of radiotracer in active glandular tissue
    - FDG uptake returns to normal within 3-4 weeks of breastfeeding cessation
  - Implants/silicone rupture
    - Leaking silicone implants or silicone granulomas: ↑ FDG uptake (typically intense)
      - □ Saline implants more rarely demonstrate FDG uptake
      - □ Dense masses anterior or superior to implant margins on mammography
      - □ MR remains modality of choice for silicone rupture
      - □ Hypointense on fat-suppressed T1 images, hyperintense on T2 images
      - □ Variable appearance on breast sonography: May range from hyper- to hypoechoic ± shadowing
    - ↑ FDG uptake at rim of calcific capsulitis
  - Infection
    - Acute or chronic, including overlying skin
    - ↑ FDG uptake 2° to mastitis, abscess, TB and fungal infections

- Reactive axillary, internal mammary, axillary lymph nodes: ↑ FDG uptake
- Activated inflammatory cells demonstrate increased glucose transporters
  - Same physiologically as malignant cells
- Trauma
  - Mild bruising or focal hematoma may show increased uptake on FDG PET for several weeks
  - Size and appearance variable dependent upon time course and extent of physical impact
- Post intervention
  - Focal ↑ FDG uptake due to core biopsy, recent surgery or radiotherapy
    - May persist for several weeks
  - Leukocyte infiltration of granulation tissue involved in wound repair
    - Resorption of necrotic debris and hematoma
- Benign breast conditions
  - Variable ↑ uptake in fibroadenomas, phyllodes tumors, fibrocystic change, and inspissated cysts
    - ↑ FDG in fibroadenomas and phyllodes tumors 2° to high proliferation and rapid growth
  - Ductal ectasia, typical/atypical hyperplasia, apocrine metaplasia
    - Often mildly ↑ FDG above normal glandular tissue
- Benign conditions without ↑ uptake on FDG PET
  - Most simple cystic lesions: No significant FDG uptake
    - Malignant lesions with cystic or mucinous components may mimic benign cysts on FDG PET (i.e., mucinous/colloid carcinoma)
  - Benign breast tumors
    - Usually decreased, but may have increased FDG uptake
  - Nonreactive intramammary nodes
    - Typically decreased FDG uptake
  - Skin thickening due to post axillary dissection lymphedema
    - Low FDG uptake

DIFFERENTIAL DIAGNOSIS

Poorly FDG-Avid Breast Cancer

- Concurrent chemotherapy or radiation treatment
  - May have decreased uptake in areas of viable tumor
  - Predictive of good response to chemotherapy/radiation
- Lobular or tubular carcinoma
  - Typically low FDG uptake 2° to low-grade tumor
  - With aggressive behavior, may show ↑ FDG uptake
- Ductal carcinoma in situ (DCIS)
  - Variable linear/branching areas of FDG uptake
    - Greater sensitivity with high-resolution positron emission mammography (PEM) units than conventional PET scanners
- Small tumors
  - Partial volume effects decrease measured SUV in tumors < 2.5 cm in diameter (false-negative)

CLINICAL ISSUES

Presentation

- Most common signs/symptoms
  - Benign breast disease often asymptomatic
    - Benign tumors, like malignant tumors, may be palpable, especially if enlarging
    - Postsurgical change and fat necrosis may also rarely be palpable secondary to associated scarring/tissue retraction
  - May have pain in areas of bruising/hematoma
  - Correlation with medical/surgical history remains key

DIAGNOSTIC CHECKLIST

Image Interpretation Pearls

- Poorly FDG avid
  - Small tumors (< 2.5 cm), DCIS, low-grade, slow-growing, noninvasive lobular and tubular carcinomas
    - Tumor size directly proportional to measured SUV
    - False-negatives with small tumor size (< 2.5 cm) and lower tumor grade
- Benign disease may be FDG-avid (although typically demonstrates milder uptake compared to breast malignancy)

SELECTED REFERENCES

1. Adejolu M et al: False-positive lesions mimicking breast cancer on FDG PET and PET/CT. AJR Am J Roentgenol. 198(3):W304-14, 2012
2. Lakhani P et al: Correlation between quantified breast densities from digital mammography and 18F-FDG PET uptake. Breast J. 15(4):339-47, 2009
3. Lim HS et al: FDG PET/CT for the detection and evaluation of breast diseases: usefulness and limitations. Radiographics. 27 Suppl 1:S197-213, 2007
4. Metser U et al: Benign nonphysiologic lesions with increased 18F-FDG uptake on PET/CT: characterization and incidence. AJR Am J Roentgenol. 189(5):1203-10, 2007
5. Berg WA et al: High-resolution fluorodeoxyglucose positron emission tomography with compression ("positron emission mammography") is highly accurate in depicting primary breast cancer. Breast J. 12(4):309-23, 2006
6. Kumar R et al: Clinicopathologic factors associated with false negative FDG-PET in primary breast cancer. Breast Cancer Res Treat. 98(3):267-74, 2006
7. Abouzied MM et al: 18F-FDG imaging: pitfalls and artifacts. J Nucl Med Technol. 33(3):145-55; quiz 162-3, 2005
8. Rosen EL et al: Detection of primary breast carcinoma with a dedicated, large-field-of-view FDG PET mammography device: initial experience. Radiology. 234(2):527-34, 2005
9. Hurwitz R: F-18 FDG positron emission tomographic imaging in a case of ruptured breast implant: inflammation or recurrent tumor? Clin Nucl Med. 28(9):755-6, 2003
10. Vranjesevic D et al: Relationship between 18F-FDG uptake and breast density in women with normal breast tissue. J Nucl Med. 44(8):1238-42, 2003
11. Avril N et al: Breast imaging with positron emission tomography and fluorine-18 fluorodeoxyglucose: use and limitations. J Clin Oncol. 18(20):3495-502, 2000
12. Bakheet SM et al: F-18 FDG uptake in breast infection and inflammation. Clin Nucl Med. 25(2):100-3, 2000

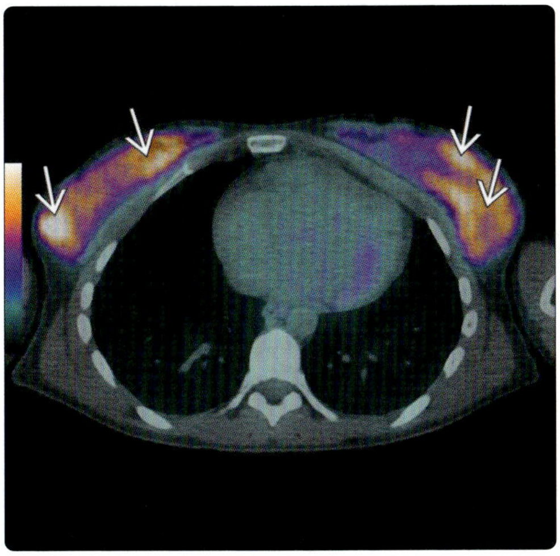

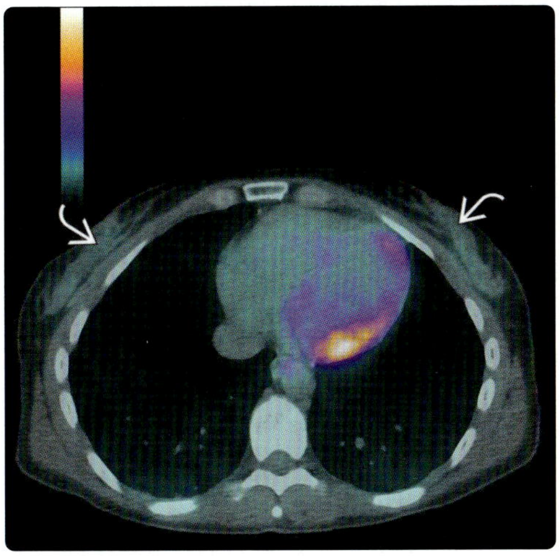

(Left) *Axial FDG PET/CT fusion image shows intense, nearly symmetric FDG uptake bilaterally, compatible with active lactation ➡. No significant FDG is secreted into the breast milk, but there is significant radiation within the breasts such that nursing should be limited immediately after the exam to reduced radiation exposure.* **(Right)** *Follow-up axial FDG PET/CT fusion image shows resolution of intense FDG uptake ➡ associated with smaller breast size when compared to prior images once the patient had ceased breast feeding.*

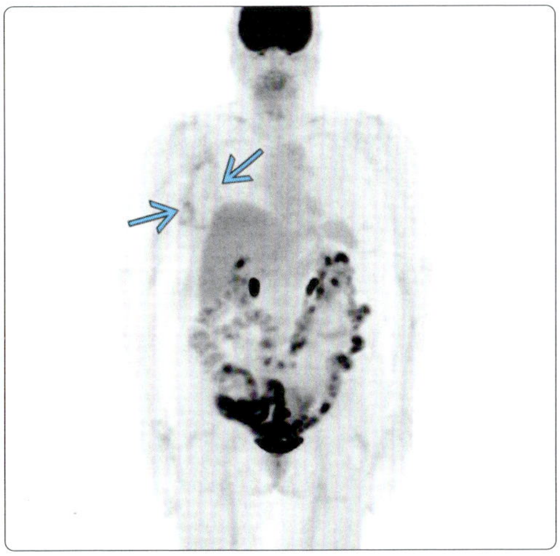

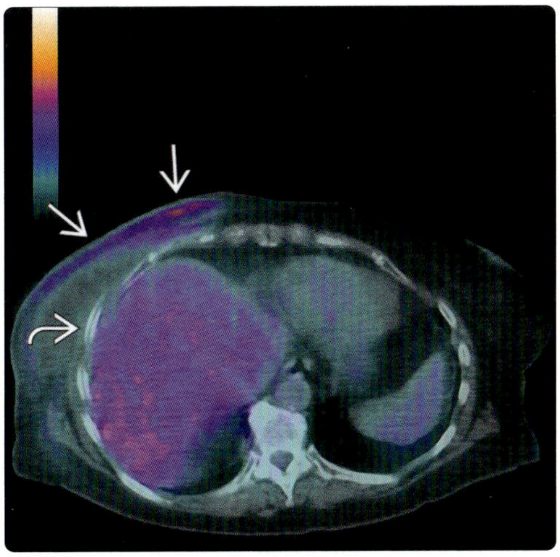

(Left) *MIP image from FDG PET shows mild linear uptake associated with recent mastectomy ➡.* **(Right)** *Axial FDG PET/CT fusion image shows mild FDG uptake within the skin overlying the right chest wall ➡, compatible with recent mastectomy. There is no significant FDG uptake within the underlying right chest wall seroma ➡. The post-mastectomy uptake resolves with time.*

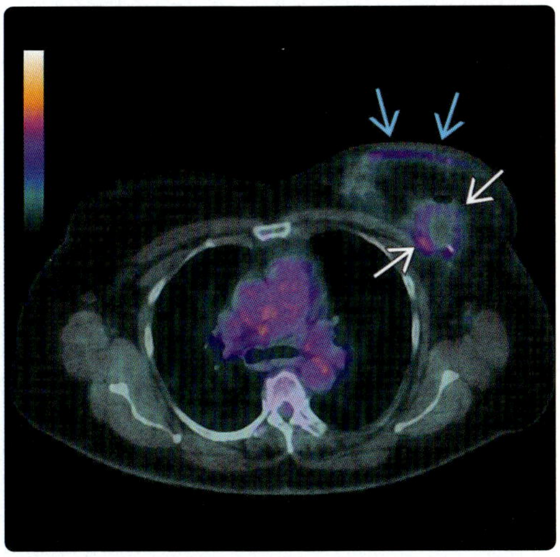

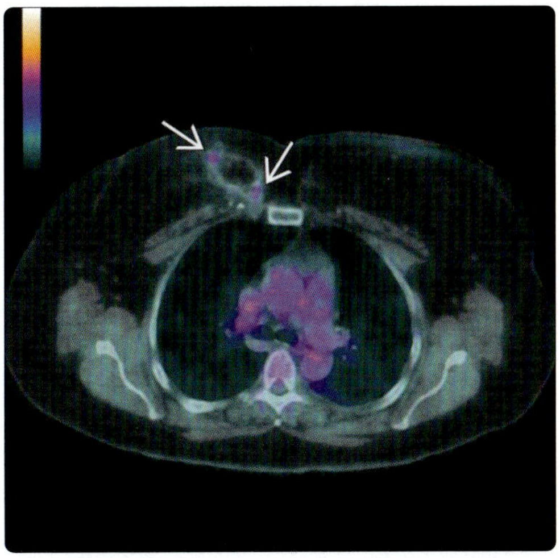

(Left) *FDG PET/CT fusion image 3 months post lumpectomy shows mild peripheral FDG uptake surrounding an ovoid fluid collection with an anterior focus of air ➡. An infected seroma should be suspected given the time interval from surgery. There is also mild uptake overlying the skin of the left breast ➡ related to recent surgery.* **(Right)** *Axial FDG PET/CT fusion image shows mild FDG activity ➡ associated with fat necrosis within the right breast from prior TRAM flap reconstruction.*

Primary Breast Cancer

KEY FACTS

IMAGING

- Primary breast carcinoma presents as focal increased activity on PET/CT, positron emission tomography (PEM), or molecular breast imaging/breast-specific gamma imaging (MBI/BSGI), and corresponds to suspicious mammographic lesion
  - These nuclear medicine imaging techniques serve as problem-solving devices when conventional breast imaging is difficult/equivocal
- Nuclear medicine imaging techniques are especially useful for women with dense breast tissue on mammography or those with equivocal MR findings
- PEM is optimized for small body parts and demonstrates higher sensitivity than PET/CT
- Sensitivity of PEM is comparable to that of breast MR
- MBI achieves greater resolution by decreasing dead space between breast and imaging surface

PATHOLOGY

- Key risk factors for breast carcinoma include increasing age, radiation exposure to chest wall, hormonal replacement therapy, early menarche, late menopause, and presence of dense breast tissue
- > 80-85% of breast cancer patients have no family history of breast carcinoma

CLINICAL ISSUES

- Breast carcinomas are often discovered by self-examination, clinical breast exam by patient's physician, or with screening mammography
- Breast carcinoma remains the most common cancer in women, with lifetime risk of 12.3% (1 in 8 women)
  - Lifetime risk for women with *BRCA* mutations is 3-7x risk of non-*BRCA* patients

(Left) *MIP PET/CT shows an intensely hypermetabolic focus over the right chest wall. No locoregional or distant metastases are seen. Lack of axillary nodal disease does not preclude sentinel node biopsy.* **(Right)** *Axial fused PET/CT in a patient shows a large, exophytic mass within the left breast, as well as an axillary metastasis and left-sided rib metastasis.*

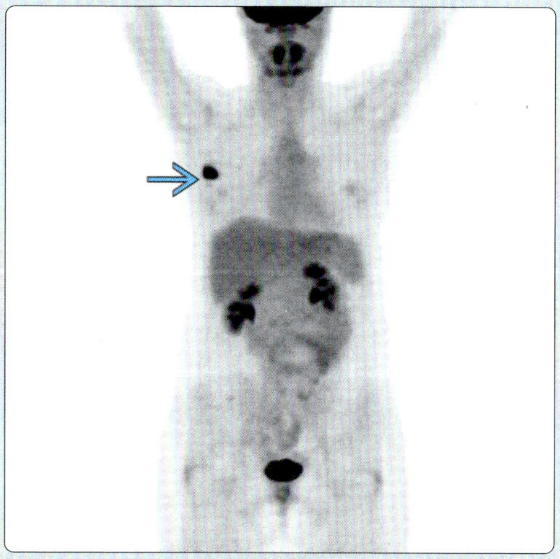

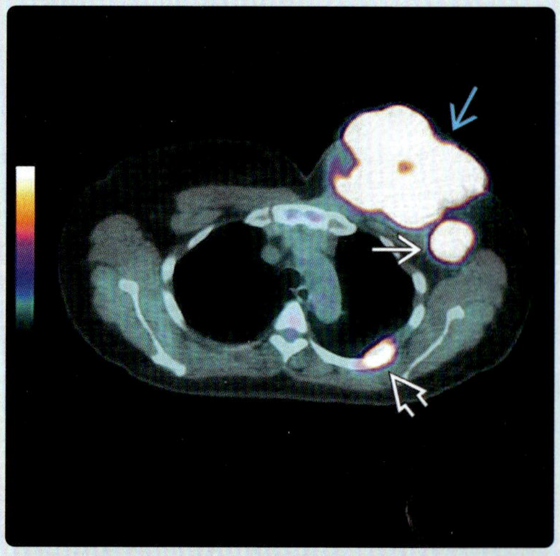

(Left) *Axial fused PET/CT shows a small, FDG-avid mass within the left breast of this male patient. Biopsy confirmed invasive ductal carcinoma. Differentiating benign gynecomastia from male breast carcinoma requires dedicated breast imaging.* **(Right)** *Axial fused PET/CT shows a single right-sided internal mammary lymph node metastasis. Detecting internal mammary nodes affects both surgical management and radiation therapy.*

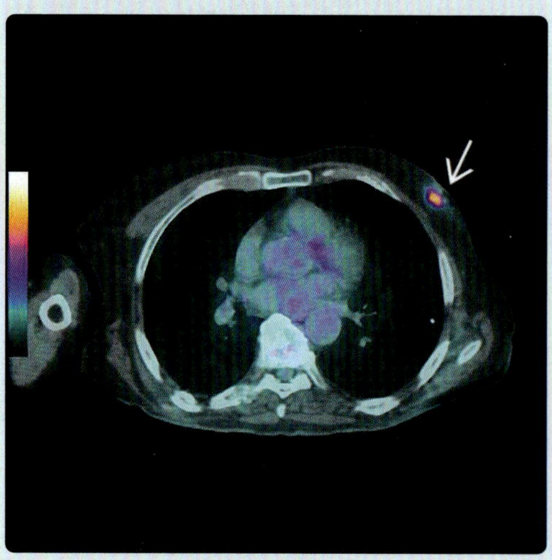

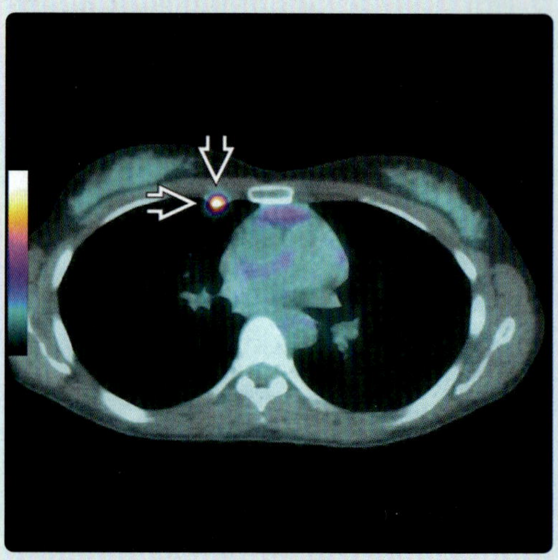

TERMINOLOGY

Definitions

- Primary malignant lesion of breast

IMAGING

General Features

- Best diagnostic clue
  - Focal increased activity on PET/CT, positron emission tomography (PEM), or molecular breast imaging/breast-specific gamma imaging (MBI/BSGI) corresponding to suspicious mammographic lesion
- Location
  - Any site within breast; overlying skin or intramammary lymph node may also demonstrate increased activity with involvement
  - Most common location for malignancy: Upper outer quadrant of breast
- Size
  - Lesions < 1-2 cm difficult to detect on whole-body PET/CT or breast scintigraphy; better seen with PEM or MBI
  - PET and breast scintigraphy performed with dedicated breast apparatus; can detect lesions as small as 4-5 mm

Nuclear Medicine Findings

- Problem-solving technique when conventional breast imaging difficult/equivocal
  - Dense breast tissue on mammography, equivocal MR findings
- PET/CT
  - Sensitivities reported in range of 79-90%; specificity 74-80%
  - 5-7 mm lesions routinely detected, especially if prone PET/CT used
  - Negative PET in breast lesion ≥ 10 mm likely benign, unless slow growing or low-grade tumor (i.e., lobular, tubular carcinoma)
  - PET may detect high-grade ductal carcinoma in situ (DCIS) if > 1.5-2 cm
  - 50% reduction in SUV on PET following 2 cycles of chemotherapy considered good response
- PEM
  - Breast-specific imaging device
  - Optimized for small body parts, with higher sensitivity than PET (1-2 mm for PEM; 4-6 mm for PET)
  - Sensitivity comparable to MR and higher than PET (93% vs. 68%)
  - High spatial resolution; can detect lesions < 2 cm
  - Not affected by breast density or hormonal/menopausal status
  - Disadvantages: Low specificity (same as PET), high radiation exposure compared to mammography
- MBI/BSGI
  - Emerging technology
  - Breast-specific imaging device
  - Achieve greater resolution by decreasing dead space between breast and imaging surface
- Tc-99m MIBI
  - No longer used due to inferior results compared to PET/CT
  - Sensitivity of 76-90%; poor sensitivity (< 50%) for small or low-grade malignancies
- Thallium (Tl)-201
  - No longer used due to higher sensitivity with modalities listed above
  - Poor sensitivity for lesions < 1.5 cm (40-60%)
  - Poor sensitivity for low-grade malignancy

Imaging Recommendations

- Best imaging tool
  - Screening: Mammography
  - Localization, tissue/mass characterization: Ultrasound
  - Sensitivity, tissue/mass characterization, extent of tumor involvement: MR
  - Problem-solving: Prone PET/CT, PEM or MBI
- Protocol advice
  - FDG PET or PET/CT
    - Lesion uptake dependent on increased utilization of glucose by cancer cells using FDG (glucose analog)
    - Prone imaging following supine study: Highest sensitivity for breast, axillary, and mediastinal lesions; separates chest wall from breast
    - Patient preparation: NPO 4-6 hours prior to PET, blood glucose < 150-200; adequate hydration
  - PEM
    - Lesion uptake dependent on increased utilization of glucose by cancer cells via FDG (similar to PET)
    - Inject 5-10 mCi (185-370 MBq) FDG IV in arm contralateral to cancer
    - 12 slices each in craniocaudal and mediolateral oblique positions, analogous to mammography
    - Patient preparation: NPO 4-6 hours prior to PEM, blood glucose < 140; adequate hydration
  - MBI/BSGI
    - Gamma-emitting radiotracer, usually Tc-99m sestamibi
    - Lesion uptake dependent on increased blood flow and transmembrane potentials
    - Uptake varies with menstrual cycle (luteal phase > follicular phase); ↑ uptake with exogenous hormones
    - Concentration in mitochondria: ↑ uptake in metabolically active cells
    - MBI: Breast compressed between 2 cadmium-zinc-telluride (CZT) detectors
    - BSGI: Breast compressed between compression paddle and single sodium iodide (NaI) detector
    - Lower dose associated with MBI (4-8 mCi) as opposed to BSGI (20 mCi); injection in arm contralateral to cancer
  - Tc-99m MIBI (scintimammography)
    - Lesion uptake dependent on increased blood flow, mitochondrial activity and concentration in tumor
    - 3 serial images (each 10 min acquisitions) beginning immediately after ~ 20 mCi (740 MBq) Tc-99m MIBI IV; prone, lateral views
  - Tl-201
    - Lesion uptake dependent on Na+/K+ pump (inactivated by ouabain) and cotransport system (inactivated by furosemide)

- 3 serial images (each 10 minute acquisitions) beginning immediately after 3 mCi (111 MBq) Tl-201 IV; prone, lateral views

DIFFERENTIAL DIAGNOSIS

Infection/Inflammation

- Usually ↓ target:background ratio than tumors of comparable size

Trauma and Surgery

- Postsurgical procedure: Frequently result in FDG uptake up to 3-6 months
- Hematoma may be FDG-avid 2° to surrounding inflammation
- Low-level FDG activity may persist in scar tissue indefinitely

Fibrocystic Disease

- Multifocal low-level FDG uptake often present

Benign Tumors

- Fibroadenoma, benign phyllodes, papilloma, etc.
- Typically ↓ FDG uptake: Higher if hypercellular or rapidly growing

Lactating Breast

- Intense FDG uptake in glandular tissue, usually fairly symmetric

Normal Breast Tissue

- FDG uptake proportional to breast density/hormonal status

PATHOLOGY

General Features

- Etiology
  - Risk factors: ↑ age, radiation exposure to chest wall (especially first 2 decades), hormonal replacement therapy, early menarche, late menopause, dense breast tissue
  - Risk reduced with early full-term pregnancy
- Genetics
  - ↑ incidence: Family history, i.e., first-degree relative (mother, sister)
    - > 80-85% breast cancer patients: No family history
  - *BRCA1*, *BRCA2* genetics indicate high likelihood for development of breast cancer

Microscopic Features

- Ductal cancers (cancers arising from ductal cells)
  - In situ: Tumor cells contained within ducts without stromal invasion by tumor cells
  - Invasive: Tumor has penetrated ductal epithelium and invaded stroma
- Lobular cancers (cancers arising from lobule cells)
  - In situ: Tumor cells contained within lobules without penetration of lobule walls
  - Invasive: Tumor cells have invaded stroma

CLINICAL ISSUES

Presentation

- Most common signs/symptoms
  - Discovered by self-examination, clinical breast exam by physician, or screening mammography
  - Nipple discharge or inverted/retracted nipple
  - Peau de orange: Inflammatory breast carcinoma

Demographics

- Epidemiology
  - Most common cancer in women (excluding skin cancer)
  - NCI new case estimates (2014): 232,670 female; 2,360 male
    - Deaths: 40,000 female; 430 male
  - Lifetime risk for breast cancer in women: 12.3% (1 in 8 women)
  - Lifetime risk in women with *BRCA* mutation: 30-80% (3-7x risk of non-*BRCA* patients)

DIAGNOSTIC CHECKLIST

Consider

- Detection is function of size, mitotic activity
- Detection enhanced by optimizing technique/choice of instrumentation: PEM/MBI > FDG PET/CT > planar MIBI > planar Tl

Image Interpretation Pearls

- Breast cancer may be multifocal/multicentric
  - Examine both breasts regardless of technique
- False-negative PET: Small (< 10 mm), in situ, low-grade cancers
- False-positive PET: Inflammation, infection, lactation, silicone rupture, fat necrosis, recent trauma or surgery

SELECTED REFERENCES

1. Fowler AM: A molecular approach to breast imaging. J Nucl Med. 55(2):177-80, 2014
2. Glass SB et al: Clinical utility of positron emission mammography. Proc (Bayl Univ Med Cent). 26(3):314-9, 2013
3. Kalles V et al: The current status of positron emission mammography in breast cancer diagnosis. Breast Cancer. 20(2):123-30, 2013
4. Ling CM et al: Breast-specific gamma imaging in the detection of atypical ductal hyperplasia and lobular neoplasia. Acad Radiol. 19(6):661-6, 2012
5. Hruska CB et al: Molecular breast imaging: use of a dual-head dedicated gamma camera to detect small breast tumors. AJR Am J Roentgenol. 191(6):1805-15, 2008
6. Berg WA et al: High-resolution fluorodeoxyglucose positron emission tomography with compression ("positron emission mammography") is highly accurate in depicting primary breast cancer. Breast J. 12(4):309-23, 2006
7. Kumar R et al: Clinicopathologic factors associated with false negative FDG-PET in primary breast cancer. Breast Cancer Res Treat. 98(3):267-74, 2006
8. Kumar R et al: Standardized uptake values of normal breast tissue with 2-deoxy-2-[F-18]fluoro-D: -glucose positron emission tomography: variations with age, breast density, and menopausal status. Mol Imaging Biol. 8(6):355-62, 2006
9. Pelosi E et al: Value of integrated PET/CT for lesion localisation in cancer patients: a comparative study. Eur J Nucl Med Mol Imaging. 31(7):932-9, 2004
10. Zangheri B et al: PET/CT and breast cancer. Eur J Nucl Med Mol Imaging. 31 Suppl 1:S135-42, 2004
11. Vranjesevic D et al: Relationship between 18F-FDG uptake and breast density in women with normal breast tissue. J Nucl Med. 44(8):1238-42, 2003
12. Bos R et al: Biologic correlates of (18)fluorodeoxyglucose uptake in human breast cancer measured by positron emission tomography. J Clin Oncol. 20(2):379-87, 2002

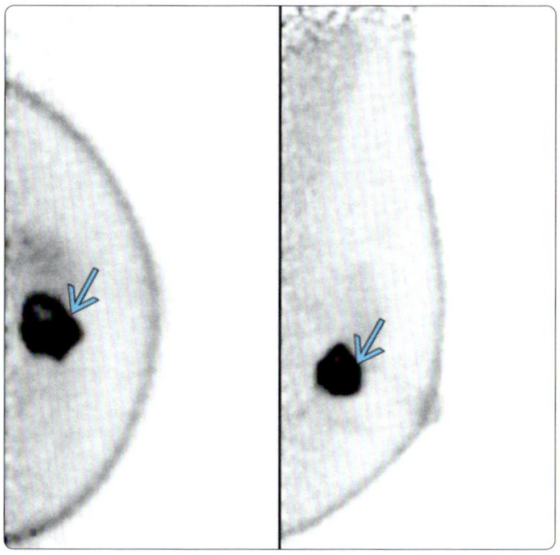

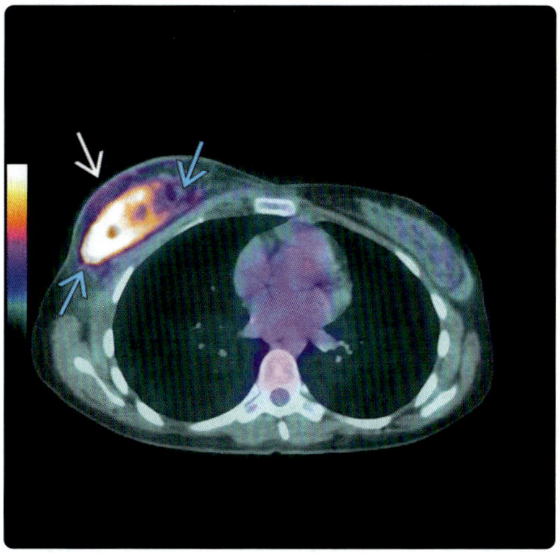

(Left) *Craniocaudal (left) and mediolateral oblique (right) images from PEM examination show an intensely hypermetabolic focus* → *within the central left breast, compatible with the patient's known primary breast carcinoma.* **(Right)** *Axial fused PET/CT in the same patient shows an FDG-avid, infiltrating mass within the right breast* →*. Low-level activity within the overlying skin is compatible with invasion of dermal lymphatics* ➡*. Note the asymmetry in breast size.*

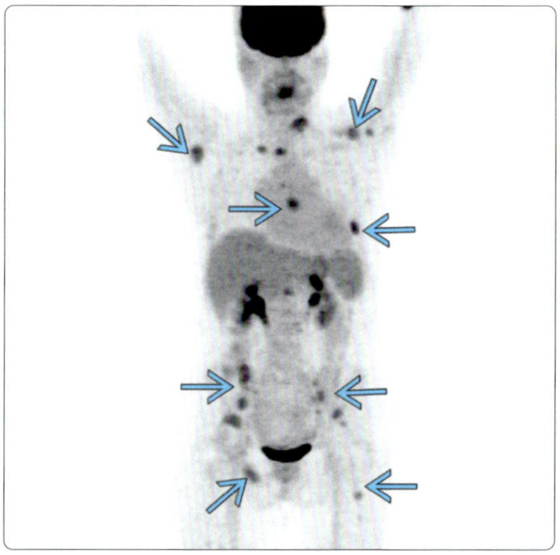

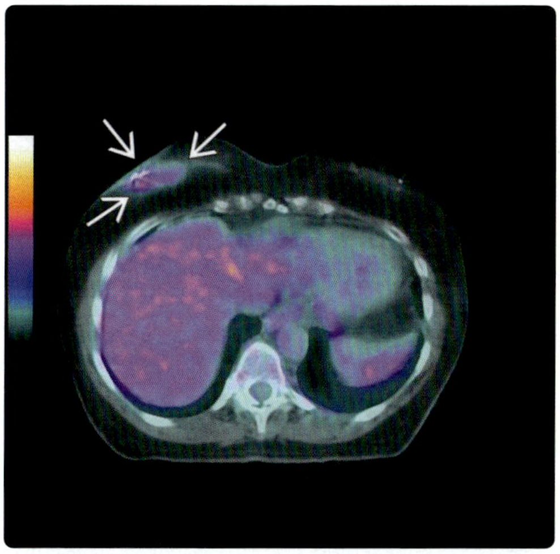

(Left) *MIP PET/CT shows multiple foci of FDG uptake* →*, compatible with multifocal lytic metastases from known lobular breast carcinoma. PET/CT advantage of whole body-imaging is evident in this case.* **(Right)** *Axial fused PET/CT shows a focus of moderately increased uptake* ➡*, compatible with recurrent invasive lobular carcinoma in reconstructed right breast (TRAM flap).*

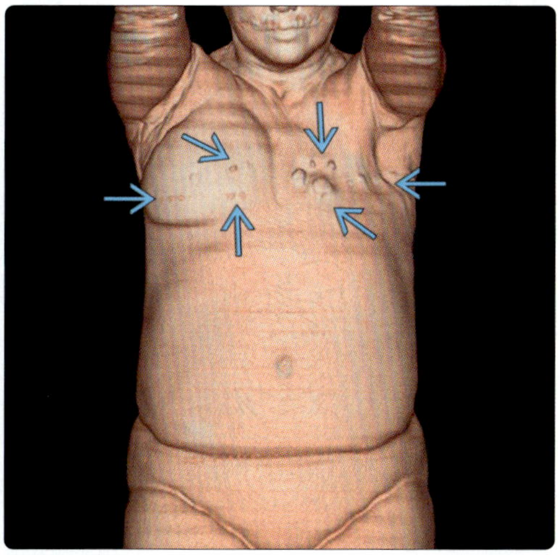

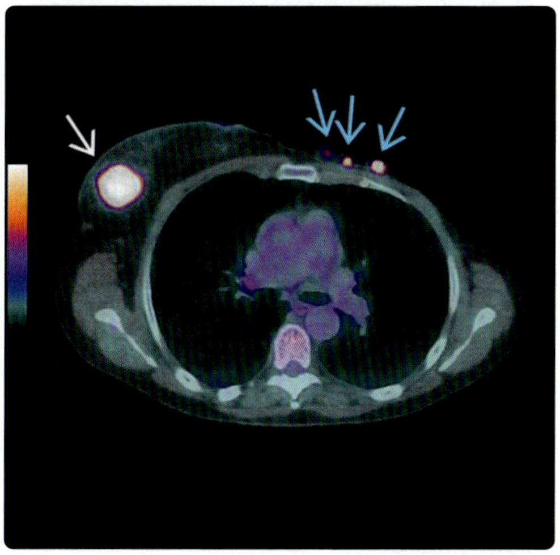

(Left) *Surface 3D reconstruction from PET/CT shows multiple chest wall cutaneous metastases* → *from the patient's known right breast carcinoma. Previous left mastectomy is noted.* **(Right)** *Axial fused PET/CT in the same patient shows an avidly enhancing mass within the lateral right breast* ➡*. Examples of cutaneous metastases are noted along the patient's left mastectomy site* →*.*

KEY FACTS

IMAGING

- On PET/CT, breast carcinoma presents as focal increased FDG uptake at primary tumor site
- Metastases may occur anywhere, but are most common in axillary and internal mammary lymph nodes, osseous structures, and liver
- PET/CT demonstrates 80-95% sensitivity for detection of distant metastases at time of initial diagnosis
- Positive predictive value is reduced by multiple false-positives: Infection, inflammation, trauma, skeletal muscle uptake, bowel activity, blood pool, physiologic uptake, and benign tumors
- Sensitivity and specificity for PET in detection of axillary metastases are dependent on multiple factors, to include lymph node size, degree of nodal replacement, and proliferative activity
- Patients harbor significantly worse prognosis with both IM and axillary nodal metastases than with axillary nodal disease alone
- Main visceral organ for distant metastases is liver
- Osseous skeleton is most common site for distant metastases in patients treated with mastectomy and adjuvant chemotherapy

PATHOLOGY

- Main risk factors for breast carcinoma include gender, increasing age, estrogen exposure, dense breast tissue, radiation and postmenopausal obesity

CLINICAL ISSUES

- Patients with metastases may notably be asymptomatic; symptoms vary by affected organ

DIAGNOSTIC CHECKLIST

- PET/CT is excellent for staging patients with potentially aggressive breast carcinoma and monitoring response to treatment
- Pertinent history, physical exam and other imaging findings are crucial elements prior to final interpretation of PET/CTs

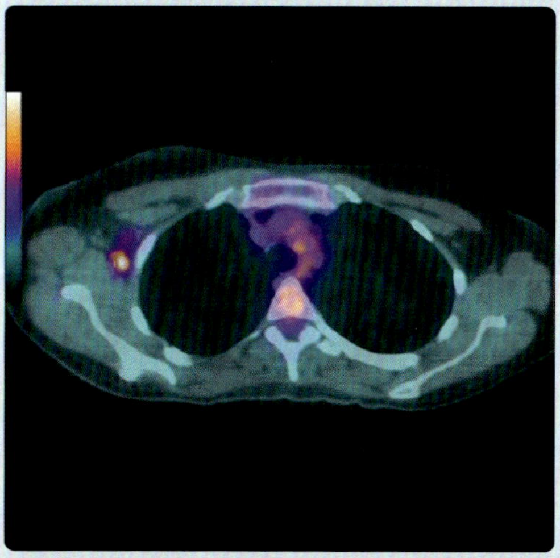

Anatomic Stage/Prognostic Groups

Stage 0	Tis	N0	M0
Stage IA	T1	N0	M0
Stage IB	T0 T1	N1mi N1mi	M0 M0
Stage IIA	T0 T1 T2	N1 N1 N0	M0 M0 M0
Stage IIB	T2 T3	N1 N0	M0 M0
Stage IIIA	T0 T1 T2 T3 T3	N2 N2 N2 N1 N2	M0 M0 M0 M0 M0
Stage IIIB	T4 T4 T4	N0 N1 N2	M0 M0 M0
Stage IIIC	Any T	N3	M0
Stage IV	Any T	Any N	M1

(Left) *Axial PET/CT fused image in a patient with left breast carcinoma (not shown) shows activity in the right axilla corresponding to a non-pathologically enlarged lymph node on CT. A large partial dosage infiltration in the right arm is noted. Lymphatic trapping most likely accounts for this contralateral lymph node activity.* **(Right)** *Table shows anatomic stage/prognostic groups for breast cancer. For full details, please see the American Joint Committee on Cancer (AJCC), 7th edition.*

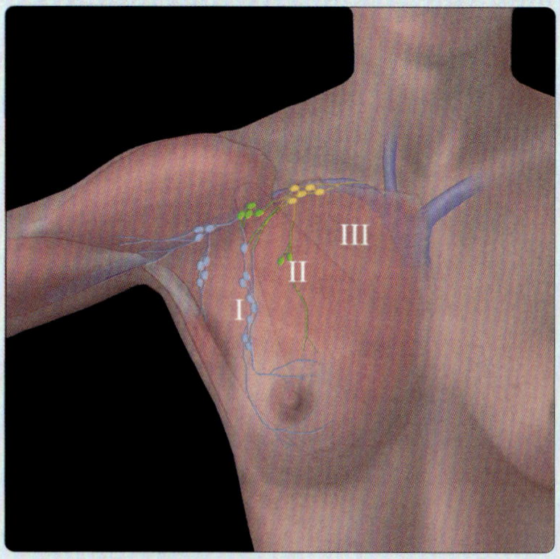

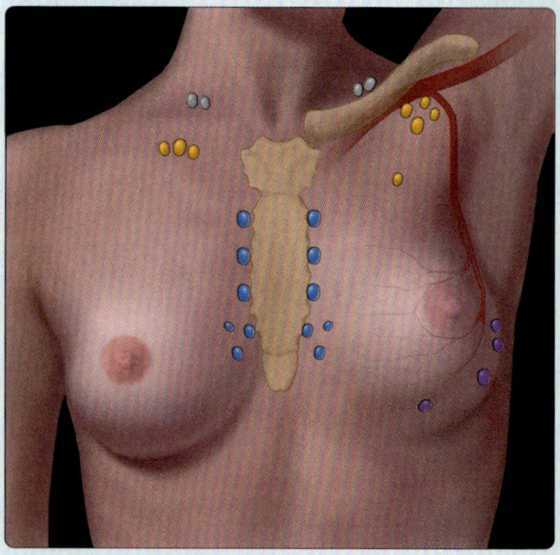

(Left) *Axillary lymph node levels are shown. Level I is the bottom level, below the lower edge of the pectoralis minor muscle. Level II is underneath the pectoralis minor muscle. Level III is above the pectoralis minor muscle.* **(Right)** *Regional nodal stations to survey for metastatic disease are shown: Silver: supraclavicular; gold: Infraclavicular; blue: Internal mammary; purple: Intramammary.*

TERMINOLOGY

Definitions

- Breast carcinoma = primary malignancy of breast

IMAGING

General Features

- Best diagnostic clue
  - PET/CT: Focal increased uptake in primary tumor, axillary/internal mammary lymph nodes (LN), and distant sites (i.e., bone, liver, lung)
  - Bone scan: Multiple sites of focally increased uptake throughout osseous structures, axial > appendicular
  - PEM/breast-specific gamma imaging (BSGI)/molecular breast imaging (MBI): Focal increased uptake in primary tumor and axillary LN
- Location
  - Metastases may occur anywhere but most common in axillary LN > internal mammary LN > bone > liver
- Staging guidelines
  - National Comprehensive Cancer Network (NCCN): Work-up for metastases in asymptomatic patients with at least stage IIIA disease and in symptomatic patients

Nuclear Medicine Findings

- PET/CT: Detection of distant metastases at time of initial diagnosis: 80-95% sensitivity
  - Negative predictive value (NPV) > 90% in evaluation of distant metastases
  - Positive predictive value (PPV) reduced by false-positives (i.e., infection, inflammation, trauma, benign tumors, etc.)
  - NPV and PPV improved with PET/CT (vs. PET alone) or fusion with MR
  - PET and PET/CT not routinely used for patients with clinical stage I/II breast carcinoma
- Axillary metastases: Sensitivity and specificity for PET dependent on multiple factors
  - Size, number of nodes
    - PET/CT: Low sensitivity (60%) for axillary metastases: Micrometastases not detected by PET
    - Limits of resolution of PET: 6-8 mm
    - SLN biopsy procedure necessary for optimal axillary staging
  - Degree of nodal replacement by metastasis and proliferative activity
  - Tumor type: Poor sensitivity for low-grade carcinomas (i.e., lobular, tubular)
  - Prior lymphadenectomy or other surgical intervention
    - PET may remain positive for 3-12 months
    - Extensive clips or sutures: Inflammation → false-positive on PET scan
- Mediastinal and internal mammary LN evaluation
  - Best detected and localized with PET/CT
  - Significantly worse prognosis with both IM and axillary nodal metastases than with axillary nodal disease alone
- Hepatic metastases
  - Main visceral organ for distant metastases
  - Generally occur later than locoregional recurrences and harbor a worse prognosis
  - Best detected with MR; PET/CT: Low-density hepatic focus with ↑ FDG uptake
  - May have positive FDG PET and negative CT; gadolinium-enhanced MR or multiphase CECT confirmation suggested
  - False-negative FDG PET: Small lesions (< 10 mm)
  - False-positive FDG PET findings: Infection/inflammation or interposed colon
- Osseous metastases
  - Most common site of distant metastases in patients treated with mastectomy and adjuvant chemotherapy
  - PET: Sensitivity high for lytic or bone marrow (BM) metastases (> 90%)
  - Bone scan: High sensitivity for detection of cortical blastic metastases
    - Low sensitivity for lytic (75-80%) or BM metastases (< 50%)
- PET has similar or higher diagnostic accuracy than conventional imaging for restaging
- PET/CT has higher sensitivity and specificity in restaging than PET alone
- SUV measurements helpful in determining adequate response to chemotherapy
  - > 50% SUV reduction at 9 weeks defined as good clinical response
  - > 55% response after 1 cycle also defined as good response
- Rise in SUV 7-10 days after antiestrogen therapy (metabolic flare) sign of good response

Imaging Recommendations

- Best imaging tool
  - SLN biopsy procedure: Optimal for axillary LN staging
  - PET/CT: Optimal for detection of disease extent, distant metastases, or assessment of response to therapy
  - Bone scan: Osseous metastases
  - MR: Brain metastases; confirmation of hepatic metastases
- Protocol advice
  - Tc-99m MDP bone scan
    - 20-30 mCi (740 MBq to 1.1 GBq) Tc-99m MDP IV
    - Planar whole-body scan 90-120 min following radiopharmaceutical administration; spot views &/or SPECT regions of interest
  - PET/CT
    - Patient preparation: NPO 4-6 hours, low carbohydrates x 12 hours prior to study; good hydration
    - 10-15 mCi (370-550 MBq) F-18 FDG IV
    - CT: ± oral contrast (2 hours prior to scan) &/or IV contrast
    - Prone breast study highly accurate for evaluation of breast, axilla, mediastinum
  - PEM
    - Also utilizes F-18 FDG
    - May be useful for imaging of primary tumor

DIFFERENTIAL DIAGNOSIS

Infection/Inflammation

- Granulomatous disease (e.g., sarcoidosis)
- Soft tissue infection (e.g., esophagitis, abscess)

- Postsurgical changes, ostomy sites
- Intramuscular injection sites
- Degenerative bone disease
- Silicone injections/leak

Trauma

- Recent rib or vertebral compression fractures
- Soft tissue trauma
- Recent biopsy/intervention

Other Malignancy

- 2nd primary neoplasm: Thyroid, lung, colon, etc.

PATHOLOGY

General Features

- Etiology
  - Risk factors: Age, estrogen exposure, dense breasts, radiation, postmenopausal obesity
- Genetics
  - ~ 85% of breast cancer sporadic
  - *BRCA1*, *BRCA2* increase likelihood of developing breast cancer
  - *BRCA1* and *BRCA2* present in ~ 0.5% of population
  - *BRCA2* may increase breast cancer risk in men

Staging, Grading, & Classification

- Stage I: Tumor < 2 cm
- Stage II: Tumor < 2 cm, 1-3 positive axillary LN; tumor 2-5 cm, negative LN or 1-3 positive LN; tumor > 5 cm, negative LN
- Stage III: Tumor < 5 cm with 4-9 positive axillary LN or positive internal mammary LN; tumor > 5 cm, positive axillary/internal mammary LN; tumor invades chest wall, ± axillary/internal mammary LN
- Stage IV: Distant metastases

CLINICAL ISSUES

Presentation

- Most common signs/symptoms
  - Patients with metastases may be asymptomatic
  - Symptoms depend on organ involved
    - Axillary: Extremity swelling, mass
    - Brain: CNS findings (i.e., dizziness, ataxia, weakness)
    - Bone: Most asymptomatic but pain is common; can be palliated with beta emitters (Sm-153, Sr-89)
    - Liver: Asymptomatic in most; may progress to hepatic failure or abdominal pain if extensive

Demographics

- Age
  - 80% of cases occur in women > 50 years
- Gender
  - Female breast cancer ~ 55x more common than male
- Epidemiology
  - 12.5% of women will develop breast cancer in their lifetime
  - *BRCA1*, *BRCA2* confers 3-7x risk of developing breast cancer compared to women without these mutations
  - 75% of recurrent breast cancer occurs within 5 years of initial diagnosis
  - Distant metastases → average survival of 1-2 years
    - 4% of patients with new diagnosis of breast carcinoma will have distant metastases at time of presentation

Natural History & Prognosis

- Mortality rate for African Americans > Caucasians
- Early stage: Survival rates ~ 98%
- Distant metastases: Remission ~ 10-20%; cure very rare

Treatment

- Surgery: Removal of primary tumor or recurrent breast tumor
- Chemotherapy: Primary therapy, adjuvant, neoadjuvant, hormonal
- Radiation therapy: Following lumpectomy; axillary &/or mediastinal radiation dependent on lymphadenopathy; treatment/palliation of metastases
- Combination of surgery, chemotherapy and radiation therapy often most effective in treatment

DIAGNOSTIC CHECKLIST

Consider

- PET/CT excellent for staging patients with potentially aggressive breast cancers/monitoring response to treatment
  - Insulin effect 2° to poor dietary preparation → potential false-negative study
  - Adequate time following injection (~ 60 min)

Image Interpretation Pearls

- Be aware of potential pitfalls and artifacts with PET/CT including motion artifact and misregistration
- Pertinent history, physical exam and other imaging findings important prior to final interpretation

SELECTED REFERENCES

1. Lee SC et al: Radiologist's role in breast cancer staging: providing key information for clinicians. Radiographics. 34(2):330-42, 2014
2. Groheux D et al: Performance of FDG PET/CT in the clinical management of breast cancer. Radiology. 266(2):388-405, 2013
3. Chung A et al: Preoperative FDG-PET for axillary metastases in patients with breast cancer. Arch Surg. 141(8):783-8; discussion 788-9, 2006
4. Zangheri B et al: PET/CT and breast cancer. Eur J Nucl Med Mol Imaging. 31 Suppl 1:S135-42, 2004
5. Eubank WB et al: Detection of locoregional and distant recurrences in breast cancer patients by using FDG PET. Radiographics. 22(1):5-17, 2002
6. Yang SN et al: Comparing whole body (18)F-2-deoxyglucose positron emission tomography and technetium-99m methylene diphosphonate bone scan to detect bone metastases in patients with breast cancer. J Cancer Res Clin Oncol. 128(6):325-8, 2002
7. Wahl RL et al: Metabolic monitoring of breast cancer chemohormonotherapy using positron emission tomography: initial evaluation. J Clin Oncol. 11(11):2101-11, 1993
8. American Joint Committee on Cancer

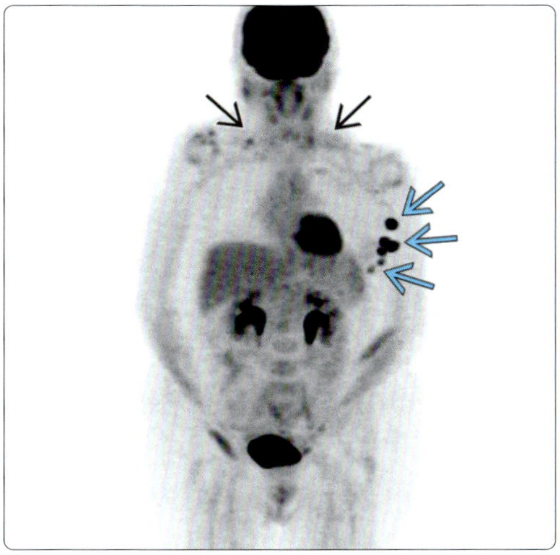

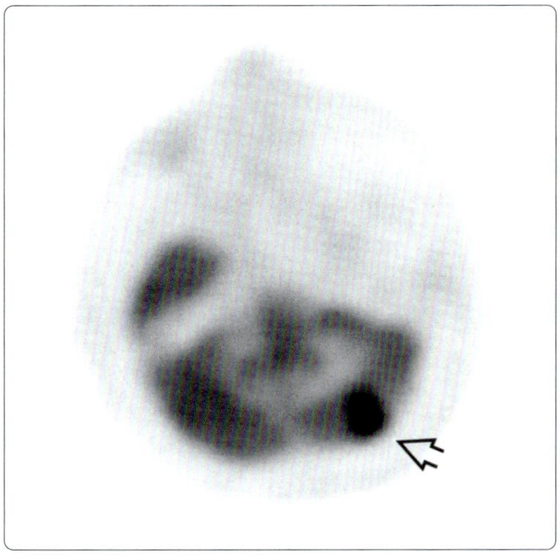

(Left) *MIP PET/CT shows multiple hypermetabolic foci in the left chest wall. Brown adipose tissue (BAT) is also noted in a symmetric distribution bilaterally. The BAT somewhat limits evaluation of underlying nodal disease.* **(Right)** *Axial PET image shows a hypermetabolic focus within the left cerebellum, compatible with metastasis. PET/CT is typically not sensitive for brain metastasis secondary to normal gray matter activity. The ordering clinician should be notified for unsuspected brain metastases.*

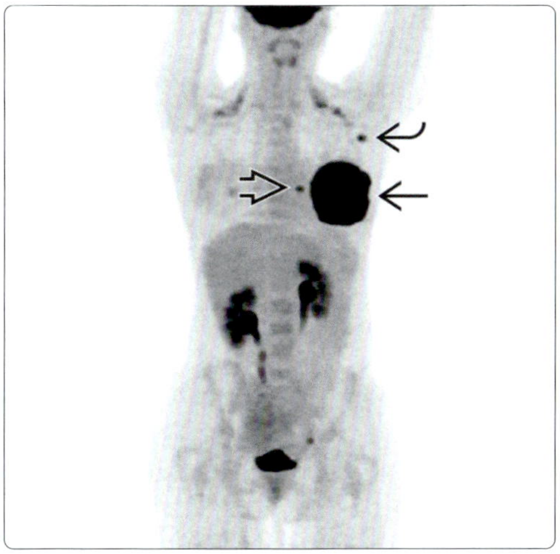

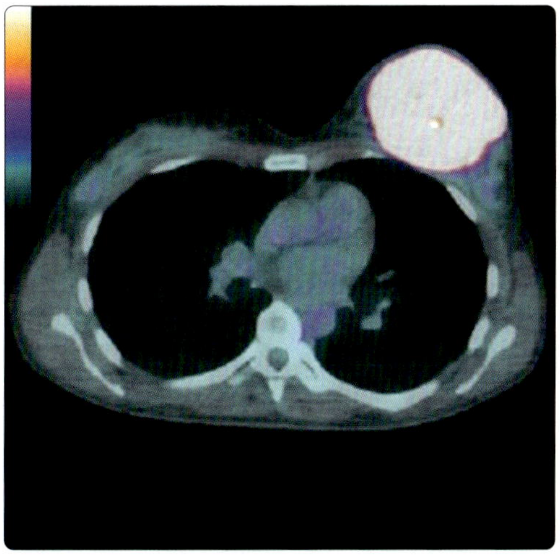

(Left) *MIP PET/CT shows an intensely hypermetabolic mass in the left breast and nodal lesions in the left axilla and left internal mammary chain.* **(Right)** *Axial PET/CT fused image in the same patient shows the primary mass to be very large and causing near-complete replacement of the left breast. Long-term patient neglect had occurred.*

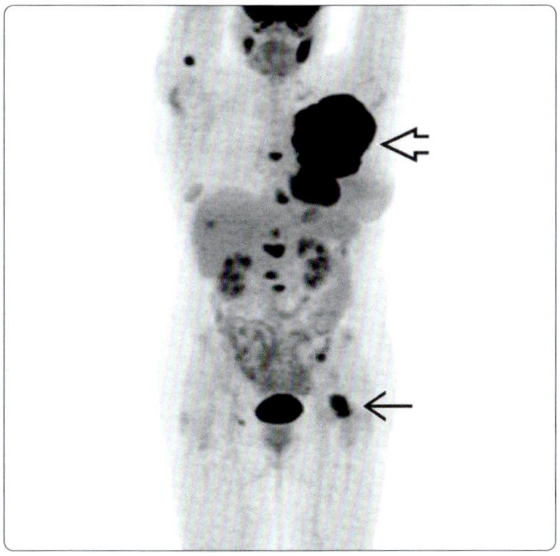

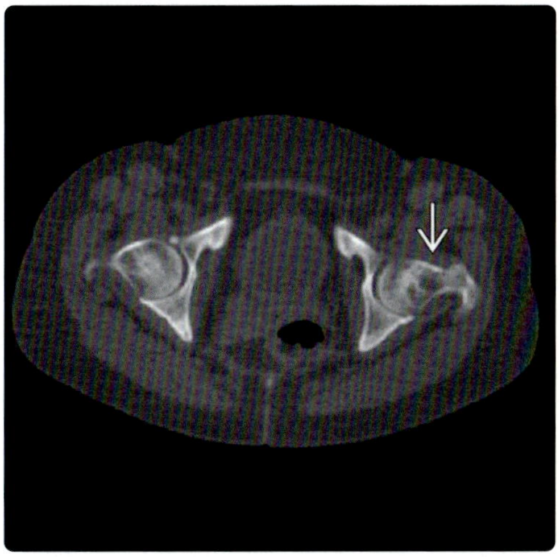

(Left) *Coronal MIP PET/CT shows a very large primary mass in the left breast with multiple metastasis including one in the left hip region. PET/CT often detects unsuspected metastasis.* **(Right)** *Axial attenuation correction CT shows a lytic, destructive lesion in the left proximal femur that is at risk for pathological fracture. The clinician should be alerted and orthopedic consultation should be suggested.*

(Left) *MIP PET/CT shows two FDG-avid foci* → *within the left axillary region in this patient status post bilateral mastectomy and chemotherapy.* **(Right)** *Axial fused PET/CT in the same patient shows an intensely FDG-avid axillary lymph node* → *that is the larger of the two FDG-avid foci on the previous MIP image, compatible with nodal recurrence post mastectomy and chemotherapy.*

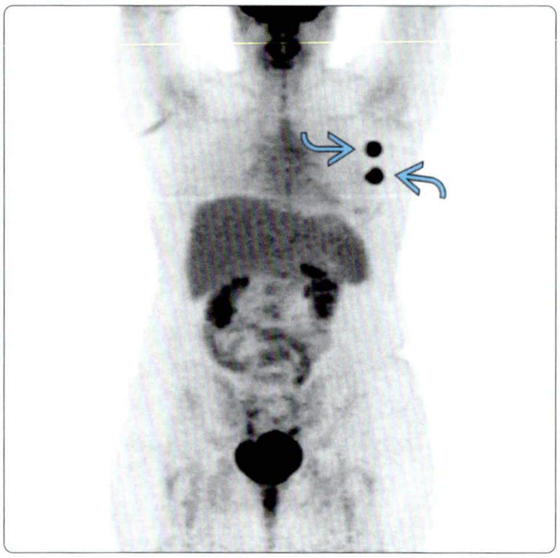

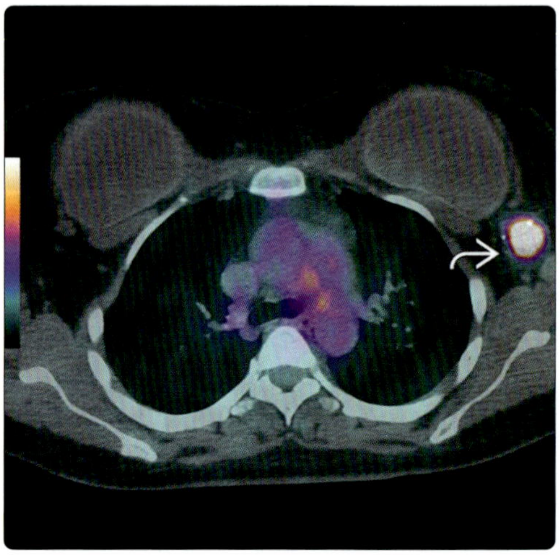

(Left) *MIP PET/CT demonstrates an intensely hypermetabolic focus within the right breast* →*, as well as a single metastatic lesion overlying the right chest wall* →*.* **(Right)** *Axial fused PET/CT shows an FDG-avid focus corresponding to a solitary right-sided rib metastasis* →*.*

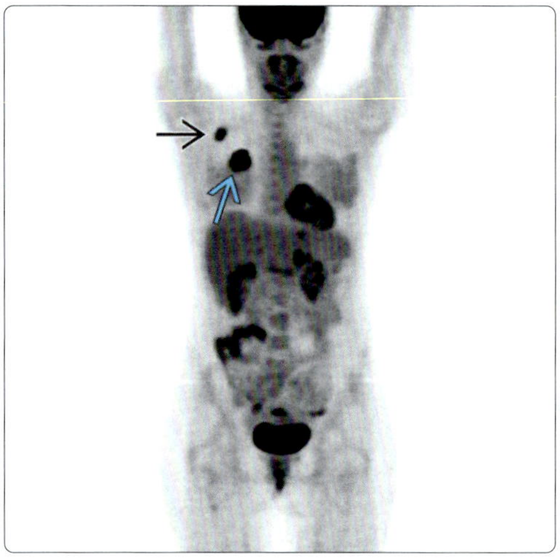

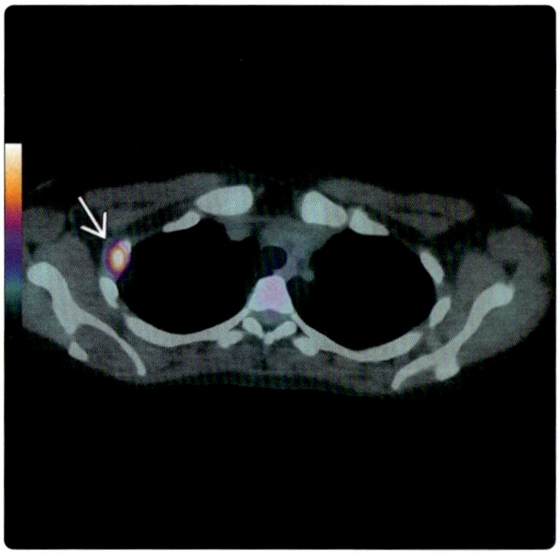

(Left) *MIP PET/CT during initial staging shows a solitary focus overlying the liver* → *without local disease. Bilateral breast MR and dedicated breast imaging would not detect unsuspected lesions such as this.* **(Right)** *Axial fused PET/CT shows a discrete hepatic lesion with uptake much greater than normal hepatic activity most compatible with a metastasis. PET/CT often upstages patients, thereby precluding unnecessary treatments.*

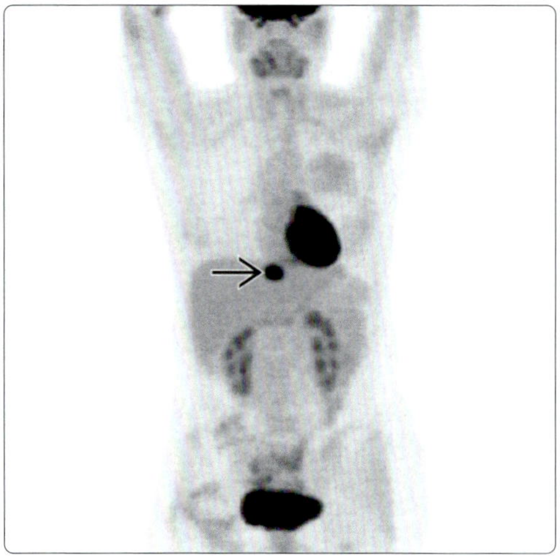

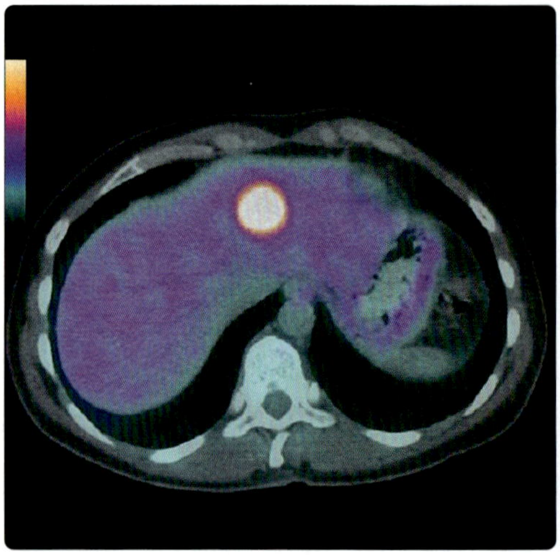

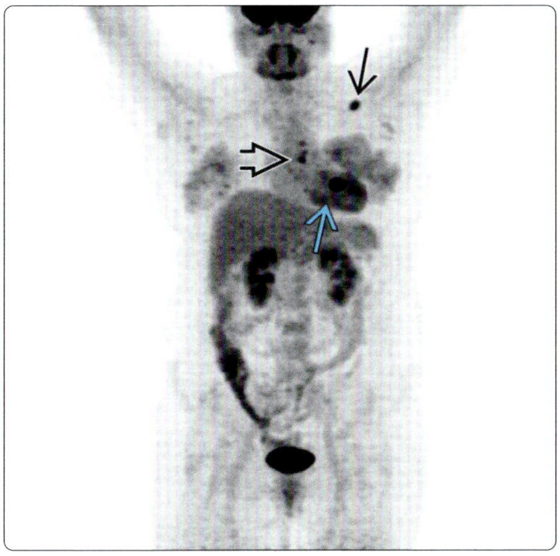

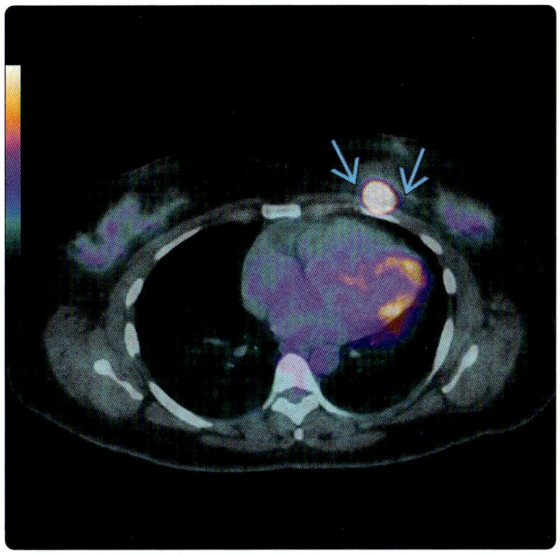

(Left) *MIP PET/CT shows an FDG-avid focus overlying the left chest , compatible with the patient's known primary breast carcinoma. Smaller hypermetabolic foci are noted within the left subpectoral and internal mammary regions.* **(Right)** *Axial fused PET/CT shows an intensely FDG-avid focus within the medial left breast , compatible with the patient's known primary breast carcinoma. Chest wall invasion is better characterized on MR.*

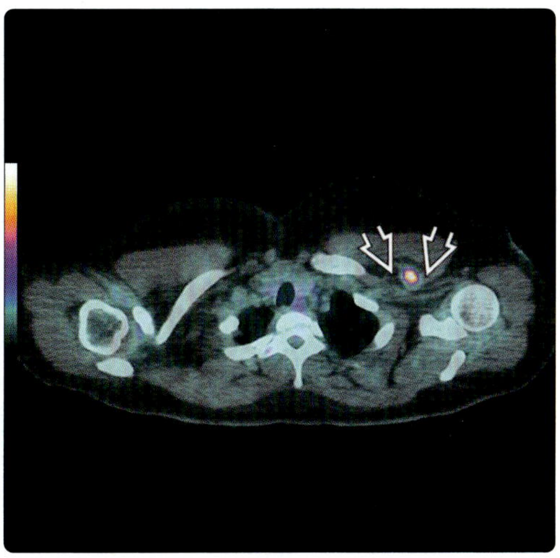

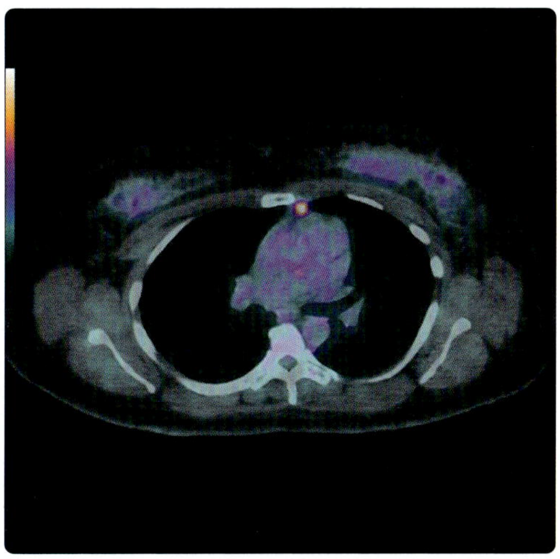

(Left) *Axial fused PET/CT shows a hypermetabolic focus within the left subpectoral region . The lymph node is not pathologically enlarged, but is significantly FDG-avid, compatible with metastatic disease.* **(Right)** *Axial fused PET/CT shows a small, hypermetabolic focus corresponding to a left internal mammary lymph node. This region is difficult to evaluate on CT and would not meet size criteria for pathological enlargement, but is suspicious for metastasis.*

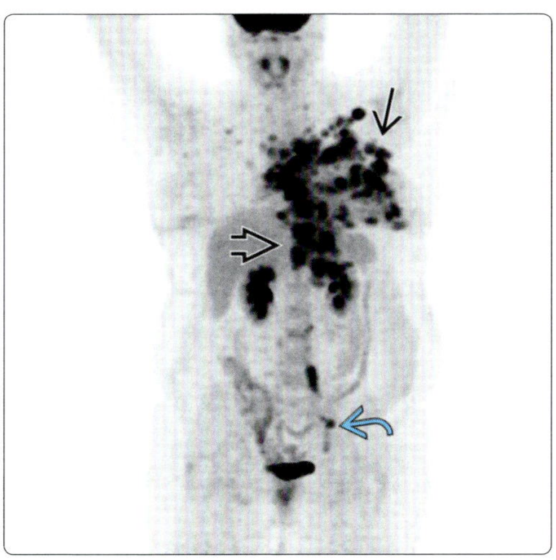

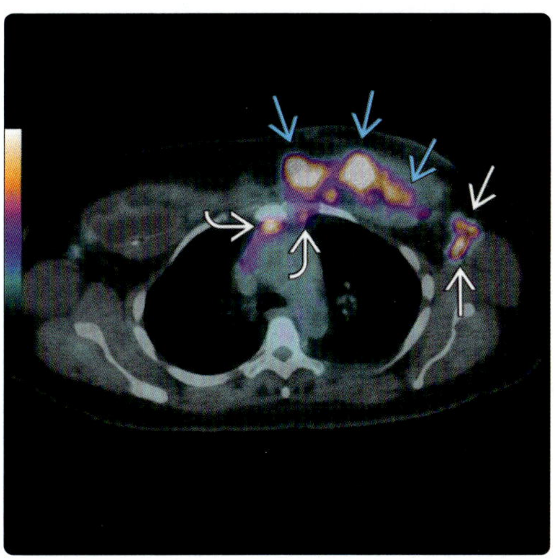

(Left) *MIP PET/CT shows extensive, locally recurrent malignancy overlying the left chest wall . Distant metastasis are shown in the retroperitoneum and left iliac nodal chain .* **(Right)** *Axial fused PET/CT shows extensive hypermetabolic left chest wall recurrence , as well as left axillary and bilateral internal mammary nodal metastases .*

KEY FACTS

IMAGING

- Contrast-enhanced MR is first-line study for diagnosis of brain metastases
- F-18 FDG PET
  - Classically hypermetabolic on F-18 FDG PET: Lung, breast, colorectal, head and neck, melanoma, thyroid
  - Classically hypometabolic on F-18 FDG PET: Mucinous adenocarcinoma, renal cell carcinoma
  - Variable uptake on F-18 FDG PET: Gliomas, lymphoma
  - Central hypometabolism suggests necrosis
- Cannot rule out small metastases due to normal brain metabolism of F-18 FDG
  - To increase sensitivity, rewindow image to make normal brain activity less intense

TOP DIFFERENTIAL DIAGNOSES

- Abscess
  - Usually hypermetabolic
  - Central hypometabolism signifies necrosis
- Cerebrovascular accident
  - Hyper- or hypometabolic
- Primary brain tumor
  - Anaplastic astrocytoma/oligodendroglioma, glioblastoma multiforme (GBM)
  - Lymphoma
- Meningioma
  - Hypometabolic
- Pituitary adenoma
  - Hypermetabolic activity near sella turcica
- Post-treatment effects
  - Hypermetabolic activity acutely (surgery, radiotherapy)
  - Hypometabolic regions correspond to treated tumor
- Epilepsy
  - Seizure activity after F-18 FDG injection can cause focal hypermetabolic activity

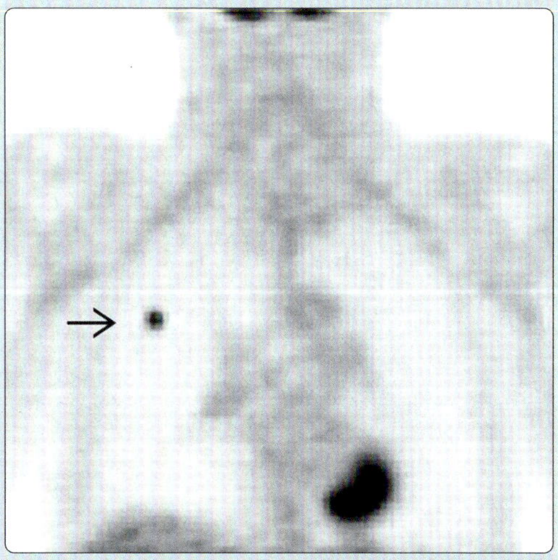

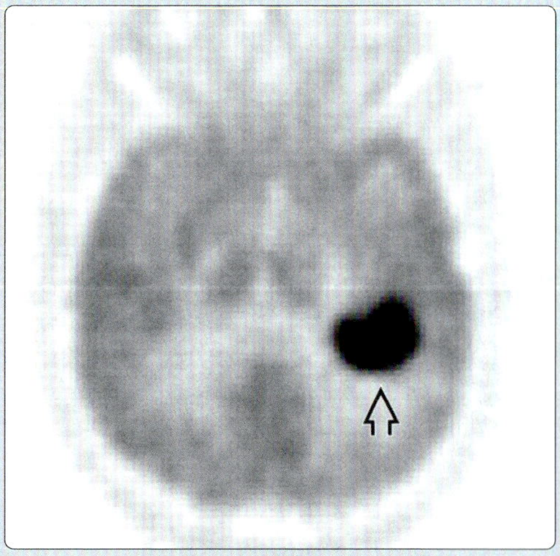

(Left) *Coronal F-18 FDG PET shows a small right lung adenocarcinoma ➡ with no lymphadenopathy.* **(Right)** *Axial F-18 FDG PET in the same patient shows a hypermetabolic brain metastasis ⇨ in the left cerebral hemisphere.*

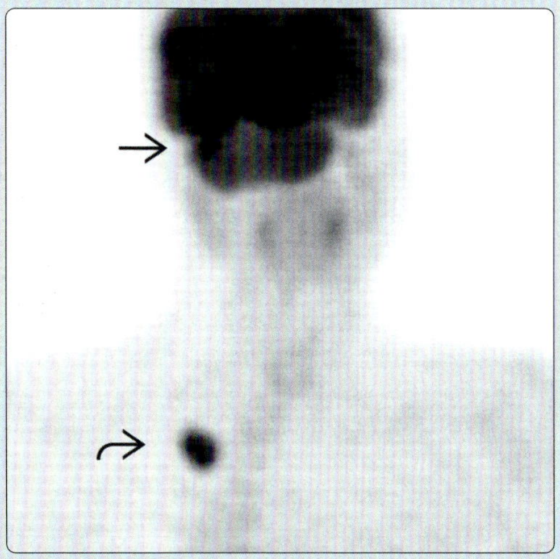

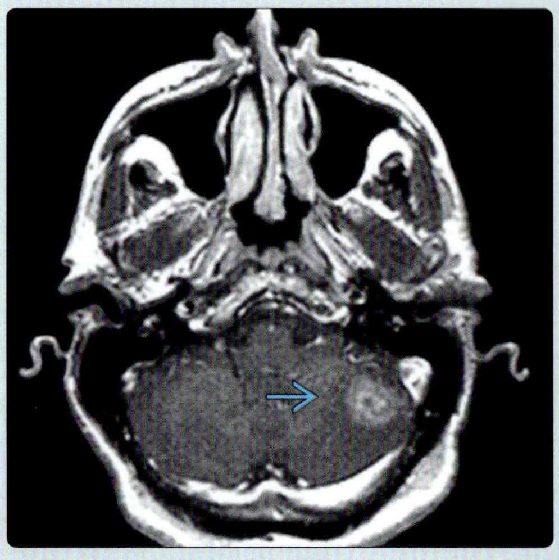

(Left) *Coronal posterior F-18 FDG PET shows a primary lung cancer ↪ in the left lung. A subtle focus of increased activity ➡ in the left cerebellum was also detected.* **(Right)** *Axial contrast-enhanced MR in the same patient shows an enhancing solitary brain metastasis ➡.*

IMAGING

Nuclear Medicine Findings

- PET
  - Although CEMR is first-line study, brain metastases are often seen incidentally on oncologic whole-body scan
  - Cannot rule out small metastases due to normal brain metabolism of F-18 FDG
  - Activity in CNS metastases depends on tumor histology
    - Classically hypermetabolic on F-18 FDG PET: Lung, breast, colorectal, head and neck, melanoma, thyroid
    - Classically hypometabolic on F-18 FDG PET: Mucinous adenocarcinoma, renal cell carcinoma
    - Variable uptake on F-18 FDG PET: Gliomas, lymphoma
    - Central hypometabolism suggests necrosis
  - Location
    - Classic
      - Cerebral hemispheres (80%)
      - Cerebellum (15%)
      - Basal ganglia (3%)
    - Less common
      - Choroid plexus, ventricular ependyma, pituitary or pineal glands, leptomeninges
    - Uncommon
      - Diffusely infiltrating tumors (carcinomatous encephalitis), perivascular or perineural spread
    - Rare
      - Brainstem

Imaging Recommendations

- Protocol advice
  - F-18 FDG PET
    - To increase sensitivity, rewindow image to make normal brain activity less intense
    - Review 3D and tomographic images

DIFFERENTIAL DIAGNOSIS

Abscess

- Usually hypermetabolic
- Central hypometabolism signifies necrosis

Cerebrovascular Accident

- Hyper- or hypometabolic

Primary Brain Tumor

- Anaplastic astrocytoma/oligodendroglioma, glioblastoma multiforme (GBM)
- Lymphoma

Meningioma

- Hypometabolic

Pituitary Adenoma

- Hypermetabolic activity near sella turcica

Post-Treatment Effects

- Hypermetabolic activity acutely (surgery, radiotherapy)
- Hypometabolic regions correspond to treated tumor

Epilepsy

- Seizure activity after F-18 FDG injection can cause focal hypermetabolic activity

CLINICAL ISSUES

Presentation

- Most common signs/symptoms
  - Neurological
    - Headache
    - Seizure
    - Confusion, obtundation
    - Ataxia
    - Nausea and vomiting
    - Vision problems
    - Papilledema
  - 10% of patients with CNS metastases are asymptomatic

Demographics

- Age
  - Incidence increases with age
    - Rare in children (skull/dura more common site than intraaxial)
    - Peak prevalence in patients over 65 years
- Gender
  - Slight male predominance
- Epidemiology
  - Number of patients with CNS metastases diagnosed annually: 100,000-500,000
  - Metastases account for ~ 50% of cerebral tumors
  - 25% of cancer patients have CNS metastases at autopsy

Natural History & Prognosis

- Overall, ~ 8% 2-year survival rate for all tumors
- Better prognosis: Single metastasis, younger age, surgical resection, whole brain radiotherapy

Treatment

- Medical management
  - Corticosteroids: Diminish effects of edema
  - Anticonvulsants: Seizure prophylaxis
  - Hyperosmolar agents: Decrease intracranial pressure
- Whole brain external beam radiotherapy
  - Prolong survival, improve neurological function
- Stereotactic radiotherapy (masses < 3 cm)
  - Prolong survival, minimally invasive, symptom palliation slower than with surgery
- Surgical resection
  - Prolong survival, symptom palliation, histopathologic tissue sample

SELECTED REFERENCES

1. Juhász C et al: Comparison of amino acid positron emission tomographic radiotracers for molecular imaging of primary and metastatic brain tumors. Mol Imaging. 13, 2014
2. Rohren EM et al: Screening for cerebral metastases with FDG PET in patients undergoing whole-body staging of non-central nervous system malignancy. Radiology. 226(1):181-7, 2003
3. Yamamoto AJ et al: Detection of cranial metastases by F-18 FDG positron emission tomography. Clin Nucl Med. 26(5):402-4, 2001

KEY FACTS

IMAGING

- Radiation necrosis
  - Radiation necrosis and recurrent brain tumor both show mass effect and contrast enhancement on CT and MR
  - High-grade tumors have more F-18 FDG uptake than low-grade tumors
  - Generally hypometabolic, F-18 FDG should not accumulate in necrotic tissue
  - Low uptake favors radiation necrosis or low-grade tumor
  - Sensitivity 75% and specificity 81% for F-18 FDG PET/CT in differentiating radiation necrosis from recurrent tumor
- Pseudoprogression
  - Subacute treatment-related effects that can mimic tumor progression
  - Early findings, 2-6 months following RT that eventually resolve
  - F-18 FDG uptake is not increased in postoperative period and is not affected by steroid therapy
- Recurrent tumor
  - Tumor cells accumulate F-18 FDG
  - High uptake favors tumor recurrence or radiation necrosis
  - High-grade primary tumors and metastases are more F-18 FDG-avid than lower grade gliomas
  - Conversion to higher grade glioma suggested by level of hypermetabolism
  - Small tumors < 6 mm may be undetectable by F-18 FDG PET/CT
- Thallium-201 or Tc-99m sestamibi SPECT
  - Radiation necrosis typically shows decreased uptake
  - Recurrent glioma typically shows increased uptake

DIAGNOSTIC CHECKLIST

- F-18 FDG PET/CT has high negative predictive value
- Lesions with no F-18 FDG uptake are likely radiation necrosis (or low-grade tumor recurrence)

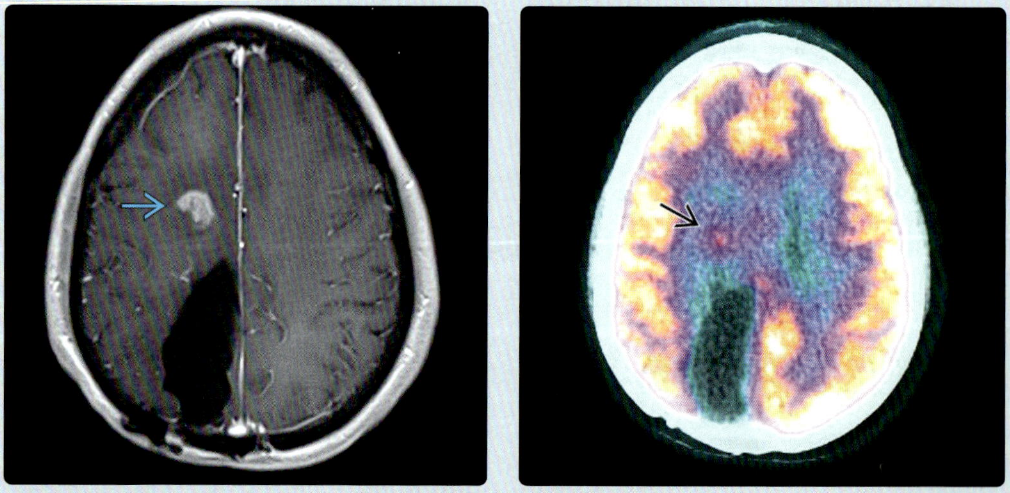

(Left) *Axial CEMR in a patient who underwent radiation therapy for glioblastoma multiforme shows focal enhancement ⇨ concerning for recurrence.* **(Right)** *Axial F-18 FDG PET/CT in the same patient shows abnormal uptake ⇨, consistent with recurrence.*

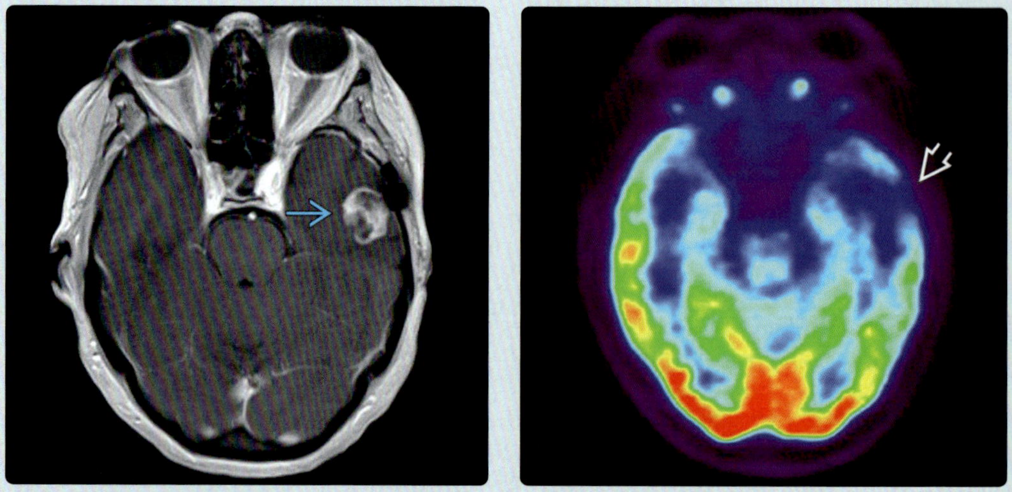

(Left) *Axial CEMR in a patient who underwent radiation therapy for glioblastoma multiforme shows region of enhancement ⇨ concerning for recurrence.* **(Right)** *Axial F-18 FDG PET shows no focal uptake in the same region ⇨, consistent with radiation necrosis.*

IMAGING

Nuclear Medicine Findings

- PET/CT
  - Radiation necrosis
    - Radiation necrosis and recurrent brain tumor both show mass effect and contrast enhancement on CT and MR
    - Generally hypometabolic, F-18 FDG should not accumulate in necrotic tissue
      - Stereotactic radiosurgery (SRS): May show inflammatory hypermetabolism, particularly around lesion perimeter, and may persist indefinitely
      - Conventionally fractionated radiation therapy (RT): Inflammatory hypermetabolism resolves by 2-3 months
    - Low uptake favors radiation necrosis or low-grade tumor
    - Sensitivity 75% and specificity 81% for F-18 FDG PET/CT in differentiating radiation necrosis from recurrent tumor
  - Pseudoprogression
    - Subacute treatment-related effects that can mimic tumor progression
    - Early findings, 2-6 months following RT that eventually resolve
    - F-18 FDG uptake is not increased in postoperative period and is not affected by steroid therapy
  - Recurrent tumor
    - Tumor cells accumulate F-18 FDG
    - High-grade tumors have more F-18 FDG uptake than low-grade tumors
    - High uptake favors tumor recurrence or radiation necrosis
    - High-grade primary tumors and metastases are more F-18 FDG avid than lower grade gliomas
      - Conversion to higher grade glioma suggested by level of hypermetabolism
    - Small tumors < 6 mm may be undetectable by F-18 FDG PET/CT
- Thallium-201 or Tc-99m sestamibi SPECT
  - Radiation necrosis typically shows decreased uptake
  - Recurrent glioma typically shows increased uptake

Imaging Recommendations

- Protocol advice
  - F-18 FDG PET/CT
    - Patient preparation
      - Patient should fast, stop IV fluids containing dextrose, stop parenteral feeding for 4-6 hours
    - Radiopharmaceutical
      - 5-10 mCi (185-370 MBq) F-18 FDG IV
    - Dosimetry
      - Brain and urinary bladder receive highest dose
    - Image acquisition
      - 2D or 3D brain images at 40-60 min

PATHOLOGY

General Features

- Epidemiology
  - Radiation necrosis in brain occurs months to years following RT for CNS or head and neck cancers; rarely follows RT for vascular lesions (e.g., AVMs)
  - Incidence of radiation necrosis in setting of CNS or head and neck radiotherapy has been estimated as 3-24%
  - Incidence of developing radiation necrosis following SRS such as gamma knife or Cyberknife estimated to be up to 68%
- Risk factors
  - Age
  - Radiation volume, radiation dose, radiation fraction size
  - Concurrent chemotherapy
  - Pretreatment cognitive dysfunction
  - Increasing survival time following RT

Microscopic Features

- Vascular effects
  - Capillary collapse with wall thickening and hyalinization of vessels leading to coagulation and liquefactive necrosis in white matter
- Local inflammatory microenvironment
  - Inflammation from direct radiation injury as well as reperfusion and other vascular injuries create chronic inflammatory environment that may contribute to necrosis
- Neural stem cells (NSC)
  - Modest doses of radiation have been shown to inhibit hippocampal NSC neurogenesis, resulting in decline in short-term memory and other cognitive effects

DIAGNOSTIC CHECKLIST

Consider

- PET imaging using new tracers is promising for the detection of malignant tumors in brain
  - Background cortical activity of brain (gray matter > white matter) results in diffuse F-18 FDG uptake
  - F-DOPA (dopamine) and C-MET (methionine) are 2 promising amino acid analogs

Image Interpretation Pearls

- F-18 FDG PET/CT, MR, Tl-201 or Tc-99m sestamibi SPECT are all options for recurrent tumor from radiation necrosis
- F-18 FDG PET/CT has high negative predictive value
  - Lesions with no F-18 FDG uptake are likely radiation necrosis (or low-grade tumor recurrence)
  - Any area with more uptake than adjacent gray/white matter is positive for tumor recurrence or radiation necrosis
- Sensitivity and specificity improved with F-18 FDG PET/CT plus MR

SELECTED REFERENCES

1. Miyatake S et al: Pathophysiology, diagnosis, and treatment of radiation necrosis in the brain. Neurol Med Chir (Tokyo). 55(1):50-9, 2015
2. Chao ST et al: The sensitivity and specificity of FDG PET in distinguishing recurrent brain tumor from radionecrosis in patients treated with stereotactic radiosurgery. Int J Cancer. 96(3):191-7, 2001

KEY FACTS

IMAGING

- Tc-99m sulfur colloid sentinel lymph node mapping
  - Recommended if thickness > 0.76 mm
  - Presence of tumor in lymph nodes is key prognostic indicator
    - 5% of patients with Breslow thickness 0.76-1.5 mm have positive SLN
    - 20% of patients with Breslow thickness 1.5-4 mm have metastasis in sentinel nodes
  - Success rate of 99% when blue dye and 2nd tracer (lymphoscintigraphy) added
  - If sentinel lymph node(s) positive, patients eligible for lymphadenectomy
- F-18 FDG PET/CT
  - Incidence of multiple primary melanomas: 1.3-8%
  - Valuable tool to detect distant metastases
  - Alters patient management in 33% of cases
- MR most sensitive modality for brain metastases, although incidental brain metastases found on F-18 FDG PET/CT if large enough

PATHOLOGY

- Staging
  - I/II: Low-risk primary melanomas (T1a-T2a) and higher risk melanomas (T2b-T4b)
  - III: Any T, N1/N2/N3, M0
  - IV: Any T, any N, any M1

DIAGNOSTIC CHECKLIST

- Most common sites of metastasis
  - Skin, subcutaneous tissue, and lymph nodes: 50-75%
  - Lungs: 70-87%
  - Liver: 54-77%
  - Brain: 36-54%
  - Bone: 23-49%
  - GI tract: 26-58%

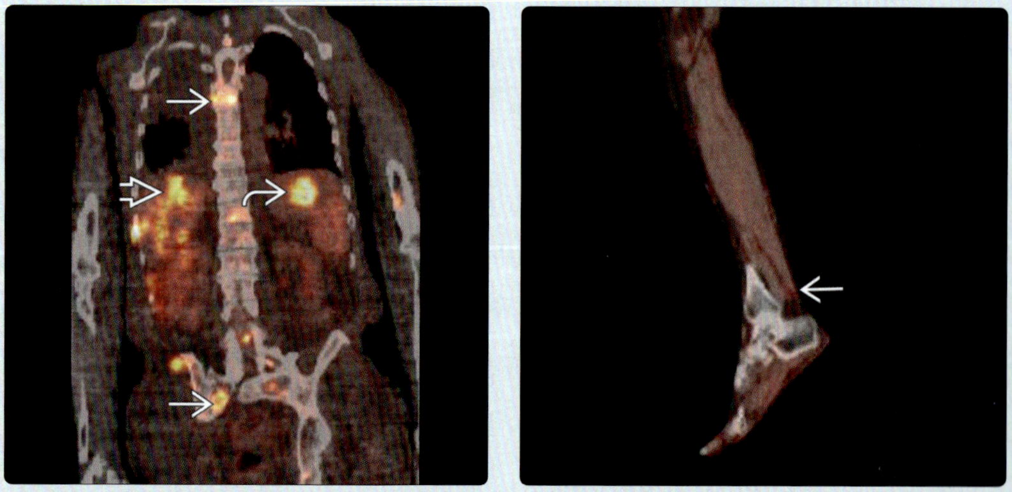

(Left) *Coronal F-18 FDG PET/CT in a 65-year-old man shows widespread osseous metastasis to axial and proximal appendicular skeleton ➡ and metastases to liver ➡ and spleen ↪.* **(Right)** *Sagittal F-18 FDG PET/CT in an 84-year-old woman shows hypermetabolic focus ➡ in left Kager's fat pad, consistent with metastatic melanoma.*

(Left) *Posterior Tc-99m filtered sulfur colloid lymphoscintigraphy shows activity around the primary lesion ➡ and a single lymphatic drainage channel ➡.* **(Right)** *Anterior Tc-99m filtered sulfur colloid lymphoscintigraphy in the same patient shows a sentinel lymph node ➡ in the left groin.*

TERMINOLOGY

Definitions

- Melanoma: Neoplasm of melanin-producing cells

IMAGING

Imaging Recommendations

- Best imaging tool
  - Tc-99m filtered sulfur colloid sentinel lymph node (SLN) mapping
    - Standard of care for intermediate-thickness (≥ 0.76 mm) melanomas without palpable lymph nodes
      - Clinically significant cutoff originally described by Breslow
      - Lymphadenectomy usually performed at time of wide local excision
      - Prognostic, staging, treatment implications if SLN positive on biopsy
    - 5% of patients with Breslow thickness 0.76-1.5 mm have positive SLN
    - 20% of patients with Breslow thickness 1.5-4 mm have SLN metastasis
  - F-18 FDG PET/CT
    - Detects occult metastatic disease in stage III and IV disease
      - 83% sensitivity and 85% specificity
      - Alters patient management in 33% of cases
    - Hypermetabolic lymphadenopathy and extranodal metastases
      - Almost any organ and unusual sites (e.g., breast)
      - Spine, lung, liver, spleen, bowel common
  - MR most sensitive modality for brain metastases, although incidental brain metastases found on F-18 FDG PET/CT if large enough
- Protocol advice
  - **Tc-99m filtered sulfur colloid SLN mapping**
    - Patient preparation
      - Patient positioned for optimal injection around primary melanoma
      - ± topical anesthetic, depending on sensitivity of area to be injected (e.g., nose)
      - Time-out procedure recommended with melanoma/biopsy site circled so correct site confirmed for surgeon
    - Radiopharmaceutical
      - 1 mCi (37 MBq) Tc-99m filtered SC in ~ 0.5 cc normal saline total
      - Inject intradermally in 4 quadrants around tumor
      - Inject 0.5-1 cm away from tumor margin/scar
      - Intradermal injection under significant pressure, risk of backsplash/spray onto personnel, equipment
      - Intradermal injection in patients with thin skin (e.g., elderly) can be difficult
      - Filtered with 0.22 millipore filter
    - Dosimetry
      - 15-18 hr after injection 0.34-0.92% of radioactivity of injected dose in sentinel node
    - Image acquisition
      - Image all possible lymph node basins to determine sentinel lymph node location
      - Some areas (head and neck; trunk) may have aberrant drainage
      - Dynamic acquisition (20 sec/frame) immediately after injection may be useful to track drainage to lymphatic basin
      - Static images of all possible lymph node basins (consider anterior/posteriors, laterals, obliques for best lymph node localization)
      - Primary melanoma may be in watershed area of lymphatic drainage to 2 lymphatic basins
      - Lateral images important to evaluate for possible in-transit nodes
      - Evaluate bilateral axillae and groin for any truncal melanoma, as unexpected drainage patterns occur
      - Head and neck melanomas can also have aberrant drainage patterns, so image all potential lymph node basins
      - Transmission source useful to outline body
      - Transmission sources can obscure superficial lymphadenopathy
      - Consider imaging with and without transmission sources when surveying lymphatic basins, particularly with head and neck melanoma
      - Cover injection site with lead if necessary to evaluate lymph node basins close to injection site
      - If possible, keep injection site just out of field of view of gamma camera
    - Marking sentinel lymph node for surgery
      - Real-time images obtained on p-scope
      - Use small amount of Tc-99m pertechnetate on Q-tip, enclosed in test tube to localize
      - Keep test tube parallel to gamma detector until lymph node localized, then move test tube toward patient in same plane
      - Confirm lymph node location in 2 planes if possible
      - Once localized, mark location with permanent marker for surgeons
    - Image processing
      - Obtain key images to aid surgeon in localization, either on hard copy with patient to surgery or on image archiving system in electronic medical record
  - **F18 FDG PET/CT**
    - Incidence of multiple primary melanomas: 1.3-8%
      - Consider extending scan to include entire body (top of skull to feet)
    - Use oncologic protocol
    - Evaluate patients for possible confounding factors: Acute infection, recent surgery, radiotherapy, chemotherapy
  - **Tc-99m MDP bone scan**
    - If clinical suspicion of bone metastases

DIFFERENTIAL DIAGNOSIS

Squamous Cell Carcinoma

- Malignant proliferation of epidermal keratinocytes
- Primary: Ulcer or reddish plaque
- 2-5% of cutaneous squamous cell carcinomas metastasize
  - F-18 FDG PET/CT sometimes used if metastases suspected

Basal Cell Carcinoma

- Locally invasive carcinoma arising from basal layer of epidermis
- Primary: Shiny, pearly nodule or red patch
- Rarely metastasizes

Merkel Cell Carcinoma

- Malignant proliferation of highly anaplastic cells, similar to neuroectodermally derived cells
  - Merkel cells: Specialized touch receptor cells of skin
  - Highly aggressive malignancy
    - 5-year survival: 50% with stage II disease, 18% with stage IV disease
- Primary: Flesh-colored, red or blue firm, painless nodule
- Tc-99m sulfur colloid sentinel lymph node mapping/biopsy and F-18 FDG PET/CT often used for staging these patients as well
  - Stage I/II: Primary lesion ≤ 2 cm or > 2 cm
  - Stage III: Regional lymph node metastases
  - Stage IV: Distant metastases

PATHOLOGY

Staging, Grading, & Classification

- TNM classification
  - Primary tumor (T)
    - T1 (thickness ≤ 1 mm); T4 (thickness > 4 mm)
    - "a" or "b" depending on ulceration and mitotic rate
  - Regional lymph node (N)
    - N0: None
    - N1: 1 node
    - N2: 2-3 nodes
    - N3: 4 or more nodes
  - Distant metastases
    - M0: No distant metastases
    - M1a: Distant skin, subcutaneous, or nodal metastases
    - M1b: Lung metastases
    - M1c: All other visceral metastases
- Staging
  - I/II: Low-risk primary melanomas (T1a-T2a) and higher risk melanomas (T2b-T4b)
  - III: Any T, N1/N2/N3, M0
  - IV: Any T, any N, any M1

Microscopic Features

- Asymmetric, poorly circumscribed nests of melanocytes
- Breslow depth
  - Millimeters from top of granular cell layer of epidermis to deepest point of penetration
- Also noted: Ulceration and mitoses/mm²

CLINICAL ISSUES

Presentation

- Most common signs/symptoms
  - Primary melanoma: Asymmetric, irregular border, color variation, diameter ≥ 5 mm, changes over time
  - Lymphadenopathy

Demographics

- Epidemiology
  - 62,480 new cases and 8,420 deaths each year
  - Occurs almost exclusively in Caucasian populations
  - Genetic risk factors: Family history, light skin, red hair, DNA repair defects (e.g., xeroderma pigmentosum)
  - Environmental risk factors: Sun exposure, tanning bed use, immunosuppression
  - Gene/environment interaction risk factors: > 100 acquired melanocytic nevi; > 5 atypical melanocytic nevi; multiple solar lentigines; personal history of cutaneous melanoma

Natural History & Prognosis

- Breslow depth = most important prognostic factor
- 5-year survival
  - Stage III: 40-78%
  - Stage IV: 9-27%

Treatment

- Surgical treatment of primary cutaneous melanoma according to thickness
  - Excision margins 0.5-2 cm
- Sentinel lymph node biopsy for tumors ≥ 0.76 mm in thickness
  - Complete lymphadenectomy if sentinel lymph node biopsy positive
- Adjuvant therapy
  - Current recommendation: Refer patients to appropriate ongoing clinical trial of adjuvant therapy

DIAGNOSTIC CHECKLIST

Consider

- Both primary lesion and post-biopsy site can be positive on PET
- Attenuation correction can smooth peripheral data: Evaluate non-attenuation corrected PET images to survey skin
- Most common sites of metastasis
  - Skin, subcutaneous tissue, and lymph nodes: 50-75%
  - Lungs: 70-87%
  - Liver: 54-77%
  - Brain: 36-54%
  - Bone: 23-49%
  - GI tract: 26-58%

SELECTED REFERENCES

1. Kauffmann RM et al: Workup and Staging of Malignant Melanoma. Surg Clin North Am. 94(5):963-972, 2014
2. Rodriguez Rivera AM et al: Value of positron emission tomography scan in stage III cutaneous melanoma: a systematic review and meta-analysis. Surg Oncol. 23(1):11-6, 2014
3. Danielsen M et al: Positron emission tomography in the follow-up of cutaneous malignant melanoma patients: a systematic review. Am J Nucl Med Mol Imaging. 4(1):17-28, 2013
4. Han D et al: Sentinel node biopsy is indicated for thin melanomas ≥0.76 mm. Ann Surg Oncol. 19(11):3335-42, 2012

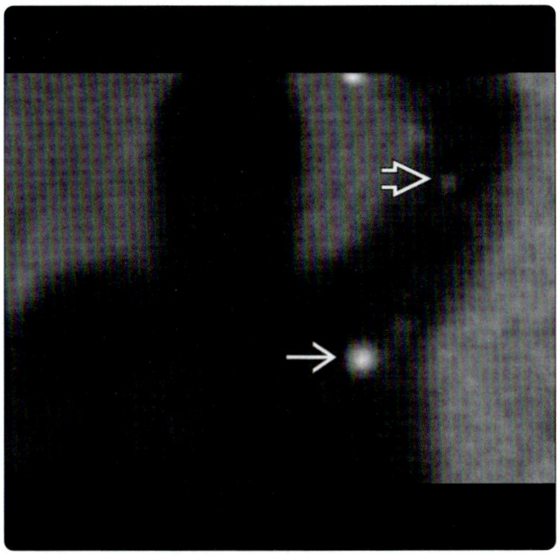

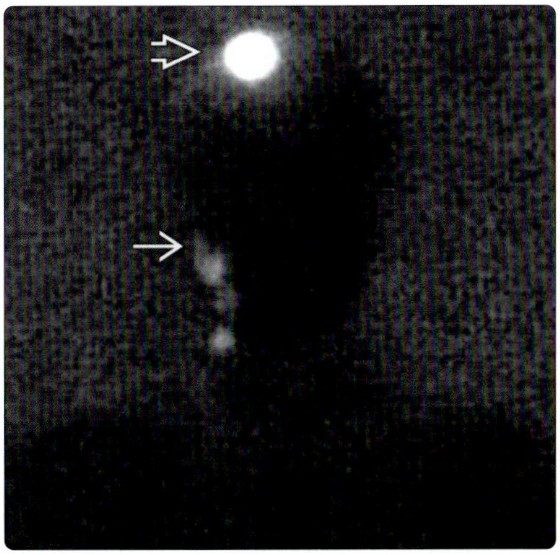

(Left) *Anterior Tc-99m filtered sulfur colloid lymphoscintigraphy in a patient with left forearm melanoma shows sentinel lymph node in the left axilla* ➡*. Note that lymphatic channels* ➡ *as well as in-transit lymph nodes can also be evident on lymphoscintigraphy.* **(Right)** *Anterior Tc-99m filtered sulfur colloid lymphoscintigraphy in a patient with a right scalp melanoma* ➡ *shows lymphatic drainage to the posterior auricular region* ➡.

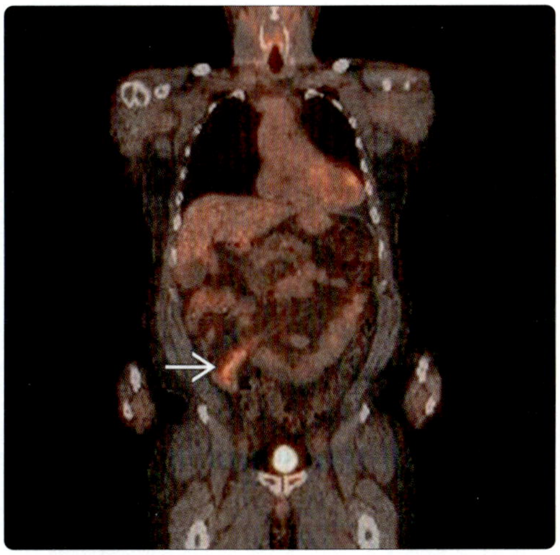

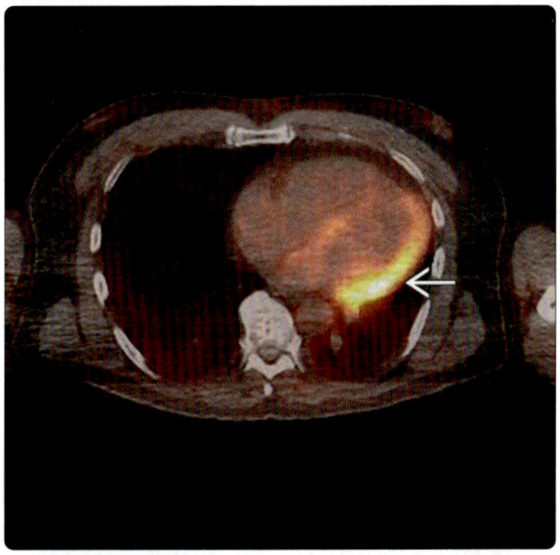

(Left) *Coronal F-18 FDG PET/CT in a 61-year-old patient with history of melanoma shows metastasis to proximal small bowel* ➡. **(Right)** *Axial F-18 FDG PET/CT in the same patient shows increased uptake in a pericardial metastasis* ➡.

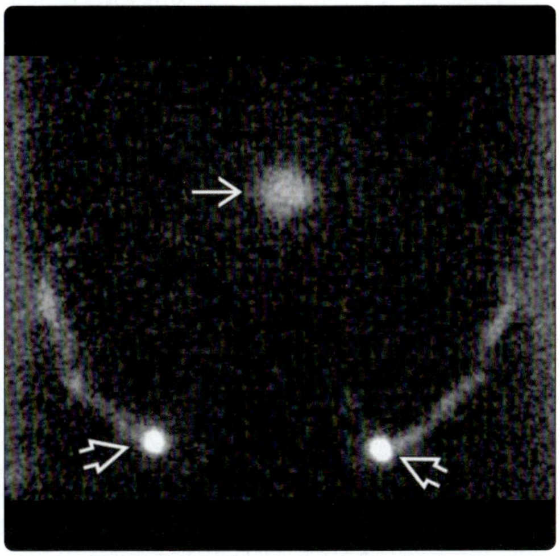

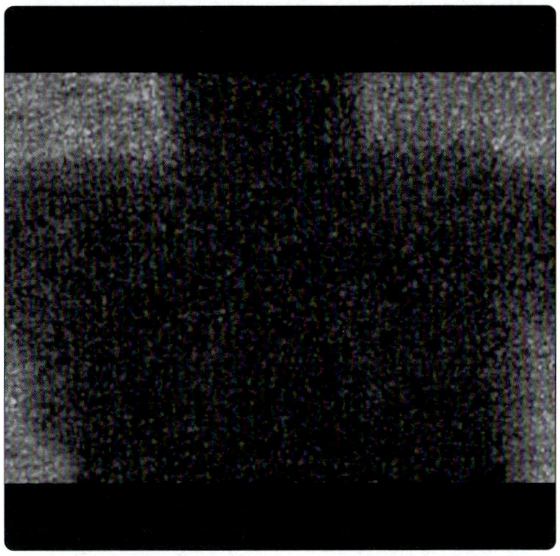

(Left) *Anterior Tc-99m filtered sulfur colloid lymphoscintigraphy in a patient with a melanoma on the central back* ➡ *shows sentinel lymph nodes in both inguinal regions* ➡. **(Right)** *Anterior Tc-99m filtered sulfur colloid lymphoscintigraphy in the same patient shows no axillary sentinel lymph nodes. Note that truncal and head & neck skin cancers can show unexpected drainage patterns.*

Esophageal Cancer

KEY FACTS

TERMINOLOGY

- Squamous cell carcinoma
  - Malignant transformation of squamous epithelium
- Adenocarcinoma
  - Arises from columnar epithelium (Barrett mucosa)

IMAGING

- **F-18 FDG PET/CT**
- Indicated for initial staging
  - High sensitivity for detection of distant metastases
  - Evaluation of response to preoperative chemoradiation therapy
  - Changes clinical management in 38.2% of cases, improving selection of patients for radical surgery
  - F-18 FDG PET/CT does not allow reliable differentiation between N0 and N1 disease: Intense uptake by primary lesion can mask adjacent lymphadenopathy
  - F-18 FDG PET/CT more accurate than CECT for detection of stage IV disease
- Indicated to evaluate response to therapy
  - After neoadjuvant therapy, prior to surgery
  - Should be done 5-6 weeks after completion of therapy
- Indicated to detect recurrence
  - High sensitivity for detection of local recurrent tumor or regional nodal disease

TOP DIFFERENTIAL DIAGNOSES

- Esophagitis
  - Inflammatory: Gastroesophageal reflux, caustic substances, radiation
  - Infectious (e.g., *Candida*, herpes simplex virus)
- Intramural primary esophageal tumor
  - Leiomyoma or fibrovascular polyp or sarcomas (rare)
- Metastatic or adjacent tumor
  - Lung cancer ± lymphadenopathy, lymphoma, melanoma

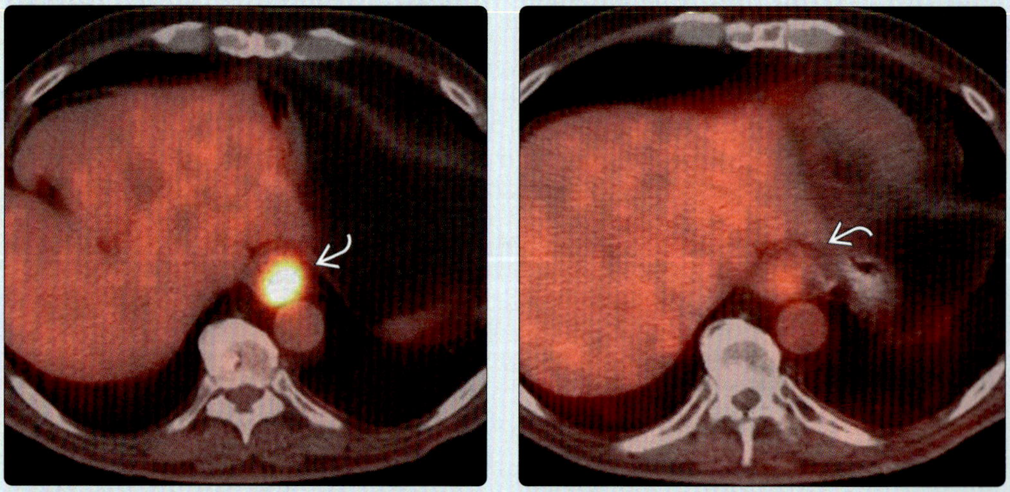

(Left) *Axial fused F-18 FDG PET/CT shows increased uptake in the distal esophagus consistent with biopsy-proven adenocarcinoma invading the adventitia (T3).* **(Right)** *Axial fused F-18 FDG PET/CT after preoperative chemoradiation therapy shows complete metabolic response.*

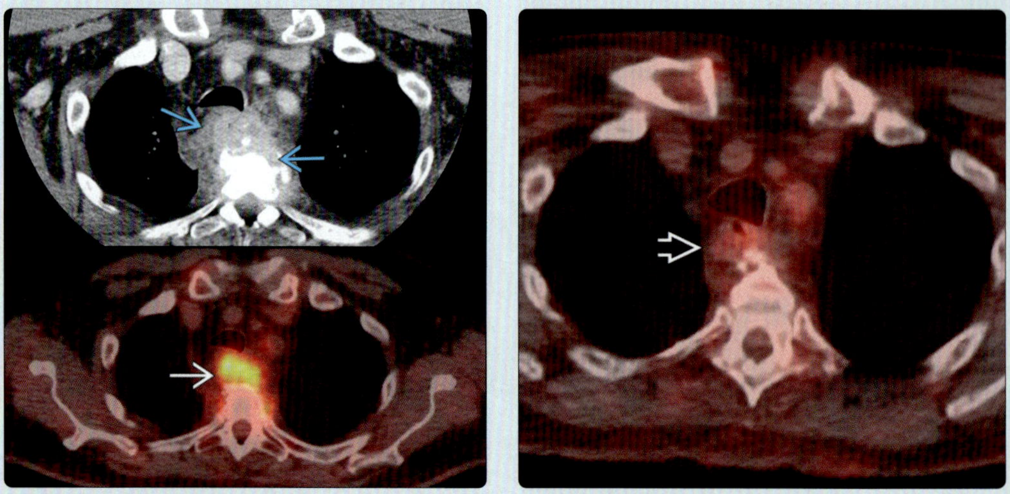

(Left) *Axial CECT after esophagectomy for squamous cell carcinoma (T2 N0) shows enhancing soft tissue mass at the anastomosis with extension and erosion of the T2 vertebral body. Axial fused F-18 FDG PET/CT shows marked increased uptake within the soft tissue mass concerning for recurrence versus infection.* **(Right)** *Axial fused F-18 FDG PET/CT in the same patient after antibiotic treatment shows resolution of what was found to be an infectious process.*

TERMINOLOGY

Definitions

- Squamous cell carcinoma
  - Malignant transformation of squamous epithelium
- Adenocarcinoma
  - Arises from columnar epithelium (Barrett mucosa)
  - Siewert tumor type should be assessed in all patient with adenocarcinoma involving the esophagogastric junction (EGJ)
    - Siewert type I: Lower esophagus, center 1-5 cm above EGJ
    - Siewert type II: Cardiac, center 1 cm above and 2 cm below EGJ
    - Siewert III: Subcardial, center 2-5 cm below EGJ; considered gastric cancer

IMAGING

Nuclear Medicine Findings

- PET
  - Local disease
    - Primary tumors: Upper 1/3 of esophagus (15%), middle 1/3 (50%), lower 1/3 (35%)
    - Adenocarcinoma and squamous cell carcinoma are F-18 FDG avid
      - F-18 FDG uptake in squamous cell carcinoma > adenocarcinoma
  - Regional nodal disease
    - Less sensitive than CECT and endoscopy ultrasound (EUS) for detection of locoregional metastatic lymph nodes
    - Does not allow reliable differentiation between N0 and N1 disease, due to intense uptake by primary lesion masking adjacent metastatic nodes
    - Regional nodes are considered to be cervical to celiac stations
    - T1-T3 ± N+ are resectable
  - Distant metastatic disease
    - More accurate than CECT for detection of stage IV disease
    - Liver, lungs, pleura, adrenal glands, kidneys, or soft tissue
  - Post neoadjuvant therapy
    - Should be done 5-6 weeks after completion of therapy
    - Useful for evaluating response to therapy
    - Complete response: Decrease in uptake > 35-45% between initial staging F-18 FDG PET/CT and post treatment
      - Patients with complete pathologic response have higher recurrence-free survival
  - Recurrence
    - High sensitivity for detection of local recurrent tumor or regional nodal disease but low specificity
    - False-positive
      - Uptake can be seen with endoscopic dilatation for stricture at anastomosis
      - Leaking/abscess formation at site of anastomosis
      - Postradiation changes
      - Postsurgical changes

Imaging Recommendations

- EUS for most accurate T and N staging
  - More accurate than CT for T (85% vs. 45%) and N (77% vs. 54%) staging
  - HER2-neu testing is recommended for metastatic adenocarcinoma
  - Possible FNA of suspicious local lymph nodes
- CECT
  - Useful for detecting locoregional metastatic nodes or staging

DIFFERENTIAL DIAGNOSIS

Esophagitis

- Focal or diffuse F-18 FDG uptake
- Inflammatory
  - Reflux esophagitis (gastroesophageal reflux disease [GERD], hiatal hernia)
  - Caustic esophagitis
  - Radiation esophagitis
- Infectious esophagitis
  - Fungal (candidiasis), viral (herpes, CMV, HIV)

Intramural Primary Esophageal Tumor

- Variable F-18 FDG uptake
- Leiomyoma or fibrovascular polyp or sarcomas (rare)

Metastatic or Adjacent Tumor

- Focal F-18 FDG uptake
- Extrinsic compression
  - Mediastinal lymphadenopathy, adjacent lung cancer, lymphoma
- Intrinsic metastasis: Melanoma

PATHOLOGY

General Features

- Etiology
  - Squamous cell carcinoma
    - Smoking, alcohol, achalasia, lye strictures
    - Celiac disease
    - Plummer-Vinson syndrome, celiac sprue, radiation
    - Prior neck or chest radiation
    - Human papillomavirus
  - Adenocarcinoma
    - Barrett esophagus
      - Risk factors: GERD, reflux esophagitis, motility disorders
- Genetics
  - Squamous cell carcinoma
    - Tylosis (nonepidermolytic palmoplantar keratosis)
    - Bloom syndrome: Early cancer (> 20 year of age)
    - Fanconi anemia
  - Adenocarcinoma
    - Familial Barrett esophagus

Staging, Grading, & Classification

- **Squamous cell carcinoma**
  - Stage 0-T1a: Tis-T1 (tumor invades lamina propia, muscularis mocosae or submucosa), grade 1 (well differentiated)

- Stage Ib: T1, grade 2-3 (moderately or poorly differentiated) or T2 (tumor invades muscularis), T3 (tumor invades adventitia), grade 1
- Stage IIA: T2-T3, grade 1-3
- Stage IIB: T2-T3, grade 2-3 or T1-T2 N1 (metastasis in 1-2 regional lymph nodes)
- Stage IIIA: T1-T2 N2 (metastasis in 3-6 regional lymph nodes) or T3 N1 or T4a (tumor invades adjacent structures but resectable)
- Stage IIIB: T3 N2
- Stage IIIC: T4a N1-2 or T4b (tumor invades adjacent structures, unresectable) or N3 (metastasis in ≥ 7 regional lymph nodes)
- Stage IV: M1 (distant metastasis)

- **Adenocarcinoma**
  - Stage 0: Tis (high-grade dysplasia), grade 1 (well differentiated)
  - Stage IA: T1 (tumor invades lamina propia, muscularis mocosae or submucosa), grade 1-2 (moderately differentiated)
  - Stage IB: T1, grade 3 (poorly differentiated) or T2 (tumor invades muscularis), grade 1-2
  - Stage IIA: T2, grade 3
  - Stage IIB: T3 (tumor invades adventitia) or T1-T2 N1 (metastasis in 1-2 regional lymph nodes)
  - Stage IIIA: T1-T2 N2 (metastasis in 3-6 regional lymph nodes) or T3 N1 or T4a (tumor invades adjacent structures but resectable)
  - Stage IIIC: T4a N1-N2 or T4b (tumor invades adjacent structures, unresectable) or N3 (metastasis in ≥ 7 regional lymph nodes)
  - Stage IV: M1 (distant metastasis)

CLINICAL ISSUES

Demographics

- Age
  - Squamous cell carcinoma and adenocarcinoma
    - > 50 years of age
- Gender
  - Squamous cell carcinoma
    - M:F = 4:1
  - Adenocarcinoma
    - M:F = 5.5:1
- Ethnicity
  - Squamous cell carcinoma
    - USA: African Americans > Caucasians (2:1)
  - Adenocarcinoma
    - USA: Caucasians > African Americans (3:1)
- Epidemiology
  - Squamous cell carcinoma
    - Central Asian belt (regions around Caspian Sea), Iran, China and India, Mediterranean countries and South Africa
  - Adenocarcinoma
    - Incidence increasing dramatically in developed countries (4-10% annually)

Natural History & Prognosis

- 5 year survival (by American Joint Committee on Cancer)
  - Localized cancer (T1-T3 N0 M0): 40%
  - Regional tumor (T4 or N1): 21%
  - Distant tumor (M1): 4%

Treatment

- Curative
  - Endoscopic resection ± ablation
    - Squamous cell carcinoma: Tis-T1a, tumors < 2 cm and well- or moderately differentiated carcinomas
    - Adenocarcinoma: Tis-T1b superficial, N0, tumors < 2 cm and well- or moderately differentiated carcinomas or high-grade dysplasia Barret esophagus
  - Esophagectomy
    - Squamous cell carcinoma ≥ T1b
    - Adenocarcinoma ≥ T1b nonsuperficial or N+
- Chemoradiation
  - Preoperative (preferred)
    - For all tumors > T2 or N+
  - Post-operative
    - With micro- or macroscopic disease present in pathology report post esophagectomy
  - Palliative
    - HER2-neu target chemotherapy for metastatic adenocarcinoma improves survival

DIAGNOSTIC CHECKLIST

Consider

- F-18 FDG PET/CT
  - Indicated for initial staging and to identify surgical candidates
  - Higher sensitivity for detection of distant metastases
  - Evaluation of response to preoperative chemoradiation therapy
  - Changes clinical management in 38.2% of cases, improving selection of patient for radical surgery
  - High sensitivity for detection of recurrence

SELECTED REFERENCES

1. Ajani JA et al: Esophageal and esophagogastric junction cancers, version 1.2015. J Natl Compr Canc Netw. 13(2):194-227, 2015
2. Calais J et al: High FDG uptake areas on pre-radiotherapy PET/CT identify preferential sites of local relapse after chemoradiotherapy for locally advanced oesophageal cancer. Eur J Nucl Med Mol Imaging. 42(6):858-67, 2015
3. Goense L et al: Diagnostic performance of 18F-FDG and PET/CT for the detection of recurrent esophageal cancer after treatment with curative intent: a systematic review and meta-analysis. J Nucl Med. ePub, 2015
4. Kukar M et al: Role of Repeat 18F-Fluorodeoxyglucose Positron Emission Tomography Examination In Predicting Pathologic Response Following Neoadjuvant Chemoradiotherapy for Esophageal Adenocarcinoma. JAMA Surg. ePub, 2015

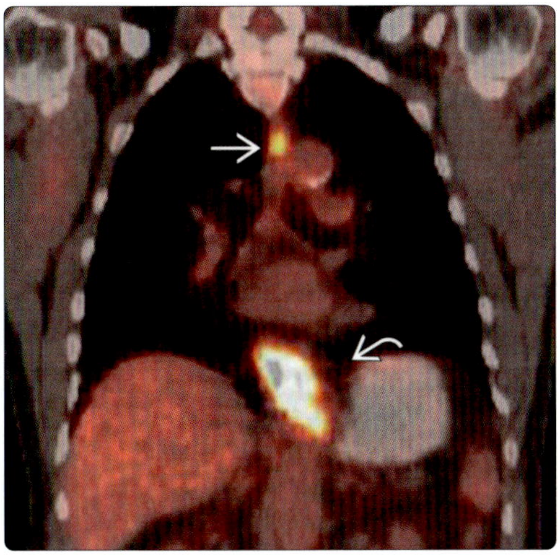

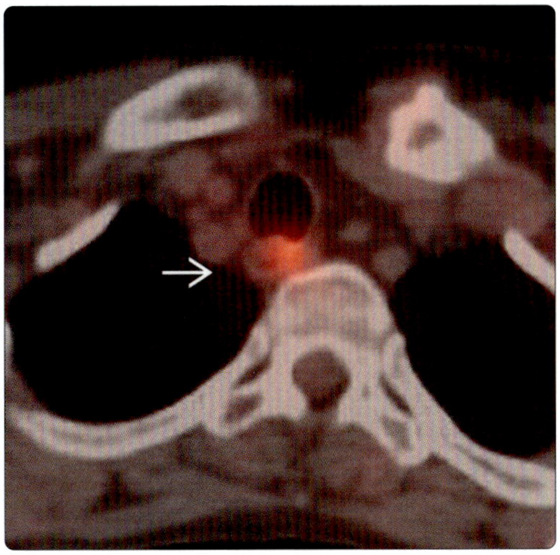

(Left) *Axial fused F-18 FDG PET/CT shows synchronous esophageal cancer with focal uptake in the upper 1/3 and lower 1/3 involving the esophagogastric junction.* **(Right)** *Axial fused F-18 FDG PET/CT demonstrates subtle focal uptake in the upper esophagus in a patient with squamous cell carcinoma.*

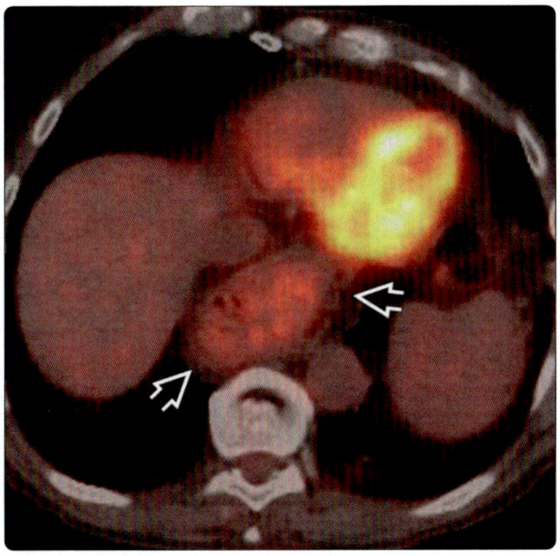

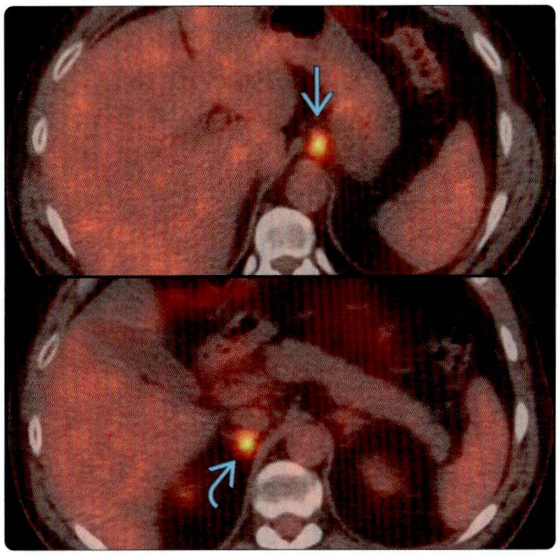

(Left) *Axial fused F-18 FDG PET/CT shows a sliding hiatal hernia in the lower mediastinum with subtle increased uptake due to gastroesophageal reflux.* **(Right)** *Axial fused F-18 FDG PET/CT in a patient with squamous cell carcinoma shows a hypermetabolic left gastric node and a metastasis in the right adrenal gland.*

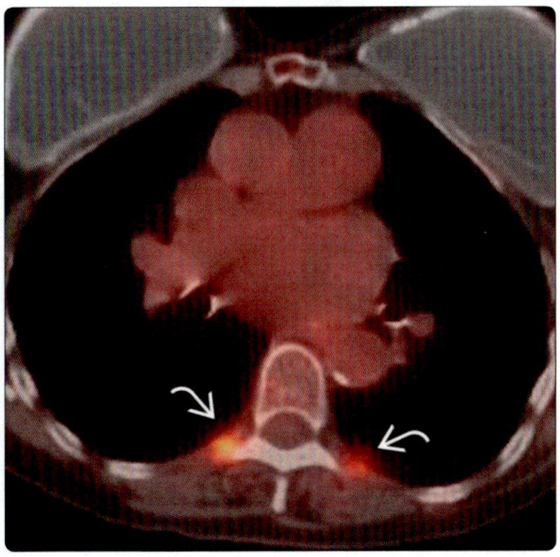

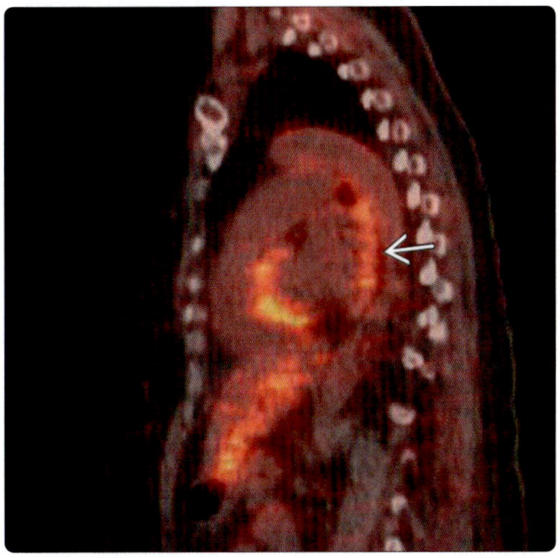

(Left) *Axial fused F-18 FDG PET/CT shows bilateral symmetric uptake at the costovertebral junctions consistent with brown fat, a common pitfall in F-18 FDG PET/CT imaging.* **(Right)** *Sagittal fused F-18 FDG PET/CT shows moderate diffuse uptake in the esophagus consistent with gastroesophageal reflux esophagitis.*

Gastric Cancer and Gastrointestinal Stromal Tumor

KEY FACTS

TERMINOLOGY

- Gastric carcinoma
  - Arises from gastric epithelial lining
- Gastrointestinal tumor (GIST)
  - Nonepithelial neoplasm, arises from interstitial cells of Cajal
  - Malignancy is based on tumor size, mitotic index rate, and presence of metastasis

IMAGING

- Evaluate extent of local disease with endoscopic ultrasound (EUS)
- Staging and resectability: CECT and F-18 FDG PET/CT
- Recurrence and response to therapy: F-18 FDG PET/CT &/or CECT

TOP DIFFERENTIAL DIAGNOSES

- Physiologic F-18 FDG activity in stomach
  - Usually low-level activity
  - Diffuse throughout stomach, nonfocal
- Gastric ulcer/gastritis
  - Usually mild to moderate F-18 FDG activity
- Gastric lymphoma
  - F-18 FDG activity variable, often hypermetabolic
  - Gastric wall thickening, may be diffuse
  - Abdominal lymphadenopathy may be present
- Crohn disease
  - Rarely affects stomach
  - Increased F-18 FDG activity in active disease

DIAGNOSTIC CHECKLIST

- F-18 FDG PET/CT for gastric carcinoma and GIST
  - For most complete preoperative staging
  - Evaluate response to therapy
  - Identify recurrence

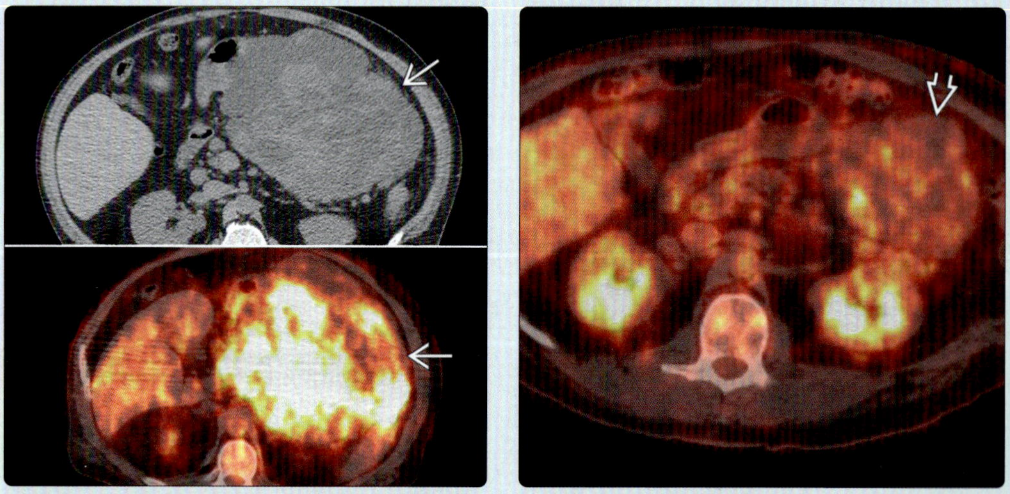

(Left) *Axial CT and fused F-18 FDG PET/CT show a hypermetabolic, 10 cm, partially necrotic mass ➔ arising from the stomach consistent with a GIST.* **(Right)** *Axial F-18 FDG PET/CT in the same patient after imatinib neoadjuvant therapy shows response to therapy, evidenced by marked reduction in size & metabolic activity of the mass ➔.*

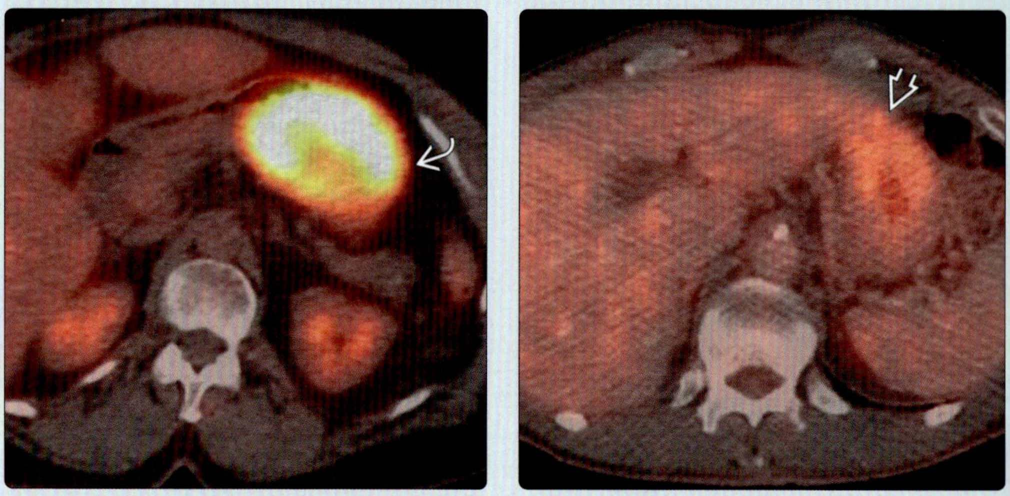

(Left) *Axial fused F-18 FDG PET/CT shows a large, hypermetabolic gastric mass ➔ that turned out to be a 10 cm adenomatous polyp with high-grade dysplasia on endoscopy.* **(Right)** *Axial fused F-18 FDG PET/CT in a patient with lung cancer shows moderate focal uptake in the gastric body ➔, which turned out to be gastritis on endoscopy.*

TERMINOLOGY

Definitions

- Gastric carcinoma
  - Arises from gastric epithelial lining
  - Siewert Classification: type III, subcardial carcinoma
    - The tumor center between 2-5 cm below the esophagogastric junction (EGJ), which may infiltrates the EGJ and lower esophagus from below
    - Siewert type I and II are considered esophageal and EGJ cancers
- Gastrointestinal tumor (GIST)
  - Nonepithelial neoplasm, arises from interstitial cells of Cajal
  - Can be benign or malignant, based on tumor size, mitotic index rate, and presence of metastasis

IMAGING

General Features

- Location
  - Gastric carcinoma: Fundus and cardia (40%); body (30%); antrum (30%)
  - GIST: Stomach (50-70%); small intestine (25-35%); anorectum (< 5%); occasionally colon, mesentery or omentum, gallbladder, duodenal ampulla, or appendix
- Size
  - Early gastric carcinoma (EGC)
    - Invasive carcinoma confined to mucosa &/or submucosa, ± lymph node metastases
  - Advanced gastric carcinoma (AGC)
    - Invades into muscularis propria or beyond
  - GIST: Variable size

Nuclear Medicine Findings

- PET
  - Local disease
    - F-18 FDG avidity varies greatly in literature, from 47-96%, with mean of 73%
    - Factors associated with high FDG uptake
      - □ Large tumor size
      - □ AGC
      - □ Non-signet ring cell carcinoma
      - □ GLUT(+) expression (17-60% frequency)
    - Unresectable
      - □ Disease infiltrating root of mesentery or encasing major vascular structures (excluding splenic vessels)
  - Regional nodal disease
    - Proximal 1/3/cardia/EG junction tumors
      - □ Perigastric, celiac, splenic hilar, porta hepatic lymph nodes
    - Middle 1/3/body tumors
      - □ Perigastric, suprapancreatic, celiac, splenic, porta hepatic, and pancreaticoduodenal lymph nodes
    - Distal 1/3/antrum/pylorus tumors
      - □ Perigastric, suprapancreatic, celiac, porta hepatic, and pancreaticoduodenal lymph nodes
    - F-18 FDG PET/CT has low sensitivity for N1 disease (56%), equally sensitive for N2-3 disease as CECT (78%)
    - Positive paraaortic lymph nodes is a criterion of unresectability
    - Survival inversely proportional to number of lymph nodes involved
  - Distant metastatic disease
    - Liver (most common)
    - Peritoneum
    - Lung
    - Bone
    - Soft tissue
    - F-18 FDG PET/CT has low sensitivity for peritoneal disease, and laparoscopy with peritoneal washout may be recommended on T3 and N+ patients
  - Assessment of tumor response and recurrence
    - F-18 FDG PET/CT can assess metabolic response to therapy
      - □ Responders have better survival and decreased rate of local recurrence
    - Surveillance often includes F-18 FDG PET/CT
      - □ Sensitivity: 70%
      - □ Negative predictive value: 60%
- GIST
  - Local disease
    - Similar performance of F-18 FDG PET/CT and CECT for staging
  - Regional nodal disease
    - Unusual and classified as stage IV if present
  - Metastatic disease
    - 50% will have metastasized by time of presentation
    - Liver > peritoneal surface > lungs
  - Response to therapy/recurrence disease
    - Important role of PET to assess early response to imatinib
      - □ Increasing chances of potentially curative total surgical resection
      - □ SUV max ≤ 2.5 after 1 month of treatment have better tumor-free survival
    - PET/CT for surveillance: 40% incidence of local recurrence

Imaging Recommendations

- Best imaging tool
  - Local disease: Endoscopic ultrasound (EUS)
    - Depth of tumor (T stage) and local abnormal lymph nodes (N1) with possibility of biopsy
    - GIST: EUS for biopsy or CT-guided biopsy to rule out lymphoma or other sarcomas
  - Staging and resectability: CECT and F-18 FDG PET/CT
  - Recurrence and response to therapy: F-18 FDG PET/CT &/or CECT
- Protocol advice
  - F-18 FDG PET/CT standard oncologic protocol

DIFFERENTIAL DIAGNOSIS

Physiologic F-18 FDG Activity in Stomach

- Usually low-level activity
- Diffuse throughout stomach, nonfocal

Gastric Ulcer/Gastritis

- Most benign ulcers located in lesser curve or posterior wall of antrum, body of stomach
- Usually mild to moderate F-18 FDG activity

Gastric Lymphoma

- F-18 FDG activity variable, often hypermetabolic
- Gastric wall thickening, may be diffuse
- Abdominal lymphadenopathy may be present

Crohn Disease

- Rarely affects stomach
- Increased F-18 FDG activity in active disease

PATHOLOGY

General Features

- Etiology
  - Gastric carcinoma
    - Dietary: High nitrates/nitrites, starch, smoked foods, salted fish/meat
    - *Helicobacter pylori*
    - Smoking
    - High alcohol intake
    - Obesity
    - Atrophic gastritis, prior gastric surgery, or gastric polyps
    - Low socioeconomic status
  - GIST
    - Sporadic
- **Gastric carcinoma staging**
  - Stage 0: Tis (intraepithelial tumor without invasion of lamina propria)
  - Stage IA: T1 (invades lamina propria, muscularis mucosae, or submucosa)
  - Stage IB: T2 N0 (invades muscularis propria) or T1 N1(metastasis in 1-2 regional lymph nodes)
  - Stage IIA: T3 (penetrates subserosal connective tissue without invasion of visceral peritoneum or adjacent structure); T2 N1 or T1 N2 (3-6+ regional lymph nodes)
  - Stage IIB: T4a (invades visceral peritoneum); T3 N1; T2 N2 or T1 N3 (> 7+ lymph nodes)
  - Stage IIIA: T4a N0; T3 N2 or T2 N3
  - Stage IIIB: T4b N0-1 (tumor invades adjacent structures); T4a N1 or T3 N3
  - Stage IIIC: T4b N1-2 or T4a N3
  - Stage IV: M1
- **GIST staging**
  - Stage IA-B: T1-3 (tumor > 5 cm but < 10 cm), low mitotic rate
  - Stage II: T1-2 (tumor < 5 cm), high mitotic rate or T3 low mitotic rate
  - Stage III: T3-4 (tumor > 10 cm), high mitotic rate
  - Stage IV: N1 or M1

CLINICAL ISSUES

Demographics

- Age
  - Gastric carcinoma: 50-70 years
  - GIST: 60 years
- Gender
  - Gastric carcinoma: M:F = 2:1
  - GIST: M = F
- Ethnicity
  - Highest incidence of gastric cancer: Eastern Asia, South America, and Eastern Europe
- Epidemiology
  - Gastric carcinoma
    - 2nd most lethal cancer worldwide
    - 4th most frequent cancer in Western countries
    - Incidence of distal intestinal-type gastric cancer has declined in USA in last century
    - Proximal gastric and GEJ cancer has increased during last 10-15 years in Western countries due to increased incidence of Barrett esophagus
  - GIST
    - 15-20 cases per million

Natural History & Prognosis

- Gastric carcinoma
  - Prognosis of early gastric carcinoma: 5-year survival > 90%, regardless of lymphadenopathy
  - Prognosis of advanced gastric carcinoma: 5-year survival > stage IIA 15-30%
- GIST
  - 60-70% benign (mostly in stomach)
  - Malignant GIST: 5-year survival: 35%
  - Recurrence: 40%

Treatment

- Gastric carcinoma
  - Surgical resection for localized disease is curative, depending on T stage
  - The more extensive the nodal dissection, better the overall survival and lower the recurrence
  - Chemotherapy and radiation increases overall survival and decreases recurrence rate
- GIST
  - Complete surgical resection
  - Imatinib mesylate and sunitinib malate for locally advanced or metastatic disease
    - Targets genetic mutations (*KIT*)
    - 80% patients with metastatic disease achieve complete, partial, or stable response

DIAGNOSTIC CHECKLIST

Consider

- F-18 FDG PET/CT for gastric carcinoma and GIST
  - For most complete preoperative staging
  - Evaluate response to therapy
  - Identify recurrence

SELECTED REFERENCES

1. Kaneko Y et al: Improving patient selection for 18F-FDG PET scanning in the staging of gastric cancer. J Nucl Med. 56(4):523-9, 2015
2. Kochhar R et al: Imaging in gastrointestinal stromal tumours: current status and future directions. Clin Radiol. 65(8):584-92, 2010
3. Gastrointestinal stromal tumor. In Edge et al. AJCC Cancer Staging Manual. 7th ed. New York, NY: Springer. 175, 2010
4. O'Sullivan PJ et al: The imaging features of gastrointestinal stromal tumours. Eur J Radiol. 60(3):431-8, 2006

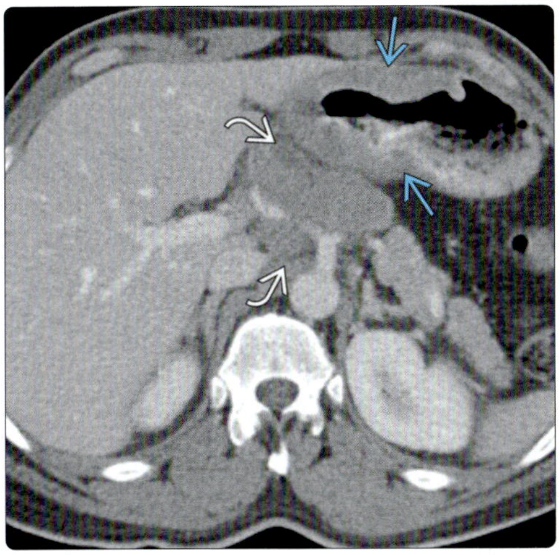

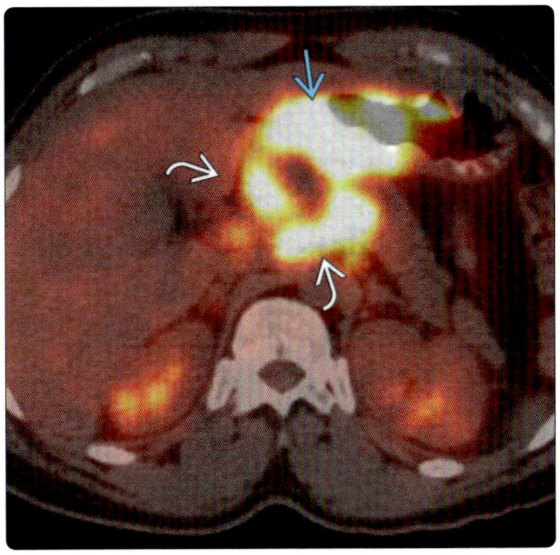

(Left) *Axial CECT shows diffuse thickening of the gastric body and antrum with associated celiac, periportal, and retroperitoneal adenopathy, suspicious for lymphoma.* **(Right)** *Axial fused F-18 FDG PET/CT in the same patient shows marked hypermetabolism in the stomach and lymphadenopathy.*

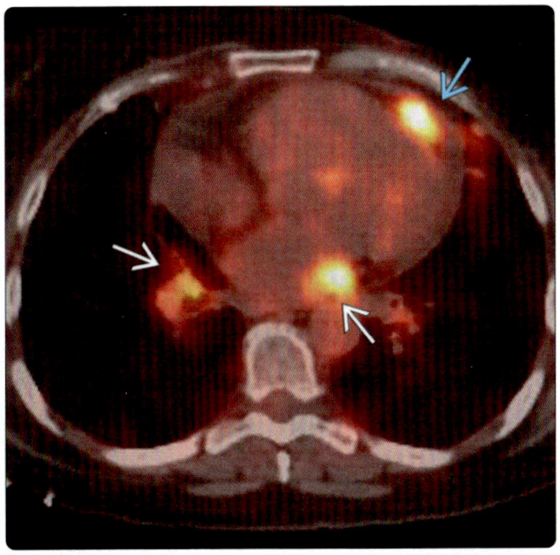

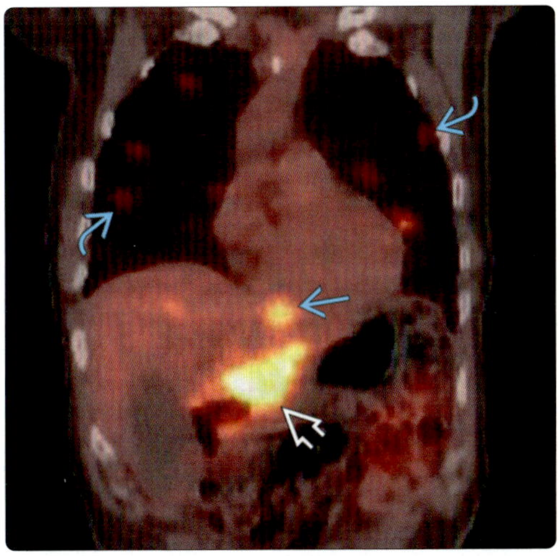

(Left) *Axial fused F-18 FDG PET/CT in this patient with gastric carcinoma demonstrates metastases involving the pericardium and bilateral hila.* **(Right)** *Coronal fused F-18 FDG PET/CT shows hypermetabolic bilateral lung and liver metastases in this patient with intestinal-type gastric carcinoma.*

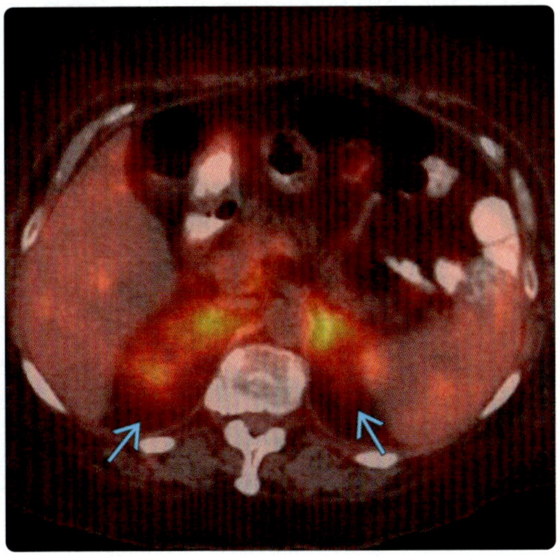

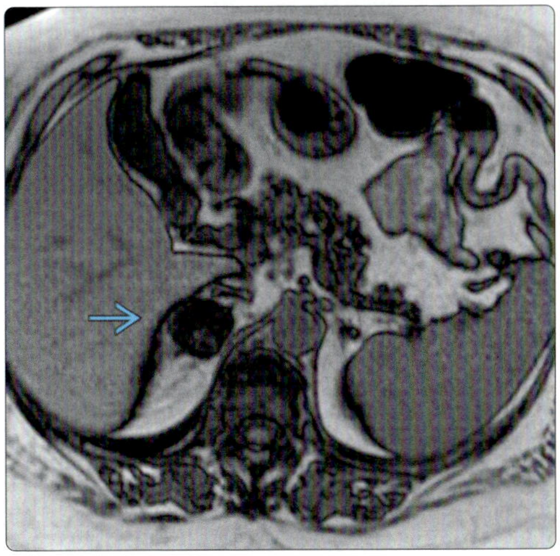

(Left) *Axial fused F-18 FDG PET/CT in this patient with gastric carcinoma shows bilateral uptake in the periadrenal regions.* **(Right)** *Chemical shift sequence on MR in the same patient demonstrates a right adrenal adenoma and no left adrenal lesion. Physiological uptake of F-18 FDG in periadrenal brown fat can cause false-positive interpretations.*

KEY FACTS

IMAGING

- F-18 FDG PET/CT
  - Valuable imaging option for initial staging, distinguishing scar vs. recurrence, evaluating response to therapy
  - Valuable for detecting occult lesions in patients with negative CECT and rising CEA
  - Focal F-18 FDG uptake in colon should be correlated with colonoscopy, even in absence of mass lesion on CT
    - May represent polyp, diverticulitis, neoplasm
  - Mucinous tumors can have low or variable 18F-FDG activity
  - Peritoneal carcinomatosis can be difficult to detect on F-18 FDG PET/CT
    - Varies from hypermetabolic nodules that are very obvious to low-level diffuse activity throughout abdomen
  - Colonic anastomoses can show increased F-18 FDG activity due to physiological uptake
  - When patients undergo F-18 FDG PET/CT, PET and CT are obtained at different times (up to 20 min apart)
    - This can lead to misregistration of anatomic and functional images
  - Anal sphincter F-18 FDG uptake can be difficult to distinguish from primary anal cancer, especially in absence of mass lesion

TOP DIFFERENTIAL DIAGNOSES

- Colorectal cancer
  - Focal F-18 FDG activity within the colon, around anastomotic site, in metastases
- Lymphoma
  - Can show diffuse or focal F-18 FDG activity within/around colon and other sites of lymphoma metastases
- Anal cancer
  - Focal F-18 FDG activity at primary site and metastases

(Left) *Axial CT in a patient with colon cancer shows presacral postsurgical soft tissue ➔ that is either a scar or recurrence.* **(Right)** *Axial fused F-18 FDG PET/CT in the same patient shows hypermetabolic activity ➔ in the soft tissue that is consistent with recurrence.*

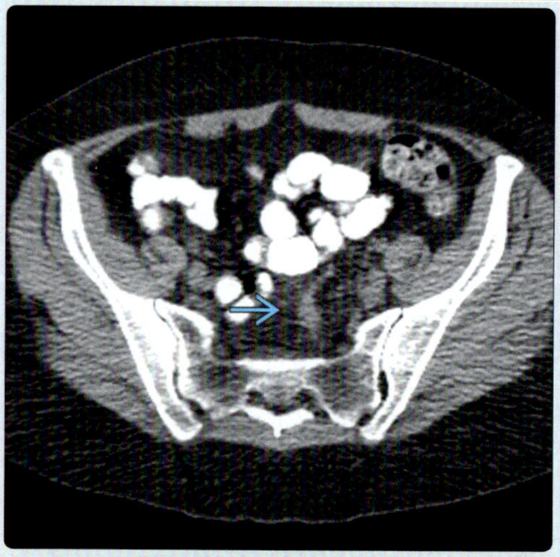

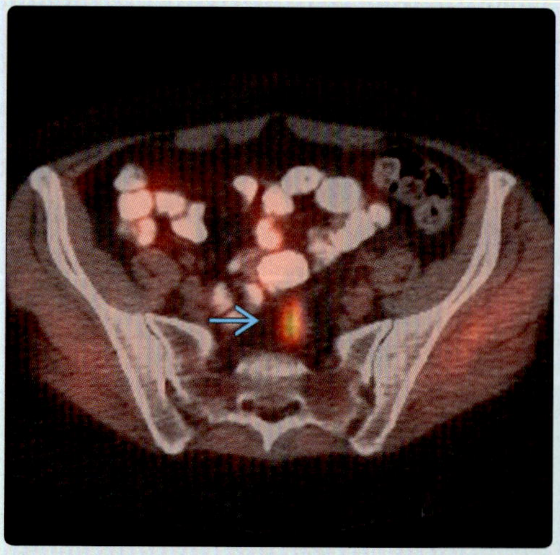

(Left) *MIP F-18 FDG PET/CT in a patient with rising CEA after surgery for colon cancer and a negative CECT shows hypermetabolic focus ➔ in the liver, consistent with metastatic disease.* **(Right)** *MIP F-18 FDG PET shows focal ➔ hypermetabolic nodules and diffuse low-level activity ➔ throughout the abdomen in this patient with peritoneal carcinomatosis.*

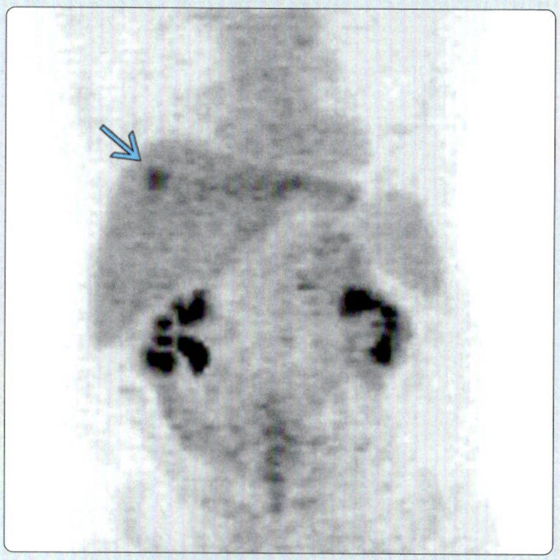

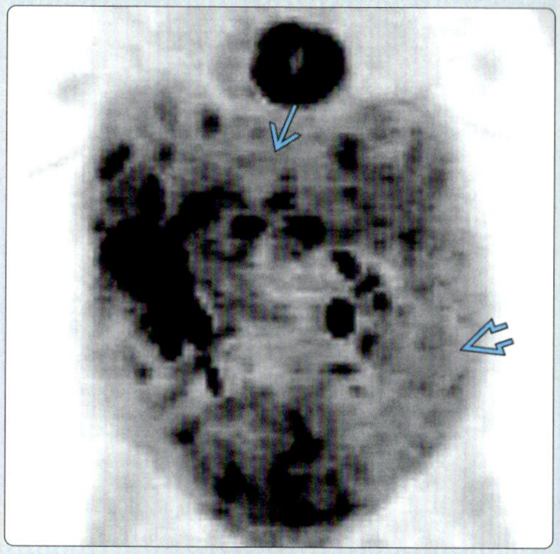

TERMINOLOGY

Definitions

- Colorectal cancer
  - Cancer that arises in colon, usually adenocarcinoma arising from adenomatous polyps
  - Cancer that arises in rectal tissue
- Anal cancer
  - Uncommon cancer of anal canal and perianal skin, strongly associated with human papilloma virus
  - Majority squamous cell carcinoma

IMAGING

General Features

- Location
  - **Colorectal cancer**
  - Primary
    - Originates in mucosa
    - Majority of lesions arise in rectosigmoid region (55%)
  - Regional
    - Invasion of adjacent structures once through serosa
  - Metastatic spread
    - Lymphatic (most common) spread follows major venous outflow from involved segment
      - Colon drains to pericolic nodes, then superior and inferior mesenteric nodes
      - Upper rectum drains to superior rectal nodes, then inferior mesenteric nodes
      - Lower rectum follows same drainage pattern as upper rectum and also middle rectal nodes, then internal iliac nodes
    - Hematogenous spread
      - Via portal system to liver (most common site for distant metastases)
      - Lung
    - Peritoneal spread
      - Direct peritoneal seeding → peritoneal carcinomatosis (diffuse peritoneal metastases)
  - Synchronous primary colorectal cancers possible
    - Synchronous primary tumors defined as 2 or more distinct primary tumors separated by normal bowel (and not due to direct spread or metastases)
    - Occurs in 3-5% of patients with colorectal cancer
  - **Anal cancer**
  - Above dentate line
    - Lymphatic drainage to perirectal and paravertebral lymph nodes
  - Below dentate line
    - Lymphatic drainage to inguinal and femoral lymph nodes

Imaging Recommendations

- Best imaging tool
  - F-18 FDG PET/CT
    - 1 of best whole-body imaging options for initial staging
    - Useful to distinguish scar vs. tumor recurrence after resection
    - Useful for detecting response to chemotherapy
    - Valuable for detect occult lesions in patients with negative CECT and rising CEA
- Protocol advice
  - Standard F-18 FDG PET/CT oncologic protocol

DIFFERENTIAL DIAGNOSIS

Colorectal Cancer

- Focal F-18 FDG activity within the colon, around anastomotic site, in metastases

Lymphoma

- Can show diffuse or focal F-18 FDG activity within/around colon and other sites of lymphoma metastases

Anal Cancer

- Focal F-18 FDG activity at primary site and metastases

PATHOLOGY

General Features

- Etiology
  - Colorectal cancer
    - Majority of colorectal carcinomas evolve from adenomatous polyps
    - Major risk factors
      - Family history
      - Personal history of polyps
      - Inflammatory bowel disease (ulcerative colitis > Crohn disease)
      - Diabetes
  - Anal cancer
    - Major risk factors
      - Human papilloma virus
      - Higher number of lifetime sexual partners
      - Genital warts
      - Cigarette smoking
      - Receptive anal intercourse
      - HIV infection
- Genetics
  - Sporadic colon cancer (70-80%)
    - Stepwise accumulation of multiple somatic mutations, termed the "adenoma-carcinoma sequence"
    - *APC* → *MMR* → *KRAS* → *P53*
    - No family history of colon cancer
    - Likely dietary and environmental factors
  - Inherited colon cancer syndromes (5-10%)
    - Results from single germline mutation
    - Divided into subtypes based on presence or absence of polyps
    - Familial adenosis polyposis
      - Autosomal dominant mutation in tumor suppressor gene *APC*
      - Hundreds of polyps seen on endoscopy beginning in 2nd decade of life
      - 100% of patients have colon cancer by age 45; average age: 39 years
    - Hereditary nonpolyposis colorectal cancer
      - Mutation in DNA mismatch repair gene *MMR* causing predisposition to cancer
      - More rapid progression of "adenoma-carcinoma sequence"

- ◻ 60% lifetime risk of colon cancer
- ◻ Also called Lynch syndrome
- – Numerous others, not all fully elucidated
- o Nonsyndromic familial colon cancer (15-20%)
  - – Family history of colon cancer
  - – Risk for developing colon cancer not as high as with inherited colon cancer syndromes

Staging, Grading, & Classification

- **TNM staging for colorectal cancer**
  - Primary tumor (T)
    - Tis: Carcinoma in situ (preinvasive; involves mucosa only)
    - T1: Extends into submucosa
    - T2: Extends into muscularis mucosa
    - T3: Extends into serosa but not through it
    - T4: Extends past serosa (visceral peritoneum)
  - Regional lymph nodes (N)
    - N0: No nodal metastasis
    - N1: Involvement of 1-3 regional lymph nodes
    - N2: Involvement of ≥ 4 regional lymph nodes
  - Distant metastasis (M)
    - M0: No distant metastasis
    - M1: Distant metastasis
  - **Stage I**: T1-T2 and N0, M0
  - **Stage II**: T3-T4 and N0, M0
  - **Stage III**: Any T, N1-N2, M0
  - **Stage IV**: Any T, any N, M1
- **TNM staging for anal cancer**
  - Primary tumor (T)
    - T0: No evidence of primary tumor
    - Tis: Carcinoma in situ
    - T1: Tumor ≤ 2 cm in greatest dimension
    - T2: Tumor > 2 cm but ≤ 5 cm in greatest dimension
    - T3: Tumor >5 cm in greatest dimension
    - T4: Tumor of any size invades adjacent organ(s), e.g., vagina, urethra, and bladder
  - Regional lymph nodes (N)
    - N0: No regional lymph node metastasis
    - N1: Metastases in perirectal lymph node(s)
    - N2: Metastases in unilateral internal iliac &/or inguinal lymph node(s)
    - N3: Metastases in perirectal and inguinal lymph nodes &/or bilateral internal iliac &/or inguinal lymph nodes
  - Distant metastasis (M)
    - M0: No distant metastasis
    - M1: Distant metastasis
  - **Stage 0-II**: Tis-T3, N0, M0
  - **Stage IIIA**: T1-3, N1, M0; T4, N0, M0
  - **Stage IIIB**: T4, N1; Any T, N2-3, M0
  - **Stage IV**: Any T, any N, M1

CLINICAL ISSUES

Presentation

- Most common signs/symptoms
  - Colon cancer
    - Early cancer often asymptomatic and found during screening colonoscopy
    - Advanced cancer presents with symptoms of abdominal pain, rectal bleeding or melena, change in bowel habits, weight loss
      - ◻ Right-sided lesions most commonly present with bleeding or unexplained iron deficiency anemia
      - ◻ Left-sided lesions more commonly present with obstructive symptoms
  - Anal cancer
    - Rectal bleeding, pain, mass

Natural History & Prognosis

- Colorectal cancer 5-year survival
  - Stage I: 70-95%
  - Stage II: 54-65%
  - Stage III: 39-60%
  - Stage IV: 0-16%
- Recurrent colorectal cancer
  - 1/2 of all CRC patients will develop recurrence, including 25% of those with stage I/II disease
  - Local recurrence rates decreasing but still common in rectal carcinoma, more likely with transanal excision
- Anal cancer 5-year survival
  - T1 and T2: 86%
  - T3: 60%
  - T4- 45%
  - N0: 76%
  - Any N: 54%

DIAGNOSTIC CHECKLIST

Image Interpretation Pearls

- F-18 FDG PET/CT
  - Decreased sensitivity in detecting small colonic lesions (5-10 mm in diameter)
  - Mucinous tumors can have low or variable 18F-FDG activity
  - Peritoneal carcinomatosis can be difficult to detect on F-18 FDG PET/CT; varies from hypermetabolic nodules that are very obvious to low-level diffuse activity throughout abdomen
  - When patients undergo F-18 FDG PET/CT, PET and CT are obtained at different times (up to 20 min apart); this can lead to misregistration of anatomic and functional images
  - Colonic anastomoses can show increased F-18 FDG activity due to physiological uptake
  - Anal sphincter F-18 FDG uptake can be difficult to distinguish from primary anal cancer, especially in absence of mass lesion
  - Focal F-18 FDG uptake in colon should be correlated with colonoscopy, even in absence of mass lesion on CT
    - May represent polyp, diverticulitis, neoplasm

SELECTED REFERENCES

1. Shin SS et al: Preoperative staging of colorectal cancer: CT vs. integrated FDG PET/CT. Abdom Imaging. 33(3):270-7, 2008

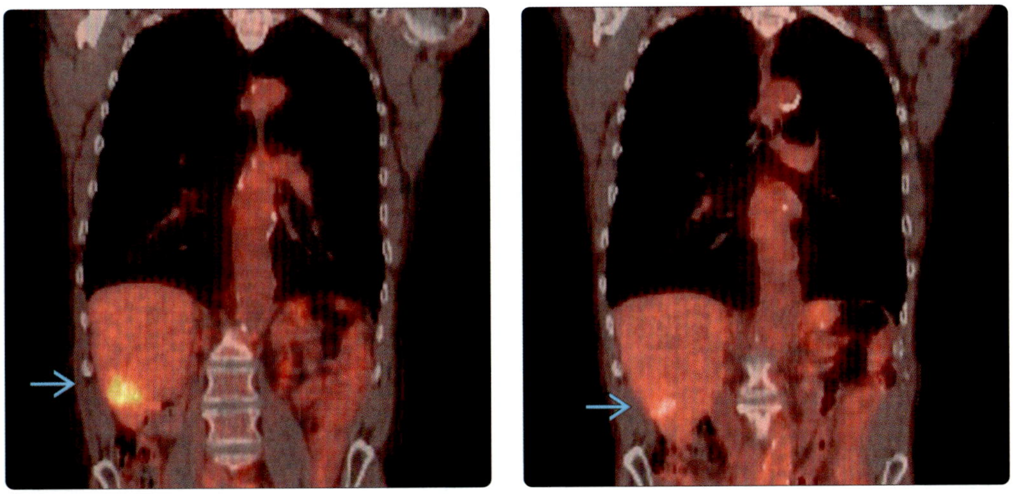

(Left) *Coronal fused F-18 FDG PET/CT in a patient with colon cancer shows a solitary hepatic metastasis →.* **(Right)** *Coronal fused F-18 FDG PET/CT in the same patient shows near complete resolution of hypermetabolic activity → after therapy.*

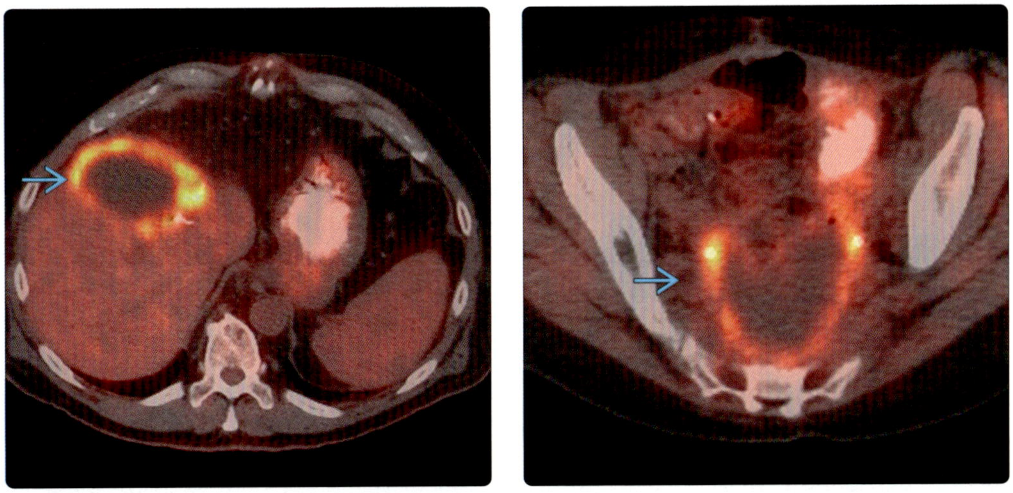

(Left) *Axial fused F-18 FDG PET/CT in a patient with colon cancer shows the typical appearance of mucinous tumor metastasis →, with a hypermetabolic rim and photopenic center.* **(Right)** *Axial fused F-18 FDG PET/CT in a patient with mucinous colon cancer shows a presacral recurrence → with a hypermetabolic rim and photopenic center. An abscess could also have this appearance.*

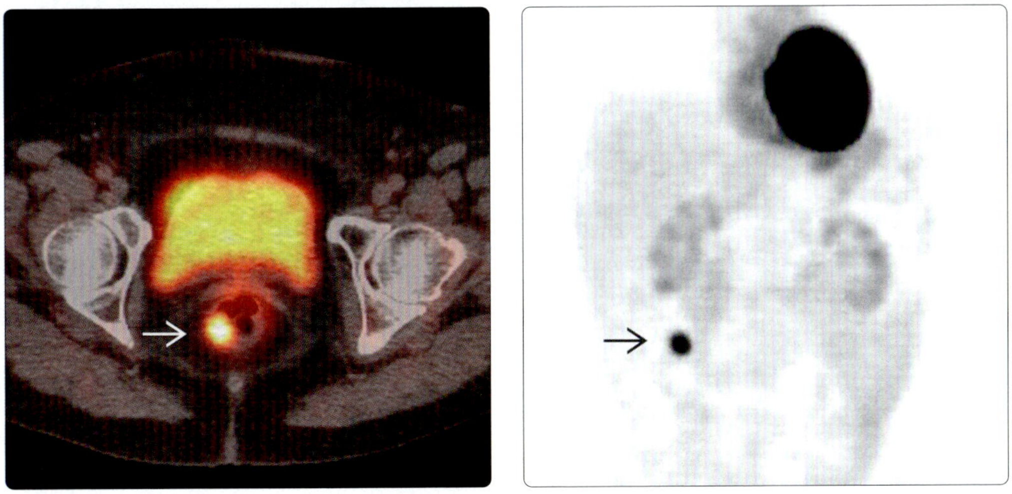

(Left) *Axial fused F-18 FDG PET/CT shows a hypermetabolic focus → and associated mass in the rectum. Focal colorectal uptake should be correlated with colonoscopy, even in the absence of CT findings.* **(Right)** *MIP F-18 FDG PET in a patient undergoing a scan for a solitary pulmonary nodule shows incidental focal colon uptake →, which was a polyp at colonoscopy.*

KEY FACTS

TERMINOLOGY

- Tumors of parotid and submandibular glands (as well as minor salivary tissue tissue) include
  - Parotid carcinoma (most common site of salivary gland cancer)
  - Benign mixed tumors or pleomorphic adenoma
  - Warthin tumor
  - Primary lymphoma

IMAGING

- F-18 FDG PET/CT
  - Cannot reliably differentiate benign vs. malignant salivary gland neoplasia
  - Hypermetabolic lesions on F-18 FDG PET/CT have ~ 30% false-positive rate for malignancy (mostly due to high uptake in Warthin tumor)
  - Any incidentally detected salivary gland neoplasm should be evaluated by otolaryngology, whether cold, warm, or hot
  - Helpful to determine response to therapy or presence of residual disease
    - After external beam radiation, neck muscles can show mildly increased, diffuse uptake
- MR and CT best for anatomic delineation of tumor and regional spread
  - Suspect malignancy if ill-defined borders, diffuse growth, surrounding soft tissue infiltration, regional lymphadenopathy

DIAGNOSTIC CHECKLIST

- Primary parotid carcinoma is almost always positive on F-18 FDG PET/CT
- Warthin tumor is commonly positive on F-18 FDG PET/CT
- Benign mixed tumors are occasionally positive on F-18 FDG PET/CT
- Squamous cell carcinoma of head and neck commonly metastasizes to parotid gland; evaluate images for separate primary tumor site outside of parotid

(Left) *Coronal fused F-18 FDG PET/CT shows a right parotid gland tumor with perineural spread* ⇒. **(Right)** *Axial fused F-18 FDG PET/CT in a patient with a solitary pulmonary nodules shows incidental hypermetabolic uptake* ➡ *in the left parotid, found at biopsy to be a benign Warthin tumor.*

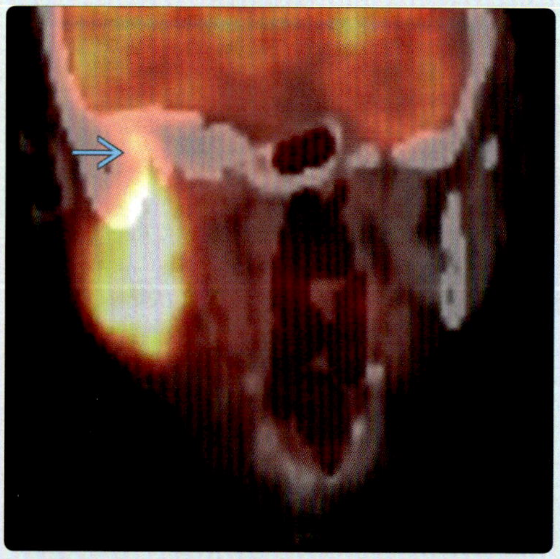

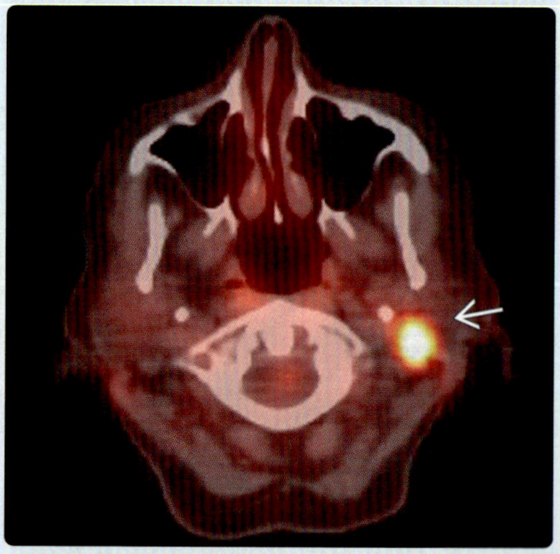

(Left) *Axial CT in a patient with a right facial mass shows an adenoid cystic lesion* ⇒. **(Right)** *Axial fused F-18 FDG PET/CT in the same patient shows mildly increased activity* ⇒ *in the adenoid cystic lesion.*

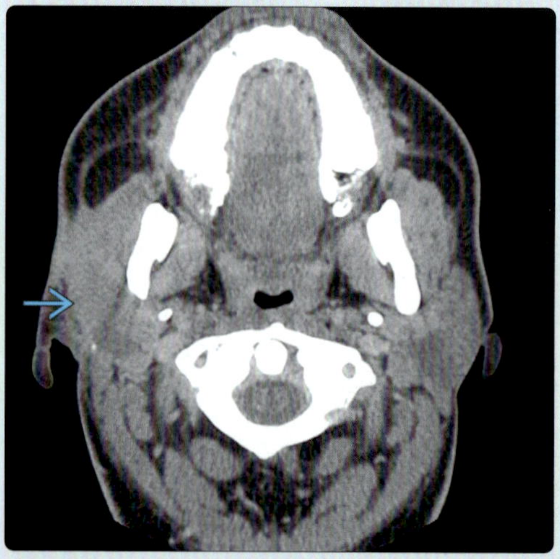

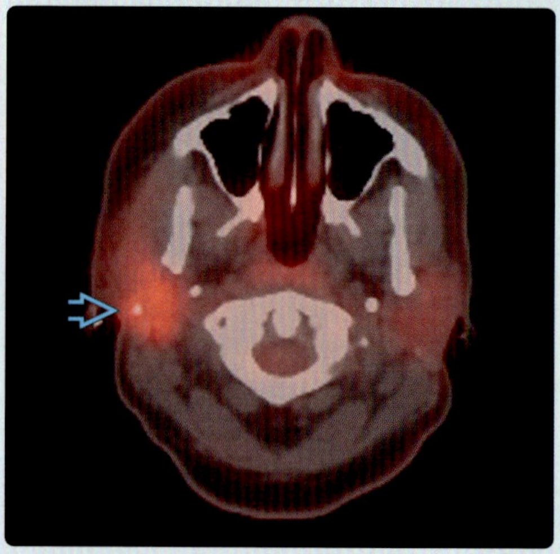

TERMINOLOGY

Definitions

- Tumors of parotid and submandibular glands (as well as minor salivary tissue) include
  - Parotid carcinoma (most common site of salivary gland cancer)
  - Benign mixed tumors or pleomorphic adenoma
  - Warthin tumor
  - Primary lymphoma

IMAGING

Nuclear Medicine Findings

- PET
  - Hypermetabolic lesions on F-18 FDG PET/CT have ~ 30% false-positive rate for malignancy (mostly due to high uptake in Warthin tumor)
  - F-18 FDG PET/CT cannot reliably differentiate benign vs. malignant salivary gland neoplasia
  - Any incidentally detected salivary gland neoplasm should be evaluated by otolaryngology, whether cold, warm, or hot on F-18 FDG PET/CT
- Ga-67 scintigraphy
  - Sensitivity of 58% and specificity of 72% for differentiation of benign from malignant parotid masses

Imaging Recommendations

- Best imaging tool
  - F-18 FDG PET/CT
    - Standard oncologic protocol
  - MR and CT best for anatomic delineation of tumor and regional spread
    - Suspect malignancy if ill-defined borders, diffuse growth, surrounding soft tissue infiltration, regional lymphadenopathy

DIFFERENTIAL DIAGNOSIS

Benign Mixed Tumor or Pleomorphic Adenoma

- Tends to be less F-18 FDG-avid than primary parotid malignancies and Warthin tumor
- Can be positive or negative on F-18 FDG PET/CT
- Frequently show small calcifications on CT
- Usually > 35 years old at presentation

Warthin Tumor

- Tend to be positive on both F-18 FDG PET/CT and Tc-99m pertechnetate salivary gland scans
- Incidence strongly correlates with smoking history
- 17% bilateral
- High incidence of multicentricity
- M > F

Primary Parotid Carcinoma

- Almost always F-18 FDG-avid
- Mucoepidermoid
  - Most common malignancy in parotid
  - Demonstrates solid and cystic components
  - F > M
- Adenoid cystic carcinoma
  - Most common carcinoma in submandibular gland
  - Often demonstrates perineural invasion
  - Commonly metastasizes to lung and bone
  - Distant metastases seen in 20% of early tumors
  - F > M
- Acinic cell
  - 15-17% of all malignant parotid tumors
  - Aggressive, with local and distant metastases common
  - F > M
- Salivary duct carcinoma
  - Uncommon, very aggressive with frequent perineural invasion
- Malignant mixed tumor
  - Frequently carcinoma ex pleomorphic adenoma (benign pleomorphic adenoma that transforms to carcinoma)
    - Over 15-year period, ~ 10% of pleomorphic adenomas develop malignant transformation
  - Typically involves parotid; high grade
- Primary squamous cell carcinoma
  - Aggressive, typically involves parotid
  - Must rule out alternate primary source
  - Exceedingly rare, most commonly metastasis to parotid (parotid is only salivary gland that has lymph nodes)
  - M > F

Non-Hodgkin Lymphoma

- Higher grade tumors more F-18 FDG-avid
- Sjögren disorder has 20-40x increased incidence of primary salivary lymphoma
- Extremely rare incidence of primary parotid lymphoma

Parotid Metastases

- F-18 FDG avidity will depend on primary lesion
- Metastases frequently originate from skin cancer primary, e.g., squamous cell carcinoma

Human Immunodeficiency Virus (HIV)

- HIV can cause fairly symmetric parotid lymphadenopathy accompanied by cystic changes in salivary glands
- Can be difficult to distinguish from lymphoma

PATHOLOGY

Staging, Grading, & Classification

- **TNM for salivary gland tumors**
- Primary tumor (T)
  - Tx: Primary tumor cannot be assessed
  - T0: No evidence of primary tumor
  - T1: Tumor ≤ 2 cm in greatest dimension without extraparenchymal extension
  - T2: Tumor ≤ 2 cm but no > 4 cm in greatest dimension without extraparenchymal extension
  - T3: Tumor > 4 cm &/or tumor having extraparenchymal extension
  - T4a: Moderately advanced disease; tumor invades skin, mandible, ear canal, &/or facial nerve
  - T4b: Very advanced disease; tumor invades skull base &/or pterygoid plates &/or encases carotid artery
- Regional lymph nodes (N)
  - NX: Regional lymph nodes cannot be assessed
  - N0: No regional lymph nodes metastasis
  - N1: Metastasis in single ipsilateral lymph node, ≤ 3 cm in greatest dimension

- N2: Metastasis in single ipsilateral lymph node, > 3 cm but no > 6 cm in greatest dimension; or in multiple ipsilateral lymph nodes, none > 6 cm in greatest dimension; or in bilateral or contralateral lymph nodes, none > 6 cm in greatest dimension
  - N2a: Metastasis in single ipsilateral lymph node, > 3 cm but no > 6 cm in greatest dimension
  - N2b: Multiple ipsilateral lymph nodes, none > 6 cm in greatest dimension
  - N2c: Bilateral or contralateral lymph nodes, none > 6 cm in greatest dimension
- N3: Metastasis in lymph node, > 6 cm in greatest dimension

- Distant metastasis (M)
  - M0: No distant metastasis
  - M1: Distant metastasis
- **Staging for salivary gland tumors**
  - Stage I
    - T1 N0 M0
  - Stage II
    - T2 N0 M0
  - Stage III
    - T3 N0 M0
    - T1-T3 N1 M0
  - Stage IVA
    - T4a N0 M0
    - T4a N1 M0
    - T1-T4a N2 M0
  - Stage IVB
    - T4b, any N, M0
    - Any T, N3, M0
  - Stage IVC
    - Any T, any N, M1

CLINICAL ISSUES

Presentation

- Most common signs/symptoms
  - Asymptomatic mass in cheek or submandibular region
  - Temporomandibular joint pain (parotid mass)
  - Dysphagia or odynophagia (submandibular or sublingual mass)
- Other signs/symptoms
  - Occasional VII nerve paralysis, which would more likely indicate high-grade lesions
  - Shortness of breath or voice changes
  - Referred otalgia

Treatment

- Submandibular or sublingual neoplasm: Gland excision
- Parotid neoplasm: Neoplasm excision with margin of normal parotid tissue
- Presurgical evaluation depends on clinical exam as well as radiologic work-up and potential evaluation for distant metastases
- Facial nerve preservation depends on intraoperative findings of nerve involvement
- Indication for postoperative radiation varies depending on tumor type and presence of nodal spread
- Additional neck dissection possible, depending on tumor histopathology and behavior

DIAGNOSTIC CHECKLIST

Consider

- Imaging type
  - MR is test of choice to evaluate primary malignancy
  - F-18 FDG PET/CT recommended for highly aggressive lesions to evaluate for distant metastases
- FNA may be most cost effective approach for evaluation of primary neoplasm
  - Sensitivity of 64-92% and specificity of 75-100%
  - Excisional biopsy not recommended due to risk of cell spillage
- Otolaryngology consultation recommended for evaluation of any incidentally detected salivary gland neoplasm evident on F-18 FDG PET/CT, even if it is not hypermetabolic

Image Interpretation Pearls

- F-18 FDG PET/CT alone is not reliable in differentiating benign vs. malignant disease
  - FNA &/or surgical excision often required to determine etiology
  - Primary parotid carcinoma is almost always positive on F-18 FDG PET/CT
  - Warthin tumor is commonly positive on F-18 FDG PET/CT
  - Benign mixed tumors are occasionally positive on F-18 FDG PET/CT
  - Squamous cell carcinoma of head and neck commonly metastasizes to parotid gland; evaluate images for separate primary tumor site outside of parotid
- F-18 FDG PET/CT for response to therapy
  - Helpful to determine response to therapy or presence of residual disease
  - After external beam radiation, neck muscles can show mildly increased, diffuse uptake
  - Focal activity in head and neck after external beam radiation suggests tumor recurrence or lymphadenopathy

SELECTED REFERENCES

1. Panwar A et al: Cancers of Major Salivary Glands. Surg Oncol Clin N Am. 24(3):615-633, 2015
2. Witt RL et al: Etiology and management of recurrent parotid pleomorphic adenoma. Laryngoscope. 125(4):888-93, 2014
3. Thoeny HC: Imaging of salivary gland tumours. Cancer Imaging. 7:52-62, 2007
4. Uchida Y et al: Diagnostic value of FDG PET and salivary gland scintigraphy for parotid tumors. Clin Nucl Med. 30(3):170-6, 2005
5. Matsuda M et al: Positron emission tomographic imaging of pleomorphic adenoma in the parotid gland. Acta Otolaryngol Suppl. 538:214-20, 1998
6. Okamura T et al: Fluorine-18 fluorodeoxyglucose positron emission tomography imaging of parotid mass lesions. Acta Otolaryngol Suppl. 538:209-13, 1998
7. Keyes JW Jr et al: Salivary gland tumors: pretherapy evaluation with PET. Radiology. 192(1):99-102, 1994
8. Beahrs O et al. American Joint Committee on Cancer (AJCC) Cancer Staging Manual. 4th ed. Chicago, IL: J. B. Lippincott, 1992

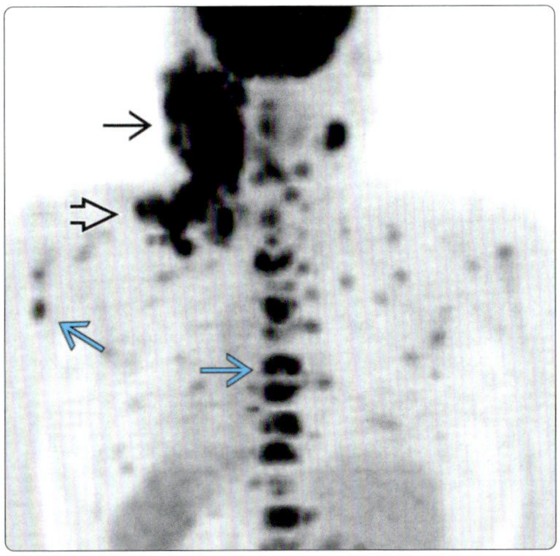

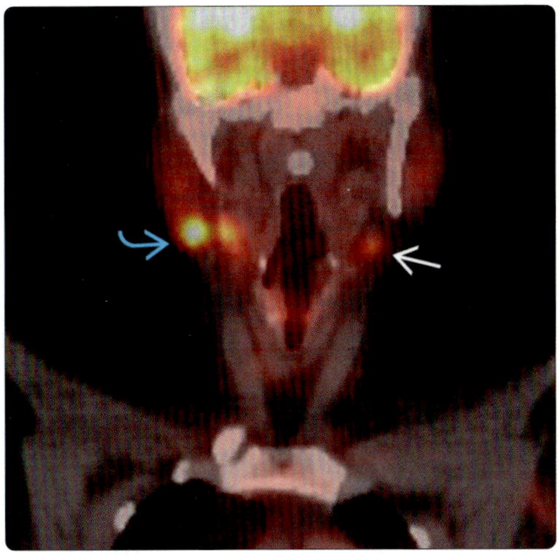

(Left) *MIP F-18 FDG PET in a patient with squamous cell carcinoma of the parotid shows lymphadenopathy and osseous metastases.* **(Right)** *Coronal fused F-18 FDG PET/CT in a patient with lymphoma shows hypermetabolic activity in the right parotid gland and contralateral cervical lymphadenopathy.*

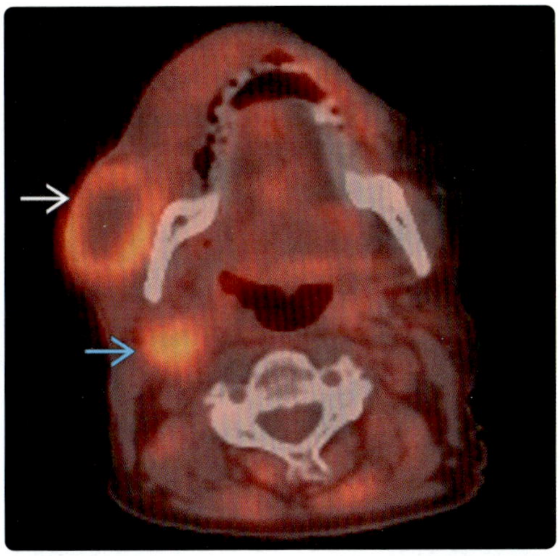

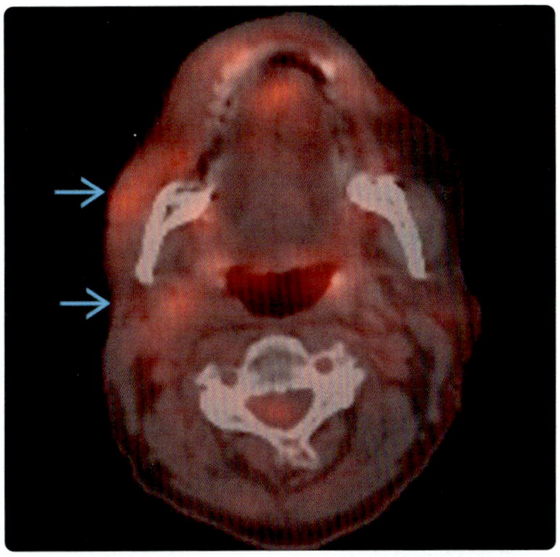

(Left) *Axial fused F-18 FDG PET/CT shows a patient with oral squamous cell carcinoma with a necrotic parotid metastasis and lymphadenopathy before treatment.* **(Right)** *Axial fused F-18 FDG PET/CT in the same patient shows decreased activity, consistent with response to therapy.*

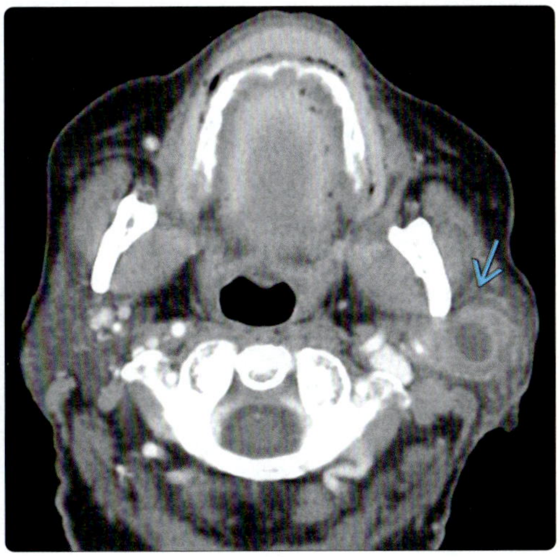

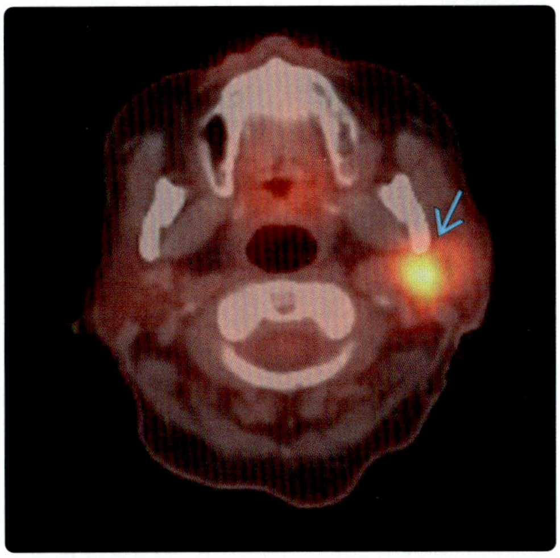

(Left) *Axial CECT in a patient with squamous cell carcinoma shows metastatic disease in the left parotid gland.* **(Right)** *Axial fused F-18 FDG PET/CT in the same patient shows hypermetabolic activity in the metastasis.*

KEY FACTS

TERMINOLOGY

- Squamous cell carcinoma (SCC) of head and neck (H&N)
  - Develops from squamous cells lining mucous membranes of H&N
  - Nasopharynx, larynx, hypopharynx, oral cavity, oropharynx, nasal cavity, paranasal sinuses, salivary glands, thyroid gland, and unknown primary

TOP DIFFERENTIAL DIAGNOSES

- Inflammatory changes/inflammatory lymph nodes (LNs)
  - LNs tend to be normal morphology to minimally enlarged, symmetrical, and low-level FDG uptake
- Metastatic disease from thyroid or melanoma
  - May look identical to SCC
- Abscess or suppurative nodes
  - Usually has central necrosis; identical in appearance to necrotic LN
- Lymphoma
  - Difficult to differentiate from H&N SCC based on imaging; associated mucosal lesion &/or necrotic nodes favor H&N SCC
- Asymmetrical muscle activity
  - Correlate PET with CT; pretreatment with benzodiazepines may reduce muscle uptake
- Brown fat
  - Warm patients before and after injection injection of F-18 FDG to reduce brown fat activity

DIAGNOSTIC CHECKLIST

- Consider F-18 FDG PET/CT for all patients with H&N SCC, particularly those
  - With high tumor (T) stage
  - Undergoing definitive radiation therapy (RT) treatment
  - With indeterminate or suspicious findings on CECT
  - With H&N SCC of unknown primary
- Know physiologic FDG uptake patterns in neck to avoid misinterpretation

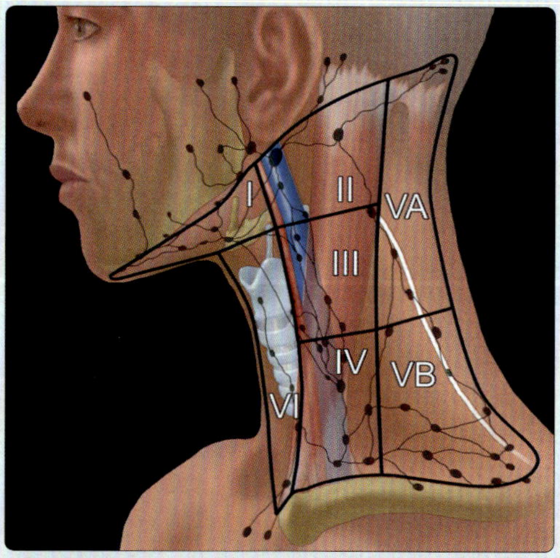

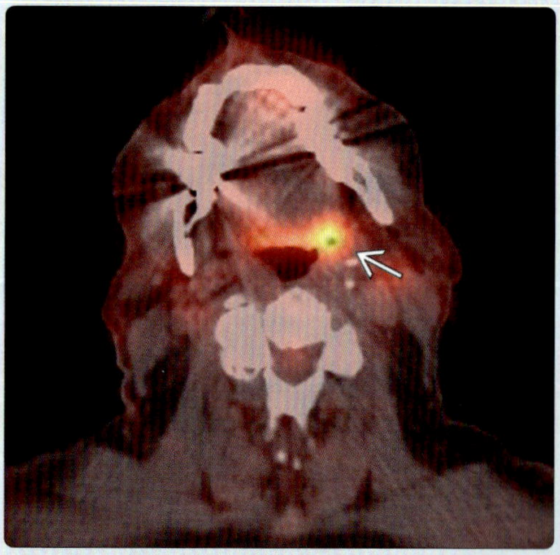

(Left) *Lateral graphic of the neck depicts nodal levels. I: Submental-submandibular; II: High jugular; III: Mid jugular; IV: Low jugular; VA and VB: High and low spinal accessory; and VI: Anterior cervical.* **(Right)** *Axial fused F-18 FDG PET/CT shows primary squamous cell carcinoma near the base of tongue. Some primary lesions are too small to be detected on F-18 FDG PET/CT.*

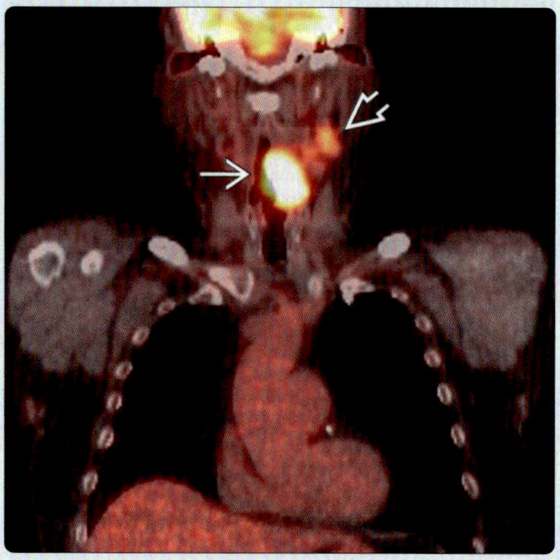

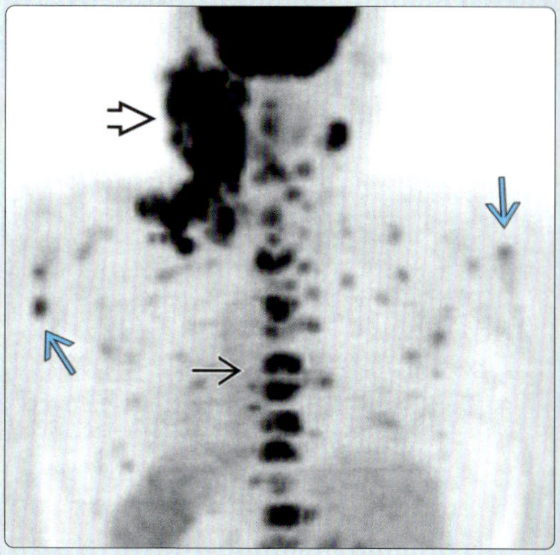

(Left) *Coronal fused F-18 FDG PET/CT shows primary oropharyngeal squamous cell carcinoma with nodal metastases. Local staging helps plan external beam radiation therapy.* **(Right)** *Maximum-intensity projection F-18 FDG PET shows extensive cervical lymphadenopathy and numerous bone metastases in spine, multiple bilateral ribs, and humeri in a patient squamous cell carcinoma.*

TERMINOLOGY

Abbreviations

- Squamous cell carcinoma (SCC)

Definitions

- SCC of head and neck (H&N)
  - Develops from squamous cells lining mucous membranes of H&N
  - Nasopharynx, larynx, hypopharynx, oral cavity, oropharynx, nasal cavity, paranasal sinuses, salivary glands, thyroid gland, and unknown primary

IMAGING

Nuclear Medicine Findings

- PET
  - Best diagnostic clue
    - Intensely FDG-avid, enlarged or necrotic lymph nodes (LNs) in neck on F-18 FDG PET/CT
  - Location
    - Look for primary lesion along mucosal surfaces and evidence for nodal or distant spread
    - LN metastases in expected drainage pattern based on primary tumor location
    - Commonly involves base of tongue, tonsils, or adenoids
  - Size
    - LN metastases may range in size from normal (< 1 cm) to several cm
    - Different CT size criteria for abnormal; ≥ 1 cm for most nodes; ≥ 1.5 cm for level I-II nodes
    - F-18 FDG PET/CT can detect smaller positive nodes
    - ~ 3-5% of H&N SCC will have subclinical primary malignancy (SCC of unknown primary)
  - Morphology
    - SCC can replace normal fatty hila with findings of mass effect, necrosis, cystic changes, calcifications, or hyperenhancement
    - Indistinct borders usually denote extranodal spread of malignancy

Imaging Recommendations

- Best imaging tool
  - F-18 FDG PET/CT may offer additional localization information and improve staging and treatment
    - Recent meta-analysis shows F-18 FDG PET/CT has sensitivity of 89.3% and specificity of 89.5%
    - F-18 FDG PET/CT is useful in detecting occult primary tumors, tumor size and stage, locoregional nodal spread, and distant nodal/organ metastases
    - Extended field F-18 FDG PET/CT staging may detect disease outside of the H&N in up to 21% of cases
- Protocol advice
  - Standard F-18 FDG PET/CT oncologic protocol
  - Whole-body F-18 FDG PET/CT is modality of choice for staging patients with T3 and T4 disease
  - Scan with arms down on F-18 FDG PET/CT to avoid beam hardening artifact; use neck immobilization device
  - F-18 FDG PET/CT is superior to conventional imaging modalities for radiation treatment planning, allowing for improved tumor coverage and sparing of normal tissues
  - F-18 FDG PET/CT is useful for monitoring treatment response and restaging, including nodal disease, distant metastasis and recurrence
  - Initial surveillance F-18 FDG PET/CT should be performed at least 8 weeks after conclusion of therapy

DIFFERENTIAL DIAGNOSIS

Inflammatory Changes/Inflammatory LNs

- LNs tend to be normal morphology to minimally enlarged, symmetrical and low-level FDG uptake
- May be associated with diffuse tonsillar uptake if recent upper respiratory or viral infection; correlate with history of recent upper respiratory infection
- Dual time F-18 FDG PET/CT (3-5 hr delay) useful in differentiating inflammatory/infectious causes from underlying recurrence
  - Cancer cells retain more FDG for longer periods of time than inflammatory tissues

Metastatic Disease From Thyroid or Melanoma

- May look identical to SCC
- Thyroid cystic metastases may have hyperintense signal on T1 MR due to thyroid protein or blood products
- Calcified LNs most commonly found with thyroid carcinoma due to psammomatous calcifications
- Well-differentiated thyroid carcinoma typically not FDG avid, dedifferentiated typically FDG avid

Abscess or Suppurative Nodes

- Usually has central necrosis; identical in appearance to necrotic LN
- F-18 FDG PET/CT not helpful for differentiation; biopsy required

Lymphoma

- Difficult to differentiate from H&N SCC based on imaging; associated mucosal lesion &/or necrotic nodes favor H&N SCC

Asymmetrical Muscle Activity

- Correlate PET with CT; pretreatment with benzodiazepines may reduce muscle uptake

Brown Fat

- Measure Hounsfield units (HU) using CT; diagnostic if HU measure -50 to -150
- Warm patients before and after injection injection of F-18 FDG to reduce brown fat activity

PATHOLOGY

General Features

- Etiology
  - Risk factors: Tobacco use, alcohol abuse, human papillomavirus
  - Age > 40-45, M > F for most primary sites
- Associated abnormalities
  - Risk factors also predispose to esophageal & lung cancer
- American Joint Committee on Cancer (AJCC) and American Academy of Otolaryngology-Head and Neck Surgery (AAO-HNS) Nodal Level Classification Scheme with Key Borders and Primary Drainage Site
  - Level IA (submental) and IB (submandibular)

    - Key borders: Hyoid bone, posterior margin of submandibular gland, anterior belly of digastric muscle
    - Primary drainage site: Anterior oral cavity, lip, sinonasal
  - Level IIA and IIB (anterior cervical or upper jugular)
    - Key borders: Inferior margin of hyoid, posterior margin of submandibular gland, and sternocleidomastoid muscle (SCM); IIA/B posterior margin of internal jugular
    - Primary drainage site: Oropharynx, posterior oral cavity, supraglottic larynx, and parotid gland
  - Level III (middle jugular)
    - Key borders: Inferior margin of hyoid, inferior margin of cricoid
    - Primary drainage site: Glottic, subglottic, and hypopharyngeal regions
  - Level IV (lower jugular)
    - Key borders: Inferior margin of cricoid, clavicle
    - Primary drainage site: Subglottic, thyroid, and cervical esophagus
  - Level V (spinal accessory)
    - Key borders: Posterior border of SCM, clavicle; VA/VB inferior margin of cricoid
    - Primary drainage site: Nasopharynx, skin (neck or occipital scalp)
  - Level VI (upper visceral nodes)
    - Key borders: Medial margins of carotid arteries, inferior margin of hyoid, superior aspect of manubrium
    - Primary drainage site: Subglottic, thyroid, and cervical esophagus
  - Level VII (superior mediastinal)
    - Key borders: Superior aspect of manubrium, innominate vein
    - Primary drainage site: Subglottic, thyroid, and cervical esophagus
  - Supraclavicular nodes
    - Key borders: At or caudal to level of clavicle and lateral to medial edge of carotid arteries
    - Primary drainage site: Any H&N cancer and cancers of thorax, abdomen, and pelvis
  - Retropharyngeal nodes
    - Key borders: Within 2 cm of skull base medial to carotid arteries
    - Primary drainage site: Nasopharynx, oral cavity, sinonasal, thyroid, and pharyngeal and laryngeal tumors with posterior wall involvement
  - Parotid
    - Key borders: Within parotid gland
    - Primary drainage site: Skin of scalp, orbit, and nasopharynx

Staging, Grading, & Classification

- General
  - Most sites of H&N use same AJCC (2010) TNM staging system, including lip, oral cavity, oropharynx, hypopharynx, larynx, and salivary glands
- Tumor (some site specific criteria for advanced staging)
  - T1: ≤ 2 cm
  - T2: > 2 cm and ≤ 4 cm
  - T3: > 4 cm
  - T4: Moderately advanced local disease
- Nodes (same for most H&N sites)
  - NX: Regional LNs cannot be assessed
  - N0: No regional LN metastases
  - N1: Single ipsilateral LN ≤ 3cm
  - N2
    - N2a: Single ipsilateral LNs, 3-6 cm in greatest dimension
    - N2b: Multiple ipsilateral LNs, ≤ 6 cm in greatest dimension
    - N2c: Bilateral or contralateral LNs, ≤ 6cm in greatest dimension
  - N3: LNs > 6 cm in greatest dimension
- Metastasis
  - M0: None
  - M1: Metastatic disease present
- Stage grouping
  - I: T1 N0
  - II: T2 N0
  - III: T3 N0, T1-3 N1
  - IVA: T4a, N2
  - IVB: T4b, N3
  - IVC: M1

CLINICAL ISSUES

Presentation

- Most common signs/symptoms
  - May present with pain associated with primary mass or neck mass
  - Other symptoms may include mouth sores, sore throat, dysphagia, otalgia, odynophagia, voice changes

Treatment

- Radiation therapy ± chemotherapy
- Radical, modified radical, or selective neck dissection
  - Radical neck dissection: Excision of levels I-V LNs, SCM, internal jugular vein and cranial nerve XI
  - Modified radical neck dissection: Excision of levels I-V LNs ± cranial nerve XI
  - Selective neck dissection: Excision of selective nodal groups

DIAGNOSTIC CHECKLIST

Consider

- Consider F-18 FDG PET/CT for all patients with H&N SCC, particularly those
  - With high tumor (T) stage
  - Undergoing definitive radiation therapy (RT) treatment
  - With indeterminate or suspicious findings on CECT
  - With H&N SCC of unknown primary

Image Interpretation Pearls

- Know physiologic FDG uptake patterns in neck to avoid misinterpretation

SELECTED REFERENCES

1. Hoang JK et al: Evaluation of cervical lymph nodes in head and neck cancer with CT and MRI: tips, traps, and a systematic approach. AJR Am J Roentgenol. 200(1):W17-25, 2013

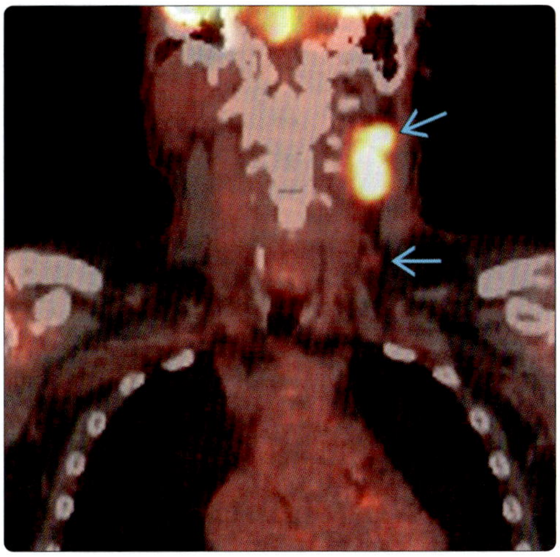

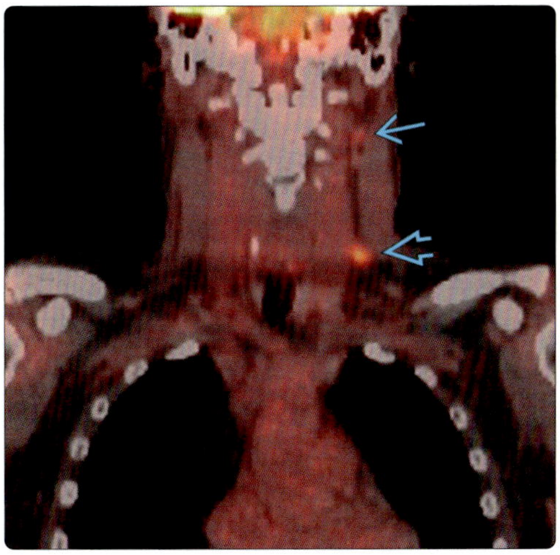

(Left) *Coronal fused F-18 FDG PET/CT in a patient with squamous cell carcinoma shows left cervical lymphadenopathy* ➙ *prior to external beam radiotherapy.* **(Right)** *Coronal fused F-18 FDG PET/CT in the same patient post therapy shows interval response to therapy with a small amount of residual disease superiorly* ➙*. Note the interval progression of inferior nodal metastasis* ➙*, which was likely outside of radiation port.*

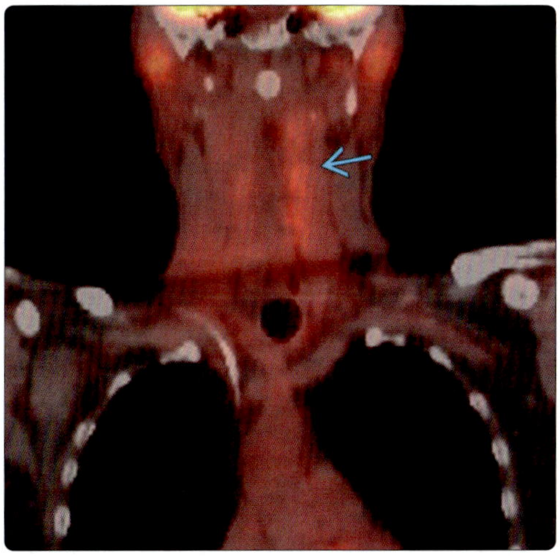

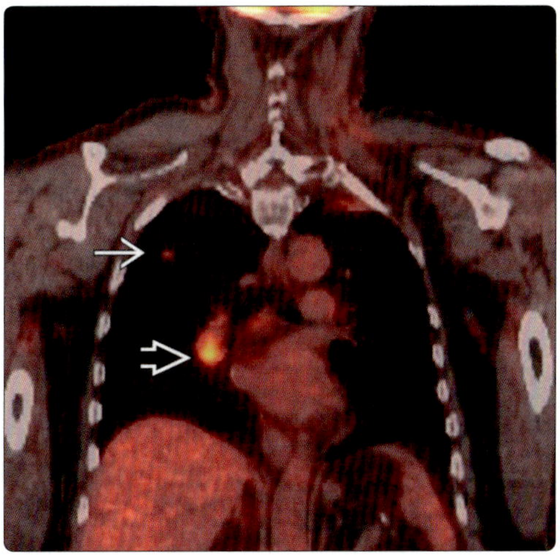

(Left) *Coronal fused F-18 FDG PET/CT shows diffuse, low-level muscle uptake* ➙ *in a patient post radiation therapy for head and neck squamous cell carcinoma, a normal post-therapy finding.* **(Right)** *Coronal fused F-18 FDG PET/CT in the same patient shows hypometabolic lung nodule* ➙ *and hilar lymphadenopathy* ➙*, concerning for metastases or primary lung carcinoma.*

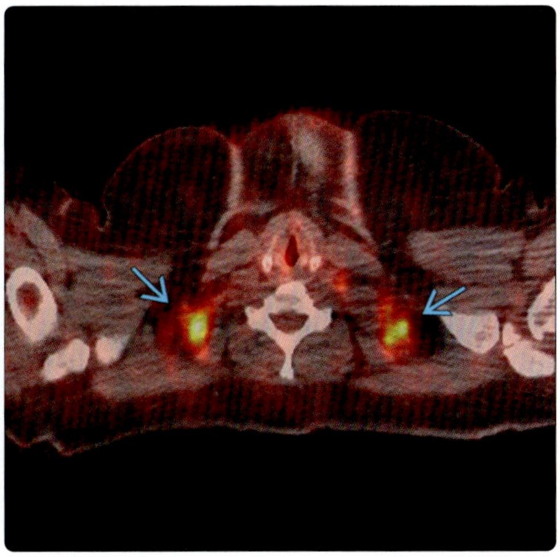

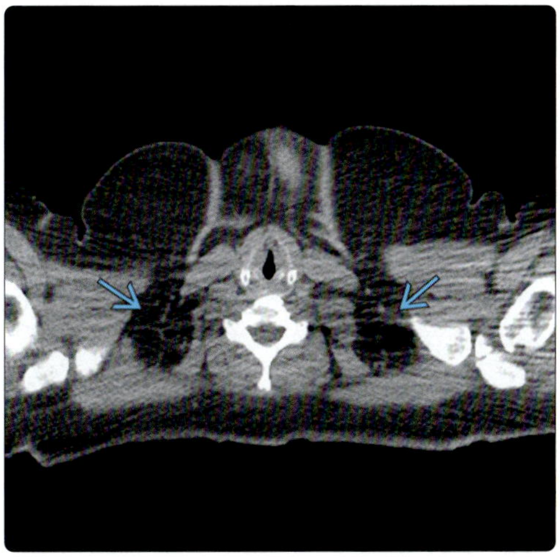

(Left) *Axial fused F-18 FDG PET/CT in a patient with head and neck squamous cell carcinoma shows increased uptake in bilateral supraclavicular regions* ➙*.* **(Right)** *Axial NECT in the same patient shows no nodal tissue in these areas* ➙*, confirming uptake of F-18 FDG in brown fat. This phenomenon limits the sensitivity and specificity of F-18 FDG PET/CT in these cases.*

(Left) *Axial fused F-18 FDG PET/CT in a patient with squamous cell carcinoma of unknown primary shows a small primary tumor in the left tonsil* . **(Right)** *Concurrent axial CECT in the same patient shows mild contour abnormality* .

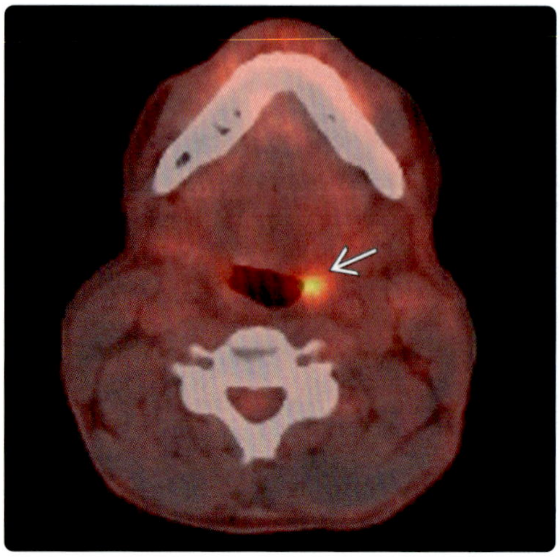

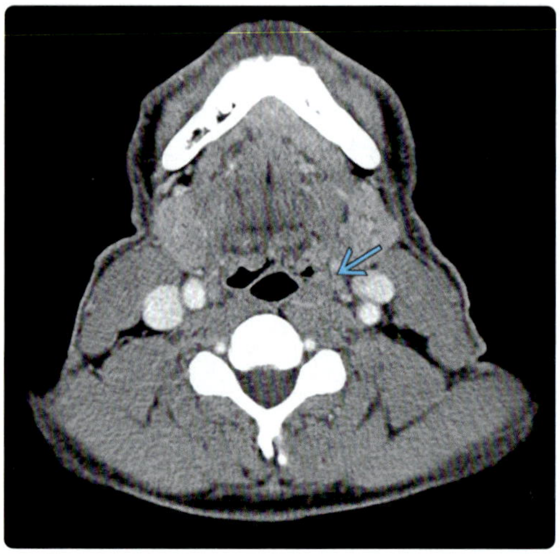

(Left) *Coronal fused F-18 FDG PET/CT in a patient with squamous cell carcinoma shows primary tumor* *and regional lymphadenopathy* . **(Right)** *Axial fused F-18 FDG PET/CT in the same patient shows a small lung metastasis* .

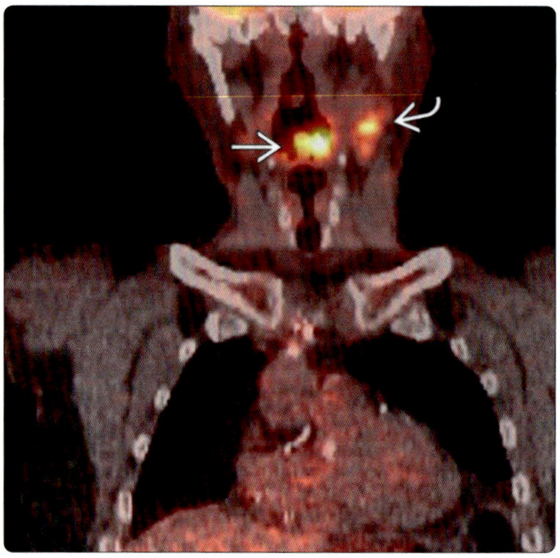

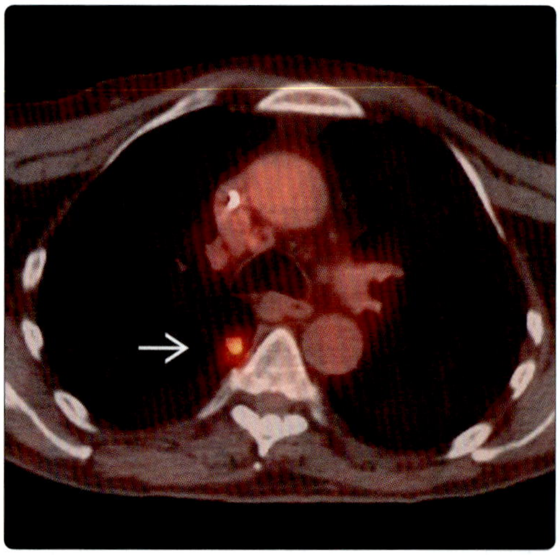

(Left) *Axial fused F-18 FDG PET/CT shows a primary tumor* *as well as hypermetabolic activity at the tip of the nose* *, most commonly artifactual.* **(Right)** *Axial fused F-18 FDG PET/CT shows misregistration* *of PET and CT data, which can cause artifactually increased uptake in tip of nose upon data reconstruction.*

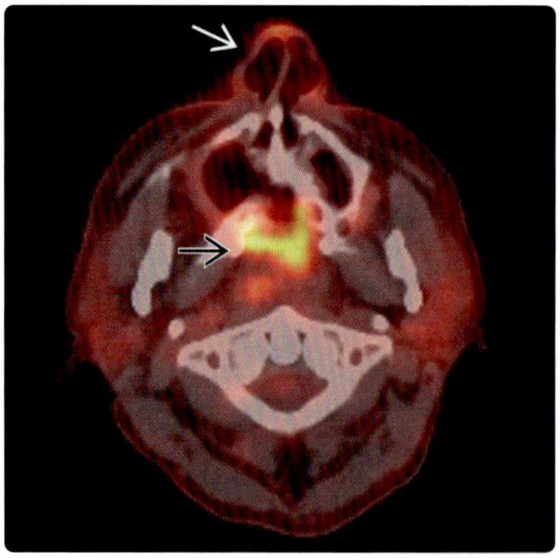

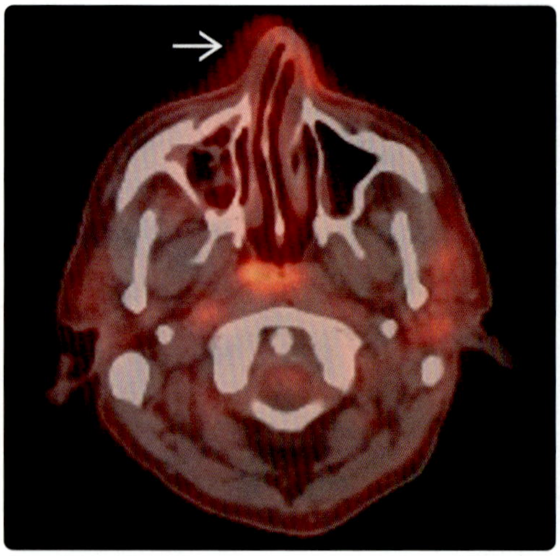

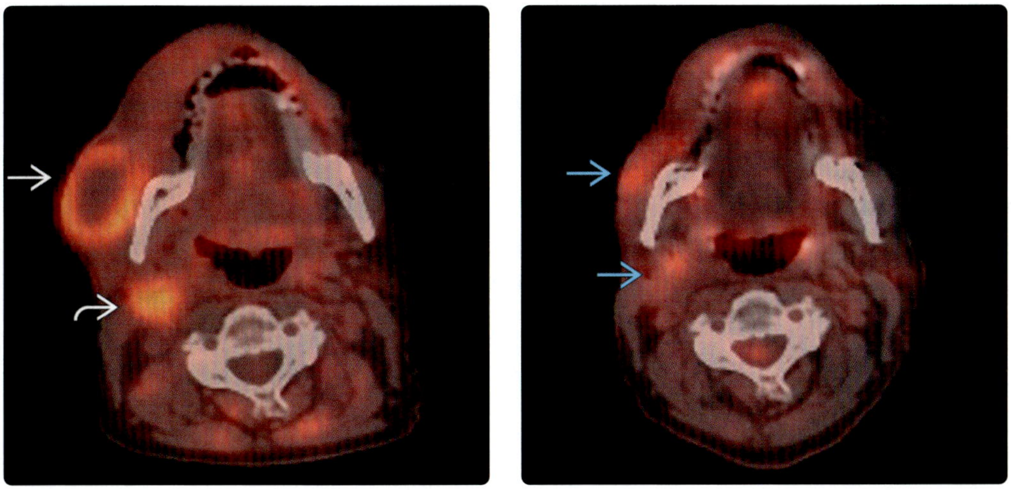

(Left) *Axial fused F-18 FDG PET/CT in a patient prior to therapy for squamous cell carcinoma shows necrotic tumor* ➡ *and lymphadenopathy* ➡. **(Right)** *Axial fused F-18 FDG PET/CT in the same patient posttherapy shows interval response to therapy with background-level activity in the same regions* ➡.

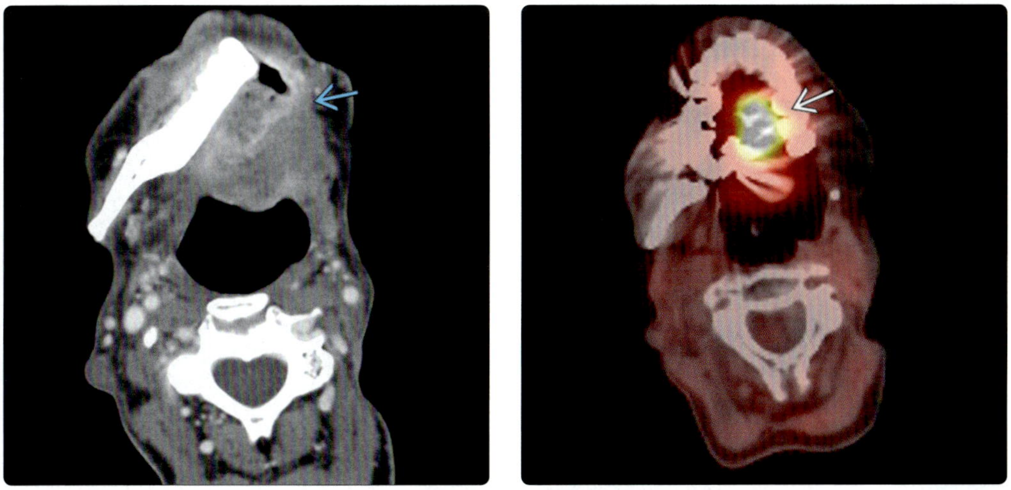

(Left) *Axial CECT in a patient with squamous cell carcinoma post resection shows enhancement in the floor of the mouth* ➡ *on follow-up.* **(Right)** *Axial fused F-18 FDG PET/CT in the same patient shows hypermetabolic activity in the recurrent tumor* ➡.

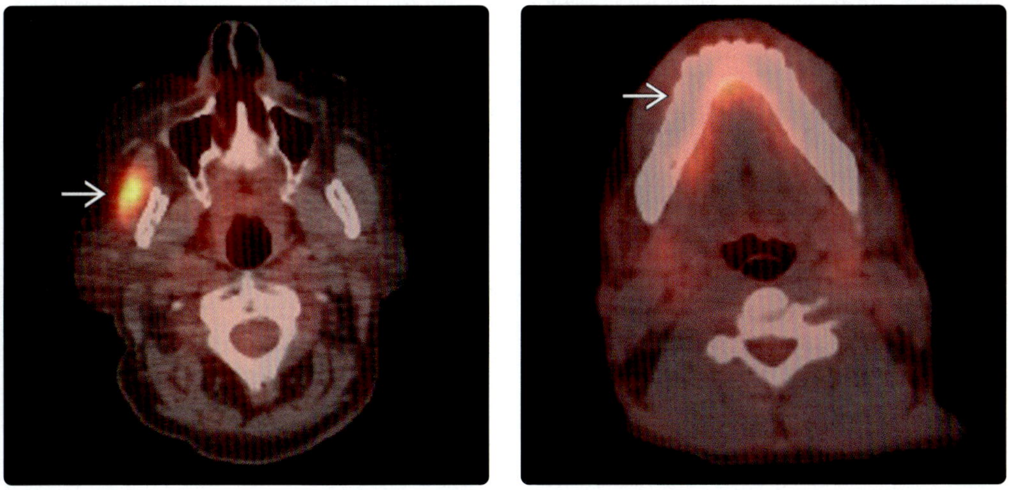

(Left) *Axial fused F-18 FDG PET/CT shows hypermetabolism in the right masseter muscle* ➡, *consistent with benign physiologic uptake.* **(Right)** *Axial fused F-18 FDG PET/CT shows increased uptake in the submental region* ➡, *a benign, physiological finding.*

Hepatobiliary Malignancy

KEY FACTS

IMAGING

- Hepatocellular carcinoma (HCC)
  - Malignant tumor of hepatocytes
- Cholangiocarcinoma (CCA)
  - Arises from simple columnar epithelium of intra-/extrahepatic biliary tree; 10% intrahepatic
- Gallbladder cancer
  - Tumors arise from simple columnar epithelium of gallbladder or cystic duct
- F-18 FDG PET/CT
  - Limited use in detection of primary lesions secondary to variable F-18 FDG uptake due to tumor size and histology
  - Cirrhosis may affect hepatocytes, F-18 FDG metabolism and consequently diagnostic performance of F-18 FDG PET/CT
  - Uptake in small tumors difficult to visualize on F-18 FDG PET/CT because of physiological F-18 FDG uptake
  - Well-differentiated HCC primary isointense to hepatic parenchyma on F-18 FDG PET/CT; higher SUV in poorly differentiated HCC
  - Variable uptake with intrahepatic CCA; lower F-18 FDG uptake may be related to arrangement of fibrous stroma and mucin pool in tumor
  - Intrahepatic CCA is usually larger than extrahepatic CAA, making diagnosis of intrahepatic tumor more sensitive
  - Higher detection of nodular subtype CCA than periductal infiltrating subtype of extrahepatic CCA
  - Low sensitivity of F-18 PET/CT for detection of metastatic nodal disease
  - F-18 FDG PET/CT may have role in detecting distant metastatic disease outside of liver with higher sensitivity than CT, making the difference in staging and treatment in 28-35%
  - Some data supporting potential role of F-18 FDG PET/CT for detecting recurrence after treatment of HCC and CCA

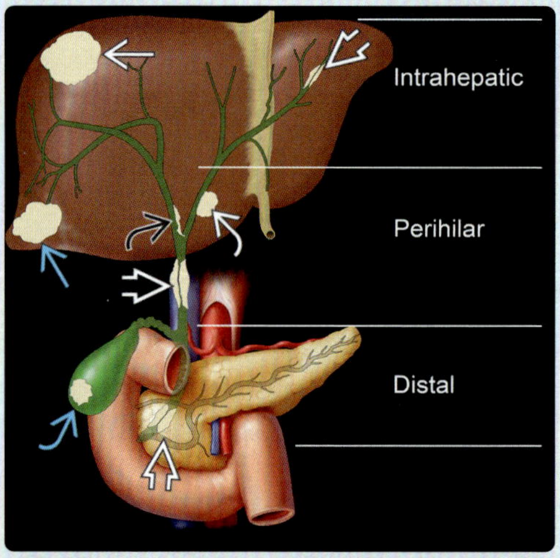

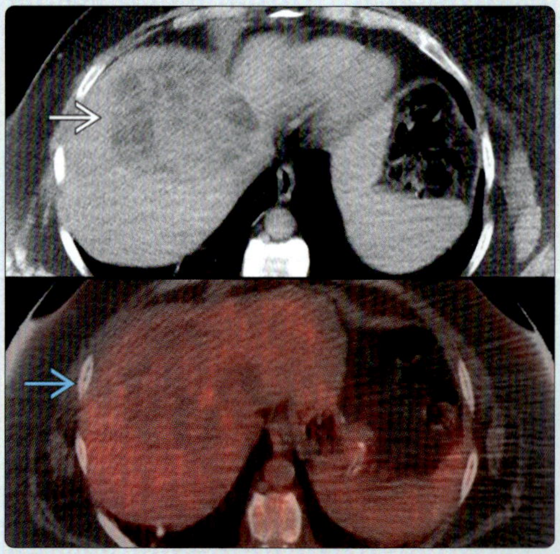

(Left) *Hepatobiliary malignancies are shown by location. Hepatocellular carcinoma and gallbladder carcinoma are noted, along with cholangiocarcinoma subtypes: Mass-forming, papillary, nodular, and periductal infiltrative.* **(Right)** *CT in a patient with hepatocellular carcinoma shows a large heterogeneous mass with focal areas of fat that are not F-18 FDG avid.*

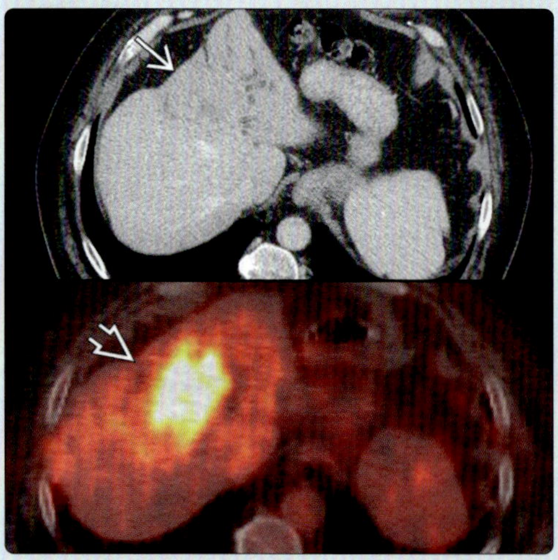

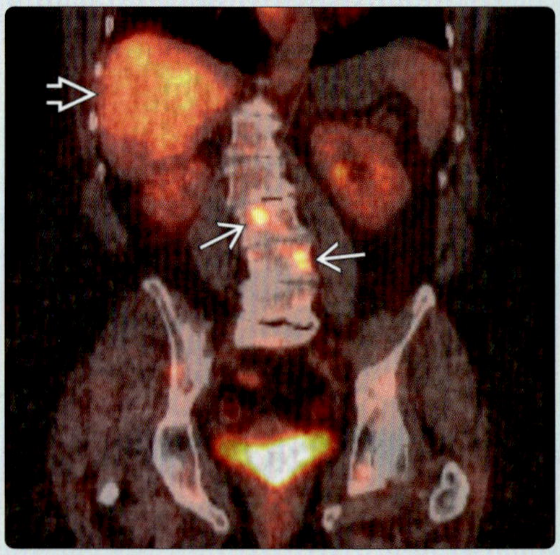

(Left) *CECT shows a mass with associated intrahepatic biliary ductal dilatation and capsular retraction, characteristic of intrahepatic CCA. Note that it is markedly hypermetabolic on F-18 FDG PET/CT.* **(Right)** *F-18 FDG PET/CT shows normal physiologic uptake in an HCC in a cirrhotic liver. Two osseous metastases are evident on F-18 FDG PET/CT and were not seen on anatomic imaging.*

IMAGING

General Features

- Location
  - Hepatocellular carcinoma (HCC)
    - Malignant tumor of hepatocytes
    - Resembles normal liver with varying degrees of hepatocellular differentiation from well-differentiated to poorly differentiated
  - Cholangiocarcinoma (CCA)
    - Arises from simple columnar epithelium of intra-/extrahepatic biliary tree
    - Intrahepatic tumors (10% of CCA) originate from distal second order bile ducts within hepatic parenchyma
      - Histopathology resembles adenocarcinoma; mass-forming subtype (most common), periductal infiltrating subtype, papillary subtype
    - Extrahepatic tumors
      - Perihilar tumors (25-50%): Arise anywhere from second order biliary ducts to common bile duct and at site of cystic duct origin (Klatskin tumor)
      - Distal tumors (40-65%): Originate between cystic duct and ampulla of Vater without its involvement
      - Histopathology subtype: Nodular, sclerosing or periductal infiltrating (most common), and papillary
  - Gallbladder cancer
    - Tumors arise from simple columnar epithelium of gallbladder or cystic duct
    - 60% from fundus, 30% from body, 10% from neck and cystic duct
    - 98% of tumors of epithelial origin, 90% adenocarcinoma
      - Remaining subtypes: Adenosquamous, squamous cell carcinoma, small cell neuroendocrine, sarcoma, lymphoma

Nuclear Medicine Findings

- PET
  - Detection of local disease
    - Limited use in detection of primary lesions secondary to variable F-18 FDG uptake due to tumor size and histology
      - Uptake in small tumors difficult to visualize on F-18 FDG PET/CT because of physiological F-18 FDG uptake
      - Well-differentiated HCC isointense to liver on F-18 FDG PET/CT (low GLUT1 and high G6Pase expression); higher SUV if poorly differentiated
      - Variable uptake with intrahepatic CCA; lower F-18 FDG uptake may be related to arrangement of fibrous stroma and mucin pool in tumor
      - Intrahepatic CCA is usually larger than extrahepatic CAA, making diagnosis of intrahepatic tumor more sensitive
      - Higher detection of nodular subtype CCA than periductal infiltrating subtype of extrahepatic CCA
    - Cirrhosis may affect hepatocytes, F-18 FDG metabolism and consequently diagnostic performance of F-18 FDG PET/CT
  - Detection of regional lymph node metastasis
    - Low sensitivity of F-18 PET/CT for detection of metastatic nodal disease
    - Metastatic nodal disease in CCA is associated with worse prognosis
    - High prevalence of lymphatic spread at time of gallbladder cancer diagnosis; however, F-18 FDG PET/CT sensitivity is poor
    - Superficial pathway of lymphatic drainage of the liver: Extensive and located beneath hepatobiliary capsule
      - Hepatoduodenal and gastrohepatic ligament pathway
      - Anterior, middle, posterior, and inferior diaphragmatic pathway
      - Falciform ligament pathway
    - Deep path of liver drainage
      - Portal pathway → hepatoduodenal ligament nodes
      - Hepatic vein pathway → juxtaphrenic and paraesophageal nodes
  - Detection of distant metastatic disease
    - F-18 FDG PET/CT may have role in detecting distant metastatic disease outside of liver with higher sensitivity than CT, making the difference in staging and treatment in 28-35%
  - Detection of recurrent disease
    - Some data supporting potential role of F-18 FDG PET/CT for detecting recurrence after treatment of HCC and CCA

Imaging Recommendations

- Best imaging tool
  - F-18 FDG PET/CT for staging distant metastases in hepatobiliary malignancy with clinical significance of 25-28%
  - Multiphase MR
    - 1st method for diagnosis of HCC
  - MRCP: Sensitivity of 71-81% for detection of CCA
  - ERCP: Could be diagnostic and therapeutic for bile obstruction in CCA
  - CECT: For staging of gallbladder or intrahepatic CCA

DIFFERENTIAL DIAGNOSIS

Hepatocellular Carcinoma (HCC)

- Can mimic intrahepatic CCA or advanced gallbladder cancer
- Most common hepatobiliary malignancy
- Associated risk factors
  - Chronic viral hepatitis B (leading cause in Asia and Africa) or C (leading cause in Europe, Japan, United States)
  - Inherited errors of metabolism: Hereditary hemochromatosis, porphyria cutanea tarda, α-1 antitrypsin deficiency, Wilson disease
  - Alcoholic cirrhosis,exposure to aflatoxin
  - Nonalcoholic steatohepatitis (NASH): US incidence 3-5%

Cholangiocarcinoma (CCA)

- Intrahepatic mass-like subtype can mimic HCC or advanced gallbladder cancer
- Second most common hepatobiliary malignancy
- Highest prevalence in Southeast Asia
- 5th-7th decade of life; M > F
- Risk factors

- Chronic biliary inflammation, primary sclerosing cholangitis (PSC), choledochal cyst
- Familial polyposis, hepatolithiasis, congenital hepatic fibrosis, fibropolycystic liver disease
- Exposure to *Opisthorchis viverrini*, *Clonorchis sinensis*, chronic typhoid carriers or Thorotrast (radiologic contrast agent used in 1960s)

Gallbladder Cancer

- Advanced presentation can mimic HCC or intrahepatic CCA
- More common in Central and South America, eastern Europe, Japan, northern India; more common in Native Americans, Hispanics
- F:M = 6:1
- Only 10% confined to gallbladder at discovery
- Incidentally found in 1-3% of cholecystectomies
- Risk factors
  - Gallstones > 3 cm, chronic cholecystitis, porcelain gallbladder, gallbladder polyps
  - PSC and congenital anomalous pancreaticobiliary duct junction
  - Obesity, diabetes, smoking

Solitary Metastasis of Unknown Primary or Liver Abscess

- Can be F-18 FDG PET/CT avid and simulate HCC or intrahepatic CCA

Hepatic Adenoma/Focal Nodular Hyperplasia/ Hepatic Epithelioid Hemangioendothelioma

- Case reports of F-18 FDG PET/CT uptake in focal nodular hyperplasia and hepatic adenoma
- Hepatic epithelioid hemangioendothelioma: Rare liver tumor with variable F-18 FDG uptake

Acute Cholecystitis/Primary Sclerosing Cholangitis/Ascending Cholangitis/Biliary Drainage or Stent

- Increased F-18 FDG uptake due to inflammatory/infectious process

Pancreatic Carcinoma/Ampullary Tumor/Duodenal Tumors

- Tumor of periampullary region can simulate a distal CCA, variable F-18 FDG uptake

PATHOLOGY

Staging, Grading, & Classification

- HCC
  - Stage I-III: Up to T4
  - Stage IVA: Any T, N1 (cystic duct, common bile duct, hepatic artery, portal vein, periaortic, pericaval, superior mesenteric artery, &/or celiac artery)
  - Stage IVB: Any T, any N, M1
- CCA
  - Intrahepatic bile ducts
    - Stage 0-III: Up to T3
    - Stage IVA: T4 or any T, N1 (cystic duct, common bile duct, hepatic artery, portal vein, periaortic, pericaval, superior mesenteric artery, &/or celiac artery)
    - Stage IVB: M1
  - Perihilar
    - Stage 0-IIIA: Up to T3
    - Stage IIIB: Up to T3, N1 (metastatic nodes along cystic duct, common bile duct, hepatic artery, portal vein)
    - Stage IVA: T4, N0-N1
    - Stage IVB: Any T, N2 (metastatic periaortic, pericaval, superior mesenteric artery, &/or celiac artery) or M1
  - Distal
    - Stage 0-IIA: Up to T3
    - Stage IIB: Up to T3, N1 (cystic duct, common bile duct, hepatic artery, portal vein, periaortic, pericaval, superior mesenteric artery, &/or celiac artery)
    - Stage III: T4, any N
    - Stage IV: M1
- Gallbladder cancer
  - Stage 0-IIIA: Up to T3
  - Stage IIIB: Up to T3, N1 (metastatic nodes along cystic duct, common bile duct, hepatic artery, portal vein)
  - Stage IVA: T4, N0-N1
  - Stage IVB: Any T, N2 (metastatic periaortic, pericaval, superior mesenteric artery, &/or celiac artery), or M1

CLINICAL ISSUES

Treatment

- HCC
  - Resectable
    - Child A: Surgical resection (surgery for Child B controversial, assess liver function)
  - Unresectable or Child C
    - Liver transplant candidate: Transplant but consider bridging therapy while waiting, e.g., ablation/transcatheter arterial chemoembolization (TACE)
    - Not liver transplant candidate, no metastasis: Ablation, TACE, stereotactic radiotherapy
    - Metastatic disease: Systemic therapy/supportive care
- CCA
  - Surgical resection: If no regional nodal or distant metastasis, no vascular or adjacent organ invasion
  - Not surgical candidate: Chemotherapy, radiotherapy, hepatic artery-based therapy for intrahepatic CCA , developing immunotherapy trials
- Gallbladder cancer
  - Surgical: Cholecystectomy (Tis-T1a), extended cholecystectomy (> T1a)
  - Locally advanced, not surgical: Chemotherapy, radiation therapy, supportive care

DIAGNOSTIC CHECKLIST

Consider

- F-18 FDG PET/CT for the detection of distant metastatic disease

SELECTED REFERENCES

1. Hennedige TP et al: Imaging of malignancies of the biliary tract- an update. Cancer Imaging. 14(1):14, 2014

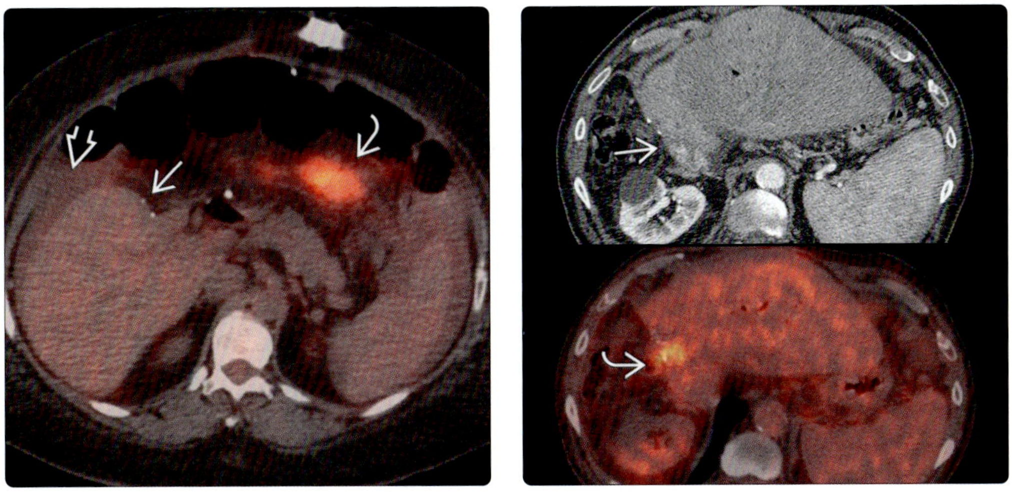

(Left) *Axial F-18 FDG PET/CT in a patient with intrahepatic CCA and partial liver resection shows no evidences of local recurrence ➔. However, hypermetabolic peritoneal implants ➔ and ascites ➔ suggests peritoneal spread of disease.* **(Right)** *Axial CECT in a patient with intrahepatic CCA and prior right hepatectomy is inconclusive for surgical margin recurrence ➔. Axial F-18 FDG PET/CT confirms local recurrence ➔.*

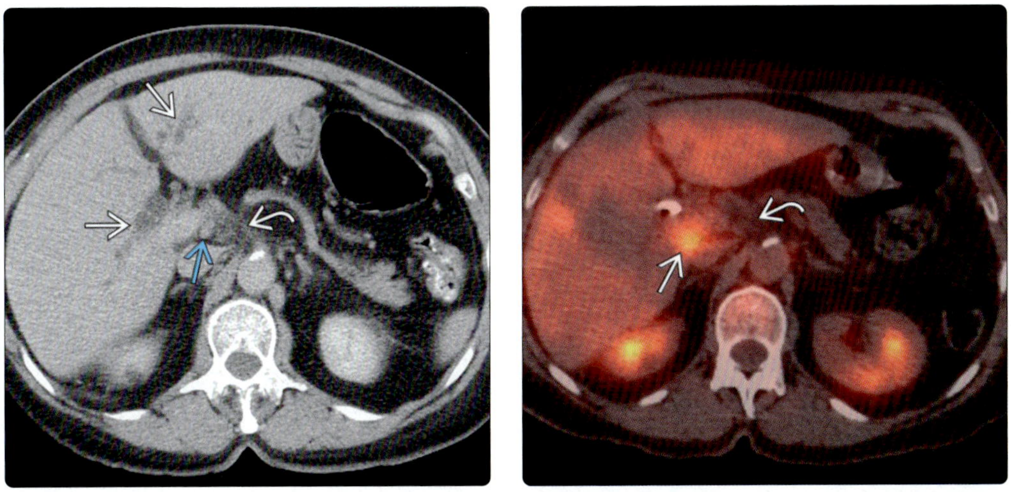

(Left) *Axial CECT shows Intrahepatic biliary ductal dilatation ➔, ill-defined soft tissue surrounding the celiac trunk ➔, and borderline-enlarged posterior periportal lymph nodes ➔. ERCP was performed and distal CCA diagnosed.* **(Right)** *Axial F-18 FDG PET/CT in the same patient shows hypermetabolic posterior portal node ➔. Note the tumor is not hypermetabolic ➔.*

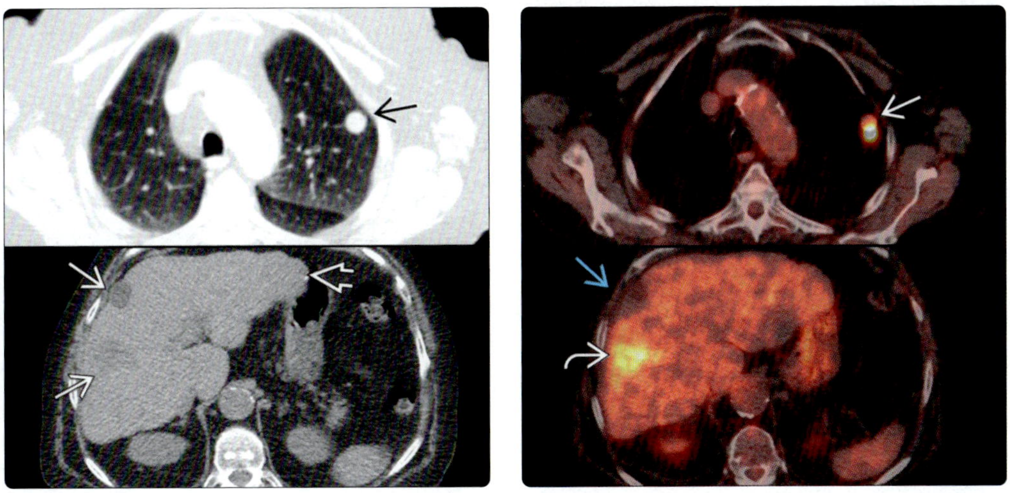

(Left) *Screening CT for lung cancer shows a pulmonary nodule ➔, subsequently proven to be adenocarcinoma. Cirrhotic morphology of the liver parenchyma ➔ and 2 liver lesions ➔ are concerning for metastases.* **(Right)** *Axial F-18 FDG PET/CT in the same patient shows hypermetabolic lung cancer ➔ and a large hypermetabolic mass ➔ shown to be poorly differentiated HCC on FNA. The 2nd lesion ➔ is benign and not hypermetabolic.*

Hodgkin Lymphoma

KEY FACTS

IMAGING

- Initial staging F-18 FDG PET/CT
  - Focal F-18 FDG uptake in lymph node (LN) or extranodal tissue spreading in contiguous fashion to other LN and viscera
  - Report findings pertinent to modified Ann Arbor staging criteria (e.g., disease above &/or below diaphragm)
    - Limited: Stage I and II ± limited extranodal disease
    - Advanced: Stage III and IV
- Interim or end-of-treatment F-18 FDG PET/CT
  - Report findings according to Deauville criteria 5-point scale
    - Score 1 and 2: Complete metabolic response (CMR)
    - Score 3: Likely CMR
    - Score 4-5: Residual disease
    - Score of 5 with no decrease in uptake or new FDG-avid disease: Treatment failure
- Recommended timing of post-treatment scan important to avoid misinterpretation of treatment-related uptake
  - 6-8 weeks after chemotherapy or surgery
  - 8-12 weeks after radiation therapy
  - 2-4 weeks after growth colony stimulating factor (G-CSF)

DIAGNOSTIC CHECKLIST

- Pitfalls in interpreting F-18 PET/CT often due to treatment-related, false-positive uptake (nonneoplastic), usually on post-therapy imaging
  - Diffuse bone marrow uptake related to administration of G-CSF or erythropoeitin
  - Flare phenomenon: FDG uptake due to inflammatory cells clearing dead tumor cells
  - Stunning of viable tumor cells (false-negative)
  - Low-level F-18 FDG uptake in enlarged thymus with post-treatment thymic rebound
  - Brown fat uptake (usually) symmetric in neck, paraspinal, supraclavicular, and mediastinal fat

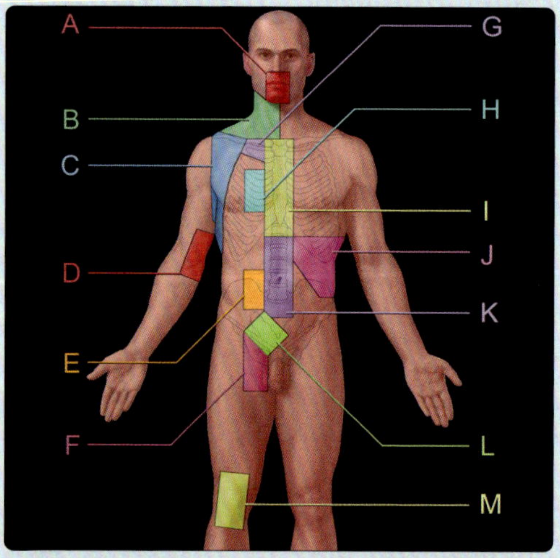

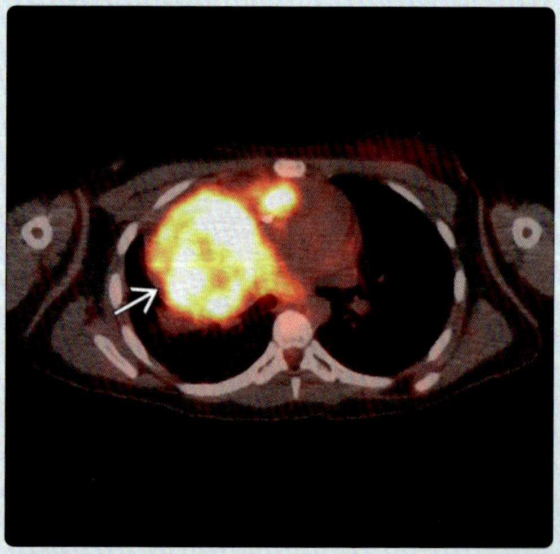

(Left) *Graphic shows lymph node regions: (A) Waldeyer ring (tonsils, base of tongue, nasopharynx), (B) cervical & supraclavicular, (C) axillary & subpectoral, (D) epitrochlear, (E) mesenteric, (F) inguinal & femoral, (G) infraclavicular, (H) hilar, (I) mediastinal, (J) spleen, (K) paraaortic, (L) iliac, (M) popliteal. Not labeled: Occipital & preauricular.* **(Right)** *Axial PET/CT of a patient with Hodgkin lymphoma (HL) shows a hypermetabolic, heterogeneous soft tissue mass ➡ in the right mediastinum.*

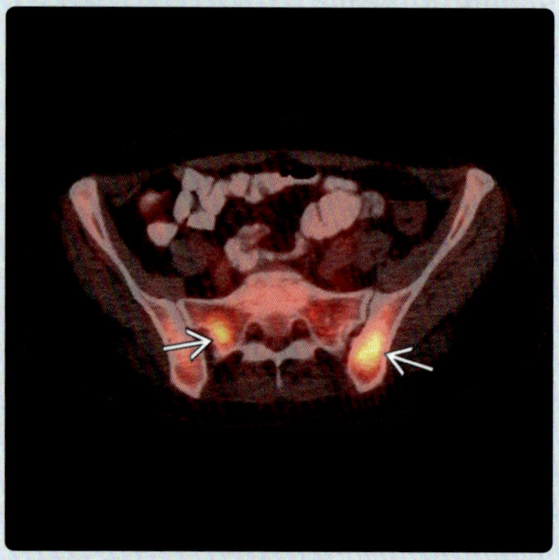

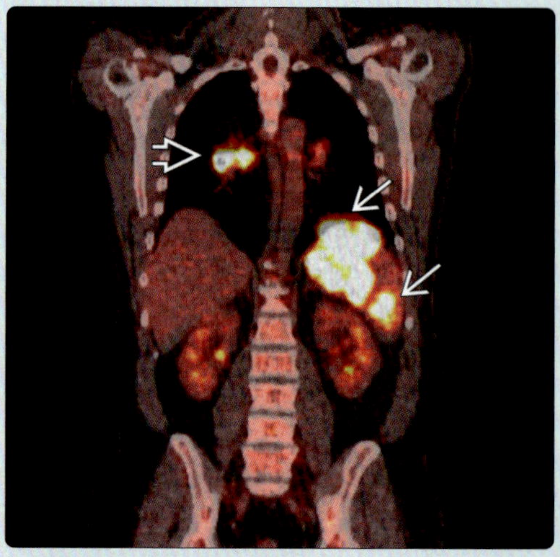

(Left) *Axial PET/CT shows multiple foci of osseous hypermetabolic activity ➡ in the pelvis in HL. These lesions did not have a correlating anatomic abnormality on the CT examination.* **(Right)** *Coronal PET/CT shows multiple areas of increased activity ➡ in the spleen and increased activity ➡ in right hilar lymph nodes compatible with stage III HL (nodal disease above and below diaphragm).*

TERMINOLOGY

Definitions

- Hodgkin lymphoma (HL): Malignancy of lymphocytes with Reed-Sternberg cells
  - Pathologic subtypes: Nodular sclerosis (most common), mixed cellularity, lymphocyte depleted, lymphocyte rich

IMAGING

General Features

- Best diagnostic clue
  - FDG PET/CT: Enlarged, hypermetabolic lymph nodes (LN) in one or more LN regions
    - Spreads in contiguous fashion to other LN, viscera, or bone marrow

Nuclear Medicine Findings

- PET/CT
  - **Initial staging PET/CT**
    - Focal uptake above physiologic background in nodal or extranodal tissue, bulky soft tissue mass ± central necrosis
    - Mediastinal blood pool is reference for background activity on attenuation corrected images
    - Report findings pertinent to modified Ann Arbor staging criteria
  - Nodal: Based on identification of uptake in LN regions in single radiation field
    - Thymus, mediastinal, internal mammary, and paravertebral LNs considered 1 region
    - Spleen and Waldeyer ring considered nodal tissue
      - Patterns of disease in spleen: Single or multifocal FDG-avid lesions, diffusely FDG avid (> liver), ± enlargement on CT
    - Femoral, inguinal, supraclavicular, infraclavicular, and cervical LN regions should be lateralized
    - Hilar LNs are separate LN regions from mediastinum and lateralized
  - Extranodal: Contiguous spread with eventual dissemination to distant sites and organs
    - Liver: Single or multiple FDG-avid lesions or diffuse uptake
    - Bone marrow: Focal site(s) of uptake or diffuse uptake often without corresponding anatomic lesion on CT
    - Unusual to have bone marrow and liver involvement without splenic disease
    - CNS: Can be missed on PET/CT due to background brain uptake and should be evaluated with MR
  - **Interim or post-therapy PET/CT: Deauville criteria**
    - Grades the most intense uptake (SUV) in initial site of disease on interim or end-of-treatment PET/CT
    - 1: No uptake
    - 2: Uptake ≤ mediastinal blood pool
    - 3: Uptake > mediastinal blood pool but ≤ liver
    - 4: Uptake moderately higher than liver
    - 5: Uptake markedly higher than liver &/or new lesions
    - X: New areas of uptake unlikely to be related to lymphoma
  - Score of 1 and 2: Complete metabolic response (CMR)
  - Score of 3: Likely a CMR
    - Considered inadequate response to avoid undertreatment in some clinical trials
  - Score 4 and 5: Residual hypermetabolic disease
    - Moderately vs. marked not yet well defined, but suggestions include
      - Moderately: Uptake > maximum SUV of normal liver
      - Marked: Uptake 2-3x > maximum SUV of normal liver
  - Score of 5 with no decrease in uptake or new FDG-avid disease: Treatment failure
  - Include SUV max of mediastinal blood pool and liver, as well as Deauville score in report

Imaging Recommendations

- Best imaging tool
  - F-18 FDG PET/CT (noncontrast, low-dose CT): More sensitive and specific than contrast CECT or PET alone for staging
    - CECT for radiation planning and anatomic delineation of cervical disease or mesenteric disease
  - Ga-67 replaced by more sensitive and specific F-18 FDG PET/CT for staging
  - MR if concern for CNS involvement
- Protocol advice
  - Knowledge of prior imaging & clinical information critical for accuracy of PET/CT interpretation
  - Initial staging exam should be performed prior to treatment
    - 1 dose of chemotherapy may decrease F-18 FDG uptake and sensitivity
  - Minimize brown fat/muscle uptake
    - Can pretreat with low-dose propranolol or diazepam
    - Keep patient warm and resting prior to and during uptake interval
  - Recommended timing of post-treatment scan important to avoid misinterpretation of nonneoplastic, treatment-related uptake
    - 6-8 weeks after chemotherapy or surgery
    - 8-12 weeks after radiation therapy
    - 2-4 weeks after G-CSF therapy

DIFFERENTIAL DIAGNOSIS

Granulomatous Process

- Infectious or noninfectious etiologies with uptake in areas of active disease on FDG PET
  - Infectious: Fungal (histoplasmosis, aspergillosis, etc.), mycobacterium TB, non-tuberculum mycobacterium
  - Noninfectious: Sarcoidosis, coal workers' pneumoconiosis

Infections

- Viral, fungal, pyogenic, parasitic, HIV-AIDS

Other Malignancy

- Lung cancer with mediastinal adenopathy, squamous cell cancer of the head and neck, etc.

Normal Lymphoid Tissue

- Normal uptake in thymic tissue or Waldeyer ring (can be mildly asymmetric)

- Thymic rebound with low-level F-18 FDG activity common after chemotherapy

Reactive Lymph Nodes

- Usually smaller than HL-affected LN

PATHOLOGY

Staging, Grading, & Classification

- **Ann Arbor staging system with Lugano modification:** Limited (stage I and II) and advanced (stage III and IV)
  - Stage I
    - 1 node or group of adjacent nodes (1 lymph node region) (I)
    - Single extranodal lesion without nodal involvement (IE)
  - Stage II
    - 2 or more nodal regions on the same side of the diaphragm (II)
    - Stage I or II by nodal extent + limited contiguous extranodal involvement (IIE)
    - Stage II "bulky": Above findings with nodal mass at least 10 cm or 1/3 of transthoracic diameter at any level
  - Stage III
    - Disease in lymph node regions on both sides of diaphragm
  - Stage IV
    - Nodal disease + noncontiguous extranodal involvement
- Modifiers
  - A or B: Absence ("A") or presence ("B") of B symptoms
  - E: Relevant only for limited extranodal disease in absence of nodal involvement (IE) or in patients with stage II disease and direct extension to a non-nodal site (IIE)

CLINICAL ISSUES

Presentation

- Most common signs/symptoms
  - Incidental mediastinal mass
  - Enlarged, nonpainful LNs &/or spleen
  - Systemic B symptoms: Unexplained fevers, drenching sweats, or weight loss
- Clinical profile
  - HIV-associated HL is aggressive and often with extranodal or bone marrow involvement
    - 10-20x increased incidence compared to non-HIV population

Demographics

- Epidemiology
  - Children and adults, but most common between 20-34 years (30% of cases annually)
  - < 1% of all cancer, ~ 9,000 new cases in USA annually, ~ 1,100 deaths/year
  - M:F ~ 3:2
  - Risk factors: Family history, history of Epstein-Barr virus infection, immunosuppression (Rx or HIV), and autoimmune disease

Natural History & Prognosis

- All stages: 5-year survival rate of 85%; localized disease (stage I) ~ 91%

Treatment

- Early stage disease (I or II): Treated with ChemoRx or ChemoRx + involved field XRT depending on case-specific prognosis
- Advanced disease (III, IV, ± II "bulky"): Usually treated with combination ChemoRx

DIAGNOSTIC CHECKLIST

Image Interpretation Pearls

- Knowledge of initial staging system and Deauville criteria critical to quality of imaging report
  - Include mediastinal blood pool and liver SUV max and Deauville score
- Pitfalls in interpreting F-18 FDG PET/CT often due to false-positive findings (nonneoplastic FDG uptake), usually on post-therapy imaging
  - Diffuse bone marrow uptake related to administration of growth colony stimulating factors (G-CSF) or erythropoeitin, which can last at least 4 weeks
  - Flare phenomenon: FDG uptake due to inflammatory cells clearing dead tumor cells
    - Can be avoided with proper timing of post-therapy exam
  - Stunning of viable tumor (false-negative): Less uptake in viable tumor cells due to altered glucose metabolism after therapy
    - Can be avoided with proper timing of post-therapy exam
  - Low-level F-18 FDG uptake in enlarged thymus with post-treatment thymic rebound
  - Brown fat uptake (usually) symmetric in neck, paraspinal, supraclavicular, and mediastinal fat
    - Benign finding that can obscure pathologic uptake in LN

SELECTED REFERENCES

1. Barrington SF et al: Role of imaging in the staging and response assessment of lymphoma: consensus of the International Conference on Malignant Lymphomas Imaging Working Group. J Clin Oncol. 32(27):3048-58, 2014
2. Cheson BD et al: Recommendations for initial evaluation, staging, and response assessment of Hodgkin and non-Hodgkin lymphoma: the Lugano classification. J Clin Oncol. 32(27):3059-68, 2014
3. Saboo SS et al: Spleen in haematological malignancies: spectrum of imaging findings. Br J Radiol. 85(1009):81-92, 2012
4. Cheson BD: Role of functional imaging in the management of lymphoma. J Clin Oncol. 29(14):1844-54, 2011
5. Paes FM et al: FDG PET/CT of extranodal involvement in non-Hodgkin lymphoma and Hodgkin disease. Radiographics. 30(1):269-91, 2010
6. Bower M et al: British HIV Association guidelines for HIV-associated malignancies 2008. HIV Med. 9(6):336-88, 2008
7. Schöder H et al: PET imaging for response assessment in lymphoma: potential and limitations. Radiol Clin North Am. 46(2):225-41, 2008
8. Raanani P et al: Is CT scan still necessary for staging in Hodgkin and non-Hodgkin lymphoma patients in the PET/CT era? Ann Oncol. 17(1):117-22, 2006
9. National Cancer Institute. SEER Stat Fact Sheets: Hodgkin Lymphoma. http://seer.cancer.gov/statfacts/html/hodg.html. Accessed July 31, 2015

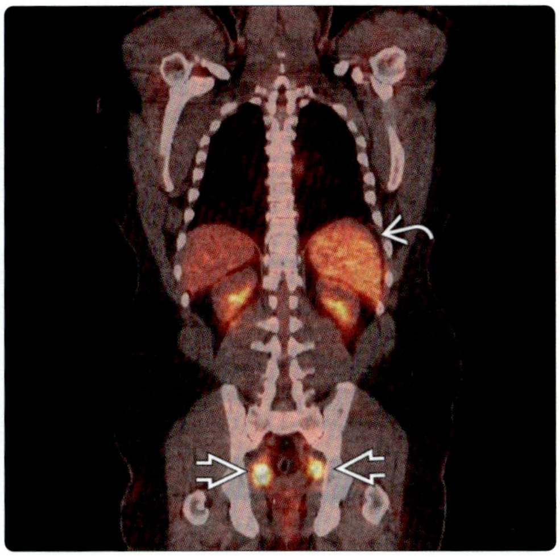

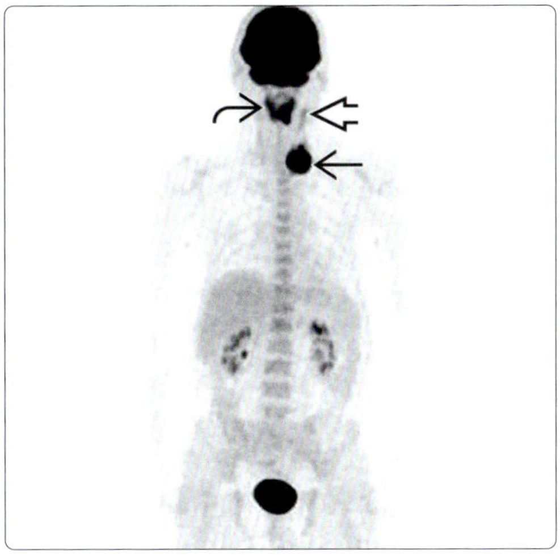

(Left) *Coronal PET/CT demonstrates diffuse uptake pattern of HL in the spleen and uptake in external iliac LNs.* **(Right)** *Anterior FDG PET shows tumor in left lower neck, Waldeyer tonsillar ring, and left upper cervical region. Multiple separate LN regions on same side of diaphragm represent stage II disease.*

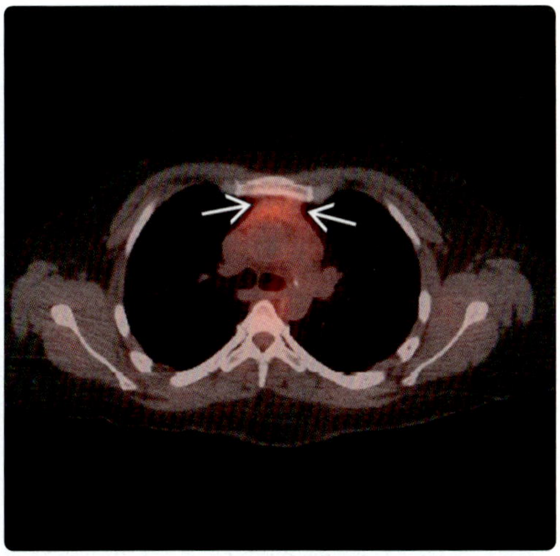

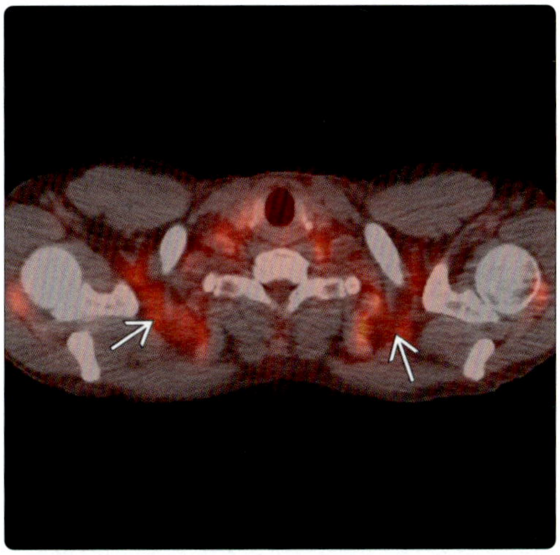

(Left) *Axial PET/CT in a 30-year-old patient shows uptake in the anterior mediastinal soft tissue, which reflected thymic rebound. Thymic uptake persisted while HL resolved on subsequent exam.* **(Right)** *Axial FDG PET/CT in a young patient with HL shows diffuse brown fat activity. This can occasionally obscure or be mistaken for malignant disease.*

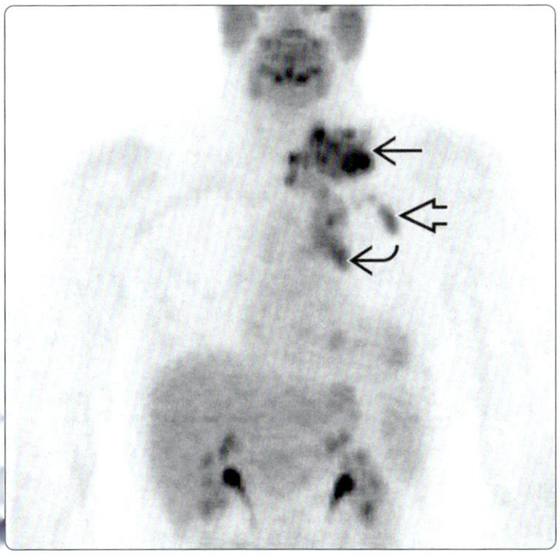

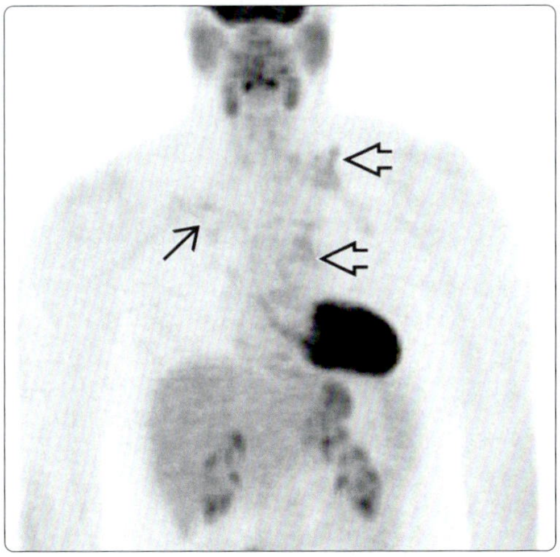

(Left) *Anterior FDG PET shows increased uptake in the left supraclavicular and cervical regions, mediastinum, and subpectoral regions compatible with stage II disease.* **(Right)** *The same patient was imaged 4 days following placement of right Port-A-Cath and single dose of ChemoRx. Tumor metabolism has dropped dramatically, showing the importance of PET/CT staging prior to any treatment. This is an example of Deauville score 3 with residual disease SUV > mediastinal blood pool and ≤ liver.*

KEY FACTS

IMAGING

- Initial staging F-18 FDG PET/CT
  - Focal F-18 FDG uptake in lymph nodes (LN) ± enlargement and involvement of extranodal tissues/organs
    - Hematogenous spread of NHL is unpredictable in comparison to contiguous spread of HL
  - Report findings pertinent to modified Ann Arbor staging criteria (e.g., disease above &/or below diaphragm)
    - Focus on limited vs. advanced disease stage for treatment guidance
- Interim or end-of-treatment F-18 FDG PET/CT
  - Report findings according to Deauville criteria (5-point scale)
    - Score 1 and 2: Complete metabolic response (CMR)
    - Score 3: Likely CMR
    - Score 4 and 5: Residual disease
    - Score 5 with no decrease in uptake or new FDG-avid disease: Treatment failure

DIAGNOSTIC CHECKLIST

- Knowledge of initial staging system and Deauville criteria critical to quality of imaging report
- PET/CT reliably detects aggressive, high-grade disease, but is less sensitive for indolent lymphoma
  - If concern exists for aggressive transformation of indolent disease, PET/CT can be useful
- Staging PET/CT must be done prior to initiation of therapy
  - Even 1 dose of ChemoRx may decrease sensitivity
- Pitfalls in interpreting PET/CT often due to false-positive findings (nonneoplastic FDG uptake), usually on post-therapy imaging
- Recommended timing of post-treatment scan important to avoid misinterpretation of nonneoplastic, treatment-related FDG uptake
  - 6-8 weeks after ChemoRx or surgery
  - 8-12 weeks after radiation therapy
  - 2-4 weeks after G-CSF therapy or erythropoietin

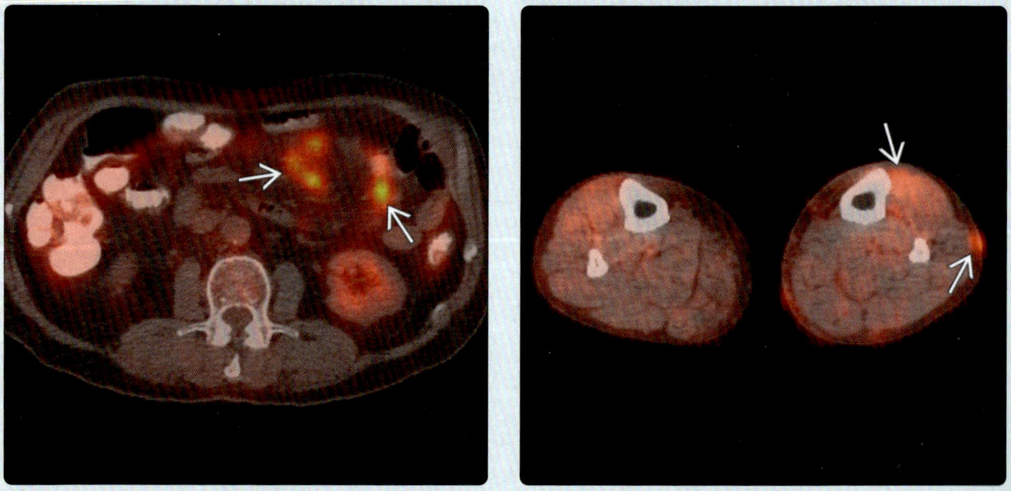

(Left) *Axial FDG PET/CT shows hypermetabolic LNs in the jejunal mesentery with → areas of ill-defined stranding or "misty mesentery" in NHL.* **(Right)** *Axial FDG PET/CT in a patient with DLBCL shows increased activity within the superficial soft tissues of the leg → consistent with extranodal involvement.*

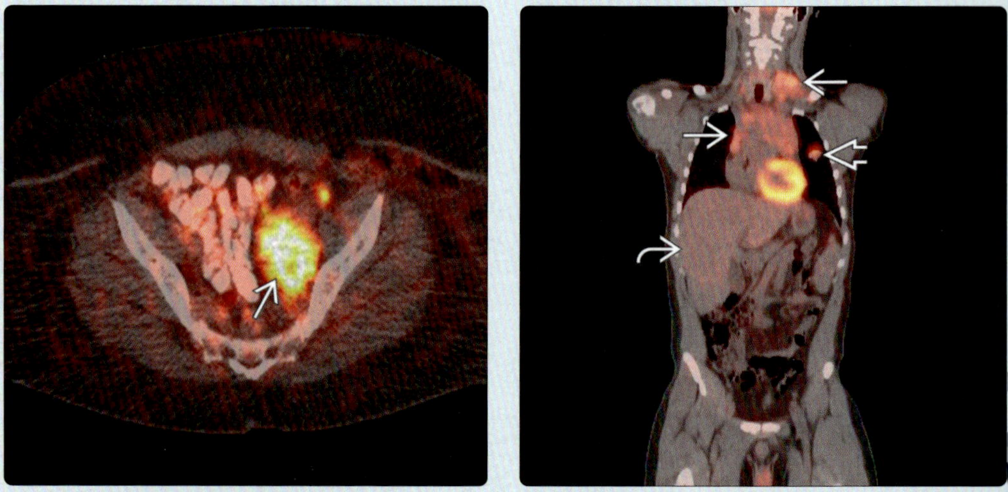

(Left) *Axial FDG PET/CT in a patient with DLBCL shows a large, hypermetabolic nodal conglomerate in the left pelvis →.* **(Right)** *Coronal FDG PET/CT shows enlarged FDG-avid mediastinal, supraclavicular, and cervical LNs → and a lung lesion → in NHL. Diffuse, increased liver uptake → and mild hepatomegaly suggests liver involvement.*

TERMINOLOGY

Definitions

- Non-Hodgkin lymphoma (NHL)
  - Broad category of T-cell and B-cell malignancies with a diverse range of disease

IMAGING

General Features

- Best diagnostic clue
  - FDG-avid lymph nodes (LN) ± enlargement and involvement of extranodal tissues/organs
- Location
  - Hematogenous spread makes NHL pattern more unpredictable than HL (usually contiguous spread)
  - ~ 1/2 present with mixed nodal and extranodal disease and ~ 1/4 present with isolated extranodal disease
  - When primarily nodal disease, extranodal involvement is often, but not exclusively, seen at certain sites: Spleen, liver, kidney, lung, bone, and bone marrow
  - Isolated extranodal disease has different range of extranodal sites: GI tract, GU (including ovaries and testes), thyroid, bone, brain, kidney, liver, breast, skin, thymus, sinonasal, Waldeyer ring, and CNS

Nuclear Medicine Findings

- PET/CT
  - Initial staging F-18 FDG PET/CT: Report findings pertinent to local or advanced disease staging (modified Ann Arbor staging criteria)
    - ↑ uptake in nodal or extranodal tissue above background
    - Mediastinal blood pool is reference for background activity on attenuation-corrected images
    - "Misty mesentery": Stranding in mesentery commonly associated with NHL ± enlarged mesenteric LNs
      - Sometimes seen after ChemoRx and limited to mesentery, which contained LNs (vs. systemic causes of mesenteric stranding)
  - Post-therapy or interim exam: Report Deauville criteria
    - Grades most intense uptake (SUV) at initial site of disease on interim or end-of-treatment PET/CT
    - 1: No uptake
    - 2: Uptake ≤ mediastinal blood pool
    - 3: Uptake > mediastinal blood pool but ≤ liver
    - 4: Uptake moderately higher than liver
    - 5: Uptake markedly higher than liver &/or new lesions
    - X: New areas of uptake unlikely to be related to lymphoma
    - Score of 1 and 2: Complete metabolic response (CMR)
    - Score of 3: Likely a CMR
      - Considered inadequate response to avoid undertreatment in some clinical trials
    - Score of 4 or 5: Residual hypermetabolic disease
    - Moderate vs. marked not yet well defined, but suggestions include
      - Moderate: Uptake > maximum SUV of normal liver
      - Marked: Uptake 2-3x > maximum SUV of normal liver
    - Score of 5 with no decrease in uptake or development of new FDG-avid disease: Treatment failure
    - Include SUV max of mediastinal blood pool and liver and Deauville score in report
  - Pitfalls in interpreting PET/CT often due to false-positive findings (nonneoplastic FDG uptake), usually on post-therapy imaging
    - Low-level FDG uptake in enlarged thymus with post-treatment thymic rebound
    - Diffuse bone marrow uptake related to administration of growth colony stimulating factor (G-CSF) or erythropoietin
    - Flare phenomenon: FDG uptake due to inflammatory cells clearing dead tumor cells
    - Stunning of viable tumor (false-negative): Less uptake in viable tumor cells due to altered glucose metabolism after therapy
    - Benign brown fat uptake (usually) symmetric in neck, paraspinal, supraclavicular, and mediastinal fat

Imaging Recommendations

- Best imaging tool
  - F-18 FDG PET/CT (noncontrast, low-dose CT) preferred for staging FDG-avid NHL over other modalities
    - Aggressive NHL is FDG-avid and reliably detected on PET/CT
    - Less sensitive for indolent lymphoma, which should be staged with CECT
    - Increased sensitivity for aggressive transformation of indolent lymphoma
      - Richter transformation: Transformation of slow-growing chronic lymphocytic lymphoma (CLL) into aggressive diffuse large B-cell lymphoma (DLBCL)
  - Ga-67 replaced by more sensitive and specific FDG PET
  - CECT used for radiation planning and anatomic delineation of cervical or mesenteric disease
- Protocol advice
  - Initial staging with PET/CT before any therapy is administered: 1 dose of chemotherapy may ↓ FDG uptake
  - Recommended timing of post-treatment scan important to avoid misinterpretation of nonneoplastic, treatment-related FDG uptake
    - 6-8 weeks after ChemoRx or surgery
    - 8-12 weeks after radiation therapy
    - 2-4 weeks after G-CSF therapy or erythropoietin
  - Minimize brown fat/muscle uptake
    - Can pretreat with low-dose propranolol or diazepam
    - Keep patient warm and resting prior to and during uptake interval

DIFFERENTIAL DIAGNOSIS

Normal Structures

- Thymus, salivary glands, muscle, tonsils, and testes can have normal, mildly asymmetric uptake

Reactive Lymph Nodes

- Usually smaller than NHL-affected lymph nodes

Other Malignancy

- Lung cancer with mediastinal adenopathy, squamous cell cancer of head and neck, etc.

Infection

- Viral, fungal, pyogenic, parasitic, HIV-AIDS

Granulomatous Process

- Infectious: Fungal (histoplasmosis, aspergillosis, etc.), mycobacterium TB, non-tuberculum mycobacterium
- Noninfectious: Sarcoidosis, coal worker's pneumoconiosis

PATHOLOGY

General Features

- Etiology
  - Unknown in most patients

Ann Arbor Staging System With Lugano Modification

- Treatment decisions based on staging with strong emphasis on categorizing as limited or advanced disease
- Limited (stage I and II)
  - 1 LN or group of adjacent LNs (LN region) (I)
  - Single extranodal lesion without nodal disease (IE)
  - 2 or more LN regions on same side of diaphragm (II)
  - Stage I or II by nodal extent + localized extranodal (IIE)
- Advanced (stage III and IV)
  - LN regions on both sides of diaphragm (III)
  - Noncontiguous extranodal disease (IV)

Classification

- Can be categorized based on FDG avidity for imaging purposes
  - High-grade, aggressive disease usually high FDG avidity
    - Diffuse large B-cell (DLBCL), Burkitt lymphoma, anaplastic large cell, natural killer/T-cell, high-grade follicular, adult T cell, peripheral T cell
  - Low-grade, indolent disease often low or variable FDG avidity
    - Chronic lymphocytic leukemia/small lymphocytic (CLL), Waldenström macroglobulinemia, cutaneous T cell (mycosis fungoides), marginal zone (MZL), mantle cell, low-grade follicular
    - Wide range of avidity in MZL in 3 distinct subtypes: Extranodal mucosa-associated lymphoid tissue (MALT) type, nodal MZL, and splenic MZL
      - MALT type: Poorly seen on PET/CT when arising from GI tract because of normal GI uptake; however, can be detected when in salivary glands, lung, thyroid, skin, etc.

CLINICAL ISSUES

Presentation

- Most common signs/symptoms
  - Highly variable and depends on aggressiveness of lymphoma
    - Aggressive: Quickly growing mass, B symptoms (unexplained persistent fever, night sweats, fatigue, weight loss)
    - Indolent: Slowly growing lymphadenopathy, hepatosplenomegaly, ± B symptoms
    - Commonly asymptomatic or incidental finding

Demographics

- Epidemiology
  - M > F; most commonly Caucasian
  - Usually age 65-74
  - < 4% of all cancer, ~ 70,000 new cases and ~ 19,000 deaths in 2014

Natural History & Prognosis

- Prognosis depends on histologic type, stage and Rx
  - 5-year survival 82% for localized vs. 62% for advanced

Treatment

- Watchful waiting: Indolent lymphomas may be followed with no Rx until B symptoms
- Can Rx early indolent NHL with radiation therapy
- Intensive combination ChemoRx can be curative with aggressive lymphoma

DIAGNOSTIC CHECKLIST

Consider

- Localized uptake to an unusual site may represent NHL, but infection/inflammation must be excluded

Image Interpretation Pearls

- Knowledge of initial staging system and Deauville criteria critical to quality of imaging report
  - Include SUV max of mediastinal blood pool and liver and Deauville score
- PET/CT reliably detects aggressive, high-grade disease, but is less sensitive for indolent lymphoma
  - If concern exists for aggressive transformation of indolent disease, PET/CT can be useful
- Staging PET/CT must be done prior to initiation of therapy: Even 1 dose of ChemoRx may decrease sensitivity

SELECTED REFERENCES

1. Barrington SF et al: Role of imaging in the staging and response assessment of lymphoma: consensus of the International Conference on Malignant Lymphomas Imaging Working Group. J Clin Oncol. 32(27):3048-58, 2014
2. Cheson BD et al: Recommendations for initial evaluation, staging, and response assessment of Hodgkin and non-Hodgkin lymphoma: the Lugano classification. J Clin Oncol. 32(27):3059-68, 2014
3. Paes FM et al: FDG PET/CT of extranodal involvement in non-Hodgkin lymphoma and Hodgkin disease. Radiographics. 30(1):269-91, 2010
4. Weiler-Sagie M et al: (18)F-FDG avidity in lymphoma readdressed: a study of 766 patients. J Nucl Med. 51(1):25-30, 2010
5. Schöder H et al: PET Imaging for Response Assessment in Lymphoma: Potential and Limitations. Radiol Clin North Am. 46(2):225-41, 2008
6. Jhanwar YS et al: The role of PET in lymphoma. J Nucl Med. 47(8):1326-34, 2006
7. Raanani P et al: Is CT scan still necessary for staging in Hodgkin and non-Hodgkin lymphoma patients in the PET/CT era? Ann Oncol. 17(1):117-22, 2006
8. SEER Stat Fact Sheets: Non-Hodgkin Lymphoma

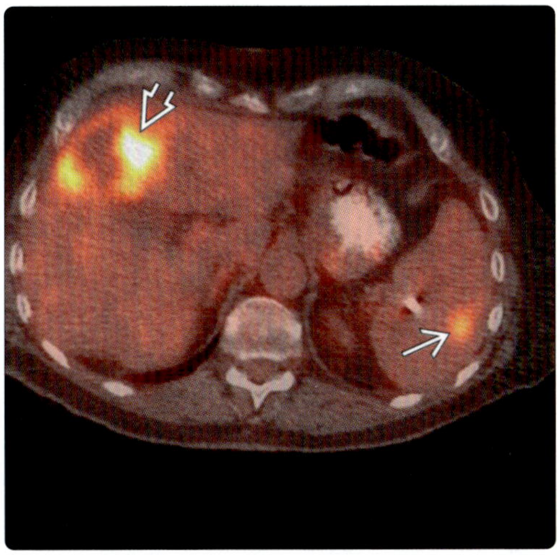

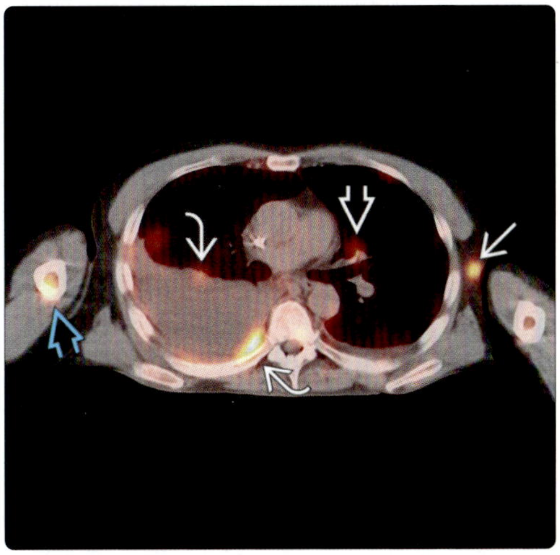

(Left) *Axial FDG PET/CT in a patient with aggressive transformation of CLL to DLBCL shows a hypermetabolic lesion in the liver and a smaller lesion in the spleen.* **(Right)** *Axial FDG PET/CT shows NHL involving the bone , pleura , axillary LN , and left hilar LN consistent with disseminated disease.*

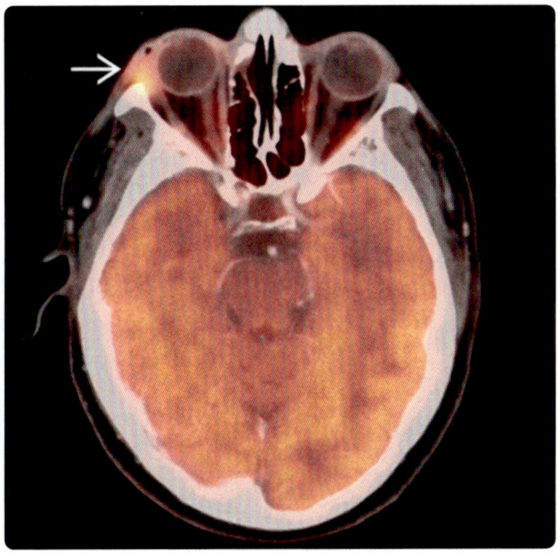

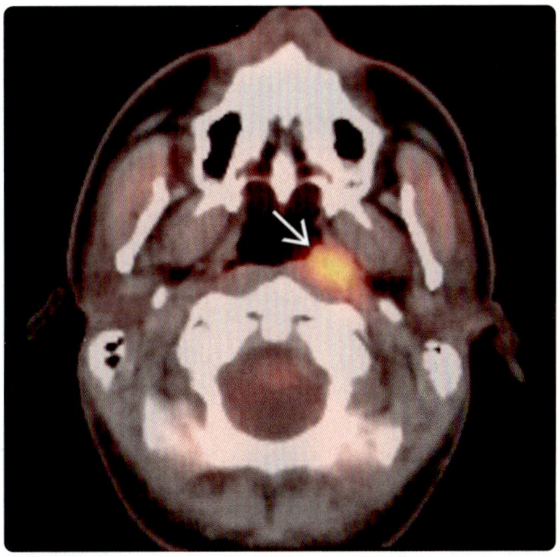

(Left) *Axial FDG PET/CT shows focal uptake and enlargement of the right lacrimal gland in a patient with NHL of the lacrimal gland.* **(Right)** *Axial FDG PET/CT shows asymmetric hypermetabolic tissue involving Waldeyer ring in MALT lymphoma.*

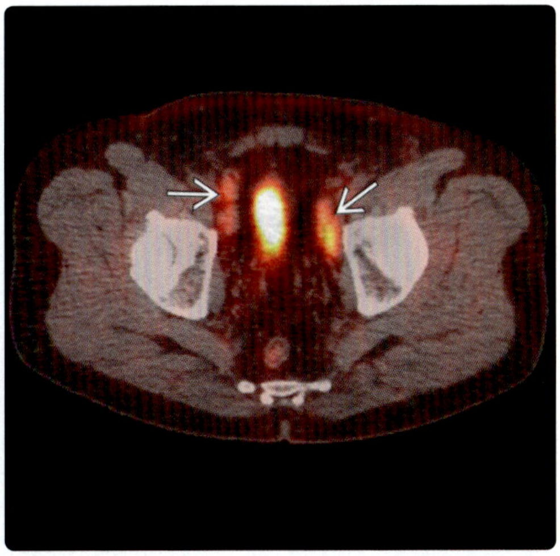

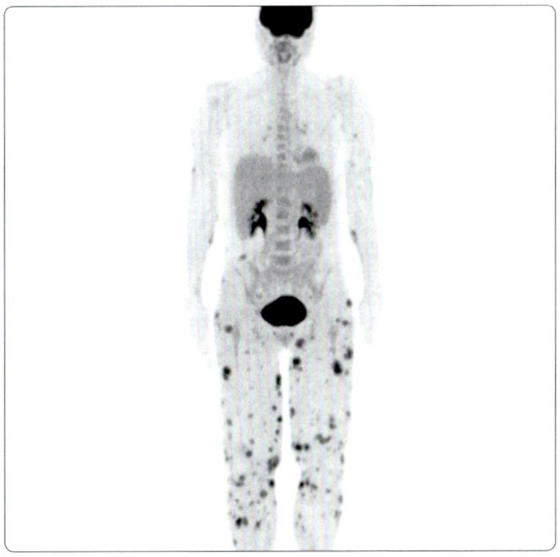

(Left) *Axial FDG PET/CT in a patient with follicular lymphoma shows bilateral hypermetabolic pelvic lymphadenopathy .* **(Right)** *Frontal MIP FDG PET demonstrates widespread subcutaneous tumor foci in a patient with peripheral T-cell lymphoma, which was FDG avid.*

Multiple Myeloma

KEY FACTS

TERMINOLOGY

- Multiple myeloma (MM): Malignant neoplasm of plasma cells in bone marrow

IMAGING

- Obtain F-18 FDG PET/CT from top of head to toes
- F-18 FDG PET/CT useful for initial diagnosis and staging (55-90% sensitivity) and restaging
- Restaging F-18 FDG PET/CT best performed ≥ 2 (preferably 4) weeks after chemotherapy cycle completion
- Limited sensitivity of F-18 FDG PET/CT in detecting diffuse bone marrow disease; MR is more sensitive

TOP DIFFERENTIAL DIAGNOSES

- Metastasis, osteopenia, osteoporosis, primary bone tumors, hematological malignancies

CLINICAL ISSUES

- Most common primary bone cancer (annual age-adjusted incidence ~ 4 cases/100,000)
- Poor prognostic factors
  - Presence of ≥ 3 lesions on baseline F-18 FGD PET/CT or ≥ 7 lesions on baseline MR, SUV max > 4.2, presence of extramedullary disease (5x higher risk), high-risk cytogenetic profile on gene expression profiling
  - Increase in number of focal lesions (not size) indicates poor prognosis
- High F-18 FDG uptake (SUV > 3.5) and diffuse or multifocal vertebral involvement by MR can indicate impending pathological fracture

DIAGNOSTIC CHECKLIST

- F-18 FDG PET/CT
  - To stage and establish baseline for monitoring therapy (especially in nonsecretory myeloma)
  - Important to localize plasmacytoma, differentiate tumor from normal structures
  - Most accurate imaging test in establishing disease activity

(Left) *Sagittal graphic shows lytic lesions in the distal femur →. Multiple myeloma may involve critical weight-bearing bones and result in pathologic fractures.* **(Right)** *Posterior MIP F-18 FDG PET in a patient with multiple myeloma shows multifocal skeletal and extraskeletal hypermetabolic activity. Note the focal lesions in the femoral necks bilaterally that are at risk for pathological fracture →.*

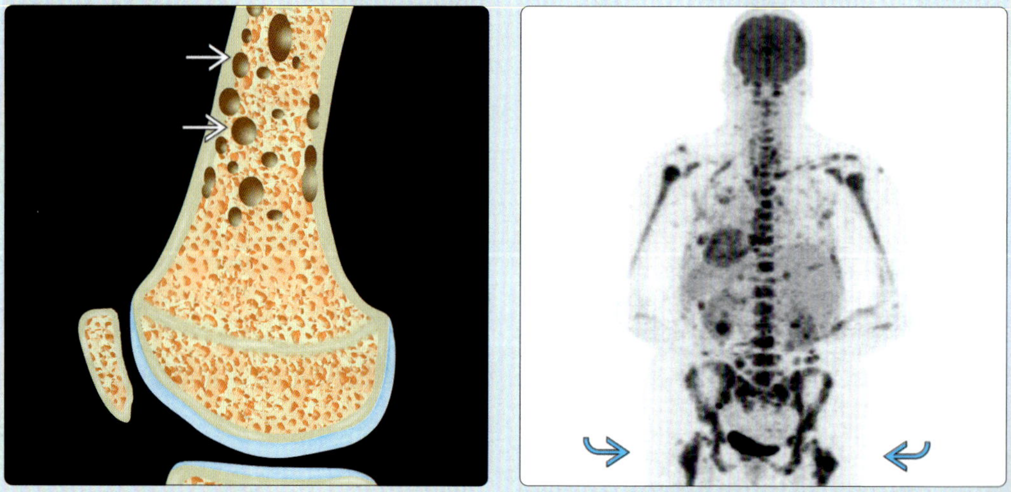

(Left) *Midline sagittal MIP F-18 FDG PET in a patient with multiple myeloma shows multifocal skeletal and extraskeletal hypermetabolic activity. Note the compression fractures of multiple vertebral bodies →.* **(Right)** *Midline sagittal fused F-18 FDG PET/CT in a patient with multiple myeloma shows multifocal skeletal and extraskeletal → hypermetabolic activity. Note the compression fractures of multiple vertebral bodies → that are better demonstrated on a fused PET/CT.*

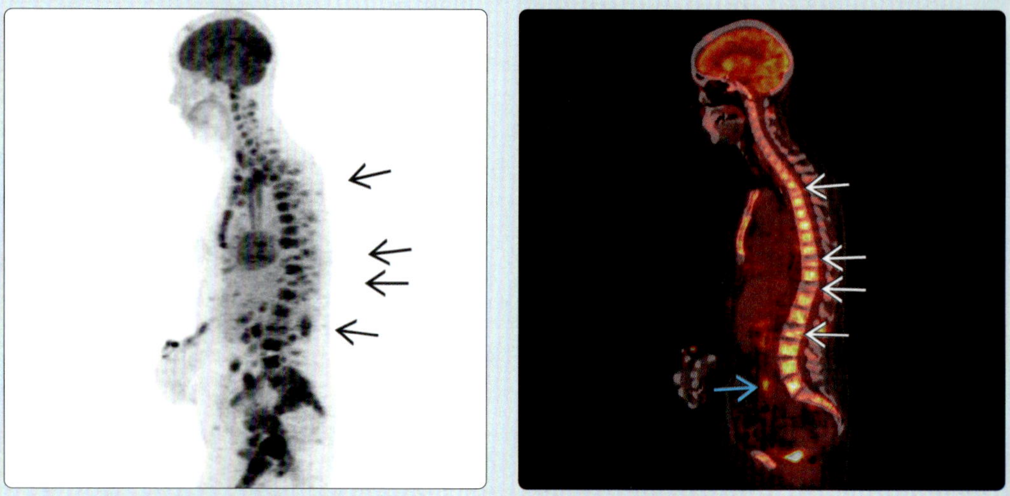

TERMINOLOGY

Definitions

- Multiple myeloma (MM): Malignant neoplasm of plasma cells in bone marrow
  - Smoldering (asymptomatic) MM
    - Elevated M-protein in serum (IgG or IgA ≥ 3 g/dL), or Bence-Jones protein ≥ 500 mg/24 &/or bone marrow clonal plasma cells 10-60%, no end-organ damage, no bone lesions, no amyloidosis
  - Active (symptomatic) MM
    - 1 or more of the following: Myeloma-related organ dysfunction (CRAB criteria), bone marrow clonal plasma cells > 60%; > 1 focal lesion (≥ 5 mm) on MR
- Diagnosis of myeloma
  - At least 10% clonal bone marrow plasma cells
  - Serum or urinary monoclonal protein
- Myeloma-related organ dysfunction (CRAB criteria)
  - Increased serum calcium (> 11.5 mg/dL), renal insufficiency (creatinine > 2 mg/dL), anemia (hemoglobin < 10 g/dL), bone disease (lytic lesions, severe osteopenia, or pathological fracture)
- Monoclonal gammopathy of undetermined significance (MGUS)
  - Elevated M-protein, bone marrow clonal plasma cells < 10%, no end-organ damage
- Solitary plasmacytoma
  - Solitary bone or soft tissue lesion without marrow clonal plasma cell proliferation, no end-organ damage

IMAGING

General Features

- Best diagnostic clue
  - Focal hypermetabolic lytic bone lesion or extramedullary site on F-18 FDG PET/CT
- Location
  - Bone marrow and bone (97%)
  - Extramedullary sites: Liver, lymph nodes, pleura, testis, skin, nasopharynx, tonsils, paranasal sinuses
  - Less common sites: Lung, spleen, liver
- Morphology
  - Diffuse marrow infiltration
  - Focal bone lesions
  - Breakout lesions: Cortical disruption of osseous lesions
  - Soft tissue extramedullary disease (EMD)

Nuclear Medicine Findings

- Tc-99m MDP bone scan
  - Sensitivity for lesion detection: 75-85%
  - Sensitivity best for cortical lesions with reactive bone formation
  - Poor sensitivity for lytic or trabecular lesions
  - False-positives in trauma, infection, degenerative disease
  - Poor test to evaluate status of disease activity
- F-18 FDG PET/CT
  - Useful for initial diagnosis and staging (55-90% sensitivity) and restaging
    - Diffuse marrow uptake on PET/CT usually indicates elevated plasma cell population
    - Negative whole-body PET/CT in patients with monoclonal gammopathy reliably identifies stable MGUS
  - Limited sensitivity in detecting diffuse bone marrow disease; MR is more sensitive
  - More sensitive as compared to MR for extramedullary disease (sensitivity: 96%, specificity: 78%)
    - Associated with advanced disease and poor prognosis
    - Clinically and radiographically detected in 10-16% patients, at autopsy in 63% patients
    - More common in younger patients
    - More aggressive myeloma types (nonsecretory myeloma, IgD myeloma, poorly differentiated), rapidly progressive, treatment resistant
    - Greater frequency with increasing duration of disease
  - Tracer uptake patterns: Focal, multifocal, diffuse, and mixed
  - Diffuse marrow hyperplasia can mimic marrow infiltration by myeloma
  - False-negative F-18 FDG PET/CT: High-dose steroid administration (within 10 days)
  - Reliable predictor of prognosis
    - Complete F-18 FDG response before stem cell transplant associated with higher overall (92%) and event-free (89%) survival
  - Assessment of treatment response
    - Functional changes (F-18 FDG uptake) precede morphological changes
    - Negative PET 60 days following stem cell transplant associated with excellent prognosis
    - Persistent F-18 FDG activity following induction therapy associated with early relapse
    - Particularly useful in nonsecretory myeloma
  - Early identification of disease recurrence or progression
    - Patients with relapse often found to have new sites of disease
    - Identification of target site for biopsy
  - Radiation therapy planning
  - PET exceptionally useful in monitoring disease activity in patients with nonsecretory myeloma
  - Detection of occult infection
  - False-negative
    - Suppression of tumor metabolism due to recent treatment

Imaging Recommendations

- Best imaging tool
  - F-18 FDG PET/CT with oral and IV CT contrast
- Protocol advice
  - Whole-body scan: Obtain PET/CT from top of head to toes
  - Use oral and IV contrast if renal function permits (creatinine < 1.5)
    - Renal dysfunction common due to high levels of proteins produced by malignant plasma cells, which affect renal tubules
  - Marrow stimulant drugs may mask underlying MM lesions
  - Restaging PET/CT best performed ≥ 2 (preferably 4) weeks after chemotherapy cycle completion

DIFFERENTIAL DIAGNOSIS

Lytic Skeletal Metastases

- Lung, breast, prostate, thyroid cancer, renal cell carcinoma

Osteopenia and Osteoporosis

- Increased radiolucency of bone, decreased bone mineral density due to number of causes

Other Bone and Soft Tissue Malignancy

- Lymphoma
- Primary bone tumors (chondrosarcoma, osteosarcoma, fibrosarcoma)

Other Hematological Malignancies

- Leukemia
- Plasma cell leukemia

PATHOLOGY

Staging, Grading, & Classification

- Durie-Salmon staging system
  - Stage I: All of the following
    - Normal metastatic bone survey (MBS) or solitary bone plasmacytoma
    - Hb >10 g/dL
    - Serum M-protein levels: < 50 g/L for IgG; < 30g/L for IgA
    - Urine light-chain M-component < 4 g/24 hour
    - Normal serum calcium (≤ 12 mg/dL)
  - Stage II: Imaging findings and laboratory values between stage I and III
  - Stage III: 1 or more of the following
    - Hb < 8.5 g/dL
    - Serum calcium > 12 mg/dL
    - ≥ 3 lytic bone lesions
    - Serum M-protein levels: > 70 g/L for IgG; > 50g/L for IgA
    - Urine light-chain M-component < 12 g/24 hour
  - A: Serum creatinine < 2.0 mg/dL
  - B: Serum creatinine ≥ 2.0 mg/dL &/or EMD on MR or F-18 FDG PET/CT
- International staging system (ISS)
  - ISS I: Albumin ≥35 g/L, beta-2 microglobulin < 3.5 mg/L
  - ISS II: Laboratory values between ISS I and ISS III
  - ISS III: beta-2 microglobulin ≥ 5.5 mg/L
- Durie-Salmon plus staging system (MR or F-18 FDG PET/CT)
  - Stage I: 0-4 focal lesions or mild diffuse marrow disease
  - Stage II: 5-20 focal lesions or moderate diffuse marrow disease
  - Stage III: > 20 focal lesions or severe diffuse marrow disease

Pathophysiology

- Complex interaction between tumor and bone microenvironment
- Osteoclast stimulation and osteoblast inhibition
- Destruction of osteoblast progenitors by Dickkopf 1 protein secreted by myeloma cells
  - Focal osteolytic myeloma lesions never heal

CLINICAL ISSUES

Demographics

- Age
  - Median age at diagnosis: 69 years
- Epidemiology
  - Most common primary bone cancer (annual age-adjusted incidence ~ 4 cases/100,000)
  - 1.4% of all new cancer cases in US
  - 1.9% of all cancer deaths in US

Natural History & Prognosis

- 10-year survival rate (patients presenting at age younger than 60): 30%
- Overall median survival: 3 years
- Relapsing or refractory patients with EMD at baseline = poor prognosis (median survival: < 1 year)
- Poor prognostic factors
  - Presence of ≥ 3 lesions on baseline F-18 FDG PET/CT or ≥ 7 lesions on base line MR, SUV max > 4.2, presence of EMD (5x higher risk), high-risk cytogenetic profile on gene expression profiling
- Increase in number of focal lesions (not size) indicates poor prognosis
  - Surrogate marker for tumor heterogeneity
  - Increased risk for development of resistance to treatment
- High F-18 FDG uptake (SUV > 3.5) and diffuse or multifocal vertebral involvement by MR can indicate impending pathological fracture

Treatment

- Usually therapy includes alkylating agents and steroids
- Thalidomide or lenalidomide often added to regimen to suppress tumor vascularity
- Stem cell transplantation
- Future directions
  - Antibody therapy may remove osteoblastic inhibition resulting in lesion healing

DIAGNOSTIC CHECKLIST

Consider

- F-18 FDG PET/CT to stage and establish baseline for monitoring therapy (especially in nonsecretory myeloma)

Image Interpretation Pearls

- Negative F-18 FDG PET/CT in patient with monoclonal gammopathy = excellent prognosis
- F-18 FDG PET/CT
  - Important to localize plasmacytoma, differentiate tumor from normal structures
  - Most accurate imaging test in establishing disease activity

SELECTED REFERENCES

1. Mesguich C et al: State of the art imaging of multiple myeloma: Comparative review of FDG PET/CT imaging in various clinical settings. Eur J Radiol. ePub, 2014
2. van de Donk NW et al: Diagnosis and Risk Stratification in Multiple Myeloma. Hematol Oncol Clin North Am. 28(5):791-813, 2014
3. Padhani AR et al: Assessing the relation between bone marrow signal intensity and apparent diffusion coefficient in diffusion-weighted MRI. AJR Am J Roentgenol. 200(1):163-70, 2013

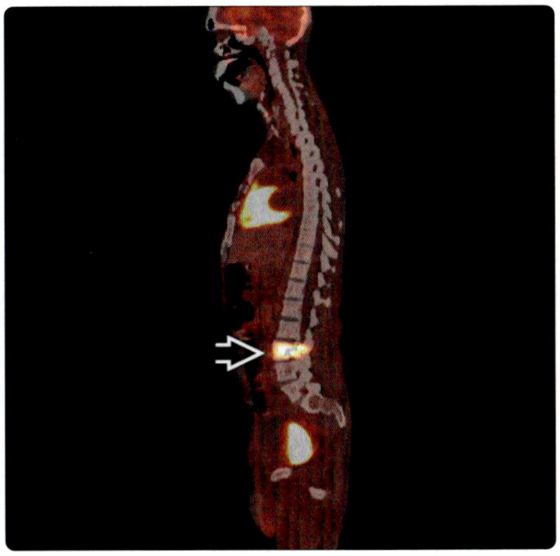

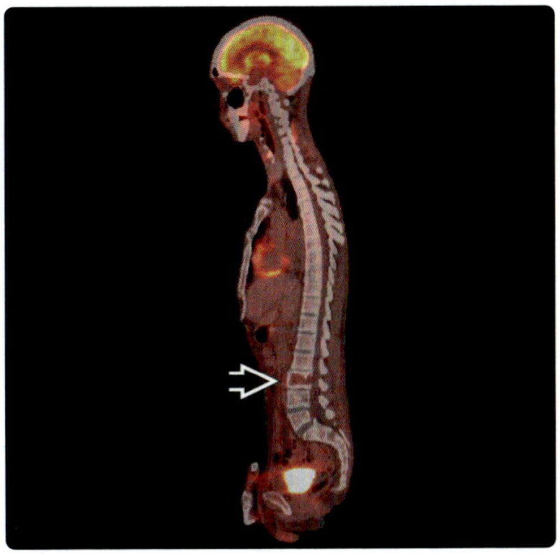

(Left) *Sagittal fused F-18 FDG PET/CT shows focal hypermetabolic activity within the lumbar vertebra ➡ that is concerning for plasmacytoma.* **(Right)** *Sagittal fused F-18 FDG PET/CT shows resolution of focal hypermetabolic activity within the lumbar vertebra ➡ after treatment with a residual lytic lesion.*

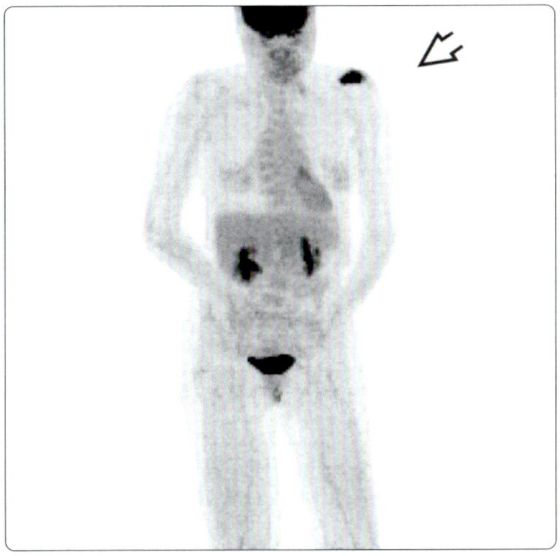

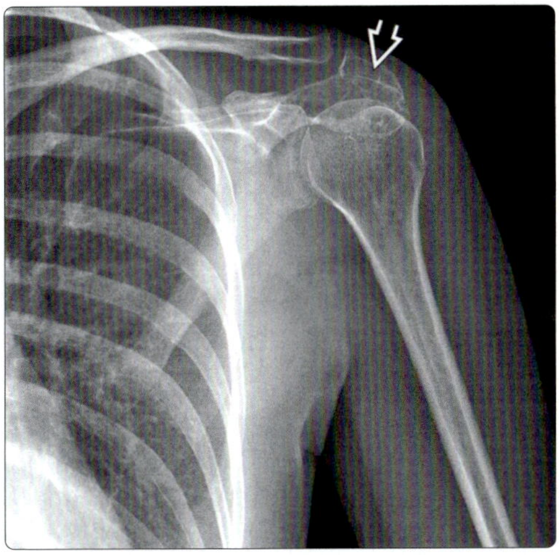

(Left) *Anterior F-18 FDG PET shows focal hypermetabolic activity within the left acromion ➡ that is concerning for plasmacytoma.* **(Right)** *Anteroposterior radiograph of the left shoulder shows a focal lytic expansile lesion within the acromion ➡.*

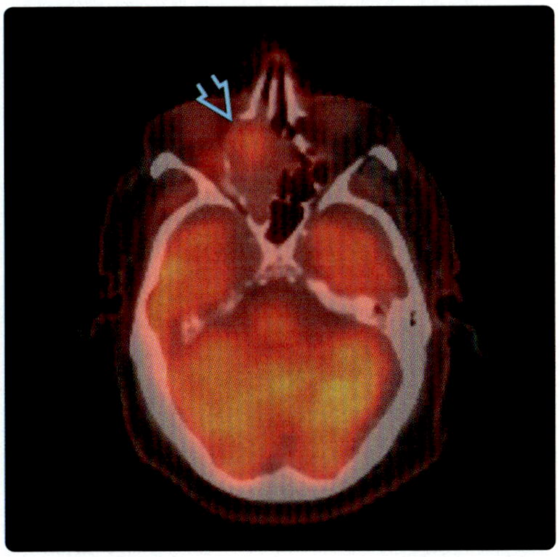

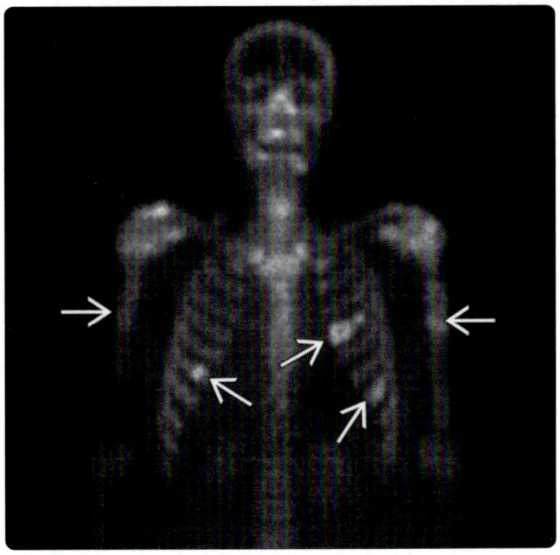

(Left) *Fused axial F-18 FDG PET/CT in a patient with multiple myeloma shows hypermetabolic soft tissue within the right maxillary sinus and right nasal cavity. Biopsy confirmed anaplastic plasmacytoma ➡.* **(Right)** *Anterior Tc-99m MDP bone scan shows focal increased tracer uptake within multiple ribs and proximal humerus bilaterally ➡.*

KEY FACTS

TERMINOLOGY

- World Health Organization (2010) uses neuroendocrine tumor (NET) or neuroendocrine neoplasm
- NET derived from enterochromaffin cells
- Carcinoid syndrome (CS): Occurs in 10% of carcinoid tumors
- Symptoms: Flushing, diarrhea, telangiectasia, and asthma
- Secretes serotonin, which is metabolized to 5-hydroxyindoleacetic acid (5-HIAA)

IMAGING

- Increased activity in bowel, lymph nodes, liver, lung, and bone by several radionuclides
- In-111 pentetreotide (Octreoscan)
- FDG PET/CT

TOP DIFFERENTIAL DIAGNOSES

- Other neuroendocrine tumors
- Lymphoma

PATHOLOGY

- NET staging, grading, and nomenclature vary by primary site with some common features

CLINICAL ISSUES

- Asymptomatic massive hepatomegaly
- Elevated serum chromogranin A (sensitivity 80%)
- Elevated 24-hour urinary 5-HIAA
- High Ki-67 labeling index implies worse patient survival
- Worse prognosis with severe carcinoid syndrome

DIAGNOSTIC CHECKLIST

- Low uptake in normal thyroid
- Moderate to high uptake in medullary carcinoma of thyroid
- Low uptake in normal pituitary
- Increased uptake in pituitary adenomas
- Normal In-111 pentetreotide localization in kidneys, bladder, liver, bowel, and spleen (highest uptake)

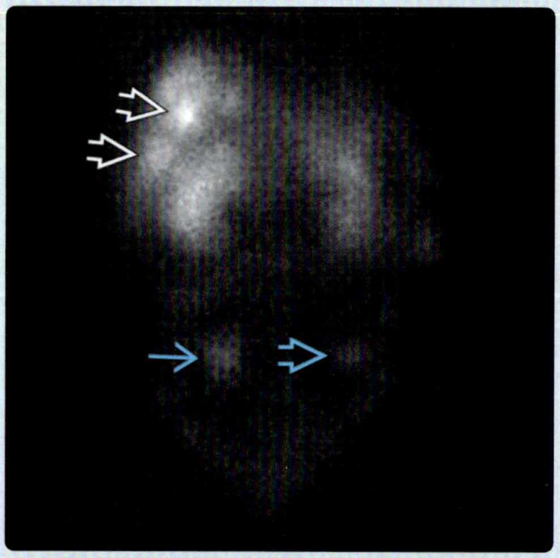

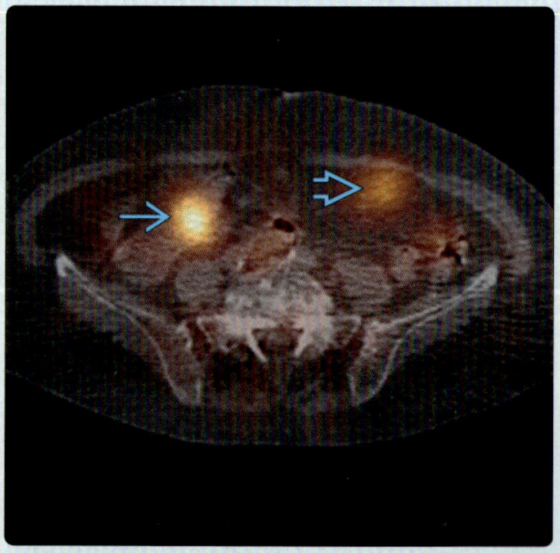

(Left) *This 75-year-old woman with well-differentiated NET liver metastases underwent staging evaluation. Avid liver masses ➔ are visible in the right lobe of the liver. Additional avid masses are demonstrated in the right → and left ⇒ lower quadrants of the abdomen.* **(Right)** *SPECT/CT shows activity in the right lower quadrant → corresponding to an ileal mass on CT (not shown). The activity in the left lower quadrant ⇒ corresponds to an enlarged mesenteric lymph node on CT (not shown).*

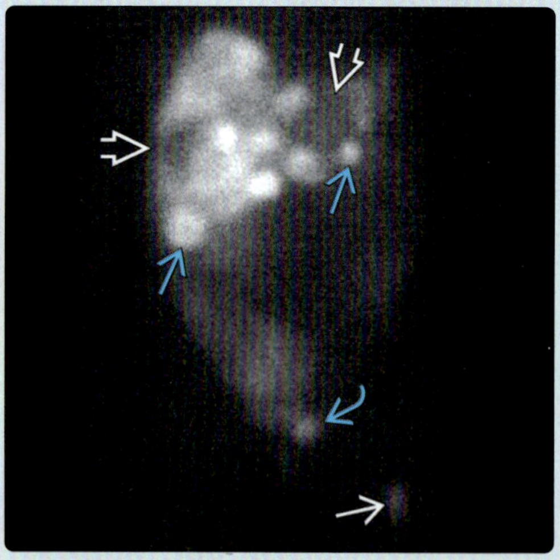

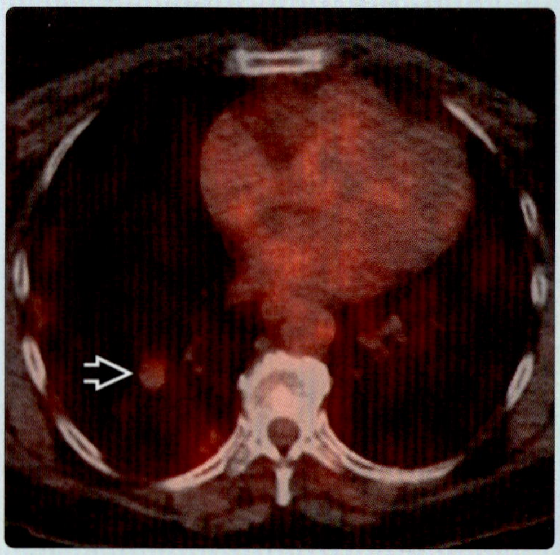

(Left) *A 60-year-old woman was seen for metastatic moderately differentiated rectal NET. There is uptake in bilobar hepatic metastases →. Foci of liver necrosis ➔ cause areas of photopenia. An area of activity in the pelvis → corresponds to residual rectal tumor. Osseous metastasis in the left femoral diaphysis ➔ demonstrates increased uptake.* **(Right)** *This 65-year-old woman underwent evaluation for slowly growing right lower lobe lung nodule. This nodule ➔ was not FDG-avid. Right lower lobectomy proved typical carcinoid.*

TERMINOLOGY

Synonyms

- World Health Organization (2010) uses neuroendocrine tumor (NET) or neuroendocrine neoplasm

Definitions

- Carcinoid
  - NET derived from enterochromaffin cells
  - Secretes serotonin, which is metabolized to 5-hydroxyindoleacetic acid (5-HIAA)
- Carcinoid syndrome (CS): Occurs in 10% of carcinoid tumors
  - Symptoms: Flushing, diarrhea, telangiectasia, and asthma

IMAGING

General Features

- Best diagnostic clue
  - CS with In-111 pentetreotide-avid mass(es) in liver, other abdominal organs, &/or lungs
  - Enhancing mass of distal ileum with partially calcified desmoplastic mesenteric infiltration on CT
  - Partially calcified endobronchial and extrabronchial mass on CT
- Location
  - Tumors of enterochromaffin origin are widely distributed
    - Gastrointestinal tract: 2/3
    - Small intestine: 42%
      - Ileum: Most common site in small bowel
    - Lung: 1/4
- Size
  - 1 mm to 15 cm
  - ≤ 2 cm = less likely malignant
- Morphology
  - Usually ovoid, but can conform to adjacent structures

Nuclear Medicine Findings

- Increased activity in bowel, lymph nodes, liver, lung, and bone by several radionuclides
  - In-111 pentetreotide (Octreoscan)
  - FDG PET/CT
  - I-131 or I-123 MIBG (used much less frequently)

Imaging Recommendations

- Best imaging tool
  - Somatostatin receptor imaging (SRI)
    - Indium-111 pentetreotide (Octreoscan)
    - Sensitivity: 88-96%; specificity: 80-95%
    - Resolution limit: ~ 1.0-1.5 cm
    - High percentage of lesions > 1.5 cm positive
    - Smaller masses less easily located, especially if in organs with normal, mild activity (e.g., liver)
  - CECT
    - Primary gastrointestinal tumor is infrequently identified on conventional CT due to small size
    - Calcified or noncalcified mesenteric lymph nodes are much more commonly seen
    - Liver metastases are typically hypervascular on arterial phase
  - MR
    - Primary tumor: Contrast-enhanced fat-suppressed T1WI is best
    - Liver: Delayed imaging with hepatocyte-specific Gd-based contrast agents
- Protocol advice
  - In-111 pentetreotide (Octreoscan)
    - Patient preparation
      - If patient not experiencing diarrhea, mild oral laxative may decrease colon accumulation
    - Radiopharmaceuticals
      - Dose: 6 mCi (222 MBq) In-111 pentetreotide IV
    - Organ receiving largest dose: Spleen
    - Protocol/image acquisition/processing
      - Empty bladder completely prior to imaging since bladder accumulation can obscure pelvic findings
      - ↑ tumor:background ratio with time
      - Delayed images may be necessary for clearance of bowel activity
      - 4 hr: Whole body anterior/posterior planar optional; consider targeted SPECT based on history and planar imaging (low bowel excretion then)
      - 24 hr: Whole body anterior/posterior planar; targeted SPECT, SPECT usually best at 24 hours
      - 48 hr: Whole body anterior/posterior planar optional; consider targeted SPECT
      - Image with large FOV at symmetric 20% energy windows over 173 keV and 247 keV photopeaks of In-111
  - Additional nuclear medicine imaging options
    - FDG PET/CT
      - 10-20 mCi (370-740 MBq) FDG IV
      - Whole-body images at 60-90 min post injection
      - Most helpful in chest
      - Sensitivity: 75%
      - Resolution limit: ~ 0.6 cm
      - Some patients are FDG-positive and In-111 pentetreotide-negative and vice-versa
    - I-131 or I-123 metaiodobenzylguanidine (MIBG)
      - 1.2-2.2 mCi (40-80 MBq) I-131 MIBG IV
      - Image with planar/SPECT at 24-48 hrs
      - I-131 MIBG: Pretreat with Lugol 1% solution (20 drops 2x/day) to block thyroid accumulation of radioactive iodine
      - Sensitivity: 55-75%; specificity: 95%
      - Small number of patients are MIBG-positive and In-111 pentetreotide-negative
      - Resolution limit: ~ 1.0-1.5 cm
      - 10.8 mCi (400 MBq) I-123 MIBG IV
      - Image with planar/SPECT at 20-24 hrs

DIFFERENTIAL DIAGNOSIS

Lymphoma

- Nodal disease in addition to bowel, liver, and lung masses
- Biopsy and lab tests distinguish
- SRI can also be positive in lymphoma

Other Neuroendocrine Tumors

- Gastrinoma
- Vasoactive intestinal polypeptide-secreting tumors (VIPomas)

- Insulinoma
- Pheochromocytoma
- Medullary carcinoma of thyroid

PATHOLOGY

General Features

- Associated abnormalities
  - Carcinoid heart disease
    - Right heart problems more common than left
    - Right heart failure 2° to severe tricuspid and pulmonary valvular dysfunction
    - Left heart symptoms may predominate with pulmonary carcinoid

Staging, Grading, & Classification

- NET staging, grading, and nomenclature vary by primary site with some common features
  - Separation of well-differentiated from poorly differentiated tumors
  - Proliferative rate: Monoclonal antigen binding to Ki-67 antigen

Gross Pathologic & Surgical Features

- Usually ovoid soft tissue masses
  - Small and large bowel primary tumor
  - Lung primary tumor
  - Metastases to lymph nodes, liver, lung, and bone

Microscopic Features

- Small cells with uniform round nuclei and stippled chromatin, without prominent nucleoli
- Growth pattern insular, trabecular, glandular, and diffuse
- Stain positive for chromogranin A or synaptophysin

CLINICAL ISSUES

Presentation

- Most common signs/symptoms
  - Asymptomatic massive hepatomegaly
  - Flushing: 85-90%; diarrhea: 70%
  - Cardiac symptoms: 35-40% (right 30%; left 10%)
  - Bowel obstruction
- Other signs/symptoms
  - Elevated 24-hour urinary 5-HIAA
    - Sensitivity: 73%; specificity: ~ 100%
  - Elevated serum chromogranin A (sensitivity 80%)
  - GI bleeding
  - Incidental finding of pulmonary or abdominal mass
  - Many are asymptomatic and likely remain occult

Demographics

- Age
  - More frequent in older adults
  - Aging population: ↑ incidence over several decades
- Gender
  - Higher in black males, slightly higher in white females
- Ethnicity
  - Higher incidence in blacks, lower in Hispanics
- Epidemiology
  - Incidence 1-5 per 100,000
  - Review of 16,294 autopsies and 44 surgical specimens
    - Incidence of 8.4 per 100,000
  - Weak association with MEN-1 syndrome (< 1%)
  - Stronger association with first-degree family member
    - 3.6 relative risk (95% confidence interval of 3.3-4.1)

Natural History & Prognosis

- High Ki-67 labeling index implies worse patient survival
- Worse prognosis with severe carcinoid syndrome
- Untreated full-blown carcinoid syndrome has poor 5-year survival (20-50%)

Treatment

- Surgery
  - Curative resection of smaller masses
  - Debulk tumor to ↓ symptoms and improve survival
- Systemic chemotherapy with alpha interferon and cytotoxic agents
- Liver metastases
  - Resection, radiofrequency ablation, cryotherapy, and chemoembolization
- Somatostatin analogs
  - Symptomatic blockade, but subject to tachyphylaxis
  - Radiolabelled analogs to target metastases

DIAGNOSTIC CHECKLIST

Consider

- If patient not experiencing frequent (at least QD) bowel movements, mild laxative can increase bowel excretion
- SPECT/CT
  - Increases contrast in smaller lesions that may not be apparent on planar images
- Normal excretory bladder activity can obscure findings

Image Interpretation Pearls

- Normal In-111 pentetreotide localization in kidneys, bladder, liver, bowel, and spleen (highest uptake)
- Thyroid uptake of In-111 pentetreotide
  - Low uptake in normal thyroid
  - Moderate to high uptake in medullary carcinoma of the thyroid
- Pituitary uptake of In-111 pentetreotide
  - Low uptake in normal pituitary
  - Increased uptake in pituitary adenomas

SELECTED REFERENCES

1. Lococo F et al: Functional imaging evaluation in the detection, diagnosis, and histologic differentiation of pulmonary neuroendocrine tumors. Thorac Surg Clin. 24(3):285-92, 2014
2. Baudin E et al: Intervention in gastro-enteropancreatic neuroendocrine tumours. Best Pract Res Clin Gastroenterol. 26(6):855-65, 2012
3. Pepe G et al: Somatostatin receptor SPECT. Eur J Nucl Med Mol Imaging. 39 Suppl 1:S41-51, 2012
4. Balon HR et al: The SNM practice guideline for somatostatin receptor scintigraphy 2.0. J Nucl Med Technol. 39(4):317-24, 2011
5. Bushnell DL et al: Standard imaging techniques for neuroendocrine tumors. Endocrinol Metab Clin North Am. 40(1):153-62, ix, 2011
6. Elsayes KM et al: Imaging of carcinoid tumors: spectrum of findings with pathologic and clinical correlation. J Comput Assist Tomogr. 35(1):72-80, 2011
7. Klimstra DS et al: The pathologic classification of neuroendocrine tumors: a review of nomenclature, grading, and staging systems. Pancreas. 39(6):707-12, 2010
8. Wong M et al: Radiopathological review of small bowel carcinoid tumours. J Med Imaging Radiat Oncol. 53(1):1-12, 2009
9. Pinchot SN et al: Carcinoid tumors. Oncologist. 13(12):1255-69, 2008

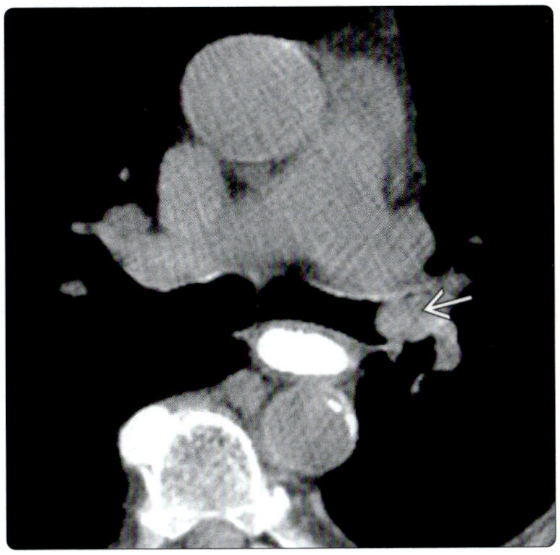

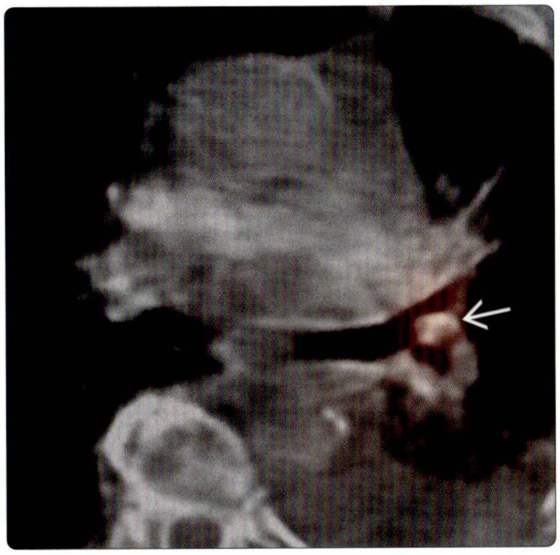

(Left) *Axial NECT in a 87-year-old man shows endobronchial atypical carcinoid of the distal left main bronchus* ➔*. No metastases were evident on this study.* **(Right)** *SPECT/CT shows focal increased activity of the endobronchial mass in the distal left main bronchus* ➔*.*

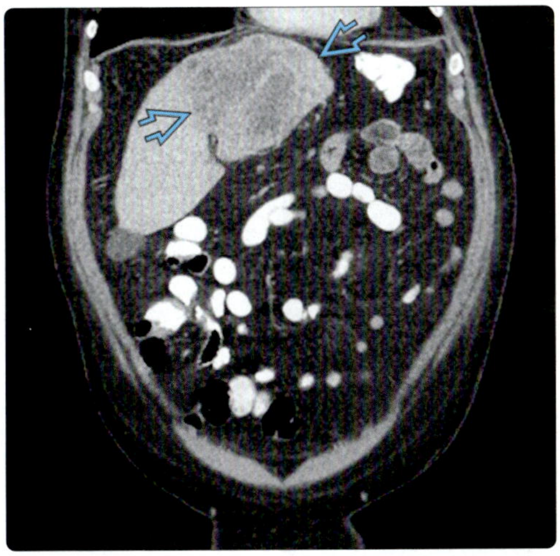

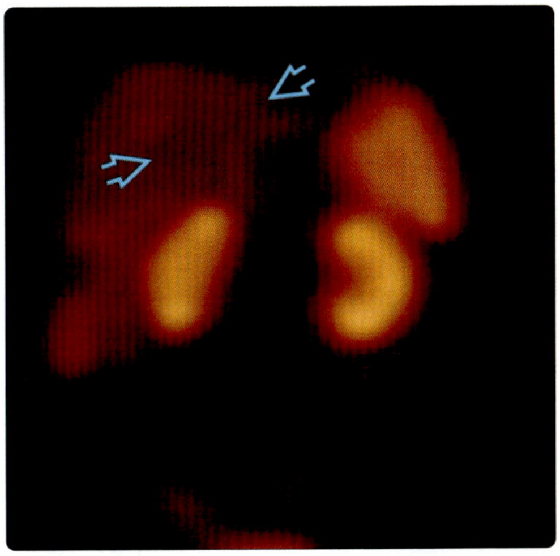

(Left) *Coronal CECT in a 54-year-old man shows a dominant mass of the left lobe of the liver* ⇨*. Liver mass biopsy showed well-differentiated NET. Primary tumor was later located in the duodenum by MR and confirmed by endoscopy.* **(Right)** *Anterior MIP of the abdomen shows no increased activity in the left lobe of the liver at the site of the known dominant mass* ⇨*. The duodenal tumor was not visible.*

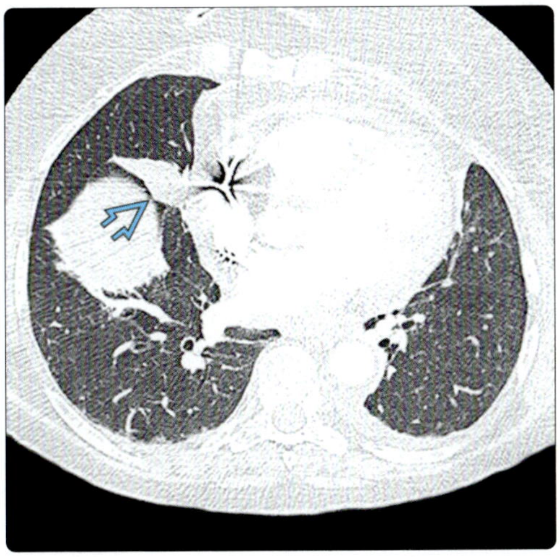

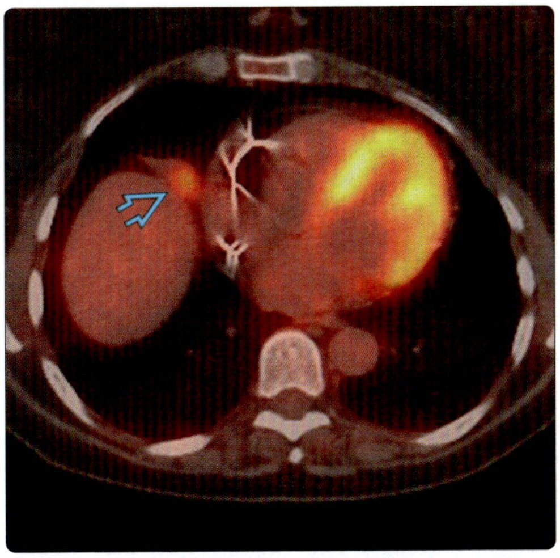

(Left) *Axial CECT shows a 61-year-old woman with right middle lobe lung nodule first detected on chest CT performed for pulmonary embolism. Initial FDG PET/CT showed mild hypermetabolism in the nodule. This nodule* ⇨ *was unchanged over 9 months and the patient was sent for follow-up FDG PET/CT.* **(Right)** *Right middle lobe nodule* ⇨ *was FDG-avid with increased activity compared to the exam 9 months earlier. CT-guided biopsy showed typical carcinoid. Octreotide scan (not shown) showed no increased activity in the nodule.*

KEY FACTS

TERMINOLOGY

- Gastroenteropancreatic neuroendocrine tumor (GEP-NET), islet cell tumors

IMAGING

- Hypervascular mass(es) in pancreas (primary) & liver (metastases)
- Pancreas (85%); ectopic (15%) in duodenum, stomach, lymph nodes (LN), ovary
- Gastrinoma triangle: Superiorly cystic & common bile duct (CBD), inferiorly 2nd & 3rd parts of duodenum, medially pancreatic neck & body
- In-111 DTPA-D-Phe octreotide (Octreoscan): Radiolabeled derivative of octreotide, binds to somatostatin receptor (subtypes 2, 5, rarely 3)
- SRS sensitivity in detection of pancreatic islet cell tumors: ~ 65%
- Many types of tumors positive on SRS: Not specific for islet cell tumors
- Consideration to discontinuing octreotide therapy for 24 hr prior to In-111 pentetreotide administration
- In patients suspected of having insulinoma, IV infusion of glucose should be prepared for the potential of inducing severe hypoglycemia
- Wide variability in sensitivity by cell type: Gastrinomas typically high, insulinomas often low (50-60%)
- In-111 Octreoscan advantage is whole-body imaging for staging and restaging
- Use of dedicated SPECT/CT camera or off-line fusion of SPECT images to CT or MR highly recommended
- Determination of somatostatin-receptor status to guide octreotide therapy
- Selection of patients with metastatic tumors for peptide receptor radionuclide therapy (PRRT)

DIAGNOSTIC CHECKLIST

- Hypervascular pancreatic tumor & liver metastases suggests islet cell/neuroendocrine tumor

(Left) *Whole-body anterior and posterior In-111 Octreoscan in a patient who had a gastrinoma resected shows focal increased uptake within the right upper abdomen ➔.* **(Right)** *SPECT/CT in the same patient shows focal increased activity localizing to the caudate lobe ➔.*

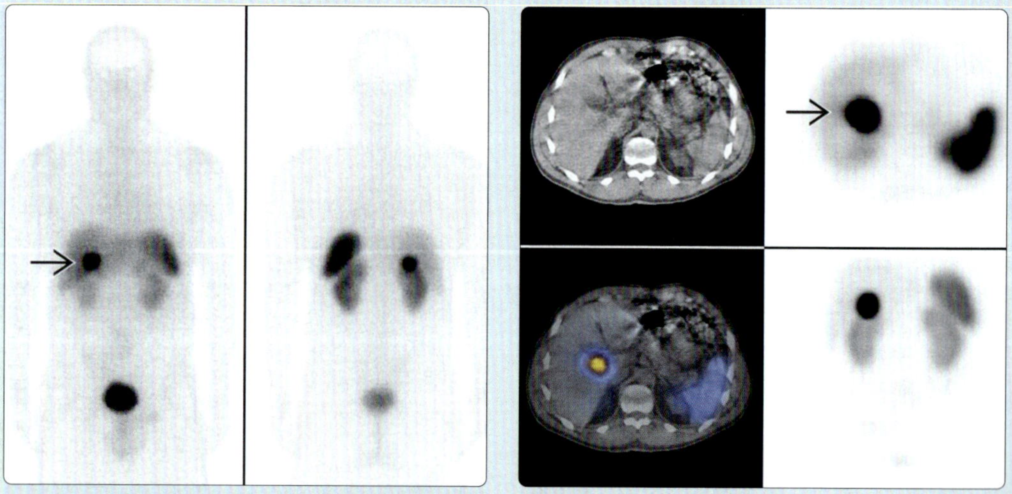

(Left) *Axial T2-weighted MR shows a hyperintense mass ➔ in the caudate lobe.* **(Right)** *Axial post-gadolinium MR shows an early enhancing mass in the caudate lobe ➔, which is a typical pattern for neuroendocrine tumor metastasis.*

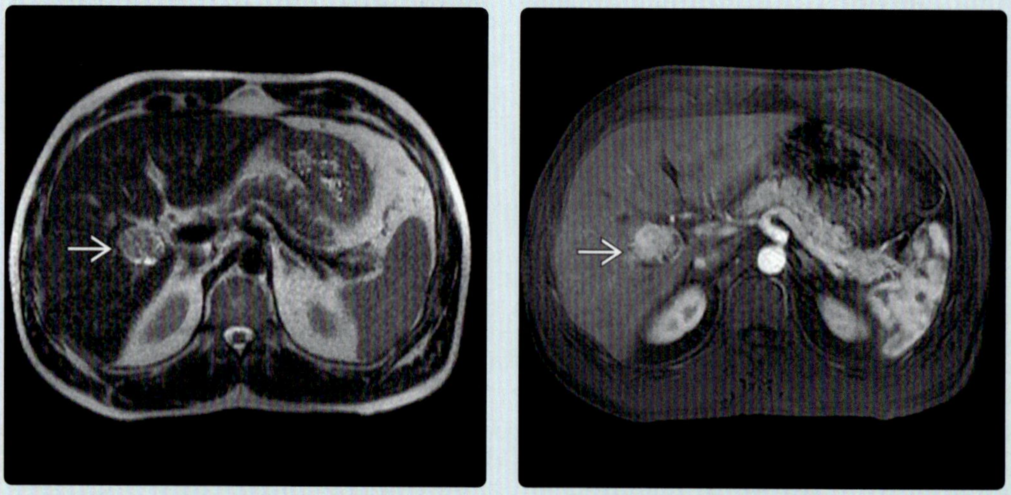

TERMINOLOGY

Synonyms

- Gastroenteropancreatic neuroendocrine tumor (GEP-NET), islet cell tumors

Definitions

- Tumors arising from pancreatic endocrine cells (islets of Langerhans)

IMAGING

General Features

- Best diagnostic clue
  - Hypervascular mass(es) in pancreas (primary) and liver (metastases)
- Location
  - Pancreas (85%); ectopic (15%) in duodenum, stomach, lymph nodes (LN), ovary
  - Gastrinoma triangle: Cystic and common bile duct junction (superiorly), junction of 2nd and 3rd portions of duodenum (inferiorly), and junction of pancreatic head and body (medially)
- Morphology
  - Rare compared to tumors of exocrine pancreas
  - Benign or malignant, single or multiple (with different cell types)
  - May be hormonally functional (85%) or nonfunctional
  - Functioning tumors can secrete multiple hormones, with dominant single defining clinical presentation
    - Insulinoma, glucagonoma, gastrinoma, somatostatinoma, VIPoma (vasoactive intestinal polypeptide), PPoma (pancreatic polypeptide), APUDoma (carcinoid clinical syndromes)
  - Nonfunctioning tumors
    - Hypofunctioning or clinically silent large tumors; larger than functioning tumors at diagnosis; cystic islet cell tumor usually non-insulin producing & nonfunctioning; high malignancy rate

Nuclear Medicine Findings

- Somatostatin receptor scintigraphy (SRS)
  - In-111 DTPA-D-Phe octreotide (Octreoscan): Radiolabeled derivative of octreotide, binds to somatostatin receptor (subtypes 2, 5, rarely 3)
  - SRS sensitivity to detect pancreatic islet cell tumors: ~ 65%
    - Wide variability in sensitivity by cell type: Gastrinomas typically high, insulinomas often low (50-60%)
  - Many types of tumors positive on SRS: Not specific for islet cell tumors
  - In-111 Octreoscan advantage is whole-body imaging for staging and restaging
  - Determination of somatostatin-receptor status to guide octreotide therapy
  - Selection of patients with metastatic tumors for peptide receptor radionuclide therapy (PRRT)
- Other SRS-avid conditions
  - Pituitary adenoma; adrenal medullary tumors; paraganglioma; benign and malignant thyroid tissue; Merkel cell; melanoma; carcinoid; small cell lung cancer; non-pancreatic neuroendocrine carcinoma; meningioma; well-differentiated glial-derived tumor; breast, prostate, renal carcinomas; lymphoma, granuloma, infection, and inflammation

CT Findings

- Functioning tumors
  - NECT: Small or large in size; calcification may be seen; small lesions usually undetectable; cystic & necrotic areas (usually non-insulin tumors)
  - CECT (arterial phase & portal venous phase): Most are hypervascular; delayed solid/ring enhancement (insulinoma); arterially enhancing metastasis in liver and LN
- Nonfunctioning tumors
  - NECT: Mixed density; usually large & complex; cystic & necrotic areas (large tumors); calcification
  - CECT: Usually hypervascular; nonenhancing cystic or necrotic areas; enhancing viable tumor and metastases; liver metastases often extensive even in relatively healthy patient
- Large functional & nonfunctional tumors: Highly malignant; calcification; local invasion; early invasion of portal vein → liver metastases

Angiographic Findings

- Hypervascular (primary & secondary); hepatic venous sampling with intraarterial stimulation → elevated hormones with functioning tumors

MR Findings

- Functional tumors
  - T1 FS: Hypointense
  - T1 C+: Solid or ring enhancement (insulinoma) on T1; hyperintense (solid enhancing lesions) on fat-saturated delayed enhanced T1 SE
  - T2 SE & STIR: Hyperintense
  - DWI useful for liver metastases
- Nonfunctioning tumors
  - T1 SE: Small tumors isointense; large tumors heterogeneous (cystic & necrotic)
  - T2 SE: Small tumors isointense; large tumors hyperintense (cystic & necrotic)
  - T1 C+: Small tumors hyperintense on fat-saturated delayed enhanced T1WI SE; large tumors nonenhancing cystic + necrotic areas

Ultrasonographic Findings

- Endoscopic ultrasound (EUS): Detects small tumors; homogeneously hypoechoic, permits transgastric Bx
- Intraoperative US: Detects small lesions; sensitivity 75-100%

Imaging Recommendations

- Best imaging tool
  - CECT with early arterial phase & delayed imaging
  - MR including dynamic contrast-enhanced imaging and MR with hepatocyte-specific contrast agent
  - SRS: Problem or equivocal cases where tumor suspected but CT, MR negative or equivocal
- Protocol advice

- Somatostatin receptor scintigraphy
  - Consideration to discontinuing octreotide therapy for 24 hr prior to In-111 pentetreotide administration
  - Consider laxative administration to reduce bowel activity; cautioned use in patients with diarrhea
  - Adult dose 6 mCi In-111 Octreoscan; slow IV push under close clinical observation
    - Hypotension may occur with neurosecretory tumors
  - 4 hr SPECT/planar images of abdomen: Visualization of lesions before normal bowel uptake
  - 24 hr SPECT/planar images of neck, chest, abdomen, pelvis: Greater sensitivity than at 4 hr, but expect bowel, bladder, gallbladder activity
  - Use of dedicated SPECT/CT camera or off-line fusion of SPECT images to CT or MR highly recommended
- Precautions
  - In patients suspected of having insulinoma, IV infusion of glucose should be prepared for potential of inducing severe hypoglycemia
  - In-111 pentetreotide should not be injected into IV lines for/together with TPN

DIFFERENTIAL DIAGNOSIS

Pancreatic Ductal Adenocarcinoma

- Hypovascular tumor; pancreatic ductal obstruction; pancreatic head (60%); obliteration or retropancreatic fat; extensive local invasion, regional mets; irregular, nodular, rat-tailed eccentric obstruction on ERCP

Mucinous Cystic Tumor of Pancreas

- Similar to cystic/necrotic islet cell tumor; tail of pancreas common; multiloculated hypodense mass on NECT; enhancement of thin internal septa & wall on CECT; cysts (hyperintense) & septations (hypointense) on T2 MR; predominantly vascular on angiography

Metastases

- Indistinguishable from islet cell tumor mets on CT, MR

Serous Cystadenoma of Pancreas

- Honeycomb or sponge appearance; pancreatic head more common; enhancing septa delineating small cysts; highly vascular on angiography; macrocystic type with thinner wall/septa than islet cell tumors

PATHOLOGY

General Features

- Etiology
  - Arise from APUD (amine precursor uptake & decarboxylation) cells
  - Nonfunctioning: Derived from α & β cells
  - Functioning tumor: Glucagonoma (α cell); gastrinoma (islet cell); insulinoma (β cell)
- Associated abnormalities
  - Gastrinoma (Zollinger-Ellison syndrome); MEN type 1

Gross Pathologic & Surgical Features

- Small tumor (encapsulated & firm); large tumor, cystic, necrotic, calcified

Microscopic Features

- Sheets of small round cells, uniform nuclei/cytoplasm: Neuron-specific enolase on electron microscopy

CLINICAL ISSUES

Presentation

- Most common signs/symptoms
  - Insulinoma: Whipple triad (hypoglycemia + low fasting glucose + relief by IV glucose)
  - Gastrinoma (Zollinger-Ellison syndrome): Peptic ulcer, increased acidity & diarrhea
  - Glucagonoma: Necrolytic erythema migrans, diarrhea, diabetes, weight loss
  - Nonfunctional: Mostly asymptomatic; pain, jaundice, variceal bleeding

Demographics

- Age
  - 4th-6th decade
- Gender
  - Insulinoma (M < F); gastrinoma (M > F)
- Epidemiology
  - 1-2% of all pancreas neoplasms
  - Insulinoma: Most common islet cell tumor; solitary benign (90%); malignant (10%)
  - Gastrinoma: 2nd common; multiple & malignant (60%); MEN1 (20-60%)
  - Nonfunctioning: 3rd common; 20-45% of islet cell tumors; malignant (80-100%)

Natural History & Prognosis

- Prognosis: Insulinoma (good); gastrinoma (poor)
- Nonfunctional: 3-year survival (60%), 5-year survival (44%); can live with metastases for many years

Treatment

- Acute phase: Octreotide (potent hormonal inhibitor)
- Insulinoma: Surgery curative
- Gastrinoma: Medical management with omeprazole, 5-fluorouracil; surgery curative in 30% cases
- Nonfunctional: Resection/embolization
- Liver metastases: Transarterial chemoembolization, radioembolization

DIAGNOSTIC CHECKLIST

Consider

- Differentiate from other solid, cystic, vascular tumors
- Correlate with clinical & biochemical information
- SRS for stage/restage or where CT, MR (-) or equivocal

Image Interpretation Pearls

- Hypervascular pancreatic tumor ± liver metastases suggests islet cell/neuroendocrine tumor
- Solid/ring-enhancement (insulinoma): Delayed scans
- Large functioning & nonfunctioning tumors: Hypervascular, complex & highly malignant
- SPECT fusion to CT or MR highly recommended for SRS

SELECTED REFERENCES

1. Mansi L et al: Diagnostic imaging in neuroendocrine tumors. J Nucl Med. 55(10):1576-7, 2014

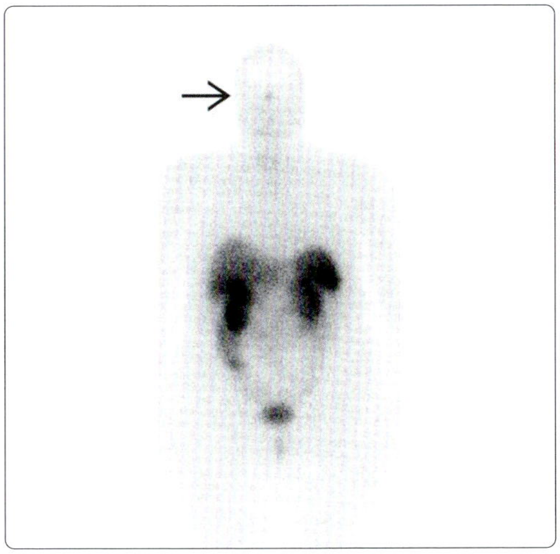

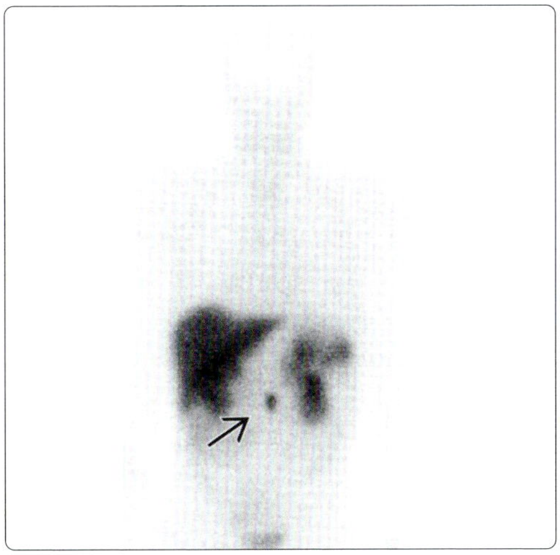

(Left) *Whole-body anterior image from an In-111 Octreoscan shows focal increased uptake of tracer in the expected location of the skull base →. This was proven to be a pituitary adenoma on MR.* **(Right)** *Whole-body anterior image from an In-111 Octreoscan shows focal increased uptake of tracer in the pancreas →. The patient underwent surgical resection, which revealed an insulinoma. In-111 Octreoscan is the least sensitive for insulinomas.*

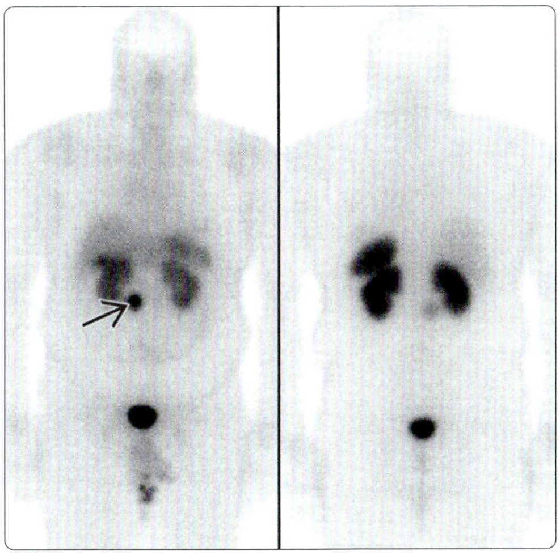

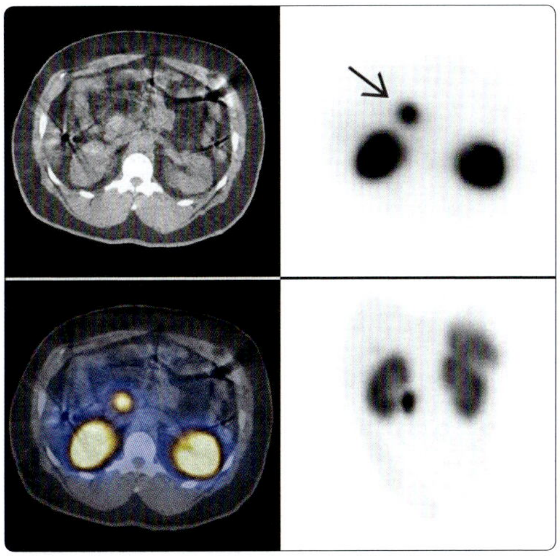

(Left) *Whole-body anterior and posterior images from an In-111 Octreoscan in a patient with Zollinger-Ellison syndrome show a single focus of activity → in the mid abdomen just right of midline.* **(Right)** *Axial images from a SPEC/CT in the same patient show the focal activity to localize to the duodenum →, which is within the gastrinoma triangle.*

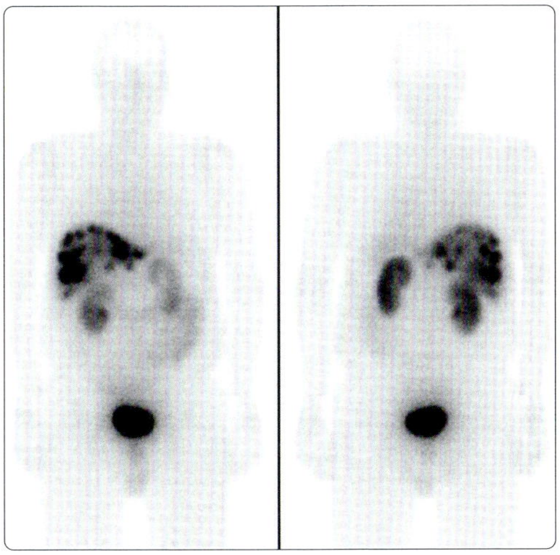

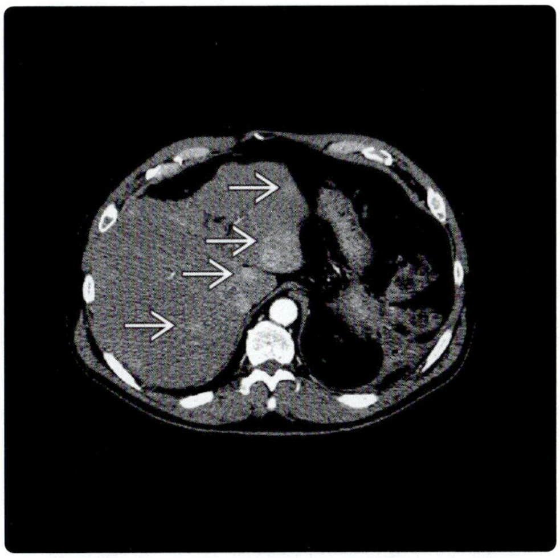

(Left) *Whole-body anterior and posterior images from an In-111 Octreoscan in a patient with elevated gastrin levels show innumerable lesions throughout the liver.* **(Right)** *Axial CECT in the arterial phase in this same patient confirms multiple early enhancing hepatic metastasis →. Metastatic gastrinoma was diagnosed upon biopsy.*

Pheochromocytoma and Paraganglioma

KEY FACTS

TERMINOLOGY

- Pheochromocytoma (pheo)
  - Catecholamine-secreting tumor arising from chromaffin cells of adrenal medulla
  - If extra-adrenal, called paraganglioma

IMAGING

- Anatomic imaging: Morphology not reliable in predicting malignant potential
- I-123 MIBG scintigraphy
  - Use for occult, ectopic, recurrent, metastatic tumors
  - Patient should discontinue drugs that interfere with MIBG for 48-72 hrs prior
- F-18 FDG PET
  - Sensitivity similar to MIBG, best for malignant pheochromocytoma/paragangliomas

PATHOLOGY

- Pheochromocytoma: The 10% tumor
  - Classically: 10% familial, 10% bilateral, 10% malignant, 10% in children, and 10% not associated with HTN
  - Newer studies indicate that ~ 30% are familial, and thus > 10% are bilateral, malignant
  - 10% with benign disease will develop recurrence, usually 5-15 years later; 50% of recurrences are metastatic
- Malignancy diagnosed by presence of metastatic deposits, **not** by presence of local invasion

DIAGNOSTIC CHECKLIST

- Most common staging system
  - Localized (benign)
  - Regional
  - Distant metastases
- Bilateral low-level adrenal uptake on I-123 MIBG scintigraphy likely normal or hyperplasia
- I-123 MIBG SPECT/CT usually performed for most complete 3D evaluation (often just SPECT in children to avoid extra radiation from CT)

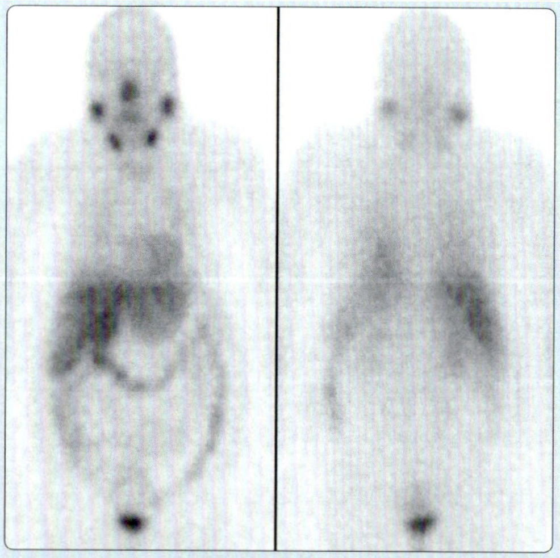

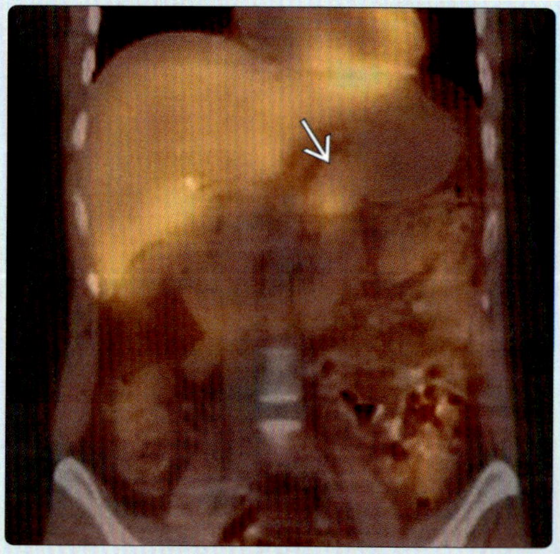

(Left) *Anterior and posterior I-123 MIBG scintigraphy in a patient post bilateral adrenalectomy for pheochromocytoma shows normal physiologic uptake of radiotracer and no evidence of recurrence. Normal, low-level adrenal activity can be visualized in up to 75% of patients on I-123 MIBG scintigraphy.* **(Right)** *Coronal fused I-123 MIBG SPECT/CT shows focal increase of tracer in an enlarged left adrenal gland ➔ consistent with pheochromocytoma.*

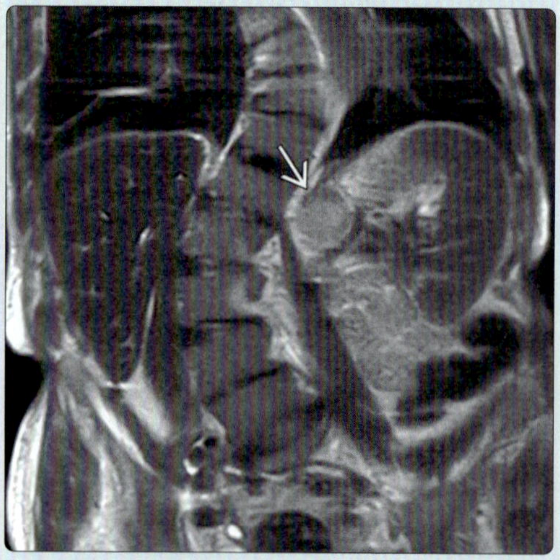

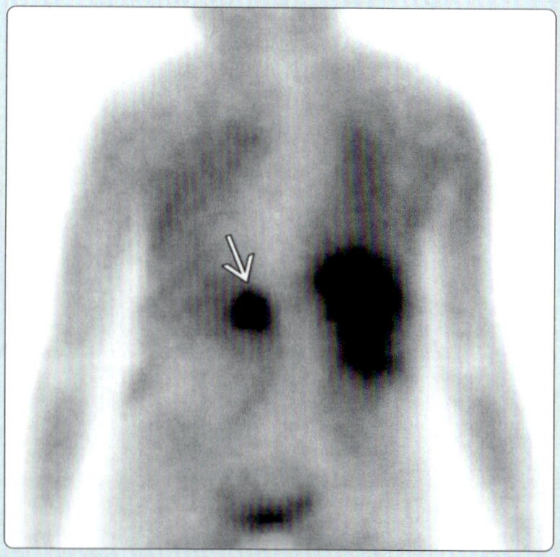

(Left) *Coronal T2WI MR shows a round, well-circumscribed, heterogeneous left adrenal mass ➔ that demonstrates T2 signal hyperintensity. This is suspicious for pheochromocytoma.* **(Right)** *Posterior I-123 MIBG scintigraphy in the same patient shows focal avid uptake of radiotracer in the left adrenal gland ➔, consistent with pheochromocytoma.*

TERMINOLOGY

Definitions

- Pheochromocytoma (pheo)
  - Tumor arising from chromaffin cells of adrenal medulla
  - Secretes epinephrine and norepinephrine
- Paraganglioma
  - Neuroendocrine tumor arising from chromoceptor/chromaffin cells of paraganglion
  - Arises from sympathetic and parasympathetic ganglion
  - May not secrete catecholamines

IMAGING

General Features

- Imaging chameleon: Morphology variable and can mimic other conditions
  - Heterogeneous mass with cystic, necrotic, calcified components, but may be solid and homogeneous
  - Typically well-circumscribed, encapsulated tumor
- Radiographic appearance not reliable in determining malignant potential
  - Highly vascular, thus prone to hemorrhage and necrosis, even if benign
  - Invasion of capsule and nearby vasculature (e.g., IVC) can be seen in benign tumors

Nuclear Medicine Findings

- PET
  - Pheochromocytoma or paraganglioma mass with increased F-18 FDG avidity
    - Adrenal mass should show F-18 FDG uptake greater than liver uptake
  - F-18 FDG sensitivity similar to meta-iodo-benzyl-guanidine (MIBG), best for malignant pheo and paraganglioma
  - Useful to monitor known pheos and paraganglioma that fail to accumulate MIBG
- MIBG scintigraphy
  - I-123 MIBG
    - Meta-iodo-benzyl-guanidine is a norepinephrine (NE) analog
    - Enters cells by active uptake via NE transporter, stored in neurosecretory granules
  - At 24-48 hrs, pheos and paragangliomas demonstrate focal and intense MIBG avidity
  - Imaging modality of choice for detecting extra-adrenal tumors and metastatic deposits at initial presentation
  - Useful for postoperative monitoring for disease recurrence
  - Good specificity (80-90%) for pheos, sensitivity 70-80%
  - Improved diagnostic accuracy if SPECT/CT done at same time

Imaging Recommendations

- Protocol advice
  - **I-123 MIBG scintigraphy**
  - Patient preparation
    - Discontinue drugs that interfere with MIBG uptake 48-72 hrs prior (may cause false-negative study)
      - Cardiopulmonary: Labetalol, calcium channel blockers, bronchodilators
      - α- and β-blockers (except labetalol) can still be used in normal doses
      - CNS: Antipsychotics, tricyclic antidepressants, sympathomimetics, stimulants
      - Neurological: Reserpine, tetrabenazine
    - Block I-123 uptake by thyroid gland 1 day prior and 2 days after I-123 MIBG injection
      - I-123 MIBG scintigraphy can induce hypothyroidism due to gamma radiation dose to thyroid on repeated studies
      - Saturated solution potassium iodide (SSKI)/Lugol 1% solution: 3 drops in water BID 1 day before I-123 MIBG administration and 2 days after
      - Capsules: 170 mg potassium iodate, 130 mg potassium iodide, or 400 mg potassium perchlorate (can be used day of injection if necessary)
      - Pediatrics (> 3 years old): 1 drop SSKI in water 1 day before I-123 MIBG administration and 2 days after
    - Patient should void prior to study as urinary bladder can mask abnormality
  - Radiopharmaceutical
    - I-123 MIBG
    - Adults: 10 mCi (370 MBq) I-123 MIBG IV slowly over 5 min
    - Children: 0.14 mCi/kg, with minimum dose of 1 mCi (37 MBq)
    - Side effects: Vomiting, tachycardia, pallor, abdominal pain (more likely if rapid IV push)
  - Dosimetry
    - Liver receives largest radiation dose
    - Thyroid blocked by potassium iodide (see above)
  - Image acquisition
    - Low-energy, high-resolution collimator
    - Anterior and posterior whole-body images at 24 hrs
      - Limited-field or spot views preferred in young children
    - SPECT/CT chest, abdomen, pelvis at 24 hrs for most complete 3D evaluation
      - In children, just perform SPECT if prior CT available for comparison
  - **F-18 FDG PET/CT**
    - Standard oncologic protocol

DIFFERENTIAL DIAGNOSIS

Other Neuroendocrine Tumors

- I-123 MIBG: Positive in neuroblastoma, ganglioneuroma, Merkel cell, carcinoid
- F-18 FDG PET/CT: Low-level, variable uptake in carcinoid, ganglioneuroma; usually high uptake in neuroblastoma, Merkel cell carcinoma

Adrenal Medullary Hyperplasia

- I-123 MIBG: Low-level uptake bilaterally, adreniform morphology
- F-18 FDG PET/CT: Mildly increased uptake bilaterally, adreniform morphology

Adrenal Adenoma/Myelolipoma

- I-123 MIBG: Negative or nonspecific low-level uptake ≤ liver
- F-18 FDG PET/CT: Uptake ≤ liver

Adrenocortical Carcinoma

- I-123 MIBG: Negative or nonspecific low-level uptake ≤ liver
- F-18 FDG PET/CT: Uptake ≥ liver

Adrenal Metastases

- I-123 MIBG: Negative or nonspecific low-level uptake ≤ liver
- F-18 FDG PET/CT: Uptake ≥ liver

Adrenal Hemorrhage

- I-123 MIBG: Negative or nonspecific low-level uptake ≤ liver
- F-18 FDG PET/CT: Negative or nonspecific low-level uptake ≤ liver

Adrenal Infection/Inflammation/Granulomatous Disease

- I-123 MIBG: Negative or nonspecific low-level uptake ≤ liver
- F-18 FDG PET/CT: Increased uptake, often ≥ liver

PATHOLOGY

General Features

- Etiology
  - The 10% tumor
    - Classically: 10% familial, 10% bilateral, 10% malignant, 10% in children, and 10% not associated with HTN
    - Newer studies indicate that ~ 30% are familial, and thus > 10% are bilateral, malignant
    - Almost all pheochromocytomas and paragangliomas are subdiaphragmatic, usually intraabdominal (98%)
    - Paragangliomas
      - Intraabdominal (85%), intrathoracic (12%), head and neck (3%)
      - Sympathetic: Organ of Zuckerkandl near aortic bifurcation, along sympathetic chain from neck to bladder
      - Parasympathetic: Carotid body, along course of vagus and glossopharyngeal nerves
- Genetics
  - Major genetic syndromes that carry an increased risk of PCC &/or PGL
    - Neurocutaneous syndromes (neurofibromatosis, von Hippel-Lindau, Sturge-Weber, tuberous sclerosis)
    - Multiple endocrine neoplasia (MEN) type IIA, type IIB (usually bilateral and rarely extra-adrenal)
    - Familial pheochromocytoma/paraganglioma syndrome (also called hereditary paraganglioma syndrome)
  - Other rare syndromes associated with paragangliomas
    - Carney-Stratakis dyad: Paraganglioma + gastrointestinal stromal tumor (GIST)
    - Carney triad: Paraganglioma + GIST + pulmonary chondroma

Staging, Grading, & Classification

- Classified by WHO as neuroendocrine tumor with tumor cells derived from neural crest
- Malignancy diagnosed by presence of metastatic deposits, not by presence of local invasion
  - Metastasis: Tumor in tissues where chromaffin cells typically absent (lymph node, liver, bone, lung)
  - Metastasis most common in liver, bone, and lung
- Most common staging system
  - Localized (benign)
  - Regional metastases
  - Distant metastases

CLINICAL ISSUES

Presentation

- Most common signs/symptoms
  - Pheochromocytoma
    - Sustained or episodic HTN (~ 90% of cases)
    - Classic triad: Paroxysms of headache, profuse sweating, tachycardia
    - Events can be spontaneous or induced: Trauma, strenuous exercise, urination (if along bladder wall)
    - Diagnosis made if compatible imaging findings + elevation of urinary or serum catecholamines
      - May be difficult to obtain laboratory evidence due to episodic nature of catecholamine excess

Natural History & Prognosis

- Pheochromocytoma
  - 90% of pheos occur in adults (average 40 years)
  - Curable if diagnosed and treated; standard treatment is surgery, regardless of stage
  - 10% with benign disease will develop recurrence, usually 5-15 years later; 50% of recurrences are metastatic
  - 5-year survival of patients with metastatic disease is 40-45%
  - Genetic counseling is recommended for all patients to evaluate risk for hereditary syndrome
  - Adrenalectomy with ligation of venous drainage (to decrease catecholamine release)
  - Requires preoperative blood pressure control
    - α-blockade 10-14 days prior, β-blockade 2-3 days prior
    - Prevents intraoperative hypertensive crisis
  - Lifelong follow-up to detect recurrent or metastatic disease

DIAGNOSTIC CHECKLIST

Image Interpretation Pearls

- Bilateral low-level adrenal uptake on I-123 MIBG scintigraphy is likely normal or hyperplasia
- I-123 MIBG SPECT/CT usually performed for most complete 3D evaluation (often just SPECT in children to avoid extra radiation from CT)

Reporting Tips

- Report should include size, location, presence of regional lymphadenopathy or distant metastases
- Report should include any limiting factors (interfering drugs that could not be discontinued, small lesion size, etc.)

SELECTED REFERENCES

1. Bombardieri E et al: 131I/123I-metaiodobenzylguanidine (mIBG) scintigraphy: procedure guidelines for tumour imaging. Eur J Nucl Med Mol Imaging. 37(12):2436-46, 2010
2. Olivier P et al: Guidelines for radioiodinated MIBG scintigraphy in children. Eur J Nucl Med Mol Imaging. 30(5):B45-50, 2003
3. Timmers HJ et al: Staging and functional characterization of pheochromocytoma and paraganglioma by 18F-fluorodeoxyglucose (18F-FDG) positron emission tomography. J Natl Cancer Inst. 104(9):700-8, 2012

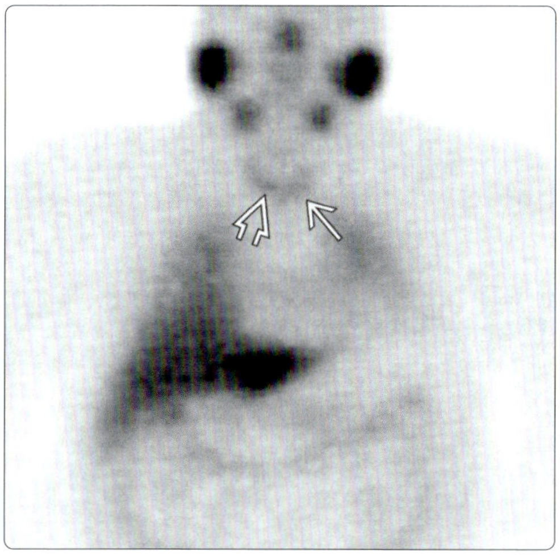

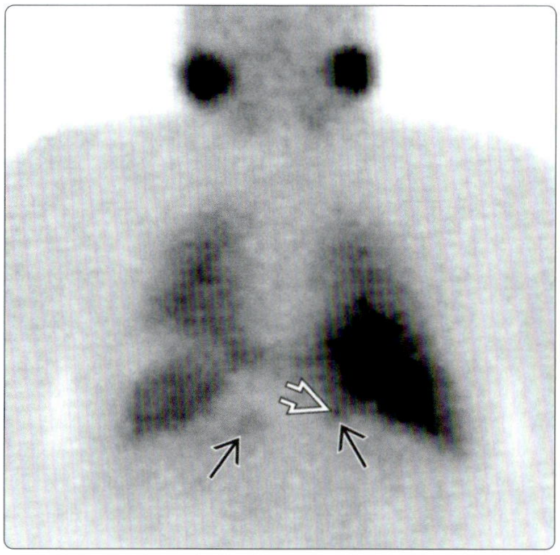

(Left) *Anterior I-123 MIBG scintigraphy in a patient with MEN syndrome shows diffuse thyroid uptake ➡ with more intense focus of uptake ➡ at the right inferior lobe, later confirmed to be malignant. Normally the thyroid will not be visualized due to blockade with potassium iodide.* **(Right)** *Posterior I-123 MIBG scintigraphy in the same patient shows bilateral adrenal uptake ➡, right ➡ greater than left, with surgical pathology confirming right adrenal pheo. Medullary hyperplasia usually causes symmetric bilateral uptake.*

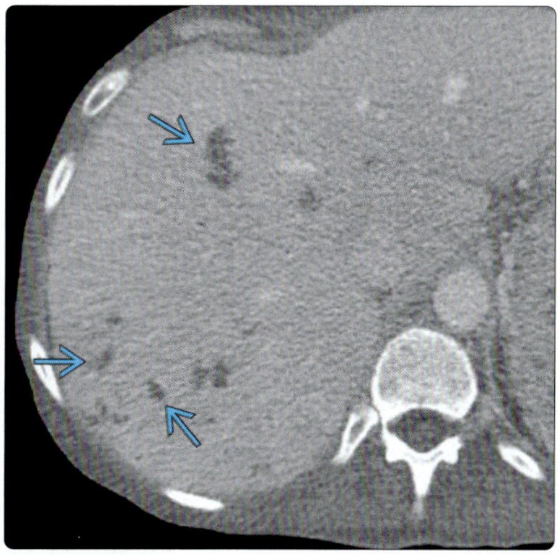

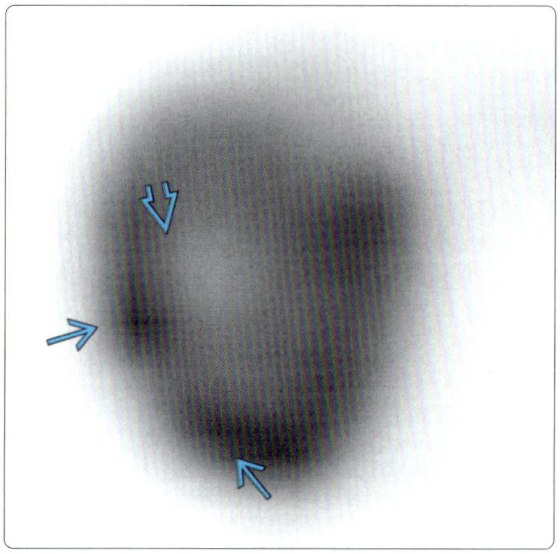

(Left) *Axial CECT in a patient with known pheo demonstrates multiple small, ill-defined lesions ➡, many of which are along the liver margins and cause contour distortion. This finding is concerning for metastatic disease.* **(Right)** *Axial I-123 MIBG scintigraphy in the same patient shows heterogeneous uptake ➡ of MIBG throughout entire liver, especially at the periphery. There is a large area of photopenia ➡ evident, consistent with necrosis. This finding is consistent with metastatic pheo.*

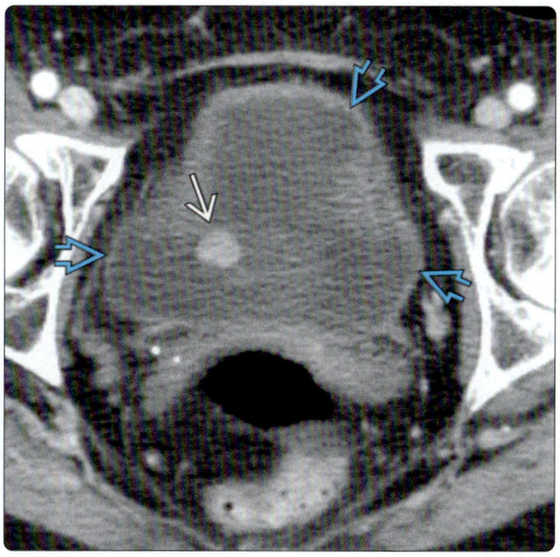

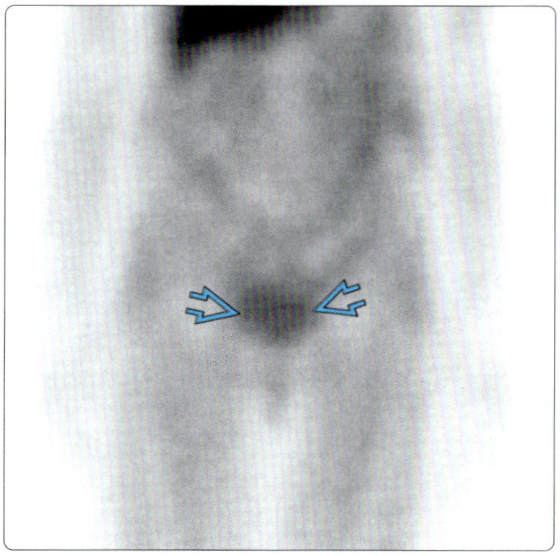

(Left) *Axial CECT in a 54-year-old woman with episodic hypertension provoked by urination shows a solid, enhancing mass ➡ in the bladder ➡. This is consistent with extra-adrenal paraganglioma.* **(Right)** *Anterior I-123 MIBG scintigraphy of the same patient fails to identify the mass due to physiologic distribution of radiotracer in the bladder ➡, which masks the paraganglioma.*

Medullary Thyroid Carcinoma

KEY FACTS

TERMINOLOGY

- Medullary thyroid carcinoma (MTC): Rare neuroendocrine malignancy arising from thyroid parafollicular C cells
  - Not radioactive iodine-avid: Scanning and treatment with radioactive iodine not effective

IMAGING

- Somatostatin receptor scintigraphy
  - Uptake in solid, usually well-circumscribed mass in thyroid gland; ± calcifications; nodal and distant metastases
  - In-111 octreotide (pentetreotide, Octreoscan): Sensitivity 25-41%, specificity 92%
- F-18 FDG PET/CT: Sensitivity 70-100%, specificity 79-90%
- Tc-99m sestamibi or tetrofosmin scintigraphy: Sensitivity 25-40%, specificity 100%
- Nuclear medicine most helpful for suspected recurrence
  - Elevated tumor markers but no gross disease on cross-sectional imaging

PATHOLOGY

- Staging system
  - Stage 0: Elevated calcitonin level on screening
  - Stage 1: T1 (< 2 cm) N0 M0
  - Stage 2: T2-T3 (> 2 cm, no extrathyroidal extension; any size tumor with extrathyroidal extension) N0
  - Stage 3: T1-T3 N1a (tracheal/laryngeal lymph nodes) M0
  - Stage 4a: T4a (spread to adjacent tissues/trachea/esophagus/larynx, recurrent laryngeal nerve) any N M0, or T1-T3 N1b (uni- or bilateral cervical or mediastinal adenopathy) M0
  - Stage 4b: T4b (spread to tissue in front of spine, surrounding carotid artery/mediastinal blood vessels) any N M0
  - Stage 4c: Any T, any N M1 (particularly lungs, bone)

(Left) *Coronal octreotide scan reveals uptake in the left thyroid lobe in this patient with medullary thyroid cancer.* **(Right)** *Coronal octreotide scan reveals uptake in the right thyroid lobe, as well as endobronchial left lung lesion in this patient with medullary thyroid cancer.*

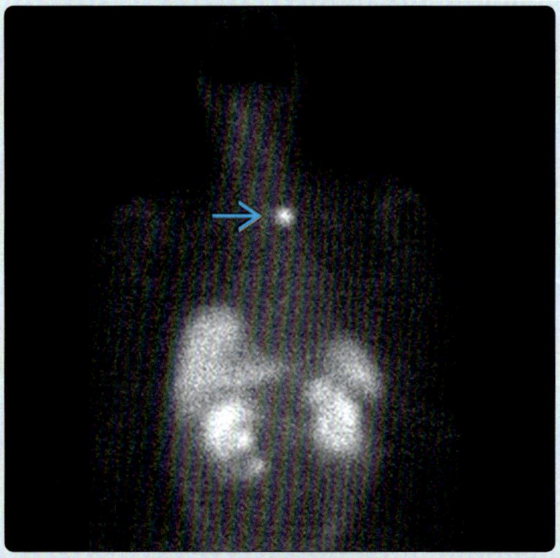

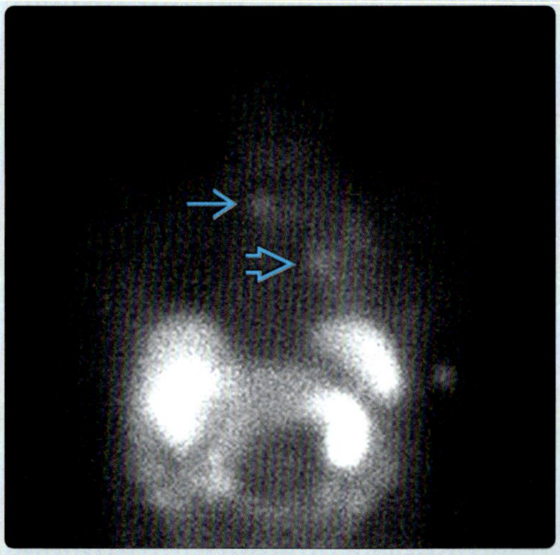

(Left) *Coronal F-18 FDG PET/CT reveals uptake in the left thyroid lobe in this patient with medullary cancer.* **(Right)** *Coronal PET reveals uptake in the bilateral thyroid lobes with diffuse uptake in the liver in this patient with advanced medullary thyroid cancer with liver metastases.*

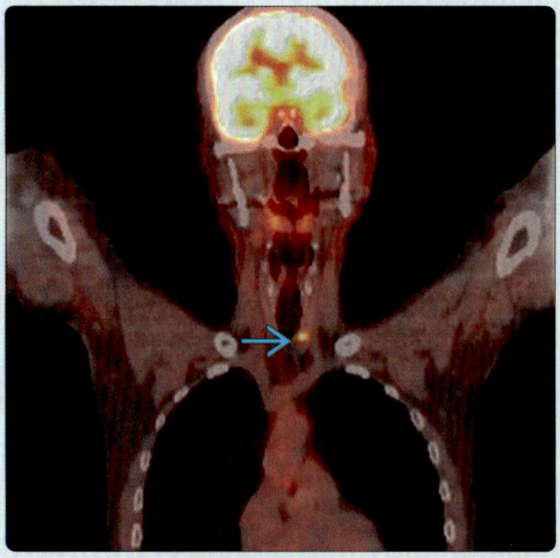

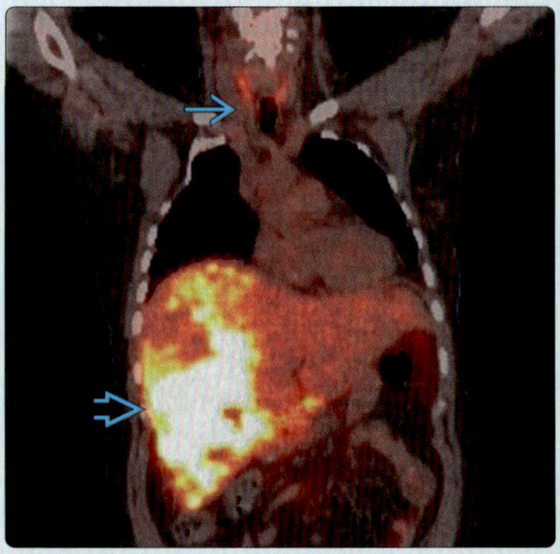

Medullary Thyroid Carcinoma

TERMINOLOGY

Definitions

- Medullary thyroid carcinoma (MTC): Rare neuroendocrine malignancy arising from thyroid parafollicular C cells

IMAGING

General Features

- Best diagnostic clue
  - Somatostatin receptor scintigraphy
    - Uptake in solid, usually well-circumscribed mass in thyroid gland; ± calcifications
      - More locally infiltrative type with familial forms
      - Frequently multifocal: 2/3 of sporadic cases, almost all familial cases
    - Uptake in nodal metastases
      - Level VI and superior mediastinum
      - Retropharyngeal nodes, levels III and IV (mid and low internal jugular chain)
    - Uptake in distant metastases

Nuclear Medicine Findings

- Methods for detection of recurrent disease when cross-sectional imaging negative
  - In-111 octreotide (pentetreotide, Octreoscan): Sensitivity 25-41%, specificity 92%
    - Also positive in many neuroendocrine tumors
  - F-18 FDG PET/CT: Sensitivity 70-100%, specificity 79-90%
    - Also positive in well-differentiated and anaplastic thyroid cancer, thyroiditis, other malignancies
  - Tc-99m sestamibi or tetrofosmin: Sensitivity 25-40%, specificity 100%
    - Also positive in thyroid and parathyroid adenomas, various malignancies
  - Tc-99m pentavalent (V) DMSA: Sensitivity 33-40%, specificity 78%
  - In same series as nuclear techniques: Sensitivity/specificity MR (82/67%), CT (50/20%)
  - I-131/I-123 methyiodobenzylguanidine (MIBG): Limited reports, can be positive in MTC
- Most helpful for suspected recurrence
  - Elevated tumor markers but no gross disease on cross-sectional imaging
- Not iodine avid: Scanning and treatment with radioiodine not effective

Imaging Recommendations

- Best imaging tool
  - High-resolution ultrasound (US) is most frequent initial tool for evaluation of thyroid nodule
    - FNA can be performed at same time
  - MR or F-18 FDG PET/CT for cases where cross-sectional imaging negative (similar performance)
  - CECT may have better performance in mediastinum than MR
- Protocol advice
  - Somatostatin receptor scintigraphy (SRS)
    - Patient preparation
      - Well-hydrate before and after injection to reduce radiation exposure
      - IV infusion of glucose on standby for patients at risk of insulinoma due to potential for inducing severe hypoglycemia
    - Radiopharmaceutical
      - In-111 pentetreotide is a conjugate of octreotide
      - Recommended administered activity is 6 mCi (222 MBq) in adults and 0.14 mCi (5.18 MBq)/kg in children
    - Dosimetry
      - Organ receiving largest dose is spleen
    - Image acquisition
      - Patient should void prior to imaging
      - Images acquired at 4 and 24 hr, or 24 and 48 hr post injection if significant bowel activity
      - Planar images acquired using large field-of-view gamma camera fitted with medium-energy collimator
      - Symmetrical 20% energy windows are centered over both photo peaks of In-111 and data from both windows is added
      - SPECT/CT if needed to localize abnormalities in three dimensions, detect small lesions

DIFFERENTIAL DIAGNOSIS

Multinodular Goiter

- Diffusely enlarged gland with multiple nodules, coarse calcifications

Follicular Adenoma

- Solitary mass without evidence of invasion, no adenopathy

Parathyroid Adenoma

- Similar features on Tc-99m sestamibi; usually extrathyroidal

Papillary Thyroid Cancer

- Painless, slow-growing mass with less frequent palpable nodal adenopathy (15-30%)

Follicular Thyroid Cancer

- Painless unifocal mass with rare nodal adenopathy, more commonly has distant metastases

PATHOLOGY

General Features

- Etiology
  - No identified exogenous cause and not related to other thyroid conditions
  - Type 2 multiple endocrine neoplasia (MEN) syndromes
    - Autosomal dominant
    - MEN 2A: Multifocal MTC, pheochromocytoma, parathyroid hyperplasia, hyperparathyroidism
    - MEN 2B: Multifocal MTC, pheochromocytoma, mucosal neuromas of lips, tongue, GI tract, conjunctiva; younger patients, more aggressive tumors
  - Familial medullary thyroid carcinoma (FMTC)
    - Autosomal dominant condition where only neoplasm is MTC
    - Later onset, more indolent course than MEN syndromes
- Genetics

- Sporadic (~ 85%) or hereditary, familial forms (15%)
- Associated with mutations of RET proto-oncogene on chromosome 10q11.2
  - Found in familial (100%) and sporadic (40-60%) cases
  - Screening for RET mutations is performed for family members of patients with MTC
- Arises from parafollicular C cells of thyroid that secrete calcitonin
  - C cells derived from ultimobranchial bodies

Staging, Grading, & Classification

- Stage 0: Elevated calcitonin level on screening
- Stage 1: T1 (< 2 cm) N0 M0
- Stage 2: T2-T3 (> 2 cm, no extrathyroidal extension; any size tumor with extrathyroidal extension) N0
- Stage 3: T1-T3 N1a (tracheal/laryngeal lymph nodes) M0
- Stage 4a: T4a (spread to adjacent tissues/trachea/esophagus/larynx, recurrent laryngeal nerve) any N M0, or T1-T3 N1b (uni- or bilateral cervical or mediastinal adenopathy) M0
- Stage 4b: T4b (spread to tissue in front of spine, surrounding carotid artery/mediastinal blood vessels) any N M0
- Stage 4c: Any T, any N M1 (particularly lungs, bone)

CLINICAL ISSUES

Presentation

- Most common signs/symptoms
  - Painless thyroid nodule
  - Other signs/symptoms
    - Less commonly dysphagia, hoarseness, pain
    - Uncommonly presents with paraneoplastic syndromes: Cushing or carcinoid syndromes
    - Rarely presents with diarrhea from elevated calcitonin, though often an associated symptom
  - Elevated serum calcitonin
    - Used as screening tool, for estimation of extent of disease and as baseline for postoperative monitoring
  - May present with the following concurrent neoplasms, if associated with MEN 2 syndromes
    - Pheochromocytoma
    - Parathyroid hyperplasia
    - Mucosal neuroma
    - Marfanoid habitus
- Clinical profile
  - Middle-aged patient with lower neck mass
  - Patient with family history of MEN with tumor on screening exam

Demographics

- Age
  - Sporadic form: Mean = 50 years
  - Familial form: Mean = 30 years
  - Can occur in children, especially with MEN 2B
- Gender
  - M < F in Caucasians and in children
- Epidemiology
  - 5-10% all thyroid gland malignancies
  - ≤ 14% thyroid cancer deaths
  - 10% pediatric thyroid malignancies (MEN 2)

Natural History & Prognosis

- Familial type almost always multifocal and bilateral
- 2/3 of sporadic cases are bilateral
- Up to 75% have lymphadenopathy at presentation
- Indicators of better prognosis
  - Female gender, younger age at surgery
  - FMTC and MEN 2A syndromes
  - Tumor < 10 cm, no nodes, early stage disease
  - Normal preoperative CEA levels, complete surgical resection
- 50-80% overall survival
- Worse prognosis if unilateral, younger age, or with metastasis

Treatment

- Prophylactic thyroidectomy performed if familial RET mutation detected
  - FMTC and MEN 2A perform thyroidectomy at age 5-6
  - MEN 2B perform thyroidectomy during infancy
- Mainstay of MTC treatment is complete resection of local and regional disease
  - Total thyroidectomy with level VI nodal dissection ± superior mediastinal nodes
  - Node levels II-V resected if positive nodes in lateral neck
- Adjuvant radiation therapy
  - XRT used if extensive soft tissue invasion or extracapsular nodal spread
- Yearly calcitonin levels to monitor for recurrence

DIAGNOSTIC CHECKLIST

Consider

- Familial syndromes with multifocal tumors/young patient

Image Interpretation Pearls

- Imaging appearance may mimic differentiated thyroid carcinoma
- F-18 FDG PET/CT and MR best performance for detection of recurrence: PET and CECT allows detection of distant mets

SELECTED REFERENCES

1. Society of Nuclear Medicine Procedure Guideline for Somatostatin Receptor Scintigraphy with In-111 Pentetreotide
2. Khan N et al: Review of fluorine-18-2-fluoro-2-deoxy-D-glucose positron emission tomography (FDG-PET) in the follow-up of medullary and anaplastic thyroid carcinomas. Cancer Control. 12(4):254-60, 2005
3. Pasha R, Golub J. Otolaryngology-Head and Neck Surgery: Clinical Reference Guide. San Diego, Ca. 4th Ed:Plural Publishing, Inc; 2013.
4. Li S et al: The radionuclide molecular imaging and therapy of neuroendocrine tumors. Curr Cancer Drug Targets. 5(2):139-48, 2005
5. de Groot JW et al: Impact of 18F-fluoro-2-deoxy-D-glucose positron emission tomography (FDG-PET) in patients with biochemical evidence of recurrent or residual medullary thyroid cancer. Ann Surg Oncol. 11(8):786-94, 2004
6. Bustillo A et al: Octreotide scintigraphy in the head and neck. Laryngoscope. 114(3):434-40, 2004
7. Massoll N et al: Diagnosis and management of medullary thyroid carcinoma. Clin Lab Med. 24(1):49-83, 2004
8. Schoder H et al: Positron emission imaging of head and neck cancer, including thyroid carcinoma. Semin Nucl Med. 34(3):180-97, 2004
9. Clayman GL et al: Medullary thyroid cancer. Otolaryngol Clin North Am. 36(1):91-105, 2003
10. Solbiati L et al: Ultrasound of thyroid, parathyroid glands and neck lymph nodes. Eur Radiol. 11(12):2411-24, 2001

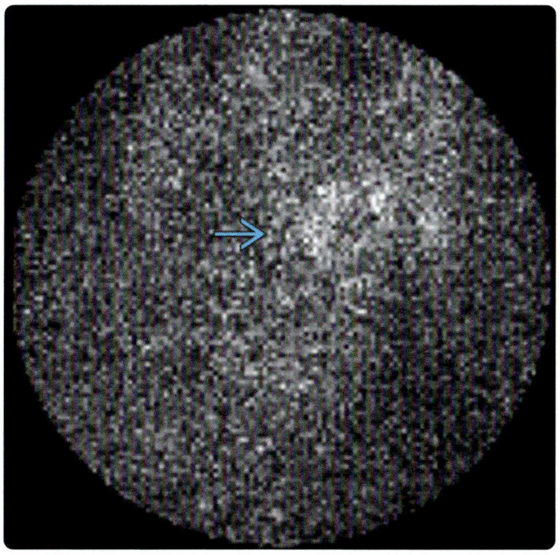

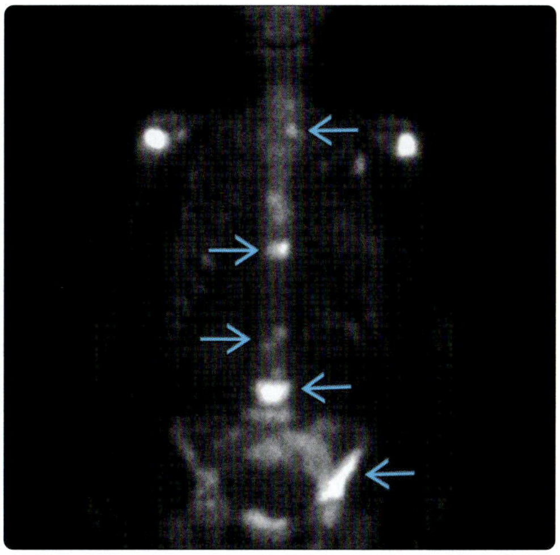

(Left) *Anterior parathyroid scan reveals uptake in the left thyroid bed → in medullary thyroid cancer status post thyroidectomy, indicating possible parathyroid adenoma. Concurrent medullary cancer and parathyroid adenoma are common findings in MEN syndromes.* **(Right)** *Anterior bone scan reveals multiple sites of bone uptake →, indicating bone metastases in this patient with medullary thyroid cancer.*

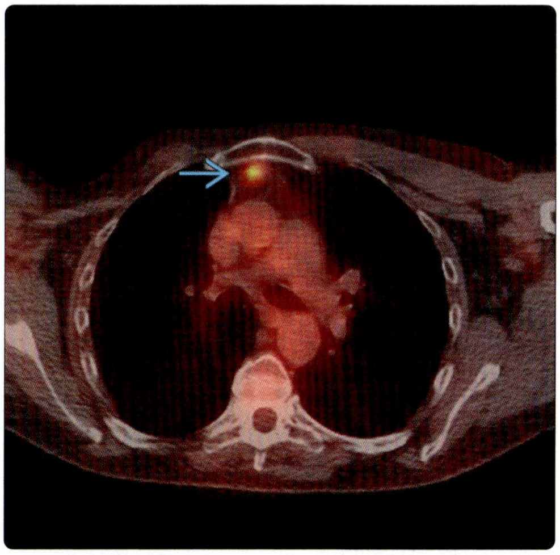

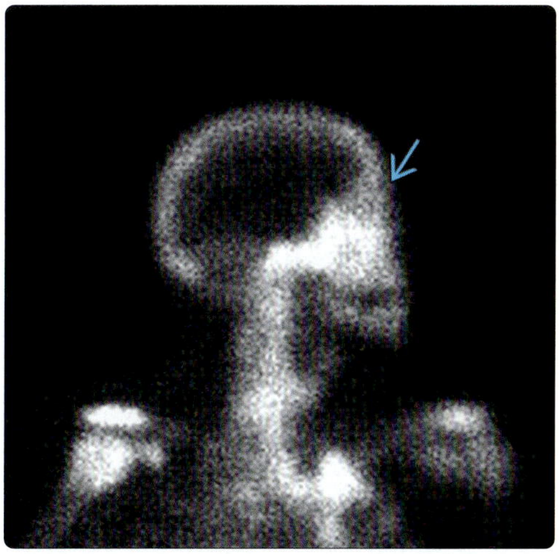

(Left) *Axial F-18 FDG PET/CT shows uptake in the mediastinum →, indicating lymph node metastasis in this patient with medullary thyroid cancer.* **(Right)** *Lateral bone scan reveals uptake within the paranasal sinuses →, raising suspicion of rare skull base metastases in this patient with medullary thyroid cancer.*

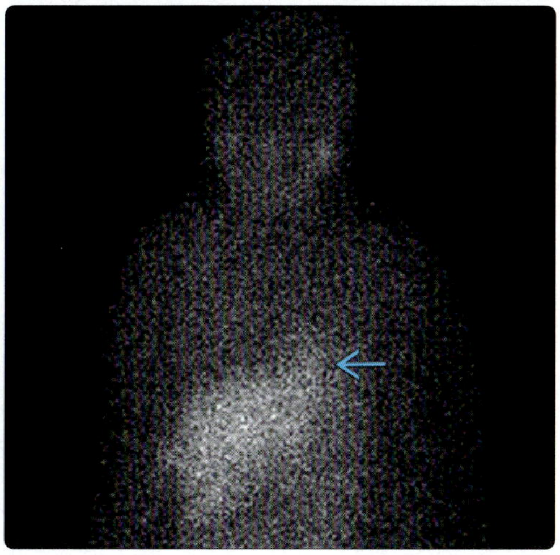

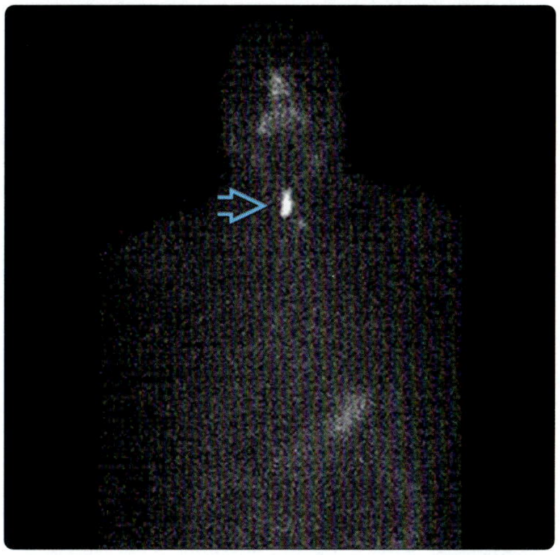

(Left) *Anterior MIBG scan shows diffuse uptake in the left adrenal gland → in a patient with elevated catecholamines, raising suspicion of pheochromocytoma. Concurrent medullary thyroid cancer and pheochromocytoma are often seen in patients with MEN syndromes.* **(Right)** *Anterior radioactive iodine scan in a patient post thyroidectomy for papillary thyroid cancer shows residual thyroid tissue →. Note medullary thyroid cancer is not followed with or treated with radioactive iodine.*

Pancreatic Adenocarcinoma

KEY FACTS

IMAGING

- Staging
  - CECT predicts resectability with ~ 70-80% accuracy
  - F-18 FDG PET/CT alters patient management in ~ 11-27% of cases
  - Sensitivity of various modalities for detecting metastatic disease
    - CECT: 57%
    - F-18 FDG PET/CT: 61%
    - F-18 FDG PET/CT + CECT: 87%
- Response to therapy
  - F-18 FDG PET/CT is useful to assess response to chemotherapy and radiation therapy

PATHOLOGY

- Staging
  - Stage 0-IB
    - T1-T2 (tumor limited to pancreas)
  - Stage IIA
    - T3 (extends beyond pancreas but without involvement of celiac axis or superior mesentery artery)
  - Stage IIB
    - T1-T3, N1 (regional lymph nodes)
  - Stage III
    - T4 (tumor involves the celiac axis or superior mesentery artery, unresectable tumor) any N
  - Stage IV
    - M1 (distant metastasis)

DIAGNOSTIC CHECKLIST

- Obtain CECT to determine resectability
- F-18 FDG PET/CT is useful in cases of borderline-resectable tumor to exclude distant metastatic disease and avoid unnecessary surgery
- F-18 FDG PET/CT can also assess response to therapy

(Left) *Axial CECT in a patient with lower abdominal pain shows a low-attenuation lesion in the pancreatic tail ➡ concerning for pancreatic adenocarcinoma.* **(Right)** *Axial fused F-18 FDG PET/CT in the same patient shows focal increase uptake in the pancreatic mass ➡. No metastatic disease was detected.*

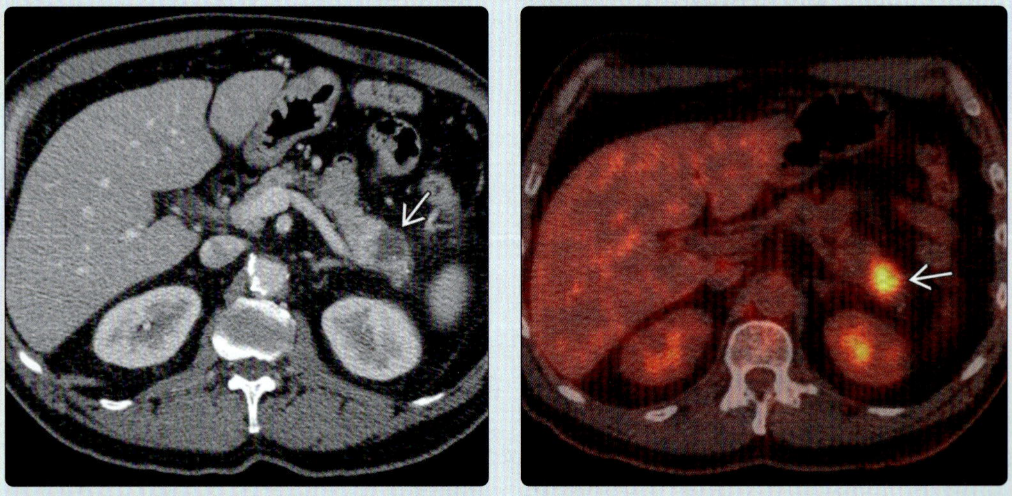

(Left) *Axial fused F-18 FDG PET/CT shows diffuse uptake throughout the pancreas ➡ in a patient with acute edematous interstitial pancreatitis.* **(Right)** *Axial CECT shows multiple cystic lesions involving the pancreatic tail and body ➡ suggestive of intraductal papillary mucinous neoplasms. Below, F-18 FDG PET/CT shows no uptake in these lesions ➡.*

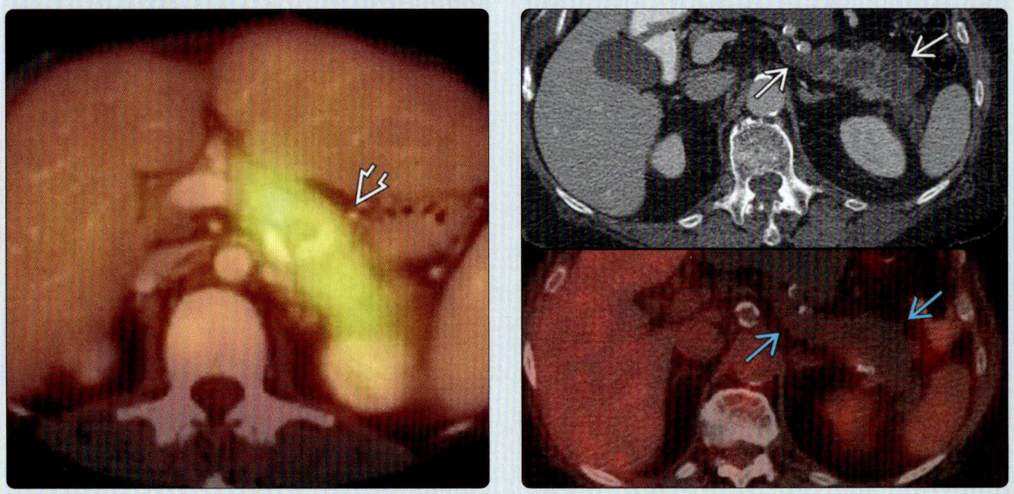

TERMINOLOGY

Definitions

- Malignant tumor of pancreas
  - Epithelial tumors
    - Exocrine
      - 95-99% of exocrine tumors arise from ductal epithelium
      - 90% are ductal adenocarcinoma
      - 10% acinar cell carcinomas, serous or mucinous cystadenocarcinoma, intraductal papillary-mucinous neoplasm, pancreatoblastoma or solid papillary carcinomas

IMAGING

Nuclear Medicine Findings

- PET
  - Local disease
    - F-18 FDG uptake in primary pancreatic tumor is variable depending on histology and size
      - Mucinous adenocarcinoma often shows low F-18 FDG uptake
      - Smaller tumors harder to detect on F-18 FDG PET/CT
  - Regional nodal disease
    - Gastroduodenal lymphatic drainage
      - Superior anterior and posterior pancreaticoduodenal nodes drain to periportal nodes
    - Inferior pancreaticoduodenal
      - Anterior and posterior pancreaticoduodenal nodes drain to superior mesenteric nodes
    - Dorsal pancreatic lymphatic drainage
      - Drain to superior mesenteric or celiac nodes
  - Distant metastatic disease
    - Liver is first solid organ to be affected
    - Tumor can show extrahepatic perineural invasion to celiac and mesenteric plexuses or intravenous spread with tumor thrombus formation
    - Tumor can spread along peritoneum or contiguous subperitoneal spaces such as mesocolon, mesentery, and peritoneal ligaments
    - Metastatic disease discover by F-18 FDG PET/CT alters patient management in 11% of cases

Imaging Recommendations

- Best imaging tool
  - Initial diagnosis
    - Endoscopic ultrasound
      - Diagnostic method of choice for pancreatic head tumors
      - Endoscopic ultrasound can be attempted for pancreatic tail tumors
      - Identifies regional nodal involvement
      - Allows nonsurgical biopsy of tumor and often lymph nodes, usually near pancreatic head or body
    - Multiphase CECT or multiphase MR + MRCP
      - Used for tumors that are difficult to access by endoscopic ultrasound
  - Staging
    - CECT predicts resectability with ~ 70-80% accuracy
    - F-18 FDG PET/CT alters patient management in approximately 11-27% of cases
    - Sensitivity of various modalities for detecting metastatic disease
      - CECT: 57%
      - F-18 FDG PET/CT: 61%
      - F-18 FDG PET/CT + CECT: 87%
  - Response to therapy
    - F-18 FDG PET/CT is useful to assess response to chemotherapy and radiation therapy
- Protocol advice
  - Utilize F-18 FDG PET/CT standard oncologic protocol

DIFFERENTIAL DIAGNOSIS

Pancreatitis

- Acute pancreatitis
  - Can cause false-positive F-18 FDG uptake secondary to increased focal uptake
  - Diffuse F-18 FDG uptake in pancreas suggests pancreatitis
- Autoimmune pancreatitis
  - Can cause mass-like appearance with increased uptake
  - Improves with corticosteroid therapy
- Chronic pancreatitis
  - Focal mass, dilated main pancreatic duct; may not be distinguishable from cancer on anatomic imaging
  - Variable F-18 FDG uptake

Islet Cell Tumor

- F-18 FDG uptake often isointense to pancreas or low-level increased uptake
- In-111 pentetreotide imaging useful for staging

Cystic Pancreatic Neoplasm

- May show mild F-18 FDG accumulation, but usually not F-18 FDG avid

Periampullary Tumors

- Adenocarcinoma of the ampulla of Vater or duodenum
- More favorable prognosis than pancreatic adenocarcinoma

Nonepithelial Tumors

- Metastases: Direct invasion or involvement of adjacent lymph nodes by many tumors including breast, melanoma, lung, renal cell carcinoma, GI tumors
- Primary pancreatic lymphoma and sarcoma are rare; usually evidence of disease elsewhere

PATHOLOGY

General Features

- Etiology
  - Risk factors
    - Diabetes, cigarette smoking, increased body mass index, heavy alcohol consumption
    - Family history of pancreatic cancer
    - Occupation exposure to chemicals such as betanasphthylamine (found in cigarettes) and benzidine (precursor of dyes and pigments)
    - Chronic pancreatitis demonstrates 7x increased risk for pancreatic cancer

- Usually sporadic
- Multiple genetic mutations identified including K-ras, *STK11*, *PRSS1*, *SPINK1*, *BRCA1*, *BRCA2*, and *CFTR*
- Peutz-Jeghers syndrome: Highly elevated risk (up to 132x)
- Familial malignant melanoma syndrome: 20-47x increased risk
- Lynch syndrome: 9-11x elevated risk
- Breast-ovarian cancer syndrome: 2.4-6x increased risk

Staging, Grading, & Classification

- Stage 0-IB
  - T1-T2 (tumor limited to pancreas)
- Stage IIA
  - T3 (extends beyond pancreas but without involvement of celiac axis or superior mesentery artery)
- Stage IIB
  - T1-T3, N1 (regional lymph nodes)
- Stage III
  - T4 (tumor involves celiac axis or superior mesentery artery, unresectable tumor) any N
- Stage IV
  - M1 (distant metastasis)
- Resectability of tumor
  - Resectable tumor
    - Stage 0-IA/B
    - No arterial or venous tumor contact
  - Borderline resectable tumor
    - Stage IIA/B
    - Solid tumor contact with arterial vessels < 180°
    - Possible vascular venous resection and reconstruction
  - Unresectable tumor
    - Stage III-IV
    - Solid tumor contact with arterial vessels > 180°
    - Unreconstructable SMV/PV due to tumor involvement or occlusion
    - Solid tumor contact with 1st jejunal SMA branch or most proximal draining jejunal branch into SMV
    - Distant metastasis

CLINICAL ISSUES

Presentation

- Most common signs/symptoms
  - Usually asymptomatic
  - Late manifestations
    - Uncontrolled diabetes mellitus or abrupt onset of diabetes
    - Pancreatic head mass may cause pancreatitis or obstructive jaundice
      - Courvoisier sign: Palpable gallbladder with painless jaundice
    - Weight loss
- Clinical profile
  - Laboratory markers: CA19-9 and CEA may be elevated

Demographics

- Age
  - 60-70 years most common at diagnosis
- Gender
  - M:F = 1:1
- Ethnicity
  - African Americans > Caucasians
- Epidemiology
  - 4th leading cause of cancer death in USA

Natural History & Prognosis

- Resectable tumor survival
  - 15-25% at 5 years
- Borderline resectable tumors
  - Neoadjuvant chemotherapy allows downstaging in approximately 30% of tumors
  - Patients who achieved complete resection defined as absence of macro- or microscopic residual tumor on resection margins
    - 15-25% survival at 5 years
- Unresectable tumor survival
  - < 5% at 5 years

Treatment

- Stage 0-IIB
  - Whipple procedure pancreatoduodenectomy
- Stage III: Borderline resectable tumor
  - Neoadjuvant chemotherapy and radiation with subsequent surgery
- Stage III-IV: Unresectable tumor
  - Chemotherapy, ongoing trials, palliative care

DIAGNOSTIC CHECKLIST

Consider

- Obtain CECT to determine resectability
- F-18 FDG PET/CT is useful in patients with borderline-resectable tumor to exclude distant metastatic disease and avoid unnecessary surgery
- F-18 FDG PET/CT is also useful to assess response to therapy

SELECTED REFERENCES

1. Raman SP et al: Cross-sectional imaging and the role of positron emission tomography in pancreatic cancer evaluation. Semin Oncol. 42(1):40-58, 2015
2. Cassinotto C et al: Locally advanced pancreatic adenocarcinoma: reassessment of response with CT after neoadjuvant chemotherapy and radiation therapy. Radiology. 273(1):108-16, 2014
3. Kim MJ et al: The value of positron emission tomography/computed tomography for evaluating metastatic disease in patients with pancreatic cancer. Pancreas. 41(6):897-903, 2012
4. Shrikhande SV et al: Multimodality imaging of pancreatic ductal adenocarcinoma: a review of the literature. HPB (Oxford). 14(10):658-68, 2012
5. Meyers MA et al. Meyers' Dynamic Radiology of the abdomen. Normal and Pathologic Anatomy, 6th Edition. Springer, 2011
6. National Comprehensive Cancer Network. Pancreatic Adenocarcinoma NCCN Guideline, Version 1.2015

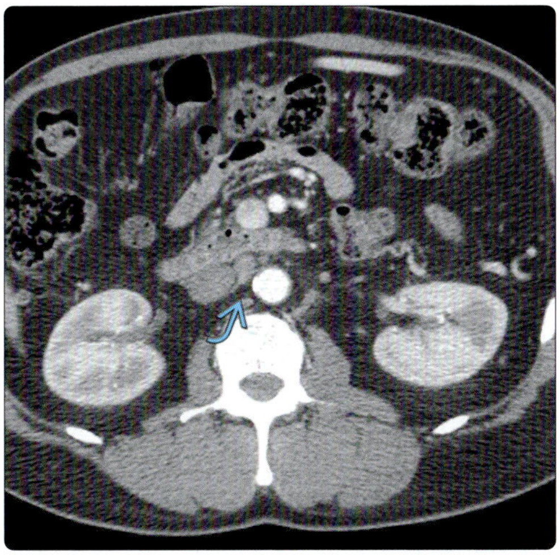

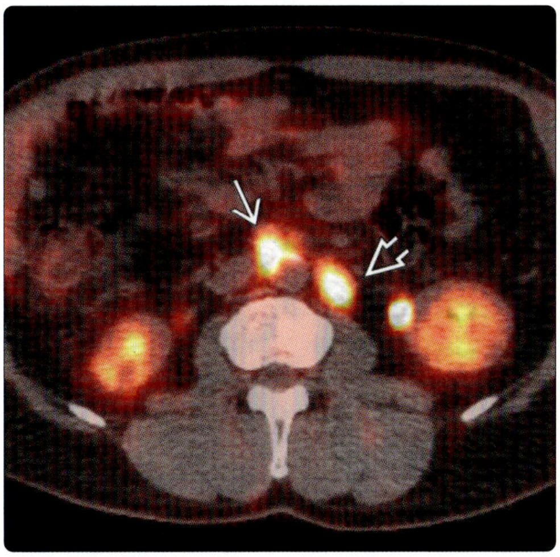

(Left) *Axial CECT performed for staging a patient with pancreatic cancer shows an enlarged retroperitoneal node* ➚. **(Right)** *Axial fused F-18 FDG PET/CT in the same patient demonstrates marked increased activity in the lymph node* ➙. *Note normal excretion of F-18 FDG in the left ureter* ➙.

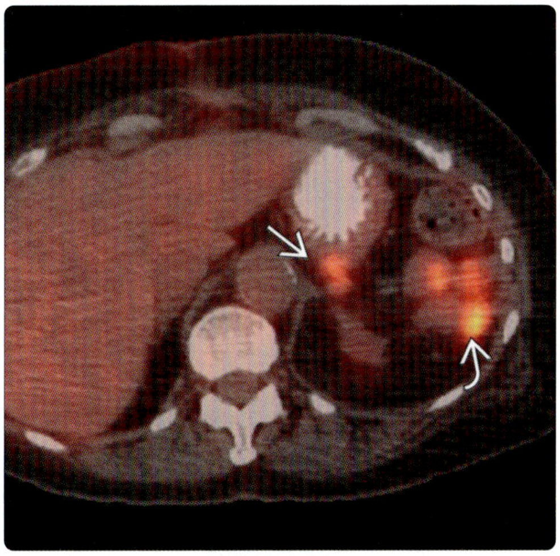

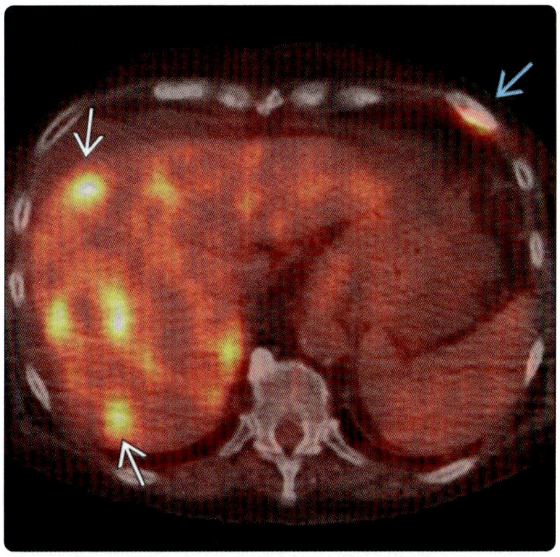

(Left) *Axial fused F-18 FDG PET/CT in a patient post partial pancreatectomy due to pancreatic tail adenocarcinoma shows hypermetabolic soft tissue suspicious for local recurrence* ➙ *and peritoneal metastases* ➚. **(Right)** *Axial fused F-18 FDG PET/CT in a patient with biopsy-proven adenocarcinoma of the pancreatic head shows hepatic* ➙ *and osseous* ➙ *metastases.*

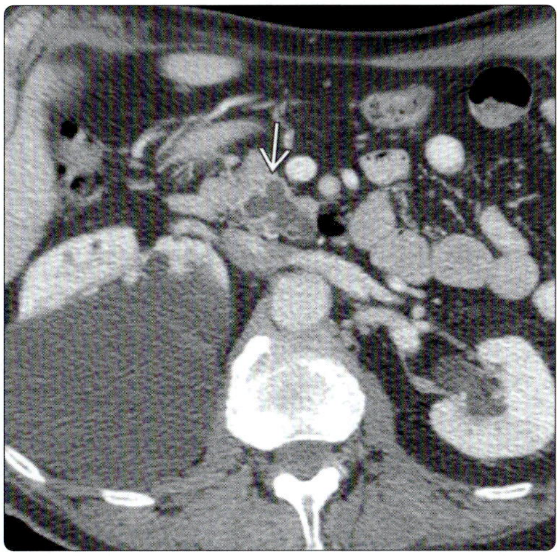

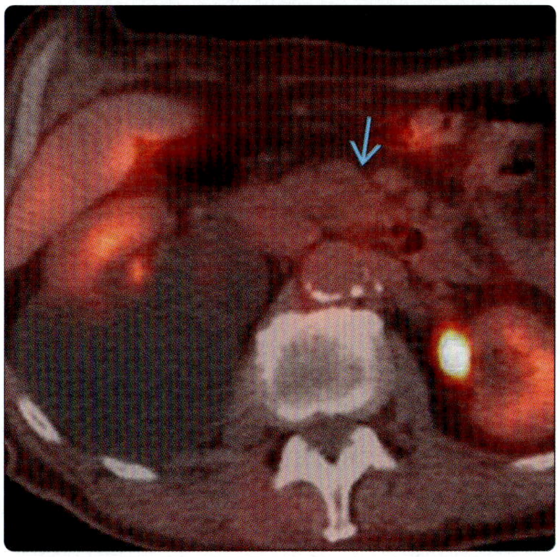

(Left) *Axial CECT shows a cystic, lobulated, nonenhancing lesion in the uncinate process* ➙ *of the pancreas.* **(Right)** *Axial fused F-18 FDG PET/CT in the same patient shows no uptake* ➙ *in this biopsy-proven mucinous neoplasm.*

Uterine and Endometrial Cancers

KEY FACTS

TERMINOLOGY

- Endometrial adenocarcinoma
  - Neoplasm of uterine glandular epithelium
  - Most common type of endometrial cancer

IMAGING

- F-18 FDG PET/CT
  - Hypermetabolic primary uterine mass
  - Hypermetabolic lymphadenopathy
    - Pelvic nodal groups
    - Common iliac
    - Paraaortic
  - Hypermetabolic distant metastases
    - Lung
    - Liver
    - Bone
  - Nonmalignant F-18 FDG uptake in younger patients who are menstruating
    - Endometrial thickness and metabolic activity varies from proliferative → secretory phase of menstrual cycle

TOP DIFFERENTIAL DIAGNOSES

- Cervical cancer
- Leiomyoma
- Endometrial sarcoma
- Endometrial polyp/hyperplasia
- Physiologic menstruation

PATHOLOGY

- Staging
  - Stage I: Confined to uterus
  - Stage II: Involvement of cervix
  - Stage III: Involvement of adjacent structures **&/or** para-aortic nodes
  - Stage IV: Invasion of bowel/bladder **&/or** inguinal nodes or distant mets

(Left) *Axial FDG PET/CT of a 72-year-old woman with endometrial cancer s/p total abdominal hysterectomy shows a hypermetabolic left supraclavicular lymph node (Virchow's node) ➡.* **(Right)** *Posterior FDG PET MIP in the same patient at left shows hypermetabolic lymphadenopathy in the iliac ➡ and paraaortic ➡ chains.*

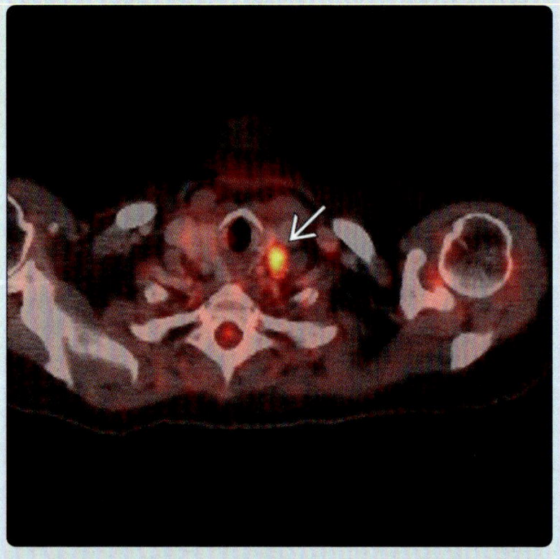

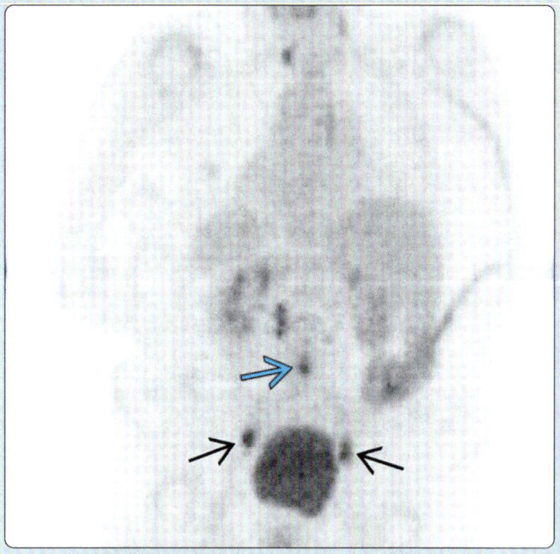

(Left) *Axial NECT in a 55-year-old woman shows a uterine mass ➡, biopsy-proven endometrial carcinoma.* **(Right)** *Anterior FDG PET MIP in the same patient shows a heterogeneous, hypermetabolic mass ➡ directly superior to the bladder ➡ and no lymphatic or distant metastases. Other foci ➡ of uptake are within the renal collecting systems bilaterally.*

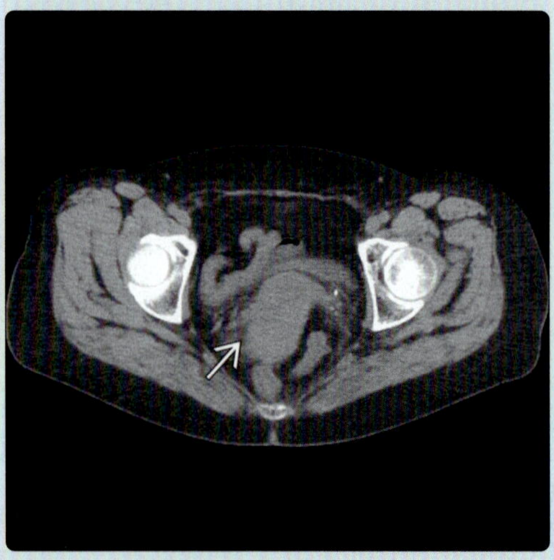

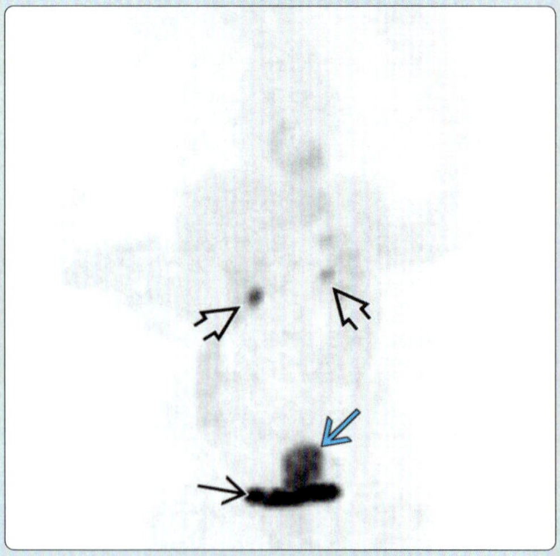

TERMINOLOGY

Definitions

- Endometrial adenocarcinoma
  - Neoplasm of uterine glandular epithelium
  - Most common type of endometrial cancer

IMAGING

General Features

- Best diagnostic clue
  - F-18 FDG PET/CT
    - Primary: Hypermetabolic primary uterine mass
      - May also see thickened endometrium on CT
      - Usually originates in glandular superior endometrium
    - Regional: Hypermetabolic invasion of adjacent structures
      - Cervix
      - Vagina
      - Bowel
      - Bladder
    - Lymphatic: Hypermetabolic lymphadenopathy
      - Pelvic nodal groups
      - Common iliac
      - Paraaortic
    - Hematogenous: Hypermetabolic lesions
      - Lung
      - Liver
      - Bone

Nuclear Medicine Findings

- PET/CT
  - Primary tumor detection
    - Superior to CT/MR in several studies
      - US is modality of choice for initial evaluation
    - Sensitivity 90%, specificity 50% for detection of primary lesions (83%, 33% for MR)
    - Extent of primary tumor can be difficult to evaluate
      - Depth of muscular invasion is critical for prognosis
  - Detection of lymph node metastases
    - Useful for preoperative staging: One study found PET/CT altered management in 48%
      - Overall diagnostic accuracy of 89.5%
    - Sensitivity 70%, specificity 90% (compared to 45% and 88% for MR)
    - Nodes missed by PET/CT usually < 1 cm
    - Detects paraaortic nodes with lower sensitivity than pelvic nodes (sensitivity 57% and specificity 83%)
    - MR is also used for local staging
  - Surveillance
    - Overall sensitivity 100%, specificity 83% in detecting recurrence
    - One study found 100% diagnostic accuracy of PET/CT in 64 asymptomatic patients
      - 100% sensitivity, specificity, PPV, NPV
    - In patients with suspected recurrence (elevated tumor markers or positive CT findings)
      - NPV 100%, PPV 95%, accuracy 96%
      - PET/CT has been found to diagnose recurrence in patients with elevated tumor markers and negative CT
    - Changed clinical decisions 21% of time
    - PET/CT role in routine surveillance not well studied

Imaging Recommendations

- Best imaging tool
  - F-18 FDG PET/CT
    - Proven efficacy for primary tumor detection, preoperative staging, detection of metastatic disease
      - Does not replace surgical staging
    - Further studies needed to determine role in post-treatment surveillance
      - Results from recent studies show high diagnostic accuracy
      - No official recommendations regarding surveillance protocols
- Protocol advice
  - Prevention of urine-associated artifact
    - Give patient 1 L of water 1 hour prior to image aquisition
    - Patient should void just prior to imaging

DIFFERENTIAL DIAGNOSIS

Neoplasms

- Cervical cancer
  - Commonly presents with vaginal bleeding
  - Hypermetabolic on F-18 FDG PET
- Leiomyoma
  - Benign smooth muscle neoplasm of uterus
  - Variable FDG uptake, difficult to distinguish on PET/CT
- Endometrial sarcoma
  - Leiomyosarcoma
    - Malignant smooth muscle neoplasm of uterus
    - Large, high-grade tumors are hypermetabolic on F-18 FDG PET
  - Carcinosarcoma
    - Malignant uterine neoplasm with both epithelial and muscle components
    - Hypermetabolic on F-18 FDG PET
- Endometrial polyp
  - Mass originating from endometrial lining
    - Pedunculated or sessile; can be premalignant
  - Can be hypermetabolic on F-18 FDG PET
- Endometrial hyperplasia
  - Proliferation of endometrial glands, can progress to endometrial carcinoma
  - Hypermetabolic on F-18 FDG PET, although typically lower SUV values than carcinoma

Uterine/Vaginal Bleeding

- Normal menstruation
- Ovulatory dysfunction
- Bleeding disorders
- Iatrogenic

PATHOLOGY

General Features

- Major risk factors

- Excess of endogenous/exogenous estrogen (main risk factor)
- Obesity
- Nulliparity
- Increasing age
- Genetic susceptibility
  - Lynch syndrome: Hereditary nonpolyposis colorectal cancer
    - DNA mismatch repair mutation carries increase risk of colon, endometrial cancer, among others
  - Cowden syndrome: Multiple hamartoma syndrome
    - Autosomal dominant, predisposition to breast, thyroid, and endometrial cancer

Staging, Grading, & Classification

- **TNM Staging**
  - Primary tumor (T)
    - Tis: Carcinoma in situ
    - T1: Confined to body of uterus
    - T2: Invasion of cervical stroma
    - T3: Involvement of adnexal structures **&/or** vagina
    - T4: Invasion of bladder **&/or** bowel
  - Regional lymph nodes (N)
    - N0: No regional mets
    - N1: Mets to pelvic nodes
    - N2: Mets to paraaortic nodes ± pelvic node involvement
  - Distant metastases (M)
    - M0: No distant mets
    - M1: Distant mets
- **Stage I**
  - T1, N0, M0
- **Stage II**
  - T2, N0, M0
- **Stage III**
  - T3 or T1-T2 with any N
- **Stage IV**
  - T4 &/or M1

CLINICAL ISSUES

Presentation

- Most common signs/symptoms
  - Premenopausal
    - May present as intermenstrual bleeding &/or menorrhagia
  - Postmenopausal
    - Any bleeding highly suspicious
- Other signs/symptoms
  - Dyspareunia
  - Nonbloody vaginal discharge
  - Pelvic pain

Demographics

- Age
  - Average at diagnosis: 61 years
  - Most cases in postmenopausal women
- Ethnicity
  - Incidence higher in Caucasians (24.8:100,000)
  - African Americans have significantly higher mortality than other ethnicities
- Epidemiology
  - 50,000 cases and 8,600 deaths each year in USA
  - Approximately 290,000 new cases worldwide in 2008

Natural History & Prognosis

- 5-year survival
  - Stage I: 85-90%
  - Stage II: 74-83%
  - Stage III: 50-66%
  - Stage IV: 20-26%

Treatment

- Surgery
  - Total extrafascial hysterectomy
  - Bilateral salpingo-oophorectomy
  - Pelvic and paraaortic lymph node dissection
- Adjuvant therapy
  - Intermediate or high-risk patients benefit from postoperative chemoradiation
- Fertility preservation
  - Women with stage I disease can be candidates for progestin therapy without surgery

DIAGNOSTIC CHECKLIST

Consider

- F-18 FDG PET/CT
  - Useful in preoperative staging
  - Lymph node detection is variable depending on size, location, and relation to other anatomic structures
  - Potential use for post-treatment surveillance
    - Recent studies have promising results
  - Limited utility in primary tumor characterization compared with CECT/MR
  - Coronal images often useful for detection of small hypermetabolic lymph nodes
  - Empty urinary bladder useful to help characterize pelvic lymphadenopathy

SELECTED REFERENCES

1. Picchio M et al: High-grade endometrial cancer: value of [(18)F]FDG PET/CT in preoperative staging. Nucl Med Commun. 31(6):506-12, 2010
2. Kitajima K et al: Accuracy of 18F-FDG PET/CT in detecting pelvic and paraaortic lymph node metastasis in patients with endometrial cancer. AJR Am J Roentgenol. 190(6):1652-8, 2008
3. Park JY et al: Clinical impact of positron emission tomography or positron emission tomography/computed tomography in the posttherapy surveillance of endometrial carcinoma: evaluation of 88 patients. Int J Gynecol Cancer.
4. Sironi S et al: Post-therapy surveillance of patients with uterine cancers: value of integrated FDG PET/CT in the detection of recurrence. Eur J Nucl Med Mol Imaging. 2006
5. Yoshida Y et al: The positron emission tomography with F18 17beta-estradiol has the potential to benefit diagnosis and treatment of endometrial cancer. Gynecol Oncol. 2006
6. Chao A et al: 18F-FDG PET in the management of endometrial cancer. Eur J Nucl Med Mol Imaging. 33(1):36-44, 2006
7. Nakamoto Y et al: Positron emission tomography application for gynecologic tumors. Int J Gynecol Cancer. 15(5):701-9, 2005

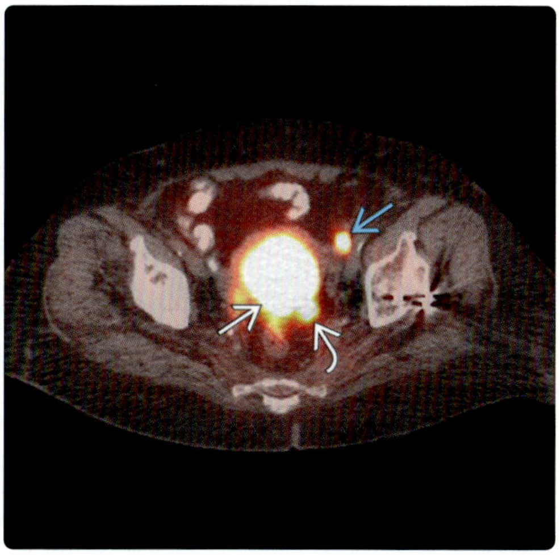

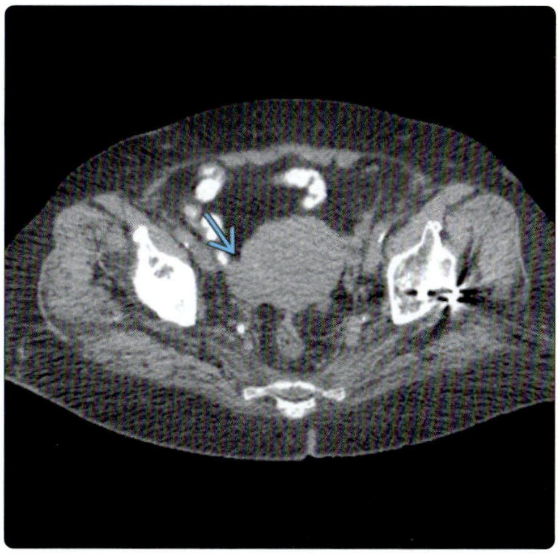

(Left) *Axial FDG PET/CT in a 73-year-old woman with endometrial cancer shows a hypermetabolic mass* ➡ *that extends to the left ovary* ➡*. A hypermetabolic left external iliac lymph node* → *is also evident.* **(Right)** *Axial NECT in the same patient shows invasion* → *of the mass into adjacent adnexal structures.*

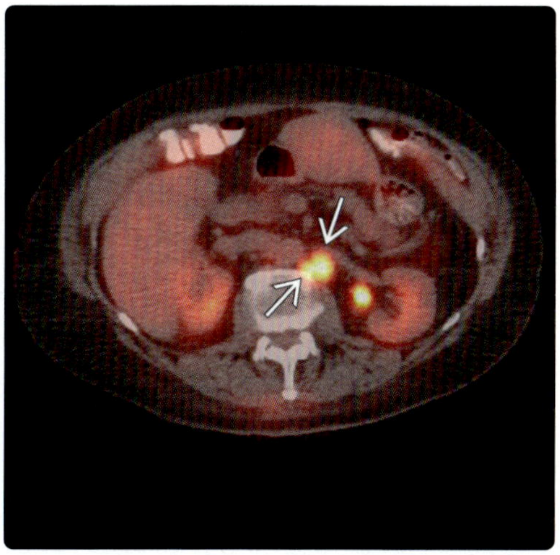

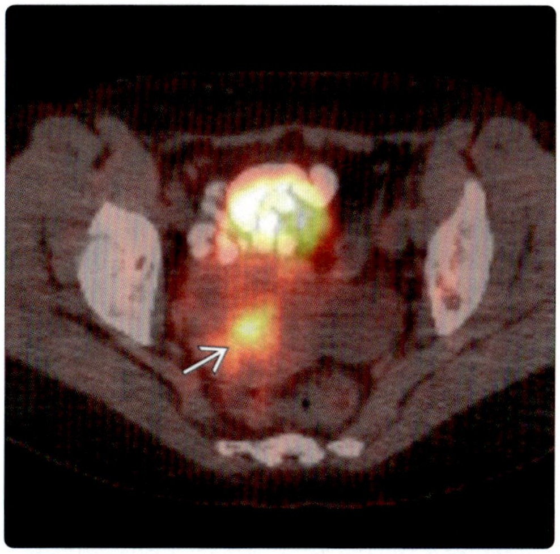

(Left) *Axial FDG PET/CT in a 73-year-old woman with endometrial cancer shows hypermetabolic paraaortic nodes* ➡ *at the level of the renal vein.* **(Right)** *Axial FDG PET/CT in a 35-year-old woman with a history of lymphoma shows a focus of activity* ➡ *(SUV: 3.7) within the uterus. This likely represents physiologic menstrual activity.*

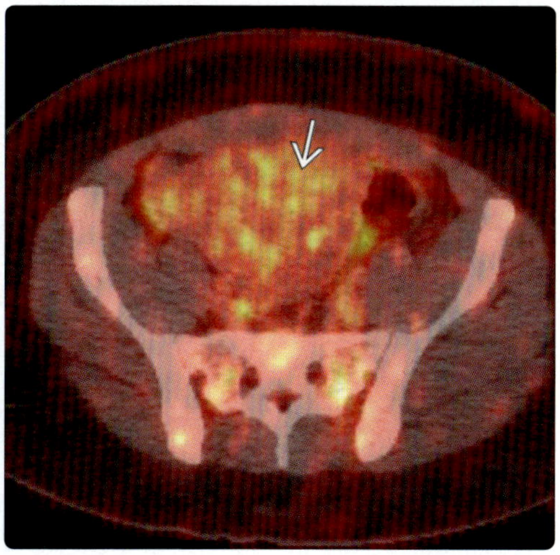

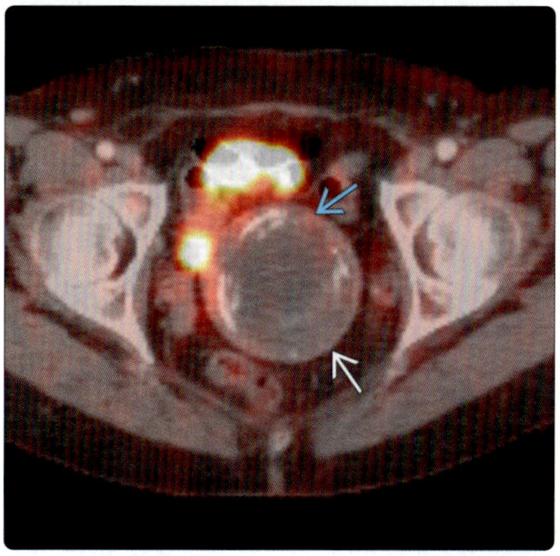

(Left) *Axial FDG PET/CT in a postpartum 38-year-old woman shows an enlarged uterus with central fluid and hypermetabolic blood products* ➡*. This can look similar to endometrial carcinoma.* **(Right)** *Axial FDG PET/CT in a 60-year-old woman with lymphoma shows a calcified, leiyomyomatous uterus* ➡*. There is mild hypermetabolic activity* → *along the periphery.*

KEY FACTS

IMAGING

- FDG PET/CT
  - Can effectively differentiate between malignant vs. benign primary tumors
    - Sensitivity 80-87%, specificity 77-100%
    - Highest specificity for lesions > 5 mm in size
    - Not effective at differentiating benign from malignant tumors with borderline uptake (SUV ~ 2)
  - Useful for preoperative evaluation, identifies late-stage patients not suitable for debulking
    - Sensitivity approaching 100%, specificity 91% in determining localized versus advanced (stage III/IV) disease
  - Highly sensitive/specific for recurrent disease in suspected patients
    - Sensitivity 89%, specificity 90%

CLINICAL ISSUES

- Stage I: Confined to ovaries/fallopian tubes
- Stage II: Extension to pelvis
- Stage III: Spread to peritoneum **&/or** regional lymph nodes
- Stage IV: Distant metastases **&/or** malignant pleural effusion

DIAGNOSTIC CHECKLIST

- Anatomic imaging most specific for primary tumor evaluation
- Consider performing study just after menstruation to avoid physiologic ovary uptake
- Report regional nodal metastases/peritoneal spread
  - Peritoneal disease can be subtle on PET
- Evaluate for distant metastases (usually liver/lung)
- Malignant pleural effusion more likely with increased FDG activity, hypermetabolic pleural nodules
- Postsurgical infection and inflammation FDG-avid on PET/CT

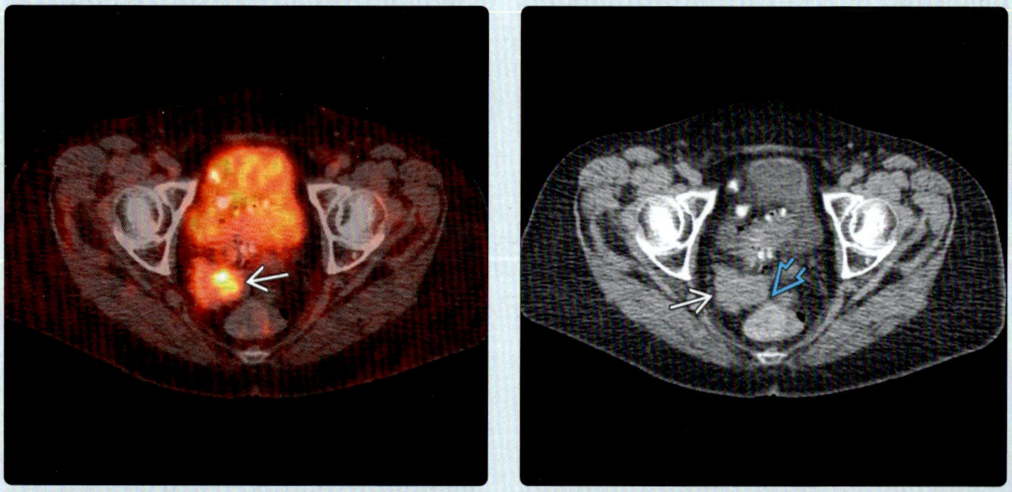

(Left) *Axial FDG PET/CT of an 82-year-old woman shows a hypermetabolic mass ➡ in the right hemipelvis, consistent with an ovarian malignancy.* **(Right)** *Axial NECT in the same patient shows the mass ➡. Note the perirectal fat plane ⇨ may be compromised and MR can best determine extent of primary tumor.*

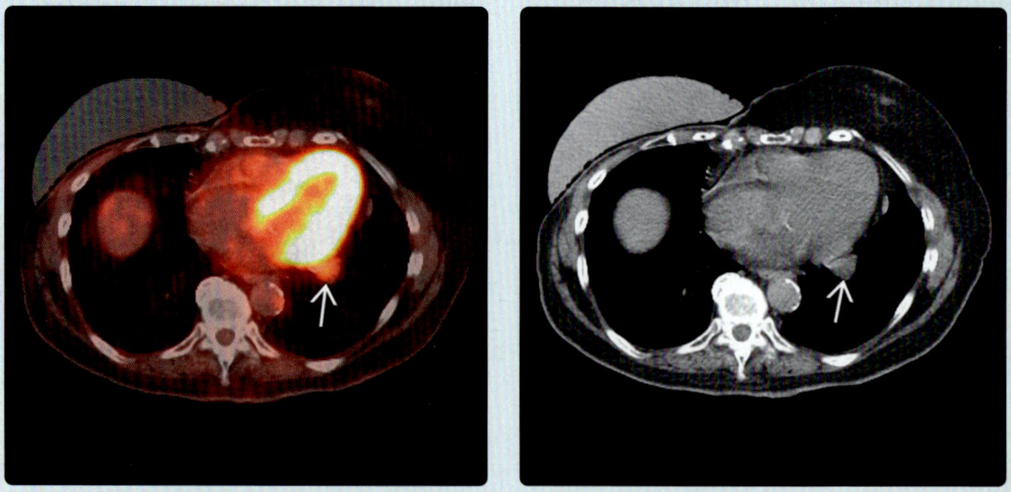

(Left) *Axial FDG PET/CT in a patient with ovarian cancer shows a hypermetabolic nodule ➡ in the left lower lobe, likely metastatic pleural disease.* **(Right)** *Axial NECT in the same patient shows this nodule ➡ abutting the pleural surface of the left hemithorax.*

IMAGING

General Features

- Best diagnostic clue
  - FDG PET/CT
    - FDG-avid ovarian mass (SUV > 3)
    - ± hypermetabolic lymphadenopathy, diffuse peritoneal involvement
    - ± distant metastases (usually liver/lung) or malignant pleural effusion
- Location
  - Primary
    - Initial mass involves ovary ± fallopian tubes
  - Spread
    - Superficially within peritoneum
      - Can lead to encasement of reproductive/abdominal organs by malignant tumor
    - Can involve pelvic &/or paraaortic nodes
    - Distant metastases include liver, lung

Nuclear Medicine Findings

- FDG PET/CT
  - Primary detection
    - Can effectively differentiate malignant vs. benign tumors
      - Sensitivity 80-87%, specificity 77-100%
    - Highest specificity for lesions > 5 mm in size
    - PET has difficulty with differentiation of benign vs. malignant w/ borderline elevated SUV
    - Physiologic uptake of ovary is highest in early secretory phase
  - Staging
    - Important tool for preoperative evaluation
    - Sensitivity approaching 100%, specificity 91% in determining early from late (stage III/IV) disease
    - Most effective at detecting peritoneal mets > 1 cm
    - Most effective at detecting lymphadenopathy > 7 mm
    - PET/CT staging accuracy 69-75% compared to 53-55% of CT alone
    - Accurately identifies late-stage patients that are not suitable for debulking
  - Surveillance
    - Effective for restaging in suspected recurrent disease
    - Sensitivity 89%, specificity 90%
    - PET/CT changes management in 44-57% of patients
    - Less sensitive for intrapelvic disease due to urinary bladder activity and postsurgical inflammation
    - No data to suggest early detection improves survival
    - Not routinely used in asymptomatic patients

Imaging Recommendations

- Best imaging tool
  - FDG PET/CT
    - Can differentiate benign vs. malignant primary tumors
    - Very useful for preoperative evaluation and staging
    - Use for evaluation in suspected recurrences

DIFFERENTIAL DIAGNOSIS

Infection

- Pelvic inflammatory disease
  - Nonspecific CT findings
- Tubo-ovarian abscess

Benign Tumors

- Complex functional cysts
  - May have intense FDG activity
- Cystadenoma
- Dermoid tumors

Physiologic Ovarian Uptake

- Most FDG-avid in secretory phase

PATHOLOGY

General Features

- Etiology
  - 3 cell types of ovarian carcinoma
    - Epithelial (90%)
      - Arises from germinal epithelium of ovary
    - Stromal (6%)
      - Arises from connective tissue
      - Low rate of metastasis
    - Germ cell (3%)
      - Teens/young women
      - Highly curable
  - Risk factors
    - BRCA mutations
    - ↑ ovulatory cycles (early menarche, late menopause)
    - Nulliparity
    - Infertility
    - Hormone therapies
    - Obesity

Staging, Grading, & Classification

- TNM staging
  - Primary tumor (T)
    - T1: Confined to ovaries/fallopian tubes
    - T2: Extension below pelvic brim or pelvic peritoneal disease
    - T3: Spread to peritoneum outside pelvis **&/or** retroperitoneal lymph nodes
  - Regional lymph nodes (N)
    - N0: No nodal mets
    - N1: Regional nodal mets
  - Distant metastases (M)
    - M0: No distant metastases
    - M1: Distant metastases **&/or** malignant pleural effusion
- **Stage I:** T1, N0, M0
- **Stage II:** T2, N0, M0
- **Stage III:** T3 **&/or** N1
- **Stage IV:** Any T, any N, M1

CLINICAL ISSUES

Presentation

- Most common signs/symptoms
  - Acute presentations
    - Pleural effusion
    - Ascites
    - Bowel obstruction
  - Subacute presentations

- Adnexal mass
- Bloating
- Urinary symptoms
- Pelvic/abdominal pain

- Other signs/symptoms
  - Postmenopausal bleeding
  - Abdominal distention

Demographics

- Age
  - Average age at diagnosis in USA: 63 years old
  - Incidence significantly increases over 50 years
- Ethnicity
  - Incidence rates
    - Highest in Caucasians
    - Lowest in Asian/Pacific Islanders
- Epidemiology
  - Incidence (USA)
    - 22,000 new cases per year
    - 14,000 cancer-related deaths per year
  - 2nd most common gynecologic malignancy in developed countries

Natural History & Prognosis

- 5-year survival
  - Stage I: 83-89%
  - Stage II: 70%
  - Stage III: 32-46%
  - Stage IV: 18%

Treatment

- Surgical debulking and staging
  - Total extrafascial hysterectomy with bilateral salpingo-oophorectomy
  - With paraaortic and lymph node dissection
- Adjuvant therapy
  - Intravenous &/or intraperitoneal chemotherapy
  - Indicated for most patients with the exception of early (stage I) disease

DIAGNOSTIC CHECKLIST

Image Interpretation Pearls

- FDG PET/CT
  - For premenopausal women, consider performing study just after menstruation to avoid physiologic ovary uptake
    - Ovarian hypermetabolic activity is often incidental finding on studies done for other indication
    - Normal ovary is spherical, discoid with smooth margins
    - Most FDG-avid in secretory phase
  - Postsurgical infection and inflammation FDG-avid on PET/CT
    - Inflammation should decrease in intensity on subsequent exams
    - Correlate with patient history and exam
  - Peritoneal disease can be subtle on PET
    - Often diffuse, low-level uptake throughout abdomen/pelvis
    - Multiple hypermetabolic nodules
  - Malignant pleural effusion
    - More likely with increased FDG activity
    - More likely if hypermetabolic pleural nodules present
  - Lung metastases
    - Multiple, bilateral hypermetabolic round nodules/masses
    - Lesions under 1 cm may not show intense hypermetabolism due to small size
  - Liver metastases
    - Hypermetabolic nodules/masses above liver background
    - Due to normal liver heterogeneity on PET/CT, small hypermetabolic nodules may be missed
    - CECT or MR more sensitive for small lesions

Reporting Tips

- Anatomic imaging most specific for primary tumor evaluation
- Report regional nodal metastases/peritoneal spread
- Report distant metastases (usually liver/lung) or evidence of malignant pleural effusion

SELECTED REFERENCES

1. Limei Z et al: Accuracy of positron emission tomography/computed tomography in the diagnosis and restaging for recurrent ovarian cancer: a meta-analysis. Int J Gynecol Cancer. 23(4):598-607, 2013
2. Palomar A et al: Value of FDG PET/CT in patients with treated ovarian cancer and raised CA125 serum levels. Mol Imaging Biol. 14(1):123-9, 2012
3. Chung HH et al: Role of [18F]FDG PET/CT in the assessment of suspected recurrent ovarian cancer: correlation with clinical or histological findings. Eur J Nucl Med Mol Imaging. 34(4):480-6, 2007
4. Mangili G et al: Integrated PET/CT as a first-line re-staging modality in patients with suspected recurrence of ovarian cancer. Eur J Nucl Med Mol Imaging. 34(5):658-66, 2007
5. Thrall MM et al: Clinical use of combined positron emission tomography and computed tomography (FDG-PET/CT) in recurrent ovarian cancer. Gynecol Oncol. 105(1):17-22, 2007
6. Kurosaki H et al: Prognostic value of FDG-PET in patients with ovarian carcinoma following surgical treatment. Ann Nucl Med. 20(3):171-4, 2006
7. Murakami M et al: Whole-body positron emission tomography and tumor marker CA125 for detection of recurrence in epithelial ovarian cancer. Int J Gynecol Cancer. 16 Suppl 1:99-107, 2006
8. Havrilesky LJ et al: FDG-PET for management of cervical and ovarian cancer. Gynecol Oncol. 97(1):183-91, 2005

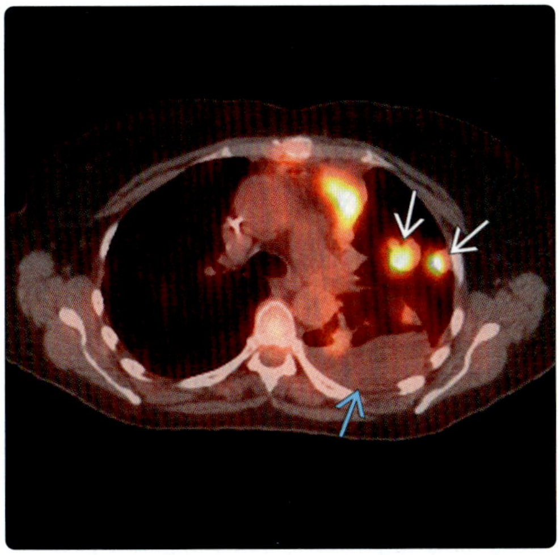

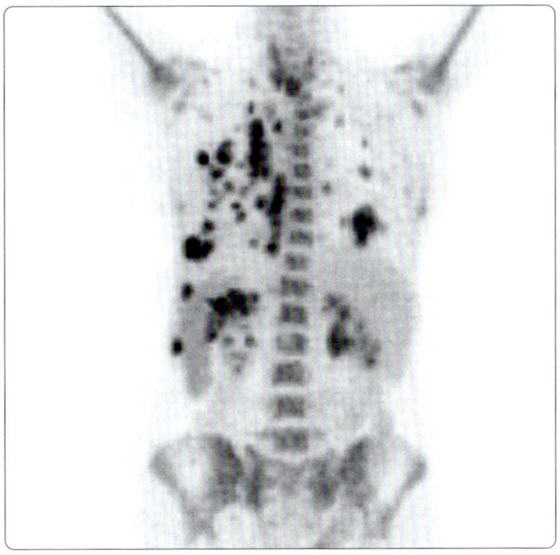

(Left) *Axial FDG PET/CT of a 68-year-old woman with ovarian cancer shows diffuse pulmonary metastatic disease with multiple hypermetabolic nodules and a left-sided loculated pleural effusion.* **(Right)** *MIP FDG PET in the same patient shows multiple bilateral pulmonary metastases.*

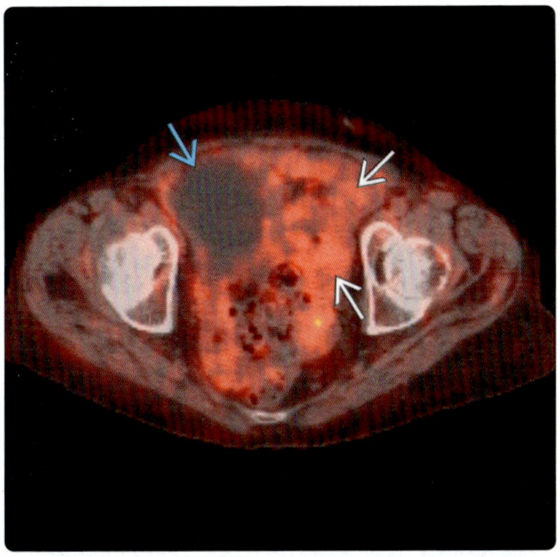

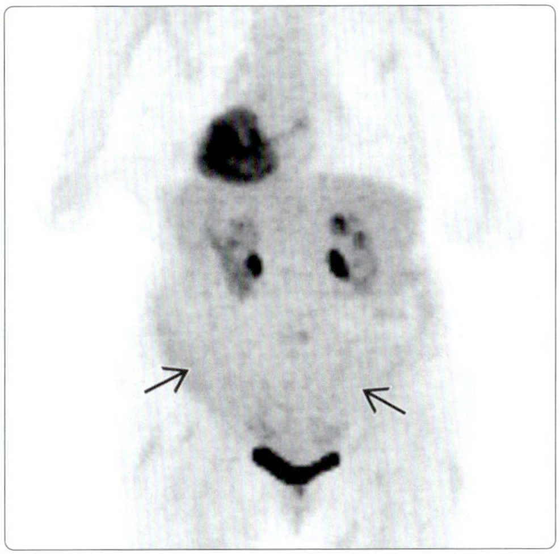

(Left) *Axial FDG PET/CT in a 73-year-old woman with history of pseudomyxoma peritonei from an ovarian primary tumor shows diffuse omental hypermetabolic activity with a large cystic lesion in the right pelvis.* **(Right)** *Coronal FDG PET in the same patient shows the diffuse, low-level hypermetabolic activity suggestive of peritoneal implants.*

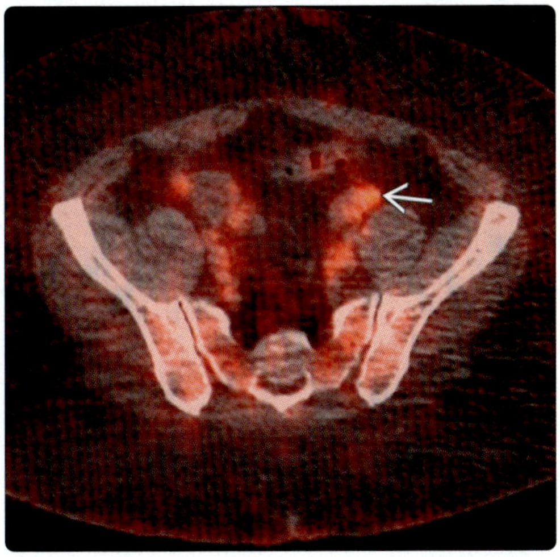

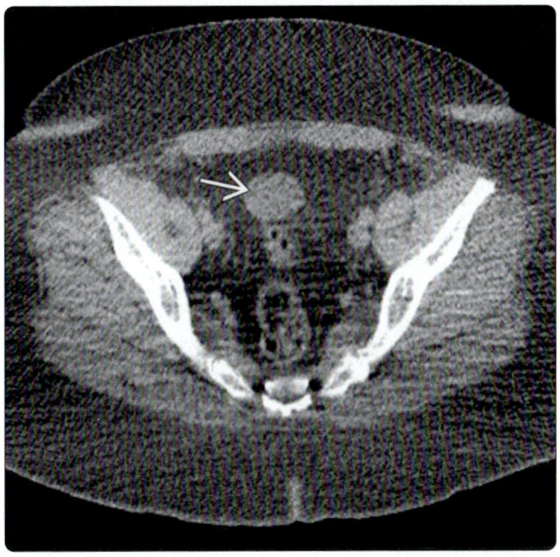

(Left) *Axial FDG PET/CT of a 36-year-old woman shows focal hypermetabolic activity within the left ovary. This is often a physiologic finding when seen in premenopausal females.* **(Right)** *Axial NECT in the same patient shows a nonhypermetabolic fluid density structure in the midline pelvis, likely a benign ovarian cyst. Ultrasound can provide specificity for both of these findings.*

Cervical Cancer

KEY FACTS

IMAGING

- FDG PET/CT
  - Modality of choice for initial staging and management of recurrent disease
  - CECT and MR best for extent of primary tumor

PATHOLOGY

- Primary originates at cervical transformation zone
- Regional invasion of adjacent structures: Uterus, vagina, bladder, rectum
- Lymphatic spread: Pelvic node groups → common iliac → paraaortic
- Hematogenous spread: Lung, liver, and bone most common

CLINICAL ISSUES

- Stage I: Confined to uterus
- Stage II: Invades beyond uterus
- Stage III: Extends to pelvic wall, lower vagina, or affects kidneys ± nodal metastases
- Stage IV: Invades other adjacent structures **&/or** distant metastases

DIAGNOSTIC CHECKLIST

- F-18 FDG excretion through ureters and urinary bladder can cause false-positives
  - p.o. patient hydration
  - Patient void prior to imaging
  - Can use diuretic FDG PET protocol
  - Can use bladder catheterization
  - CECT can assist in PET interpretation to distinguish ureter from lymphadenopathy
- Involved nodal groups can have variable F-18 FDG uptake
  - Subcentimeter pelvic and paraaortic lymphadenopathy can show mild F-18 FDG activity
  - SUV underestimated due to small size of lymph nodes and limits of scanner resolution

(Left) *Axial FDG PET/CT in a 79-year-old woman with advanced-stage cervical cancer shows a large, heterogeneous, markedly hypermetabolic mass ➡ arising from the lower cervix.* **(Right)** *Axial noncontrast CT in the same patient shows the mass ➡ contacting the posterior aspect of the bladder. There is extensive lymphadenopathy ⇨ along the iliac chains bilaterally.*

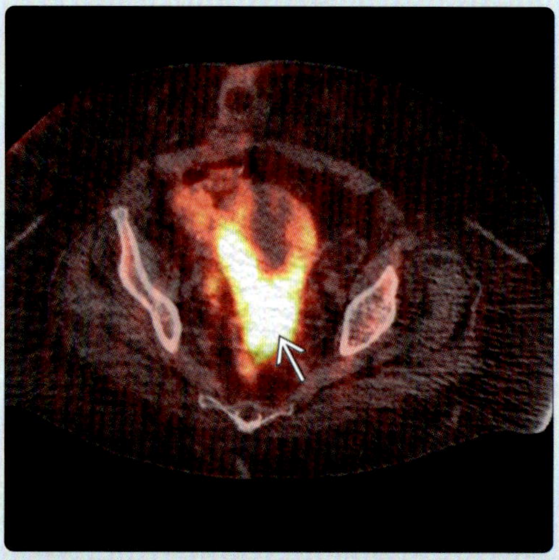

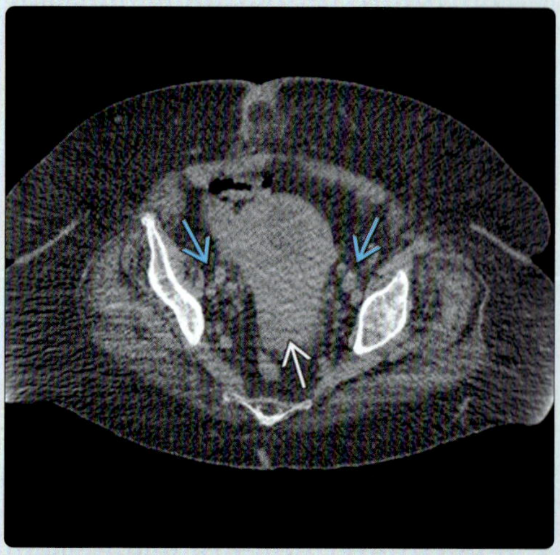

(Left) *Axial FDG PET/CT in the same patient shows hypermetabolic osseous metastases ➡ involving the iliac bones bilaterally.* **(Right)** *Axial FDG PET/CT in the same patient shows another osseous metastasis: An expansile mixed sclerotic/lytic lesion ➡ within the manubrium.*

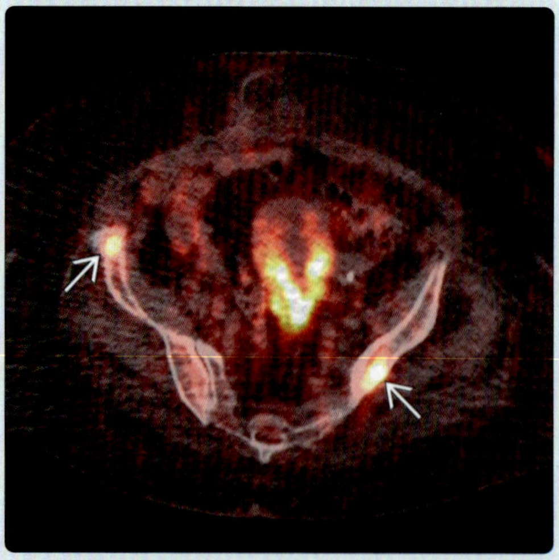

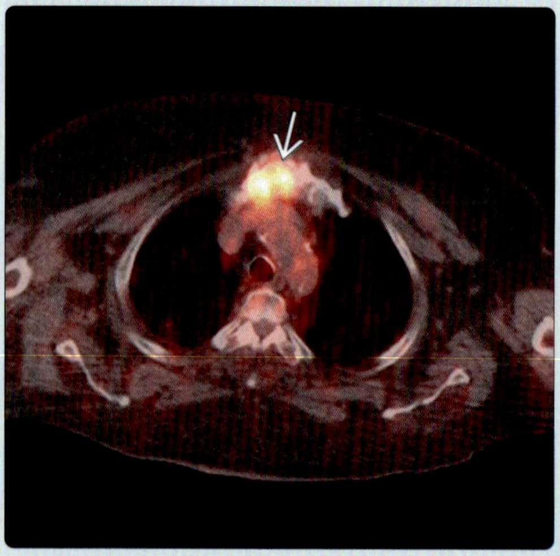

IMAGING

General Features

- Best diagnostic clue
  - FDG PET/CT
    - Intense FDG activity in primary cervical mass
    - Variable uptake in uterus, vagina, and parametria, depending on spread
    - Pelvic and paraaortic FDG-avid lymphadenopathy
    - Distant metastases in lung, liver, bone
- Location
  - Primary
    - Originates at cervical transformation zone (transition from glandular to squamous epithelium)
  - Regional
    - Invasion of adjacent structures
      - Uterus
      - Vagina
      - Bladder
      - Rectum
  - Spread
    - Lymphatic
      - Pelvic node groups → common iliac → paraaortic
    - Hematogenous
      - Most common sites: Lung, liver, and bone

Nuclear Medicine Findings

- PET/CT
  - FDG PET/CT
    - Detection of local disease
      - Primary detection usually based on clinical examination alone
      - CECT and pelvic MR more commonly used, helpful for preoperative planning
      - If lymph nodes are suspicious, PET/CT is used for further evaluation
    - Detection of lymph node metastases
      - Commonly used for initial staging
      - PET/CT proven superior (sensitivity 75%, specificity 98%) compared to MR (56%, 93%) and CT (58%, 92%)
      - PET/CT performs best at detection of paraaortic nodes (sensitivity 84%, specificity 95%), some limitations with detection of pelvic nodes
      - In patients with positive pelvic nodes, PET detection of paraaortic nodes has 12-22% false-negative rate
    - Detection of recurrent disease
      - Indicated in work-up of symptomatic patients or those with abnormal findings (sensitivity 93%, specificity 95%)
      - Often impacts therapeutic decisions
      - Not currently recommended as surveillance strategy in post-treatment patients

Imaging Recommendations

- Best imaging tool
  - FDG PET/CT
    - Modality of choice for initial staging and for management of recurrent disease
  - CECT
    - Commonly used for post-treatment surveillance

Artifacts and Quality Control

- F-18 FDG excretion through ureters and urinary bladder can cause false-positives
  - p.o. patient hydration
  - Patient void prior to imaging
  - Can use diuretic F-18 FDG PET protocol
    - 40 mg furosemide IV with oral fluid intake of 1.5-2 L
    - Void 2-3x to excrete majority of F-18 FDG, then hold urine for bladder distention prior to imaging
  - Can use bladder catheterization
    - ± continuous bladder infusion with 3-way flushing catheter during imaging

DIFFERENTIAL DIAGNOSIS

Other Neoplasms

- Endometrial cancer
- Ovarian cancer
- Leiomyoma: Variable FDG uptake

Physiologic F-18 FDG Activity

- Menstruation
  - F-18 FDG activity in endometrium
- Urine contamination
  - F-18 FDG activity in vagina
- Ureter and urinary bladder excretion
  - CECT may be useful to distinguish ureter from lymphadenopathy
  - Urinary bladder may be indistinguishable from primary tumor, may obscure adjacent lymphadenopathy

Postsurgical and Post-Radiation Uptake

- Abscess
  - Intense F-18 FDG activity
- Seroma
  - Usually diffuse, mild F-18 FDG activity
- Tumor/surrounding structures (particularly muscle)
  - Mild activity within radiation port

PATHOLOGY

General Features

- Etiology
  - Cervical cancer: Neoplasm that commonly arises from epithelial or glandular cells of cervix
    - Squamous cell carcinoma (SCC) most common
    - 99.7% of cervical cancers are associated with HPV
      - HPV-16 and HPV-18 most common
  - Major risk factors
    - Early sexual activity
    - Many sexual partners
    - History of STD
    - Immunosuppression
    - Low socioeconomic status
    - Cigarette smoking (SCC only)

Staging, Grading, & Classification

- TNM staging
  - Primary tumor (T)
    - Tis: Carcinoma in situ (preinvasive)
    - T1: Confined to uterus

  - T2: Invades beyond uterus, but **not** to pelvic wall or lower 1/3 of vagina
  - T3: Extends to pelvic wall or lower 1/3 of vagina, **&/or** causes hydronephrosis or renal failure
  - T4: Invades bladder/rectum **&/or** extends beyond true pelvis
- Regional lymph nodes (N)
  - N0: No nodal metastases
  - N1: Regional nodal metastases
- Distant metastasis (M)
  - M0: No distant metastases
  - M1: Distant metastases

- **Stage I:** T1 and N0, M0
- **Stage II:** T2 and N0, M0
- **Stage III:** T3 and any N, M0
- **Stage IV:** T4 and any N, any M

CLINICAL ISSUES

Presentation

- Most common signs/symptoms
  - Early cervical cancer (stage I)
    - Frequently asymptomatic (screening important)
  - Common presentations
    - Irregular/heavy vaginal bleeding
    - Postcoital bleeding
  - Advanced stage
    - Pelvic pain
    - Low back pain
    - Bowel/urinary symptoms

Demographics

- Age
  - Mean at diagnosis: 48 years
  - Incidence increases substantially in patients > 30 years
- Epidemiology
  - In 2008
    - 530,000 new cases worldwide
    - 275,000 deaths worldwide
  - 12,000 new cases of invasive cancer with 4,000 deaths every year in USA

Natural History & Prognosis

- 5-year survival
  - Stage I: 80-90%
  - Stage II: 60%
  - Stage III: 35%
  - Stage IV: 15%

Treatment

- Microinvasive disease
  - Cervical conization (preserves fertility) or extrafascial hysterectomy
- Advanced/invasive disease
  - Radical hysterectomy ± lymphadenectomy
- Recurrent disease or risk of recurrence
  - Chemotherapy
  - Pelvic radiation

DIAGNOSTIC CHECKLIST

Consider

- FDG PET/CT
  - Hypermetabolic mass in region of cervix/uterus
    - CECT and MR best for evaluation of extent of primary tumor
  - Regional pelvic and paraaortic lymph nodes frequently involved
  - Distant metastatic locations include bone, liver, and lungs

Image Interpretation Pearls

- FDG PET/CT
  - Involved nodal groups can have variable FDG uptake
    - Subcentimeter pelvic and paraaortic lymphadenopathy can show mild F-18 FDG activity
      - SUV underestimated due to small size of lymph nodes and limits of scanner resolution
      - Use coronal images to evaluate for subcentimeter lymphadenopathy
  - Physiologic bladder activity can obscure primary tumor and local lymphadenopathy
    - Consider patient hydration, diuretic protocol, urinary bladder catheterization
  - CECT can assist in PET interpretation to distinguish ureter from lymphadenopathy

SELECTED REFERENCES

1. Delbke D et al: Procedure Guideline for Tumor Imaging with 18F-FDG PET/CT 1.0*. Society of Nuclear Medicine and Molecular Imaging: Practice Guidelines. http://snmmi.files.cms-plus.com/docs/jnm30551_online.pdf. Approved February 11, 2006. Accessed August 26, 2014
2. Leblanc E et al: Accuracy of 18-fluoro-2-deoxy-D-glucose positron emission tomography in the pretherapeutic detection of occult para-aortic node involvement in patients with a locally advanced cervical carcinoma. Ann Surg Oncol. 18(8):2302-9, 2011
3. Showalter TN et al: 18F-fluorodeoxyglucose-positron emission tomography and pathologic tumor size in early-stage invasive cervical cancer. Int J Gynecol Cancer. 19(8):1412-4, 2009
4. Amit A et al: The role of hybrid PET/CT in the evaluation of patients with cervical cancer. Gynecol Oncol. 100(1):65-9, 2006
5. Chou HH et al: Low value of [18F]-fluoro-2-deoxy-D-glucose positron emission tomography in primary staging of early-stage cervical cancer before radical hysterectomy. J Clin Oncol. 24(1):123-8, 2006
6. Chung HH et al: Clinical impact of FDG-PET imaging in post-therapy surveillance of uterine cervical cancer: from diagnosis to prognosis. Gynecol Oncol. 103(1):165-70, 2006
7. Chung HH et al: Clinical impact of integrated PET/CT on the management of suspected cervical cancer recurrence. Gynecol Oncol. 2006
8. Lin CT et al: Role of [18F]fluoro-2-deoxy-D-glucose positron emission tomography in re-recurrent cervical cancer. Int J Gynecol Cancer. 16(6):1994-2003, 2006
9. Sironi S et al: Lymph node metastasis in patients with clinical early-stage cervical cancer: detection with integrated FDG PET/CT. Radiology. 238(1):272-9, 2006
10. Grosu AL et al: Positron emission tomography for radiation treatment planning. Strahlenther Onkol. 181(8):483-99, 2005
11. Havrilesky LJ et al: FDG-PET for management of cervical and ovarian cancer. Gynecol Oncol. 97(1):183-91, 2005
12. Park W et al: The usefulness of MRI and PET imaging for the detection of parametrial involvement and lymph node metastasis in patients with cervical cancer. Jpn J Clin Oncol. 35(5):260-4, 2005
13. Roh JW et al: Role of positron emission tomography in pretreatment lymph node staging of uterine cervical cancer: a prospective surgicopathologic correlation study. Eur J Cancer. 41(14):2086-92, 2005

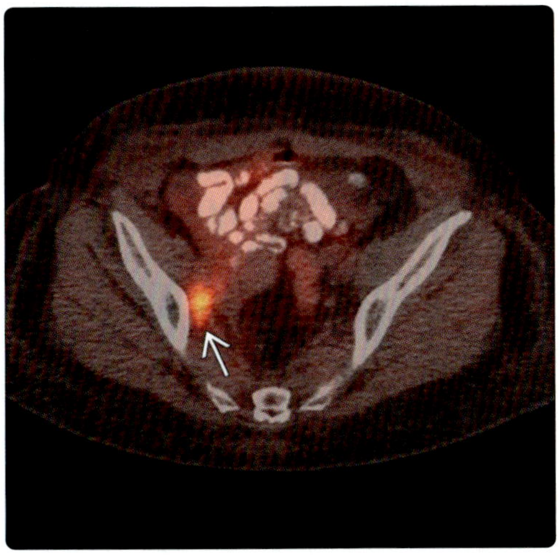

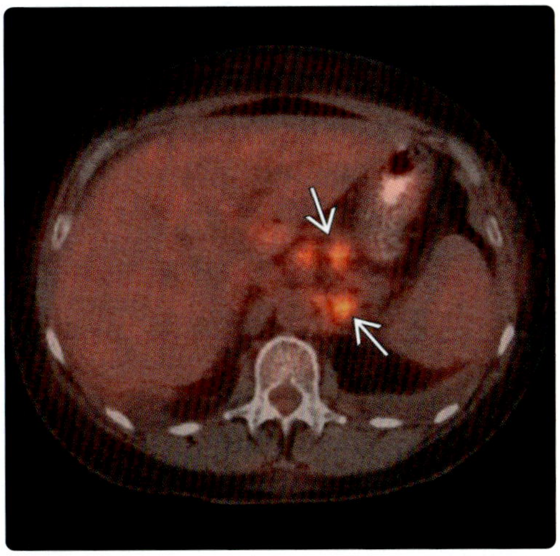

(Left) *Axial FDG PET/CT of a 56-year-old woman with recurrent cervical cancer status post radical hysterectomy shows a hypermetabolic node involving the pelvic sidewall, concerning for regional nodal disease.* **(Right)** *Axial FDG PET/CT in the same patient shows hypermetabolic paraaortic and gastrohepatic lymphadenopathy, a common route of lymphatic spread.*

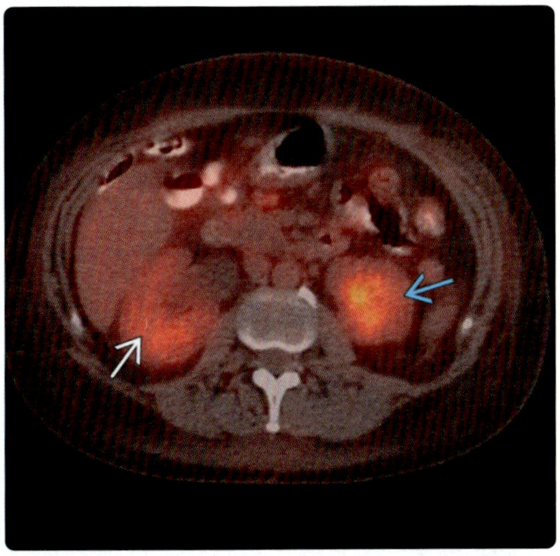

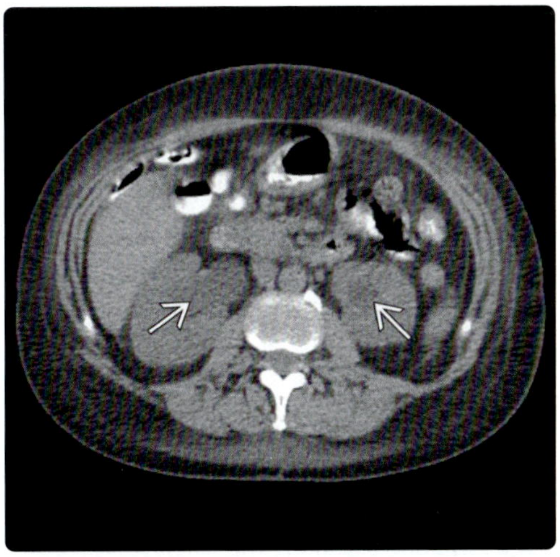

(Left) *Axial FDG PET/CT in the same patient shows bilateral hydronephrosis, right greater than left, a poor prognostic factor in metastatic cervical cancer.* **(Right)** *Axial noncontrast CT in the same patient shows bilateral hydronephrosis with no focal obstruction identified.*

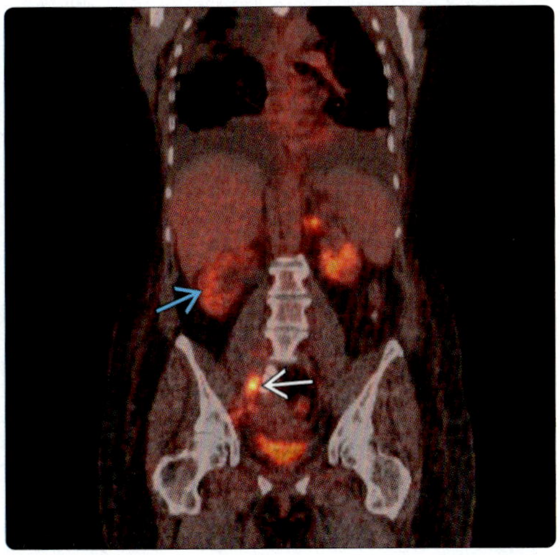

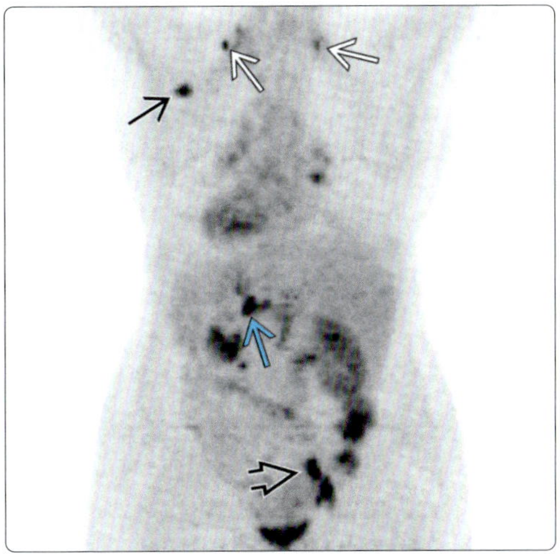

(Left) *Coronal FDG PET/CT shows right hydronephrosis and lymphadenopathy vs. ureter activity within the right hemipelvis.* **(Right)** *Posterior MIP FDG PET shows bilateral supraclavicular, left axillary, mesenteric, and right pelvic sidewall hypermetabolic lymphadenopathy.*

Vulvar and Vaginal Cancer

KEY FACTS

IMAGING

- F-18 FDG PET/CT for vulvar cancer
  - Highly sensitive for detection of primary lesion and adjacent deposits
    - FDG-avid vulvar lesion ± inguinofemoral hypermetabolic lymphadenopathy
  - Can be used for staging and preoperative evaluation of disease
- F-18 FDG PET/CT for vaginal cancer
  - High sensitivity in primary tumor detection and nodal evaluation
    - FDG-avid vaginal lesion ± local extension, lymphadenopathy

DIAGNOSTIC CHECKLIST

- Vulvar cancer
  - Primary tumor: Most often labia majora; other sites include labia minora, perineum, clitoris, mons
  - Regional spread: Involvement of adjacent structures (vagina, urethra, anus)
  - Lymphatic spread: Inguinal-femoral nodes initially, then pelvic nodes
  - Hematogenous spread: Rare, only in advanced disease; lung most common
- Vaginal cancer
  - Primary tumor: Superficially within vaginal wall
    - Lesion in middle or lower 1/3 of vagina is poor prognostic factor
  - Regional spread: Invasion of paravaginal tissues, parametria, bladder and rectal mucosa
  - Lymphatic spread: Upper 1/3 → pelvic, lower 2/3 → inguinal, posterior tumors → deep pelvic
  - Hematogenous spread: Lung most common, less frequently liver and bone

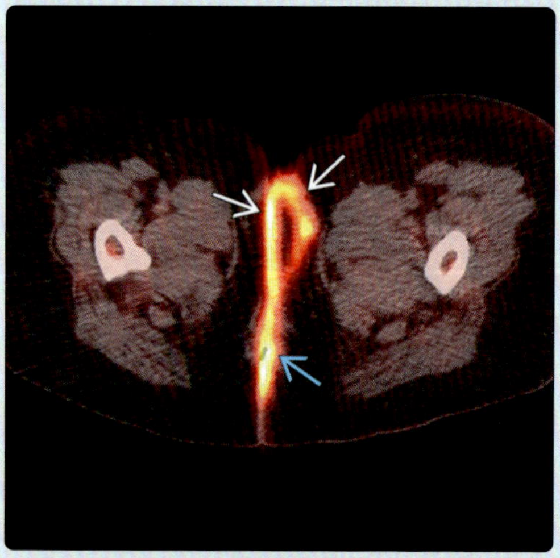
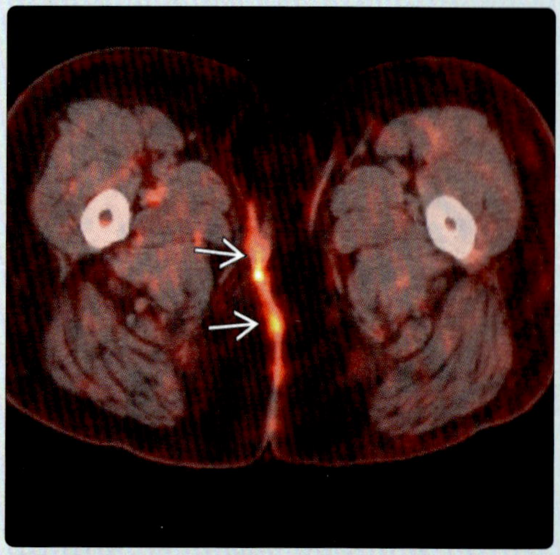

***(Left)** Axial F-18 FDG PET/CT in a 50-year-old woman shows hypermetabolic activity in the vulvar region ➡ consistent with primary vulvar carcinoma. The activity extends to the perianal area ➡ as well. **(Right)** Axial F-18 FDG PET/CT in the same patient after vulvectomy shows hypermetabolic activity in the postoperative site ➡ with associated thickening of the soft tissue margins, concerning for disease recurrence.*

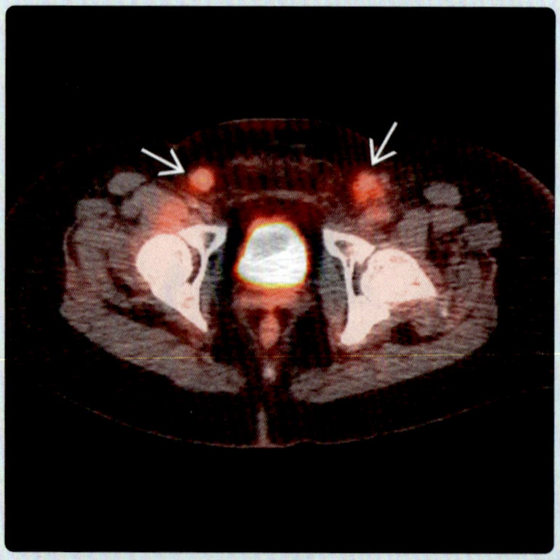
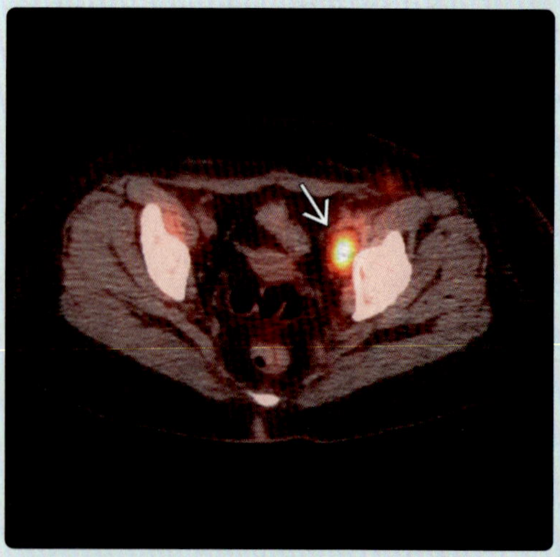

***(Left)** Axial F-18 FDG PET/CT of the same patient shows bilateral hypermetabolic inguinal lymphadenopathy ➡, a common site of regional lymphatic spread. **(Right)** Axial PET/CT in the same patient shows an additional hypermetabolic left iliac node ➡.*

IMAGING

General Features

- Best diagnostic clue
  - F-18 FDG PET/CT
    - Vulvar cancer: FDG-avid vulvar lesion ± inguinofemoral hypermetabolic lymphadenopathy
    - Vaginal cancer: FDG-avid vaginal lesion ± local extension, lymphadenopathy
- Location
  - Primary
    - Vulvar: Most often labia majora; other sites include labia minora, perineum, clitoris, mons
    - Vaginal: Superficially within vaginal wall
      - Lesion in middle or lower 1/3 of vagina is poor prognostic factor
  - Regional
    - Vulvar: Involvement of adjacent structures (vagina, urethra, anus)
    - Vaginal: Invasion of paravaginal tissues, parametria, bladder and rectal mucosa
  - Spread
    - Lymphatic
      - Vulvar: Inguinal-femoral nodes initially, then pelvic nodes
      - Vaginal: Upper 1/3 → pelvic, lower 2/3 → inguinal, posterior tumors → deep pelvic
    - Hematogenous
      - Vulvar: Rare, only in advanced disease; lung most common
      - Vaginal: Lung most common, less frequently liver and bone

Nuclear Medicine Findings

- F-18 FDG PET/CT
  - Detection of primary lesions
    - 100% sensitivity for squamous cell cancers, 60% for nonsquamous in 1 study
    - Effective in detecting metastatic vulvar deposits secondary to primary tumor
    - Urine contamination can lead to false-positives or mask primary tumor
  - Staging
    - Useful as adjunct to sentinel lymph node biopsy &/or dissection
    - Sensitivity 80%, specificity 90%, PPV 80%, NPV 90% for detection of local nodal metastases
    - PET/CT has high specificity and accuracy for detection of extranodal disease
    - One study found that PET/CT changed therapeutic management in 61.5% of cases
  - Surveillance
    - No recommendations for or against routine PET/CT imaging
    - PET/CT may be useful at identifying distant recurrent disease in high-risk patients

Imaging Recommendations

- Best imaging tool
  - F-18 FDG PET/CT
    - Useful to detect nearby metastatic vulvar deposits not evident on physical exam
    - Effective for planning prior to nodal dissection
    - Best at detecting extranodal metastases

DIFFERENTIAL DIAGNOSIS

Neoplasms

- Melanoma
  - 2nd most common vulvar malignancy
- Verrucous carcinoma
- Bartholin gland adenocarcinoma
  - Metastatic disease common
- Basal cell carcinoma
- Sarcoma
- Extramammary Paget disease
  - Similar in appearance to breast disease
- Cervical cancer
- Uterine cancer
- Vaginal lymphoma
  - Secondary vaginal involvement from diffuse disease

Vulvar Dermatoses

- Lichen sclerosis
- Lichen planus
- Vulvar intraepithelial neoplasia

Endometriosis

- Discrete foci of FDG activity within pelvis

Physiologic

- Urine contamination: Patients w/ incontinence may have FDG activity in vulvar area
- Menstruation: FDG activity reported in vaginal tampons
  - Poorly understood, suggests tracer may be within sloughed blood products
  - Urine contamination of tampons possible as well

PATHOLOGY

General Features

- Etiology
  - Vulvar: Squamous cell carcinoma most common
  - Vagina: Squamous cell carcinoma most common
    - Also: Adenocarcinoma, sarcoma, melanoma

Staging, Grading, & Classification

- **Vulvar carcinoma TNM staging**
  - Primary tumor (T)
    - T1: Confined to vulva
    - T2: Extension to adjacent perineal structures ± positive inguinal nodes
    - T3: Extension to any of the following: Urethra, vagina, bladder, rectum, pelvic bone
  - Regional lymph nodes (N)
    - N0: No nodal mets
    - N1: 1 lymph node met ≥ 5 mm **or** up to 2 lymph node mets < 5 mm
    - N2: ≥ 2 lymph node mets ≥ 5 mm **or** ≥ 3 lymph node mets < 5 mm
    - N3: Fixed or ulcerated regional lymph node mets
  - Distant metastases (M)

- M0: No distant metastasis
- M1: Distant metastasis (including pelvic lymph node mets)
- **Stage**
  - **Stage I:** T1, N0, M0
  - **Stage II:** T2, N0, M0
  - **Stage III:** T1 **or** T2, N1 **or** N2, M0
  - **Stage IV:** Any T, N3 **&/or** M1
- **Vaginal carcinoma TNM staging**
  - Primary tumor (T)
    - T1: Confined to vagina
    - T2: Invasion of paravaginal tissues
    - T3: Extension to pelvic wall
    - T4: Invasion of bladder/rectum **or** extension beyond true pelvis
  - Regional lymph nodes (N)
    - N0: No regional node mets
    - N1: Regional node mets (pelvic or inguinal)
  - Distant metastases (M)
    - M0: No distant mets
    - M1: Distant mets
  - **Stage**
    - **Stage I:** T1, N0, M0
    - **Stage II:** T2, N0, M0
    - **Stage III:** T3 **or** T1-T3 with N1
    - **Stage IV:** T4 **or** M1 with any T, N

CLINICAL ISSUES

Presentation

- Most common signs/symptoms
  - Vulvar carcinoma: Vulvar mass, plaque, or ulcer; pruritus; bleeding, discharge, dysuria
  - Vaginal carcinoma: Postmenopausal vaginal bleeding; vaginal discharge; urinary/GI symptoms

Demographics

- Age
  - Vulvar carcinoma: Mean age at diagnosis: 60-65 years
  - Vaginal carcinoma: Mean age at diagnosis: 60 years; in patients < 20 years, adenocarcinoma most common
- Epidemiology
  - Vulvar carcinoma
    - 5% of all female genitourinary malignancies
    - Incidence (USA): 4,900 new cases each year
  - Vaginal carcinoma
    - 3% of all female genitourinary malignancies
    - Incidence (USA): 3,000 new cases each year

Natural History & Prognosis

- **Vulvar carcinoma**
  - Risk factors
    - HPV-16 and -33 responsible for 55% of vulvar cancers
    - Cigarette smoking
    - Vulvar dystrophy
    - Immunodeficiency syndromes
  - 5-year survival
    - Stage I: 78%
    - Stage II: 58%
    - Stage III: 43%
    - Stage IV: 13%
  - Inguinal &/or femoral node involvement is most important prognostic factor
- **Vaginal carcinoma**
  - Risk factors
    - HPV-16 or-18 associated with > 50% of cases in one study
    - Many lifetime sexual partners
    - Smoking
    - In utero DES exposure is major risk factor for adenocarcinoma
  - 5-year survival
    - Stage I: 92%
    - Stage II: 68%
    - Stage III: 44%
    - Stage IV: 13%

Treatment

- **Vulvar carcinoma**
  - Stage I or II disease
    - Surgical excision ± adjuvant chemoradiation
  - Locally advanced disease
    - Surgical excision when possible ± inguinofemoral node evaluation and chemoradiation
  - Metastatic disease
    - Primary chemoradiation
- **Vaginal carcinoma**
  - Stage I disease
    - Radical hysterectomy, upper vaginectomy, bilateral pelvic lymphadenectomy
    - Intracavitary radiation therapy
  - Stage II disease
    - Neoadjuvant chemotherapy then surgery ± radiation
  - Late-stage disease
    - Chemoradiation
    - Surgery if possible

DIAGNOSTIC CHECKLIST

Consider

- F-18 FDG PET/CT for vulvar cancer
  - Highly sensitive in primary lesion detection
  - Useful for preoperative evaluation and planning of radiation therapy
  - May be used for surveillance in high-risk patients
- F-18 FDG PET/CT for vaginal cancer
  - Sensitivity approaches 100% for detection of primary vaginal tumors
  - Shown effective in inguinal, pelvic, and paraaortic node evaluation
  - No recommendations regarding staging or surveillance

SELECTED REFERENCES

1. Basu S et al: PET and PET-CT imaging of gynecological malignancies: present role and future promise. Expert Rev Anticancer Ther. 9(1):75-96, 2009
2. Stehman FB et al: Carcinoma of the vulva. Obstet Gynecol. 107(3):719-33, 2006
3. Yen TC et al: Positron emission tomography in gynecologic cancer. Semin Nucl Med. 36(1):93-104, 2006

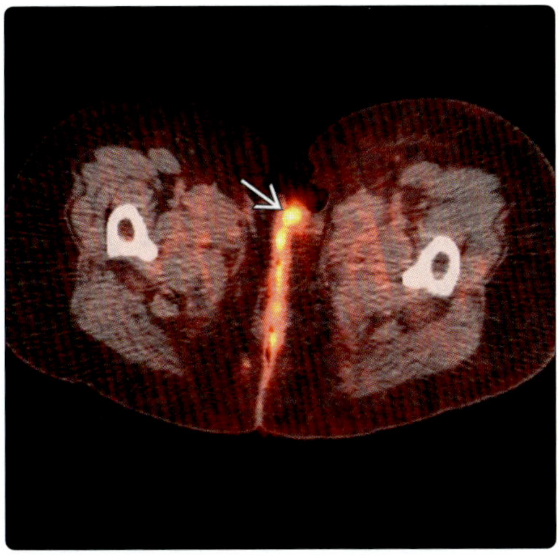

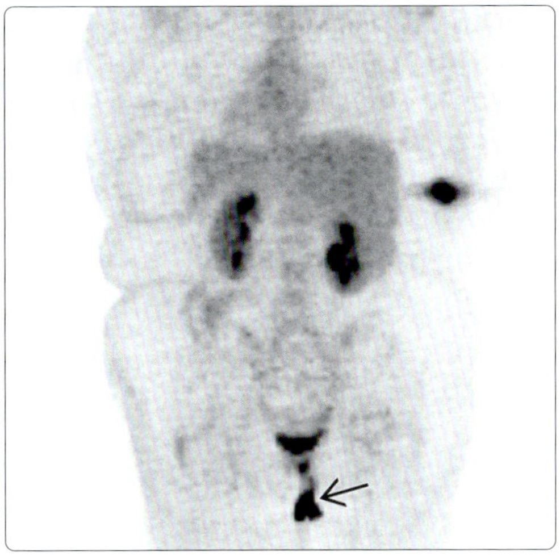

(Left) *Axial F-18 FDG PET/CT of a 58-year-old woman with a history of vulvar cancer shows significant hypermetabolic activity* ➡ *but it is difficult to discern from urinary contamination.* **(Right)** *MIP FDG PET in the same patient shows significant external urinary contamination* ➡*, which can make evaluation of the perineum difficult.*

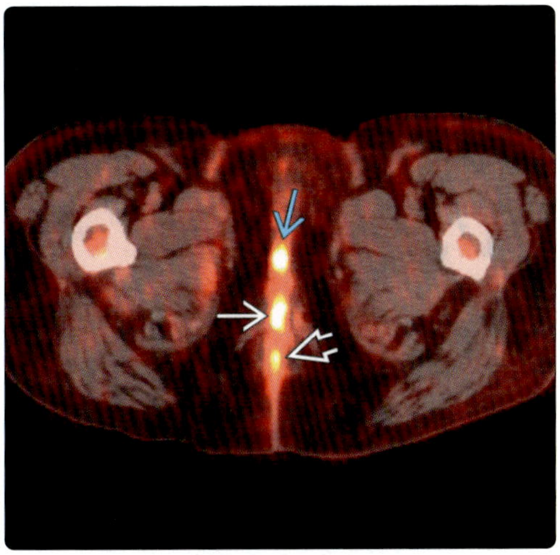

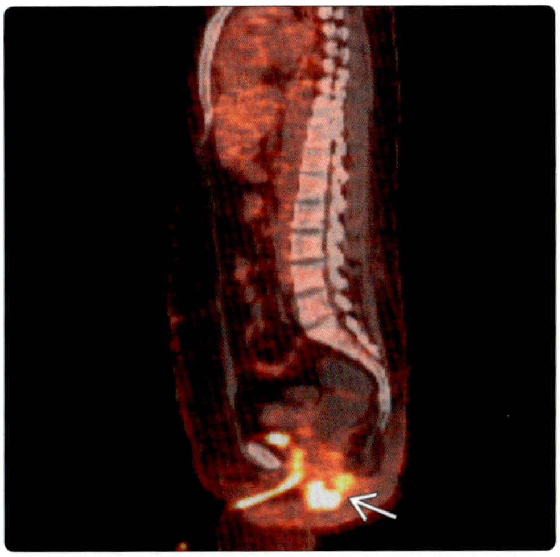

(Left) *Axial F-18 FDG PET/CT of a 36-year-old woman with a history of vulvar cancer shows hypermetabolic activity in the perineum* ➡ *and anal* ➡ *regions as well as physiologic activity in a urinary catheter* ➡*.* **(Right)** *Sagittal F-18 FDG PET/CT in the same patient shows hypermetabolic soft tissue in the area of the anus and rectum* ➡*, concerning for recurrent disease.*

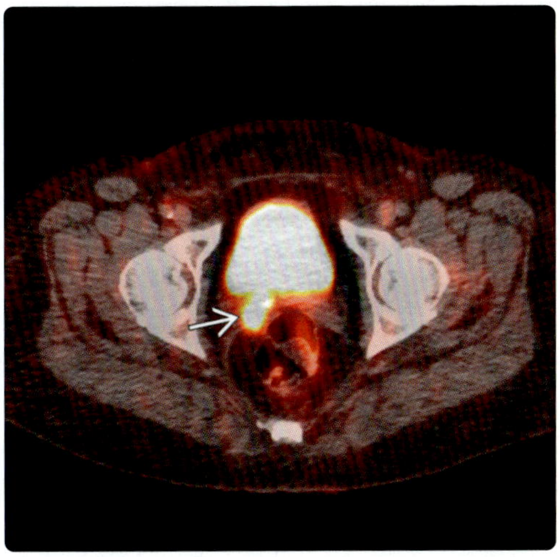

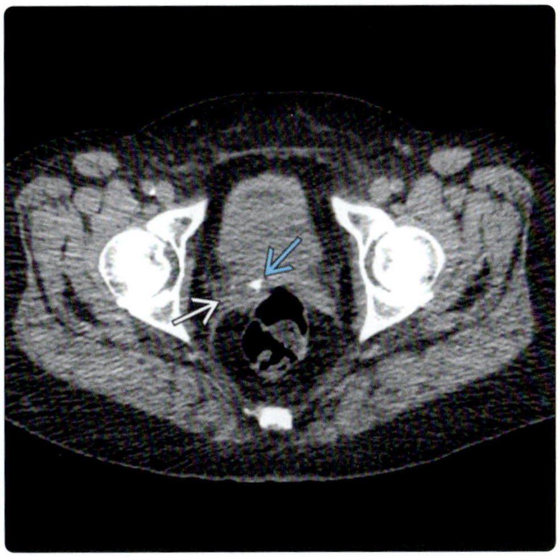

(Left) *Axial F-18 FDG PET/CT of a 53-year-old woman with suspected vaginal cancer shows a hypermetabolic mass* ➡ *along the right vaginal cuff, highly suspicious for vaginal carcinoma. FDG-avid masses within the vagina can often be obscured by FDG excretion.* **(Right)** *Axial noncontrast CT of the same patient shows thickening of the right vaginal wall* ➡*. There is adjacent high-density material* ➡ *that is likely silver nitrate, used for hemostasis after biopsy.*

KEY FACTS

TERMINOLOGY

- Prostate cancer: > 95% is adenocarcinoma, characterized by small, infiltrating glandular tissue with prominent nucleoli

IMAGING

- FDG PET/CT
  - Primary tumor can appear as hypermetabolic focus commonly located in peripheral zone of prostate
  - Not sensitive enough to confidently detect primary tumor
  - Lymph nodes and bone metastases most common
- Tc-99m MDP bone scan or FDG NaF PET
  - Intense uptake in variably sized, multifocal skeletal lesions
  - Metastases are usually axial, then follow distribution of red bone marrow
  - Vertebra and rib involvement common due to tumor cell dissemination from prostate through Batson venous plexus
  - Over time, metastases can become confluent and yield superscan on bone scan

TOP DIFFERENTIAL DIAGNOSES

- **Primary tumor**
  - Benign prostatic hypertrophy
  - Postsurgical inflammation
  - Prostatitis
- **Bone metastatic disease**
  - Fracture
  - Osteoarthritis
  - Paget disease

DIAGNOSTIC CHECKLIST

- Correlate uptake in weight-bearing areas with plain films to evaluate for impending pathologic fracture
- Uptake on Tc-99m MDP bone scan has low specificity for metastatic disease when PSA < 10 ng/mL in patient not on antiandrogen therapy

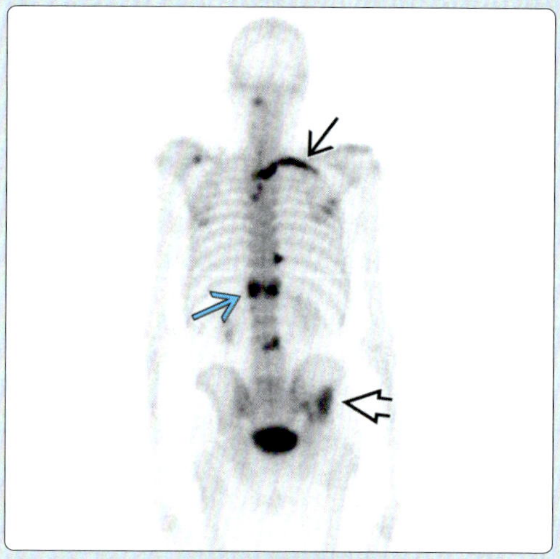

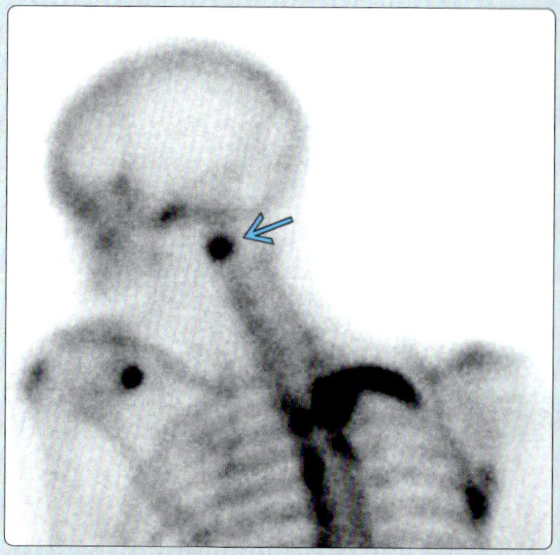

(Left) *Posterior Tc-99m MDP bone scan in a man with prostate cancer shows multifocal osseous metastases involving the ribs →, vertebral bodies →, and pelvis →.* **(Right)** *Left lateral Tc-99m MDP bone scan in the same patient shows involvement of cervical spine →.*

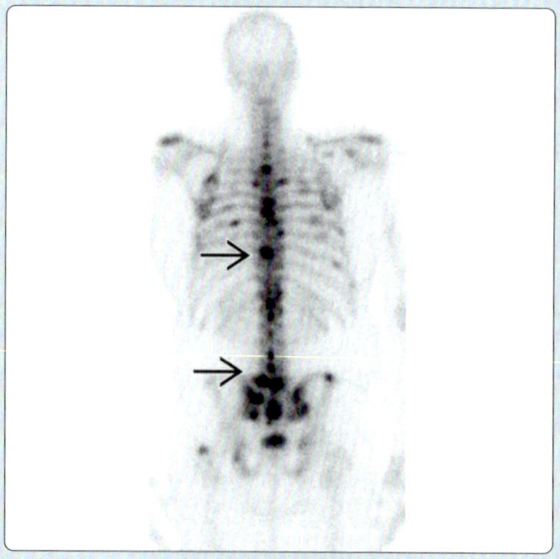

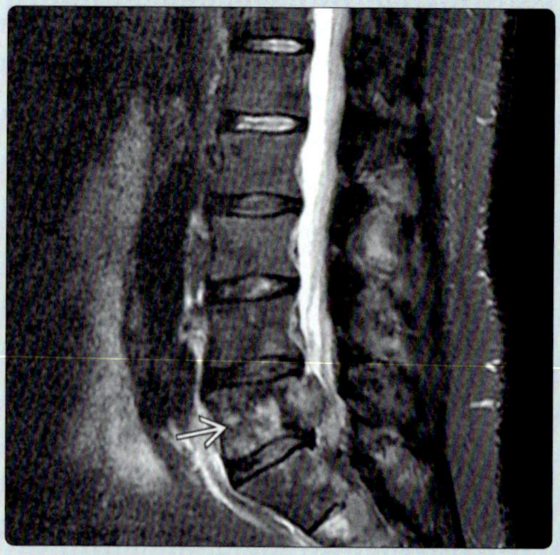

(Left) *Posterior Tc-99m MDP bone scan in a patient with prostate cancer shows characteristic axial skeleton distribution of metastases. Prostate cancer metastases are often found in vertebral bodies →, as prostate cancer cells travel through Batson venous plexus.* **(Right)** *Sagittal T2 MR in the same patient shows metastatic involvement of the L5 vertebral body →. This patient had developed neurologic symptoms likely due to compromise of the spinal canal and nerve roots at this level.*

TERMINOLOGY

Definitions

- Prostate cancer: > 95% is adenocarcinoma, characterized by small, infiltrating glandular tissue with prominent nucleoli

IMAGING

General Features

- Best diagnostic clue
  - FDG PET/CT
    - F-18 FDG-avid primary mass with hypermetabolic lymphadenopathy and axial bone lesions
      - Primary tumor can appear as hypermetabolic focus commonly located in peripheral zone of prostate
      - FDG PET/CT not sensitive enough to confidently detect primary tumor
    - F-18 FDG-avid metastatic disease
      - Lymph nodes and bone metastases most common
  - Bone scan
    - Tc-99m MDP bone scan or FDG NaF PET
      - Intense uptake in variably sized, multifocal skeletal lesions
      - Metastases are usually axial, then follow distribution of red bone marrow
      - Vertebra and rib involvement common due to tumor cell dissemination from prostate through Batson venous plexus
      - Over time, metastases can become confluent and yield superscan on bone scan

Nuclear Medicine Findings

- Bone scan
  - Tc-99m MDP bone scan
    - Use as 1st line to detect metastases in high-risk patient
    - Routine scans in conjunction with PSA measurements are recommended to follow metastatic disease and response to treatment
    - Detection of bony metastases
      - Sensitivity 51-57%, specificity 56-82%
      - More sensitive than plain film, detects 10% change in bone turnover
      - Recommended for symptomatic patients or asymptomatic patients at risk for occult metastases
      - Patients considered at risk for occult metastases include those with PSA > 20 ng/mL **or** PSA > 10 with T2-T4 primary **or** Gleason score > 8
      - Bone scan is of limited value when PSA < 10 ng/mL for detection of metastases but can serve as useful baseline examination for comparison on follow-up
      - Uptake on Tc-99m MDP bone scan has low specificity for metastatic disease when PSA < 10 ng/mL in patient not on antiandrogen therapy
    - Limitations
      - Bone scan can have nonspecific uptake in degenerative changes, inflammation, Paget disease, and trauma, mimicking metastases
      - Flare phenomenon: Uptake due to increased osteoblastic bone healing after therapy can mimic disease progression
      - Findings of mixed response suggest flare phenomenon: Some lesions improve, some lesions more conspicuous, some new lesions
      - Follow-up bone scan often required to confirm diagnosis of flare phenomenon
  - NaF PET/CT
    - Detection of bony metastases
      - Highly effective: Sensitivity 96-100%, specificity 98-100%
      - High therapeutic impact, found to change management in 44-52% of patients
      - Proven superior to other modalities at detection of bony metastases: Identifies bony metastases earlier and with more accuracy than any other modality
    - Most expensive and least available modality
      - No cost-effective analysis to date
      - May be useful as 2nd line in equivocal cases
- PET/CT
  - Detection of primary lesions on FDG PET/CT
    - Limited efficacy in localized disease due to variable cellular uptake and close proximity to bladder
    - BPH, inflammation, prostatitis, and post-therapy changes can have hypermetabolic activity
  - Detection of metastatic disease on FDG PET/CT
    - Variable sensitivity and specificity
    - Sclerotic metastases commonly have low FDG uptake
  - Other PET/CT radiotracers
    - F-18 FDG choline and C-11 acetate have shown efficacy in research setting

DIFFERENTIAL DIAGNOSIS

Hypermetabolic Activity in Prostate on FDG PET

- Prostate cancer
- Prostatitis
- Postsurgical inflammation

Focal Uptake on Tc-99m MDP Bone Scan

- Osseous metastases
- Paget disease
- Osteoarthritis
- Post-traumatic, postsurgical

PATHOLOGY

General Features

- Etiology
  - Prostatic intraepithelial neoplasia is likely precursor
    - Major risk factors
      - Increasing age
      - Family history in 1st-degree relatives
      - Obesity
      - High testosterone

Staging, Grading, & Classification

- TNM staging
  - Primary tumor (T)
    - T1: Clinically inapparent tumor (neither palpable nor visible on imaging) **but** identified by biopsy
    - T2: Tumor confined within prostate
    - T3: Tumor extends through prostate capsule

- T4: Tumor invades adjacent structures, can include rectum, bladder, pelvic wall
- Regional lymph nodes (N)
  - NX: Lymph nodes not assessed
  - N0: No regional nodal metastases
  - N1: Metastases to regional nodes
- Distant metastases (M)
  - M0: No distant metastases
  - M1: Distant metastases
    - M1a: Metastases to nonregional lymph nodes
    - M1b: Metastases to bone
    - M1c: Metastases to other site(s)
- Gleason score
  - Pathologic grading system, ranges 2-10
  - Higher score = poorer differentiation
- **Stage I**: T1-T2, N0, M0, PSA < 10, Gleason score < 7
- **Stage IIA**: T1-T2, N0, M0, PSA < 20, Gleason score < 8
- **Stage IIB**: T1-T2, N0, M0, any PSA, any Gleason score
- **Stage III**: T3, N0, M0, any PSA, any Gleason score
- **Stage IV**: T4 **or** N1 **or** M1

CLINICAL ISSUES

Presentation

- Most common signs/symptoms
  - Primary tumors
    - Urinary frequency, urgency, nocturia, and hesitancy common but nonspecific
  - Metastatic disease
    - Bone pain
    - Pathologic fracture
- Other signs/symptoms
  - Hematuria and hematospermia are less common but should prompt consideration

Demographics

- Age
  - 99% of patients diagnosed with prostate cancer are > 50 years old
- Ethnicity
  - African American men have 58% higher incidence than Caucasian men
- Epidemiology
  - Prevalence: 1.1 million cases worldwide in 2012
  - Mortality: 307,000 deaths worldwide in 2012

Treatment

- Surgery
  - Radical prostatectomy
    - Indicated for regionally localized disease and locally advanced disease without tumor fixation or lymph node involvement
    - Usually insufficient for management of high-risk disease; need adjuvant therapy
- Systemic therapies
  - Androgen deprivation therapy
  - Chemoradiation
- Radium-223
  - Indicated for castration-resistant disease w/ symptomatic bony metastases
  - Taken up by bone, similar to calcium
  - Uses mostly α radiation to selectively treat bone lesions
    - α emission (95.3%; energy range: 5.0-7.5 MeV)
    - β emission (3.6%; average energies: 0.445 MeV and 0.492 MeV)
    - γ emission (1.1%; energy range: 0.01-1.27 MeV)
  - Shown to improve overall survival (median 14.9 months compared with 11.3 months for placebo)

DIAGNOSTIC CHECKLIST

Consider

- Bone scan
  - Useful in high-risk disease and to serve as baseline for lower-risk disease
  - Serial bone scans are necessary to follow known metastases
  - FDG NaF PET is most sensitive modality but more expensive and less clinically available compared with Tc-99m MDP bone scan

Image Interpretation Pearls

- Correlate uptake in weight-bearing areas with plain films to evaluate for impending pathologic fracture
- Uptake on Tc-99m MDP bone scan has low specificity for metastatic disease when PSA < 10 ng/mL in patient not on antiandrogen therapy
- Findings of mixed response suggest flare phenomenon: Some lesions improve, some lesions more conspicuous, some new lesions

SELECTED REFERENCES

1. Parker C et al: Alpha emitter radium-223 and survival in metastatic prostate cancer. N Engl J Med. 369(3):213-23, 2013
2. Mackiewicz-Wysocka M et al: Progress in the treatment of bone metastases in cancer patients. Expert Opin Investig Drugs. 21(6):785-95, 2012
3. Saad F et al: The current role of circulating tumor cells in the diagnosis and management of bone metastases in advanced prostate cancer. Future Oncol. 8(3):321-31, 2012
4. Jadvar H: Prostate cancer: PET with 18F-FDG, 18F- or 11C-acetate, and 18F- or 11C-choline. J Nucl Med. 52(1):81-9, 2011
5. Ibrahim T et al: Pathogenesis of osteoblastic bone metastases from prostate cancer. Cancer. 116(6):1406-18, 2010
6. Saylor PJ et al: Bone health and prostate cancer. Prostate Cancer Prostatic Dis. 13(1):20-7, 2010
7. Messiou C et al: Imaging metastatic bone disease from carcinoma of the prostate. Br J Cancer. 101(8):1225-32, 2009
8. Logothetis CJ et al: Understanding the biology of bone metastases: key to the effective treatment of prostate cancer. Clin Cancer Res. 14(6):1599-602, 2008
9. Tu SM et al: Current trials using bone-targeting agents in prostate cancer. Cancer J. 14(1):35-9, 2008
10. Storey JA et al: Bone metastases in prostate cancer: a targeted approach. Curr Opin Oncol. 19(3):254-8, 2007
11. Saad F et al: Natural history and treatment of bone complications in prostate cancer. Eur Urol. 49(3):429-40, 2006

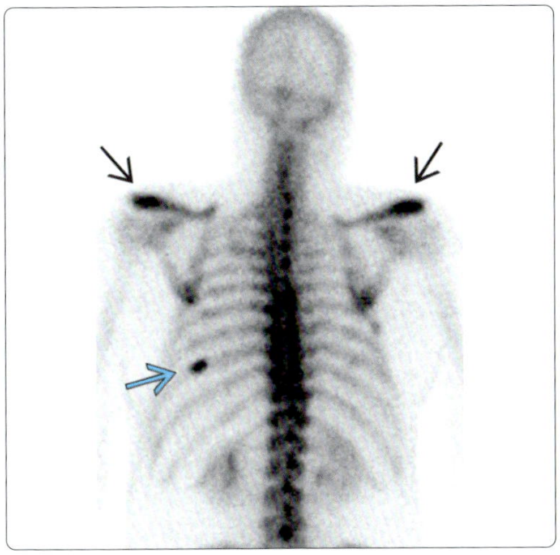

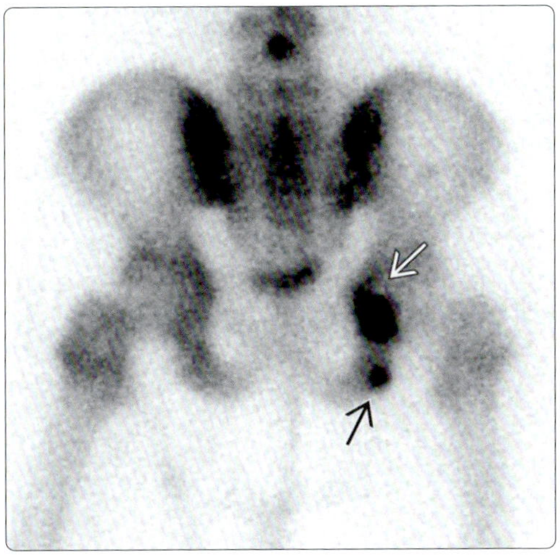

(Left) *Posterior Tc-99m MDP bone scan in a patient with prostate cancer shows solitary bone metastasis in a rib* →. *Symmetric, bilateral shoulder uptake* → *is degenerative in nature.* **(Right)** *Posterior Tc-99m MDP bone scan in a patient with prostate cancer shows asymmetrically increased activity in the right acetabulum* ➡ *and ischium* →.

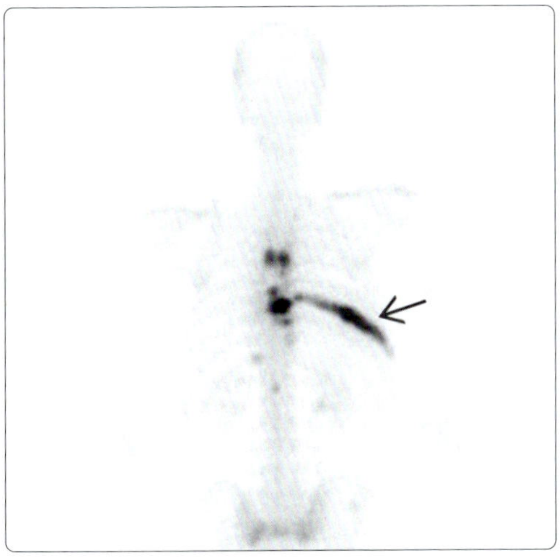

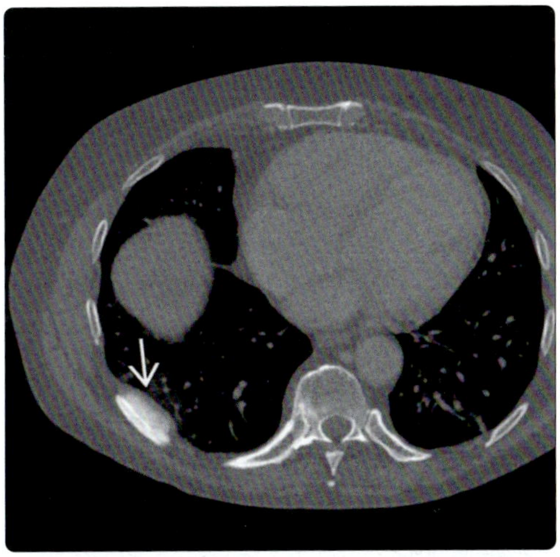

(Left) *Posterior Tc-99m MDP bone scan of a 65-year-old man with metastatic prostate cancer shows multiple areas of involvement, including the posterolateral right 9th rib* →. **(Right)** *Corresponding axial chest CT shows the expansile sclerotic lesion of the right 9th rib* ➡, *indicating osteoblastic response.*

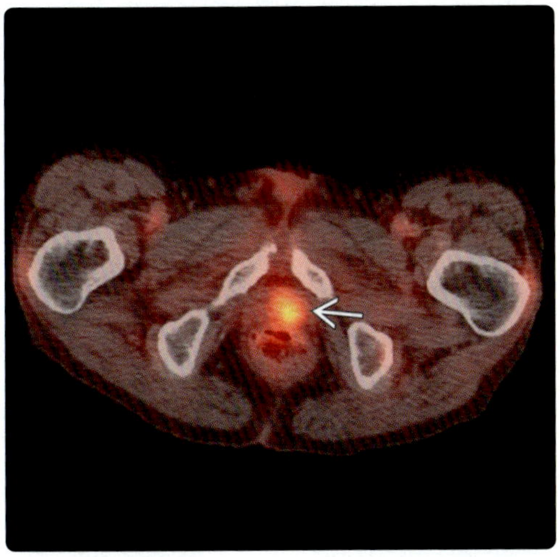

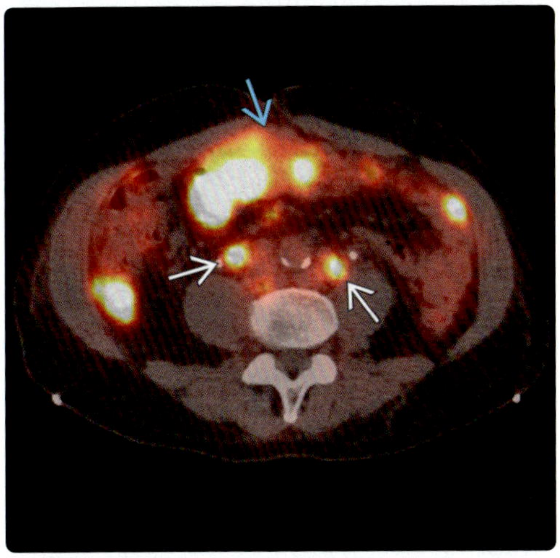

(Left) *Axial FDG PET/CT of an 80-year-old man with a history of prostate cancer shows focal enlargement of the prostate gland with hypermetabolic activity* ➡. *This is nonspecific but could indicate disease recurrence.* **(Right)** *Axial FDG PET/CT of a 65-year-old man with metastatic prostate cancer shows hypermetabolic paraaortic* ➡ *nodes (SUV: 6) and an omental mass* → *with adjacent bowel activity.*

Testicular Cancer

KEY FACTS

TERMINOLOGY

- Germ cell tumors
  - Seminomas
  - Nonseminomatous

TOP DIFFERENTIAL DIAGNOSES

- Testicular neoplasm
  - Other germ cell/non-germ cell tumors
  - Lymphoma
  - Metastases
- Infection/inflammation
  - Orchitis
  - Torsion/infarct
- Other GU cancers
  - Prostate
  - Bladder

PATHOLOGY

- 95% of testicular tumors are malignant germ cell
- Staging
  - Stage I: Local, confined to testes or surrounding structures
  - Stage II: Regional metastases
  - Stage III: Distant metastases

DIAGNOSTIC CHECKLIST

- F-18 FDG PET/CT
  - Used primarily to look for metabolic activity inside residual masses
    - Most effective with masses > 3 cm
- Tc-99m bone scan
  - More sensitive than CT
  - Bone metastases are rare; use in symptomatic individuals only
  - Increased uptake in axial skeleton, commonly lumbar spine

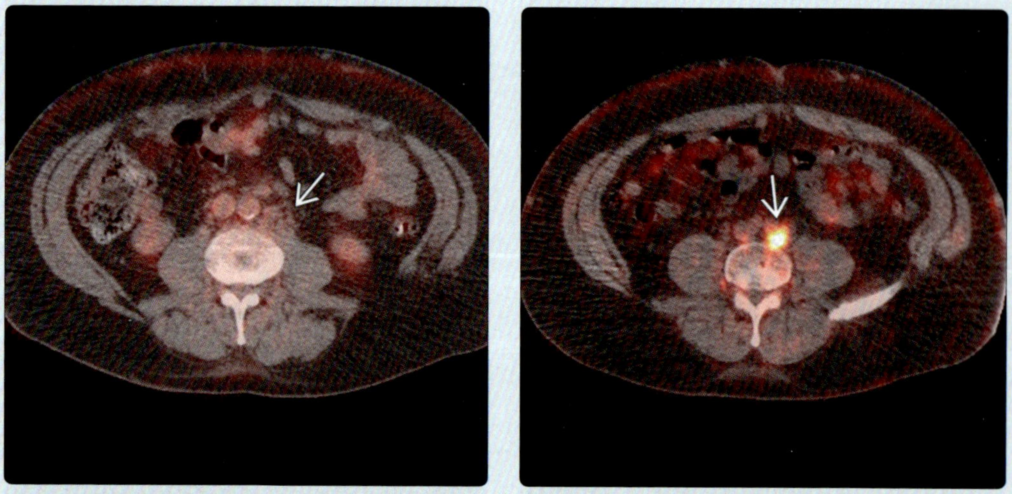

(Left) *Axial FDG PET/CT of a 41-year-old man s/p right orchiectomy for seminoma shows multiple enlarged aortoilliac nodes without hypermetabolic activity* ➡. **(Right)** *Axial FDG PET/CT of the same patient 2 years later shows a hypermetabolic (SUV: 11.6) node in this aortoilliac region* ➡*, consistent with recurrent metastatic disease. This SUV is fairly high, which is atypical for testicular cancer, where nodal disease typically has lower values.*

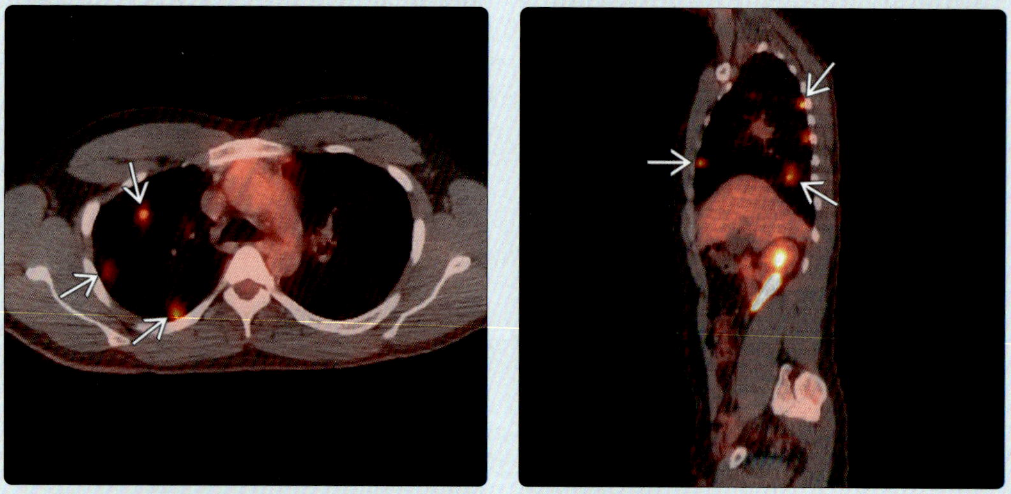

(Left) *Axial FDG PET/CT of a 24-year-old man s/p left orchiectomy for embryonal carcinoma shows numerous hypermetabolic nodules* ➡ *in both lungs, consistent with metastatic disease.* **(Right)** *Corresponding sagittal view shows many hypermetabolic nodules* ➡ *within the right lung.*

IMAGING

General Features

- Best diagnostic clue
  - F-18 FDG PET/CT
    - Primary tumor can have variable FDG uptake, SUV often < 3
    - FDG-avid metastases are first seen in retroperitoneal lymph nodes
  - Tc-99m MDP bone scan
    - Axial involvement, most commonly lumbar spine
- Location
  - Primary tumor
    - Intratesticular, within tunica albuginea
  - Metastases
    - Regional lymph nodes
    - Lung
    - Brain
- Morphology
  - Germ cell tumors: Heterogeneous, solid mass
    - Seminomas: No cystic areas or calcification
    - Nonseminomatous: Variable cystic elements, calcification, necrosis/hemorrhage
    - Any size can be malignant
  - Non-germ cell tumors: Well circumscribed, round to lobulated
    - Malignant usually > 5 cm

Nuclear Medicine Findings

- Bone scan
  - Tc-99m bone scan
    - Only indicated in symptomatic patients
      - □ Can detect bone lesions before CT
      - □ Bony metastases rare: 3% of patients with metastatic disease have bone involvement
      - □ Isolated bone metastases extremely uncommon
- PET/CT
  - F-18 FDG PET/CT
    - Useful modality to monitor post-chemotherapy residual disease in malignant seminoma
      - □ Differentiates viable masses from necrosis, fibrosis, or scar tissue
      - □ Effective at detecting viable tumor within residual masses > 3 cm: Sensitivity 80%, specificity 100%, PPV 100%, NPV 96%
      - □ Cannot reliably detect viable tumor within residual masses < 3 cm
      - □ Residual tumor resection can be avoided with lesions > 3 cm **and** negative PET
    - FDG PET offers no advantage over CT in initial staging of germ cell tumors
      - □ Risk of false-negatives: Mature teratomas (cold), micrometastases (undetectable)
      - □ Risk of false-positives: Inflammatory masses (hot), sarcoidosis
      - □ Can be used when CT is equivocal
    - Limited published experience with FDG PET in evaluation of malignant non-germ cell tumors
    - Significant risk of late relapse after negative FDG PET
      - □ Longitudinal follow-up required

Imaging Recommendations

- Best imaging tool
  - F-18 FDG PET/CT: Superior for detection of viable residual disease
    - No advantage in initial staging of germ cell tumors compared to CT
    - Limited data in evaluation of non-germ cell tumors
  - Tc-99m bone scan: Symptomatic patients, axial involvement most common

DIFFERENTIAL DIAGNOSIS

Testicular Neoplasm

- Other germ cell/non-germ cell tumors
- Lymphoma
  - Older age group
  - 50% bilateral
  - Often higher FDG uptake than primary testicular cancer
- Metastases
  - From prostate most common, followed by lung, melanoma

Infection/Inflammation

- Torsion/infarct
  - Acute infarct commonly FDG avid due to associated hemorrhage and inflammation
- Orchitis

Other GU Cancers

- Prostate
- Bladder

PATHOLOGY

General Features

- Etiology
  - 95% of testicular tumors are malignant germ cell
- Genetics
  - Family history ↑ risk of of germ cell tumors
  - Peutz-Jeghers, Carney syndromes; Kleinfelter syndrome: Non-germ cell tumors
- Associated abnormalities
  - Germ cell tumors: Gynecomastia, prepubescent virilization, cryptorchidism, testicular microlithiasis, family history
  - Non-germ cell tumors: Prepubescent virilization, feminization, stigmata of Kleinfelter syndrome; Peutz-Jeghers and Carney syndromes

Staging, Grading, & Classification

- Stage IA: Tumor confined to testis and epididymis, may extend to tunica albuginea
- Stage IB: Tumor either involves tunica vaginalis, involves spermatic cord or scrotum, or has local vascular/lymphatic invasion
- Stage IS: Any of the above plus positive serum tumor markers
- Stage II: Mets to regional nodes, can have tumor marker class of S1
  - Stage IIA: Regional node mets < 2 cm (5 cm^3)
  - Stage IIB: Regional node mets 2-5 cm (10 cm^3)
  - Stage IIC: Regional node mets > 5 cm

- Stage III: Distant mets
  - Stage IIIA: Nonregional nodal or pulmonary mets
  - Stage IIIB: Nonregional nodal or pulmonary mets **or** any met with tumor marker class of S2
  - Stage IIIC: Any met with tumor marker class of S3 **or** distant mets to areas other than lymph nodes or lung
- Serum tumor markers: Required for staging
  - S0: Levels within normal limits
  - S1: LDH < 1.5 x upper limit of normal **and** hCG < 5,000 **and** AFP < 1,000
  - S2: LDH 1.5-10 x upper limit of normal **or** hCG 5,000-50,000 **or** AFP 1,000-10,000
  - S3: LDH > 10 x upper limit of normal **or** hCG > 50,000 **or** AFP >10,000
- In metastatic disease, the two most important prognostic factors
  - Size of retroperitoneal lymph nodes
  - Degree of vascular infiltration

Definitions

- Germ cell tumors: Neoplasm derived from germ cell elements
  - Seminomas: Originate in germinal epithelium of seminiferous tubules
  - Nonseminomatous tumors: Originate from embryonal stem cells; commonly exist in "mixed" type, containing more than one of the types below
    - Choriocarcinoma
    - Teratomas: Several types
      - Can contain tissue or organ components within the tumor
      - Dermoid cyst
      - Monodermal teratoma
    - Embryonal carcinoma
    - Yolk sac tumor
  - Non-germ cell tumors: Usually benign from non-germ cell elements
    - Leydig cell tumors (LCT): From interstitial cells
    - Sertoli cell tumors (SCT): From sustentacular cells lining seminiferous tubules
    - Granulosa cell tumors: Rare benign tumors
    - Gonadoblastoma: Contains both non-germ cell and germ cell elements

CLINICAL ISSUES

Presentation

- Most common signs/symptoms
  - Painless testicular enlargement; dull/acute pain in < 30%
- Other signs/symptoms
  - Germ cell tumors: ↑ serum markers (beta-HCG, alpha-fetoprotein, LDH)
  - Precocious virilization, gynecomastia, ↓ libido/impotence (adults)

Demographics

- Epidemiology
  - Germ cell tumors: Most common cancer in 15-34 year olds; 1% of all cancers in men
    - Seminomas: Most common in 35-39 year olds; rare < 10 years
  - Non-germ cell tumors: Age 30-60 years; 25% before puberty; malignant LCT only in adults; SCT in all ages (1/3 < 12 years)
  - Lymphoma: Most common testicular tumor > 50 years

Natural History & Prognosis

- 5-year survival
  - All stage I: 99%
  - All stage II **or** stage III without distant mets: 96%
  - Stage III with distant spread: 74%

Treatment

- Germ cell tumors: Radical orchiectomy; retroperitoneal nodal dissection for nonseminomatous tumor; XRT, chemotherapy for metastatic
- Non-germ cell tumors: Orchiectomy or testis-sparing surgery; same as germ cell tumors if metastatic disease

DIAGNOSTIC CHECKLIST

Consider

- Primary tumor: Variable uptake on PET
- Metastatic disease: Moderately FDG avid on PET
  - Initial retroperitoneal nodal spread
  - Lungs, liver, brain, bones

Reporting Tips

- F-18 FDG PET/CT
  - Include any hypermetabolic foci
    - Primary or residual masses
    - Local or regional lymph nodes
    - Distant foci of uptake
  - Include extent of primary tumor
    - Important for initial staging
  - Include tumor response
    - Complete metabolic response: SUVmax < 2.5 or equivalent to background
    - Partial response: Decrease in SUVmax ≥ 25%
    - Progressive disease: Increase in SUVmax ≥ 25%
- Tc-99m bone scan
  - Discuss any osseous lesions suspicious for metastatic disease
    - Usually axial

SELECTED REFERENCES

1. Becherer A: PET in testicular cancer. Methods Mol Biol. 727:225-41, 2011
2. Tiemstra JD et al: Evaluation of scrotal masses. Am Fam Physician. 78(10):1165-70, 2008
3. Becherer A et al: FDG PET is superior to CT in the prediction of viable tumour in post-chemotherapy seminoma residuals. Eur J Radiol. 54(2):284-8, 2005
4. De Santis M et al: 2-18fluoro-deoxy-D-glucose positron emission tomography is a reliable predictor for viable tumor in postchemotherapy seminoma: an update of the prospective multicentric SEMPET trial. J Clin Oncol. 22(6):1034-9, 2004
5. Lassen U et al: Whole-body FDG-PET in patients with stage I non-seminomatous germ cell tumours. Eur J Nucl Med Mol Imaging. 30(3):396-402, 2003
6. Sanchez D et al: 18F-fluoro-2-deoxyglucose-positron emission tomography in the evaluation of nonseminomatous germ cell tumours at relapse. BJU Int. 89(9):912-6, 2002
7. Spermon JR et al: The role of (18)fluoro-2-deoxyglucose positron emission tomography in initial staging and re-staging after chemotherapy for testicular germ cell tumours. BJU Int. 89(6):549-56, 2002

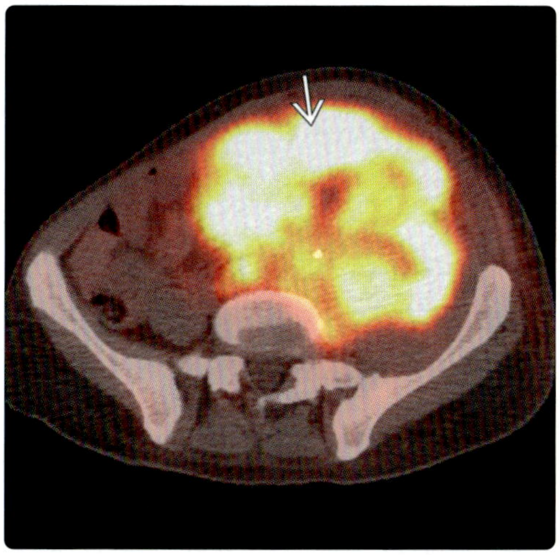

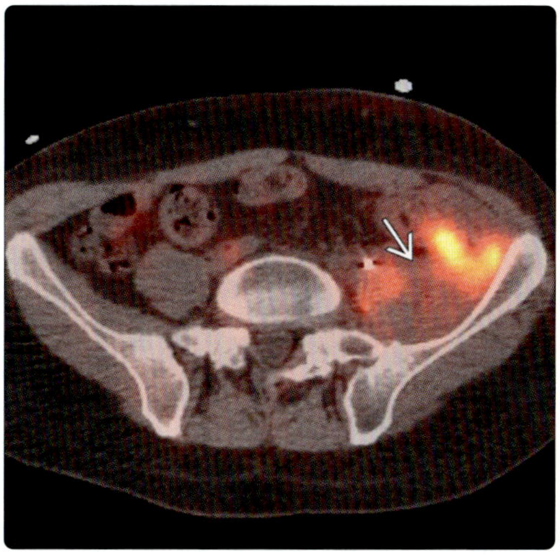

(Left) *Axial FDG PET/CT of a 36-year-old man s/p left orchiectomy for testicular seminoma shows large nodal conglomerate in the left iliac fossa with malignant-range hypermetabolic activity* ➔*.* **(Right)** *Axial FDG PET/CT 1 year later shows interval decrease in the size and metabolic activity of this mass* ➔*. This patient had received several cycles of chemotherapy along with pelvic radiotherapy.*

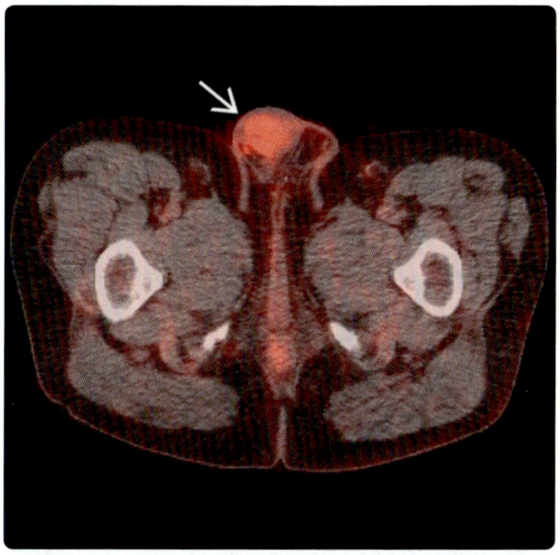

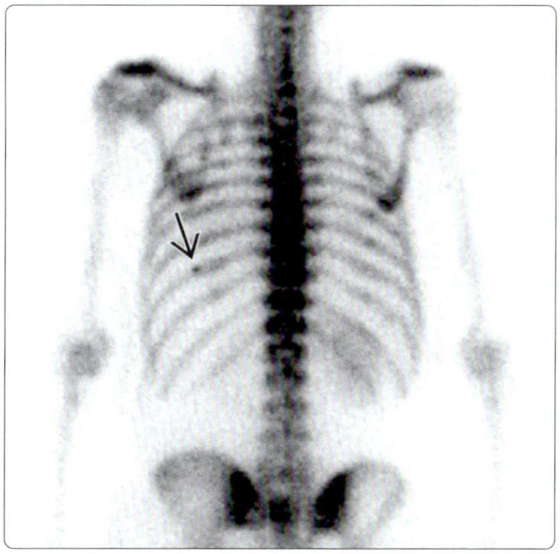

(Left) *Axial FDG PET/CT of a 54-year-old man with B-cell non-Hodgkin lymphoma shows increased activity within the right testicle* ➔*, which can mimic primary testicular malignancy.* **(Right)** *Posterior bone scan of a 37-year-old man with a history of testicular seminoma and new-onset rib pain shows a solitary focus of increased uptake within the posterior aspect of the left 9th rib* ⇨*, which was considered indeterminate for malignancy.*

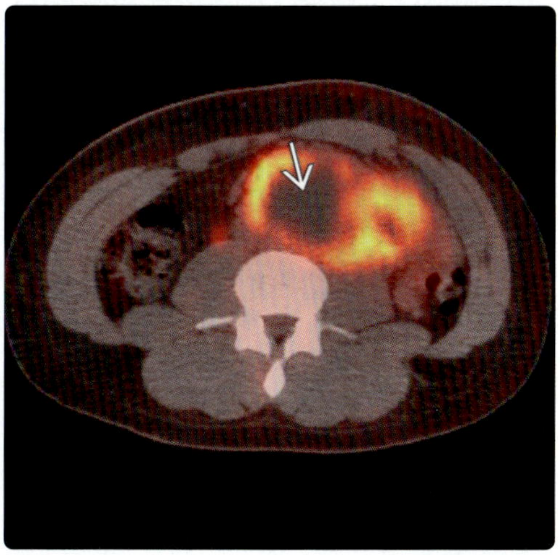

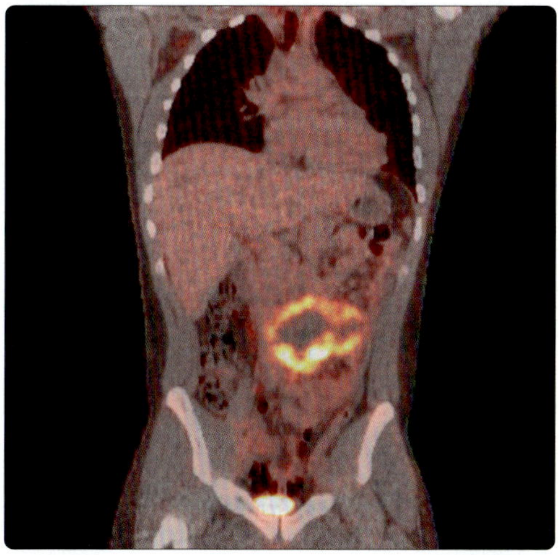

(Left) *Axial FDG PET/CT of a 20-year-old man s/p left orchiectomy for seminoma shows a hypermetabolic left paraaortic mass with central necrosis* ➔*.* **(Right)** *Corresponding coronal FDG PET/CT is shown. Even large nodal masses can be very responsive to chemotherapy and radiation.*

Malignant Pleural Mesothelioma

KEY FACTS

TERMINOLOGY

- Malignant tumor that originates from mesothelial surface of pleura

IMAGING

- CECT
  - Constricted hemithorax with pleural effusion and lobular pleural masses &/or foci of pleural thickening, often diffuse
  - Associated signs of metastatic disease, such as invasion of chest wall, diaphragm, or mediastinum; lymphadenopathy, ascites, peritoneal implants, or skeletal metastases
  - Evidence of asbestos exposure, such as pleural calcifications, contralateral pleural plaques, or bibasilar pulmonary fibrosis from asbestosis
- F-18 FDG PET/CT
  - Directs biopsy to hypermetabolic pleural plaques
  - Most complete staging when compared with CT
  - Talc pleurodesis incites pleural inflammation and can cause lymphadenopathy, all of which can be hypermetabolic and decrease specificity of F-18 FDG PET/CT
  - Higher uptake associated with shorter survival time

PATHOLOGY

- Strong association with asbestos and erionite exposure
- 3 histologic cell types: Epithelioid (best prognosis), sarcomatoid (worst prognosis), biphasic

DIAGNOSTIC CHECKLIST

- For best interpretation of F-18 FDG PET/CT
  - Review patient's occupational history
  - Review pleurodesis status before interpreting examination
  - Check along sites of pleural intervention for seeding

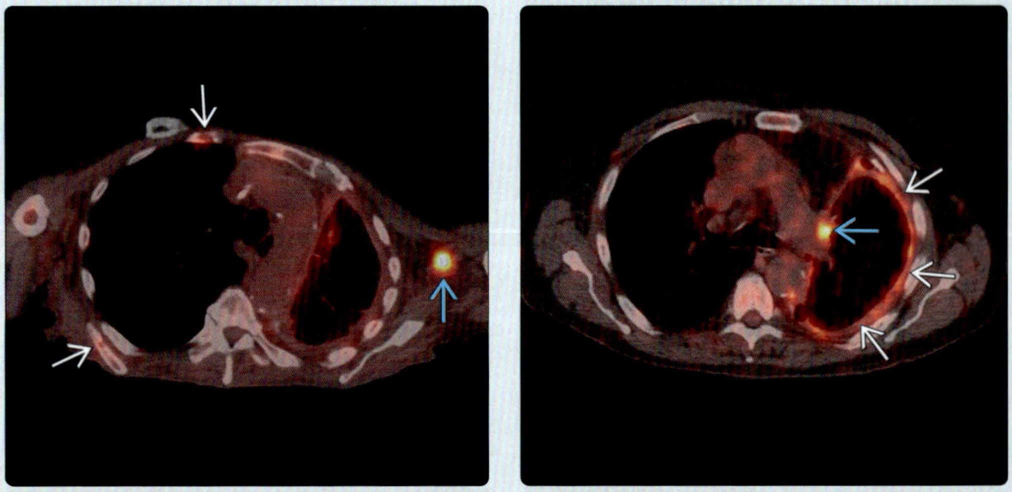

(Left) *Axial fused F-18 FDG PET/CT in an 86-year-old man with malignant left pleural mesothelioma shows focal intense uptake in a left axillary lymph node metastasis ➡ and in a partially imaged skeletal metastasis ➡.* **(Right)** *Axial fused F-18 FDG PET/CT in the same patient shows intense, diffuse pleural activity ➡ and a metastatic left hilar lymph node ➡. At times, hilar lymph node activity cannot be distinguished from generalized pleural activity.*

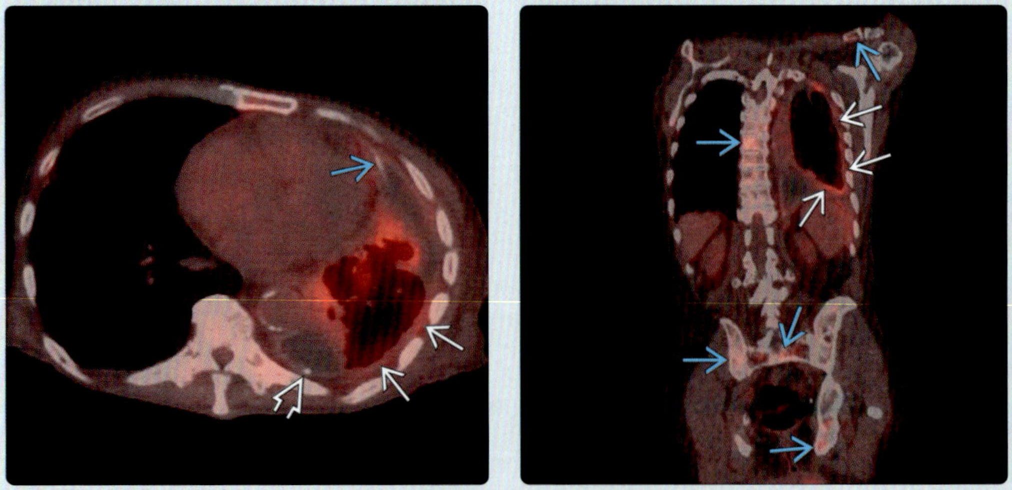

(Left) *Axial fused F-18 FDG PET/CT shows high-density material in the left anterior pleural space ➡ after talc pleurodesis. Related diffuse pleural thickening with mild hypermetabolic activity ➡ is present. A small calcified plaque is seen posteriorly ➡.* **(Right)** *Coronal fused F-18 FDG PET/CT shows multifocal hypermetabolic skeletal metastases ➡. Generalized left pleural thickening and increased activity ➡ is due to talc pleurodesis.*

TERMINOLOGY

Abbreviations

- Malignant pleural mesothelioma (MPM)

Definitions

- Malignant tumor that originates from mesothelial surface of pleura

IMAGING

Nuclear Medicine Findings

- PET/CT
  - Hypermetabolic pleural masses &/or pleural rind with associated pleural effusion
  - Can be associated with hypermetabolic evidence of direct invasion or distant metastatic disease

Imaging Recommendations

- Best imaging tool
  - CECT: For initial evaluation
  - F-18 FDG PET/CT
    - For staging when planning definitive surgery
    - Sensitive for follow-up after surgical resection when considering metastatic disease
    - Helpful in assessing chemotherapy response
    - Useful for further evaluation when other imaging is equivocal
- Protocol advice
  - Standard F-18 FDG PET/CT oncology protocol

General Features

- Best diagnostic clue
  - Constricted hemithorax with pleural effusion and lobular pleural masses &/or foci of pleural thickening, often diffuse
  - Associated signs of metastatic disease, e.g., invasion of chest wall, diaphragm, or mediastinum; lymphadenopathy, ascites, peritoneal implants, or skeletal metastases
  - Evidence of asbestos exposure, such as pleural calcifications, contralateral pleural plaques, or bibasilar pulmonary fibrosis from asbestosis
  - Mesh replacement of hemidiaphragm in patients who have undergone extrapleural pneumonectomy

Image-Guided Biopsy

- CT-guided core biopsy for patients with demonstrable pleural mass or thickening on imaging
  - F-18 FDG PET/CT can direct to most hypermetabolic lesion for biopsy
- Video-assisted thoracoscopy-guided biopsy: For patients with only pleural effusion visible

DIFFERENTIAL DIAGNOSIS

Inflammatory Disease

- Asbestos-related pleural disease
- Talc pleurodesis
- Chronic organized empyema
- Tuberculous pleural involvement

Other Neoplasms

- Solitary fibrous tumor of pleura
- Pleural metastases
- Lymphoma
- Fibrosarcoma

PATHOLOGY

General Features

- Etiology
  - Strong association with asbestos and erionite exposure
    - Associated with exposure in 80% of cases
    - Latency period of up to 50 years
    - Incidence in asbestos workers is 10%
- Genetics
  - Tumor suppressor genes: Neurofibromatosis type 2, BRCA1-associated protein-1
- Associated abnormalities
  - Asbestosis, asbestos-related pleural plaques (calcified and noncalcified), and asbestos-related pleural effusion

Staging, Grading, & Classification

- Most commonly used staging system is TNM
- Stage I: T1 N0 M0
  - Unilateral pleural involvement
  - No nodal disease or distant sites
- Stage II: T2 N0 M0
  - Unilateral involvement
  - Has grown into diaphragm or lung
- Stage III: T1 or T2, N1 or N2, M0 **or** T3, N0 to N2, M0
  - Regional lymph node involvement
    - N1: Ipsilateral hilar or bronchial nodes
    - N2: Ipsilateral nodes to include subcarinal, mediastinal, internal mammary nodes, or peridiaphragmatic nodes
  - T3: Into 1st layer of chest wall, fatty tissue of mediastinum, single place in deeper layers of chest wall, or surface of pericardium
- Stage IV: T4, any N, M0 **or** any T, N3, M0 **or** any T, any N, M1
  - T4: To more than one place in deeper levels of chest wall, through diaphragm into peritoneum, any organ in mediastinum, spine, to contralateral pleura, through pericardium, or into heart
  - N3: Supraclavicular lymph nodes or contralateral hilar or mediastinal nodes
  - M1: Distant nodes or organs
    - Contralateral lung, pleura, liver, bone, or adrenal
  - Unresectable

Gross Pathologic & Surgical Features

- Diagnosis may be difficult
  - Pleural fluid cytology and closed pleural biopsy have relatively low yield
  - Video-assisted thoracoscopy allows larger sampling and is more sensitive
- Initially, can present with multiple nodules more pronounced on parietal side of pleura
  - Soft gelatinous, pinkish-gray appearance
- More advanced disease forms thick tumor rind
  - Visceral and parietal pleura can be fused
- 3 histologic cell types
  - Epithelioid

- Best prognosis
- Sarcomatoid
  - Worst prognosis
- Biphasic

- Local invasion common
  - Chest wall
  - Diaphragm
  - Interlobar fissure
  - Pericardium
  - Mediastinum
- Tends to seed along sites of pleural intervention

CLINICAL ISSUES

Presentation

- Most common signs/symptoms
  - Pulmonary symptoms appear as pleural space is obliterated
    - Chest pain
    - Dyspnea
    - Cough
  - Can invade thoracic structures
    - Dysphagia
    - Hoarseness
    - Spinal cord compression
    - Brachial plexopathy
    - Horner syndrome
    - Superior vena cava syndrome
- Other signs/symptoms
  - Fatigue
  - Weight loss
- Clinical profile
  - Unilateral dullness to percussion
  - Can have scoliosis toward side of disease

Demographics

- Age
  - Average at diagnosis: 69
- Gender
  - > 80% male
- Epidemiology
  - Strong association with asbestos exposure
    - Used in shipbuilding, automotive brake linings, and ceiling tiles
    - Incidence decreasing in countries with good workplace safety controls
      - 3,000 cases/year in USA
    - Long latency period
      - Average latency up to 50 years after exposure

Natural History & Prognosis

- Tumor begins in parietal pleura
- Poor prognosis
- Surgically managed patients
  - Median survival dependent on cell type
    - Epithelioid: 19 months
    - Biphasic: 13 months
    - Sarcomatoid: 8 months
  - Median survival times of patients treated surgically with curative intent
    - Stage I: 21 months
    - Stage II: 19 months
    - Stage III: 16 months
    - Stage IV: 12 months
- Most die of respiratory failure
- Better prognosis: Young, female, no weight loss, and no chest pain

Treatment

- Options, risks, complications
  - Talc pleurodesis incites pleural inflammation and can cause lymphadenopathy, affecting staging
- Chemotherapy
  - Pemetrexed and cisplatin are a commonly used combination chemotherapy for MPM
- Surgery
  - Best surgical results: Patients with epithelioid tumors, limited extent, and no lymph node involvement
  - Pleurectomy/decortication can help control pleural effusion
  - Role of extrapleural pneumonectomy is controversial
- Radiotherapy
  - Pain relief
  - Prophylaxis at intervention and incision sites
- Increasing use of multimodality treatment

DIAGNOSTIC CHECKLIST

Consider

- Patient's occupational history when interpreting exams

Image Interpretation Pearls

- CECT
  - Pleural masses or rind
  - Unilateral volume loss
- F-18 FDG PET/CT
  - Can help differentiate malignant vs. benign pleural disease
  - Can help identify best biopsy target within rind: Foci with most hypermetabolism are good biopsy targets
  - Review pleurodesis status before interpreting examination: Pleurodesis can cause hypermetabolic pleural plaques
  - Check along sites of pleural intervention for seeding
  - Higher uptake associated with shorter survival time

SELECTED REFERENCES

1. American College of Radiology: ACR-SPR practice parameter for performing FDG-PET/CT in oncology. Published 2014. Accessed July 2015.
2. Sekido Y: Molecular pathogenesis of malignant mesothelioma. Carcinogenesis. 34(7):1413-9, 2013
3. Neumann V et al: Malignant pleural mesothelioma: incidence, etiology, diagnosis, treatment, and occupational health. Dtsch Arztebl Int. 110(18):319-26, 2013
4. van Zandwijk N et al: Guidelines for the diagnosis and treatment of malignant pleural mesothelioma. J Thorac Dis. 5(6):E254-307, 2013
5. Truong MT et al: Malignant pleural mesothelioma: role of CT, MRI, and PET/CT in staging evaluation and treatment considerations. Semin Roentgenol. 48(4):323-34, 2013
6. Mott FE: Mesothelioma: a review. Ochsner J. 12(1):70-9, 2012
7. Rusch VW et al: Initial analysis of the international association for the study of lung cancer mesothelioma database. J Thorac Oncol. 7(11):1631-9, 2012

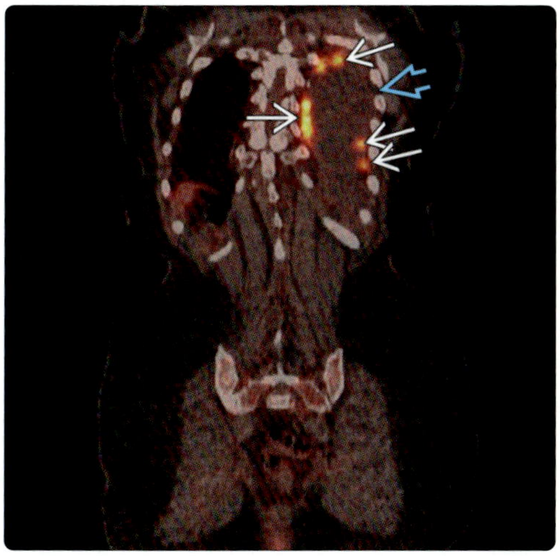

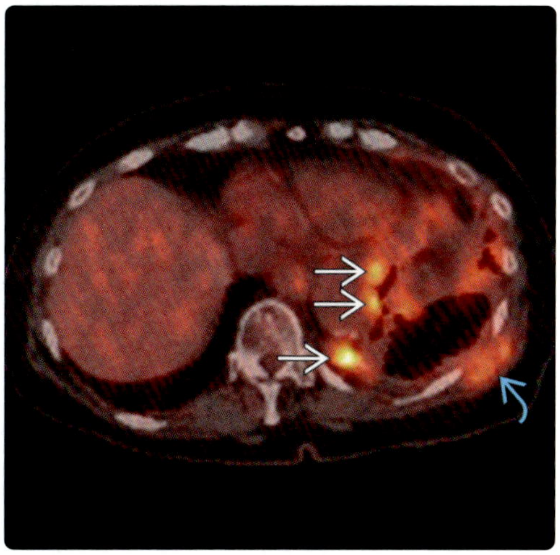

(Left) *Coronal F-18 FDG PET/CT in an 82-year-old woman with malignant left pleural mesothelioma shows a left pleural effusion* ➩. *Multiple hypermetabolic pleural metastases* ➡ *line the pleural space.* **(Right)** *Axial fused F-18 FDG PET/CT in the same patient shows multifocal pleural metastases* ➡. *Focal increased activity in the left chest wall* ➩ *corresponds to the tract of a recently removed chest tube. Note that tumor seeding can occur along a chest tube tract.*

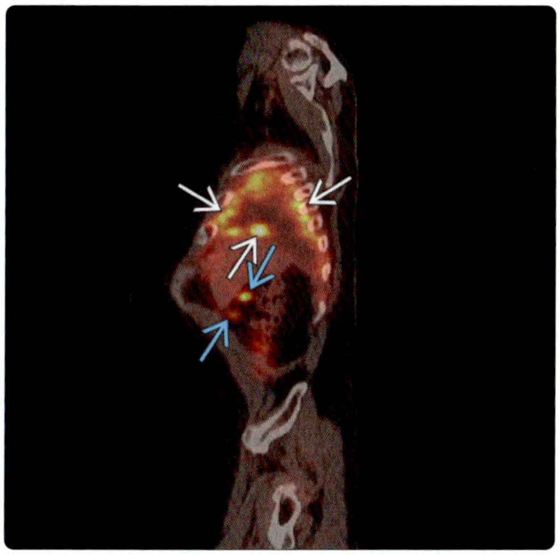

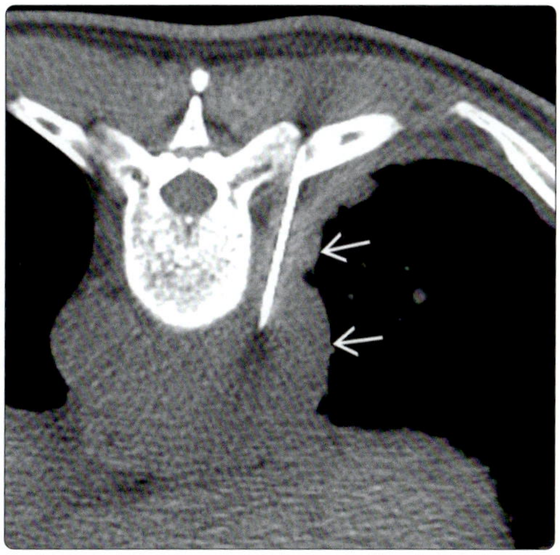

(Left) *Sagittal fused F-18 FDG PET/CT in an 83-year-old man with malignant pleural mesothelioma shows multiple pleural metastases* ➡ *and 2 peritoneal implants* ➩. **(Right)** *Axial CT-guided biopsy in prone position shows a right pleural mass* ➡. *F-18 FDG PET/CT can direct pleural biopsy to the most suspicious pleural mass.*

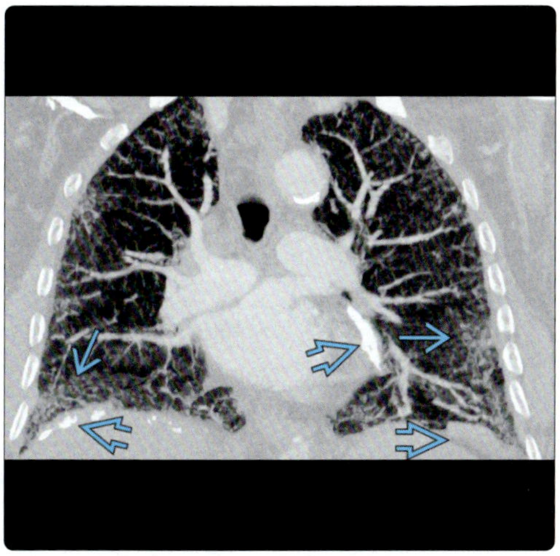

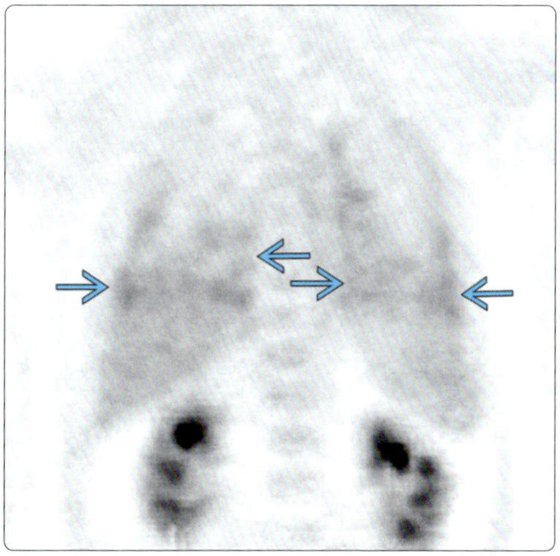

(Left) *Coronal MIP CECT in a man with asbestosis and asbestos-related pleural plaques shows predominantly basilar and peripheral fibrosis* ➩. *Bilateral pleural plaques* ➩ *are visible, some of which are calcified.* **(Right)** *Coronal F-18 FDG PET in the same patient shows diffuse bibasilar low-level uptake* ➩ *without focal hypermetabolic activity to suggest malignancy.*

Non-Small Cell Lung Cancer

KEY FACTS

IMAGING

- PET has established role in staging
  - FDG PET avoids unnecessary thoracotomy in 20% by detecting occult distant disease
- PET useful in determining response to therapy
- Adenocarcinoma, carcinoid and small (< 1 cm) tumors may not have hypermetabolic activity

TOP DIFFERENTIAL DIAGNOSES

- Granulomatous disease
  - Symmetrical mildly FDG-avid hilar & mediastinal nodes
- Pneumonia
  - FDG uptake can be high, but more rapid temporal change
- Mediastinal mass
  - Consider small cell lung cancer, lymphoma
- Hamartoma
  - Typically low FDG activity, popcorn calcification
- Pulmonary infarct
  - FDG uptake as great as with lung cancer
- Carcinoid
  - May not be highly FDG avid
- Small cell carcinoma
  - Requires biopsy to differentiate

DIAGNOSTIC CHECKLIST

- F-18 FDG PET/CT
  - Respiratory motion makes localization more difficult, particularly in lung bases
  - Smaller the nodule, SUV spuriously low
  - Necrosis may show lack of activity centrally
  - Image with arms up when possible
  - Adenocarcinoma in situ may not demonstrate increased FDG uptake
  - Carcinoid may have low FDG uptake
  - High glucose levels or high insulin levels may cause decreased FDG uptake

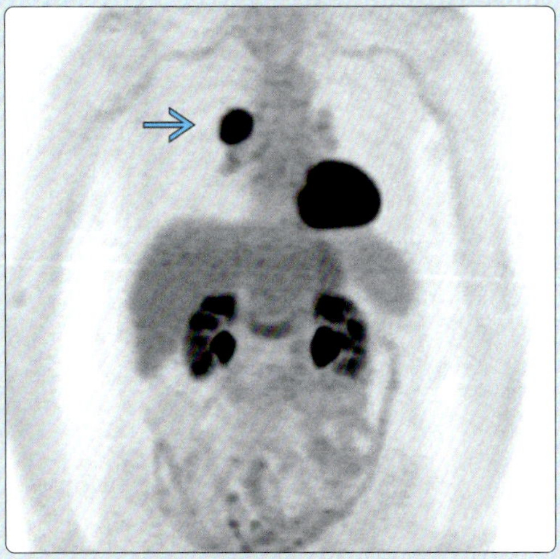
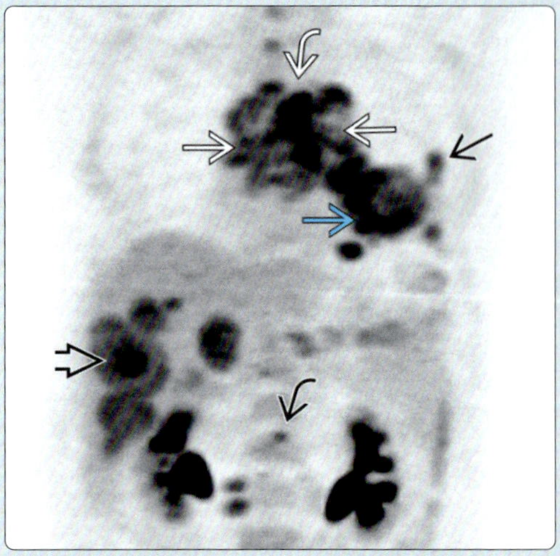

(Left) *MIP F-18 FDG PET shows right upper lobe hypermetabolic mass ➡ without evidence of hilar, mediastinal, or distant metastases. The patient was treated surgically.* **(Right)** *MIP F-18 FDG PET shows a patient presenting with advanced lung cancer. Note the large left lower lobe mass ➡, bilateral hilar ➡ and mediastinal ➡ adenopathy, and pleural ➡, bone ➡, and liver ➡ metastases.*

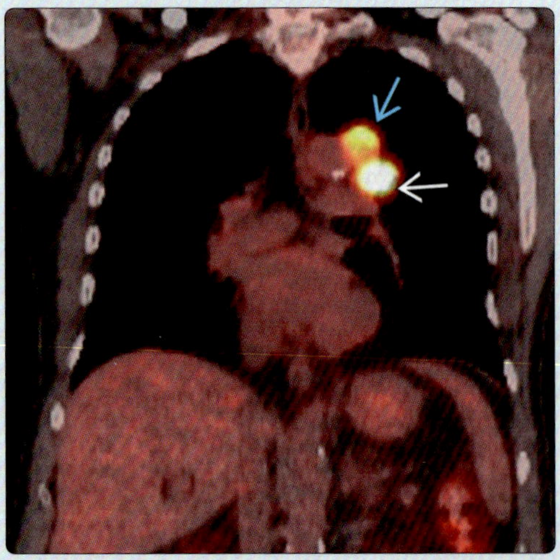
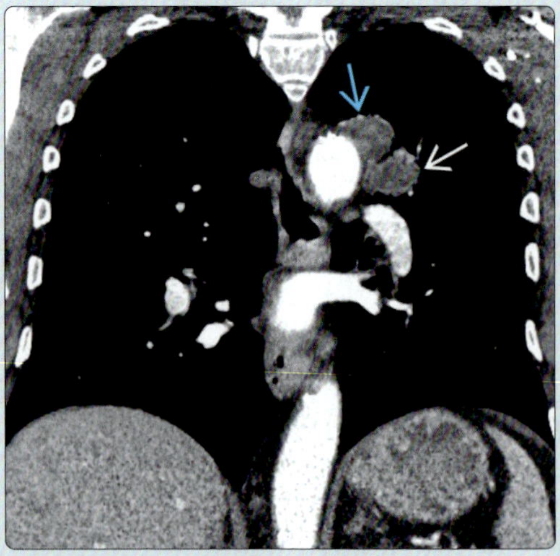

(Left) *Coronal fused F-18 FDG PET/CT in a patient presenting with T2 N1 M0 lung cancer shows left suprahilar ➡ tumor with left hilar ➡ adenopathy.* **(Right)** *Coronal CECT in the same patient shows a suprahilar mass ➡ abutting the mediastinum with adjacent hilar ➡ adenopathy.*

TERMINOLOGY

Definitions

- Non-small cell lung cancer (NSCLC)
  - Group of lung cancers arising from secretory cells
  - Accounts for 85% of all lung cancers
  - Squamous cell carcinoma, large cell carcinoma, adenocarcinoma, and adenocarcinoma in situ

IMAGING

General Features

- Best diagnostic clue
  - Irregular mass in bronchus or lung parenchyma
    - Squamous cell carcinomas tend to be more central in location
    - Adenocarcinomas tend to occur more peripherally
    - Large cell carcinomas tend to be peripheral

Nuclear Medicine Findings

- Bone scan
  - No longer routinely used in initial staging when F-18 FDG PET/CT available
  - May find extremity lesions missed on other studies
- PET
  - F-18 FDG PET/CT avoids nontherapeutic thoracotomy in 20% by detecting previously occult distant disease
  - Negative FDG PET: Does not exclude microscopic disease; does not preclude mediastinal/hilar surgical staging
  - FDG PET/CT increasingly used in simulations for radiation treatment planning
  - Early glucose metabolic response predicts long-term patient survival
  - Prognostic data from FDG PET: ↑ SUV associated with aggressive neoplasm, poorer prognosis
  - Useful for monitoring response to cytotoxic and biologic therapy
- False (-) PET: Tumor with low metabolic rate (low-grade adenoCA, adenocarcinoma in situ, carcinoid), tumor < 10 mm, "stunned" tumor post therapy, high serum glucose (competition)
- False (+) PET: Nonmalignant metabolically active conditions (active inflammation, infectious, granulomatous disease)

Imaging Recommendations

- Protocol advice
  - F-18 PET
    - Skull base to proximal thigh
    - Optimal positioning is with arms overhead

DIFFERENTIAL DIAGNOSIS

Granulomatous Disease

- Symmetrical mildly FDG-avid hilar & mediastinal nodes

Mediastinal Mass

- Consider small cell lung cancer, lymphoma

Hamartoma

- Typically low FDG activity, popcorn calcification

Carcinoid

- Centrally located
- May not be highly FDG avid

Pneumonia

- FDG uptake can be high, but more rapid temporal change

Pulmonary Infarct

- FDG uptake as great as with lung cancer

Small Cell Carcinoma

- Requires biopsy to differentiate

PATHOLOGY

General Features

- Etiology
  - Tobacco: Responsible for 85% of cancer cases
  - Asbestos
  - Environmental toxins
    - Radon, beryllium, nickel, copper, inorganic arsenic, cadmium and atmospheric pollution
    - Exposure to ionizing radiation

Microscopic Features

- Squamous cell
  - High mitotic rate, irregular nucleoli, intracellular bridging
  - Keratin stain
- Adenocarcinoma
  - Gland formation (acinar, papillary, bronchoalveolar, mucus-secreting)
  - Lepidic growth
- Large cell
  - Round or polygonal cells, prominent nucleoli, pale cytoplasm

CLINICAL ISSUES

Presentation

- Most common signs/symptoms
  - Early often asymptomatic
  - Advanced may present with hemoptysis, dyspnea, postobstructive pneumonitis, cough, recurrent infections
  - Systemic disease: Malaise, weight loss, fever, fatigue
  - Metastases can result in bone pain, spinal cord compression, or neurologic symptoms including headache, seizures and weakness, and numbness of limbs
- Other signs/symptoms
  - Pancoast tumor
    - Located in lung apex
    - Horner syndrome: Compression of sympathetic ganglion
      - Ipsilateral ptosis; miosis (pupil constriction), enophthalmos, anhidrosis (loss of sweating)
    - Severe pain from brachial plexus involvement
  - Involvement of recurrent laryngeal nerve: Hoarseness
  - Superior vena cave syndrome
    - Obstruction of blood flow to heart from head/neck region and upper extremities from mediastinal mass

- Facial edema, neck vein distension, dusky skin coloration, upper extremity edema

Demographics

- Age
  - Most frequently 50-70; continues to peak after 70
- Gender
  - More common in men
    - In Western countries, rates are increasing in women and in younger ages
- Ethnicity
  - Higher incidence in African American men compared to white men
  - Similar incidence in African American women compared to white women
  - Incidence is expected to rise in China and India over next decades following increased smoking rates
- Epidemiology
  - Most commonly diagnosed cancer worldwide
    - 1.5 million new cases diagnosed worldwide in 2007
    - 1.35 million deaths related to lung cancer
  - In USA, 215,000 new cases/year
    - Approximately 161,000 deaths due to lung cancer

Natural History & Prognosis

- Progression to advanced cancer and metastasis
  - Spread by local extension and lymphatic or hematogenous extension
- Prognosis related to stage at presentation
  - Most present late due to lack of symptoms early on
  - At initial diagnosis, 20% have localized disease, 25% have regional metastasis, and 55% of patients have distant metastases
- 5-year survival rates
  - Stage 1A: 75%
  - Stage 1B: 55%
  - Stage IIA: 50%
  - Stage IIB: 40%
  - Stage IIIA: 10-35%
  - Stage IIIB: < 5%
  - Stage IV: < 5%
- In USA, 5-year overall survival rate is 15.7%
  - Slightly improved from 1975 (12.5%)
- Worldwide overall 5-year survival rate is 8%

Treatment

- Stage I & II: Surgery, then adjuvant chemotherapy in selected patients
- Stage IIIA: Neoadjuvant chemoradiation, then surgery in selected patients; stage IIIB: Chemoradiation, then surgery in selected T4N0
- Stage IV: Chemotherapy, palliative radiation in selected; solitary brain mets: Resection of brain met and primary if possible
- Radiation or RFA: Symptomatic nonoperable lesions

Surgery

- Preoperative assessment of resectability includes high-resolution CT, PET/CT as well as assessment of cardiopulmonary reserve and perioperative risk
- Video-assisted thoracoscopic surgery (VATS)
  - Minimally invasive, more easily tolerated in elderly patients or those with comorbid conditions
  - No significant difference in recurrence rates in comparison to open thoracotomy
  - Low perioperative mortality
- Wedge resection/segmentectomy
  - Sublobar resection
- Lobectomy: Helps preserve pulmonary function
- Pneumonectomy: May be necessary for hilar and more proximal tumors
  - Higher perioperative morbidity/mortality (6%)

Combined Chemoradiation

- Combination of platinum-based chemotherapy and radiation
- Used in unresectable stage III cancer

Systemic Therapy

- Chemotherapy
  - NSCCL is only moderately sensitive to chemotherapy
  - Not used as front line therapy
    - May be given as neoadjuvant or adjuvant therapy
  - Cisplatin + another chemotherapeutic agent common
- Biologics
  - Uses molecular targets based on mutation identification
  - Current agents include gefitinib, erlotinib, cetuximab

Radiation Therapy

- May be used as local therapy in stage I and II in patients who are not surgical candidates
- Use complex radiotherapy in stage III patients who are not candidates for chemotherapy
- Stereotactic body radiotherapy targets high doses of radiation to tumor, limiting dose and toxicity to surrounding organs
- Role of postoperative radiation controversial, may be used in patients with positive margins
- Radiofrequency ablation option in patients with peripheral tumors < 3 cm in size

DIAGNOSTIC CHECKLIST

Image Interpretation Pearls

- F-18 FDG PET/CT
  - Respiratory motion makes localization more difficult, particularly in lung bases
  - Smaller the nodule, SUV spuriously low
  - Necrosis may show lack of activity centrally
  - Image with arms up when possible
  - Adenocarcinoma in situ may not show ↑ FDG uptake
  - Carcinoid may have low FDG uptake
  - High glucose levels or high insulin levels may cause decreased FDG uptake

SELECTED REFERENCES

1. Detterbeck FC et al: Screening for lung cancer: Diagnosis and management of lung cancer, 3rd ed: American College of Chest Physicians evidence-based clinical practice guidelines. Chest. 143(5 Suppl):e78S-92S, 2013

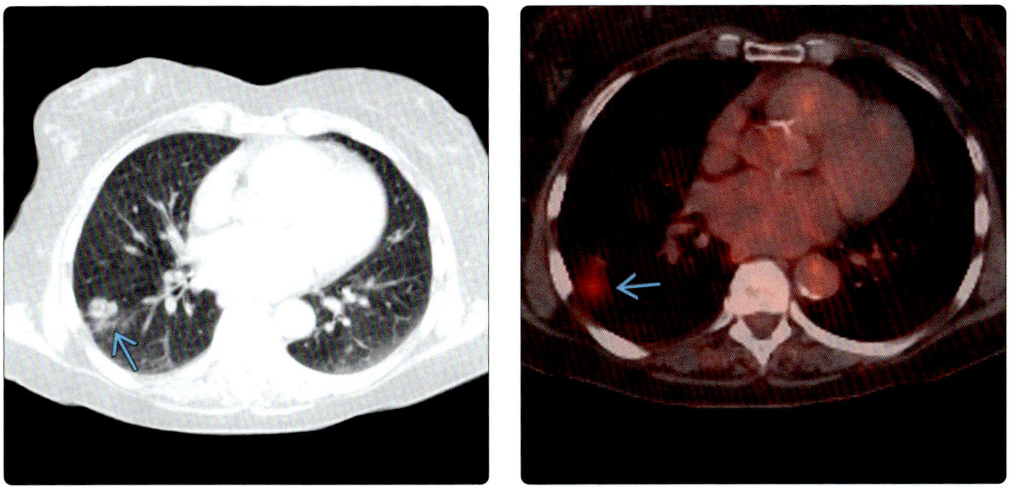

(Left) *Axial CT shows a solid lung mass with surrounding ground-glass opacity →.* **(Right)** *Axial fused F-18 FDG PET/CT shows relatively low uptake → in the solid portion of tumor. Regions of ground-glass opacity on CT show no uptake. Areas of adenocarcinoma in situ may not exhibit increased F-18 FDG activity.*

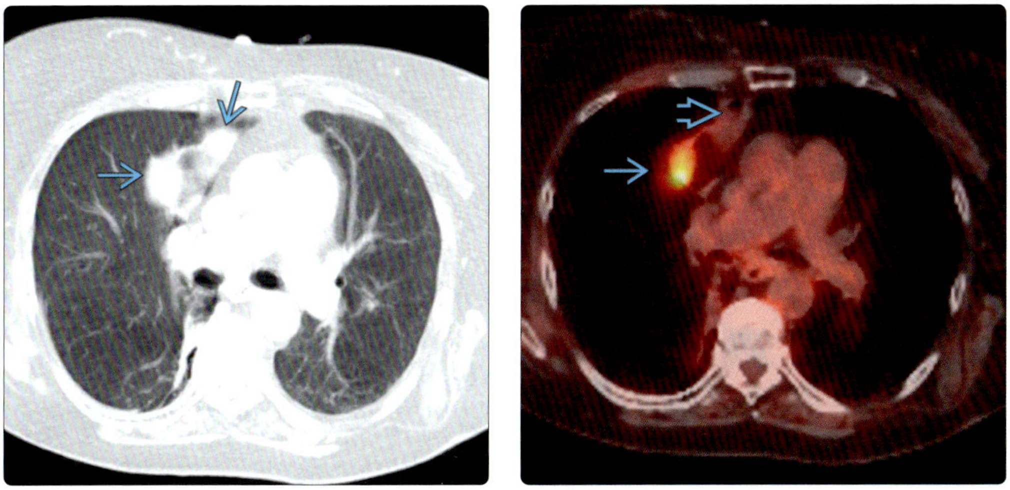

(Left) *Axial CT demonstrates two masses → in a patient with previously treated lung tumor.* **(Right)** *Axial fused F-18 FDG PET/CT demonstrates uptake in recurrent disease → but no uptake at the site of treated tumor ⇒.*

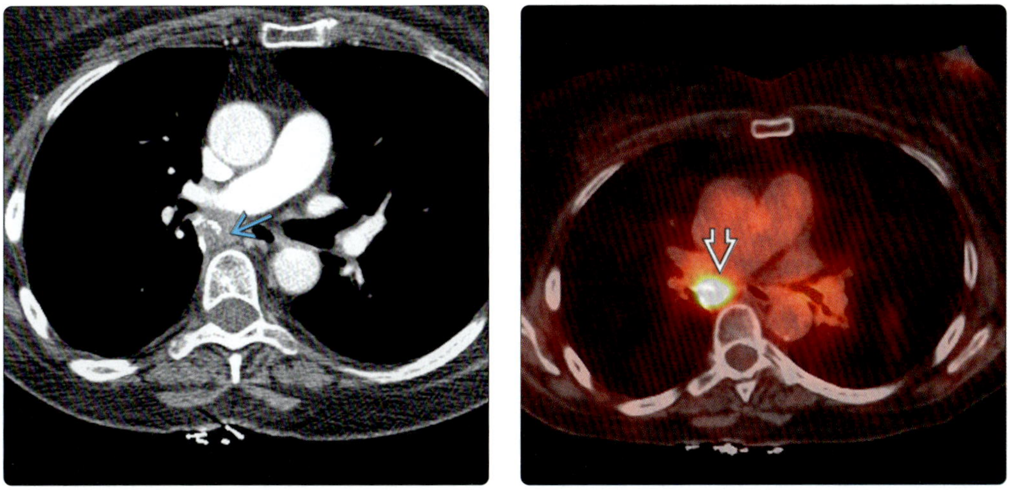

(Left) *Axial CT in a patient post surgery for lung cancer shows soft tissue adjacent to surgical sutures ⇒.* **(Right)** *Axial fused F-18 FDG PET/CT in the same patient shows marked uptake ➡ at the site of soft tissue, indicating postsurgical tumor recurrence.*

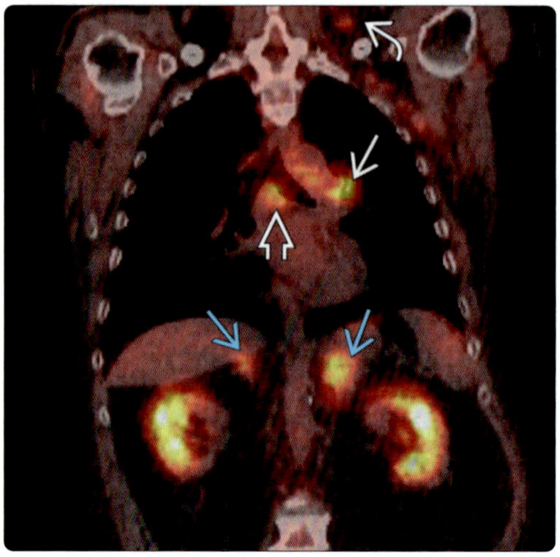

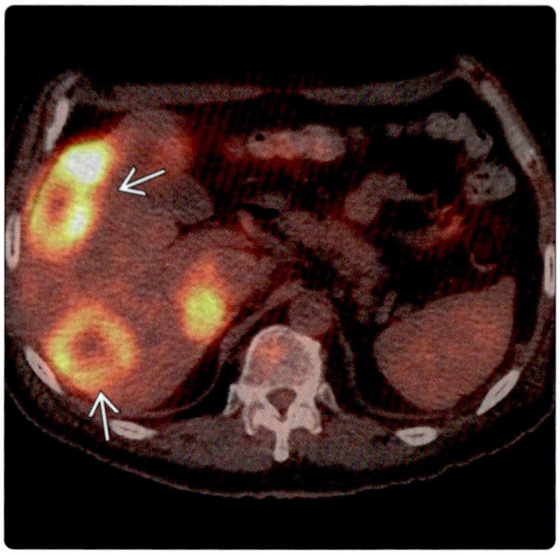

(Left) *Coronal fused F-18 FDG PET/CT shows N3 M1 disease, including supraclavicular lymphadenopathy ➡ and bilateral adrenal metastases ➡. Hilar ➡ and subcarinal ➡ lymphadenopathy is also present.* **(Right)** *Axial fused F-18 FDG PET/CT shows necrotic liver metastases ➡ from squamous cell lung primary.*

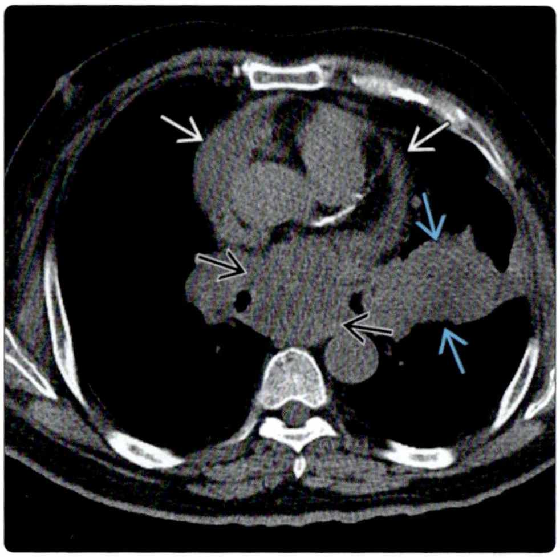

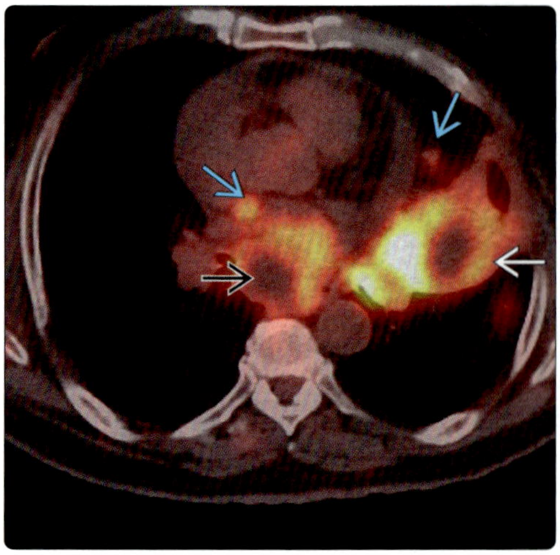

(Left) *Axial CT in a patient with lung cancer shows bulky subcarinal nodes ➡ and left hilar tumor ➡. A pericardial effusion ➡ is also present.* **(Right)** *Axial fused F-18 FDG PET/CT in the same patient shows lack of uptake in portions of adenopathy ➡ and primary tumor ➡, corresponding to necrosis. Histology revealed squamous cell tumor, which is often associated with necrosis. Note uptake in metastatic pericardial nodes ➡. Lack of uptake in the pericardial effusion does not exclude tumor.*

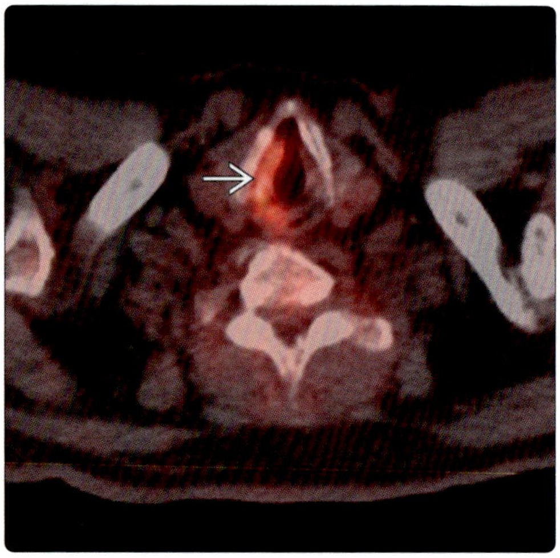

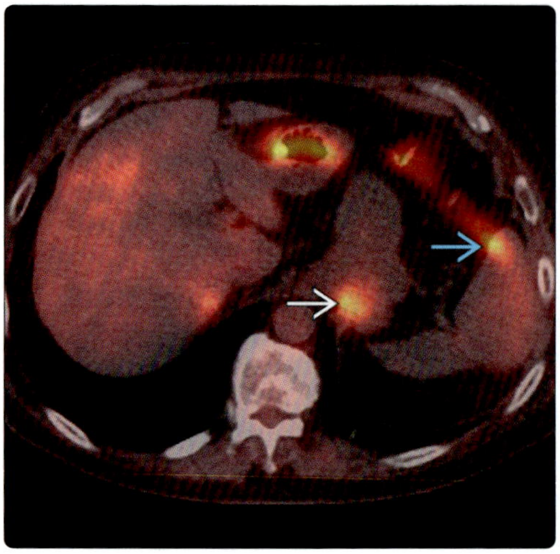

(Left) *Axial fused F-18 FDG PET/CT in the same patient shows unilateral uptake in the right vocal cord ➡. Lack of uptake in the left vocal cord is due to paralysis from left hilar tumor.* **(Right)** *Axial fused F-18 FDG PET/CT shows a common pitfall in fused imaging. Bowel uptake ➡ appears to be in spleen and adrenal uptake ➡ appears to be in stomach. This is caused by mismatch from the CT images and PET images and may be identified by viewing in all planes.*

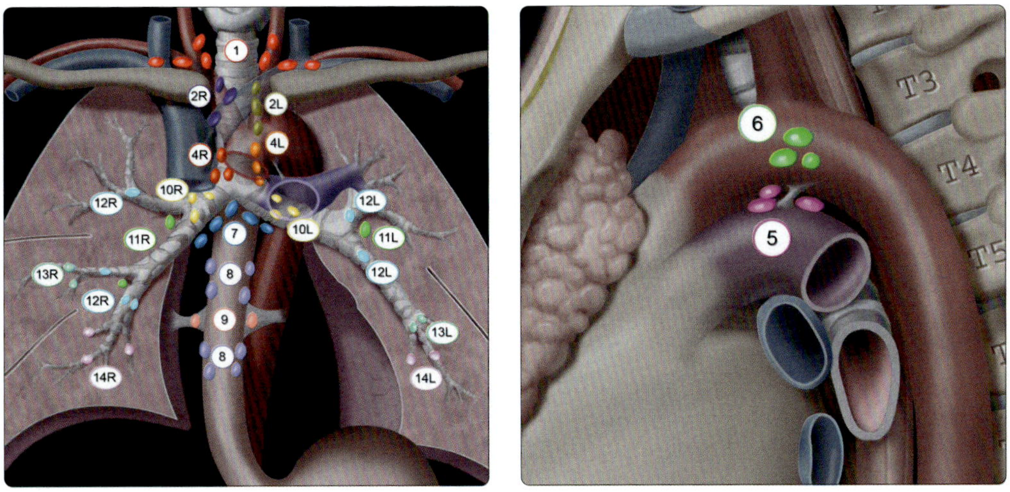

(Left) *Coronal graphic depicts the International Association for the Study of Lung Cancer lymph node stations.* **(Right)** *Sagittal graphic depicts AP window (lymph nodes: 5) subaortic and 6) paraaortic (ascending aorta or phrenic).*

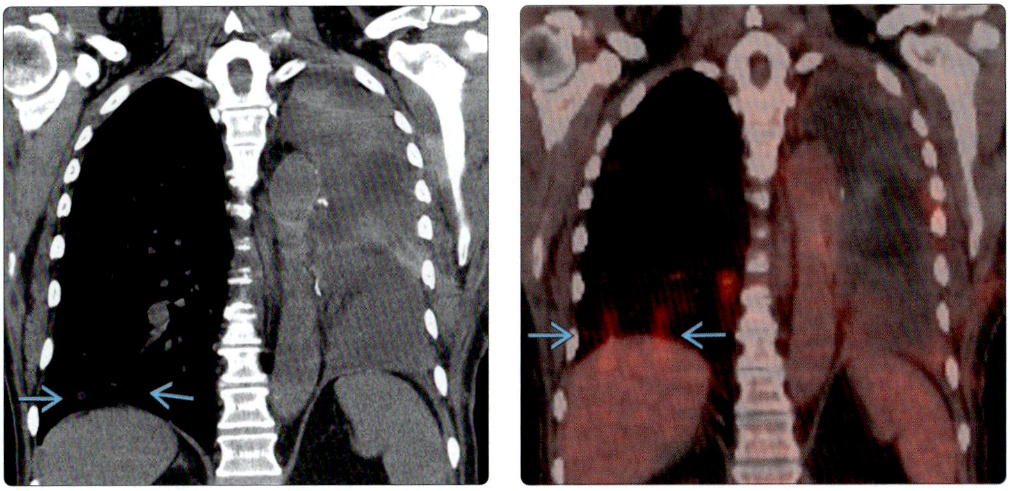

(Left) *Coronal CT shows pulmonary nodules* ➔ *in the right lung base in a patient post pneumonectomy.* **(Right)** *Coronal fused F-18 FDG PET/CT in the same patient shows the effects on respiratory motion on evaluation of pulmonary nodules. Note linear uptake corresponding to pulmonary nodules* ➔*. The SUV is underestimated in these nodules.*

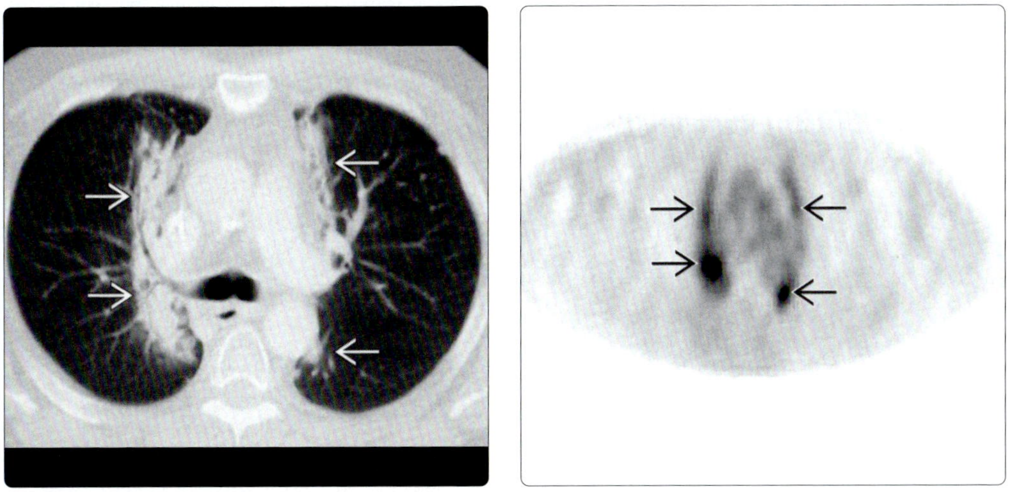

(Left) *Axial CT following mediastinal radiation shows fibrotic changes within radiation field* ➔. **(Right)** *Axial F-18 FDG PET in the same patient shows hypermetabolism in region of post-radiation fibrosis* ➔*, a finding that can persist, but most often decreases over time.*

KEY FACTS

IMAGING

- Anatomic imaging
  - Hilar mass with bulky mediastinal adenopathy
  - Often infiltrates submucosa, obstructs bronchus
  - May have small primary tumor
- PET/CT for most complete staging
- MR required for brain metastases

TOP DIFFERENTIAL DIAGNOSES

- Non-small cell lung carcinoma
- Lymphoma
- Metastatic cancer
- Granulomatous disease
- Infection

CLINICAL ISSUES

- Primary tumor: Rapid doubling time
- Early development of metastases
  - Liver, adrenal, bone, brain
- Treatment
  - Limited
    - Chemotherapy plus radiation
    - May have complete response (but relapse with median duration of 6-8 months)
  - Extensive
    - Combination chemotherapy
    - May include prophylactic brain irradiation

DIAGNOSTIC CHECKLIST

- Limited stage
  - Confined to ipsilateral thorax and regional nodes
  - Contained in single radiation portal
- Extensive stage
  - Malignant pleural effusion
  - Malignant pericardial effusion
  - Contralateral lymphadenopathy
  - Distant metastases
  - Not contained in single radiation portal

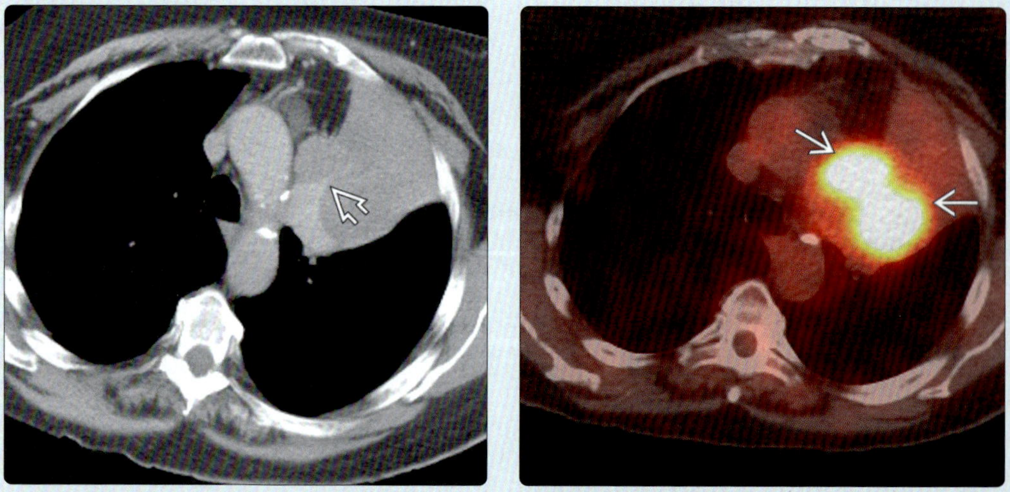

(Left) *Axial CT shows small cell lung cancer (SCLC) ➔ encasing and narrowing the pulmonary artery. It is difficult to differentiate tumor from postobstructive collapse.* **(Right)** *Axial fused PET/CT shows obstructing hilar mass with peripheral lung collapse ➔. The hypermetabolic activity delineates tumor from the area of collapse.*

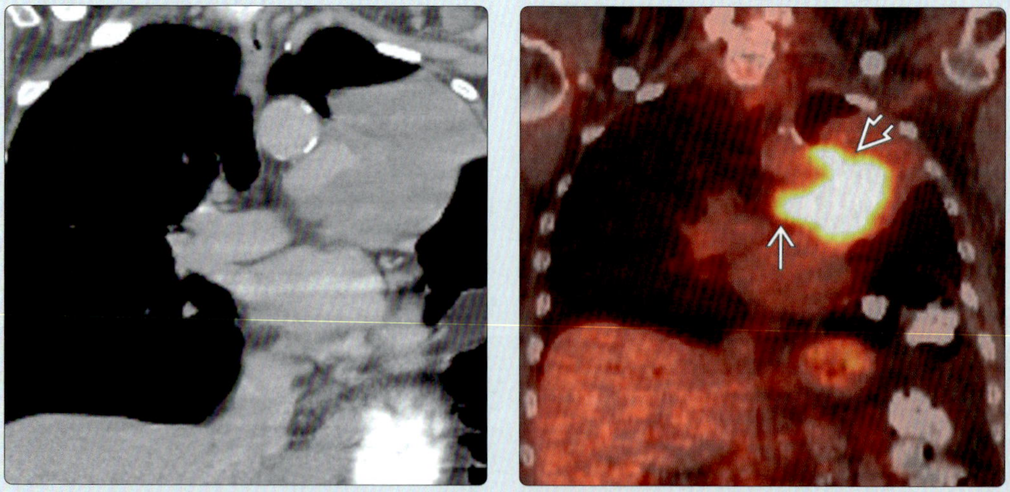

(Left) *Coronal PET/CT demonstrates a large mass, but cannot differentiate the tumor from distant collapse.* **(Right)** *Coronal fused PET/CT demonstrates a bulky mass extending into the mediastinum ➔ and radiating out from the hilum ➔. Postobstructive collapse extends to hila.*

TERMINOLOGY

Definitions

- Small cell lung cancer (SCLC), a.k.a. oat cell carcinoma
  - Originates from epithelial cells
  - Neuroendocrine tumor
  - 15% of all lung cancers

IMAGING

General Features

- Best diagnostic clue
  - Hilar mass with bulky mediastinal adenopathy
    - Often infiltrates submucosa, obstructs bronchus
    - May have small primary tumor

Imaging Recommendations

- Best imaging tool
  - PET/CT for most complete staging, but does not differentiate cell types
  - MR required for brain metastases

DIFFERENTIAL DIAGNOSIS

PET-Positive Lesions

- Infections
- Granulomatous disease
- Small cell and non-small cell lung carcinoma
- Metastatic cancer

PET-Negative Lesions

- Small tumor size, < 1 cm
- Neuroendocrine tumors, carcinoid, adenocarcinoma in situ
- Imaging in postprandial state can compete with tumors for F-18 FDG uptake

PATHOLOGY

Staging, Grading, & Classification

- Limited
  - Confined to ipsilateral thorax and regional nodes
  - Contained in single radiation portal
- Extensive
  - Malignant pleural/pericardial effusion, contralateral nodes, distant metastases
  - Not contained in single radiation portal

Microscopic Features

- Small cells: Sparse cytoplasm, fine chromatin, nuclear molding, blue on H&E
- Immunoreactive for keratin, epithelial membrane antigen
- Tumors may contain several cell types, including NSCLC and SCLC

CLINICAL ISSUES

Presentation

- Most common signs/symptoms
  - Local tumor burden: Cough, dyspnea, chest pain, hemoptysis, SVC compression
  - Metastases: Fatigue, weight loss, headache, neurologic symptoms, paraneoplastic syndromes
- Other signs/symptoms
  - Most common malignancy associated with paraneoplastic endocrine syndromes
    - Antidiuretic hormone: Hyponatremia
    - Adrenocorticotrophic hormone: Cushing disease
    - Nervous system hormones: Neuromuscular disorders

Demographics

- Epidemiology
  - Proportion of lung cancers classified as SCLC decreasing
    - 1986: 17%
    - 2002: 13%
  - Very high association with smoking
  - Associated with p53 mutations, loss of retinoblastoma gene and haploinsufficiency, other mutations
  - Increasing incidence in women

Natural History & Prognosis

- Rapid doubling time
- Early development of metastases
  - 70% of patients present with metastasis
  - Liver, adrenal, bone, brain
- Survival rates
  - Limited: 15-20 months
  - Extensive: 8-13 months
  - Short survival time without treatment

Treatment

- Limited: Chemotherapy plus radiation
  - May have complete response
  - Relapse with median duration of 6-8 months
  - Chemotherapy: Platinum based
- Extensive: Combination chemotherapy
  - May include prophylactic brain irradiation

DIAGNOSTIC CHECKLIST

Image Interpretation Pearls

- Anatomic appearance key to diagnosis
  - Small peripheral tumor
  - Hilar mass
  - Bulky mediastinal adenopathy

Reporting Tips

- Report limited vs. extensive disease
  - Limited: Confined to ipsilateral thorax and regional nodes
    - Contained in single radiation portal
  - Extensive: Malignant pleural/pericardial effusion, contralateral nodes, distant metastases

SELECTED REFERENCES

1. Pillai RN et al: Small cell lung cancer: therapies and targets. Semin Oncol. 41(1):133-42, 2014
2. Chheang S et al: Lung Cancer Staging: Clinical and Radiologic Perspectives. Semin Intervent Radiol. 30(2):99-113, 2013
3. Sharma P et al: Positron emission tomography-computed tomography in the management of lung cancer: An update. South Asian J Cancer. 2(3):171-178, 2013
4. Gaspar LE et al: Limited-stage small-cell lung cancer (stages I-III): observations from the National Cancer Data Base. Clin Lung Cancer. 6(6):355-60, 2005

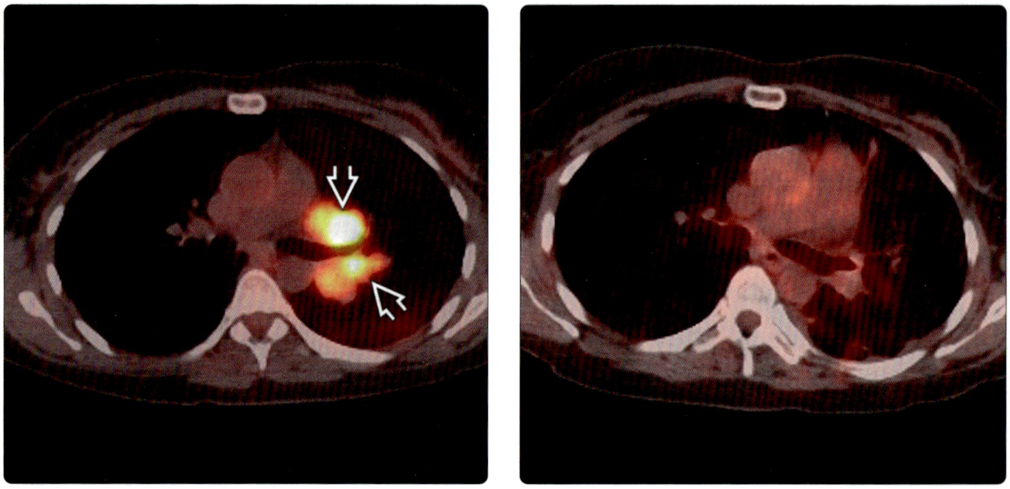

(Left) *Axial fused PET/CT at initial presentation demonstrates bulky left hilar nodes ➡ encircling bronchus.* **(Right)** *Axial fused PET/CT obtained post therapy demonstrates complete metabolic response to radiation/chemotherapy with no uptake above blood pool.*

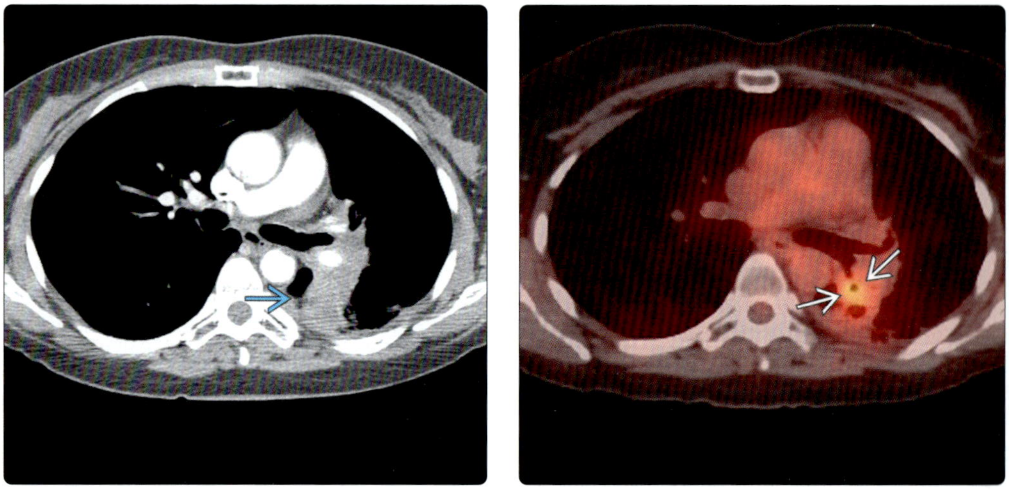

(Left) *Axial CECT in the same patient several months later shows increasing collapse in the irradiated field → but does not clearly delineate recurrent tumor.* **(Right)** *Axial fused PET/CT demonstrates new uptake ➡ above background in previously irradiated field, corresponding to site of relapse.*

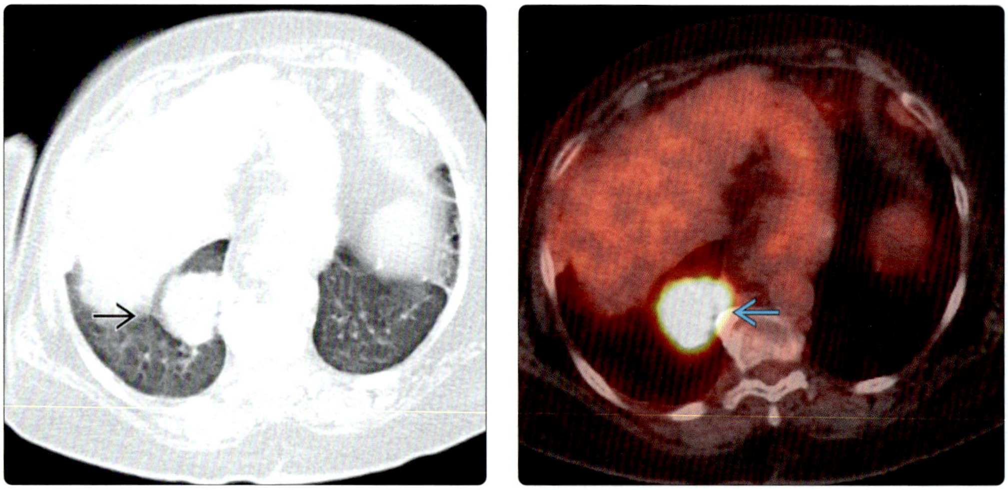

(Left) *Axial CT shows a large mass in the right lower lung →. There is no evidence of contact with bone.* **(Right)** *Axial fused PET/CT in the same patient shows activity overlapping bone →. Because of the lesser spatial resolution of PET, involvement of structures adjacent to tumor must be confirmed on anatomic images.*

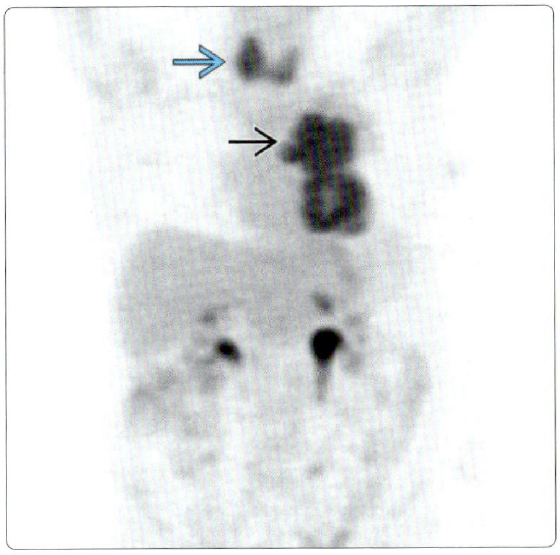

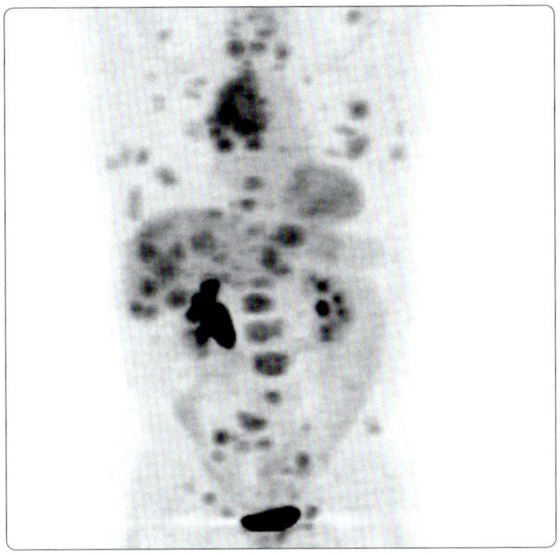

(Left) *MIP PET shows limited extent of disease, with activity limited to 1 hemithorax. Diffuse thyroid activity is due to thyroiditis, not metastases.* **(Right)** *MIP F-18 FDG PET demonstrates extensive stage of disease, involving liver and bone as well as mediastinal nodes.*

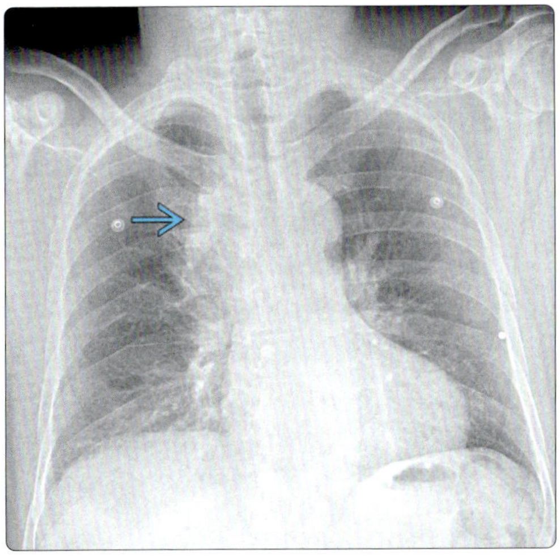

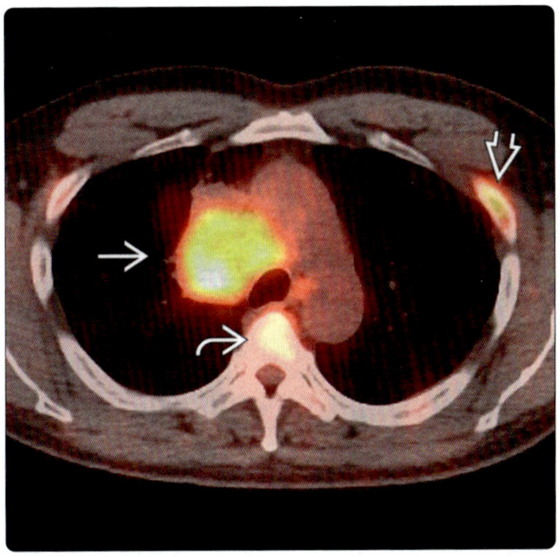

(Left) *PA radiograph demonstrates widened mediastinum in a patient with initial diagnosis of SCLC. Patients often present with advanced disease that produces symptoms from contact with mediastinal structures.* **(Right)** *Axial fused PET/CT shows a bulky mediastinal mass, a rib metastasis, and a vertebral body metastasis, making this extensive-stage disease.*

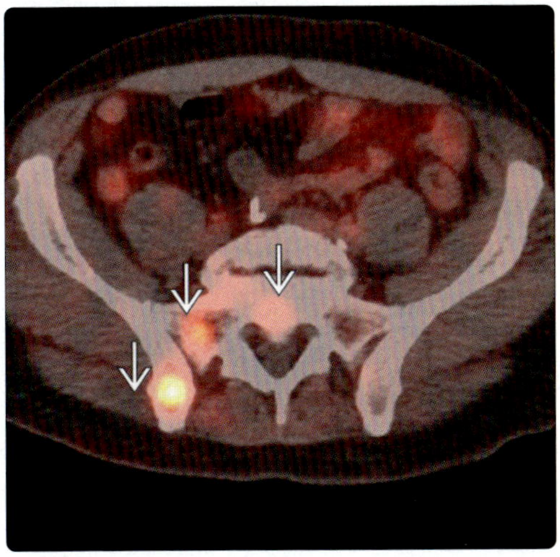

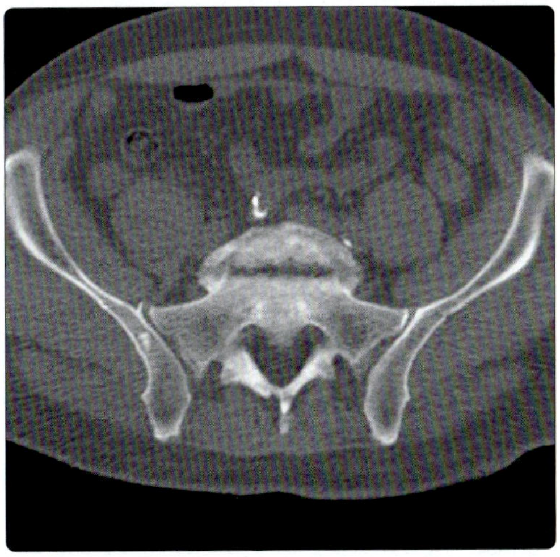

(Left) *Axial fused F-18 FDG PET/CT shows multiple sites of osseous metastatic disease in this patient presenting with advanced stage disease.* **(Right)** *Axial CT in the same patient shows that osseous metastases are not well delineated.*

KEY FACTS

TERMINOLOGY

- Thymic neoplasms: Continuum of low-grade to cancerous thymic diseases
  - Thymoma
    - Low-risk thymoma: Types A, AB, and B1
    - High-risk thymomas: Types B2 and B3
  - Thymic carcinoma
    - Thymoma type C

IMAGING

- F-18 FDG PET/CT
  - Imaging features that suggest aggressive disease
    - Local infiltration, extensive areas of necrosis and calcification, metastases
  - Low-level F-18 FDG uptake in low-risk thymomas
  - Higher level F-18 FDG uptake in high-risk thymomas and thymic carcinoma
  - F-18 FDG PET/CT cannot distinguish high-risk thymomas from thymic carcinoma
  - F-18 FDG PET/CT useful to identify lymph node and distant metastases
  - CECT first line to evaluate after surgical resection
    - F-18 FDG PET/CT may yield additional information about recurrence in difficult cases

PATHOLOGY

- Stage I: No capsular invasion
- Stage II
  - IIA: Microscopic invasion through tumor capsule
  - IIB: Macroscopic invasion through tumor capsule into adjacent fatty tissue
- Stage III: Tumor invasion into pericardium, mediastinal pleura, or lung; potentially resectable
- Stage IV
  - IVA: Wide invasion into pleura or pericardium
  - IVB: Spread to distant organs (lymphatic or hematogenous)

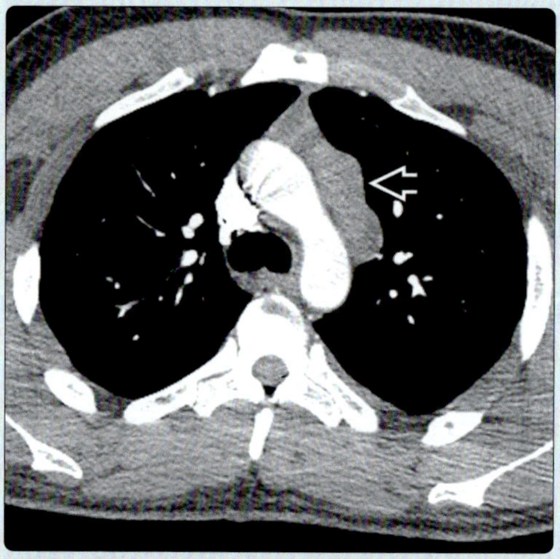

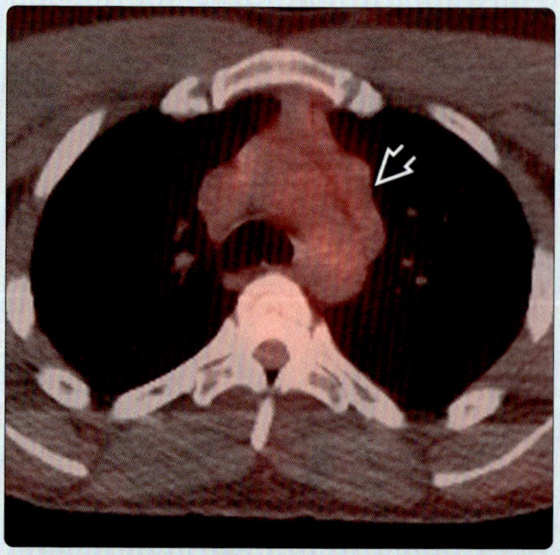

(Left) *Axial CECT demonstrates the undulating border of a well-encapsulated thymoma, outlining anatomic boundaries of the anterior mediastinum. The tumor abuts the adjacent pleura; however, imaging cannot determine invasion.* **(Right)** *Axial PET/CT demonstrates uptake similar to blood pool background in low-risk thymoma.*

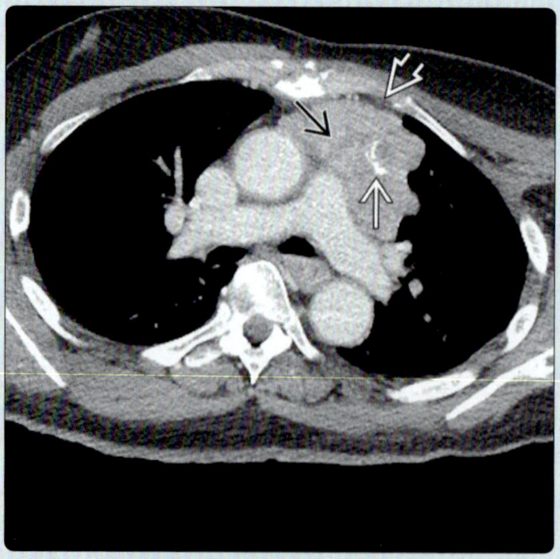

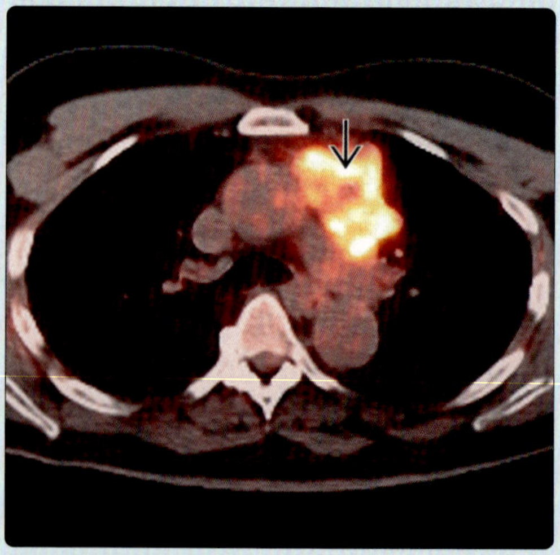

(Left) *Axial CECT demonstrates area of calcification and necrosis in high-risk thymoma. This tumor has more extensive contact with pleura, but fat plane is maintained.* **(Right)** *Axial PET/CT demonstrates heterogeneous uptake of F-18 FDG that far exceeds blood pool activity in patient with high-risk thymoma. Photopenic area corresponds to area of necrosis.*

TERMINOLOGY

Definitions

- Thymic neoplasms: Continuum of low-grade to cancerous thymic diseases
  - Thymoma
    - Low-risk thymoma: Types A, AB, and B1
    - High-risk thymomas: Types B2 and B3
  - Thymic carcinoma
    - Thymoma type C
- In some tumors, there is a continuum of differentiation from thymoma to carcinoma

IMAGING

General Features

- Best diagnostic clue
  - Thymoma
    - Encapsulated neoplasm: Fibrous saccule
      - Cystic components may be present
    - May have invasive components
    - Can be adherent to adjacent structures
  - Thymic carcinoma
    - Large, firm, infiltrating mass
    - Cystic component common
- Location
  - Most common: Anterior mediastinal mass
  - Rare ectopic location from submandibular region to cardiophrenic angle
    - Neck
    - Thyroid gland
    - Other regions of mediastinum
    - Pulmonary hilum
    - Lung
    - Pleura
- Morphology
  - Normal thymus in anterior mediastinum
    - In young children (< 5 years of age): Quadrilateral shape with convex borders
      - Subsequently becomes triangular with straight or concave borders
    - Thymus involutes at puberty
      - Fatty involution
      - Residual thymus may appear as islands of soft tissue density within areas of fat
  - Thymic hyperplasia
    - Thymic tissue after puberty, e.g., post chemotherapy
    - Can be associated with Graves disease
  - Thymoma and thymic carcinoma
    - Stages I-II
      - Sharp/smooth mass with preservation of mediastinal fat planes
      - Homogeneous soft tissue attenuation
      - Mild to moderate enhancement
    - Stages III-IV
      - Larger size
      - Surrounding fat obscured
      - Lobular or irregular margins
      - Calcifications
      - Low-density areas: Hemorrhage, necrosis, cystic change
      - Heterogeneous enhancement
      - Pleural seeding can be unilateral or bilateral
      - Pericardial seeding
      - Can cross diaphragm into abdomen and retroperitoneal space

Nuclear Medicine Findings

- PET/CT
  - Low-level uptake in thymus is normal in children and adults < 40 years
  - Thymoma
    - Low risk: Background-level F-18 FDG activity
    - High risk: Increased F-18 FDG activity
  - Thymic carcinoma
    - Variable F-18 FDG activity, but generally higher than thymoma
    - Larger mass
    - Irregular or lobular borders
    - Areas of necrosis and calcification
    - No well-defined capsule
    - Surrounding vessel invasion
    - Mediastinal adenopathy
    - Pleural/pericardial effusion
    - Extrathoracic metastases

DIFFERENTIAL DIAGNOSIS

Substernal Thyroid

- May contain cysts or calcifications

Germ Cell Tumors

- Teratoma
- Seminoma
- Yolk sac tumor
- Embryonal cell tumor
- Choriocarcinoma
- Mixed cell type

Lymphoma

- Hodgkin lymphoma
- Non-Hodgkin lymphoma

Thymic Cyst

- Low density
- No FDG uptake

Thoracic Aortic Aneurysm

- F-18 FDG uptake equal to blood pool

Thymic Hyperplasia

- F-18 FDG uptake may be background to increased
- Clinical correlation essential (e.g., recent chemotherapy, Graves disease)

PATHOLOGY

Staging, Grading, & Classification

- Stage I
  - No capsular invasion
- Stage II
  - IIA: Microscopic invasion through tumor capsule

- IIB: Macroscopic invasion through tumor capsule into adjacent fatty tissue
- Stage III
  - Tumor invasion into pericardium, mediastinal pleura, or lung
  - Potentially resectable
- Stage IV
  - IVA: Wide invasion into pleura or pericardium
  - IVB: Spread to distant organs
    - Lymphatic or hematogenous

Gross Pathologic & Surgical Features

- Thymoma
  - Fibrous capsule
  - Circumscribed, firm, tan mass
  - Higher grades may be invasive
- Thymic carcinoma
  - Large, firm, infiltrating mass
  - Low-grade and high-grade subsets
  - Areas of cystic change and necrosis common
- Diagnosis difficult on frozen section
- All cystic areas should be examined closely for tumor foci

CLINICAL ISSUES

Presentation

- Most common signs/symptoms
  - Strong association with myasthenia gravis
    - 30-40% of cases of thymomas, rare with thymic carcinoma
      - Thymectomy will decrease symptoms
    - Autoimmune disorder of neuromuscular junction
      - Muscle weakness
  - Lesser association with other paraneoplastic syndromes
  - If invasive, symptoms due to compression of adjacent organs
    - Chest pain
    - Dyspnea
    - Phrenic nerve palsy
- Other signs/symptoms
  - Immunodeficiency
    - Hypogammaglobulinemia
  - Multiorgan autoimmune disease
- May be asymptomatic
  - Discovered incidentally on thoracic imaging
- Patients at risk for 2nd primary tumors
  - 17-28% following thymectomy

Natural History & Prognosis

- Prognosis depends on stage of disease, resectability, and histologic type
- Thymic carcinoma metastases
  - Kidney
  - Lymph nodes
  - Liver
  - Brain
  - Adrenals
  - Thyroid
  - Bone
- 5-year survival
  - Stage I: 94-100%
  - Stage II: 86-95%
  - Stage III: 56-69%
  - Stage IV: 11-50%
- Invasion is most important prognostic factor
  - Best determined surgically
  - May be adherent without being invasive

Treatment

- Stage I: Surgical resection
  - Follow with CT/MR yearly
- Stage II
  - Negative margins: Consider postoperative XRT
  - Residual disease: Adjuvant XRT
- Stages III and IVA: Potentially resectable
  - Multimodality therapy may include neoadjuvant chemotherapy and adjuvant radiation
- Stage IV
  - Chemotherapy
    - If positive response, may undergo surgical resection
  - Radiation therapy

DIAGNOSTIC CHECKLIST

Consider

- Differential diagnosis for anterior mediastinal mass
  - Thymoma, thymic carcinoma, thymic hyperplasia, lymphoma, substernal thyroid, germ cell tumor

Image Interpretation Pearls

- Higher uptake of F-18 FDG with thymic carcinomas in comparison to thymomas
- Thymic carcinoma has more heterogeneous uptake
- Thymic rebound may have increased F-18 FDG uptake
- F-18 FDG PET/CT can identify lymph node and distant metastases
- F-18 FDG PET/CT particularly useful to evaluate for recurrence

Reporting Tips

- Degree of F-18 FDG uptake important, as this may signify low- vs. high-risk features
- Mention homogeneous vs. heterogeneous F-18 FDG uptake

SELECTED REFERENCES

1. Priola AM et al: Imaging of thymus in myasthenia gravis: from thymic hyperplasia to thymic tumor. Clin Radiol. 69(5):e230-45, 2014
2. Seki N et al: ^{18}F-fluorodeoxyglucose positron emission tomography for evaluation of thymic epithelial tumors: utility for World Health Organization classification and predicting recurrence-free survival. Ann Nucl Med. 28(3):257-62, 2014
3. Viti A et al: Is a positron emission tomography-computed tomography scan useful in the staging of thymic epithelial neoplasms? Interact Cardiovasc Thorac Surg. Epub ahead of print, 2014

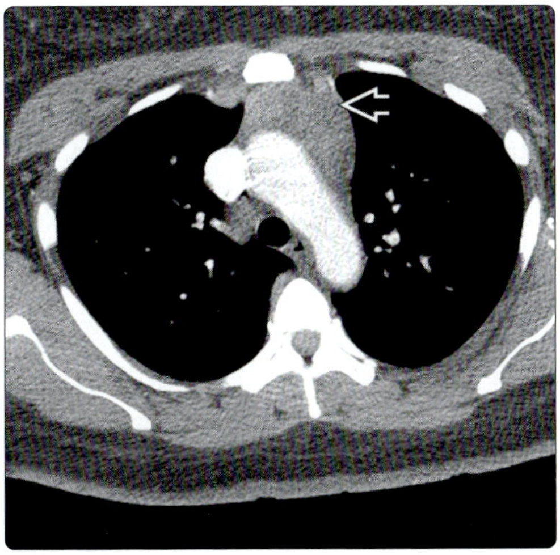
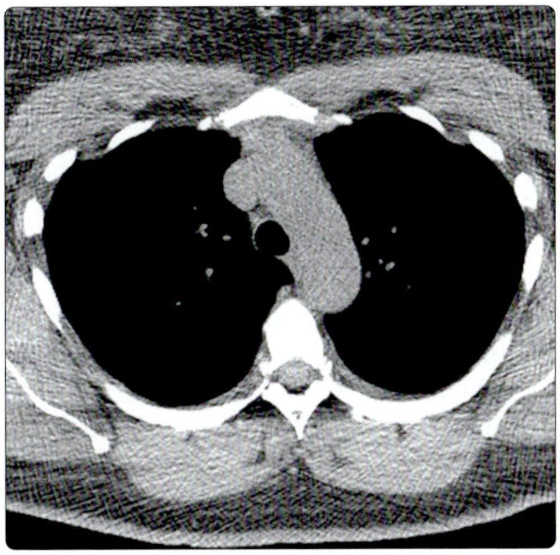

(Left) *Axial CECT demonstrates a well-defined anterior mediastinal mass ➔ in a patient presenting with Graves disease. Thymic hyperplasia can be seen in association with Graves disease.* **(Right)** *Axial NECT in the same patient following I-131 treatment of Graves disease shows that thymic rebound has resolved.*

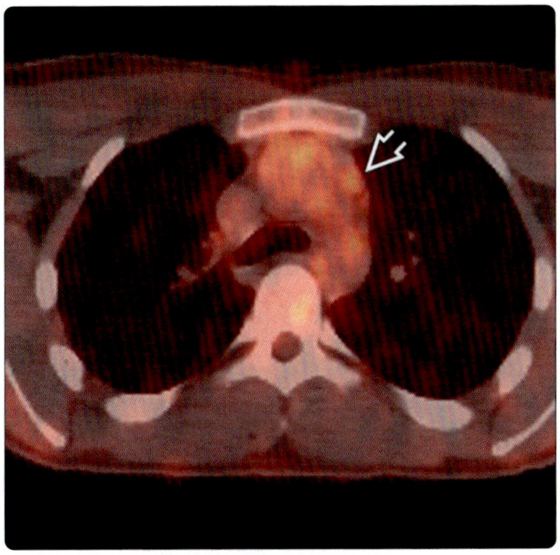
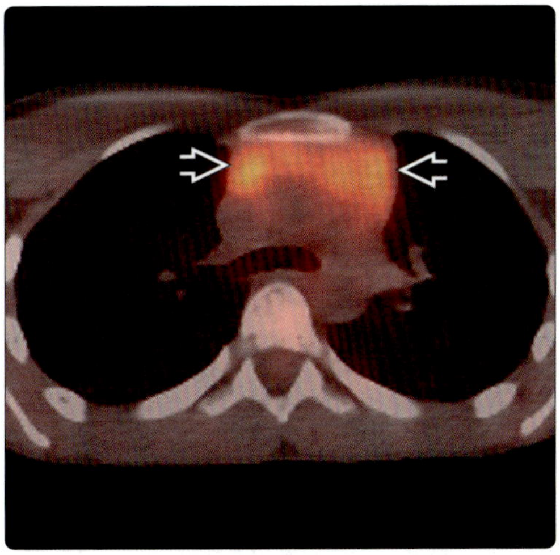

(Left) *Axial PET/CT demonstrates mild thymic rebound with low-level FDG ➔ uptake following chemotherapy.* **(Right)** *Axial PET/CT shows high degree of F-18 FDG uptake in the anterior mediastinum ➔ in a 14-year-old boy following chemotherapy. Findings represent thymic rebound in this case with diffusely increased uptake above blood background.*

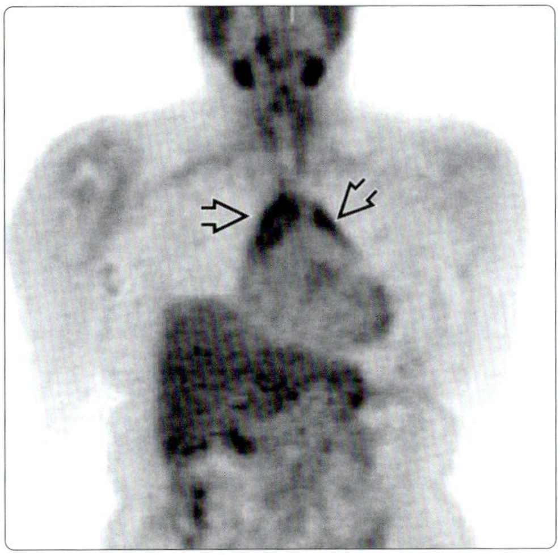
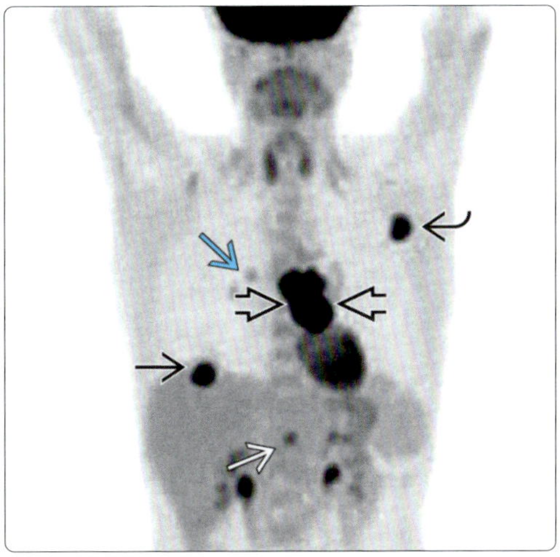

(Left) *Coronal PET in an adult patient shows thymic rebound ➔ following chemotherapy. Thymus has a triangular shape seen in infants, but normally involutes at puberty.* **(Right)** *Coronal PET demonstrates marked F-18 FDG uptake in thymic carcinoma ➔, as well as axillary ➔, lung ➔, hilar ➔, and abdominal ➔ metastases.*

KEY FACTS

TERMINOLOGY

- Solitary pulmonary nodule (SPN)
  - Single, small (< 3 cm) solid or subsolid parenchymal opacity
  - Differential diagnosis include neoplasm, infection, inflammation, vascular, and congenital etiologies

TOP DIFFERENTIAL DIAGNOSES

- **F-18 FDG positive**
  - Malignant
    - Primary lung cancer: Bronchogenic; small cell, large cell, adenocarcinoma, and squamous cell carcinoma
    - Metastatic disease: Most nonmucinous adenocarcinoma, sarcoma, lymphoma, melanoma
  - Benign
    - Infection: TB, fungal, bacterial; inflammation (sarcoid, granulomatosis with polyangiitis, rheumatoid)
    - Other: Bronchiolitis obliterans organizing pneumonia, pulmonary infarction, round atelectasis, lymph node, mucoid impaction
- **Variable to low F-18 FDG uptake**
  - Malignant
    - Primary lung cancer: Adenocarcinoma in situ, carcinoid (typically endobronchial but approximately 20% present as peripheral, well-circumscribed SPNs)
    - Metastatic disease: Highly mucinous adenocarcinoma, testicular, renal cell, prostate, hepatocellular carcinoma
- **Usually F-18 FDG negative**
  - Benign
    - Inactive granulomatous disease, bronchogenic cyst, hamartoma, pleural plaque
    - Other: Lipoma, fibroma, AVM, pulmonary varix, congenital cystic adenomatoid malformation

(Left) *Axial CECT shows a mildly spiculated, solid solitary pulmonary nodule ➡ in the left upper lobe in a smoker, concerning for primary lung cancer.* **(Right)** *Axial CECT shows a ground-glass solitary pulmonary nodule ➡. Note that the normal parenchymal structure can be visualized through a subsolid nodule.*

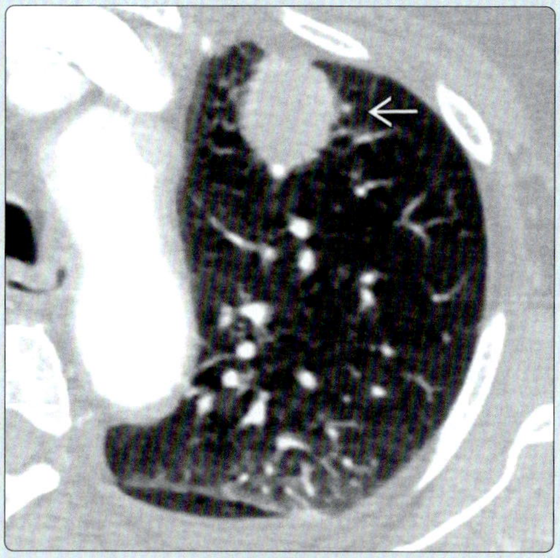

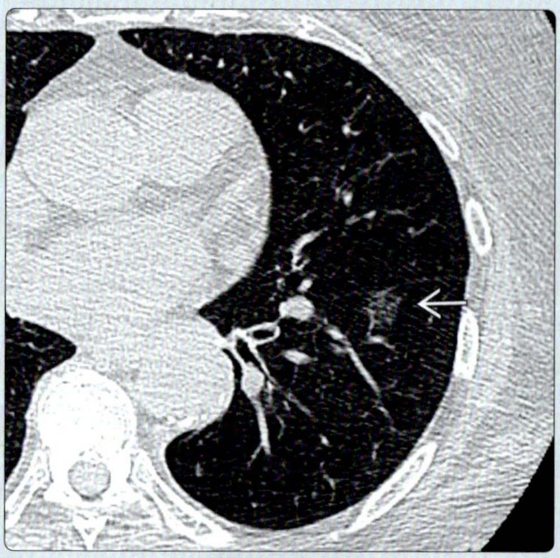

(Left) *Graphic shows benign calcification patterns that can occur in solitary pulmonary nodules: A: diffuse/homogeneous, B: central, C: popcorn, and D: laminated/concentric.* **(Right)** *Axial CT shows a mixed solid ➡ and subsolid ➡ solitary pulmonary nodule in the left upper lobe. Since this lesion is over 8 mm, appropriate management includes F-18 FDG PET/CT or biopsy.*

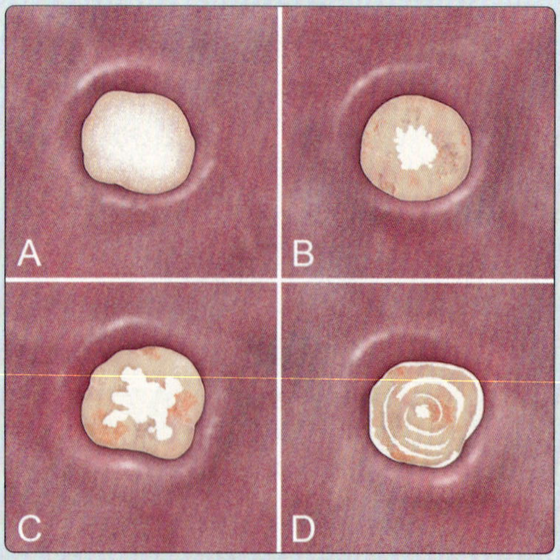

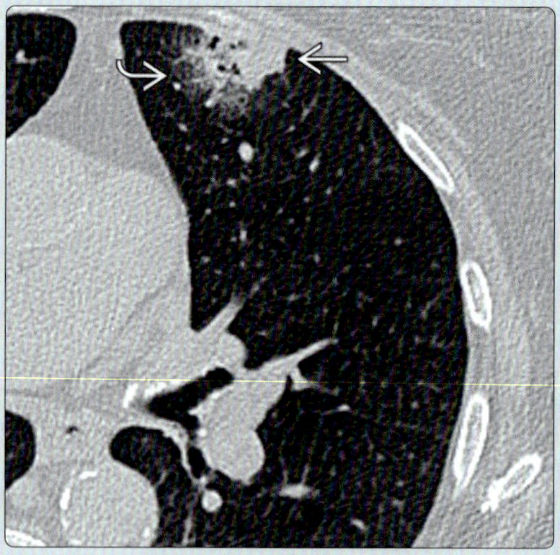

TERMINOLOGY

Definitions

- Solitary pulmonary nodule (SPN)
  - Single, small (< 3 cm), solid or subsolid parenchymal opacity
  - Differential diagnosis includes neoplasm, infection, inflammation, vascular, and congenital etiologies

IMAGING

Nuclear Medicine Findings

- PET
  - F-18 FDG PET/CT has sensitivity of ~ 95% and specificity of ~ 80% in detecting malignant SPNs > 1 cm in diameter
  - F-18 FDG avidity measured by standardized uptake value (SUV)
    - No strict cutoff value exists, although SUV > 2.5 is suggested as general marker of malignancy in clinical practice
    - Most likely benign: Smooth border, no FDG uptake; however, requires CT follow-up
    - Most likely malignant: Spiculated; SUV > 2.5
    - Any detectable F-18 FDG activity higher than background (> mediastinal blood pool) for SPNs < 15 mm is concerning for malignancy
      - F-18 FDG uptake is underestimated in small lesions
  - Metabolically active nonmalignant conditions can have high SUVs
    - Infection/inflammation (pneumonia, mycobacterial disease, rheumatoid nodules, sarcoidosis)
  - Less metabolically active tumors can have low SUVs
    - Adenocarcinoma in situ, mucinous adenocarcinoma, carcinoid
    - Size < 15 mm and subsolid lesions (critical mass of metabolically active malignant cells required for detection by F-18 FDG PET/CT)
    - Uncontrolled hyperglycemia or recent insulin response, which hinders F-18 FDG uptake in tumor

CT Findings

- Location
  - Primary lung cancer SPN: 2/3 in upper lobes
  - Metastatic SPN: 2/3 of metastases occur in lower lobes
- Size: Risk of malignancy rises with increasing size
  - < 1 cm 35%
    - 1-2 cm 50%
    - 2-3 cm 80%
    - > 3 cm 97%
- Growth
  - Likely benign if solid nodule is stable in size over 2 years
  - Likely benign if subsolid nodule is stable in size over 3 years
  - Volume doubling time (VDT)
    - VDT < 20 days
      - Benign: Infection, infarction
      - Malignant: Lymphoma or fast-growing metastases
    - VDT between 20-400 days
      - Likely malignant for solid nodules
    - VDT > 400 days
      - Likely benign; however note that subsolid nodules are more likely to be seen with early or low-grade adenocarcinoma, which has slower average VDT
- Margins
  - Most likely benign: Well-circumscribed, smooth borders
    - However, 20% of smoothly/sharply marginated nodules are malignant (e.g., carcinoid)
  - Most likely malignant: Ill-defined, irregular borders
    - Scalloped (60%), spiculated (90%), corona radiata (95%)
- Attenuation
  - Solid: Typically dense and homogeneous
  - Subsolid: Poor attenuation on imaging, such that normal parenchymal structure (airways, vessels) can be visualized through them
    - Assess for presence of solid component (part solid)
    - Less amenable to functional imaging/biopsy
  - Fat or water density within lesion: Most likely benign
  - Enhancement: More typical of malignancy
- Calcifications
  - Benign calcification patterns: Diffuse/homogeneous, central, popcorn, laminated/concentric
  - Eccentric calcification: Indeterminate/suggestive of malignancy

DIFFERENTIAL DIAGNOSIS

F-18 FDG Positive

- Malignant
  - Primary lung cancer: Neuroendocrine; adenocarcinoma; small cell, large cell, and squamous cell carcinoma
  - Metastatic disease: Most nonmucinous adenocarcinoma, sarcoma, lymphoma, melanoma
- Benign
  - Infection: (TB, fungal, bacterial); inflammation (sarcoid, granulomatosis with polyangiitis, rheumatoid)
  - Other: Bronchiolitis obliterans organizing pneumonia, pulmonary infarction, round atelectasis, lymph node, mucoid impaction

Variable to Low F-18 FDG Uptake

- Malignant
  - Primary lung cancer: Adenocarcinoma in situ, carcinoid (typically endobronchial but ~ 20% present as peripheral, well-circumscribed SPNs)
  - Metastatic disease: Highly mucinous adenocarcinoma, testicular, renal cell, prostate, hepatocellular carcinoma
- Benign
  - Inactive granulomatous disease, bronchogenic cyst, hamartoma, pleural plaque
  - Other: Lipoma, fibroma, AVM, pulmonary varix, congenital cystic adenomatoid malformation

PATHOLOGY

General Features

- Epidemiology
  - 150,000 SPNs detected annually in USA
    - Malignancy incidence, 10-70%; depends on population under study (e.g., age, smoking status, referral pattern, study location)
  - Important features in patient history

Management of Subsolid Solitary Pulmonary Nodules

Average of Length and Width	Management Recommendation
> 5 mm	CT at 3 months to confirm persistence; if persistent, annual CT for 3 years minimum
Solitary part-solid nodules	CT at 3 months to confirm persistence; if persistent and solid component < 5 mm, annual CT for 3 years minimum; if persistent with solid component > 5 mm, then biopsy or surgical resection

Adapted from Recommendations for the Management of Subsolid Pulmonary Nodules Detected at CT: A Statement from the Fleischner Society. Radiology, 266(1):304-317, 2013 Jan (suggested management for patients > 35 years).

Management of Solid Solitary Pulmonary Nodules

Average of Length and Width	No/Minimal Smoking, No Other Risk Factors	Smoking History, Other Risk Factors
≤ 4 mm	No follow-up	CT at 12 months; if stable, no further follow-up
> 4-6 mm	CT at 12 months; if stable, no further follow-up	CT at 6-12 months; if stable, again at 18-24 months
> 6-8 mm	CT at 6-12 months; if stable, again at 18-24 months	CT at 3-6 months; if stable, again at 9-12 and 24 months
> 8 mm	CT at 3, 9, and 24 months to evaluate stability or CECT, F-18 FDG PET, &/or biopsy	CT at 3, 9, and 24 months to evaluate stability or CECT, F-18 FDG PET, &/or biopsy

Adapted from Guidelines for Management of Small Pulmonary Nodules Detected on CT Scans: A Statement from the Fleischner Society. Radiology, 237(2):395-400, 2005 Nov (suggested management for patients > 35 years).

    - Age: Risk of malignancy 3% at 35-39 years, 15% at 40-49 years, 43% at 50-59 years, > 50% at 60+ years
    - History of smoking, malignancy, TB
    - Pulmonary mycosis or travel to regions endemic to mycosis
    - Occupational risk factors for malignancy (asbestos, radon, nickel, chromium, vinyl chloride, polycyclic hydrocarbons)

CLINICAL ISSUES

Presentation

- Most common signs/symptoms
  - Most SPNs asymptomatic, incidental finding
  - SPN in setting of another primary (breast, head and neck, colon, etc.) is most often primary bronchogenic carcinoma

Natural History & Prognosis

- Low-risk population: If no risk factors, clinical history, prior imaging, or concerning imaging features to suggest high-risk patient
  - Current recommendations are to prove stability over 2-year period (for solid SPN) and 3-year period (for subsolid SPN) with follow-up imaging
- High-risk population: Depends on clinical scenario
  - Management may include
    - Interval CT follow-up
    - Percutaneous biopsy, bronchoscopic/transesophageal biopsy
    - Bronchoscopic washings
    - Video-assisted thoracoscopic surgery
    - Resection of nodule

DIAGNOSTIC CHECKLIST

Image Interpretation Pearls

- Hypermetabolic pulmonary nodules may reflect neoplastic, infectious, or inflammatory disease
- If nodule has imaging features of adenocarcinoma in situ or carcinoid, a negative F-18 FDG PET/CT does not rule out malignancy
- For small nodules (< 1.5 cm) hypermetabolic activity may be underestimated
  - Any nodule with F-18 FDG activity higher than background or mediastinal blood pool remains concerning for malignancy
- SUV may be underestimated with nodules in lung bases due to linear motion artifact from respiratory motion
- Recognize calcification patterns in lung nodules that correlate with benign disease to decrease false-positive interpretations on F-18 FDG PET/CT

Reporting Tips

- Continue CT follow-up for F-18 FDG PET/CT negative solid and semisolid nodules

SELECTED REFERENCES

1. Naidich DP et al: Recommendations for the management of subsolid pulmonary nodules detected at CT: a statement from the Fleischner Society. Radiology. 266(1):304-17, 2013
2. Lowe VJ et al: Prospective investigation of positron emission tomography in lung nodules. J Clin Oncol. 16(3):1075-84, 1998
3. Erasmus JJ et al: Solitary pulmonary nodules: Part I. Morphologic evaluation for differentiation of benign and malignant lesions. Radiographics. 20(1):43-58, 2000
4. Erasmus JJ et al: Solitary pulmonary nodules: Part II. Evaluation of the indeterminate nodule. Radiographics. 20(1):59-66, 2000

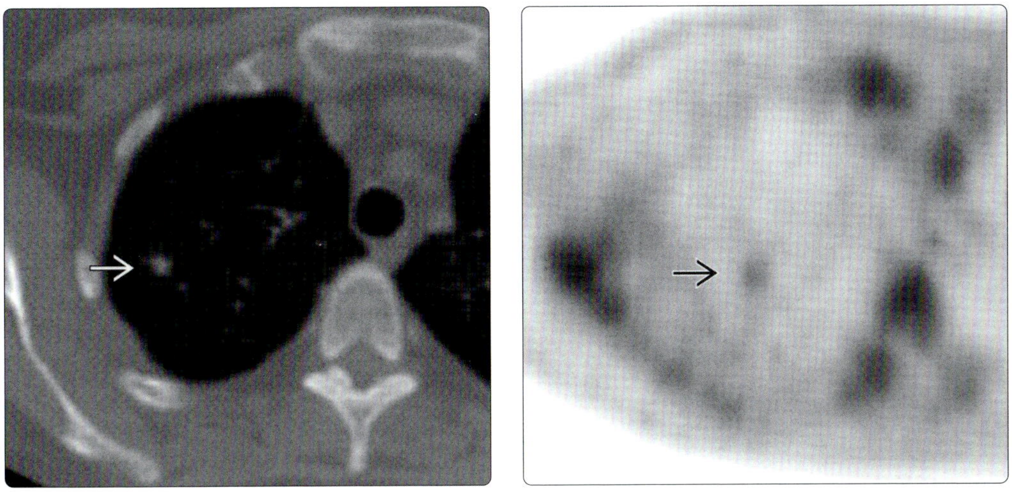

(Left) *Axial CT shows a subcentimeter solitary pulmonary nodule* ➡ *in the right upper lobe.* **(Right)** *Axial F-18 FDG PET/CT in the same patient shows hypermetabolic activity associated with the nodule* ⇨*, a biopsy-proven primary lung cancer.*

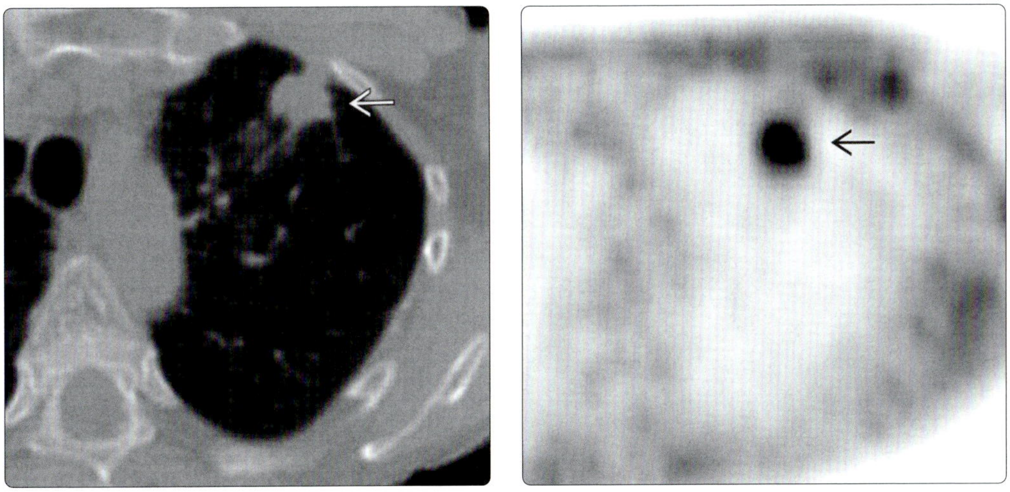

(Left) *Axial CT shows a spiculated solitary pulmonary nodule* ➡ *in the left upper lobe.* **(Right)** *Axial F-18 FDG PET/CT in the same patient shows hypermetabolic activity in the nodule* ⇨*, a biopsy-proven granuloma.*

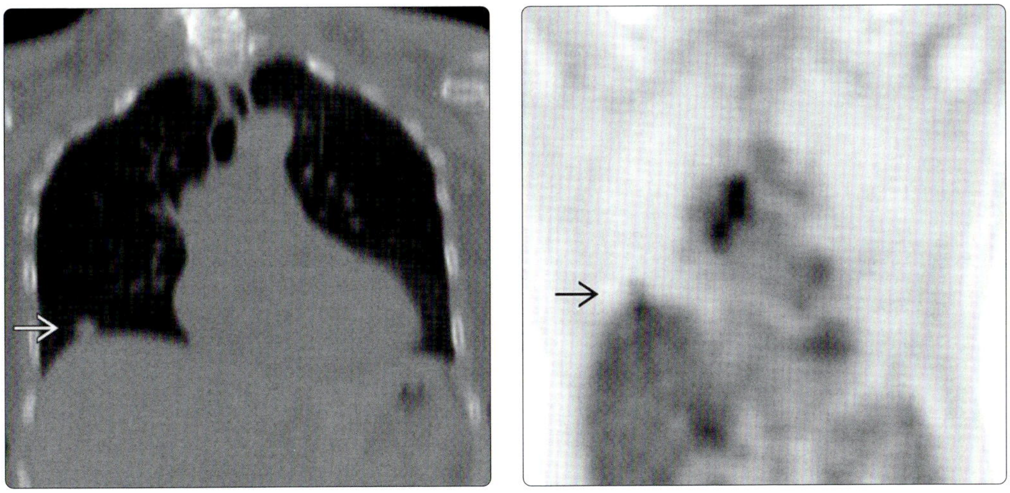

(Left) *Coronal CT shows a solitary pulmonary nodule* ➡ *in the right lung base in close proximity to the right hemidiaphragm.* **(Right)** *Coronal F-18 FDG PET in the same patient shows linear FDG activity* ⇨ *at the site of the nodule, an artifact due to respiratory motion. This results in underestimation of the standard uptake value (SUV) in the nodule.*

(Left) *Axial CT shows a ground-glass nodule ➡ in the right upper lobe.* **(Right)** *Axial F-18 FDG PET/CT in the same patient shows low-level FDG uptake in the right upper lobe ground-glass nodule ⇨, biopsy-proven adenocarcinoma.*

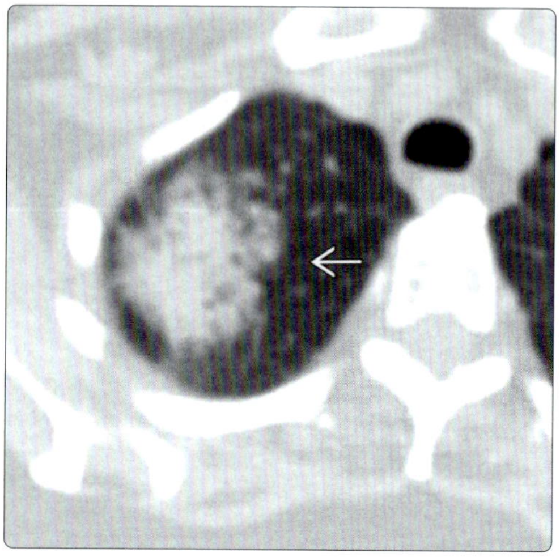

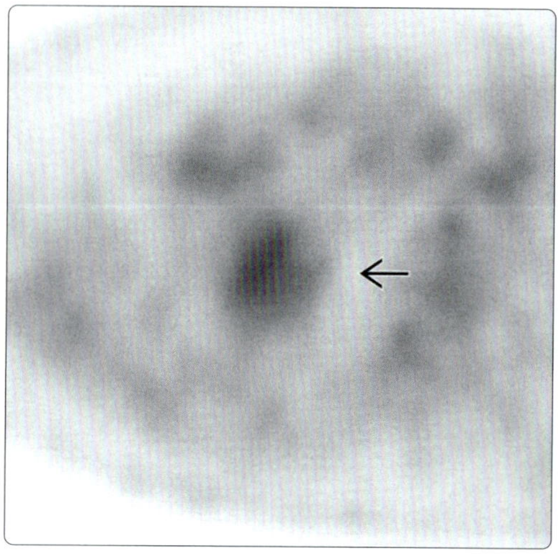

(Left) *Axial CT shows a well-circumscribed solitary pulmonary nodule ➡ in the right lung base. Carcinoids are most commonly round on CT.* **(Right)** *Axial F-18 FDG PET/CT in the same patient shows hypermetabolic activity ⇨ in the nodule, a biopsy-proven carcinoid. Unlike this case, carcinoids often show little to no uptake on PET.*

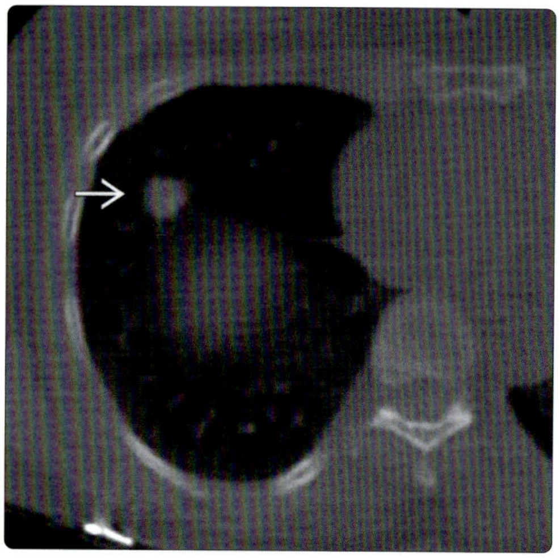

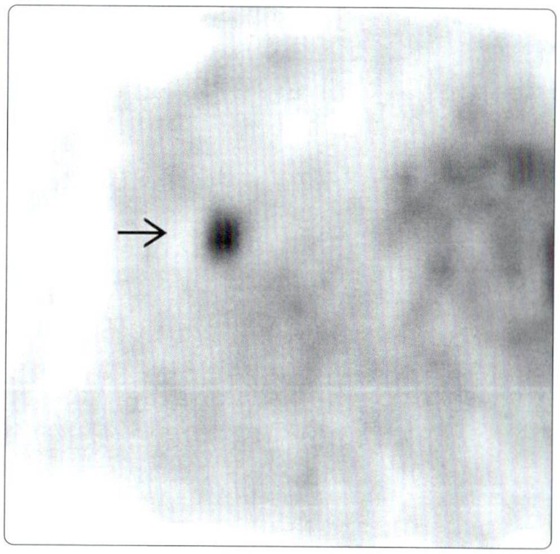

(Left) *Axial CT shows a solitary large ground-glass opacity ➡ in the right lower lobe.* **(Right)** *Axial F-18 FDG PET/CT in the same patient shows hypermetabolic activity associated with the mass ⇨, biopsy-proven mucosa-associated lymphoid tissue (MALT) lymphoma.*

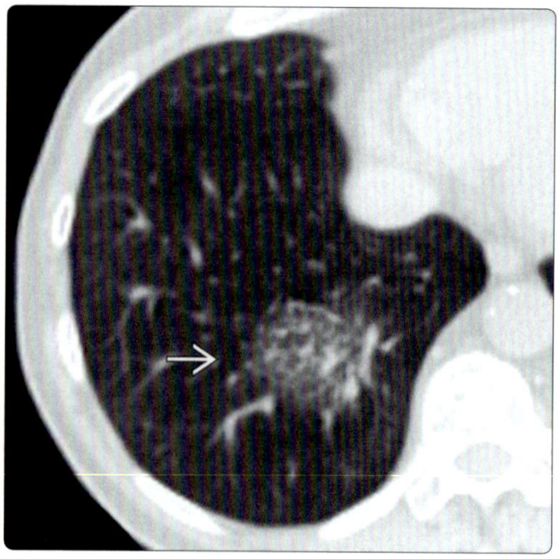

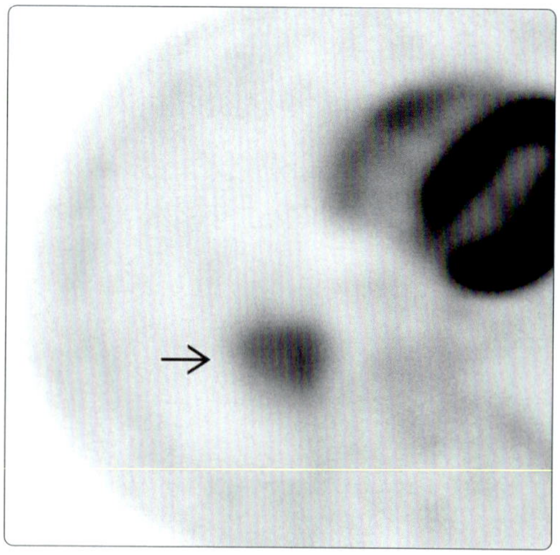

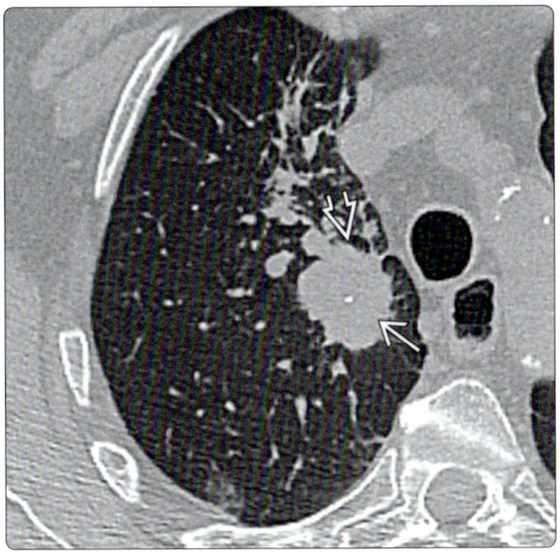

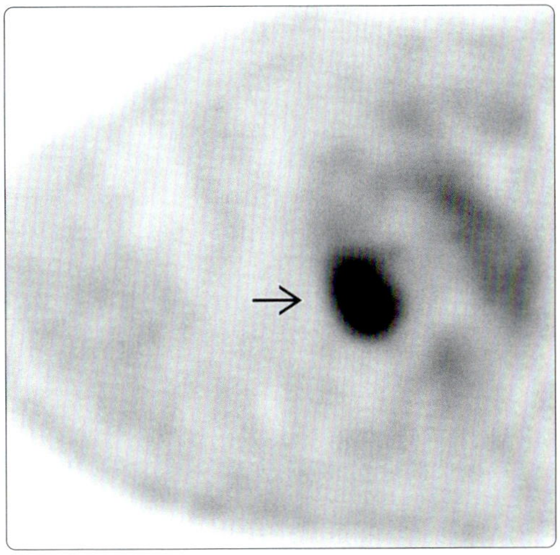

(Left) *Axial NECT shows a pulmonary nodule with punctate central calcification, a finding that suggests benign etiology; however, the large solid component and spiculations are concerning for malignancy.* **(Right)** *Axial F-18 FDG PET/CT in the same patient shows hypermetabolic activity associated with the nodule, a biopsy-proven adenocarcinoma enveloping a granuloma.*

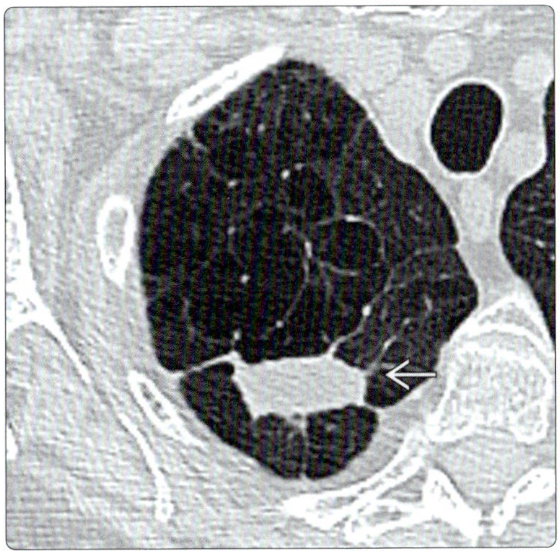

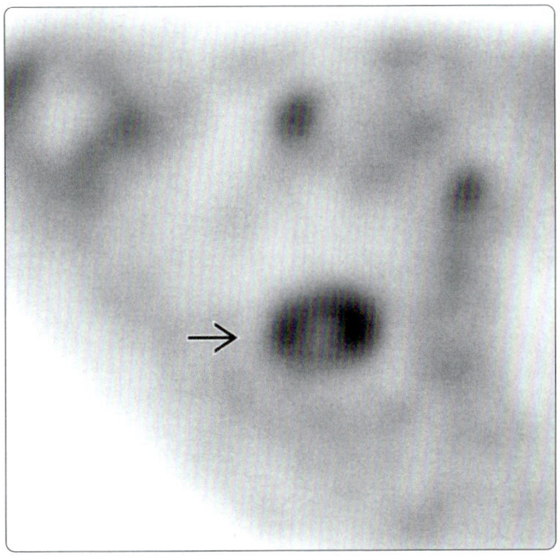

(Left) *Axial CT in a long-term smoker shows a spiculated right upper lobe mass.* **(Right)** *Axial F-18 FDG PET/CT in the same patient shows that the mass has a hypermetabolic rim with central photopenia, suggesting central necrosis, a typical feature of squamous cell carcinoma due to its rapid growth; however, biopsy showed a fungal infection.*

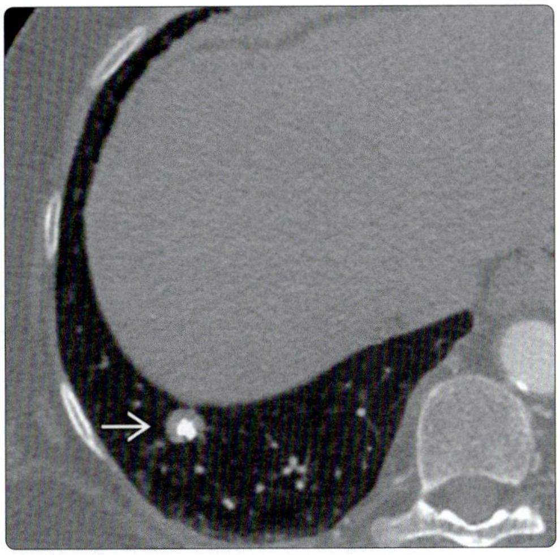

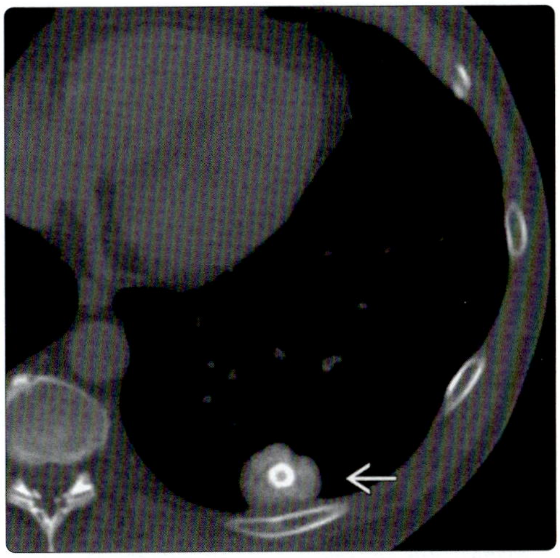

(Left) *Axial NECT shows a solitary pulmonary nodule with internal popcorn calcification, characteristic of a benign calcification pattern.* **(Right)** *Axial CT shows a solitary pulmonary nodule with a laminated internal calcification, characteristic of a benign calcification pattern.*

KEY FACTS

IMAGING

- **I-123 whole-body scan**
  - I-123 localizes to thyroid tissue that transports and organifies iodine
  - Detects thyroid remnant, lymphadenopathy, and distant metastatic or recurrent disease
  - 159 keV gamma rays more optimal for LEAP collimators
  - Physiologic uptake in salivary glands, stomach, lactating breasts
  - Renal excretion
- **F-18 FDG PET/CT**
  - Uptake of radioactive glucose analogue into thyroid tissue through GLUT1 transporter
  - Can be used to evaluate patients with tumors that are not iodine avid and have elevated thyroglobulin levels (> 10 ng/mL)
- **Tc-99m MDP bone scan**
  - Can be used for skeletal survey if bone metastases suspected

CLINICAL ISSUES

- **I-123 whole-body scan**
  - Patient needs elevated TSH
    - Thyroid hormone withdrawal for 3 weeks: Goal TSH > 30 mU/L
    - Thyrogen stimulation: Thyrogen (human recombinant TSH) stimulation with 0.9 mg IM on 2 consecutive days
  - Low-iodine diet: Usually followed for 7-14 days to increase uptake of radioactive iodine by thyroid tissue
- Lactating women
  - If I-123 scan absolutely necessary during lactation, pump and discard milk for 2-3 days (4 half lives)
  - No I-131 therapy in lactating women as iodine taken up and excreted by breasts (must cease lactation for 1-2 months prior)

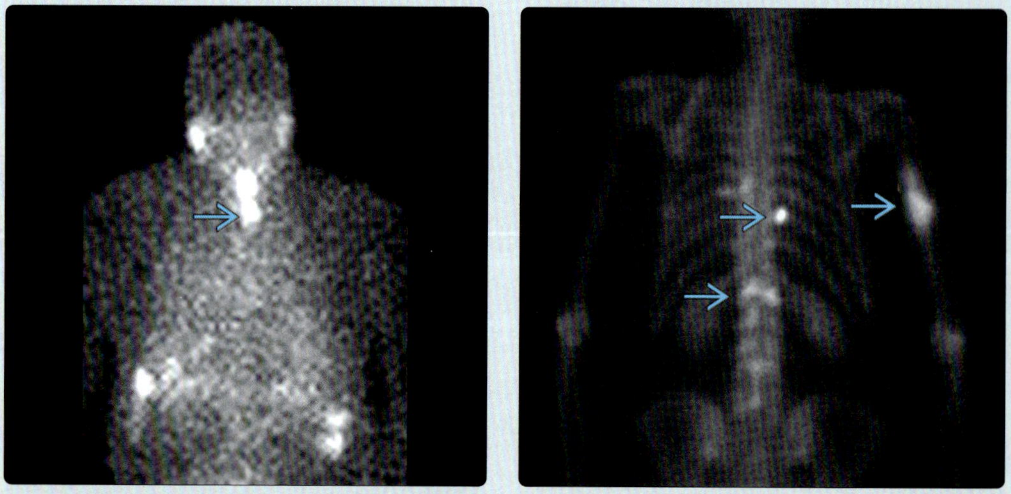

(Left) *Anterior I-123 whole-body scan in a patient post thyroidectomy for thyroid cancer shows remnant thyroid tissue in the native thyroid bed as well as substernally →.* **(Right)** *Posterior bone scan shows multifocal bone metastases → in a patient with papillary thyroid cancer.*

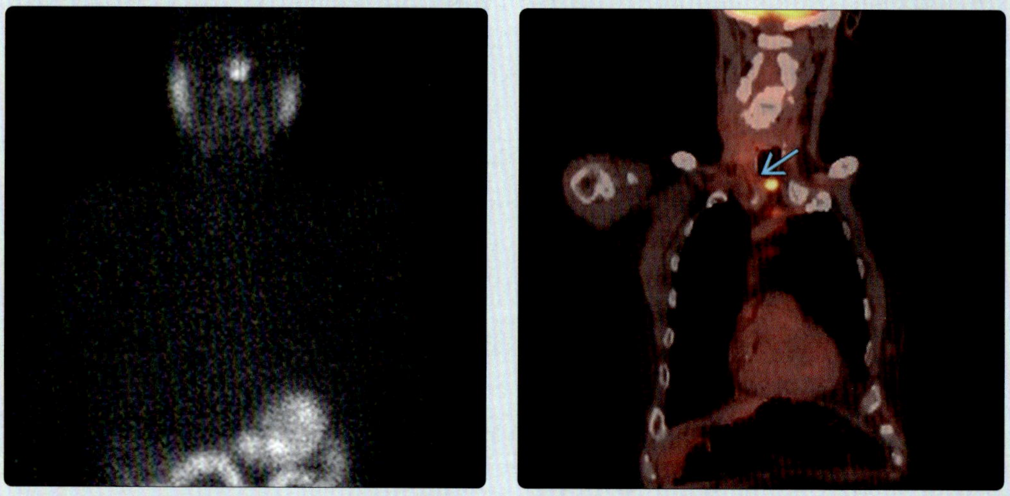

(Left) *Anterior post-thyroidectomy radioactive iodine scan in patient with rising thyroglobulin shows no abnormal activity in thyroid bed, lungs, or bones.* **(Right)** *Coronal F-18 FDG PET/CT in the same patient shows hypermetabolic soft tissue in the thyroid bed →. Non-radioactive iodine-avid disease can be detected on F-18 FDG PET/CT.*

IMAGING

Nuclear Medicine Findings

- **I-123 whole-body scan**
  - I-123 localizes to thyroid tissue that transports and organifies iodine
  - Detects thyroid remnant, lymphadenopathy, and distant metastatic or recurrent disease
  - Physiologic uptake in salivary glands, stomach, lactating breasts
  - Renal excretion
  - 159 keV gamma rays more optimal for LEAP collimators
- **I-131 whole-body scan**
  - I-131 is gamma (364 keV) and beta (0.606 MeV) emitter
  - Higher radiation burden as compared to I-123
  - Possible risk of thyroid stunning prior to I-131 ablation due to high-energy beta
  - Imaging characteristics not as good as I-123
- **F-18 FDG PET/CT**
  - Uptake of radioactive glucose analogue into thyroid tissue through GLUT1 transporter
  - GLUT1 has been found to be overexpressed in thyroid carcinomas, thus increased uptake of tracer suggests carcinoma
  - Minimal data to suggest should be part of initial work-up of those with indeterminate or nondiagnostic FNA
  - Can be used to evaluate patients with tumors that are not iodine avid and have elevated thyroglobulin levels (> 10 ng/mL)
    - Studies suggest that it can detect metastatic disease in 70% of these patients
    - Sensitivity increases when TSH elevated (thyroid hormone withdrawal or Thyrogen stimulation prior)
    - Tumors that are radioiodine-negative and F-18 FDG-positive are associated with less favorable prognosis
- **Tc-99m MDP bone scan**
  - Can be used for skeletal survey if bone metastases suspected

Imaging Recommendations

- Protocol advice
  - **I-123 whole-body scan**
    - TSH stimulation
      - Thyroid hormone withdrawal for 3 weeks (goal TSH > 30 mU/L); concomitant serum thyroglobulin, anti-thyroglobulin antibody assays, and TSH can be drawn prior to I-123 administration
      - Thyrogen stimulation: Thyrogen (human recombinant TSH) stimulation with 0.9 mg IM on 2 consecutive days
      - Thyrogen stimulation: Serum thyroglobulin, anti-thyroglobulin antibody assays drawn on day 5 after first injection, usually not after I-131 therapy because blood radioactive; mostly on follow-up scans
    - Low-iodine diet: Usually followed for 7-14 days to increase uptake of radioactive iodine by thyroid tissue
    - Lactating women
      - If I-123 scan absolutely necessary during lactation, pump and discard milk for 2-3 days (4 half-lives)
      - No I-131 therapy in lactating women as iodine taken up and excreted by breasts (must cease lactation for 1-2 months prior)
    - Radiopharmaceutical
      - 2-5 mCi (74-185 MBq) I-123
      - Images obtained 6-48 hours following the administration
    - Dosimetry
      - Bladder wall receives largest radiation dose
    - Image acquisition
      - 159 keV with 20% window
      - Patient supine with neck extended
      - Low-energy collimator and large-field-of-view camera preferred
      - Anterior and posterior images from top of skull through femurs
      - Spot neck images can be obtained; 10-15 min per image
      - Whole-body images take approximately 40 min per pass or 4-5 cm/min
      - SPECT/CT may be useful to evaluate for lymphadenopathy, indeterminate lesions on whole-body anterior and posterior scan

DIFFERENTIAL DIAGNOSIS

Papillary Thyroid Cancer

- Papillae with neoplastic cells surrounding fibrovascular stalk
  - Typically unencapsulated
  - Follicular variant of papillary thyroid cancer
- Poor prognostic indicators include tumors > 1.5 cm and extracapsular spread, age > 45 years
- Lymph node involvement common
- Most commonly spreads via lymphatics to lungs (also bones)
- Radioactive iodine-avid

Follicular Thyroid Cancer

- Typically unifocal follicular cells with extension outside capsule and vascular invasion
  - Hurthle cell variant: Considered to have poorer prognosis than follicular; poor radioactive iodine avidity
  - Insular variant: Poorly differentiated follicular; commonly invasive with regional/distant metastases
- Lymph node involvement less common than papillary
- Most commonly spreads hematogenously to bone
- 3x more common in women
- Radioactive iodine-avid

Medullary Thyroid Cancer

- Neuroendocrine tumor of parafollicular/C-cell origin
- Frequently found with concurrent neck, brain, or abdominal masses
- Surgery for primary tumor and metastases
- Not radioactive iodine-avid

Anaplastic Thyroid Cancer

- Undifferentiated tumor of thyroid follicular epithelium
- Typically advanced with soft tissue invasion at time of presentation
- Palliative surgery
- Rapid clinical course with ~ 100% disease-specific mortality

- Not radioactive iodine-avid

PATHOLOGY

General Features

- Risk factors
  - Radiation exposure
  - Family history of thyroid disorder
  - Age < 20 or > 50 years
  - Male gender
- Autopsy studies indicate 60% of Americans have thyroid nodules
- 5-15% malignancy rate for every thyroid nodule
- Distant metastases rate of < 10%
- 25% of recurrences/metastases are non-iodine avid
  - Require other imaging modalities such as F-18 FDG PET/CT, MR
  - Treatment options include external-beam or intraoperative radiation therapy, systemic chemotherapy considered for more advanced disease

Staging, Grading, & Classification

- Tumor-node-metastases classification
  - Primary tumor (T)
    - T1: Tumor size ≤ 2 cm
    - T2: Tumor size 2-4 cm
    - T3: Tumor size > 4 cm, no spread outside thyroid
    - T4a: Tumor of any size extending beyond thyroid capsule to invade adjacent structures
    - T4b: Tumor invades prevertebral fascia or encases carotid artery or mediastinal vessels
  - Regional lymph nodes (N)
    - N0: No lymphatic spread
    - N1a: Metastasis to level VI (pretracheal, paratracheal, and prelaryngeal/Delphian lymph nodes)
    - N1b: Metastasis to unilateral, bilateral, or contralateral cervical (levels I-V), retropharyngeal, or superior mediastinal lymph nodes (level VII)
  - Distant metastasis (M)
    - M0: No distant metastasis
    - M1: Distant metastasis
  - Staging
    - PTC/FTC, < 45 years
      - Stage 1: Any T, any N, M0
      - Stage 2: Any T, any N, M1
    - PTC/FTC, > 45 years
      - Stage 1: T1 N0 M0
      - Stage 2: T2 N0 M0
      - Stage 3: T3 N0 M0, or T1-T3 N1a M0
      - Stage 4a: T4a, any N M0, or T1-T3 N1b M0
      - Stage 4b: T4b, any N M0
      - Stage 4c: Any T, any N M1

CLINICAL ISSUES

Presentation

- Most common signs/symptoms
  - Slow-growing, painless solitary thyroid nodule (50% present with hoarseness due to local invasion)
  - With advanced disease, exam may demonstrate hard, fixed mass; pain; lymphadenopathy; vocal fold paresis

Demographics

- Epidemiology
  - In USA, ~ 62,980 new cases of thyroid cancer and ~ 1,890 deaths from thyroid cancer each year

Natural History & Prognosis

- 5-year survival
  - Papillary thyroid cancer: 95%
  - Follicular thyroid cancer: 70-85%
  - Hurthle cell carcinoma: 50%

Treatment

- ATA recommends US for contralateral lobe and cervical lymph nodes for all patients undergoing thyroidectomy for malignant cytologic findings on biopsy
  - Macrometastases in cervical lymph nodes in 20-50%, with micrometastases approaching 90%
  - US can identify suspicious cervical adenopathy in 20-31% of cases; however, identifies only 1/2 of lymph nodes found at surgery due to overlying thyroid
- Total thyroidectomy ± lymphadenectomy for clinical nodal disease
- Postoperative radioactive iodine, depending on primary tumor characteristics/whole-body RAI scan
- Long-term thyroid hormone suppression
  - Low risk: TSH 0.1-0.5 mU/L
  - Intermediate and high risk: TSH 0.1 mU/L
- Screen with ultrasound plus serum thyroglobulin levels for recurrence
  - Whole-body radioactive iodine scan if clinical suspicion for recurrence high

DIAGNOSTIC CHECKLIST

Image Interpretation Pearls

- Thymus may show up on pre- and post-therapy scans
- Must distinguish lymphadenopathy from asymmetric salivary gland uptake (e.g., prior salivary gland surgery/external beam radiation, radioactive iodine damage)

SELECTED REFERENCES

1. Qiu ZL et al: Comparison of the diagnostic and prognostic values of 99mTc-MDP-planar bone scintigraphy, 131I-SPECT/CT and 18F-FDG-PET/CT for the detection of bone metastases from differentiated thyroid cancer. Nucl Med Commun. 33(12):1232-42, 2012
2. American Thyroid Association. Cooper DS, et al. Revised ATA Management Guidelines for Patients with Thyroid Nodules and Differentiated Thyroid Cancer. From ATA Guidelines Taskforce on Thyroid Nodules and Differentiated Thyroid Cancer. http://www.thyroid.org/thyroid-guidelines/revised/taskforce. 2010
3. ACR–SNM–SPR Practice guideline for the performance of thyroid scintigraphy and uptake measurements. http://snmmi.files.cms-plus.com/docs/Thyroid_Scintigraphy_1382732120053_10.pdf. Created October 1, 2009. Accessed July 31, 2015
4. Society of Nuclear Medicine. Procedure Guideline for Scintigraphy for Differentiated Papillary and Follicular Thyroid Cancer. http://snmmi.files.cms-plus.com/docs/Scintigraphy%20for%20Differentiated%20Thyroid%20Cancer%20V3%200%20%289-25-06%29.pdf.

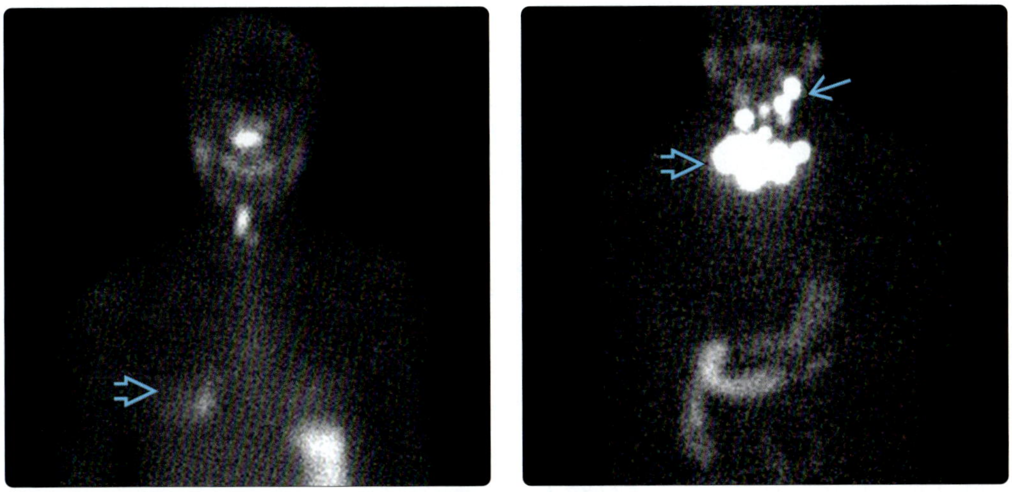

(Left) *Anterior radioiodine scan shows breast uptake* ⇨ *in a patient post thyroidectomy for thyroid cancer who ceased lactation 1 month prior. Radioactive iodine therapy is contraindicated in lactating patients.* **(Right)** *Anterior radioiodine scan shows residual cervical* → *and thoracic inlet* ⇨ *lymphatic metastases in a patient with papillary thyroid cancer s/p total thyroidectomy. Further surgical lymphadenectomy was performed prior to radioactive iodine therapy.*

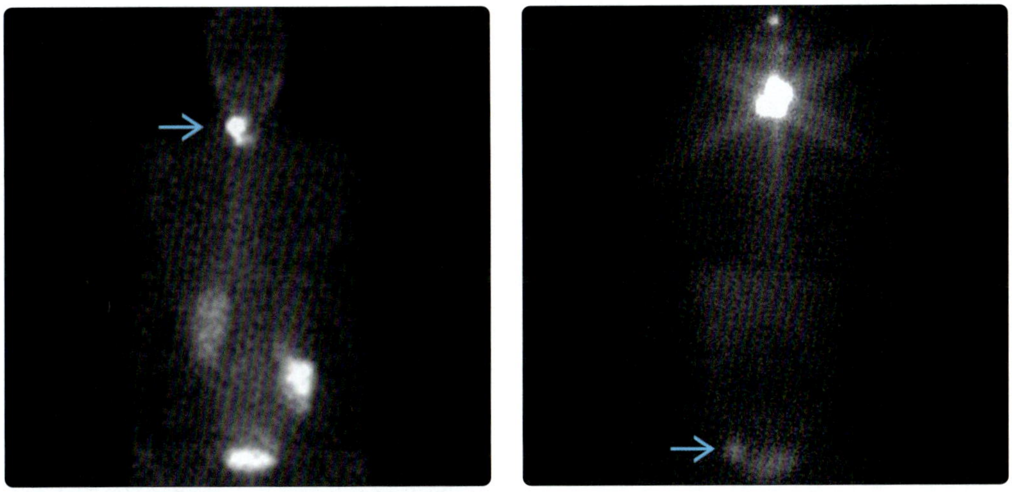

(Left) *Anterior radioiodine scan shows thyroid bed activity* → *without distant metastasis.* **(Right)** *Anterior post-therapy I-131 scan in the same patient shows abnormal activity in the pelvis* →*. The differential diagnosis includes bladder diverticulum versus adnexal mass.*

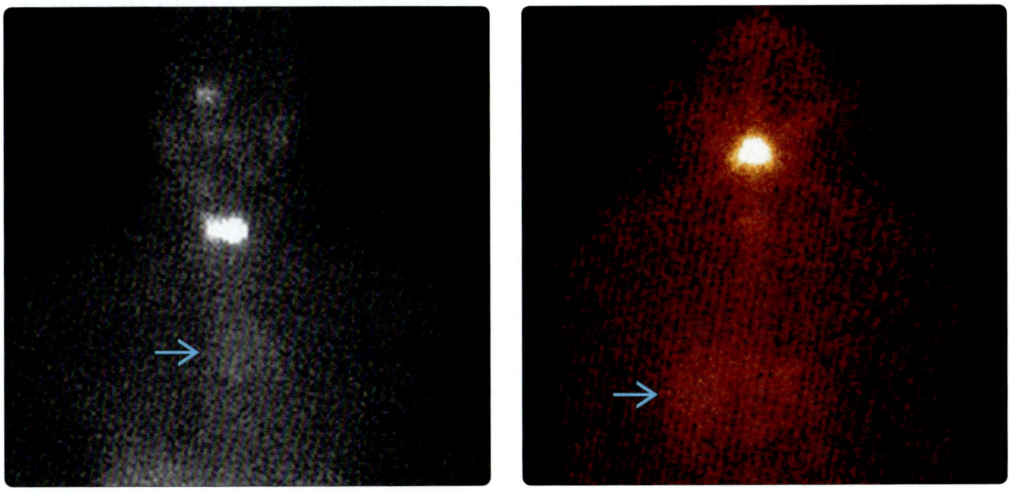

(Left) *Anterior radioiodine scan in a young patient with follicular thyroid cancer shows faint mediastinal uptake* →*, which can be seen in normal thymus.* **(Right)** *Anterior post-therapy radioiodine scan shows homogeneous hepatic uptake* →*, a normal physiological finding as the liver processes radioactive iodine incorporated into normal thyroid hormone.*

Renal Cell Carcinoma

KEY FACTS

TERMINOLOGY

- Renal cell carcinoma (RCC): Carcinoma of renal tubular epithelium

IMAGING

- F-18 FDG PET: Isointense or hypermetabolic renal mass ± lymphadenopathy, metastases
  - Used for postoperative surveillance and detection of metastatic disease
- Bone scan: Use in symptomatic patients, high serum alkaline phosphatase or late-stage disease

TOP DIFFERENTIAL DIAGNOSES

- Renal oncocytoma
- Transitional cell carcinoma
- Lymphoma, infection, metastases

PATHOLOGY

- **TNM staging**
  - Primary tumor (T)
    - T1: Tumor ≤ 7 cm, limited to kidney
    - T2: Tumor > 7 cm, limited to kidney
    - T3: Extension into major veins or perinephric tissues
    - T4: Extension into ipsilateral adrenal &/or Gerota fascia
  - Regional lymph nodes (N)
    - N0: No nodal mets
    - N1: Nodal mets present
  - Distant metastasis (M)
    - M0: No distant metastasis
    - M1: Distant metastasis
- **Stage**
  - **Stage I:** T1, N0, M0
  - **Stage II:** T2, N0, M0
  - **Stage III:** T3 **&/or** N1
  - **Stage IV:** T4 **&/or** M1

CLINICAL ISSUES

- Common symptoms: Hematuria (60%), flank pain (40%)

(Left) *Anterior bone scan of a 65-year-old woman shows multiple areas of increased uptake, including the skull and left iliac wing. There is a pathologic fracture of the right tibial plateau. Note the photopenic mass in the abdomen.* **(Right)** *Corresponding axial CECT shows a large right renal cell carcinoma with central necrosis. Note the circumscribed left abdominal mass with peripheral calcification, likely a benign tumor.*

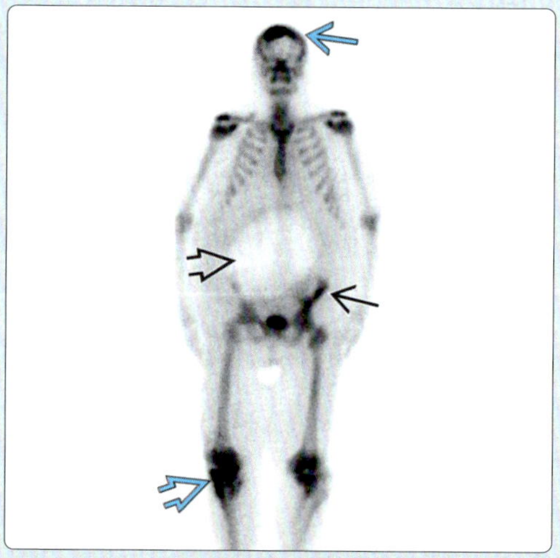

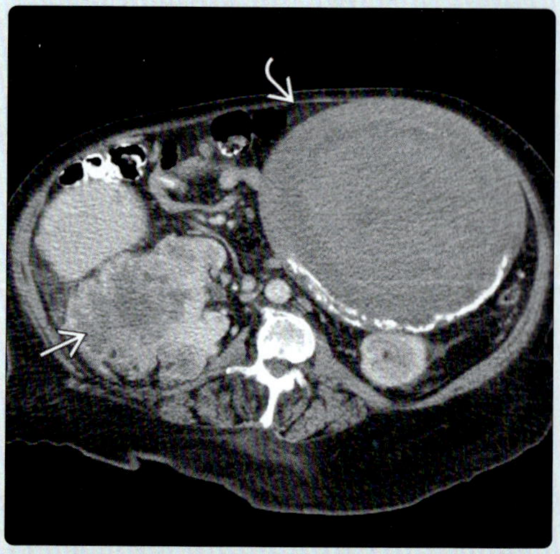

(Left) *Anterior bone scan of a 71-year-old man with RCC post right nephrectomy shows increased uptake in the proximal right humerus consistent with metastatic disease.* **(Right)** *Corresponding axial CECT of the same patient prior to nephrectomy shows a cortically based, enhancing right renal mass consistent with primary RCC.*

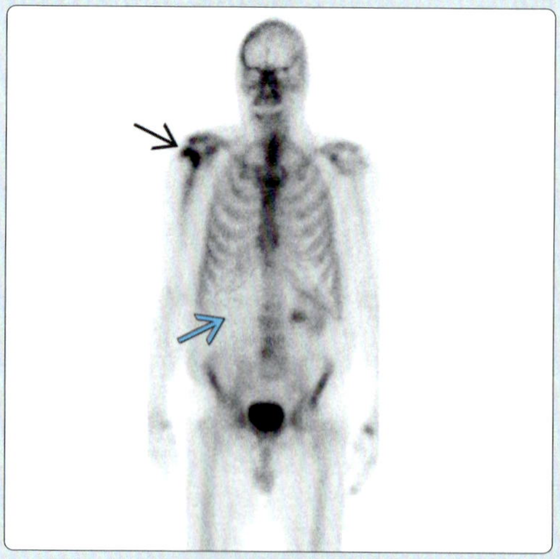

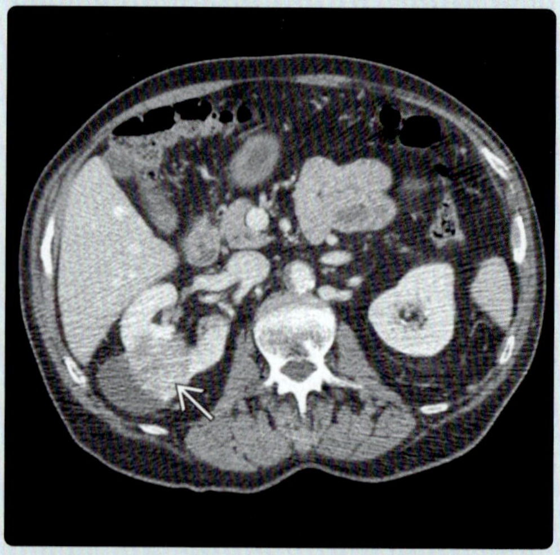

TERMINOLOGY

Abbreviations

- Renal cell carcinoma (RCC)

Definitions

- Carcinoma of renal tubular epithelium

IMAGING

General Features

- Best diagnostic clue
  - F-18 FDG PET/CT
    - Isointense or hypermetabolic mass in renal cortex
    - Lymphadenopathy
    - Distant metastases
  - Bone scan
    - Multifocal bone lesions
    - Axial lesions most common
  - CECT
    - Enhancing mass that disrupts renal contour
- Location
  - Commonly renal cortex
  - Exophytic
    - Originates from lining of proximal convoluted tubule
  - Can be bilateral (2%)
    - Especially individuals with genetic syndromes (von Hippel-Lindau)
- Size
  - Variable depending on time of diagnosis
- Morphology
  - 10% calcified, often irregular
  - 2-5% cystic

Nuclear Medicine Findings

- F-18 FDG PET/CT
  - Low sensitivity for primary tumor detection
    - Sensitivity 60%, specificity 100%
    - Many RCCs are isointense to renal parenchyma
    - Urine excretion can mask tumor adjacent to collecting system, ↑ false-negatives
  - Lymphadenopathy
    - Regional nodal metastases usually hypermetabolic
  - Distant metastases
    - Most common
      - Lung
      - Liver
      - Bone
      - Brain
    - Usually F-18 FDG avid
    - Sensitivity 64-90%, specificity 75-100%
      - Useful for postoperative surveillance and restaging
      - Can miss mets in liver and brain due to physiologic F-18 FDG uptake
    - Prognostic value unclear
      - SUV has not been shown to correlate with histologic type or nuclear grade
      - No difference in survival time of PET-positive vs. PET-negative patients
- Bone scan
  - Detection of metastatic disease
    - Sensitivity 94%, specificity 86%
    - Bone scan unnecessary in asymptomatic patients with T1-T3 tumors
      - Most patients with bone metastases are symptomatic (96% in one study)
      - Bone metastases rare in patients with early stage disease
  - Findings
    - Axial lesions most common
      - Pelvis and ribs (48%)
      - Spine (42%)
    - Lesions predominantly osteolytic (~ 70%)
      - Can be photopenic or hot on bone scan

Imaging Recommendations

- Best imaging tool
  - F-18 FDG PET/CT
    - Helpful in staging and monitoring for relapse in high-risk patients
    - Not commonly used for diagnostic evaluation of primary RCC
    - Useful to characterize indeterminate lesions on CT, MR, bone scan
  - Bone scan
    - Patients with bone pain
    - Patients with elevated serum alkaline phosphatase
    - Large or aggressive tumor
  - CECT
    - Pre-contrast, post-contrast, nephrographic phase
    - Indicated for diagnosis/evaluation of size and extent of primary tumor
    - If contraindication, MR superior to NECT

DIFFERENTIAL DIAGNOSIS

Renal Neoplasm

- Renal oncocytoma
  - Can be indistinguishable on PET, especially chromophobe type
- Urothelial carcinoma
  - Often confined to renal pelvis and ureters although can be diffusely infiltrative
- Renal angiomyolipoma
  - Benign neoplasm
  - Composed of vascular, smooth muscle, and fat elements
- Lymphoma
  - Homogeneous and diffusely infiltrative
- Metastases from other primary
  - Breast, colon, lung, pancreas most common
- Renal adenoma
  - Benign solid renal tumor
- Renal cyst
  - Simple = benign
  - Complex
    - Increased risk of malignancy, depending on characteristics

Infection

- Pyelonephritis → lobar nephronia → abscess
  - Lobar nephronia appears as mass-like wedge of affected parenchyma

PATHOLOGY

Staging, Grading, & Classification

- **TNM staging**
  - Primary tumor (T)
    - T1: Tumor ≤ 7 cm, limited to kidney
    - T2: Tumor > 7 cm, limited to kidney
    - T3: Extension into major veins or perinephric tissues
    - T4: Extension into ipsilateral adrenal &/or Gerota fascia
  - Regional lymph nodes (N)
    - N0: No nodal mets
    - N1: Nodal mets present
  - Distant metastasis (M)
    - M0: No distant metastasis
    - M1: Distant metastasis
- **Stage**
  - **Stage I:** T1, N0, M0
  - **Stage II:** T2, N0, M0
  - **Stage III:** T3 **&/or** N1
  - **Stage IV:** T4 **&/or** M1

CLINICAL ISSUES

Presentation

- Most common signs/symptoms
  - Symptomatic triad occurs in 9% of patients
    - Hematuria (60%)
    - Flank pain (40%)
    - Flank/abdominal mass (30-40%)
  - Many RCCs discovered incidentally on CT
- Other signs/symptoms
  - Fever
  - Nausea
  - Weight loss
  - Paraneoplastic syndromes (humoral factors)
    - Anemia
    - Hypercalcemia (PTHrP)
    - Hepatic dysfunction (↑ alkaline phosphatase [alk phos]) = Stauffer syndrome

Demographics

- Age
  - Generally 50-70 years, with wide distribution
- Gender
  - M > F (2:1)
- Epidemiology
  - Incidence
    - ~ 64,000 new cases each year in USA
    - 14,000 deaths each year in USA
  - Extent at diagnosis
    - 62%: Localized to kidney
    - 38%: Regional or distant mets

Natural History & Prognosis

- Over last 50 years, 5-year survival has increased from 34% to 71% (2008)
- Prognosis worse for larger, marginated, or necrotic tumors, which tend to be ↑ grade
- Major risk factors
  - Smoking
  - Hypertension
  - Obesity
  - Chemical exposure (DES, cadmium, asbestos, etc.)

Treatment

- Localized disease
  - Nephrectomy curative in majority of patients
  - Adjuvant immunotherapy or molecular agents also used
- Advanced disease
  - Usually unresectable
  - Molecularly targeted agents most often used
  - Immunotherapy less common

DIAGNOSTIC CHECKLIST

Consider

- **NECT** followed by **CECT** for primary evaluation
  - **US** to differentiate hyperdense cyst from mass if CT is unclear
- **MR**
  - Can be helpful for indeterminate lesions on CT or US
- **F-18 FDG PET/CT**
  - Can be useful for staging, postoperative surveillance, and response to therapy evaluation
- **Bone scan**
  - Use in symptomatic patients, high serum alkaline phosphatase or late-stage disease

Image Interpretation Pearls

- Primary RCC has variable uptake on F-18 FDG PET, often isointense to renal parenchyma
- Physiologic F-18 FDG excretion can mask tumors adjacent to collecting system

SELECTED REFERENCES

1. ACR Appropriateness Criteria: renal cell carcinoma staging. Agency for Healthcare Research and Quality, National Guideline Clearinghouse. http://www.guideline.gov/content.aspx?id=35153. Accessed September 24, 2014
2. Nakatani K et al: The potential clinical value of FDG-PET for recurrent renal cell carcinoma. Eur J Radiol. 79(1):29-35, 2011
3. Kumar R et al: Role of FDG PET-CT in recurrent renal cell carcinoma. Nucl Med Commun. 31(10):844-50, 2010
4. Lawrentschuk N et al: Positron emission tomography (PET), immuno-PET and radioimmunotherapy in renal cell carcinoma: a developing diagnostic and therapeutic relationship. BJU Int. 97(5):916-22, 2006
5. Ak I et al: F-18 FDG PET in detecting renal cell carcinoma. Acta Radiol. 46(8):895-9, 2005
6. Ide M et al: The detection of renal cell carcinoma with adrenal and para-aortic lymph node metastases by FDG-PET. Eur J Nucl Med Mol Imaging. 32(10):1246, 2005
7. Nguyen BD: Positron emission tomography imaging of renal vein and inferior vena cava tumor thrombus from renal cell carcinoma. Clin Nucl Med. 30(2):107-9, 2005
8. Kang DE et al: Clinical use of fluorodeoxyglucose F 18 positron emission tomography for detection of renal cell carcinoma. J Urol. 171(5):1806-9, 2004
9. Schoder H et al: Positron emission tomography for prostate, bladder, and renal cancer. Semin Nucl Med. 34(4):274-92, 2004
10. Watanabe N et al: A case of renal pelvic tumor visualized by 18F-FDG-PET imaging. Ann Nucl Med. 18(2):161-3, 2004
11. Jadvar H et al: Diagnostic role of [F-18]-FDG positron emission tomography in restaging renal cell carcinoma. Clin Nephrol. 60(6):395-400, 2003

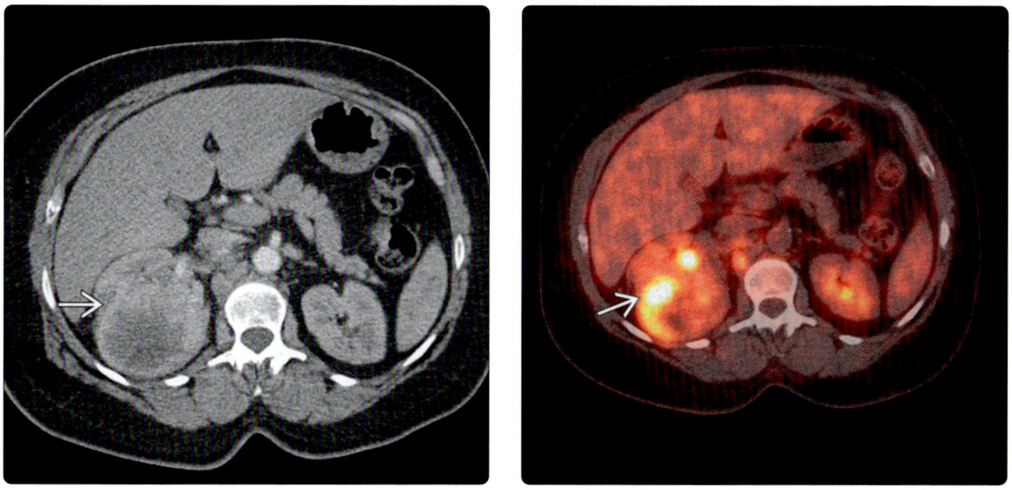

(Left) *Axial CECT in a 50-year-old woman with metastatic RCC shows the large, ill-defined right renal mass* ➔ *with areas of central necrosis.* **(Right)** *Corresponding F-18 FDG PET/CT shows patchy areas* ➔ *of increased metabolic activity. Primary tumors can be iso- or hyperintense to renal parenchyma.*

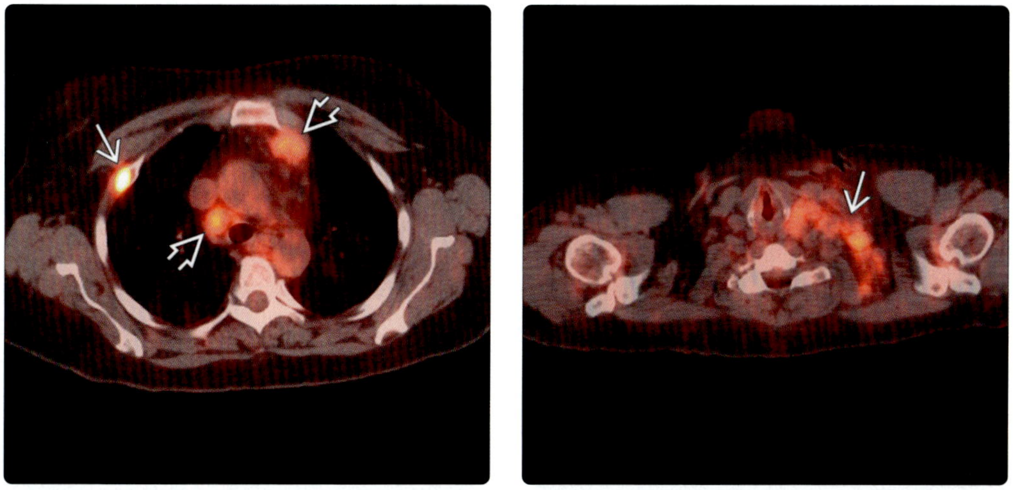

(Left) *Axial F-18 FDG PET/CT in the same patient shows an expansile lytic lesion of the right 3rd rib with increased metabolic activity* ➔ *consistent with metastatic disease. Note the hypermetabolic mediastinal lymphadenopathy* ➔. **(Right)** *F-18 FDG PET/CT of the same patient shows diffuse supraclavicular adenopathy* ➔ *with hypermetabolic activity.*

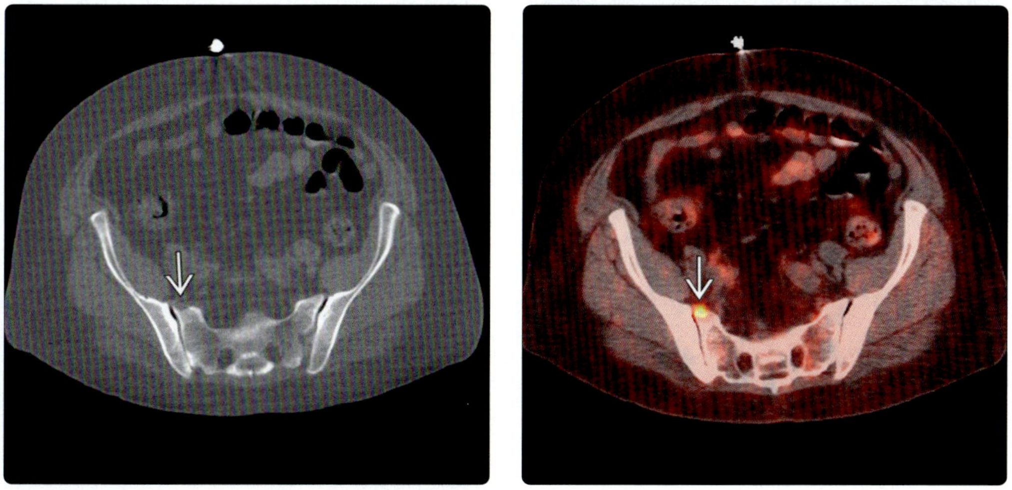

(Left) *Axial CT of the same patient shows a lytic lesion in the superior right sacrum* ➔. **(Right)** *Corresponding F-18 FDG PET/CT in the same patient shows hypermetabolic activity* ➔.

Transitional Cell Carcinoma

KEY FACTS

TERMINOLOGY

- Transitional cell carcinoma (TCC)
  - Usually involves urinary bladder but can arise from urethra, ureter, or renal pelvis

IMAGING

- F-18 FDG PET/CT
  - Focal increased FDG activity in primary tumor, regional nodes, distant metastases
  - Diuretic and oral hydration prior to imaging improves visualization
  - Important to evaluate muscle-invasive disease; high likelihood of metastases
- Bone scan
  - Multifocal sites of increased uptake, most common axially
  - Indicated in symptomatic patients &/or rising alkaline phosphatase
  - Bone metastases present in only 3% of patients at diagnosis, but risk increases with ↑ stage
  - > 60% of patients with bone metastases have invasive detrusor muscle disease

PATHOLOGY

- **Stage I:** No muscular invasion, N0, M0
- **Stage II:** Muscular invasion, N0, M0
- **Stage III:** T3 or T4 (without pelvic/abdominal wall involvement), N0, M0
- **Stage IV:** T4 (with pelvic/abdominal wall invasion) **or** M1 with any T, any N

CLINICAL ISSUES

- Treatment for early stage
  - Transurethral resection of bladder tumor (TURBT), intravesical chemotherapy
- Treatment for late stage
  - Radical cystectomy, neoadjuvant chemotherapy

(Left) *Axial F-18 FDG PET/CT in a 72-year-old female with multifocal transitional cell carcinoma shows a focal area of increased activity involving the left ureter ➡. Evaluation of metabolic activity is severely limited due to excreted tracer.* **(Right)** *Axial NECT in the same patient shows diffuse urothelial thickening ➡, concerning for malignancy.*

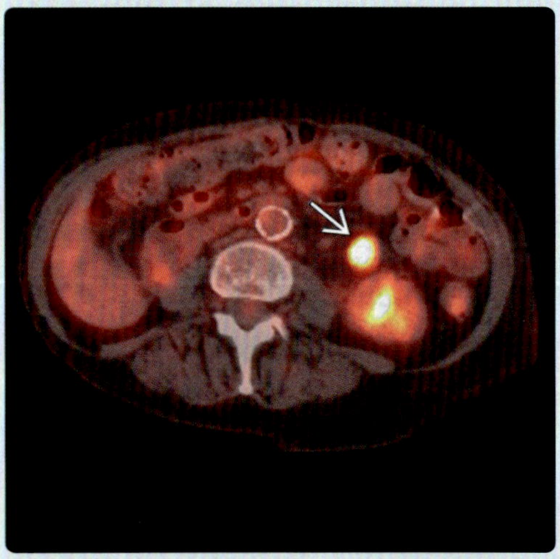

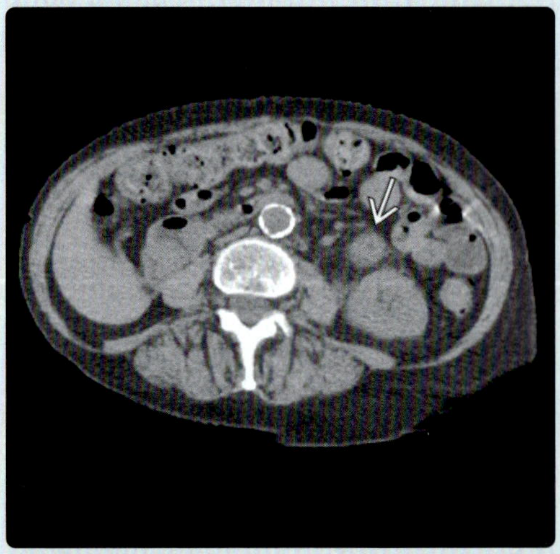

(Left) *Posterior MIP F-18 FDG PET in the same patient shows large left ureter ⇨ with hypermetabolic activity in a paraaortic node ⇨ and a liver metastasis ⇨.* **(Right)** *Corresponding coronal F-18 FDG PET/CT shows excreted radiotracer in the dilated left hydroureter ➡ and a hypermetabolic paraaortic node ⇨.*

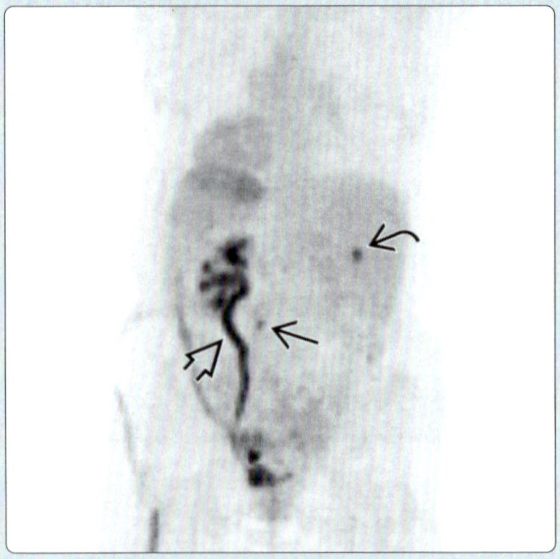

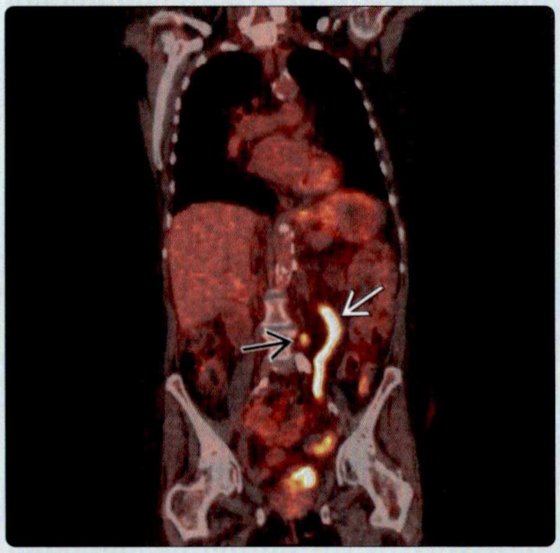

TERMINOLOGY

Definitions

- Transitional cell carcinoma (TCC)
  - Most common malignancy of urinary system
  - Usually involves urinary bladder but can arise from urethra, ureter, or renal pelvis

IMAGING

General Features

- Best diagnostic clue
  - Tc-99m bone scan
    - Multiple scattered foci of increased activity in skeleton, axial > appendicular
  - F-18 FDG PET/CT
    - Focal increased FDG activity in primary tumor, regional nodes, and distant metastases
    - Best for staging and monitoring for recurrence
- Location
  - Primary
    - Bladder wall/lumen most common
    - Other sites include ureter, renal pelvis, urethra
  - Regional
    - Local invasion into detrusor muscle, prostate, uterus, vagina
  - Spread
    - Lymphatic: Regional pelvic, retroperitoneal, paraortic nodes
    - Hematogenous: Bone (axial most common), lung, liver
- Morphology
  - Important for prognosis
    - Superficial (70-80%)
      - Confined to mucosa, lamina propria
      - Project into bladder lumen (papillary)
      - Usually low grade
    - Invasive (20-30%)
      - Within detrusor muscle
      - Solid, infiltrating
      - Usually high grade

Nuclear Medicine Findings

- Bone scan
  - Tc-99m bone scan
    - Findings
      - Multifocal sites of increased uptake, most common axially
      - Bony metastases present in 3% of patients at time of diagnosis
    - Indications
      - Symptomatic patients &/or those with elevated serum alkaline phosphatase
      - Bone scan not commonly used for diagnosis or preoperative staging
    - Risk of bone metastases increases with tumor grade and stage
      - Over 60% of patients with bone metastases have invasive detrusor muscle disease
      - Potential routine use for patients with advanced disease
- PET
  - F-18 FDG PET/CT
    - Primary diagnosis/staging
      - Initial clinical staging most often involves CECT or MR
      - PET/CT not routinely used for primary detection due to urinary FDG excretion
      - PET/CT with diuretic protocol: Sensitivity of 96% for primary tumor and sensitivity of 78% for regional nodes
      - Comprehensive pathologic staging (cystectomy + regional lymphadenectomy) is gold standard for bladder tumors
    - Detection of distant metastases
      - Sensitivity 70-87%, specificity 88-94%
      - Muscle-invasive primary tumor (T2) → higher likelihood of metastases
      - SUV typically in moderate range (~ 5)
      - Bone lesions are predominantly sclerotic
      - Potential role in directing therapy and preoperative planning
      - One study found that PET/CT changed preoperative treatment in 47% of patients
    - Surveillance
      - Emerging role as surveillance tool
      - PET/CT found to have 2x sensitivity of CT for nodal metastases, similar specificity
    - Visualization of tumor and regional nodes limited by urinary F-18 FDG excretion
      - Primary tumor staged with delayed images obtained after diuretic administration and oral hydration improve detection of tumor
      - Continuous bladder irrigation and immediate postvoid images not as effective at reducing intravesical F-18 FDG activity

Imaging Recommendations

- Best imaging tool
  - F-18 FDG PET/CT
    - Proven efficacy for detection of primary tumor, local disease, and distant metastases
    - Consider use when diagnostic/staging CT equivocal
    - Effective surveillance tool
  - Tc-99m bone scan
    - Indicated in symptomatic patients &/or those with rising alkaline phosphatase
    - Consider use in patients with invasive disease

Artifacts and Quality Control

- Diuretic F-18 FDG PET/CT
  - For primary tumor detection and optimal staging
    - 40 mg furosemide IV + oral fluid intake of 1.5-2 L
    - Void 2-3x, then hold urine for bladder distention prior to imaging

DIFFERENTIAL DIAGNOSIS

Cystitis

- Infection (acute or chronic)
- Radiation or chemotherapy-induced
- Hemorrhagic cystitis

Neoplasms

- Prostate cancer
- BPH
  - Can be FDG avid
- Nonurothelial bladder cancers
  - Squamous cell carcinoma: Schistosomiasis exposure
  - Adenocarcinoma
  - Sarcomas
- Metastases
- Endometriosis

PATHOLOGY

General Features

- Etiology
  - Risk factors
    - Cigarette smoking (most significant risk factor)
    - Radiation exposure, aniline dyes
    - Chemical carcinogens
    - Chronic UTI
  - High daily fluid intake (> 2.5 L) found to be protective

Staging, Grading, & Classification

- Most important prognostic factor: Depth of invasion of primary tumor
  - Primary tumor (T)
    - Ta: Noninvasive papillary carcinoma
    - Tis: Carcinoma in situ
    - T1: Invasion into subepithelial tissue
    - T2: Invasion into muscularis propria
    - T3: Invasion into perivesical tissue
    - T4: Invasion of adjacent organs, including prostate, seminal vesicles, uterus, vagina, pelvic wall
  - Regional lymph nodes (N)
    - N0: No lymph node metastasis
    - N1: Single lymph node metastasis in pelvis
    - N2: Multiple lymph node metastasis in pelvis
    - N3: Lymph node metastasis to common iliac nodes
  - Distant metastasis (M)
    - M0: No distant metastasis
    - M1: Distant metastasis
- **Stage I**: T1, N0, M0
- **Stage II:** T2, N0, M0
- **Stage III:** T3 or T4 (without pelvic/abdominal wall involvement), N0, M0
- **Stage IV:** T4 (with pelvic/abdominal wall invasion) **or** M1 with any T, any N

CLINICAL ISSUES

Presentation

- Most common signs/symptoms
  - Typical presentation is painless hematuria
    - 10-20% of patients with gross painless hematuria eventually diagnosed with bladder cancer
  - Can present with voiding symptoms
    - Frequency
    - Urgency
- Other signs/symptoms
  - Pain in flank, suprapubic, and abdominal areas suspicious for tumor invasion/metastases
  - Constitutional symptoms signify advanced disease

Demographics

- Age
  - Usually older adults (55-80 years)
  - Median age at diagnosis: 69 years
- Gender
  - M:F = 4:1
- Ethnicity
  - Caucasians:African Americans = 2:1
- Epidemiology
  - In USA: ~ 75,000 new cases and 16,000 deaths every year
  - Worldwide: 386,000 new cases of bladder cancer in 2008

Natural History & Prognosis

- From 1975 to 1996, 5-year survival increased slightly from 75% to 81%
  - Most patients have recurrences

Treatment

- Early stage
  - Transurethral resection of bladder tumor (TURBT)
  - Intravesical chemotherapy
- Late stage
  - Radical cystectomy
  - Neoadjuvant chemotherapy
  - Nephroureterectomy for renal pelvis/ureter tumors

DIAGNOSTIC CHECKLIST

Consider

- F-18 FDG PET/CT
  - Best used for detection of metastases
  - Diuretic protocol shown to significantly improve primary tumor detection, staging, and surveillance
  - Important to evaluate muscle-invasive disease; high likelihood of metastases
- Tc-99m bone scan
  - Bone metastases present in only 3% of patients at diagnosis, but risk increases with ↑ stage
  - Not for use in routine surveillance

SELECTED REFERENCES

1. Nayak B et al: Diuretic 18F-FDG PET/CT imaging for detection and locoregional staging of urinary bladder cancer: prospective evaluation of a novel technique. Eur J Nucl Med Mol Imaging. 40(3):386-93, 2013
2. Anjos DA et al: 18F-FDG PET/CT delayed images after diuretic for restaging invasive bladder cancer. J Nucl Med. 48(5):764-70, 2007
3. Setty BN et al: State-of-the-art cross-sectional imaging in bladder cancer. Curr Probl Diagn Radiol. 36(2):83-96, 2007
4. Jana S et al: Nuclear medicine studies of the prostate, testes, and bladder. Semin Nucl Med. 36(1):51-72, 2006
5. Kamel EM et al: Forced diuresis improves the diagnostic accuracy of 18F-FDG PET in abdominopelvic malignancies. J Nucl Med. 47(11):1803-7, 2006
6. Liu IJ et al: Evaluation of fluorodeoxyglucose positron emission tomography imaging in metastatic transitional cell carcinoma with and without prior chemotherapy. Urol Int. 77(1):69-75, 2006
7. Drieskens O et al: FDG-PET for preoperative staging of bladder cancer. Eur J Nucl Med Mol Imaging. 32(12):1412-7, 2005

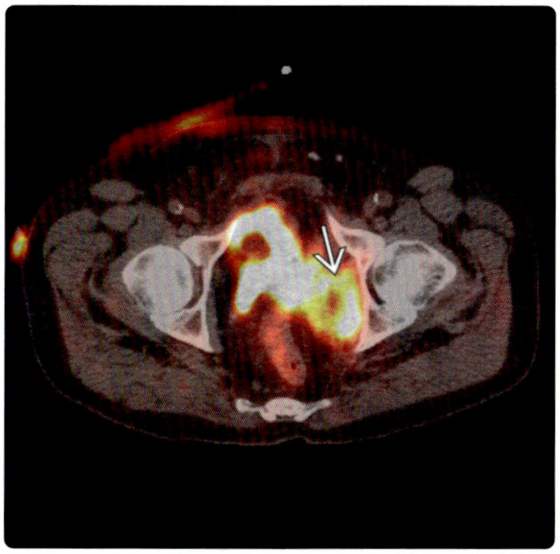
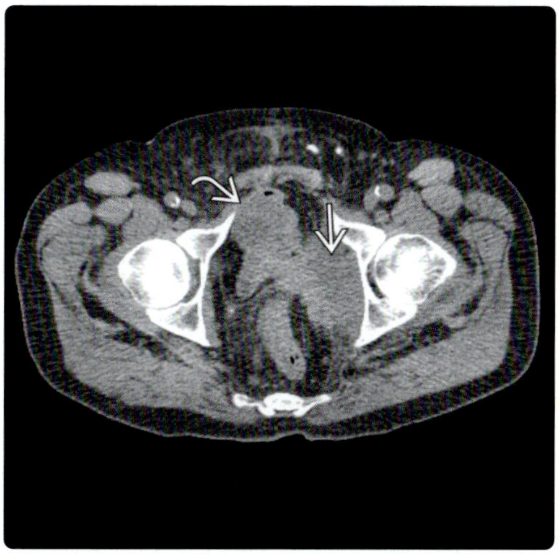

(Left) *Axial F-18 FDG PET/CT of a 53-year-old man with recurrent TCC shows a large, hypermetabolic soft tissue mass in the left anatomic pelvis* → *consistent with malignancy.* **(Right)** *Corresponding axial CT shows the soft tissue mass* →*. This patient had a prior TURBT and construction of a neobladder* ↪*.*

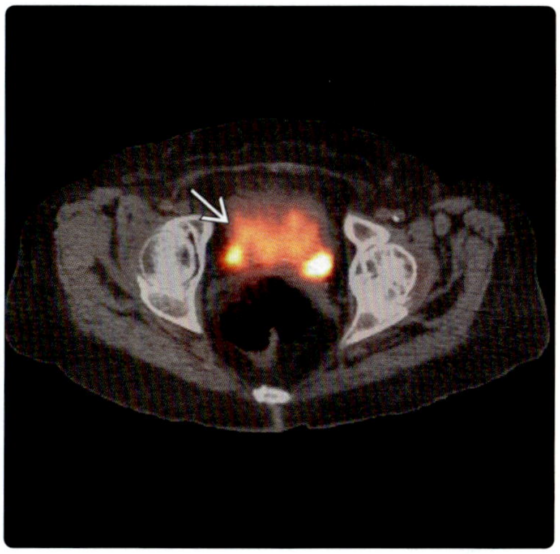
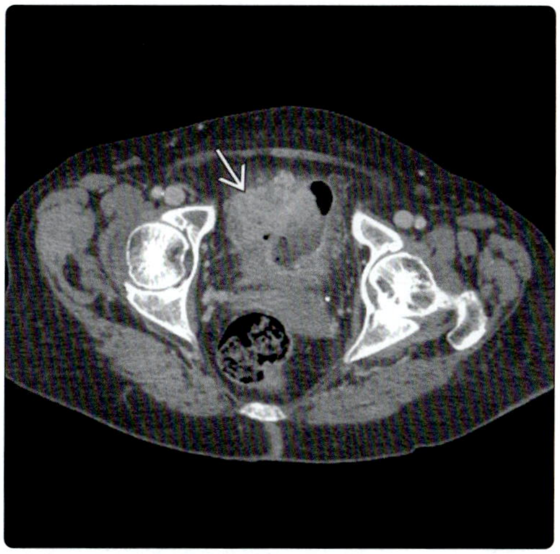

(Left) *Axial F-18 FDG PET/CT of an 86-year-old woman shows an infiltrative bladder mass involving the anterolateral wall* →*. Renally excreted F-18 FDG limits visualization.* **(Right)** *Corresponding axial CECT in the same patient better delineates the extent of this mass* →*.*

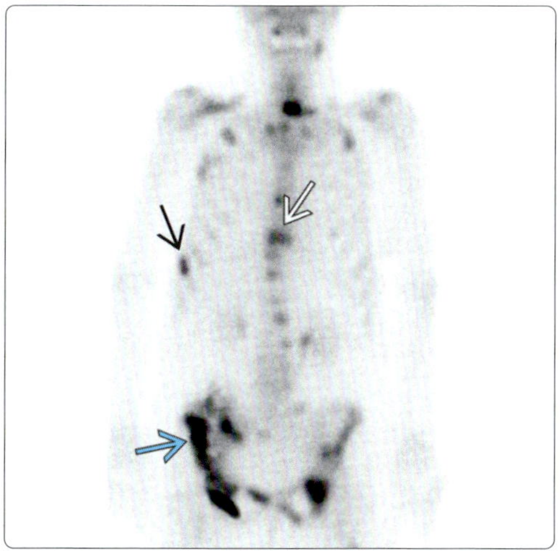
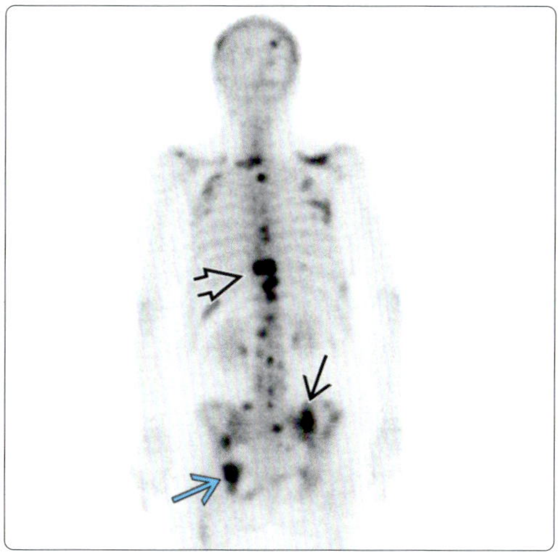

(Left) *Anterior bone scan of a 67-year-old woman with metastatic transitional cell carcinoma shows multifocal sites of increased uptake involving the vertebrae* →*, ribs* →*, and right hemipelvis* →*.* **(Right)** *Posterior bone scan in the same patient shows sites at risk of pathologic fracture in the mid thoracic spine* ⇨*, right sacroiliac joint* →*, and left acetabulum* →*.*

Ewing Sarcoma

KEY FACTS

TERMINOLOGY

- Majority have translocation between EWSR1 (chromosome 22) and ETS transcription factor

IMAGING

- Destructive osseous lesion with associated soft tissue mass
- Femur is single most common site (~ 20%)
- > 85% in pelvis, extremities and ribs
- Askin tumor: Aggressive chest wall/pleural mass with associated effusion
- Tc-99m MDP bone scan shows increased uptake in tumor in all phases, but is not adequate for local staging (poor sensitivity for "skip lesions")
- Tc-99m MDP bone scan 71% sensitive for osseous metastases (may miss lytic metastases)
- FDG PET/CT
  - Defines primary tumor better than MDP bone scan
  - Superior to bone scintigraphy for identification of osseous metastatic disease (may miss sclerotic metastases)
  - Useful to assess response to neoadjuvant chemotherapy
  - 90% accurate at detecting recurrence
- MR best characterizes extent (intraosseous and soft tissue) of disease and identifies "skip lesions"
- Chest CT for staging/identification of lung metastases

TOP DIFFERENTIAL DIAGNOSES

- Osteosarcoma

CLINICAL ISSUES

- 2nd most common primary malignant bone tumor in children and young adults
- Presence of metastases at diagnosis = key prognostic indicator

(Left) *Lateral radiograph in a 17-year-old male with right mid diaphyseal femur Ewing sarcoma shows an expansile, permeative, destructive lesion → with aggressive margins (wide zone of transition) and aggressive periosteal reaction (Codman triangles) →.* **(Right)** *Whole-body Tc-99m MDP bone scan in the same patient shows radiotracer uptake associated with the femoral Ewing sarcoma →. Foci of abnormal uptake in the left femoral neck → and left aspect of the T6 vertebra reflect metastatic disease →.*

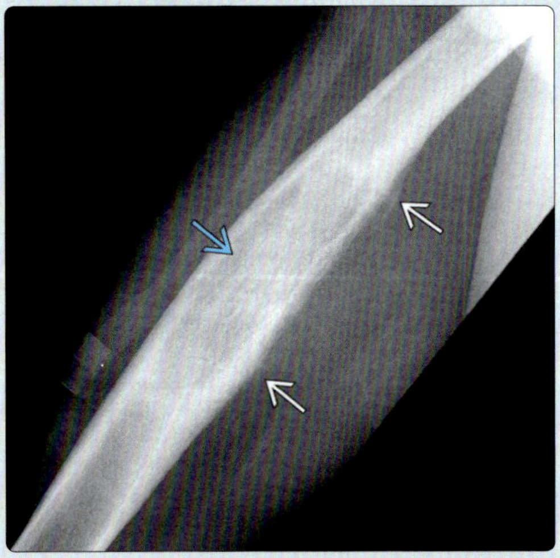

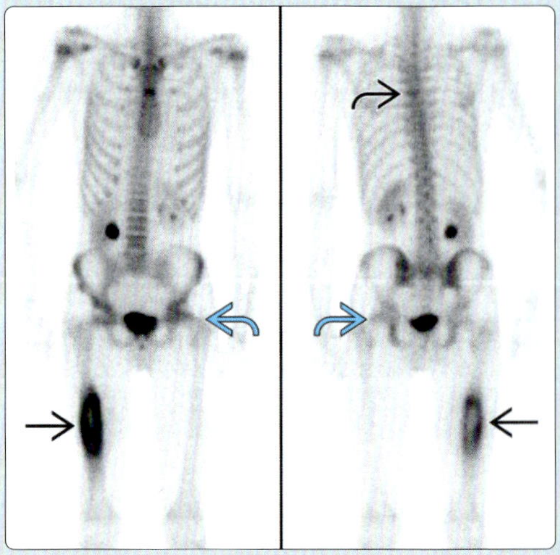

(Left) *FDG PET in a 20-year-old man with right upper arm extraosseous Ewing sarcoma shows heterogeneous FDG uptake throughout the soft tissue mass →. There is no abnormal FDG uptake in the underlying humerus.* **(Right)** *Axial T1-weighted C+ MR in the same patient shows a heterogeneously enhancing mass in the soft tissue of the posterior arm →. Tumor extends along the superficial fascia of the underlying muscle →.*

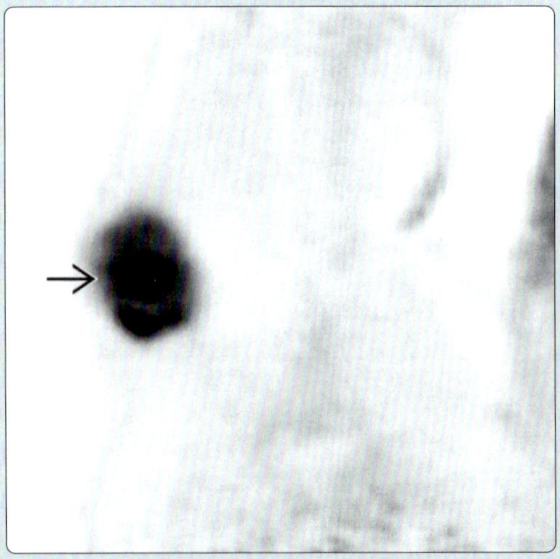

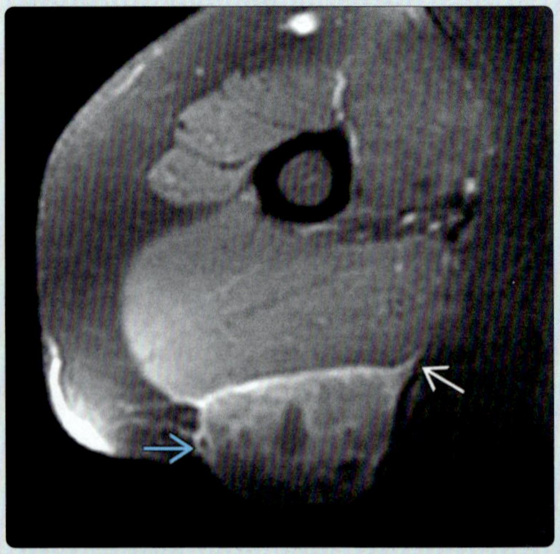

TERMINOLOGY

Abbreviations

- Ewing sarcoma (ES)

Definitions

- Ewing sarcoma family of tumors
  - Osseous Ewing sarcoma
  - Extraosseous Ewing sarcoma
  - Askin tumor
  - Primitive neuroectodermal tumor (PNET)
- Malignant small round cell tumor
- Majority have translocation between EWSR1 (chromosome 22) and ETS transcription factor

IMAGING

General Features

- Best diagnostic clue
  - Osseous ES
    - Destructive lesion with associated soft tissue mass
      - Generally less mineralized than osteosarcoma
    - FDG-avid osseous and soft tissue components
    - Radionuclide (Tc-99m MDP, gallium-67) uptake in soft tissue mass and reactive bone
  - Askin tumor
    - Aggressive chest wall/pleural mass with associated effusion
    - Rib destruction in majority
- Location
  - Osseous ES
    - Femur single most common site (~ 20%)
    - > 85% in pelvis, extremities, and ribs
    - Lower > upper extremity
    - Long bones
      - Metadiaphyseal > diaphyseal
      - Proximal > distal
    - Originate in medullary canal, spread outward
  - Extraosseous ES
    - Paravertebral and lower extremity most common (~ 30% each)
  - Askin tumor
    - Chest wall/pleura
  - Metastases (15-30% at diagnosis)
    - Lung
    - Bone
    - Liver

Nuclear Medicine Findings

- Bone scan
  - Primary osseous ES and Askin tumor
    - Increased uptake in tumor in all phases
    - Greatest uptake on delayed phase at sites of mineralization or reactive bone formation
      - Soft tissue mass may only show low-level uptake on delayed phase
      - Areas of photopenia may reflect more aggressive tumor or tumor necrosis
    - Not adequate for local staging; poor sensitivity for "skip lesions"
    - May show decreasing uptake on delayed phase with response to therapy
  - Primary extraosseous ES
    - Radionuclide uptake more apparent in flow and pool phases
    - Uptake in delayed phase related to tumoral calcification or adjacent osseous remodeling
  - Metastases (71% sensitive)
    - Foci of uptake on delayed phase
    - May miss purely lytic metastases
- **FDG PET/CT**
  - Primary
    - Intraosseous and soft tissue components of tumor all show uptake
    - Better defines local extent of tumor than MDP bone scan
    - Mineralization/bone formation and soft tissue mass visible by CT
    - Useful to assess response to neoadjuvant chemotherapy
      - Various measures described in literature: Percent change in SUV, maximal SUV thresholds, reduction in metabolic tumor volume (MTV)
      - Decrease in soft tissue mass suggests response to therapy
    - 90% accurate in detecting recurrence
  - Metastases
    - Superior to bone scintigraphy for identification of osseous metastatic disease
    - May miss sclerotic metastases

Imaging Recommendations

- Best imaging tool
  - Local disease/primary tumor
    - Radiography: First step in work-up of suspected bone lesion
    - MR: Best characterizes local extent (intraosseous and soft tissue), identifies noncontiguous medullary lesions in same bone as primary ("skip lesions")
    - FDG PET/CT: Defines primary tumor better than MDP bone scan, can be used to assess response to therapy
  - Metastases
    - CT for lung metastases
    - FDG PET/CT for metastatic disease outside of lung
  - Surveillance
    - Radiograph or chest CT for lung recurrence
    - FDG PET/CT for local and distant recurrence: Does not suffer from hardware artifacts
    - MR can be used for local recurrence but may be limited by hardware artifact

DIFFERENTIAL DIAGNOSIS

Malignant Bone Tumors

- Osteosarcoma
  - Generally more mineralized except when aggressive
- Primary bone lymphoma
  - Generally older patients
  - Similar permeative appearance in bone
  - Much less soft tissue mass
- Mesenchymal chondrosarcoma (rare)

- Predominately lytic ± chondral calcifications
- Acute leukemia

Benign Bone Lesions

- Eosinophilic granuloma
- Giant cell tumor

Osteomyelitis

- Similar systemic symptoms (fever, elevated erythrocyte sedimentation rate can occur with ES)
- Subperiosteal fluid collections, sequestrum, substantial inflammatory response favor osteomyelitis

Fracture

- Healing fracture can occasionally have bizarre appearance (follow-up radiograph or MR can help distinguish)
- Take care not to miss an underlying lesion leading to pathologic fracture

Bone Metastases (Rhabdomyosarcoma, Neuroblastoma, etc.)

- Generally multifocal
- ± history of primary malignancy

PATHOLOGY

General Features

- Etiology
  - Neuroectodermal origin
- Genetics
  - 90% have translocation between chromosome ESWR1 (22q12) and one of the ETS transcription factors
    - ESWR1-FLI1 (11q24) is most common (85%)
    - ESWR1-ERG (21q22) is 2nd most common

Gross Pathologic & Surgical Features

- Osseous ES
  - Gray-white-tan, soft with osseous and soft tissue components

Microscopic Features

- 3 subtypes
  - Classical ES (majority)
    - Small round blue cells
  - Primitive neuroectodermal tumor (PNET)
    - Homer Wright rosettes
  - Atypical ES
- Immunohistochemistry
  - Membranous staining by CD99: Sensitive but not specific
  - Nuclear staining by FLI-1: Sensitive but not specific
  - Markers of neural differentiation: Indicative of PNET

CLINICAL ISSUES

Presentation

- Most common signs/symptoms
  - Pain, swelling at tumor site
- Other signs/symptoms
  - Palpable mass
  - Constitutional symptoms (fever, fatigue, weight loss)
  - Pathologic fracture (rare)

Demographics

- Age
  - Osseous ES
    - Highest incidence in 2nd decade
    - Rare < 5 years or > 30 years of age
  - Extraosseous ES
    - Majority between 20 months and 30 years
  - Askin tumor
    - 4 months to 20 years
- Ethnicity
  - Majority (95%) of cases occur in Caucasians
  - Rare in African Americans
- Epidemiology
  - Osseous ES
    - 2nd most common primary malignant bone tumor in children and young adults
    - 1-3 cases per 1 million children per year
    - 3% of pediatric cancers

Natural History & Prognosis

- Metastases in 15-30% at diagnosis
- Presence of metastases at diagnosis = key prognostic indicator
  - Overall survival 63-82% for localized disease
  - Overall survival 25-39% for metastatic disease
- Prognosis for Askin tumor worse than rest of Ewing sarcoma family
- Poor prognostic factors
  - < 90% necrosis with neoadjuvant chemotherapy
  - Tumor > 8 cm
  - Pelvic tumor
  - Older age at presentation
  - Elevated serum lactate dehydrogenase (LDH)
- Recurrence
  - Majority occur within 5 years
    - Prognosis following local recurrence is poor (10% survival)

Treatment

- Neoadjuvant chemotherapy, followed by local control, followed by adjuvant chemotherapy
  - > 90% necrosis considered good response
  - Surgery favored over radiation for local control

SELECTED REFERENCES

1. Choi EY et al: Ewing sarcoma. Semin Diagn Pathol. 31(1):39-47, 2014
2. Cote GM et al: Update in treatment and targets in Ewing sarcoma. Hematol Oncol Clin North Am. 27(5):1007-19, 2013
3. Grohar PJ et al: Prospects and challenges for the development of new therapies for Ewing sarcoma. Pharmacol Ther. 137(2):216-24, 2013
4. Murphey MD et al: From the radiologic pathology archives: ewing sarcoma family of tumors: radiologic-pathologic correlation. Radiographics. 33(3):803-31, 2013
5. Ross KA et al: The biology of ewing sarcoma. ISRN Oncol. 2013:759725, 2013
6. Treglia G et al: Diagnostic accuracy of ^{18}F-FDG-PET and PET/CT in patients with Ewing sarcoma family tumours: a systematic review and a meta-analysis. Skeletal Radiol. 41(3):249-56, 2012
7. Eary JF et al: Imaging in sarcoma. J Nucl Med. 52(12):1903-13, 2011
8. Maheshwari AV et al: Ewing sarcoma family of tumors. J Am Acad Orthop Surg. 18(2):94-107, 2010

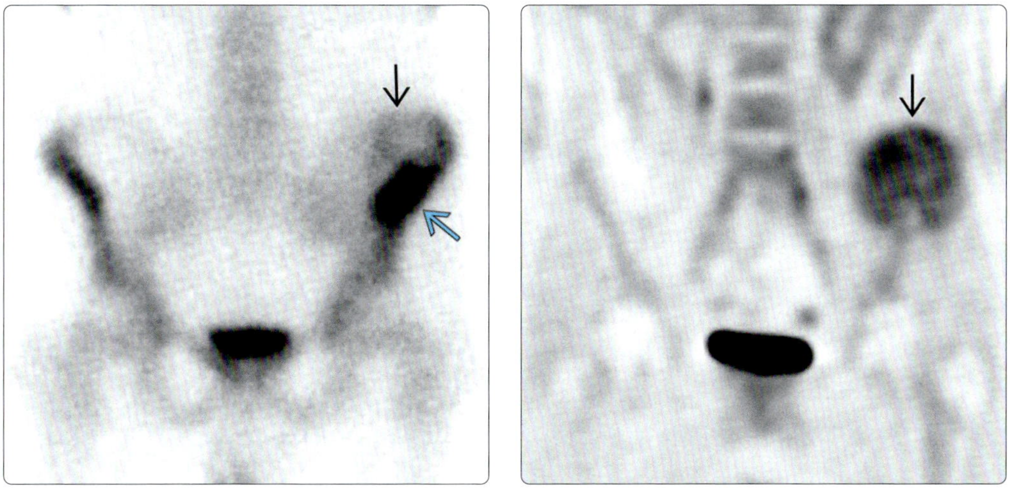

(Left) *Anterior image of the pelvis from a Tc-99m MDP bone scan in a 22-year-old man with left iliac Ewing sarcoma shows uptake in the anterior ileum related to reactive bone formation* ➡*. There is more subtle uptake of radiotracer in the tumor mass* ➡*.* **(Right)** *FDG PET in the same patient shows heterogeneous uptake of FDG throughout the tumor mass* ➡*. FDG PET more clearly defines the tumor than does the MDP bone scan.*

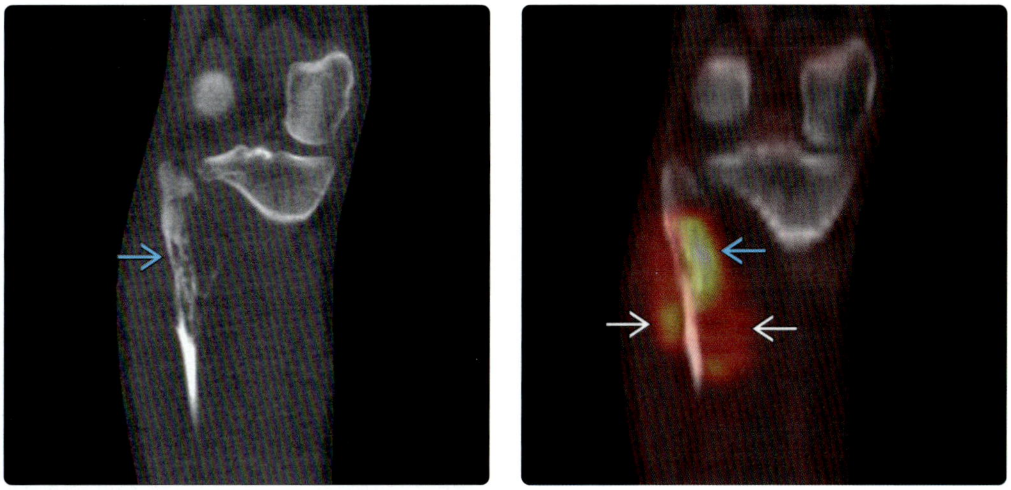

(Left) *Coronally reformatted CT in a 17-year-old male with right proximal fibular Ewing sarcoma shows an expansile, destructive lesion in the proximal fibula* ➡*.* **(Right)** *Fused coronal PET/CT in the same patient shows uptake of FDG in the intraosseous* ➡ *and soft tissue components of the tumor* ➡*.*

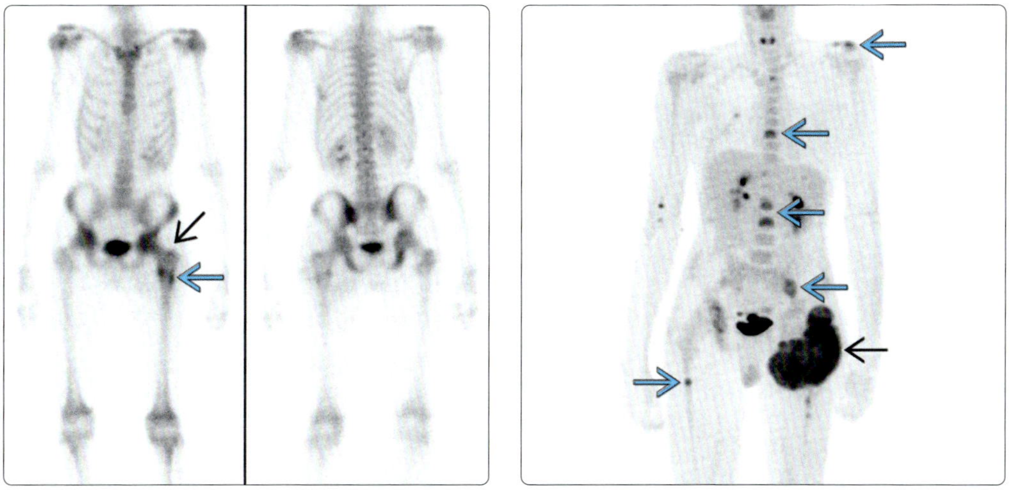

(Left) *Whole-body Tc-99m MDP bone scan in a 20-year-old man with left proximal femoral Ewing sarcoma shows diffusely increased uptake in the proximal femur* ➡ *with more focal uptake in reactive bone at the level of the proximal metadiaphysis* ➡*. There are no findings of osseous metastatic disease.* **(Right)** *MIP FDG PET in the same patient shows FDG uptake in a large tumor mass in the left thigh* ➡ *with multiple foci of osseous metastatic disease* ➡ *that were not visible by bone scan.*

KEY FACTS

TERMINOLOGY

- Embryonic tumor derived from primitive neural crest cells along peripheral sympathetic chain

IMAGING

- MIBG avidity is key imaging finding (≥ 90% specificity for disease)
- I-123 MIBG favored over I-131 MIBG due to dose profile, resolution, imaging characteristics
- Pretreat with SSKI and hold interfering medications (many) prior to MIBG imaging
- MIBG uptake in bone is **never** normal (indicative of metastatic disease)
- Consider SPECT ± CT to clarify planar imaging findings or better define disease
- Tc-99m MDP bone scan as good as MIBG to determine ± metastatic disease but will not identify all lesions seen by MIBG
- FDG uptake seen in most neuroblastomas
- CT or MR for assessment of tumor relationship to anatomic structures

PATHOLOGY

- Now staged based on INRGSS: Presurgical staging scheme based on extent of disease and image-defined risk factors
- "Favorable" or "unfavorable" histology based on degree of neuroblast differentiation, nuclear morphology (mitosis-karyorrhexis index), age
- Tumors with MYCN amplification are more aggressive with poorer prognosis

CLINICAL ISSUES

- ~ 50% have distant metastases at diagnosis
- Treatment depends on INRG risk strata: Ranges from observation, to surgery only, to chemotherapy plus surgery, to intensive multimodality therapies

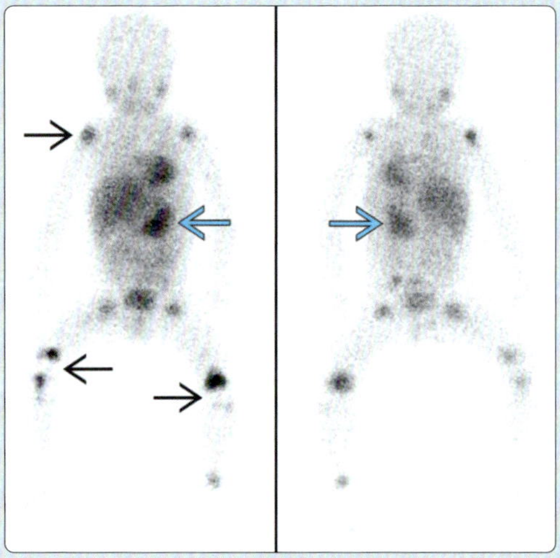

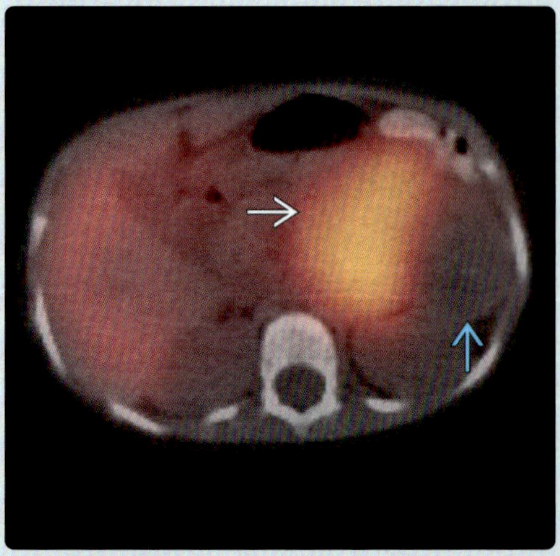

(Left) *Anterior and posterior projection images from a whole-body I-123 MIBG scan in a 3-year-old boy with metastatic neuroblastoma show an MIBG-avid left upper quadrant mass → and multiple sites of osseous metastatic disease, predominately in the long bone metaphyses →.* **(Right)** *Axial I-123 MIBG SPECT/CT in the same patient shows uptake in part of the left upper quadrant mass →. A necrotic portion of the mass is non-MIBG-avid →.*

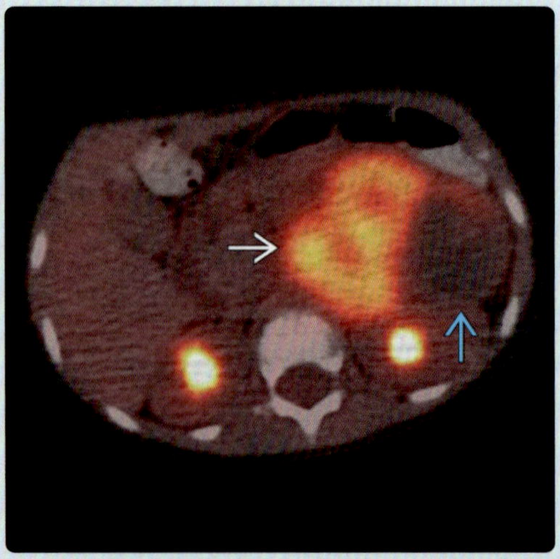

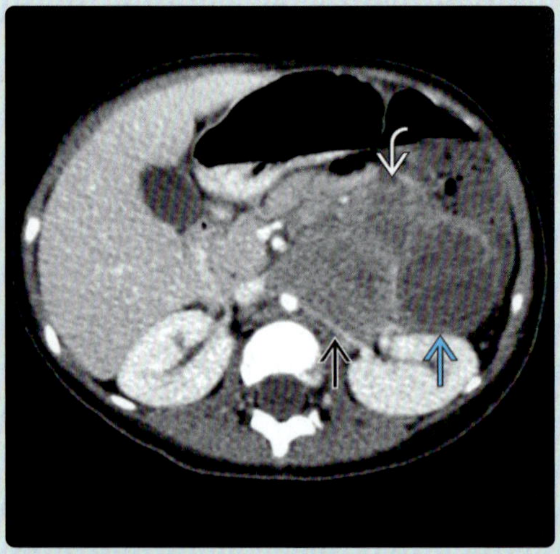

(Left) *Axial fused FDG PET/CT in the same patient shows a similar pattern of uptake in the left upper quadrant mass to what was seen on the MIBG study. FDG uptake is present in the medial solid portion of the mass → without substantial uptake in the lateral necrotic portion →.* **(Right)** *Axial CT in the same patient shows the infiltrative retroperitoneal mass → that encases the renal arteries →. The necrotic portion of the tumor is hypoattenuating →.*

TERMINOLOGY

Definitions

- Neuroblastoma: Embryonic tumor derived from primitive neural crest cells along peripheral sympathetic chain

IMAGING

General Features

- Best diagnostic clue
  - I-123 metaiodobenzylguanidine (MIBG) scintigraphy
    - Suprarenal mass with typical calcifications or infiltrative retroperitoneal mass that shows I-123 MIBG avidity
- Location
  - Primary tumor: Along sympathetic chain
    - ~ 30% adrenal medulla
    - ~ 60% abdominal paraspinal ganglia
  - Metastases: Bone, lymph nodes, liver, lung, brain, soft tissue
- Morphology
  - Highly variable depending on tumor location
  - Tends to infiltrate and surround; extends into neural foramina, encases vessels
  - Variable calcification, tends to further calcify with therapy

Nuclear Medicine Findings

- Bone scan
  - Primarily for identification of osseous metastatic disease
    - May see soft tissue uptake or uptake in calcification of primary tumor (~ 75%)
  - Metastases appear as foci of radiotracer uptake, often at metaphysis
  - As good as MIBG for overall diagnosis of presence or absence of metastatic disease
  - Less sensitive at individual lesion level
  - May be positive when MIBG scan is negative
- **I-123 MIBG scintigraphy**
  - ≥ 90% specificity for disease
  - MIBG
    - Structurally similar to norepinephrine, taken up by neuroendocrine transporter
    - Normal distribution: Salivary glands, thyroid, myocardium, liver, renal collecting systems and bladder (excretion), bowel (excretion)
    - May see uptake in normal adrenal gland after unilateral adrenalectomy
  - False-negatives: Interfering medications, overlap with physiologic structures (planar imaging), small foci of disease, tumor maturation
  - Imaging scoring systems have been defined: Predictive value still being investigated
- **I-131 MIBG scintigraphy**
  - Generally only performed post I-131 therapy (due to dose considerations)
  - Additional physiologic uptake seen in basal ganglia and cerebellum
- **FDG PET/CT**
  - FDG uptake seen in most neuroblastomas
  - Clinical role uncertain: May have value in MIBG negative cases

Imaging Recommendations

- Best imaging tool
  - MIBG for assessment of disease burden and activity (highly specific)
  - CT or MR for assessment of tumor relationship to anatomic structures
- Protocol advice
  - I-123 label favored over I-131 due to dose profile, resolution, imaging characteristics
  - Patient preparation
    - SSKI pretreatment to protect thyroid from free radioiodide
    - Interfering medications (long list) must be withdrawn
  - Scan technique
    - Medium energy collimation reduces image noise, increases lesion conspicuity
    - Generally only need to image at 24 hours after radiopharmaceutical administration
      - 48 hour imaging for problem solving: Higher tumor:background ratio, normally further clearance from background tissue
      - SPECT can obviate 48 hour imaging
    - Spot lateral images of head/neck helpful to define calvarial/facial disease
    - Consider SPECT ± CT to clarify planar imaging findings or better define disease

DIFFERENTIAL DIAGNOSIS

Other MIBG-Positive Lesions

- Ganglioneuroblastoma: Part of spectrum of neural crest tumors, intermediate malignancy
- Ganglioneuroma: Part of spectrum of neural crest tumors, most benign
- Pheochromocytoma
- Paraganglioma
- Adrenal hyperplasia

Wilms Tumor

- Arises from kidney
- Tends to push rather than infiltrate and surround normal anatomic structures

Multifocal/Diffuse Bone Lesions

- Metastatic rhabdomyosarcoma
- Langerhans cell histiocytosis (LCH)
- Leukemia

Lymphoma

- Generally older population

PATHOLOGY

General Features

- Etiology
  - Arise from primitive neural crest cells along peripheral sympathetic chain
- Genetics
  - Extensive molecular heterogeneity without single causative mutation

  - Family history in 1-2%
- Important genetic drivers
  - MYCN: Transcription factor
  - Anaplastic lymphoma kinase (ALK) activation: Receptor tyrosine kinase
  - Paired-like homeobox 2B (PHOX2B): Transcription factor
- Chromosomal abnormalities
  - Ploidy: ~ 55% of neuroblastoma are triploid/near-triploid
  - 1q deletions: ~ 30% of neuroblastoma
  - 11q deletions: ~ 40% of neuroblastoma

Staging, Grading, & Classification

- Previously staged based on International Neuroblastoma Staging System (INSS): Surgical staging scheme reflective of disease extent
- Now staged based on International Neuroblastoma Risk Group Staging System (INRGSS): Presurgical staging scheme based on extent of disease and image-defined risk factors
  - L1: Localized tumor without imaging-defined risk factors
  - L2: Locoregional tumor with imaging-defined risk factor(s)
  - M: Distant metastatic disease
  - MS: Metastatic disease limited to skin, liver &/or bone marrow in children > 18 months
- INRG pretreatment classification scheme: Very low risk, low risk, intermediate risk, high risk
  - Based on INRG stage, age, histology, tumor differentiation, MYCN status, 11q loss of heterozygosity, ploidy

Gross Pathologic & Surgical Features

- Circumscribed or infiltrative mass without a capsule
- Soft, tan, ± hemorrhage and calcification

Microscopic Features

- Neuroblasts in varying degrees of schwannian stroma
- "Favorable" or "unfavorable" histology based on degree of neuroblast differentiation, nuclear morphology (mitosis-karyorrhexis index), age

CLINICAL ISSUES

Presentation

- Most common signs/symptoms
  - Abdominal mass/distention
  - Constitutional symptoms: Fever, weight loss, fatigue

Demographics

- Age
  - Median at diagnosis ~ 20 months
    - 90% < 5 years, 30% within 1st year
- Gender
  - Slight male preponderance
- Ethnicity
  - Slight preponderance in Caucasians
- Epidemiology
  - Most common extracranial solid tumor in children
  - 8-10% of all childhood cancers
  - ~ 10 cases per million children (0-14) per year in USA
    - 500-700 new cases per year
  - ~ 50% of cases are high risk at presentation
  - ~ 50% have distant metastases at diagnosis

Natural History & Prognosis

- Broad spectrum of behavior ranging from spontaneous regression, maturation to benign ganglioneuroma, or aggressive fatal metastatic disease
- INRG risk strata reflect prognosis
  - > 90% event-free survival (EFS) in non-high-risk patients
  - 78% vs. 90% 5-year EFS in stage L2 vs. L1 disease
- Degree of tumor differentiation important prognostic factor
- 15% of cancer-related deaths in children

Treatment

- Depends on INRG risk strata: Ranges from observation, to surgery only, to chemotherapy plus surgery, to intensive multimodality therapies including chemotherapy, surgery, radiation, stem-cell transplant, I-131 MIBG therapy, and immunotherapy

DIAGNOSTIC CHECKLIST

Consider

- FDG PET/CT when MIBG scan is negative

SELECTED REFERENCES

1. Louis CU et al: Neuroblastoma: Molecular Pathogenesis and Therapy. Annu Rev Med. ePub, 2014
2. Mueller WP et al: Nuclear medicine and multimodality imaging of pediatric neuroblastoma. Pediatr Radiol. 43(4):418-27, 2013
3. Davidoff AM: Neuroblastoma. Semin Pediatr Surg. 21(1):2-14, 2012
4. Colon NC et al: Neuroblastoma. Adv Pediatr. 58(1):297-311, 2011
5. Cohn SL et al: The International Neuroblastoma Risk Group (INRG) classification system: an INRG Task Force report. J Clin Oncol. 27(2):289-97, 2009
6. Monclair T et al: The International Neuroblastoma Risk Group (INRG) staging system: an INRG Task Force report. J Clin Oncol. 27(2):298-303, 2009
7. Ilias I et al: New functional imaging modalities for chromaffin tumors, neuroblastomas and ganglioneuromas. Trends Endocrinol Metab. 16(2):66-72, 2005
8. Kushner BH: Neuroblastoma: a disease requiring a multitude of imaging studies. J Nucl Med. 45(7):1172-88, 2004
9. Juweid ME et al: 111In-pentetreotide versus bone scintigraphy in the detection of bony metastases of neuroblastoma. Nucl Med Commun. 23(10):983-9, 2002
10. Lonergan GJ et al: Neuroblastoma, ganglioneuroblastoma, and ganglioneuroma: radiologic-pathologic correlation. Radiographics. 22(4):911-34, 2002
11. Minard V et al: Adverse outcome of infants with metastatic neuroblastoma, MYCN amplification and/or bone lesions: results of the French society of pediatric oncology. Br J Cancer. 83(8):973-9, 2000
12. Perel Y et al: Clinical impact and prognostic value of metaiodobenzylguanidine imaging in children with metastatic neuroblastoma. J Pediatr Hematol Oncol. 21(1):13-8, 1999
13. Shulkin BL et al: Current concepts on the diagnostic use of MIBG in children. J Nucl Med. 39(4):679-88, 1998
14. Leung A et al: Specificity of radioiodinated MIBG for neural crest tumors in childhood. J Nucl Med. 38(9):1352-7, 1997
15. Shulkin BL et al: Iodine-131-metaiodobenzylguanidine and bone scintigraphy for the detection of neuroblastoma. J Nucl Med. 33(10):1735-40, 1992

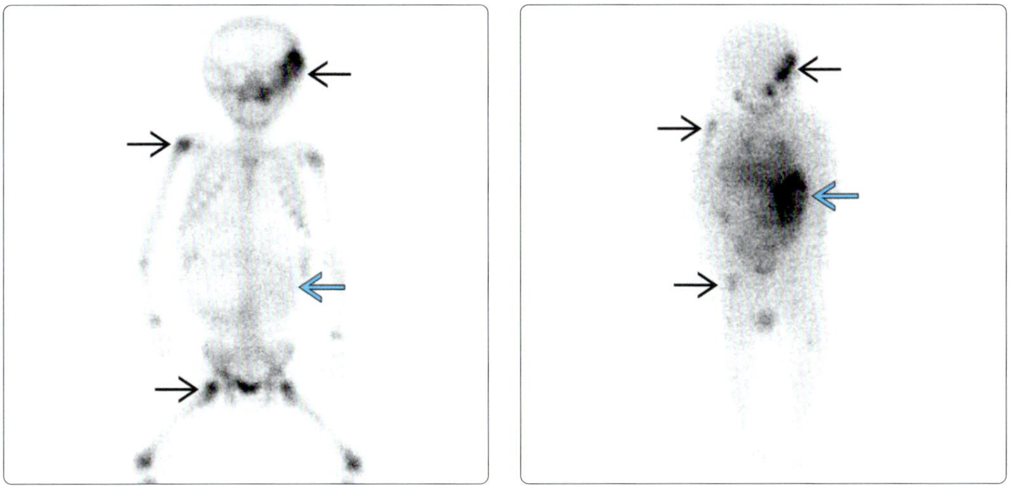

(Left) *Tc-99m MDP bone scan in a 14 month old with metastatic neuroblastoma shows multiple foci of abnormal radiotracer uptake due to metastatic disease →. There is faint uptake in a LUQ mass →.* **(Right)** *MIBG scan in the same patient shows abnormal uptake at the sites of osseous metastatic disease seen by Tc-99m bone scan → and at other sites not well seen by bone scan. The left upper quadrant mass → is better defined on this MIBG scan. Note the noise in this image obtained with a low-energy collimator.*

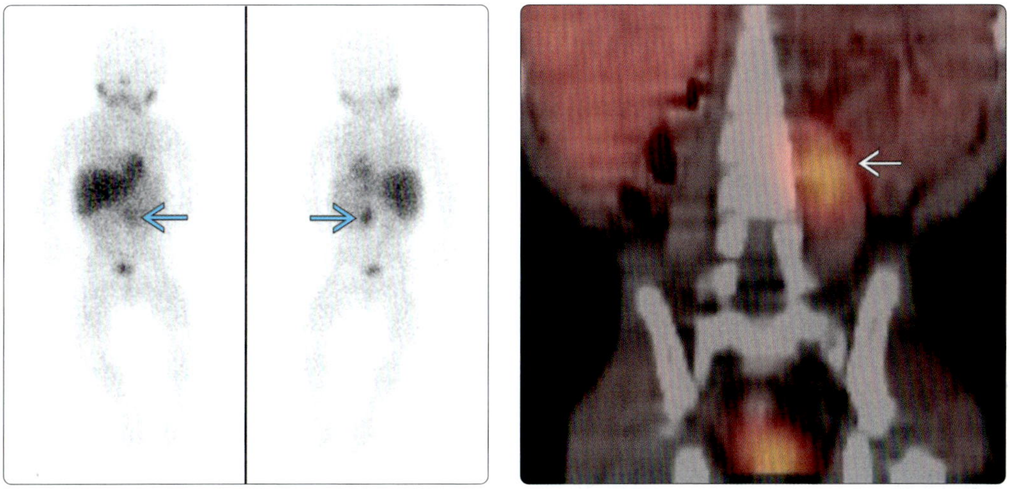

(Left) *Anterior and posterior whole-body images from an MIBG scan in a 11-month-old boy with left paraspinal neuroblastoma show focal left paraspinal uptake →. There is no metastatic disease.* **(Right)** *MIBG SPECT/CT in the same patient localizes the uptake to the patient's paraspinal mass →.*

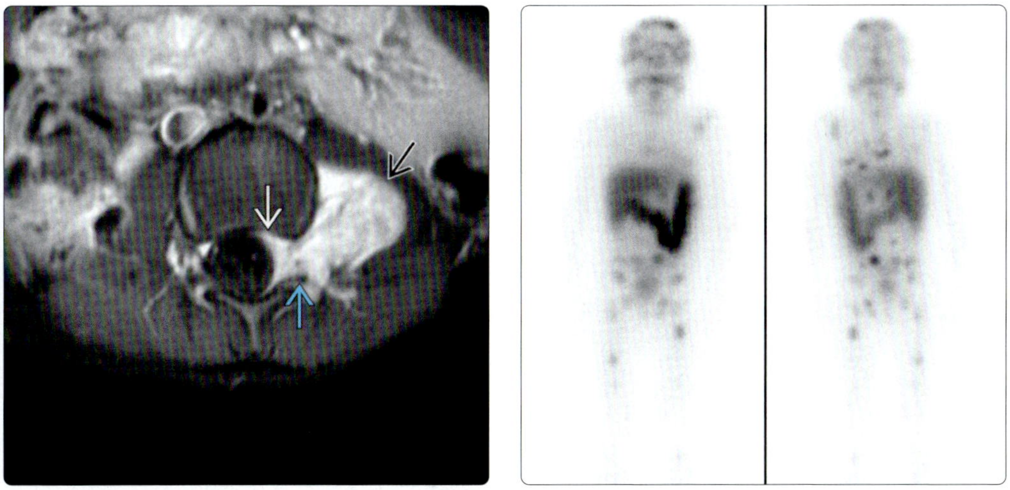

(Left) *Axial post-contrast fat-saturated T1-weighted MR in the same patient shows heterogeneous enhancement of the mass →, which infiltrates the neural foramen → and extends into the spinal canal →.* **(Right)** *Post-therapy I-131 MIBG scan in a 7-year-old girl with widely metastatic neuroblastoma shows numerous foci of abnormal MIBG uptake reflecting osseous metastatic disease. Note the decreased resolution due to the high-energy collimator and the haze caused by septal penetration.*

Osteosarcoma

KEY FACTS

TERMINOLOGY

- Primary malignant tumor of bone (mesenchymal origin) whose cells produce osteoid

IMAGING

- ~ 90% of conventional OS are metaphyseal
- Majority of OS (regardless of subtype) occur in femur (40-70%)
- FDG PET/CT better defines (relative to MDP bone scan) areas of tumor that are not producing substantial osteoid but may miss sclerotic metastases
- FDG PET/CT useful for therapy response assessment
- MR: Best characterizes tumor structure (e.g., identifying cystic spaces of telangiectatic OS), best assessment of local extent of disease, best assessment for skip metastases
- CT for screening for lung metastases

TOP DIFFERENTIAL DIAGNOSES

- Ewing sarcoma

PATHOLOGY

- Osteoid is most important histologic finding to make diagnosis of osteosarcoma

CLINICAL ISSUES

- Associated with periods of rapid growth
- Uncommonly occur in background of benign bone disease and can occur in prior radiation field
- Treatment is neoadjuvant chemotherapy, followed by local control and resection of lung metastases, followed by adjuvant chemotherapy
  - Response to chemotherapy (> 90% considered good) is most important prognostic factor
  - Limb salvage procedures favored for local control
- Osteosarcoma is radioresistant

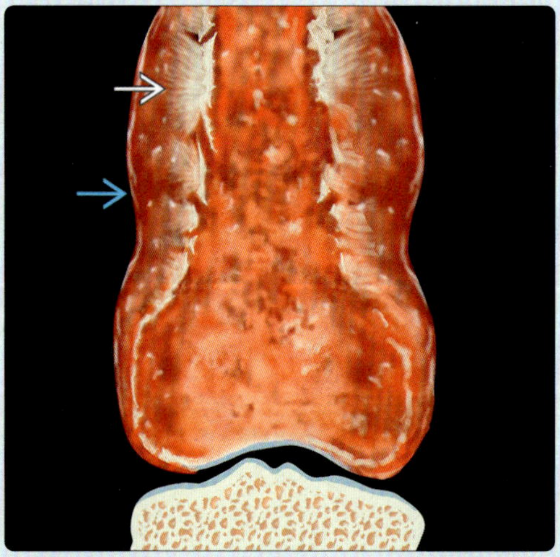

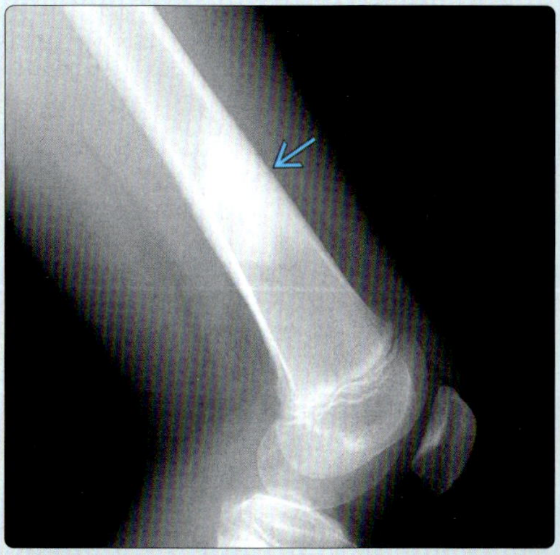

(Left) *Graphic of conventional osteosarcoma shows a large tumor centered in the distal femoral metaphysis (most common location for conventional osteosarcoma) and extending through the cortex into the soft tissue. Aggressive periosteal new bone formation is present.* **(Right)** *Lateral radiograph of the distal femur in a 13-year-old boy with left distal femoral conventional osteosarcoma shows a sclerotic mass centered in the metadiaphysis.*

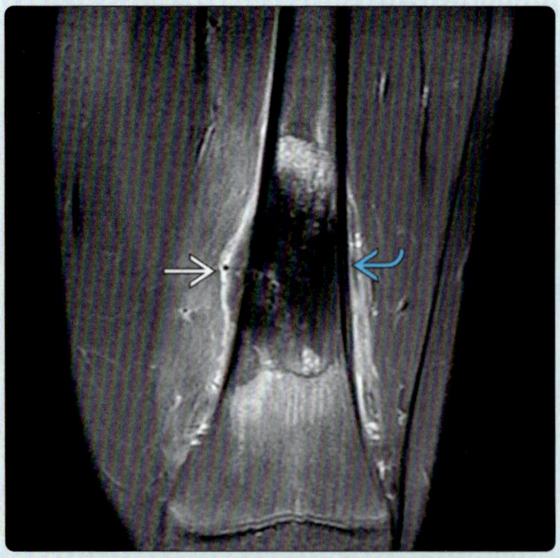

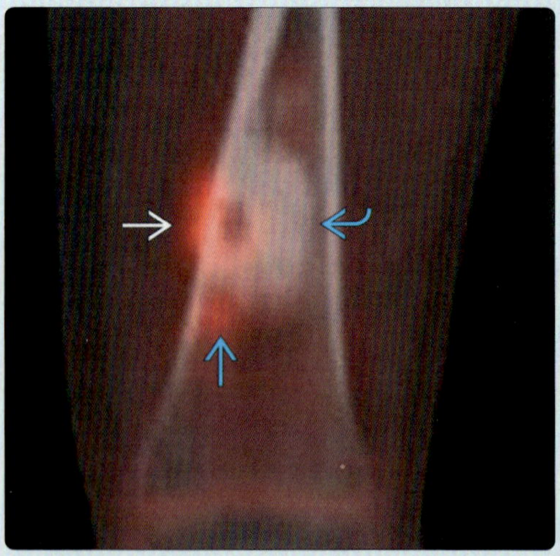

(Left) *Coronal STIR MR in the same patient shows an intramedullary tumor with extension through the medial cortex. Low signal within the tumor reflects the osteoid matrix seen on the radiograph.* **(Right)** *Fused FDG PET/CT in the same patient shows the osteoid tumor matrix with FDG uptake associated with both the intraosseous and soft tissue components of the tumor.*

TERMINOLOGY

Abbreviations

- Osteosarcoma (OS)

Synonyms

- Osteogenic sarcoma
- Telangiectatic osteosarcoma: Hemorrhagic OS, malignant bone aneurysm, aneurysmal bone cyst-like OS
- Low-grade central osteosarcoma: Low-grade intramedullary OS, well-differentiated intramedullary OS, low-grade intraosseous-type OS
- Parosteal osteosarcoma: Juxtacortical OS, juxtacortical low-grade OS, low-grade surface OS

Definitions

- Primary malignant tumor of bone (mesenchymal origin) whose cells produce osteoid
- Subtypes (World Health Organization)
  - Conventional osteosarcoma: Most common (~ 75%)
  - Telangiectatic osteosarcoma (5-7%)
  - Secondary osteosarcoma
  - Small-cell osteosarcoma (1-2%)
  - Low-grade central osteosarcoma (1-2%)
  - Surface osteosarcoma
    - Parosteal osteosarcoma (5%)
    - Periosteal osteosarcoma (1-2%)
    - High-grade surface type (1%)

Associated Syndromes

- Predisposition with
  - Retinoblastoma gene mutation
  - Li-Fraumeni syndrome
  - Rothmund-Thompson syndrome
  - Mutations of p53 and MDM2 (murine double minute oncogene)
  - Chromosomal heterozygosity at 3q, 13q, and 18q

IMAGING

General Features

- Best diagnostic clue
  - Aggressive metaphyseal lesion/mass with osteoid formation
  - FDG-avid metaphyseal mass with osteoid formation
  - Metaphyseal mass with Tc-99m MDP uptake
- Location
  - Appendicular >>> axial skeleton (~ 10%)
  - ~ 90% of conventional OS are metaphyseal
    - ~ 75% of periosteal OS are diaphyseal
  - Majority of OS (regardless of subtype) occur in the femur (40-70%)
    - Proximal tibia (16-25%) and proximal humerus (5-15%) are next most common for conventional OS
  - Rarely soft tissue primary
  - Metastases (10-20% at diagnosis)
    - Lung
    - Bone
    - Lymph nodes

Nuclear Medicine Findings

- Bone scan
  - Uptake associated with tumor matrix and areas of reactive bone formation
    - Telangiectatic osteosarcoma may show central photopenia
  - Metastases typically show radiotracer uptake
- FDG PET/CT
  - Uptake in primary tumor and metastases
    - Better defines (relative to MDP bone scan) areas of tumor that are not producing substantial osteoid
    - May miss sclerotic metastases
  - Useful for therapy response assessment
    - Multiple measures described in literature: 2012 meta-analysis favored SUVmax < 2.5 after treatment and > 50% decrease in SUVmax with treatment as most prognostically significant

Imaging Recommendations

- Best imaging tool
  - Local disease/primary tumor
    - Radiography: 1st step in work-up of any bone lesion
    - MR: Best characterizes tumor structure (e.g., identifying cystic spaces of telangiectatic OS), best assessment of local extent of disease, best assessment for skip metastases
    - FDG PET/CT: Defines primary tumor better than MDP bone scan, can be used to assess response to chemotherapy
  - Metastases
    - CT for lung metastases
    - FDG PET/CT or Tc-99m MDP bone scan for other metastases
  - Surveillance
    - Radiograph or chest CT for lung recurrence
    - FDG PET/CT or Tc-99m MDP bone scan for local and distant recurrence (do not suffer from hardware artifacts)
    - MR can be used for local recurrence but may be limited by hardware artifact

DIFFERENTIAL DIAGNOSIS

Malignant Bone Tumors

- Ewing sarcoma
  - Generally less mineralized than OS (unless aggressive OS)
  - More likely axial in location

Benign Bone Lesions

- Aneurysmal bone cyst
- Eosinophilic granuloma
- Giant cell tumor

Fracture

- Healing fracture can occasionally have a bizarre appearance (follow up radiograph or MR can help distinguish)
- Take care not to miss an underlying lesion leading to pathologic fracture

Osteomyelitis

- May mimic OS if extensive bone involvement
- Systemic symptoms
- Subperiosteal fluid collections, sequestrum, substantial inflammatory response favor osteomyelitis

Bone Metastases (Rhabdomyosarcoma, Neuroblastoma, etc.)

- Generally multifocal
- ± history of primary malignancy

PATHOLOGY

General Features

- Etiology
  - Mesenchymal origin
  - Uncommonly occur in background of benign bone disease
    - Paget disease (older patients), chronic osteomyelitis, fibrous dysplasia (generally Albright syndrome), bone infarct
  - Can occur in prior radiation field

Gross Pathologic & Surgical Features

- Conventional OS
  - Fleshy, firm tumor arising in central medullary space of metaphysis
- Surface osteosarcomas
  - Generally prominently mineralized
  - Periosteal osteosarcoma by definition does not involve medullary space
- Telangiectatic osteosarcoma
  - Cysts partially filled with blood clots

Microscopic Features

- Osteoid is most important histologic finding to make diagnosis of osteosarcoma
- Conventional osteosarcoma
  - Variable cellular content including: Osteoid, cartilage, fibrous tissue
    - Cell type comprising > 50% of tumor defines tumor type (e.g., osteoblastic, chondroblastic, fibroblastic)

CLINICAL ISSUES

Presentation

- Most common signs/symptoms
  - Pain, swelling at tumor site
    - Except parosteal subtype: More commonly painless
- Other signs/symptoms
  - Limitation of joint movement
  - Pathologic fracture: More common with proximal humeral disease

Demographics

- Age
  - Bimodal distribution
    - 75% < 20 years; 15-20% > 65 years
  - Associated with periods of rapid growth
- Gender
  - Conventional osteosarcoma more common in males (2:1)
  - Periosteal osteosarcoma more common in males (2:1)
  - Parosteal osteosarcoma more common in females (1.3:1)
- Ethnicity
  - Slightly higher incidence in African Americans than Caucasians (5/million/year vs. 4.2/million/year)
- Epidemiology
  - 5% of childhood cancers
  - 4-5 cases/million/year in people < 20 years old
  - Most common primary malignant bone tumor in children and adolescents

Natural History & Prognosis

- Metastases in 10-20% at diagnosis
  - Lung most common
  - Skip metastases in 1-7%
- ~ 60% 5-year survival
- Prognostic factors
  - Response to chemotherapy (> 90% considered good) most important
  - Primary tumor location
    - Worse with axial location
    - Worse with proximal humeral tumors
  - Disease stage
  - Tumor pathologic subtype
  - Age at diagnosis
  - Race
- Recurrence
  - 30-40% of patients with localized disease
  - 90% occur in lung
  - Usually in 1st 2-3 years

Treatment

- Classic osteosarcoma
  - Neoadjuvant chemotherapy, followed by local control and resection of lung metastases, followed by adjuvant chemotherapy
  - Limb salvage procedures favored for local control
  - Radiation generally reserved for unresectable disease or palliation
    - Osteosarcoma is radioresistant
- Parosteal and periosteal osteosarcoma
  - Chemotherapy generally not indicated

SELECTED REFERENCES

1. Green JT et al: Osteogenic tumors of bone. Semin Diagn Pathol. 31(1):21-9, 2014
2. Luetke A et al: Osteosarcoma treatment - where do we stand? A state of the art review. Cancer Treat Rev. 40(4):523-32, 2014
3. Fox MG et al: Osteosarcoma: review of the various types with emphasis on recent advancements in imaging. Semin Musculoskelet Radiol. 17(2):123-36, 2013
4. Hongtao L et al: 18F-FDG positron emission tomography for the assessment of histological response to neoadjuvant chemotherapy in osteosarcomas: a meta-analysis. Surg Oncol. 21(4):e165-70, 2012
5. Cui J et al: Epigenetic changes in osteosarcoma. Bull Cancer. 98(7):E62-8, 2011
6. Kaste SC: Imaging pediatric bone sarcomas. Radiol Clin North Am. 49(4):749-65, vi-vii, 2011
7. Gorlick R: Current concepts on the molecular biology of osteosarcoma. Cancer Treat Res. 152:467-78, 2009
8. Ottaviani G et al: The etiology of osteosarcoma. Cancer Treat Res. 152:15-32, 2009
9. Hayden JB et al: Osteosarcoma: basic science and clinical implications. Orthop Clin North Am. 37(1):1-7, 2006

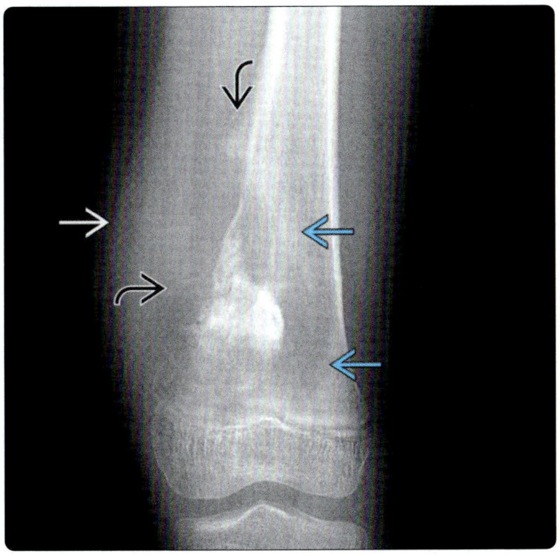

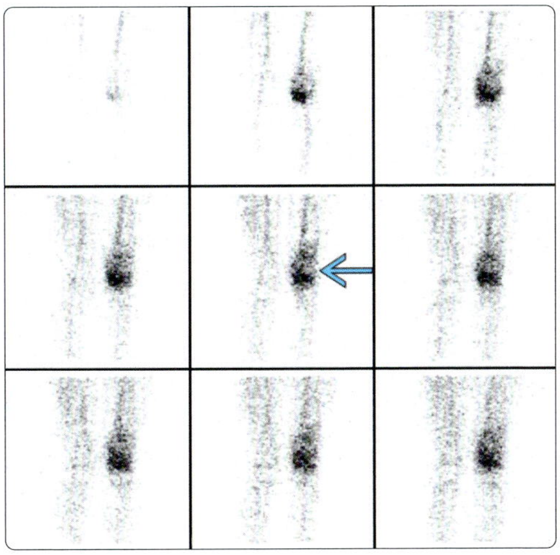

(Left) *Frontal radiograph in an 8-year-old girl with left distal femoral conventional osteosarcoma shows an aggressive, mixed lytic and osteoid-forming lesion arising from the metaphysis →. There is an associated soft tissue mass → and aggressive periosteal new bone formation →.* **(Right)** *Blood flow images from a Tc-99m MDP bone scan in the same patient show increased flow to the tumor →.*

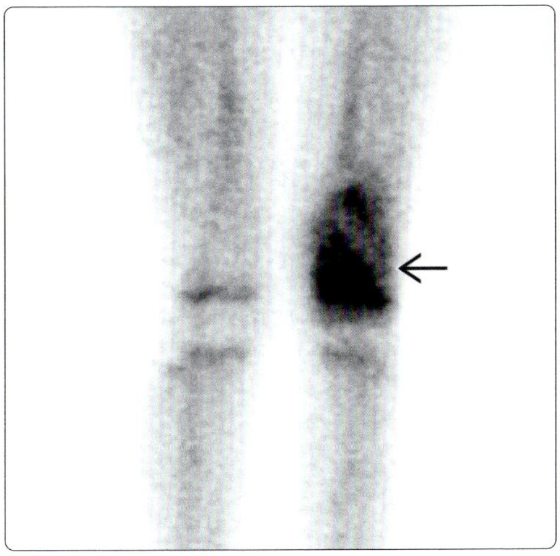

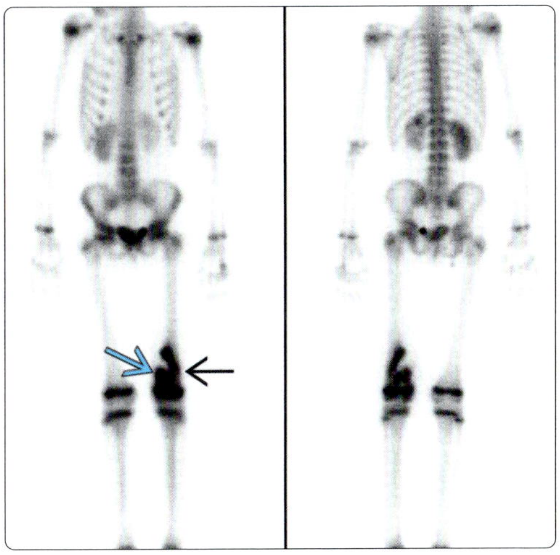

(Left) *Blood pool image from the same Tc-99m MDP bone scan shows increased radiotracer uptake in both the osseous and soft tissue components of the tumor →.* **(Right)** *Delayed phase whole-body images from the same Tc-99m MDP bone scan show radiotracer uptake along the margins of the tumor → and associated osteoid production → and periosteal new bone formation.*

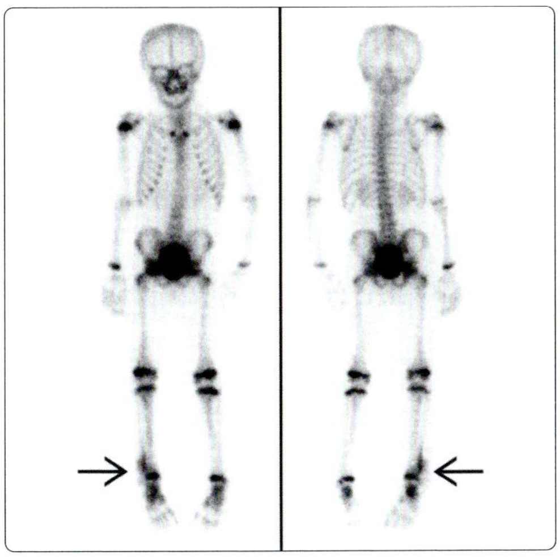

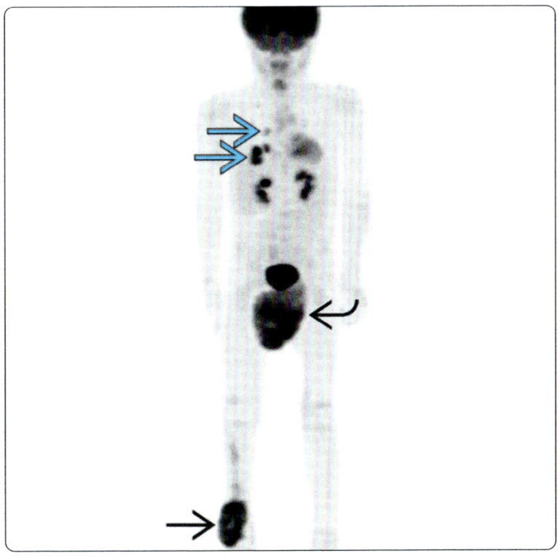

(Left) *Delayed phase whole-body Tc-99m bone scan in a 5-year-old girl with right distal fibular osteosarcoma shows accumulation of radiotracer within the distal fibular tumor →. There are no scintigraphic findings of metastatic disease.* **(Right)** *FDG PET in the same patient shows more extensive uptake associated with the soft tissue components of the distal fibular tumor →. There are multiple FDG-avid lung metastases → that are not seen on the MDP bone scan. Groin activity is excreted FDG in a diaper →.*

(Left) *Frontal radiograph of the knee in a 15-year-old male with telangiectatic osteosarcoma shows an aggressive lytic lesion arising from the lateral femoral metaphysis →. A soft tissue mass is also present →.* **(Right)** *Axial T2-weighted MR of the distal femur in the same patient shows an expansile metaphyseal mass with internal cystic spaces with fluid-fluid levels →. Posteriorly, the lesion extends through the cortex →.*

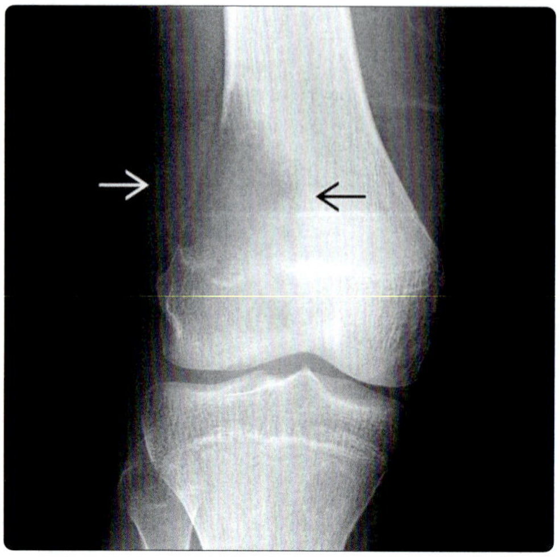

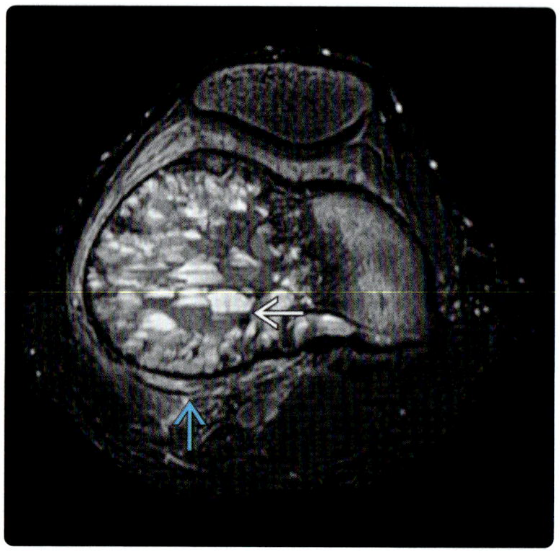

(Left) *Delayed phase Tc-99m MDP bone scan in the same patient shows the characteristic rim of radiotracer uptake with central photopenia → seen with telangiectatic osteosarcoma.* **(Right)** *Fused FDG PET/CT in the same patient shows a rim of abnormal FDG uptake around the lytic distal femoral and soft tissue mass →.*

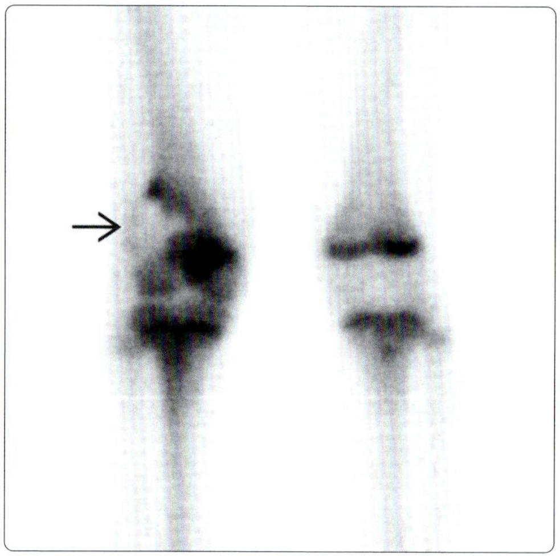

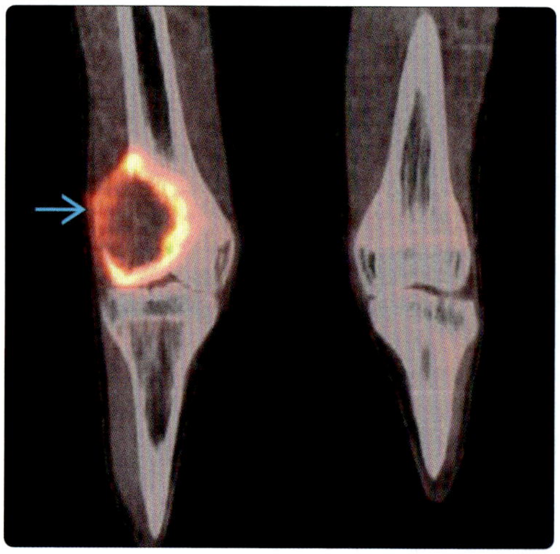

(Left) *Delayed phase whole-body Tc-99m MDP bone scan in a 14-year-old male with thoracic spinal osteosarcoma shows focal, mass-like accumulation of radiotracer at the level of the mid thoracic spine →. There is abnormal, long segment uptake along adjacent ribs reflecting extension of disease →.* **(Right)** *Axial CT in the same patient shows an infiltrative mass with internal osteoid matrix arising from a thoracic vertebra →. Tumor extends along adjacent ribs → and into the spinal canal →.*

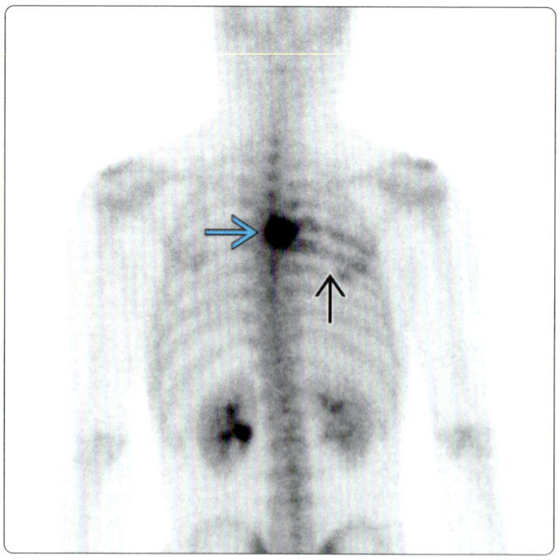

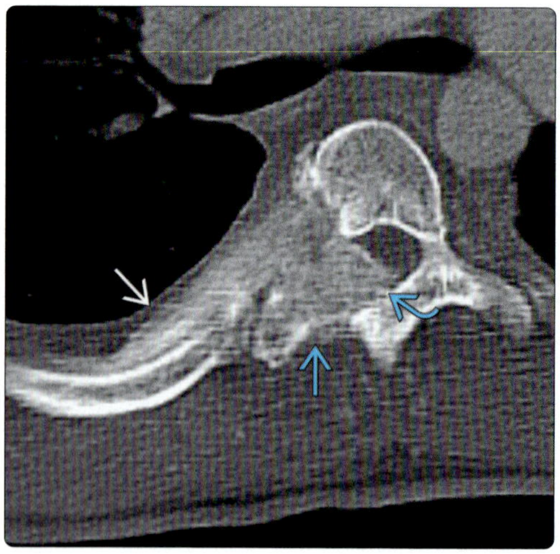

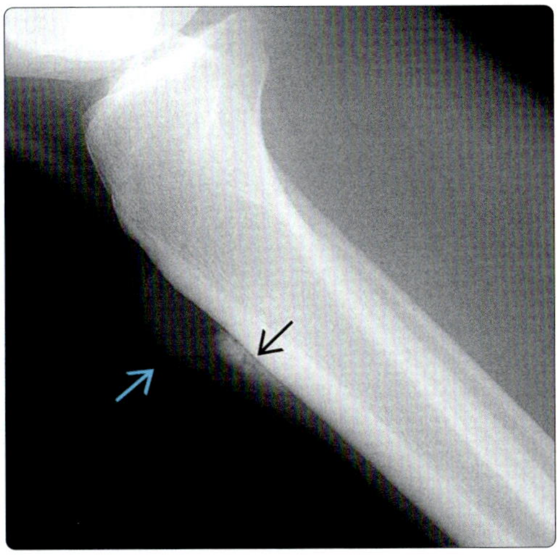
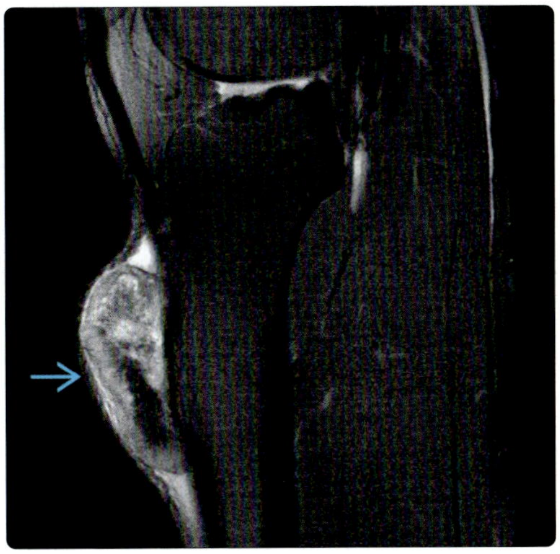

(Left) *Lateral radiograph of the knee in a 26-year-old man with proximal tibial periosteal osteosarcoma shows a pretibial soft tissue mass* → *with internal osteoid matrix* →. *There is subtle scalloping of the underlying tibia, which is otherwise normal.* **(Right)** *Sagittal T2-weighted fat-saturated MR in the same patient shows the pretibial mass* → *to be intimately associated with the surface of the tibia. There is no abnormality within the medullary space.*

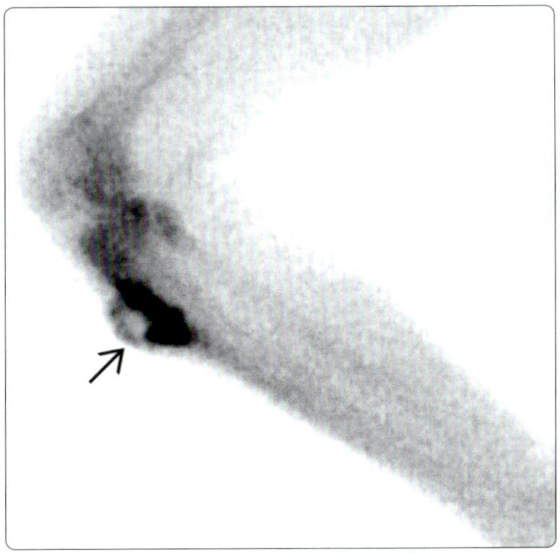
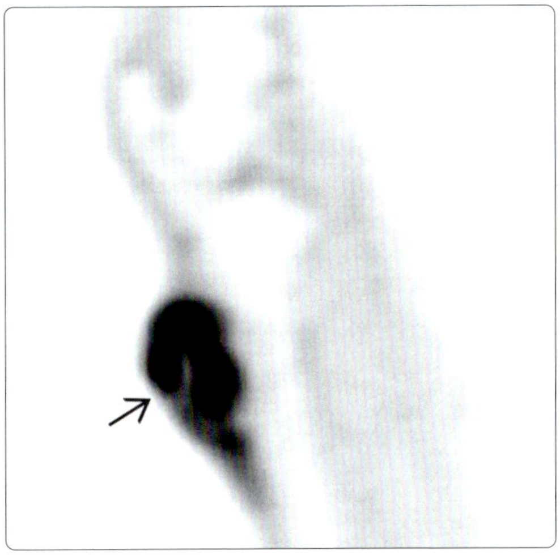

(Left) *Lateral delayed phase Tc-99m MDP bone scan in the same patient shows radiotracer uptake associated with the pretibial mass* → *without abnormal uptake in the medullary space.* **(Right)** *Sagittal FDG PET in the same patient shows FDG uptake in the pretibial mass* → *without abnormal uptake in the medullary space.*

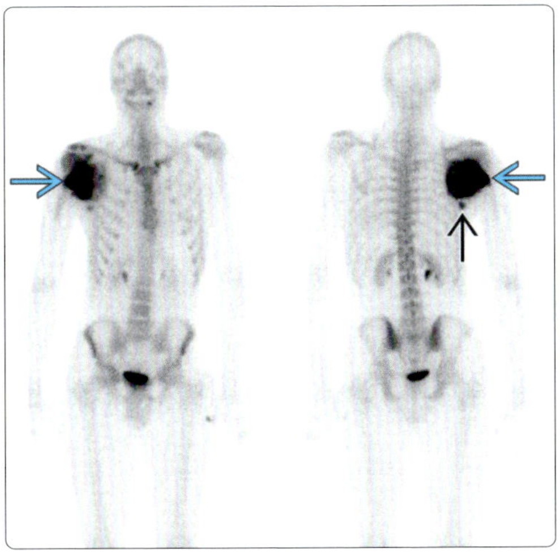
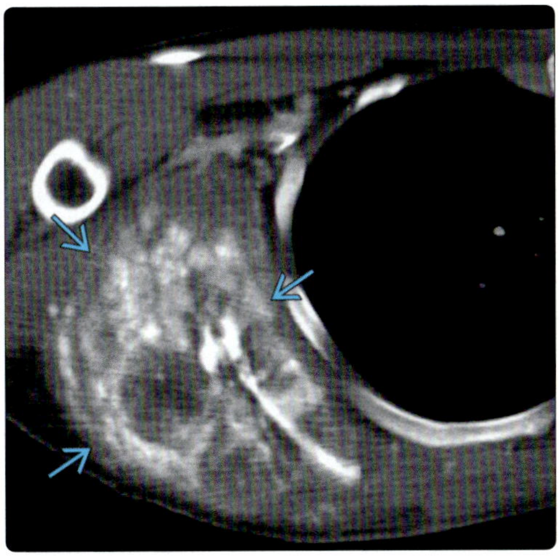

(Left) *Delayed phase whole-body Tc-99m MDP bone scan in a 21-year-old man with right scapular osteosarcoma shows tumoral uptake of radiotracer in the large right scapular mass* →. *A separate, more caudal focus represents a satellite lesion* →. **(Right)** *Axial CT in the same patient shows a large mass with internal osteoid matrix arising from the right scapula* →.

SECTION 12

Nuclear Medicine Therapy

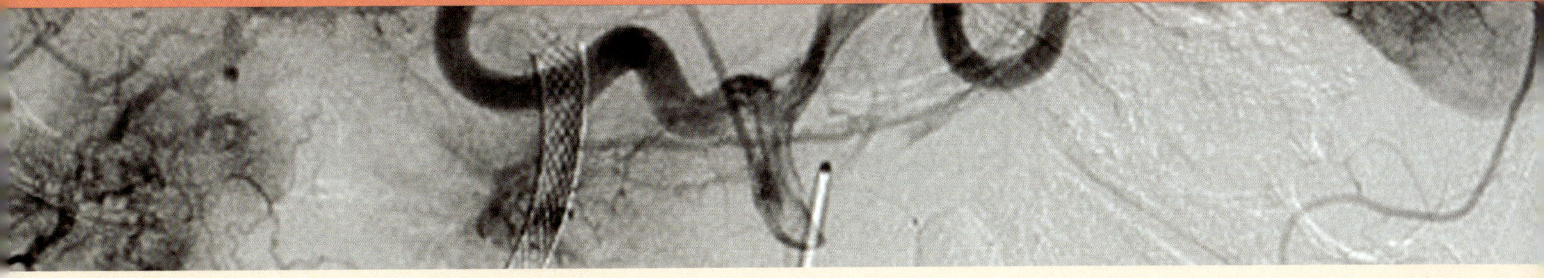

I-131 Therapy for Thyroid Cancer

KEY FACTS

TERMINOLOGY

- Radioactive iodine (RAI) treatment with I-131
  - I-131 ablates residual thyroid gland and thyroid cancer with high-energy beta emissions (0.606 MeV)
  - Effective for papillary and follicular thyroid cancers and their variants
  - Anaplastic and medullary thyroid cancers: Not RAI-avid

PROCEDURE

- Determine dose of I-131; practice patterns vary
  - Low risk, post thyroidectomy: 50-100 mCi (1.8-3.7 GBq)
  - Intermediate/high risk, post thyroidectomy: 100-150 mCi (3.7-5.5 GBq)
  - Lymphadenopathy: 125-175 mCi (4.6-6.5 GBq)
  - Recurrent/residual disease: 150-200 mCi (5.5-7.4 GBq)
  - Bone metastases: 200 mCi (7.4 GBq)
  - Lung metastases: 200 mCi (7.4 GBq), keeping total dose to lung < 80 mCi (2.9 GBq)
  - Occasionally treat with > 200-300 mCi (7.4-11.1 GBq) for recurrent, aggressive disease
  - For I-131 doses ≥ 200 mCi (7.4 GBq)
    - May need to check pre- and post-therapy CBCs, particularly in elderly
    - Dosimetry studies can be used to determine patient-specific RAI excretion over time and allow for maximum tolerated I-131 dose
- Other therapies
  - Consider surgery ± I-131 for recurrent disease in neck
  - External beam radiation
    - Considered for gross tumor therapy when surgery, I-131 not effective (non-RAI-avid disease)
    - Palliation of bone metastases causing pain, pathologic fracture, neurologic compromise

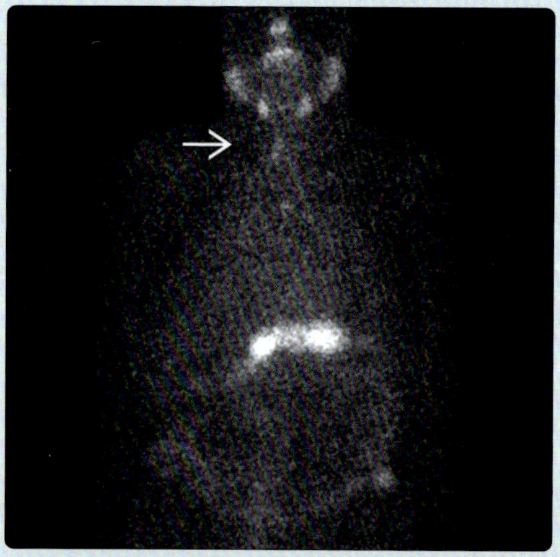
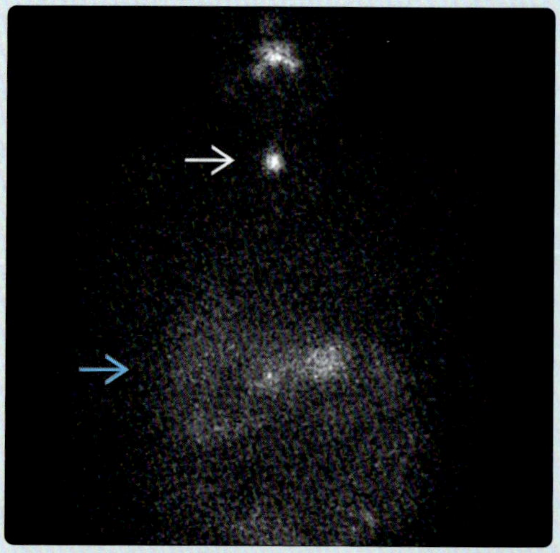

(Left) *Anterior I-123 scan in a patient post thyroidectomy for thyroid cancer shows a small amount of residual thyroid tissue in the thyroid bed ➡. The patient received 100 mCi (3.7 GBq) I-131 for ablation.* **(Right)** *Anterior scan in the same patient one week after I-131 therapy shows focal uptake in remnant thyroid tissue ➡ and no lymphadenopathy or distant metastases. Note the liver shows diffuse activity → due to its normal physiologic processing of radioactive thyroid hormone.*

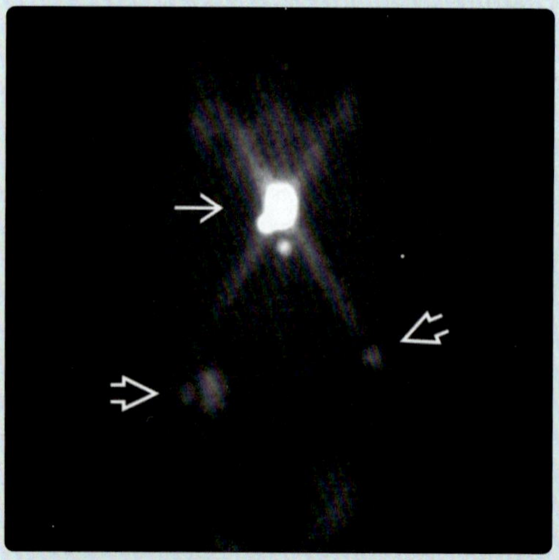
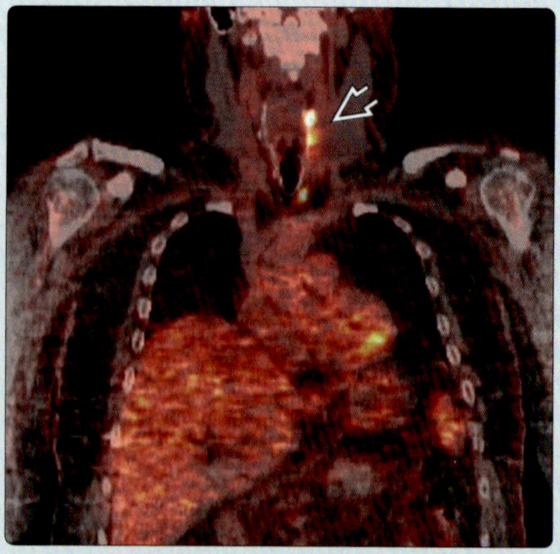

(Left) *Anterior post-therapy I-131 scan in a thyroid cancer patient post remote thyroidectomy and RAI ablation with subsequent suboptimal thyroid hormone suppression. Note large amount of thyroid tissue in thyroid bed ➡ as well as pulmonary metastases ⇨.* **(Right)** *Coronal F-18 FDG PET/CT in a thyroid cancer patient who had rising thyroglobulin and a negative I-123 scan shows F-18 FDG-avid disease in the left thyroid bed ⇨. Non-RAI-avid disease can be treated surgically or with external beam radiotherapy.*

TERMINOLOGY

Definitions

- Radioactive iodine (RAI) treatment with I-131
  - I-131 ablates residual thyroid gland and thyroid cancer with high-energy beta emissions (0.606 MeV)
  - Effective for papillary and follicular thyroid cancers and their variants
  - Anaplastic and medullary thyroid cancers are not RAI-avid

PREPROCEDURE

Indications

- I-131 therapy decreases risk of death
  - In patients > 45 years and T3 disease
  - Primary tumor with gross extrathyroidal extension (T4)
  - M1 disease
  - Conflicting data, possible decreased risk of death
    - In patients > 45 years and nodal disease
- I-131 therapy decreases risk of recurrence
  - In patients > 45 years and T3 disease
  - Primary tumor with gross extrathyroidal extension (T4)
  - M1 disease
  - Conflicting data, possible decreased risk of recurrence
    - Any age, nodal disease present
    - In patients < 45 years with T3 disease
    - Any age, 1-4 cm intrathyroidal tumors
  - Inadequate data
    - Any size, any age, minimal extrathyroidal extension
- I-131 therapy facilitates initial staging and follow-up
  - All patients with thyroid cancer
  - Generally administered within 6 months post thyroidectomy
  - Serum thyroglobulin levels should be ≤ 2 ng/mL if ablation successful
  - Recurrence suspected if thyroglobulin levels rise over time, particularly if > 10 ng/mL
    - Thyroglobulin not specific for thyroid cancer, however; it is made by normal thyroid tissue as well
  - If thyroglobulin > 10 ng/mL and whole-body RAI scan negative, consider F-18 FDG PET/CT

Contraindications

- Pregnancy
  - I-131 crosses placenta
  - If pregnant patient given therapeutic dose of I-131 prior to 10-12 weeks gestation, fetus gets unacceptable radiation dose due to urinary bladder excretion of I-131
  - If pregnant patient given therapeutic dose of I-131 after 10-12 weeks gestation, fetal thyroid is present, will be ablated, and fetus gets unacceptable radiation dose due to urinary bladder excretion of I-131
  - Also, avoiding pregnancy within 6 months is recommended for both men and women undergoing I-131 therapy due to urinary bladder excretion of I-131 during active gamete formation
- Lactation within 2 months of treatment
  - I-131 concentrated in lactating breasts due to increased sodium-iodide symporter activity
  - Delivers inappropriate radiation dose to breasts
- Inability to follow radiation safety precautions after I-131 administration
  - Often dementia, incontinence, inability to care for oneself interferes with radiation safety guidelines

Getting Started

- Patient preparation
  - Confirm no recent iodine load
    - Wait 4-6 weeks after IV contrast to begin RAI scan and therapy
    - Amiodarone
    - High dietary iodine (e.g., sea kelp supplements)
  - Most experts recommend low-iodine diet 1-2 weeks prior to whole-body scan and therapy
    - Foods to avoid
      - Iodized salt, sea salt
      - Ocean fish and shellfish
      - Dairy products: Milk, cheese, yogurt, ice cream, butter (cow udders often cleaned with iodine-containing solution)
      - Commercial baked goods (many use iodate dough conditioners)
      - Iodine-containing supplements and medications (e.g., sea kelp, red dye #3)
      - Salted commercial foods (e.g., cured meats, canned goods)
      - Meals you do not prepare yourself (e.g., restaurant, prepackaged meals from grocery)
      - Any food made with red dye #3
  - Elevate TSH prior to whole-body scan and RAI therapy
    - Levothyroxine (Synthroid) withdrawal for 3 weeks in adults, 2 weeks in children
      - Increased RAI uptake in tumor cells when TSH > 30 mU/L
      - > 95% of patients in one study had TSH > 30 mU/L after 2.5 weeks of levothyroxine withdrawal
      - Short-term (~ 3 weeks) thyroid hormone withdrawal found to be well tolerated
    - Stimulation with human recombinant TSH (Thyrogen)
      - Useful to avoid hypothyroid symptoms (e.g., elderly patients, patients with psychiatric illnesses)
      - 3-day protocol (IM injection on days 1 and 2, day 3 scan and RAI therapy)
      - More expensive than withdrawal
  - Urine pregnancy test in women
  - Draw thyroglobulin and thyroglobulin antibody assays as desired
- Pre-therapy RAI whole-body scan
  - Useful to evaluate for nodal, distant metastases, confirm RAI-avid disease in recurrence (> 1 cm), determine dose of I-131 therapy
  - Can use I-123 or I-131 for whole-body scan; however, I-123 has better imaging characteristics than I-131
- RAI thyroid uptake measurement
  - Usually 1-5%
  - Consider lower therapy dose if ≥ 5% uptake in remnant
  - If hemithyroidectomy, standard of care is completion thyroidectomy, no RAI ablation of remaining lobe
    - Occasionally, patients who cannot tolerate 2nd surgery undergo RAI ablation of remaining lobe; may require 2 doses of I-131 6 months apart

Papillary and Follicular Thyroid Cancer Staging

- **TNM classification**
  - Tumor
    - T1: 2 cm or smaller, includes microscopic multifocal tumors
    - T2: > 2-4 cm, intrathyroidal
    - T3: > 4 cm, intrathyroidal or minimal extrathyroidal extension
    - T4: Gross extrathyroidal extension
  - Nodes
    - N0: No metastatic nodes
    - N1a: Metastases to level VI nodes
    - N1b: Metastases to any cervical, superior mediastinal nodes
  - Metastases
    - M0: No distant metastases
    - M1: Distant metastases
- **Staging**
  - **< 45 years old**
    - Stage 1: Any T, any N, M0
    - Stage 2: Any T, any N, M1
  - **> 45 years old**
    - Stage 1: Tumor < 2 cm (T1), N0, M0
    - Stage 2: Tumor 2-4 cm (T2), N0, M0
    - Stage 3: Tumor > 4 cm, no spread outside thyroid (T3), N0, M0 or T1-T3, N1a, (level VI) M0
    - Stage 4a: Tumor of any size extending beyond the thyroid capsule to invade adjacent structures (T4a), any N, M0 or T1-T3, N1b, M0
    - Stage 4b: Tumor invades prevertebral fascia or encases carotid artery or mediastinal vessels (T4b), any N, M0
    - Stage 4c: Any T, any N, M1
- **Risk stratification also considered**
  - Low-risk patients
    - No local/distant metastases
    - Complete tumor resection
    - No tumor invasion of regional structures
    - Nonaggressive histology
    - No vascular invasion
    - Whole-body scan post thyroidectomy shows no nodal or distant metastases
  - Intermediate-risk patients
    - Microscopic perithyroidal tissue invasion
    - In patients post RAI ablation, cervical lymphadenopathy or uptake outside thyroid bed on follow-up radioactive iodine scan
    - Aggressive histology (e.g., tall cell, insular cell, columnar cell, Hurthle cell)
    - Vascular invasion
  - High-risk patients
    - Macroscopic tumor invasion
    - Incomplete tumor resection
    - Distant metastases
    - High thyroglobulin levels

PROCEDURE

Equipment Preparation

- I-131
  - Beta and gamma emissions
    - High-energy beta emissions (0.606 MeV) travel 0.8 mm and destroy thyroid tissue
    - Gamma emissions (364 KeV) travel ~ 6 feet and need to be considered for post-therapy radiation safety precautions to avoid radiation dose to people in close proximity to patient
  - T 1/2: 8.06 days
  - Can take 1-3 months for ablation

Procedure Steps

- Determine dose of I-131; practice patterns vary
  - Low risk, post thyroidectomy: 50-100 mCi (1.8-3.7 GBq)
  - Intermediate and high risk, post thyroidectomy: 100-150 mCi (3.7-5.5 GBq)
  - Lymphadenopathy: 125-175 mCi (4.6-6.5 GBq)
  - Recurrent/residual disease: 150-200 mCi (5.5-7.4 GBq)
  - Bone metastases: 200 mCi (7.4 GBq)
  - Lung metastases: 200 mCi (7.4 GBq), keeping total dose to lung < 80 mCi (2.9 GBq) to decrease risk of radiation fibrosis in patients with miliary disease
  - Occasionally treat with > 200-300 mCi (7.4-11.1 GBq) for recurrent, aggressive disease
  - For I-131 doses ≥ 200 mCi (7.4 GBq)
    - Check pre- and post-therapy CBCs, particularly in elderly
    - Dosimetry studies can be used determine patient-specific RAI excretion over time and allow for maximum tolerated I-131 dose
  - If patient has consecutive rising thyroglobulin levels (> 10 ng/mL) and negative RAI scan, may give empiric dose of 200 mCi (7.4 GBq) I-131
    - RAI-avid disease may be evident on post I-131 therapy whole-body scan
    - If RAI-avid disease that is below detection limits of RAI scan is present, thyroglobulin level should decrease over time
    - For thyroglobulin levels over 10 ng/mL, F-18 FDG PET/CT may show disease amenable to surgery or external beam radiotherapy
  - Consider lower doses
    - Elderly patients
    - Renal insufficiency/dialysis patients
- If patient unable to swallow I-131 capsule, liquid I-131 administered via straw or feeding tube
  - Stringent radiation safety precautions required to avoid contaminating personnel with volatile liquid
- Obtain informed consent
  - Inform of side effects including temporary sore throat, neck &/or salivary gland swelling and pain, nausea
  - Increased risk of secondary cancers caused by I-131 therapy is controversial
    - Very low increased risk of secondary cancer in patients with differentiated thyroid cancer
      - Breast, colon, and lung most common 2nd primary malignancy, whether or not I-131 given
      - May be due to genetic predisposition that caused primary thyroid cancer instead of I-131 therapy
    - High cumulative doses of I-131 likely related to secondary primary malignancies

    - Salivary, breast, bladder, gastrointestinal cancers theoretically influenced
    - Occur 2-10 years after I-131, prevalence of ~ 0.5%
  - Although risk low, requires close follow-up for diagnosis of 2nd primary cancers
- Some institutions perform time-out procedure to avoid medical events (misadministrations)
- Patient NPO 3-4 hrs prior to treatment
- Give 48-72 hrs post-procedure instructions to patient
  - Resume low-iodine diet 2 hrs following I-131
    - Normal diet may be resumed in 48-72 hrs
  - Encourage fluid intake
    - Frequent urination → lower radiation dose to genitourinary tract
  - Begin using sour candy, gum 24 hrs post treatment
    - Reduces stasis of I-131 in salivary glands
    - Reported increased salivary damage if given earlier than 24 hrs
  - Ibuprofen 600 mg 3x a day for neck/salivary pain, swelling
  - Resume thyroid hormone 48-72 hrs post RAI therapy; continue thyroid hormone if rhTSH used
- Radiation safety precautions
  - Any I-131 not taken up by thyroid tissue will be excreted in tears, mucus, saliva, sweat, menstrual blood, urine, and feces
    - Avoid sharing items that contact mouth, such as eating utensils, kitchenware, toothbrushes
    - Sit while urinating, flush toilet twice with lid down
    - Change incontinence or menstrual pads 2x normal frequency and place in trash outside
    - Bathe daily
    - Wash patient's clothes, linens separately
    - Avoid open-mouth kissing, sexual intercourse
  - I-131 that remains in thyroid gland will emit low-level radiation
    - Stay 6 feet from other people
    - Avoid children and pregnant (or potentially pregnant) women
    - Stay out of public places, including hotels, public transportation, public events, workplaces
    - Sleep alone in bed separate from other people
  - Amount of time patients follow these precautions vary, mostly based on practitioner opinions
    - Range of 3-11 days most common
- **Radiation Safety Release Requirements (Per NRC Regulatory Guide 8.39)**
  - I-131 doses > 33 mCi (1.1 GBq)
    - Patient may be released to outpatient setting after written radiation safety precaution instructions given **and**
    - Calculation based on radiopharmaceutical t1/2, excretion rates, and dose to ensure estimated dose to bystanders is < 500 mrem (≤ 5 mSv)

Findings and Reporting

- Include specific dose of I-131 administered, that patient received written radiation safety instructions and estimated dose to bystanders release calculation

Alternative Procedures/Therapies

- Consider surgery ± I-131 for recurrent disease in neck
- External beam radiation
  - Considered for gross tumor therapy when surgery, RAI not effective (non-RAI-avid disease)
  - Palliation of bone metastases causing pain, pathologic fracture, neurologic compromise
- Chemotherapy: Little data to support use

POST PROCEDURE

Things To Do

- Post-therapy whole body scan
  - 4-10 days following RAI therapy
  - Detects additional sites of disease in ≤ 26% of patients
  - If additional sites of disease detected, may change follow-up

Side Effects

- Nausea
  - Common and can last 3-5 days (prescribe antiemetic)
  - Vomiting rare
- Sore throat
  - Due to local radiation dose from thyroid bed
  - Throat lozenges, ibuprofen for symptomatic relief
- Salivary gland complications
  - Sialadenitis, xerostomia, salivary calculi
  - Sour candy and gum used to increase salivary excretion of RAI; may prevent salivary gland complications
- Change in sense of taste
  - Usually returns to normal in 1-6 months
  - Patients commonly complain of metallic taste
- Radiation thyroiditis
  - Mild neck pain that increases over time
  - More common with significant residual thyroid
  - Treat with nonsteroidal anti-inflammatory medication or corticosteroid taper

OUTCOMES

Complications

- Most feared complication(s)
  - Xerostomia
    - Salivary glands take up I-131, fibrosis/scar can occur
  - Radiation lung fibrosis
    - If diffuse pulmonary metastases, consider dosimetry to keep total dose to lungs < 80 mCi (2.9 GBq)
  - Bone marrow suppression
    - Consider dosimetry for very large doses, especially in children, elderly or renal insufficiency
  - Secondary malignancies
    - Very low risk, may not be from I-131, but from genetic predisposition that caused primary thyroid cancer
    - Data more firm for patients with high cumulative doses of I-131

SELECTED REFERENCES

1. ATA Guidelines Taskforce on Thyroid Nodules and Differentiated Thyroid Cancer et al: Revised American Thyroid Association management guidelines for patients with thyroid nodules and differentiated thyroid cancer. Thyroid. 19(11):1167-214, 2009

I-131 Therapy for Hyperthyroidism

KEY FACTS

PREPROCEDURE

- Indications for I-131 therapy
  - Graves disease
  - Toxic adenoma, toxic multinodular goiter
- Contraindications to I-131 therapy
  - Pregnancy
  - Lactation within past 2 months
  - Patient unable to follow radiation safety precautions

PROCEDURE

- I-131 taken up by thyroid gland in proportion to thyroid uptake determination
  - High-energy beta emissions (0.606 MeV) travel 0.8 mm and destroy thyroid tissue
  - Gamma emissions (364 KeV) travel ~ 6 feet and need to be considered in radiation safety precautions to avoid radiating people in close proximity to patient
- I-131 doses for Graves disease
  - Typically 15-20 mCi (555-740 MBq) I-131 po
  - 15 mCi (555 MBq) minimum advocated in children to reduce risk of giving sublethal dose of radioactivity to thyroid (increases future risk of malignancy)
- I-131 doses for toxic nodular disease (toxic adenoma, multinodular goiter)
  - 20-30 mCi (740 MBq to 1.1 GBq) I-131 po, sometimes 40 mCi (1.4 GBq)
  - Larger I-131 doses required due to relatively lower thyroid uptake compared with Graves disease

POST PROCEDURE

- Hypothyroidism is goal of I-131 therapy
  - Often patients are undertreated with I-131 therapy if goal of clinician is to achieve euthyroidism
- Radiation thyroiditis can occur after treatment
  - Continued pain and swelling in thyroid gland
  - Often needs steroid taper to reduce inflammation & pain

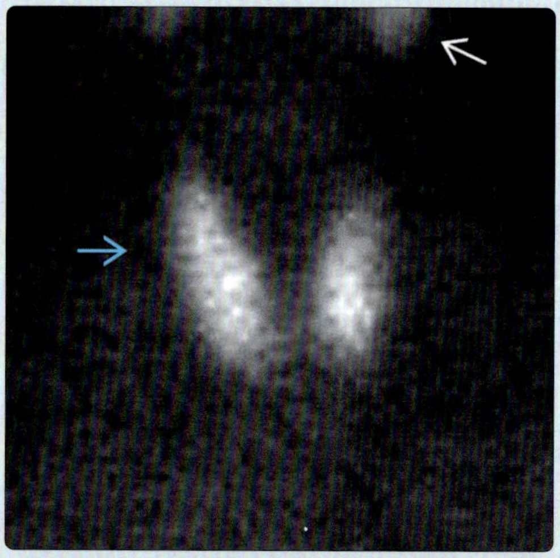
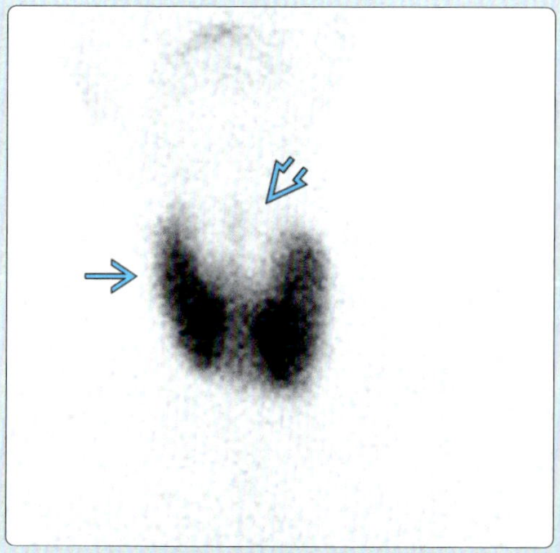

(Left) *Anterior Tc-99m pertechnetate thyroid scan shows a normal thyroid gland ➡. Note normal salivary gland uptake ➡.* **(Right)** *Anterior Tc-99m pertechnetate thyroid scan shows a homogeneously enlarged thyroid gland ➡ and no salivary gland uptake in this patient with Graves disease. Note the pyramidal lobe ➡ is visible.*

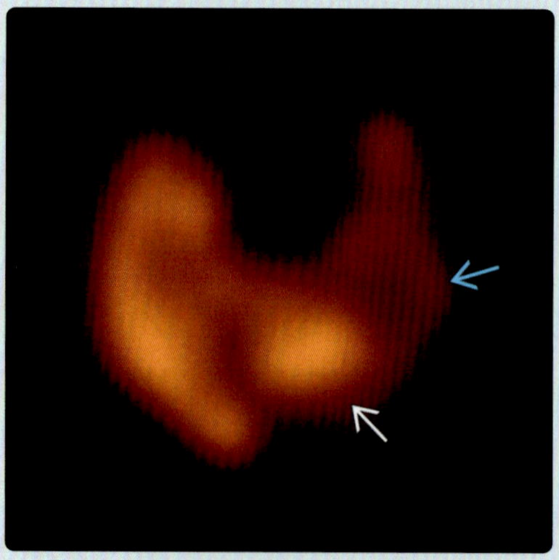
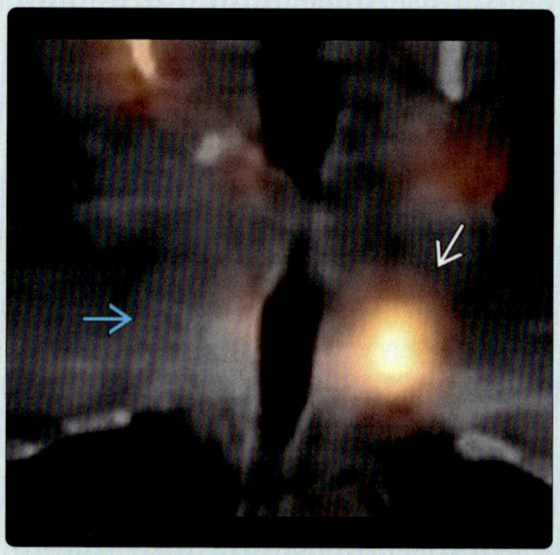

(Left) *Anterior Tc-99m pertechnetate thyroid scan in a patient with hyperthyroidism shows multiple hot ➡ and cold ➡ nodules throughout an enlarged thyroid gland, consistent with toxic multinodular goiter.* **(Right)** *Coronal Tc-99m pertechnetate thyroid SPECT/CT shows a focal hot nodule ➡ and suppressed uptake ➡ in the remainder of the thyroid gland, consistent with a toxic adenoma.*

I-131 Therapy for Hyperthyroidism

PREPROCEDURE

Indications

- Hyperthyroidism
  - Graves disease
    - Autoimmune hyperthyroidism induced by thyroid-stimulating antibodies
    - Thyroid functions autonomously, independent of pituitary thyrotropin-stimulating hormone (TSH)
    - Most common cause of hyperthyroidism in children, often confused with signs of attention deficit hyperactivity disorder
  - Toxic adenoma and multinodular goiter
    - Autonomously functioning nodule causes hyperthyroidism
    - May or may not suppress function in remainder of thyroid gland

Contraindications

- Pregnancy
  - I-131 crosses placenta
    - If pregnant patient given therapeutic dose of I-131 prior to 10-12 weeks gestation, fetus gets unacceptable radiation dose due to urinary bladder excretion of I-131
    - If pregnant patient given therapeutic dose of I-131 after 10-12 weeks gestation, fetal thyroid is present, will be ablated, and fetus gets unacceptable radiation dose due to urinary bladder excretion of I-131
  - Also, avoiding pregnancy within 6 months is recommended for both men and women undergoing I-131 therapy due to urinary bladder excretion of I-131 during active gamete formation
- Lactation within past 2 months
  - Lactating breasts take up radioactive iodine
  - Delivers inappropriate radiation dose to breasts
  - In hyperthyroid patient who is lactating, patient required to cease lactation for 2 months prior to therapy
- Inability to follow radiation safety precautions after I-131 administration
  - Often dementia, incontinence, inability to care for oneself interferes with radiation safety guidelines

Preprocedure Imaging

- I-131 or I-123 thyroid uptake determination at 24 hours
  - Toxic adenoma or multinodular goiter: Normal or mildly elevated
  - Graves disease: > 50%, often 70-90%
  - Subacute, painless, and postpartum thyroiditis will have low I-131 uptake values (< 5% at 24 hrs)
    - I-131 therapy not indicated for these etiologies
- Thyroid scintigraphy
  - Toxic adenoma or multinodular goiter: Solitary hot nodule or multinodular thyroid gland with varying degrees of uptake; ± enlargement
  - Graves disease: Homogeneous uptake of radiotracer in diffusely enlarged thyroid gland

Getting Started

- Things to Check
  - Confirm hyperthyroidism with recent TSH value
  - Urine pregnancy test
  - No IV contrast in 4-6 weeks
  - Off anti-thyroid medications
  - No interfering medications or high-iodine supplements (e.g., amiodarone, sea kelp supplements)
  - Patient ability to follow radiation safety precautions
  - Low-iodine diet not needed for treatment of benign thyroid disease

PROCEDURE

Patient Positions/Location

- Best procedure approach
  - Obtain informed consent
    - Include expected risk of hypothyroidism
    - Include possible need for repeat I-131 therapy
    - Inform of side effects including temporary sore throat, swelling, pain
    - Inform of rare risk of radiation thyroiditis induced by I-131
  - Some institutions perform time-out procedure to avoid medical events (misadministrations)
  - Explain post procedure radiation safety precautions to patient
    - Any I-131 not taken up by thyroid will be excreted in tears, mucus, sweat, saliva, menstrual blood, urine, and feces
      - Avoid sharing items that contact mouth, such as eating utensils, kitchenware, toothbrushes
      - Sit while urinating, flush toilet twice with lid down
      - Change incontinence or menstrual pads twice normal frequency and place in trash outside
      - Bathe daily
      - Wash patient's clothes, linens separately
      - Avoid open-mouth kissing, sexual intercourse
    - I-131 that remains in thyroid gland will emit low-level radiation
      - Stay 6 feet from other people
      - Stay out of public places, including hotels, public transportation, public events, workplaces
      - Sleep alone in bed separate from other people
      - Avoid children and pregnant (or potentially pregnant) women
    - Amount of time patients should follow these recommendations vary, mostly based on practitioner opinions
      - Range of 3-11 days most common

Equipment Preparation

- I-131
  - Na I-131 taken up by thyroid gland in proportion to thyroid uptake determination
  - Beta and gamma emissions
    - High-energy beta emissions (0.606 MeV) travel 0.8 mm and destroy thyroid tissue
    - Gamma emissions (364 KeV) travel ~ 6 feet and need to be considered for post-therapy radiation safety precautions to avoid radiation dose to people in close proximity to patient
  - T 1/2: 8.06 days
  - Can take 1-3 months to ablate thyroid
  - Dosimetry

- Adult hyperthyroid
  - Target organ (thyroid): 7.0 rad/mCi (1.9 mGy/MBq)
  - Effective dose: 0.28 rem/mCi (0.075 mSv/MBq)
- Child (5 year old) hyperthyroid
  - Target organ (thyroid): 36 rad/mCi (9.8 mGy/MBq)
  - Effective dose: 1.3 rem/mCi (0.45 mSv/MBq)

Procedure Steps

- Determine dose of I-131; practice patterns vary
  - Empiric standard dose or calculated dose both equally effective based on studies
  - Calculate dose based on uptake measurement and thyroid size
    - 8-10 mCi (296-370 MBq) into thyroid gland (# mCi I-131 desired divided by 4- or 24-hr uptake value)
- Graves disease
  - Typically 15-20 mCi (550-740 MBq) I-131 po
  - 15 mCi (550 MBq) minimum advocated in children to reduce risk of giving sublethal dose of radioactivity to thyroid (increases future risk of malignancy)
- Toxic nodular disease
  - 20-30 mCi (740 MBq to 1.1 GBq) I-131 po, sometimes 40 mCi (1.4 GBq)
  - Larger I-131 doses required due to relatively lower thyroid uptake compared with Graves disease
- Consider higher doses for large goiter, low thyroid uptake values, repeat I-131 therapy

Findings and Reporting

- Reporting should include specific dose of I-131 administered
- Reporting should include that patient received written radiation safety instructions
- Reporting should include estimated dose to bystanders calculation if > 33 mCi (1.2 GBq) I-131 administered

Alternative Procedures/Therapies

- Surgical
  - Thyroidectomy is procedure of choice for multinodular goiter if large, substernal, or compressing trachea/vascular structures
- Other
  - Anti-thyroid drugs
    - Methimazole
      - Used most commonly
      - Once daily dosing, rapid onset of action
      - Side effects: Blood dyscrasias and hepatic toxicity
    - Propylthiouracil
      - Side effects: Blood dyscrasias and hepatic toxicity
      - Used during 1st trimester of pregnancy in pregnant patients
  - Beta blockers for tachycardia

Radiation Safety Release Requirements (Per NRC Regulatory Guide 8.39)

- I-131 doses < 7 mCi (259 MBq)
  - No radiation safety precautions required, although this dose would usually be too low for I-131 therapy
- I-131 doses < 33 mCi (1.2 GBq)
  - Patient may be released to outpatient setting after written radiation safety precaution instructions given
- I-131 doses > 33 mCi (1.2 GBq)
  - Patient may be released to outpatient setting after written radiation safety precaution instructions given **and**
  - Calculation based on radiopharmaceutical t1/2, excretion rates, and dose is performed prior to release to ensure estimated dose to bystanders is < 500 mrem (≤ 5 mSv)

POST PROCEDURE

Expected Outcome

- Hypothyroidism is goal of I-131 therapy
  - Essentially, thyroidectomy without risks of surgery
    - Infection
    - Bleeding
    - Recurrent laryngeal nerve damage
    - Scar on neck
    - Anesthesia risks
  - Often patients are undertreated with I-131 therapy if goal of clinician is to achieve euthyroidism
  - Hypothyroidism more common after I-131 therapy for Graves disease compared with toxic nodular disease

OUTCOMES

Complications

- Immediate/periprocedural complication(s)
  - Radiation thyroiditis
    - Continued pain and swelling in thyroid gland, not relieved within 1-2 weeks or increasing pain not controlled with anti-inflammatory medications
    - Often requires steroid taper to reduce inflammation and pain
- Other complications
  - Ophthalmopathy exacerbation in patients with Graves disease who smoke cigarettes
    - I-131 therapy is not recommended in these patients

SELECTED REFERENCES

1. Bahn RS et al: Hyperthyroidism and other causes of thyrotoxicosis: management guidelines of the American Thyroid Association and American Association of Clinical Endocrinologists. Endocr Pract. 17(3):456-520, 2011
2. Rivkees SA et al: An optimal treatment for pediatric Graves' disease is radioiodine. J Clin Endocrinol Metab. 92(3):797-800, 2007
3. Tuttle WK 3rd et al: Applying Nuclear Regulatory Commission guidelines to the release of patients treated with sodium iodine-131. J Nucl Med Technol. 28(4):275-9, 2000

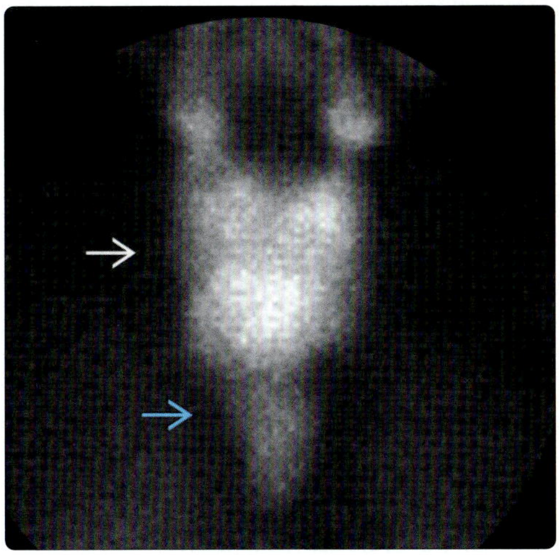

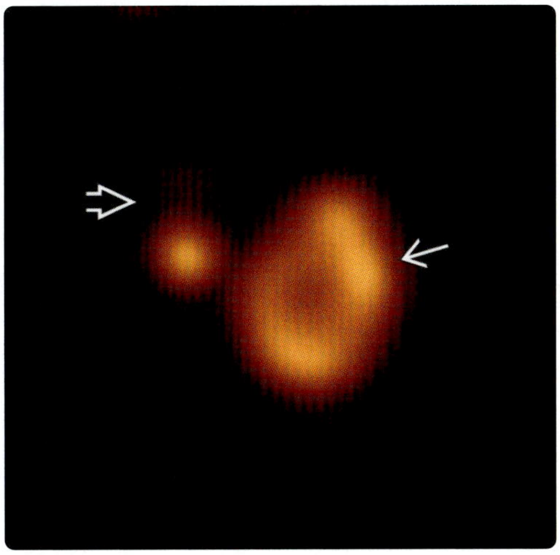

(Left) *Anterior Tc-99m pertechnetate thyroid scan shows massively enlarged multinodular goiter* ➡ *with substernal extension* ➡*. Surgery is the preferred treatment for a goiter this large.* **(Right)** *Anterior Tc-99m pertechnetate thyroid scan shows an enlarged, hot nodule with a photopenic center* ➡ *and suppression of most of the remainder of the thyroid gland* ➡*, consistent with a degenerating toxic adenoma. This patient could be followed with medical management, as the adenoma may resolve spontaneously.*

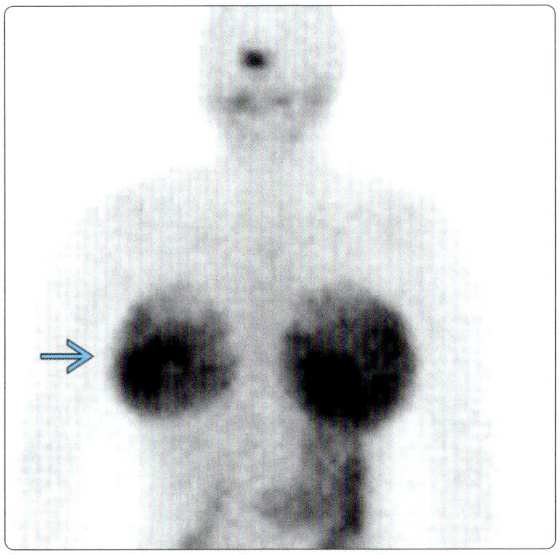

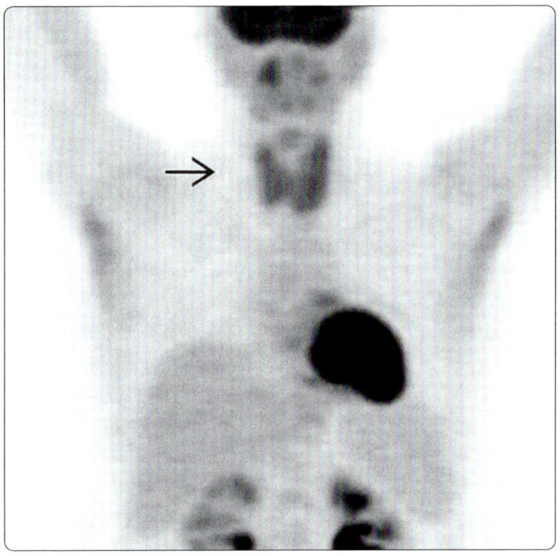

(Left) *Anterior I-123 whole-body thyroid scan in a patient post thyroidectomy for thyroid cancer shows radioactive iodine uptake in lactating breasts* ➡*. Women need to cease lactation two months prior to I-131 therapy to avoid an unacceptable radiation dose to the breasts.* **(Right)** *MIP F-18 FDG PET shows diffuse, heterogeneous uptake in the thyroid gland* ➡*. This suggests a diffuse thyroid process such as thyroiditis or Graves disease.*

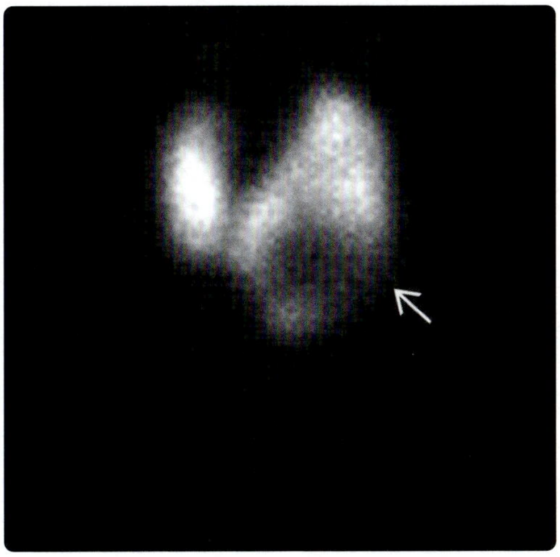

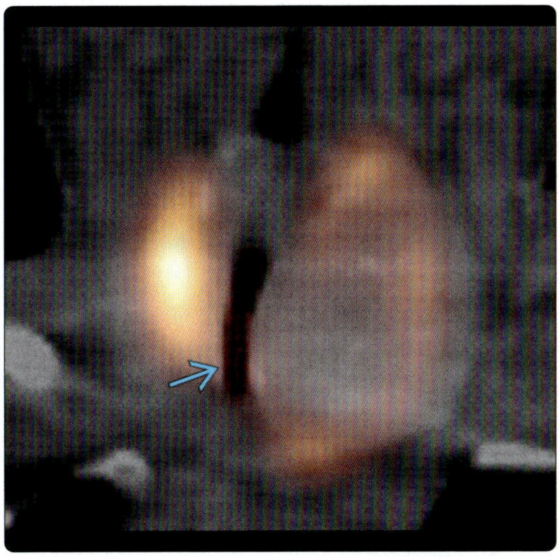

(Left) *Anterior Tc-99m pertechnetate thyroid scan in a patient with hyperthyroidism shows an enlarged left thyroid lobe with a dominant cold nodule* ➡*. This would need correlation with ultrasound to evaluate for malignancy prior to I-131 therapy.* **(Right)** *Coronal fused Tc-99m pertechnetate thyroid SPECT/CT in the same patient shows tracheal compression* ➡*. Most commonly, this finding favors surgical treatment instead of I-131 therapy.*

Lymphoma Therapy

KEY FACTS

TERMINOLOGY

- Radioimmunotherapy (RIT): Targeted therapy delivering localized radiation to tumor via monoclonal antibody (anti-CD20)
  - Labeling anti-CD20 with radionuclide allows for 2 therapeutic mechanisms
    - Anti-CD20 promotes cellular apoptosis and delivers radionuclide to tumor
    - Emission of β particle from radionuclide provides local radiation to tumor cells
- Yttrium-90 ibritumomab tiuxetan (Zevalin): Only RIT currently available in USA
- Rituximab (Rituxan): Serves as a "predose" agent for RIT, administered as "cold" antibody before radiolabeled antibody
  - Saturates CD20 binding sites of B-cells in circulation and in spleen and promotes better binding of therapeutic dose to tumor

PREPROCEDURE

- Indications: Relapsed or refractory low-grade or follicular B-cell lymphoma during or after initial treatment with rituximab and standard chemotherapy; previously untreated follicular lymphoma with partial or complete response to 1st-line therapy

PROCEDURE

- Predose (day 1): Infusion of rituximab
  - Whole-body biodistribution dose and imaging no longer required by FDA
- Therapeutic dose (day 7, 8, or 9): Infusion of 2nd round of rituximab followed by infusion of Y-90 ibritumomab
  - Dose based on platelet count and weight

OUTCOMES

- Overall response rate of ~ 80% and complete response rate of ~ 30% in refractory or relapsed disease
- Complications: Neutropenia, thrombocytopenia

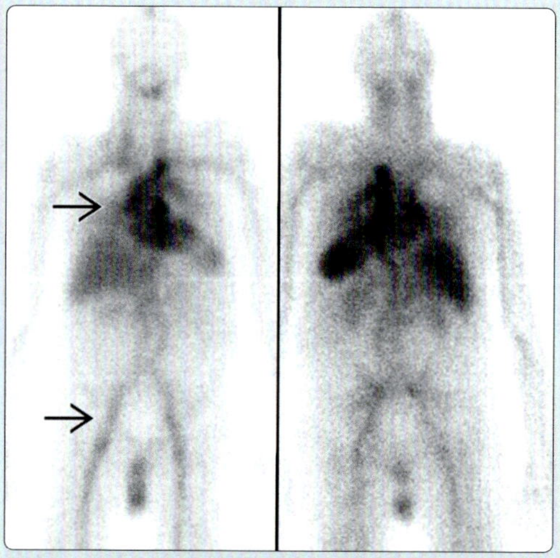

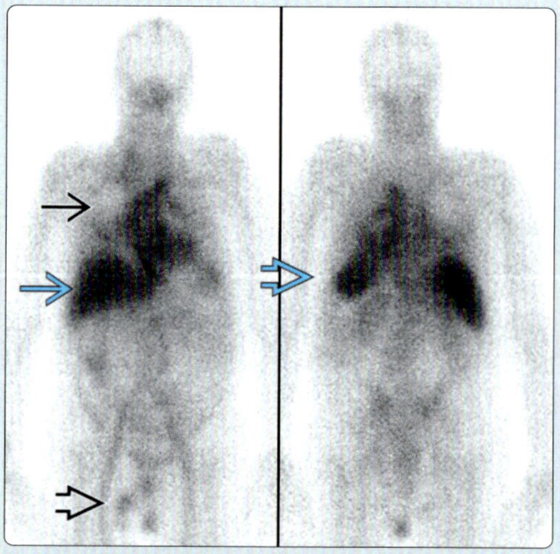

(Left) *Normal blood pool activity → is shown after 5 mCi (185 MBq) In-111 ibritumomab tiuxetan on anterior and posterior 4-hr biodistribution images.* **(Right)** *Decreasing blood pool activity → and normal amount of liver → and spleen ⇨ activity are shown on anterior and posterior 48-hr biodistribution images after 5 mCi (185 MBq) In-111 ibritumomab tiuxetan in the same patient. Activity is evident in right groin lymphadenopathy ⇨.*

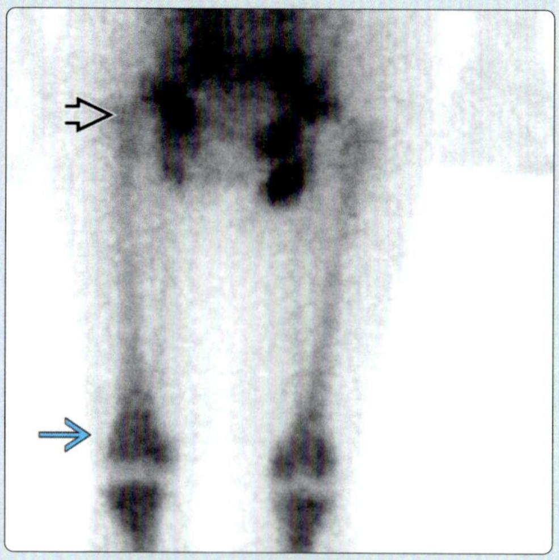

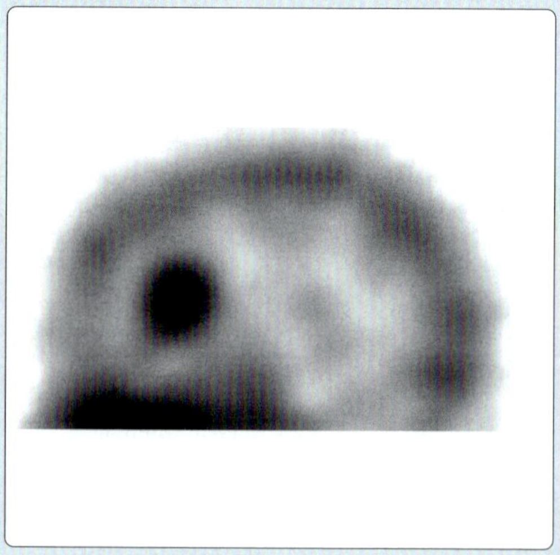

(Left) *Biodistribution image after 5 mCi (185 MBq) In-111 ibritumomab tiuxetan shows bilateral groin lymphadenopathy ⇨ and diffuse activity in the bone marrow →, a relative contraindication to therapy due to bone marrow suppression.* **(Right)** *Sagittal SPECT biodistribution image after 5 mCi (185 MBq) In-111 ibritumomab tiuxetan shows uptake in a focus of CNS lymphoma.*

TERMINOLOGY

Definitions

- Radioimmunotherapy (RIT): Targeted therapy delivering localized radiation to tumor via monoclonal antibody (anti-CD20)
  - Epitope CD20 often expressed on B-cells of non-Hodgkin lymphoma (NHL), pre-B-cells, and mature B-cells, but not plasma cells
  - Labeling anti-CD20 with radionuclide allows for 2 therapeutic mechanisms
    - Anti-CD20 promotes cellular apoptosis and delivers radionuclide to tumor
    - Emission of β particle from radionuclide provides local radiation to tumor cells
- Yttrium-90 ibritumomab tiuxetan (Zevalin)
  - Physical t1/2 of 2.7 days; β decay, particle energy 2.3 MeV; particle path length 5.3 mm
  - Ibritumomab: Murine monoclonal antibody (anti-CD20), which binds to cells with CD20(+)
  - Tiuxetan: Metallic stabilizing agent used to link Y-90 and ibritumomab
- Other RIT drug, I-131 tositumomab (Bexxar), discontinued in 2014 for commercial reasons, partly due to projected decline in sales
- Rituximab (Rituxan)
  - Chimeric anti-CD20 monoclonal antibody (non-radiolabeled) primarily used as single agent or in combination with chemotherapy for lymphoma
  - Serves as "predose" agent for RIT: Administered as "cold" antibody before radiolabeled antibody
    - Saturates CD20 binding sites of B-cells in circulation and in spleen and promotes better binding of therapeutic dose to tumor

PREPROCEDURE

Indications

- Relapsed or refractory low-grade or follicular B-cell lymphoma during or after initial treatment with rituximab and standard chemotherapy
- Previously untreated follicular lymphoma with partial or complete response to 1st-line therapy

Getting Started

- Things to Check
  - Confirm initial biopsy has CD20 expression
  - Confirm bone marrow biopsy < 25% involvement
  - Complete blood count for platelets and ANC
  - Review allergies and medications

Precautions

- No pregnancy or breastfeeding
- Treatment not recommended if
  - Absolute neutrophil count (ANC) < 1,500 cells/mm³
  - Platelets < 100,000/mm³
  - > 25% bone marrow involvement

PROCEDURE

Equipment Preparation

- IV placement
- Oral antipyretic and antihistamine prophylaxis for infusion reaction before rituximab

Procedure Steps

- Y-90 ibritumomab tiuxetan (Zevalin)
  - Predose (day 1)
    - Infusion of rituximab
    - Whole-body biodistribution dose and imaging (bioscan) no longer required by FDA
      - Was performed to confirm normal biodistribution and exclude abnormal pharmacokinetics
      - Performed with infusion of 5 mCi (185 MBq) In-111 ibritumomab after rituximab on day 1
      - Normal: Uptake in cardiac blood pool, great vessels, liver, ± lymph nodes, mild spleen, minimal renal
      - Post-marketing surveillance found bioscan to be an unreliable predictor of altered biodistribution with many false-positives
  - Therapeutic dose (day 7, 8, or 9)
    - Infusion of 2nd round of rituximab followed by infusion of Y-90 ibritumomab
    - Dose of Y-90 ibritumomab based on platelet count and weight

POST PROCEDURE

Expected Outcome

- Overall response rate of ~ 80% and complete response rate of ~ 30% in refractory or relapsed disease

Things To Do

- General radiation safety precautions to avoid contamination of others with body fluids without specified time duration

Things To Avoid

- NSAIDs and aspirin given risk of cytopenias, thrombocytopenia

OUTCOMES

Problems

- Complications: Anaphylaxis (most feared), prolonged neutropenia, thrombocytopenia

SELECTED REFERENCES

1. Prasad V: The withdrawal of drugs for commercial reasons: the incomplete story of tositumomab. JAMA Intern Med. 174(12):1887-8, 2014
2. Chamarthy MR et al: Radioimmunotherapy of non-Hodgkin's lymphoma: from the 'magic bullets' to 'radioactive magic bullets'. Yale J Biol Med. 84(4):391-407, 2011
3. Goldsmith SJ: Radioimmunotherapy of lymphoma: Bexxar and Zevalin. Semin Nucl Med. 40(2):122-35, 2010
4. Wahl RL: Tositumomab and (131)I therapy in non-Hodgkin's lymphoma. J Nucl Med. 46 Suppl 1:128S-40S, 2005
5. Zevalin Dosing and Administration. Spectrum Pharmaceuticals, 2014

Hepatic Metastases Therapy

KEY FACTS

TERMINOLOGY

- Yttrium-90 radioembolization for hepatic metastases therapy → pure beta emitter, tissue penetration ~ 2.5 mm, t1/2 = 64.2 hrs
- Targeted delivery of Yttrium-90 microparticles allows destruction of unresectable hepatic tumors, sparing normal liver

PREPROCEDURE

- Indications: Unresectable primary liver malignancy or metastatic disease with liver predominant tumor burden **and** life expectancy > 3 months
- Contraindications: Disseminated extrahepatic metastases, liver failure, excessive lung shunt fraction on Tc-99m MAA scan, unavoidable extrahepatic perfusion

PROCEDURE

- Tc-99m MAA embolization scan
    - Calculate lung shunt fraction, detect extrahepatic perfusion, calculate Yttrium-90 dose
    - Intraarterial injection of 3-5 mCi (111-185 MBq) Tc-99m MAA
    - Freshly eluted Tc-99m, inject < 30 min after prep
- Tc-99m MAA imaging
    - Anterior/posterior static images of thorax/abdomen
    - SPECT or SPECT/CT images of upper abdomen
- Yttrium-90 injected 1-2 weeks later
    - Sir-sphere empirical dose: % liver involved → 20% = 2 GBq; 25-50% = 2.5 GBq; > 50% = 3 GBq
    - Therasphere dose: A = (D • M)/(50 Gy • kg • GBq^{-1})

POST PROCEDURE

- Prophylactic medications: Nausea → antiemetics, gastritis → PPI or H1 blocker, post-embolization syndrome (fever, malaise, lethargy) → tapering steroids
- Post-therapy imaging: PET shows response to therapy sooner than CT/MR, DWI-MRI more accurate for assessing response

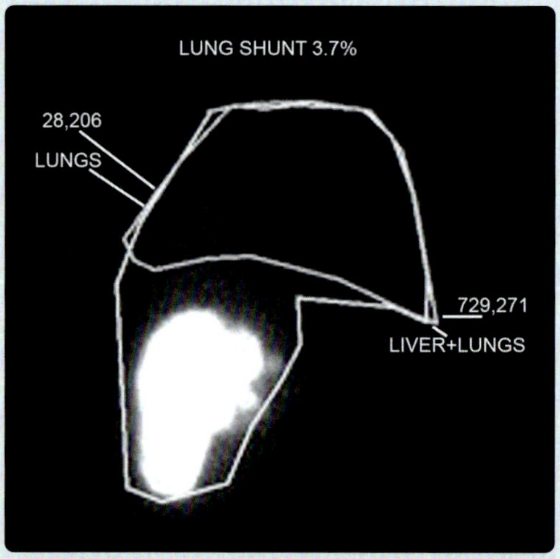

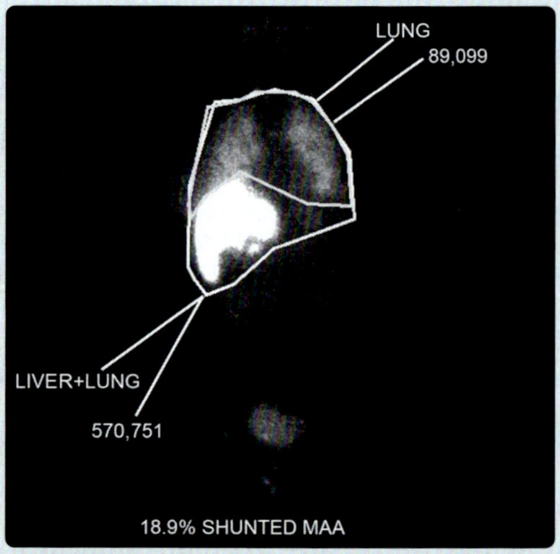

(Left) *Anterior static planar image demonstrates normal lung shunt fraction (~ 3.7%) with right hepatic intraarterial infusion of Tc-99m MAA. Lung shunt fraction = [lung counts/(lung + liver counts)] * 100.* **(Right)** *Anterior static planar image demonstrates 19% lung shunt fraction with infusion of Tc-99m MAA. Adjust dose for lung shunting: < 10%, no reduction; 10-15%, ↓ dose 20%; 15-20%, ↓ dose 40%; > 20%, no treatment.*

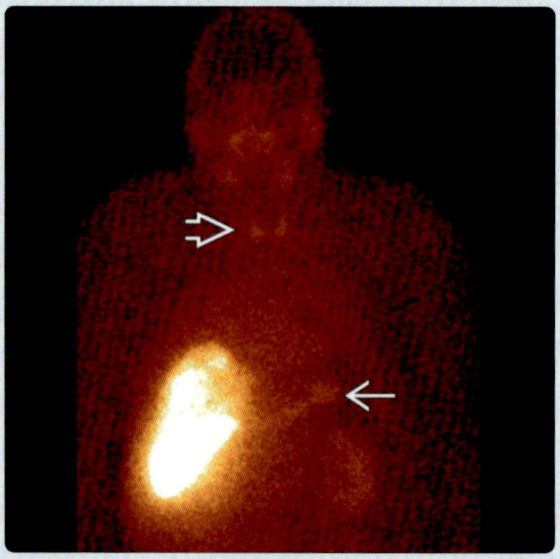

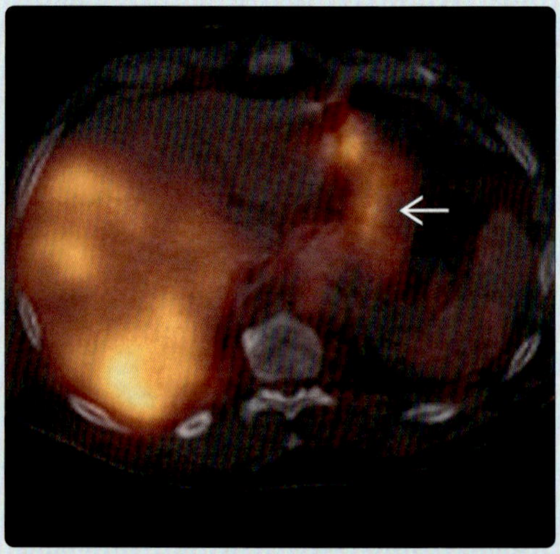

(Left) *Anterior static planar image demonstrates activity within the stomach ➡ and thyroid gland ➡ consistent with free pertechnetate. Using freshly eluted Tc-99m MAA and injecting < 30 min after preparation reduces false-positive activity.* **(Right)** *Axial fused SPECT/CT from the same patient after Tc-99m MAA right hepatic artery infusion shows diffuse uptake within the stomach ➡. This differs from extrahepatic perfusion which is more likely focal. Correlation with angiographic findings is often required.*

TERMINOLOGY

Definitions

- Yttrium-90 radioembolization for hepatic metastases therapy
- Pure beta emitter (mean: 2.28 MeV); tissue penetration ~ 2.5 mm, t1/2 = 64.2 hrs
- 2 radiopharmaceuticals: Yttrium-90 resin microparticles (SirSpheres) and glass microparticles (TheraSpheres)

Concept

- Liver malignancies derive ~ 90% of blood supply from hepatic arteries, normal parenchyma 70% from portal vein
- Targeted delivery of Yttrium-90 microparticles allows destruction of tumor cells while sparing normal liver

PREPROCEDURE

Indications

- Unresectable 1° liver malignancy or metastatic disease with liver predominant tumor burden **and** life expectancy > 3 months

Contraindications

- Resectable liver cancer
- Disseminated extrahepatic metastases
- Excessive lung shunt fraction on Tc-99m MAA
    - Sir-Sphere: > 20% lung shunting
    - TheraSphere: > 16.5 mCi (610 MBq) of Yttrium-90 delivery to lungs
- Unavoidable extrahepatic perfusion: Contraindicated if treatment results in nontarget embolization of viscera
- ± portal vein thrombosis
- ± liver failure: ↑ AST or ALT > 5x normal, bilirubin > 2 mg/dL

Preprocedure Imaging

- CECT/MR of abdomen/pelvis: Evaluate tumor volume, liver volume, resectability and portal vein patency
- F-18 FDG PET/CT: Assess extent of disease or presence of metastases
- Arteriography and Tc-99m MAA lung shunting study
    - Delineate vascular anatomy and identify congenital variants
    - Empiric coil embolization of right gastric, gastroduodenal &/or cystic artery to prevent nontarget treatment
    - Coil embolize extrahepatic vascularity arising from hepatic arteries, e.g., falciform artery
    - Inject Tc-99m MAA

Getting Started

- Things to Check
    - History, physical examination, assessment of performance status
    - Laboratory tests (CBC, BMP, LFTs, PT/INR)
    - Tumor marker assay (carcinoembryonic antigen [CEA], α-fetoprotein [AFP])

PROCEDURE

Procedure Steps

- Tc-99 macroaggregated albumin (MAA)
    - Calculate lung shunt fraction to determine risk of radiation pneumonitis
    - Detect extrahepatic perfusion arising from injected vascular territory to ascertain risk of nontargeted radioembolization
    - Calculate Yttrium-90 microsphere dose to be delivered
    - Confirm deposition at sites of tumor
- Tc-99m MAA injection protocol
    - Last step of angiography
    - Position catheter within hepatic artery supplying involved liver segment
    - Gently agitate syringe to resuspend MAA particles
    - Hand inject of 3-5 mCi (111-185 MBq) Tc-99m MAA suspended in normal saline under sterile conditions
    - Use freshly eluted Tc-99m, inject < 30 min after preparation (reduces false positive activity from free pertechnetate)
    - Inject slowly to avoid reflux
- Tc-99m MAA imaging
    - Image in nuclear medicine department as soon as practical after angiography procedure, usually within 1-2 hours after injection
    - Planar scan: Anterior or anterior/posterior images of thorax + abdomen in whole-body mode
    - Calculate lung shunt fraction
        - Draw single region of interest (ROI) around both lungs and a separate ROI around liver and lung
        - Lung shunt fraction = [lung counts/(lung + liver counts)] * 100
        - If anterior and posterior views are obtained, geometric mean of counts used
    - SPECT/CT of upper abdomen strongly recommended
        - Confirm hepatic segments embolized with MAA correspond with malignancy
        - Detect evidence of extrahepatic perfusion; common sites include stomach, gallbladder, peripancreatic, 2nd portion of duodenum and periumbilical
        - Free pertechnetate can create false-positive mimic of extrahepatic gastric perfusion
            - If thyroid activity is also present, then etiology is free
            - Focal gastric uptake favors extrahepatic perfusion, whereas free pertechnetate more likely involves entire stomach
- Yttrium-90 administered dose
    - Sir-sphere
        - Empirical method (historical) based on % liver involved: 20% = 54 mCi (2 GBq); 25-50% = 68mCI (2.5 GBq); > 50% = 81 mCI (3 GBq)
        - Adjust dose for lung shunting: < 10% no reduction; 10-15% ↓ dose 20%; 15-20% ↓ dose 40%; >20% no treatment
        - Partition model (more accurate): Complex calculation based upon body surface area, liver volume to be treated and % of volume involved by tumor with corrections for lung shunt
        - Online calculator provides convenient dose calculation: http://apps01.sirtex.com/smac
    - Therasphere
        - Goal: 80-150 Gy to liver
        - $A = (D \bullet M)/(50\ Gy \bullet kg \bullet GBq^{-1})$
            - A is activity of Yttrium-90 required (GBq), D is nominal target dose (Gy), M is liver mass (kg)

Yttrium-90 Resin and Glass Microsphere Comparison

Parameters	Sirspheres	Theraspheres
FDA approval	Metastatic colorectal as neoadjuvant therapy or pretransplant	Unresectable hepatocellular carcinoma
Diameter	20-60 μm	20-30 μm
Activity per particle	50 Bq	2500 Bq
Number of microspheres per 3 GBq vial	40-80 x 10^6	1.2 x 10^6
Material	Resin microsphere	Glass microsphere

POST PROCEDURE

Expected Outcome

- Postembolization syndrome: Fever, malaise, lethargy
  - Cytokine effect from radiation injury to tumor and regeneration/neovascularization of normal liver
  - Treatment: Oral steroid taper unless contraindicated
- Nausea, gastric irritation: Due to radiation from adjacent liver
  - Commence antiemetics morning of procedure
  - Proton pump inhibitor or H1 blocker 1 week prior to 4 weeks after
- Transient rise in LFTs posttherapy; should subside in 1-2 weeks
- Effective duration of treatment ~ 92.4 hrs (94% of radiation delivered in 11 days)

Post-Therapy Imaging

- F-18 FDG PET/CT shows treatment response sooner than CT/MR for metastases; utility for nonhypermetabolic HCC or cholangiocarcinoma limited
- DWI MR more accurate than CT/MR for assessing response
- Size criteria alone is imperfect evaluation of response
  - Tumors may increase in size (pseudoprogression from edema, necrosis, or hemorrhage)
  - Avoid early posttreatment CT, may misinterpret findings for progression
- Most common CT appearance after therapy: ↓ attenuation in treated parenchyma; liver edema, congestion, microinfarction; incidental, self-limited reversible process
- Post Yttrium-90 bremsstrahlung scan
  - Broad-spectrum secondary gamma-ray emissions produced by interaction of high-energy beta emissions with tissue
  - Commonly performed to delineate hepatic distribution of microspheres and to detect unexpected extrahepatic deposition
  - Planar scintigraphy &/or SPECT/CT within 30 hrs of infusion (dual-head gamma camera with medium-energy collimators)

OUTCOMES

Complications

- Most feared complication(s)
  - Progressive pulmonary insufficiency secondary to radiation pneumonitis: Very rare but fatal complication
  - Radiation pneumonitis occurs with > 30 Gy in a single treatment, 50 Gy cumulative
  - Meticulous planning required to avoid Yttrium-90 therapy in patients with hepatopulmonary shunting
- Delayed complication(s)
  - Cholecystitis: Microspheres through patent cystic artery
    - Usually self-limited, rarely requires cholecystectomy
    - Avoid by infusing distal to cystic artery origin, empiric coil embolization
  - Gastritis, duodenitis or esophagitis: Inadvertent intestinal microsphere deposition
    - Can progress to chronic ulceration, bleeding and perforation
    - Minimized with empiric gastroduodenal artery coil embolization
  - Radiation dermatitis: Failure to empirically embolize falciform artery
  - Radiation-induced pancreatitis
- Other complications
  - Radioembolization-induced liver disease (REILD): Rare complication of Yttrium-90 microsphere treatment
    - Manifests as varying degrees of hepatic decompensation with development of jaundice and ascites
    - High-dose steroids traditionally used to decrease intrahepatic inflammation

SELECTED REFERENCES

1. Uliel L et al: From the angio suite to the γ-camera: vascular mapping and 99mTc-MAA hepatic perfusion imaging before liver radioembolization--a comprehensive pictorial review. J Nucl Med. 53(11):1736-47, 2012
2. Dezarn WA et al: Recommendations of the American Association of Physicists in Medicine on dosimetry, imaging, and quality assurance procedures for 90Y microsphere brachytherapy in the treatment of hepatic malignancies. Med Phys. 38(8):4824-45, 2011
3. Ibrahim SM et al: Radiologic findings following Y90 radioembolization for primary liver malignancies. Abdom Imaging. 34(5):566-81, 2009
4. Kennedy A et al: Recommendations for radioembolization of hepatic malignancies using yttrium-90 microsphere brachytherapy: a consensus panel report from the radioembolization brachytherapy oncology consortium. Int J Radiat Oncol Biol Phys. 68(1):13-23, 2007
5. Keppke AL et al: Imaging of hepatocellular carcinoma after treatment with yttrium-90 microspheres. AJR Am J Roentgenol. 188(3):768-75, 2007
6. Miller FH et al: Response of liver metastases after treatment with yttrium-90 microspheres: role of size, necrosis, and PET. AJR Am J Roentgenol. 188(3):776-83, 2007
7. Gulec SA et al: Dosimetric techniques in 90Y-microsphere therapy of liver cancer: The MIRD equations for dose calculations. J Nucl Med. 47(7):1209-11, 2006
8. Bienert M et al: 90Y microsphere treatment of unresectable liver metastases: changes in 18F-FDG uptake and tumour size on PET/CT. Eur J Nucl Med Mol Imaging. 32(7):778-87, 2005
9. Murthy R et al: Yttrium-90 microsphere therapy for hepatic malignancy: devices, indications, technical considerations, and potential complications. Radiographics. 25 Suppl 1:S41-55, 2005
10. Covey AM et al: Variant hepatic arterial anatomy revisited: digital subtraction angiography performed in 600 patients. Radiology. 224(2):542-7, 2002

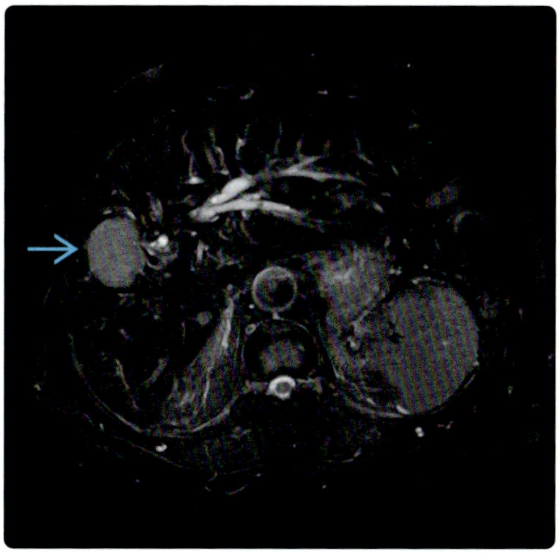

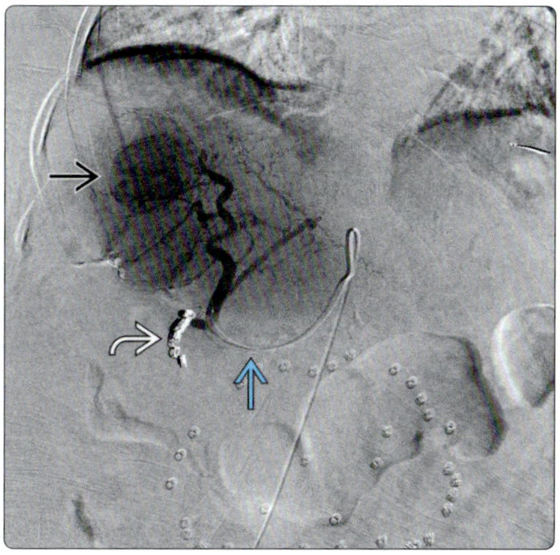

(Left) *Axial T2 FS MR demonstrates a 4 cm metastatic carcinoid tumor within segment 8 of the right hemiliver →.* **(Right)** *Planning right hepatic arteriogram shows a microcatheter ⇨ prior to Yttrium-90 therapy. Angiogram demonstrates a 4 cm hypervascular metastatic neuroendocrine tumor in segment 8 →. Empiric embolization of the gastroduodenal artery has been performed ↪.*

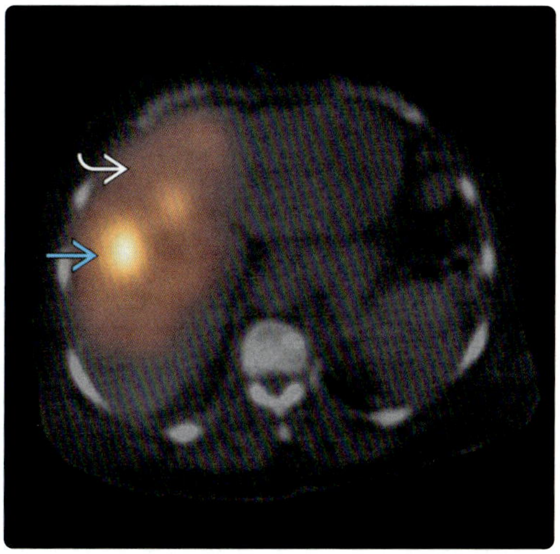

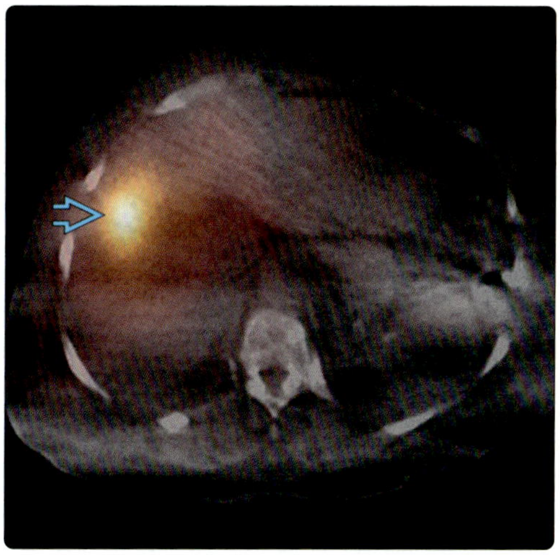

(Left) *Axial fused SPECT/CT in the same patient obtained after right hepatic arterial infusion of 2.5 mCi (92 MBq) of Tc-99m MAA is shown. Diffuse uptake is noted throughout segment 8 ↪ with more focal uptake within a carcinoid metastasis →.* **(Right)** *Axial SPECT/CT post Yttrium-90 therapy demonstrates focal uptake within the segment 8 carcinoid metastasis ⇨.*

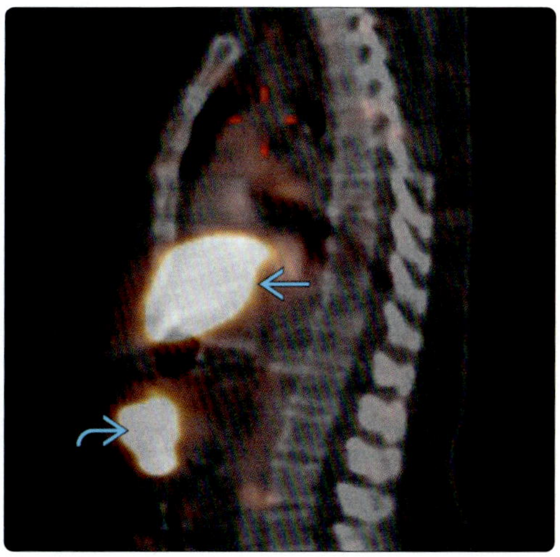

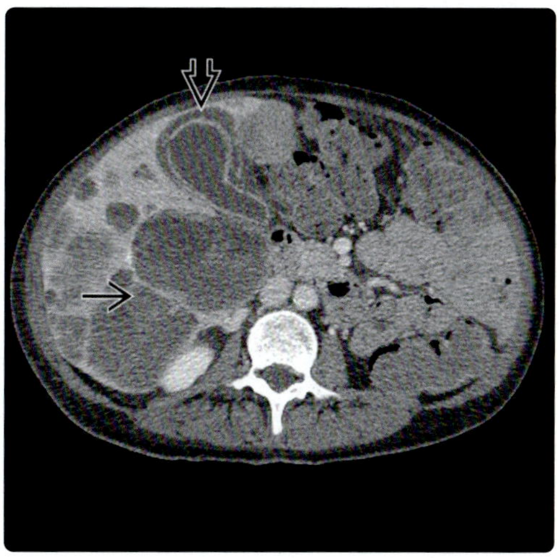

(Left) *Left sagittal fused SPECT/CT following hepatic arterial Tc-99m MAA infusion → shows significant abnormal periumbilical radiotracer uptake ↪. Inability to cannulate and empirically coil the falciform artery excluded this patient from receiving Yttrium-90 therapy.* **(Right)** *Post-contrast axial CT after Yttrium-90 therapy in a different patient shows metastatic neuroendocrine cancer →. Inadvertent radioembolization via cystic artery collaterals resulted in acute perforated radiation cholecystitis ⇩.*

Metastatic Bone Tumor Therapy

KEY FACTS

TERMINOLOGY

- Palliative radiopharmaceutical treatment of metastatic bone pain refractory to analgesics
- Radium-223 (Ra-223) (Xofigo, formerly Alpharadin)
    - 1st α-particle therapy approved in United States
    - 1st radiopharmaceutical therapy that extends survival in patients with bone metastasis
    - 3.6 month median survival advantage compared to placebo
- ALSYMPCA (ALpharadin in SYMptomatic Prostate CAncer patients) trial showed survival benefit of Ra-223 treatment in castration-resistant prostate cancer (CRPC) patients
- No specific radiation safety restrictions regarding contact with other people

PREPROCEDURE

- Recent Tc-99m MDP bone scan (< 8 weeks) with metastases
- Complete blood count with differential within 7 days before treatment
- Exclude contraindications

PROCEDURE

- IV access required with isotonic saline flush before and after injection
- Slow IV injection (usually over 1 min)
- Ra-223 dose: 1.3 μCi (50 kBq)/kg at 4 week intervals for 6 doses
- For maximum survival benefit, treating physician must plan for patient to receive all 6 cycles of Ra-223 treatment
- Pain relief is not a surrogate marker for treatment efficacy and failure of pain relief should not prompt treatment discontinuation

POST PROCEDURE

- CBC with differential every 3 weeks for evidence of hematopoietic recovery
- Ra-223: Up to 70% of patients show improvement in pain (20% complete pain response)
- May take 2-3 infusions (up to 3 months) for pain relief

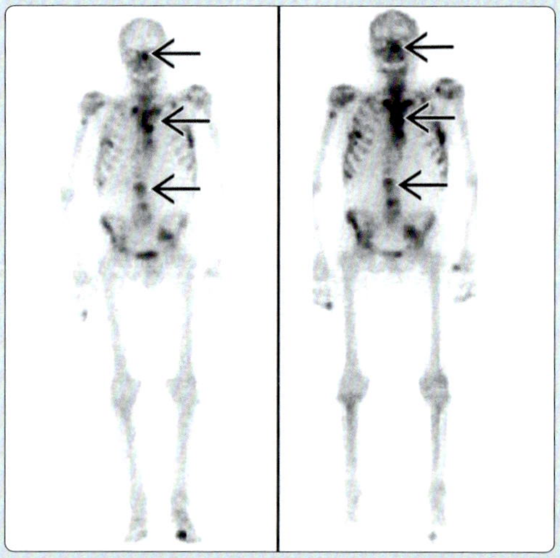

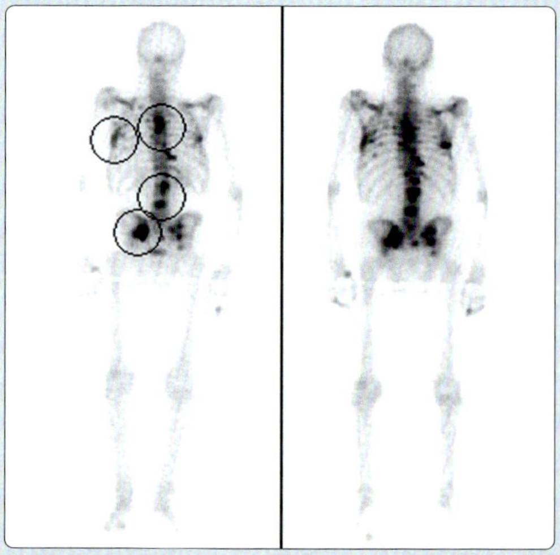

(Left) *Anterior bone scan with Tc-99m MDP (left) and Sm-153 (right) shows matching increased activity in a patient with diffuse bone pain from metastatic prostate cancer. (Courtesy Cytogen Corp.)* **(Right)** *Pain map in the same patient shows Tc-99m MDP (left) and tracer localization in the same regions with Sm-153 (right), predicting good response. (Courtesy Cytogen Corp.)*

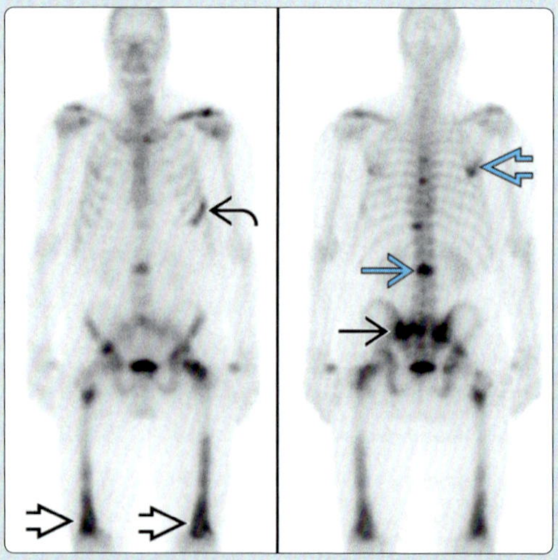

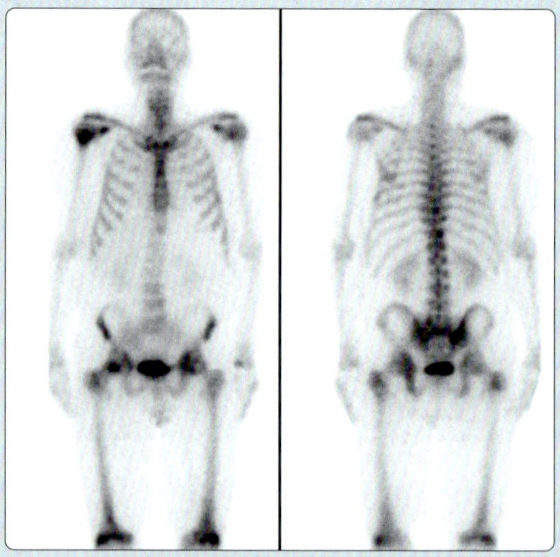

(Left) *Anterior and posterior Tc-99m MDP bone scan in a patient with metastatic prostate cancer shows multifocal tracer uptake in the spine, rib, scapula, pelvis, and femora.* **(Right)** *After Ra-223 treatment, anterior and posterior Tc-99m MDP bone scan in the same patient shows decreased tracer uptake. This patient had a decrease in pain after Ra-223.*

TERMINOLOGY

Definitions

- Bone pain is a cardinal symptom of bone metastases
  - Initially intermittent pain of variable intensity; progresses to chronic pain with breakthrough acute episodes
  - Major impact on quality of life
  - Mechanical allodynia (normal, nonpainful activities become painful, e.g., coughing)
- Metastatic bone tumor therapy
  - Radiopharmaceutical treatment of metastatic bone pain refractory to analgesics
    - **Alpha emitter: Radium-223** (Ra-223) (trade name Xofigo; formerly known as Alpharadin)
      - ALSYMPCA (ALpharadin in SYMptomatic Prostate CAncer patients) trial showed survival benefit of Ra-223 treatment in castration-resistant prostate cancer (CRPC) patients
      - Median survival advantage of 3.6 months as compared to placebo
      - 30% ↓ in risk of death compared to placebo
    - **Beta emitters: Samarium-153, strontium-89**
      - Considered palliative: Usually do not affect survival

Alpha Emitter

- **Radium-223 (Xofigo)**
  - 1st α-particle therapy approved in United States
  - 1st radiopharmaceutical therapy that extends survival in patients with bone metastases
  - Bone-seeking α emitter mimicking calcium, 4 α-particles generated for each decay
  - Produced from Ra-223 extraction generator (parent isotopes Ac-227 and Th-227)
  - t1/2: 11.43 days
  - Alpha emission (95.3%; energy range: 5-7.5 MeV), beta emission (3.6%; average energies: 0.445 MeV and 0.492 MeV), gamma emission (1.1%; energy range: 0.01-1.27 MeV)
  - Greater biological effectiveness due to high linear energy transfer
  - Less hematological toxicity due to shorter path length (60-100 μm) of α-particles
  - Rapid blood clearance (< 1% blood activity at 24 hours), no significant redistribution
  - Decreases bone specific alkaline phosphatase (ALP), marker for tumor response in CRPC
  - Excretion: Gastrointestinal (52% activity in bowel at 24 hours), minimal urinary excretion (< 5%)
  - **Mechanism of action**
    - Increased uptake and complex formation with hydroxyapatite at sites of increased bone turnover
    - α-particle-induced double-stranded DNA breaks
  - **Benefits**
    - Survival benefit in symptomatic and progressive metastatic CRPC (2 or more skeletal metastases, no visceral metastases) regardless of disease extent, previous treatment with docetaxel and current treatment with bisphosphonates (ALSYMPCA trial)
      - 16% of patients showed ≥ 30% drop in PSA at 12 weeks
      - Delayed onset of first symptomatic skeletal event (symptomatic pathological bone fracture)
      - Pain relief
      - Improved quality of life
      - Delayed increase in ALP and PSA

Beta Emitters

- **Sm-153 (Lexidronam/Quadramet)**
  - t1/2: 1.9 days
  - Dose: 1 mCi (37 MBq)/kg maximum
  - Mixed beta and gamma emitter
  - 640, 710, and 810 keV beta emissions (mean: 0.23 MeV); average path length: 0.6 mm
  - Can image 103 keV gamma emissions (28% abundance)
  - Labeled to bisphosphonate ethylenediamine tetramethylene phospate (EDTMP) (↑ bone-seeking properties)
  - Urinary excretion: Complete ~ 6 hrs after administration
  - < 1% activity in blood 5 hrs after injection
- **Sr-89 (Metastron)**
  - t1/2: 50.5 days
  - Dose 40-60 uCi (1-1.6 MBq)/kg up to 4 mCi (148 MBq); dose can be repeated after 3-4 months
  - Pure beta emitter (1.49 MeV maximum energy; mean: 0.58 MeV), maximum path length: 8 mm; average path length: 2.4 mm
  - Bremsstrahlung imaging possible, but not practical
  - Physiologic distribution mimics calcium
  - Excretion: Mainly urinary (80%), partially fecal (20%)
  - Used in patients with moderate pain, reasonable life expectancy (> 3 months) due to long response duration
- **Mechanism of action**
  - Not well understood
  - Localized radiation to metastatic sites
  - May ↓ tumor volume
  - Likely ↓ in circulating cytokine, humoral factors that sensitize and stimulate nerve endings

PREPROCEDURE

Indications

- **Alpha emitters**
  - Skeletal metastases in CRPC, symptomatic bone metastases, and no known visceral metastatic disease or malignant lymphadenopathy exceeding 3 cm
    - Not currently receiving or scheduled to receive concurrent chemotherapy
    - Not currently receiving or scheduled to receive hemibody external beam radiotherapy
  - Skeletal metastases for other types of cancer not yet approved/reimbursed
- **Beta emitters**
  - Metastatic bone pain due to CRPC and visceral metastases, metastatic bone pain palliation in patients with osteoblastic metastases from primaries other than prostate cancer
    - Treatment can be repeated
      - Duration of response may decrease
      - Risk of myelotoxicity generally increases

Contraindications

- **Alpha emitters**

- Pregnancy (however, not currently indicated for use in women currently)
- **Beta emitters**
  - Patient at high risk for pathologic fracture/cord compression (surgical, radiotherapy emergencies)
  - Hemoglobin < 90 g/L or 9 g/dL
  - White blood cells < 3,500 cells/mm^3
  - Platelets < 600,000/mm^3
  - Pregnancy, breast-feeding, and women of child-bearing age
  - Life expectancy < 3 months (especially for long T½ agents)
  - Disseminated intravascular coagulation (DIC)
  - Acute or chronic renal failure (glomerular filtration rate < 30 mL/min)
  - Urinary incontinence/obstruction (not absolute contraindication)
    - Consider catheterization, stenting prior to treatment

Getting Started

- Things to check
  - **Alpha emitters**
    - 1st dose: Blood counts prior to treatment initiation
      - ANC ≥ 1.5 x 10^9/L, platelet count ≥ 100 x 10^9/L, and hemoglobin ≥ 10 g/dL
    - Subsequent doses (doses 2-6): Blood count prior to treatment, order blood counts 1 week prior to therapy
      - ANC ≥ 1 x 10^9/L and platelet count ≥ 50 x 10^9/L (hemoglobin > 8 g/dL was threshold in clinical trial)
    - Close monitoring of patients with compromised bone marrow reserves; provide supportive care (e.g., transfusions, G-CSF therapy) as indicated
    - Discontinue if hematologic values do not recover within 6-8 weeks after last administration despite supportive care
- **Beta emitters**
  - Recent Tc-99m MDP bone scan (< 8 weeks) showing metastases (radiographs demonstrating osteosclerotic lesions not adequate)
    - Most predictable response to treatment in bone scan positive lesions
    - Symptoms can be mapped to bone scan to confirm pain caused by lesions
    - Superscan or diffuse proximal long bone activity indicates extensive marrow involvement; may predict myelotoxicity
  - No myelosuppressive chemotherapy for 6 weeks before and 12 weeks after treatment
  - No external beam hemibody radiotherapy for 2-3 months before treatment
  - Complete blood count within 7 days before treatment
  - Exclude contraindications
  - Dose reduction may be needed for renal failure
  - Exclude spinal cord compression

PROCEDURE

Procedure Steps

- **Alpha emitters**
  - Outpatient treatment after informed consent and discussion of radiation safety precautions
  - Fasting not required
  - 1.36 uCi/kg (50 kBq/kg) IV at 4 week intervals for 6 total doses
  - Flush IV line or cannula with isotonic saline before and after Ra-223 injection
  - IV injection of radiopharmaceutical over 1 min
  - If dose infiltrates, stop and treat as if iodinated contrast extravasation; new IV to complete dose administration if necessary; most of dose will be absorbed and delivered to metastases
  - No dose adjustment currently recommended for patients with renal or hepatic impairment
  - No known effect of concurrent bisphosphonates or calcium channel blockers administration on safety and efficacy of Ra-223
  - Concomitant administration of Ra-223 and chemotherapy (outside clinical trials) is not recommended due to additive bone marrow suppression
- **Beta emitters**
  - Outpatient treatment after informed consent and discussion of radiation safety precautions
    - Informed consent should include discussion of transient pain increase ("flare"), leukocytopenia with increased risk of infections, and thrombocytopenia with increased risk of bleeding
  - Fasting not required, good patient hydration
  - Running IV access essential as dose infiltration can cause soft tissue necrosis
  - Slow IV injection of radiopharmaceutical (usually over 1 min) followed by saline flush
  - Plastic syringe shield decreases bremsstrahlung radiation
  - If Sm-153 used, can perform whole-body imaging
  - Stop bisphosphonates for 48 hours after treatment, consider bone scan to confirm uptake if bisphosphonates used within 2 weeks preceding treatment
  - Although not essential, imaging can verify uptake in painful lesions

POST PROCEDURE

Expected Outcome

- **Alpha emitters**
  - Pain relief is not a surrogate marker for treatment efficacy; failure of pain relief should not prompt treatment discontinuation
  - Mean duration of pain relief: 44 days
  - Overall pain response rate: 52%, 60%, and 56% of patients at 1, 4, and 8 weeks after therapy, respectively
  - For maximum survival benefit, recommended that patient receives all 6 Ra-223 treatments
- **Beta emitters**
  - 25-80% probability of subjective pain response
  - Pain reduction may take 1-3 weeks; treatment failure should not be assumed until 4 weeks
  - Overall pain response rates
    - Sm-153: 62-74%
    - Sr-89: 60-84%
  - Duration of response
    - Sm-153: Mean of 8 weeks (4-35 weeks)

  - Sr-89: Mean of 6 months (≤ 14 months)

OUTCOMES

Problems

- **Alpha emitters**
  - Transient pain increase may occur after treatment (flare response), most commonly in 1st week after treatment
  - Radiation safety and other precautions
    - Low tissue penetrating power of α-particles (absorbed by dead outer layer of skin)
    - Low γ emission from Ra-223 decay
    - No specific restrictions regarding contact with other people
    - Good personal hygiene, particularly with bowel movements and urination
      - Flush toilet several times after each use
    - Body fluid handling: Gloves and hand washing to protect caregivers
    - Soiled clothing should be washed promptly and separately
    - For skin or eye contact: Affected area should be washed immediately with water
    - Sexually active males should use condoms, and their female partners should use contraception and avoid pregnancy for 6 months after completion of treatment with Ra-223
- **Beta emitters**
  - Most common reason for treatment failure = poor patient selection
    - Positive bone scan mapped to bone pain = highest likelihood of response
  - Transient increased pain (painful flare) may occur 2-3 days (up to 21 days) after treatment
    - Usually self-limited (2-5 days)
    - Most prominent with Sr-89 treatment, rare with Sm-153
    - May suggest good therapeutic response
  - Response less predictable in patients with primarily osteolytic lesions
  - Post treatment monitoring
    - Leukocyte and platelet counts 2 weeks after injection, subsequently every 1-2 weeks for 12-16 weeks
  - Radiation safety and other precautions
    - Maximum (80-90%) urinary excretion during first 48 hours
    - Good personal hygiene particularly with urination
      - Avoid soiling underclothing or area around toilet bowl
      - Wash soiled underclothes separately
      - Sit down to urinate
      - Flush toilet twice after use
      - Wash hands thoroughly after urination
    - Body fluid handling: Gloves and gown to protect caregivers
    - Incontinent patients: Bladder catheterization or condom drainage, absorbent undergarments, plastic mattress covers

Complications

- Most feared complication(s)
  - **Alpha emitters**
  - Systemic complications
    - Hematological toxicity
      - Bone marrow failure or pancytopenia (2% of patients)
      - Grade 3-4 lymphocytopenia (20%), anemia (6%), leukopenia (3%), thrombocytopenia (3%), neutropenia (2%)
    - Nonhematological toxicity
      - More common, usually transient
      - Nausea (36%), diarrhea (25%), vomiting (19%)
      - Grade 3-4 peripheral edema (2%)
      - Grade 3-4 renal failure and impairment (1%)
      - Dehydration (3%)
      - Potential increased risk of fertility impairment, secondary malignant neoplasms (osteosarcoma, lymphoma, and mammary gland carcinoma in rats) and hereditary defects
  - Local complications
    - Toxicity: Injection site erythema, pain, edema (1%)
  - **Beta emitters**
  - Systemic complications
    - Myelotoxicity
      - Critical organ: Bone marrow
      - Most patients typically develop transient myelosuppression 4-8 weeks after therapy (for Sm-152 nadir at 3-4 weeks, recovery by 8 weeks)
      - Duration and severity variable depending on radionuclide, dose, and bone marrow reserve
      - Myelotoxicity may be cumulative for repeat treatments
      - Toxicity can be more severe in patients with subclinical disseminated intravascular coagulation (10-20% of patients with advanced prostate cancer)
  - Local complications
    - Dose infiltration
      - Beta-emitting radiopharmaceutical delivered to skin/tissues around IV site
      - Can cause skin and muscle necrosis requiring surgical intervention
      - Ensure properly working IV before administration
  - Other complications
    - Transient ↑ in pain with Sr-89
      - Increased dose of breakthrough analgesics often required
    - Musculoskeletal complaints
    - Nausea/vomiting, diarrhea
    - Bleeding
    - Case reports of leukemia following treatment with Sr-89 (causal relationship not established)

SELECTED REFERENCES

1. Abi-Ghanem AS et al: Radionuclide therapy for osseous metastases in prostate cancer. Semin Nucl Med. 45(1):66-80, 2015
2. Shore ND: Radium-223 Dichloride for Metastatic Castration-resistant Prostate Cancer: The Urologist's Perspective. Urology. 85(4):717-724, 2015
3. Maini CL et al: 153Sm-EDTMP for bone pain palliation in skeletal metastases. Eur J Nucl Med Mol Imaging. 31 Suppl 1:S171-8, 2004
4. Pandit-Taskar N et al: Radiopharmaceutical therapy for palliation of bone pain from osseous metastases. J Nucl Med. 45(8):1358-65, 2004

SECTION 13

Physics

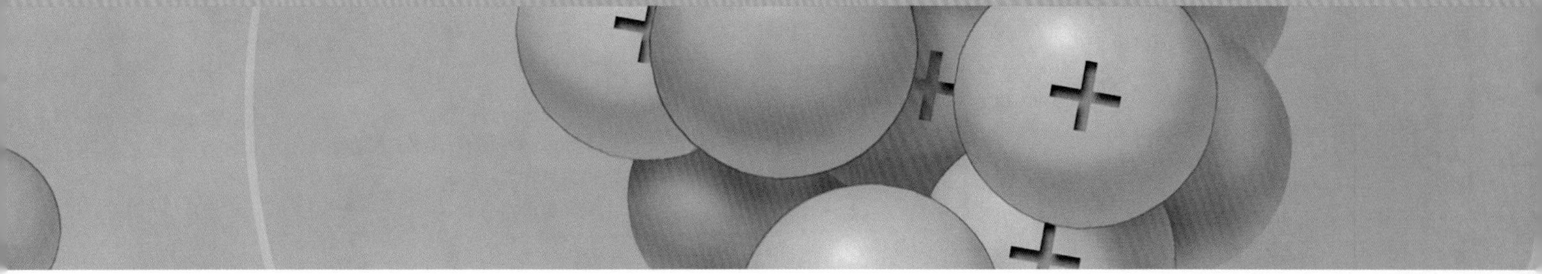

KEY FACTS

ISOTOPE IDENTIFICATION

- X = element name
- A = total number of protons and neutrons
- Z = total number of protons
  - Also called atomic number
- t1/2 (half-life) = amount of time for half of any sample of unstable isotope to change its energy state/decay

TERMINOLOGY

- Alpha particle (α)
  - Essentially helium nucleus (2 protons, 2 neutrons)
  - Emitted in decay of heavier isotopes (atomic mass unit > 106)
  - Alpha particles are very ionizing (energy ~ 5 MeV) and have very low tissue penetration (20-40 μm)
- Beta particle (β)
  - Electron ejected from nucleus with excess neutrons (higher than normal n/p ratio)
- Positron particle (β+)
  - Positively charged electron ejected from nucleus with excess protons (lower than normal n/p ratio)
  - Due to abundance of electrons (antiparticle to positrons), positron very quickly annihilates when combining with electron, emitting 2 diametrically opposed gamma rays
- Electron capture (ε-)
  - Occurs when proton-rich nucleus captures electron and converts proton to neutron and ejects neutrino
- Gamma particle (γ)
  - High-energy photon emitted from nucleus that has excess energy
  - Can be created when positron and electron collide and annihilate
- Neutron (n)
  - Decay occurs with heavy isotopes of smaller elements and in fission of large nuclei
  - Not generally used in nuclear medicine

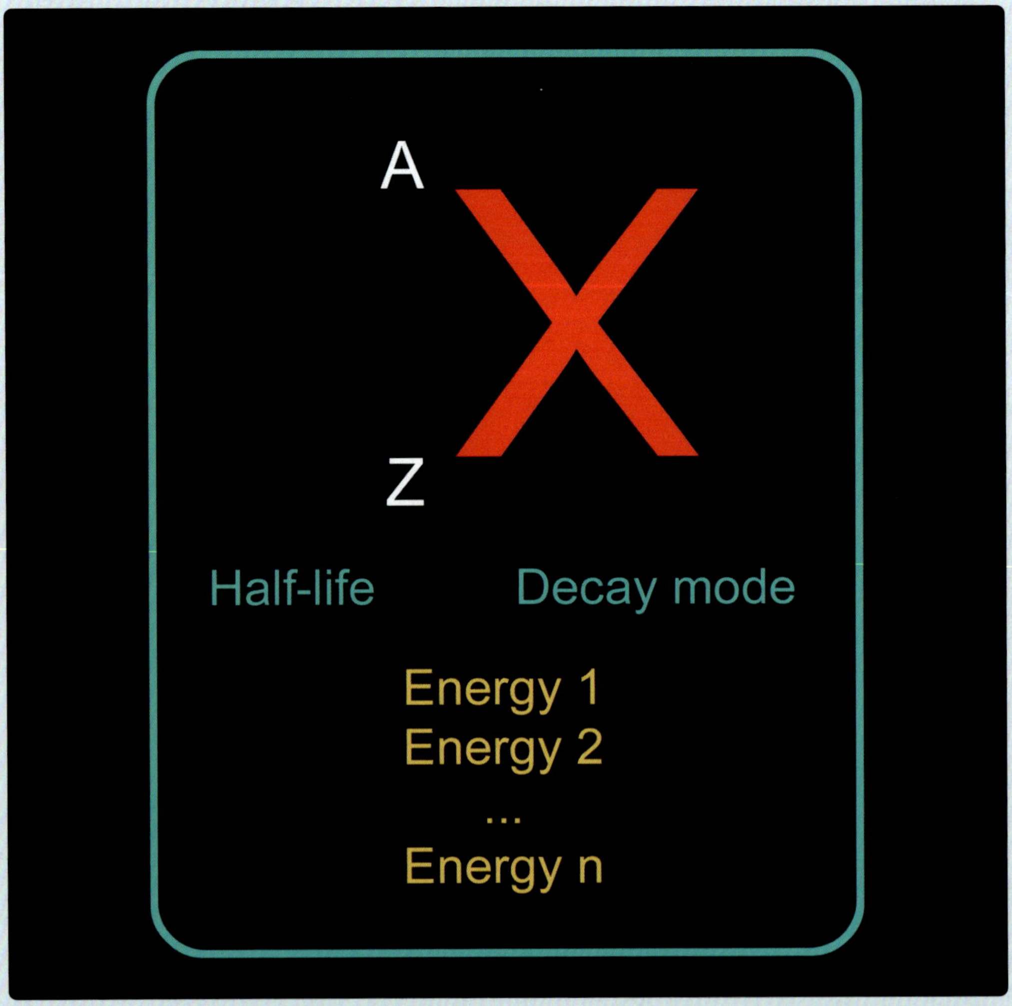

Isotope identification is shown. X represents the element. A (atomic mass) represents total number of protons and neutrons (~ 1 amu each). Z represents total number of protons (atomic number). Half-life indicates the time for half the particles in a sample to decay. Decay mode indicates the primary mode of radioactive decay for the isotope. The energies represent the energy of particles that emerge as a result of the decay.

TERMINOLOGY

Definitions

- Atom
  - Collection of protons and neutrons in nucleus with orbiting electrons
  - Bohr model simplification is adequate for nuclear medicine, though atoms actually have quantum orbitals
  - Atomic number: Number of protons
  - Atomic mass: Number of protons + neutrons
    - Proton: 1.00728 atomic mass unit (amu)
    - Neutron: 1.00867 amu
    - Electron: 0.000549 amu (much smaller than proton or neutron and thus not significant part of atomic mass)
- Isotope
  - One of multiple forms of atom (equal in proton count; variable number of neutrons)
  - Stable isotopes have similar numbers of neutrons and protons and are not radioactive
    - Most elements (up to Pb) have > 1 stable isotope
  - Unstable isotopes (all isotopes of elements beyond Pb) have higher number of neutrons and are radioactive
    - Larger elements require more neutrons to hold nucleus together
    - Neutron-to-proton (n/p) ratio is > 1
- Radiation
  - In general, radiation is any emission of energy or energetic particle
  - Specific particles emitted from unstable elements that are used in nuclear medicine include alpha (α), beta (β), positron (β+), and gamma (γ) radiation
  - X-rays are also created from secondary interactions with electron shell of atom
  - X-rays are lower energy subset of gamma rays
- Radioactive decay
  - Unstable radionuclides try to become stable by releasing particle or emission of high-energy photon
  - For lighter nuclides, stable nuclides have approximately same number of neutrons and protons
  - For heavier nuclides, stable nuclides have approximately 1.5x as many neutrons as protons
  - Becquerel (Bq) (Standard International (SI) unit) = 1 disintegration per second (dps)
  - Curie (non-SI unit) = 37 trillion dps = 37 billion Bq; 1 mCi = 37 MBq

RADIOACTIVE DECAY

General Concepts

- Nucleus decays when unstable parent isotope emits photon &/or particle and produces daughter isotope of lower energy
  - Electronvolt (eV): Amount of energy gained or lost by charge of single electron that is moved across electric potential difference of 1 volt
  - Units of emitted particle energies in nuclear medicine: kilo-electron volts (keV) and mega-electron volts (MeV)
  - 1 eV = 1.6×10^{-19} joules
- t1/2 (half-life)
  - Physical t1/2
    - Amount of time for half of any sample of unstable isotope to change its energy state/decay
      - Probability of decay of any specific unstable nucleus is fixed
      - Collection of particles decays at constant logarithmic rate
  - Biologic t1/2
    - Amount of time half of radioactive compound is eliminated from body
    - Elimination is typically via urine, feces, exhalation
  - Effective t1/2
    - Amount of time half of radioactive compound is eliminated from body via radioactive decay **and** biological excretion
    - 1/effective t1/2 = 1/physical t1/2 + 1/biologic t1/2

Modes of Decay

- Alpha decay (α)
  - Alpha particle is effectively helium nucleus (2 protons and 2 neutrons)
  - Alpha particles are emitted in decay of heavier isotopes (atomic mass unit > 106)
  - Alpha particles are very ionizing (energy ~ 5 MeV) and have very low tissue penetration (20-40 μm)
    - Alpha particles can be stopped by layer of skin or few cm of air
    - Very dangerous if ingested, as surface mucosa of GI tract is very sensitive to alpha radiation damage
  - Alpha particles are used to deliver radiation to specific local area, sparing adjacent tissues
- Beta decay (β-)
  - Occurs in neutron-rich nuclei
  - Beta particle is electron ejected from nucleus with excess neutrons (higher than normal n/p ratio)
    - In decay, neutron is transformed into proton, electron, and antineutrino
  - Atomic mass does not change (A; protons + neutrons) but atomic number (Z; number of protons) increases by 1
  - Because of low mass and high speed, beta particles have medium tissue penetration (0-1 cm), but can be stopped by few mm of metal shielding
  - Beta particles are very ionizing and when decelerated can give off secondary x-rays (bremsstrahlung radiation)
- Positron decay (β+)
  - Occurs in proton-rich nuclei
  - Positron particle is positively charged electron ejected from nucleus with excess protons (lower than normal n/p ratio)
    - In decay, proton is transformed into neutron, positron, and neutrino
  - Atomic mass does not change (A; protons + neutrons) but atomic number (Z; number of protons) decreases by 1
  - Due to abundance of electrons (antiparticle to positrons), positron very quickly annihilates when combining with electron, emitting 2 diametrically opposed gamma rays
- Electron capture (ε-)
  - Electron capture occurs when proton-rich nucleus captures electron and converts proton to neutron and ejects neutrino

- Alternate decay path when insufficient energy to eject positron (ΔE of < 1.022 MeV [combined rest mass of positron and electron])
- Gamma decay (γ)
  - Gamma particles can be emitted from nucleus that has excess energy
    - No change in A number or Z number of isotope, simply change in energy state
  - Gamma particles can be created when positron and electron collide and annihilate
    - 2 gamma particles of energy 0.511 MeV along oppositely directed vectors
  - Lower energy gamma particles can be created when decelerating charged particle
    - For example, decelerating electrons create bremsstrahlung radiation
- Neutron decay (n)
  - Occurs with heavy isotopes of smaller elements and in fission of large nuclei
  - Not generally used in nuclear medicine

RADIOPHARMACEUTICAL PRODUCTION

Radionuclides

- Typically short t1/2 of min to days
- Emit energies that are reasonable to stop efficiently with 3/8" NaI crystal (such as Tc-99m that emits gamma ray at 140 keV)
- Ideally decay to stable isotope
- Radionuclides can be created by
  - Adding neutron (n) to atom
    - Fission in nuclear reactor (source of thermal neutrons to bombard atom)
    - Xe-132 + ^{1}n → Xe-133 + γ
      - Xe-133 gas is used for lung ventilation scans
    - Mo-98 + ^{1}n → Mo-99 + γ
      - Mo-99 is parent product of Tc-99m
  - Adding charged particle to atom
    - Accelerator or cyclotron, which accelerates speed of charged particle to bombard atom
    - ^{16}O + ^{3}He → F-18 + p
      - F-18 is positron emitter commonly used in PET/CT imaging (e.g., F-18 FDG)
  - Allowing parent radionuclide to decay, producing daughter radionuclide from generator system
    - Decay-growth relationship of parent to daughter radionuclide
      - Long-lived parent radionuclide produces short-lived daughter radionuclide (t1/2 parent > t1/2 daughter)
      - Parent and daughter radionuclides must be different so that they can be separated chemically
      - As parent radionuclide decays, daughter is formed until equilibrium is reached
      - Frequent milking of generator produces more daughter radionuclide (will continue to try to reach equilibrium)
      - At equilibrium, daughter radionuclide appears to have same t1/2 as parent radionuclide
    - Example: Tc-99m generator: TC-99m is product of Mo-99 decay
      - ^{99}Mo → ^{99m}Tc → ^{99}Tc → ^{99}Ru (t1/2: 67 hrs → 6 hrs → long → stable)
      - Molybdate (MoO_4^{2-}) is absorbed onto acid alumina column
      - As Mo-99 decays to Tc-99 by beta decay, loss of electron in pertechnetate (TcO_4^-) causes it to be more loosely bound to alumina
      - Normal saline dissolves loose pertechnetate, leaving parent Mo-99 on column
      - Generator is milked to extract Na-99 mTcO_4 solution

Radiopharmacy

- Labeling radiopharmaceuticals with Tc-99m
  - Most radiopharmaceuticals are prepared with kit by radiopharmacy to tag pharmaceutical agent to radionuclide
  - Tc-99m most common radionuclide tag due to its low physical t1/2, low radiation dose to patient with relatively high mCi doses, and ideal gamma camera imaging characteristics of 140 keV gamma ray

Quality Control

- Radionuclide purity
  - Assess for desired radionuclide without impurity
  - Must have < 0.15 μCi (0.00555 MBq) of Mo-99/mCi of Tc-99m
  - Use moly breakthrough test in dose calibrator to assess
- Radiochemical purity
  - Assessing correct chemical form of sample
  - Thin layer chromatography (TLC) used to assess free pertechnetate or hydrolyzed reduced form of Tc-99m
- Chemical purity
  - Aluminum in eluate of Tc-99m assessed with colorimetric test
- Sterility
  - Absence of contaminating microorganisms including spores
  - Test by culturing samples
- Apyrogenicity
  - Assess for pyrogens that produce fever
  - Limulus amoebacyte lysate test used

SELECTED REFERENCES

1. Cherry et al. Physics in Nuclear Medicine. Saunders, 2012

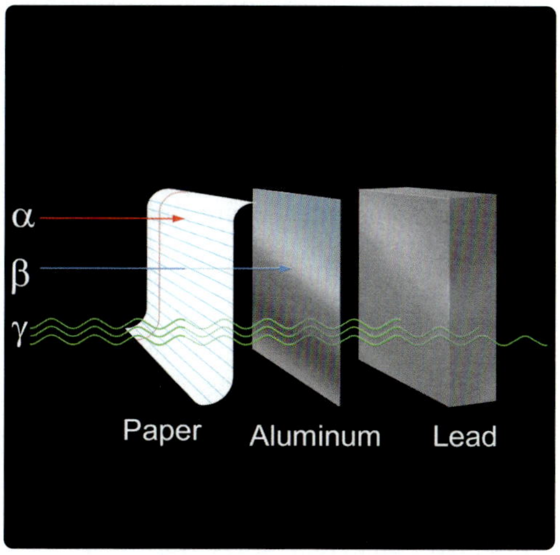

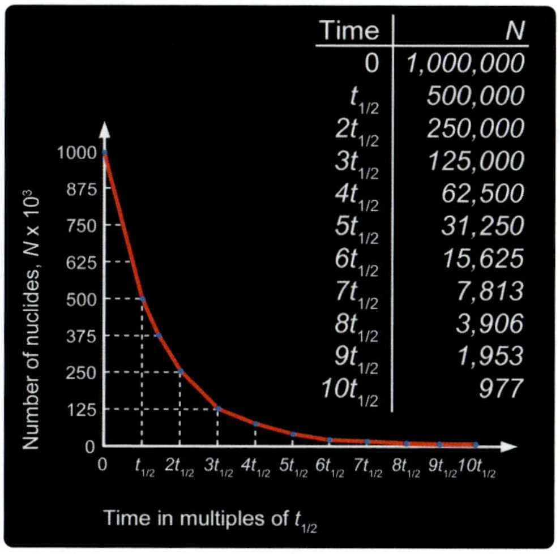

(Left) *Alpha particles are large and will only penetrate to a shallow depth. Beta particles can penetrate deeper, but are easily attenuated by a few centimeters of water or a thin metal sheet. Gamma rays easily pass through tissue, are moderately attenuated by dense tissues like bone, and require thick lead shielding for protection.* **(Right)** *The exponential law of decay states that for each t1/2 time, the number of atoms that decayed is half of what remains after the last t1/2 time. This produces an exponential pattern.*

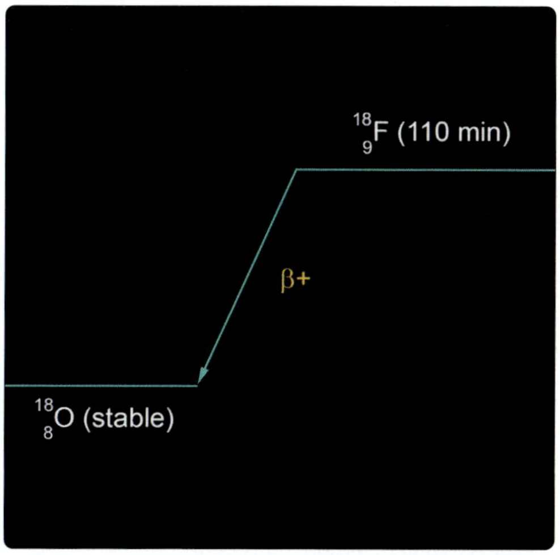

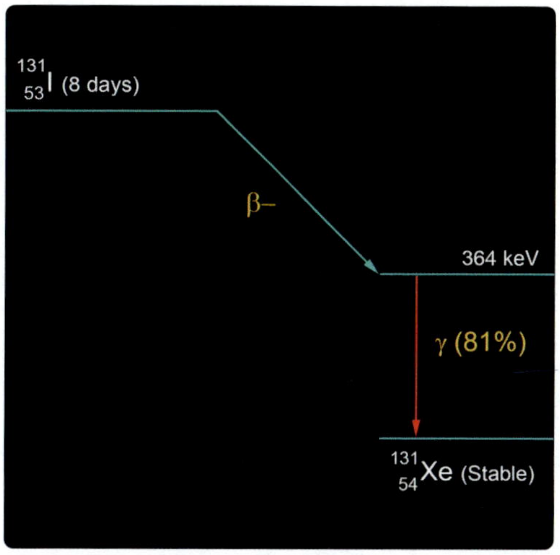

(Left) *Fluorodeoxyglucose-18 (^{18}F) decays via positron emission (β^+) to stable oxygen 18 (^{18}O) with a t1/2 of 110 min. ^{18}F tagged to FDG (fluorodeoxyglucose; a sugar) is used in most PET imaging.* **(Right)** *Iodine (^{131}I) decays to stable xenon (^{131}Xe) via beta minus (β^-) decay and gamma (γ) emissions with a t1/2 of 8 days. ^{131}I NaI is used to treat hyperthyroidism and thyroid cancer. The β^- component kills the thyroid cells while the γ allows for gamma camera imaging of the localization.*

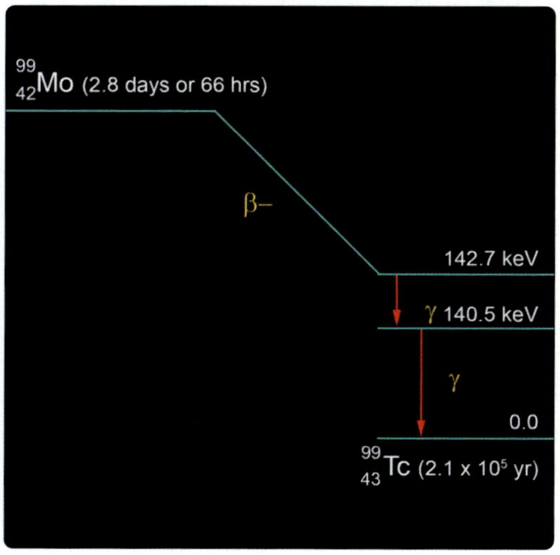

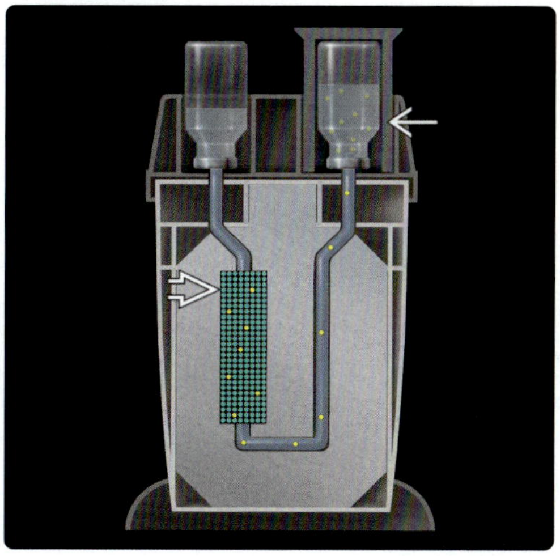

(Left) *Molybdenum (^{99}Mo) decays to technetium (^{99}Tc) via beta minus (β^-) decay and gamma (γ) emissions with a t1/2 of 67 hrs. ^{99}Mo is placed in a generator to allow for decay to ^{99m}Tc, which will then be eluted.* **(Right)** *Molybdenum (^{99}Mo) ➨ generator that produces technitium-99m (^{99m}Tc) ➨ is shown.*

KEY FACTS

PERSONAL DOSIMETERS

- Monitor cumulative radiation dose in individual to ensure they are not exceeding safe exposure limits

DOSE CALIBRATORS, WELL COUNTERS, THYROID PROBES, AND AREA MONITORS

- Gas-filled vs. crystal scintillator
  - Gas-filled detectors
    - For general use in ionizing radiation detection
    - Cannot discern type or energy spectrum of radiation (for dose calibrator, must select button for each radionuclide is used)
    - Examples include Geiger Müller (GM) detector and dose calibrator (argon-filled detector)
    - Contains inert gas (such as helium, argon, or neon) with atoms ionized by radiation exposure (electrons knocked out of orbit)
    - Knocked-out electrons either create pulse (GM) or current stream of electrons (ion chamber or dose calibrator) that can be calibrated to set dose display (such as counts per minute or mR per hour [GM] or mCi or MBq [dose calibrator])
  - Scintillation detectors
    - Some systems, especially wells and probes, can resolve energy spectrum or limit detection to set energy window
    - Contains crystal (typically NaI with Tl doping) that converts gamma or x-ray radiation to light energy that is collected by photomultiplier (PMT) tube
    - Scintillator crystal is fragile and can easily be damaged by rapid changes in temperature, rough handling, or exposure to humidity
    - Nonimaging examples: Handheld detector, thyroid probe, or well counter
    - Imaging example: Gamma camera crystal

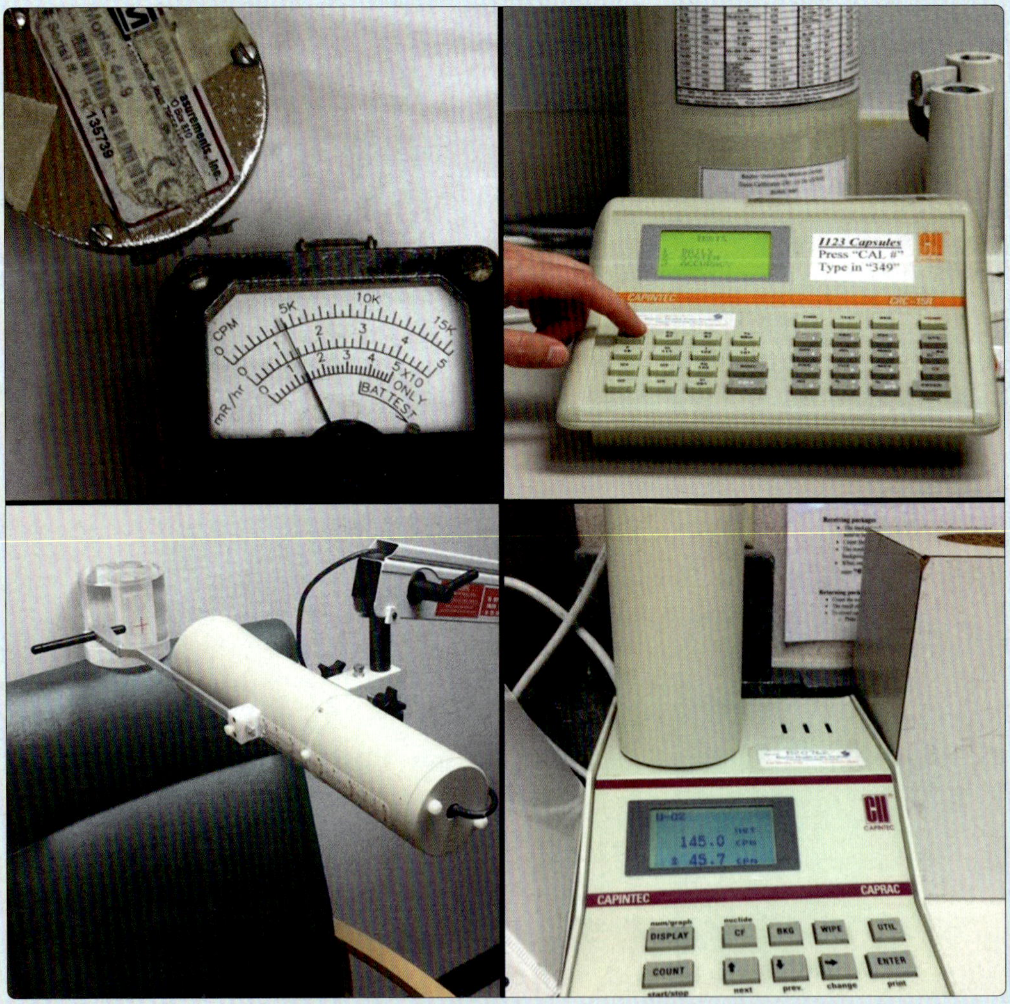

Gas-filled and scintillation detectors are shown: Geiger Müller (GM) gas-filled detector (top left) reads out in units of mR/hr; dose calibrator gas-filled detector (top right) typically reads out in mCi or MBq; thyroid uptake probe scintillation detector (bottom left) reads out in disintegration per minute (dpm); and well counter scintillation detector (bottom right) reads out in counts per minute (cpm) or distintegrations per minute (dpm) when radionuclide efficiency is taken into account.

TERMINOLOGY

Definitions

- Used to detect ionizing radiation for diagnostic/therapeutic as well as radiation safety purposes

NONIMAGING DETECTOR TYPES

Personal Dosimeters

- Monitor cumulative radiation dose in individual to ensure they are not exceeding safe exposure limits
  - Detects gamma rays, x-rays, beta particles, neutron radiation
- **Thermoluminescent dosimeter**
  - Uses materials that release light when heated (thermoluminescence) in response to previously stored radiation exposure
  - Measures intensity of visible light emitted from crystal when heated
  - Reusable after processing
- **Optically stimulated luminescence (OSL)**
  - Thin strip of aluminum oxide between multiple filters in small, sealed package (e.g., Landauer's Luxel+)
  - Aluminum oxide crystalline detector, when stimulated with laser, releases light in response to previously absorbed radiation
  - Filters in package help determine energy of absorbed radiation and thus better estimate correct exposure based on radiation quality
  - Also contains unique grid-like filter that helps determine if dose was static or dynamic for exposures > 500 mrem
  - Worn on torso/chest to monitor exposure to vital organs
  - Reusable after processing
  - Results expressed in deep dose equivalent (DDE), lens dose equivalent (LDE), and skin dose equivalent (SDE)
- **Film badge dosimeters**
  - Photographic or dental x-ray film in holder
  - Silver film emulsion sensitive to radiation; can have multiple emulsion coatings to detect wide range of exposures
  - Once developed, exposed areas blacken in response to previously absorbed radiation; can also darken if exposed to heat or light leakage into package, thus not reusable
  - Holder has filters that attenuate radiation so that types of radiation and energy can be distinguished upon developing film
  - Worn on torso or chest to monitor exposure to vital organs
  - Results expressed in DDE, LDE, and SDE
- **Electronic personal dosimeter**
  - Similar to Geiger-Müller (GM) counters or silicon solid-state detectors
  - Monitors exposure to radiation in real time; electronic version may have alarm capabilities
  - Can be locally reset and reused but should be sent out for calibration for accurate readings

Dose Calibrators, Well Counters, Thyroid Probes, and Area Monitors

- **Gas-filled detectors**
  - Gas contents are typically inert gas like argon or helium, which is easily ionized
  - Radiation (high-energy photon or particle) impacts gas particle in tube, ejecting electron
  - Free electron is accelerated through tube by voltage applied across gas
  - Accelerated electron impacts electrode at end of tube, creating temporary current
  - Current is detected and delivers signal to output device (visible or audible)
  - Ion chambers
    - Contains inert gas (such as helium, argon, or neon) with atoms ionized by radiation exposure (electrons knocked out of orbit) and produces current of electrons
    - Dose calibrators are used in nuclear medicine hot labs to verify total dose in mCi or MBq of radioisotope before administering to patient
    - Handheld ion chambers are used to measure patient exposure (e.g., for I-131 therapy patient prior to release with instructions on how to reduce exposure to others); e.g., Cutie Pie
  - Geiger-Müller counters
    - Contains gas (inert gas such as helium, argon or neon) with atoms ionized by radiation exposure (electrons knocked out of orbit); pulse of signal with each detection that can be audible or silent
    - GM meters are useful in radiation safety by detecting location and relative intensity of contamination; used for daily surveys
    - Daily battery check should be performed
- **Scintillation detectors**
  - Detects ionizing radiation using fluorescent material (crystal scintillator) and photomultiplier (PMT)
  - Fluorescent material (scintillation crystal) used will vary based on type of ionizing radiation to be detected
    - Gamma ray detectors (primary scintillation detector in NM) use high Z inorganic crystals, which have higher gamma detection cross sections; sodium iodide (NaI) doped with thallium (Tl) impurity is commonly used detection material
  - After interaction with ionizing particle, scintillation crystal emits light photon
  - PMT converts light to electrons and dynodes in PMT multiplies electrons and thus amplifies signal
  - Examples of nonimaging scintillation detectors include handheld meters, thyroid probes, and well counters
  - Well counters are used to do tests of contamination: Weekly wipe tests and daily package wipes
  - Scintillation counters are commonly used in thyroid uptake scans, detecting gamma radiation from I-123 or I-131 NaI
  - Handheld scintillation counters are more sensitive to radiation than GM detectors and are often required for measuring radioactive waste at background after 10 t1/2 decay-in-storage (for radionuclides with < 120 day t1/2)
- Detector geometry: Detector efficiency increases if detector can better surround source (e.g., dose calibrator and well counter)

SELECTED REFERENCES

1. Cherry SR et al. Physics in Nuclear Medicine, 4th edition. Saunders, 2012

KEY FACTS

TERMINOLOGY

- Gamma camera (Anger camera)
  - Detection device capable of capturing and counting gamma rays
  - Sodium iodide crystal (scintillator) + array of photomultiplier tubes (PMTs)
    - Thallium-doped sodium iodide crystal produces light when stimulated by gamma or x-ray photons
    - PMTs gather light and convert it to electronic signal near location it was detected
  - Collimator
    - Designed as series of holes that allow gamma rays through inside metal honeycomb pattern
    - Designed to eliminate photons that would degrade image (scattered or off-angle)
    - Parallel hole (most common type of collimator): Hole columns are all parallel to each other and perpendicular to gamma camera crystal
      - Only allows gamma photons that are perpendicular to face of camera to reach crystal
  - Gamma camera quality control
    - Daily flood: Uniformly flood camera with radioactive source and look for any nonuniformities
      - Intrinsic flood (with collimators removed): Point source is set at distance away from camera head
      - Extrinsic flood (with parallel hole collimators on): Flat uniform source (large rectangle or disc)
    - Weekly bars: Bar phantom is placed on camera head and imaged as test of detail resolution

(Left) *Collimators are designed to eliminate photons that would degrade image (e.g., scattered or off-angle). Here, parallel hole collimator (most often used) is shown, where the detector image size matches the object size.* **(Right)** *Diverging collimator is shown, where the detector image size is smaller than the object size.*

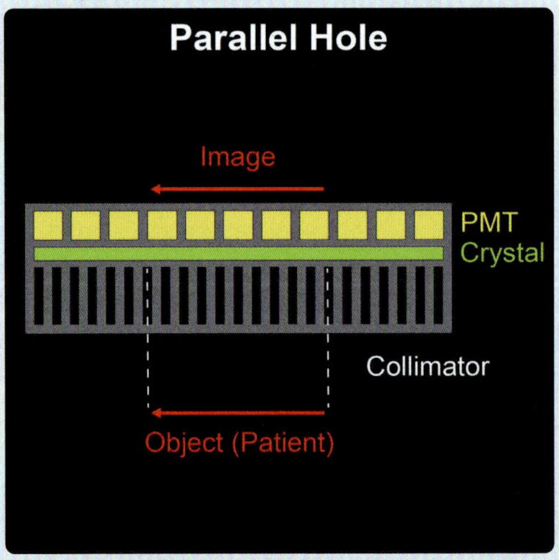

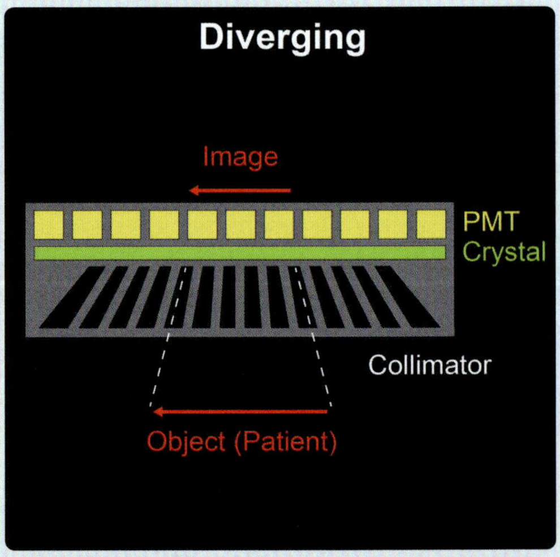

(Left) *Converging collimator is shown, where the detector image size is larger than object size.* **(Right)** *Pinhole collimator is shown, where the detector image size is larger and reversed.*

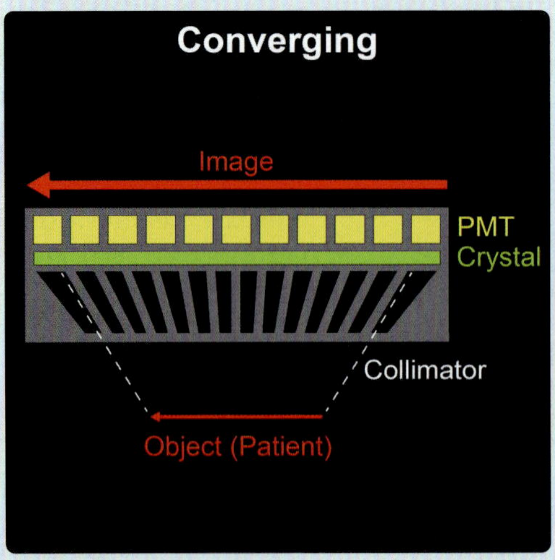

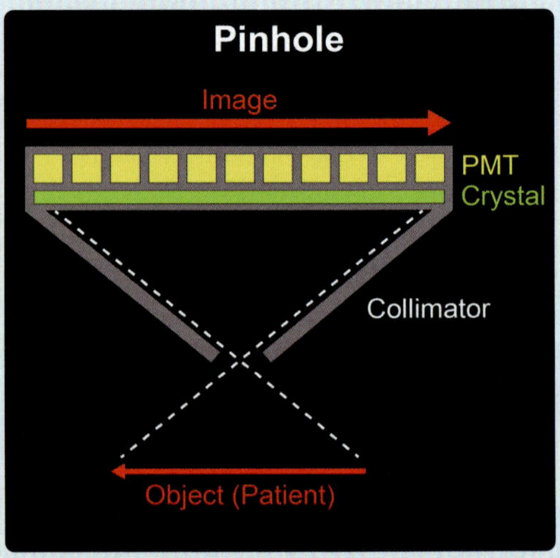

TERMINOLOGY

Definitions

- Gamma radiation
  - Electromagnetic radiation that has high enough energy to knock electron out of orbit or more (ionizing radiation)
  - Originates from nucleus of atom, usually from radioactive decay
  - Appear like x-rays at same energy but x-rays are produced by interactions with electron shells of atom
- Gamma camera (Anger camera)
  - Detection device capable of capturing and counting gamma rays
  - Uses solid crystal, which energizes or ejects electrons when interact with gamma ray photon
  - Sodium iodide crystal (scintillator) + array of photomultiplier tubes (PMTs)
    - Thallium-doped sodium iodide crystal produces light when stimulated by gamma or x-ray photons
      - Thicker crystal is more sensitive (more counts stopped) but has lower resolution
      - Thickness typically 3/8" based on primary use of Tc-99m (140 keV)
    - PMTs gather light and convert it to electronic signal near location it was detected
      - Includes set of dynodes that amplify signal
  - As electron falls back to lower energy level, low-energy photon (typically in visible spectrum) is emitted, detected, and counted by PMT
- Collimator
  - Device attached to gamma camera crystal front that only allows gamma photons perpendicular to face of camera to reach camera crystal
  - Designed as series of holes that allow gamma rays through inside metal honeycomb pattern
  - Designed to eliminate photons that would degrade image (e.g., scattered or off-angle)
  - Protects crystal face; typically designed with pressure sensor to prevent impact with patient or other objects
  - Collimators by shape
    - Parallel hole (most common type): Hole columns are all parallel to each other and perpendicular to gamma camera crystal
      - Only allows gamma photons perpendicular to face of camera to reach crystal
    - Diverging: Hole columns are arranged like a "V" with camera at narrow end and body at wider end; resulting images on camera are smaller than real size
    - Converging: Hole columns are arranged like a "V" with camera at wide end and body at narrow end; resulting images on camera are larger than real size
    - Pinhole: Exaggerated version of converging collimator where there is only 1 hole that converges out to width of camera to capture enlarged image
  - Collimators by energy and resolution (LEHR, MEGP, etc.)
    - Low energy (LE): Thin; used with Tc-99m or Tl-201
    - Medium energy (ME): Medium thickness; used with Ga-67 or In-111
    - High energy (HE): Thickest; used with I-131
    - High resolution (HR): Many holes and thick walls between hole columns; lower counts but increased image quality
    - Ultra high resolution (UHR): Many holes and thickest walls between hole columns; lower counts but increased image quality
    - General purpose (GP): Medium number of holes and medium thickness of walls; average between high resolution and high sensitivity
    - High sensitivity (HS): Thin walled between hole columns to allow for higher counts

Planar Imaging

- Camera is placed in fixed position or single view over patient
  - Acquires image of radionuclide position in body from one orientation

Radionuclides Used for Gamma Camera Imaging

- t1/2 short enough to see biological function
- Primarily gamma-only emitter
  - Beta or alpha emitters better for radiation therapy than imaging
- Preferably single energy or only a few energies between 100 and 300 keV
- Best example: Tc-99m 140 keV, 6 hour t1/2
- Affordable and readily available

IMAGING ANATOMY

General Anatomic Considerations

- Closer proximity of detector improves resolution and reduces radiation dose

CLINICAL IMPLICATIONS

Clinical Importance

- In contrast to SPECT and PET, gamma camera imaging produces 2-dimensional, planar image
- In contrast to radiography, gamma camera imaging places radiation source inside body and is more useful for measuring physiological function rather than anatomy
- Radiotracer selection and dosing should consider tracer t1/2, organ uptake, elimination routes and rates, and time required to collect adequate count levels for diagnosis

SELECTED REFERENCES

1. Cherry SR et al. Physics in Nuclear Medicine. Saunders, 2012
2. Christian PE et al. Nuclear Medicine and PET: Technology and Techniques, 5th Edition. Mosby, 2004
3. Karesh SM et al. Questions and Answers in Nuclear Medicine. Mosby, 1999

Intrinsic (collimators removed) uniformity QC test is shown with a point source → (10 uCi Tc-99m) placed at a distance < 5 field of views (FOVs) to allow irradiation of both camera heads simultaneously.

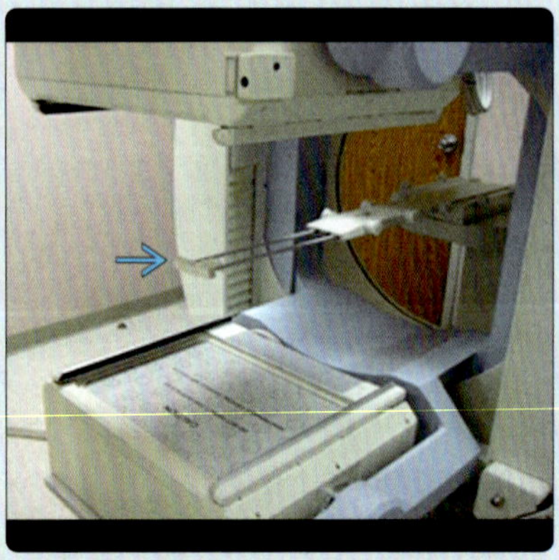

Intrinsic (collimators removed) uniformity QC test is shown with a point source → placed at a distance > 5 FOVs to allow irradiation of both camera heads simultaneously. Intrinsic uniformity tests can be done with ~ 0.5 mCi of any clinically used radionuclide.

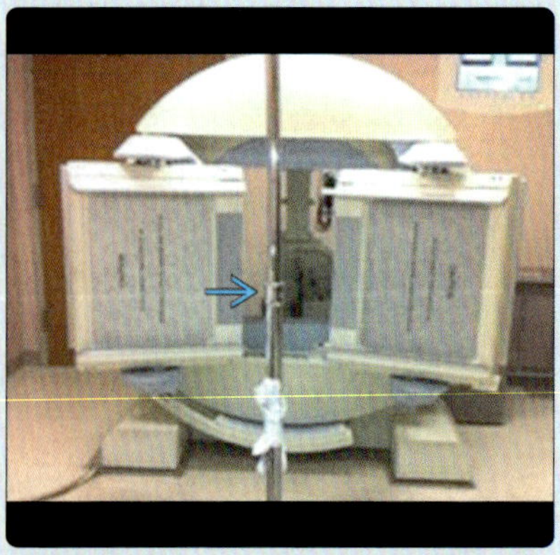

Extrinsic (parallel hole collimators on) uniformity QC test is shown with a Co-57 flood source → placed at a position half-way between camera heads to allow irradiation of both simultaneously. One head at a time may also be done at a closer distance.

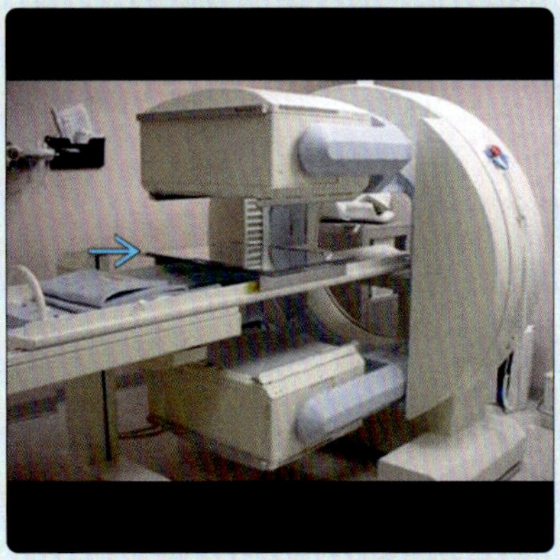

Extrinsic uniformity image of Co-57 flood source is shown. This test helps to look for camera and collimator issues. It is thus also called a system uniformity test.

Nonuniform image shows intrinsic imaging with point source < 5 FOVs from camera head. Curvature or dome correction is required to correct for nonuniformity based on known distance to source.

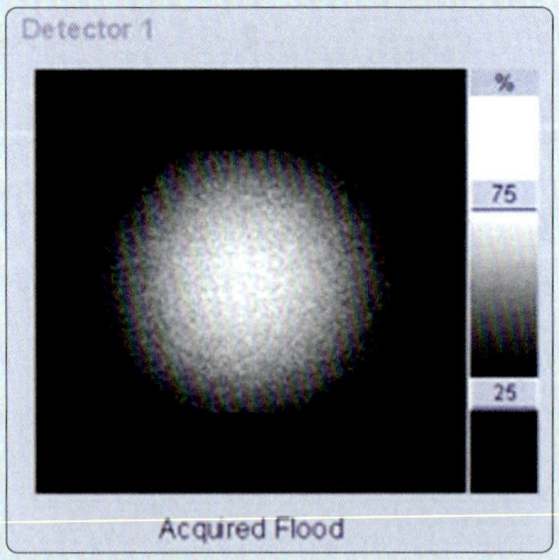

Intrinsic uniformity image after dome correction is shown; however, the intrinsic uniformity image acquired with point source at > 5 FOVs would also look the same.

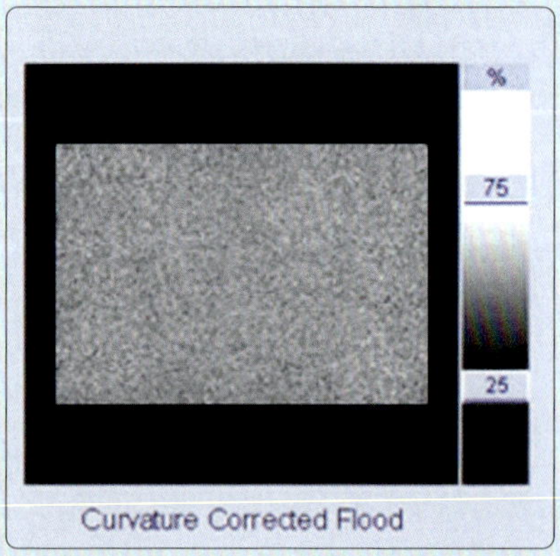

Bars image resolution test is done intrinsically (collimators removed) with bar phantom on top of camera and Tc-99m point source (0.5 mCi) at 5 FOV. It may also be done extrinsically (collimator on) with flood source placed on top of bars.

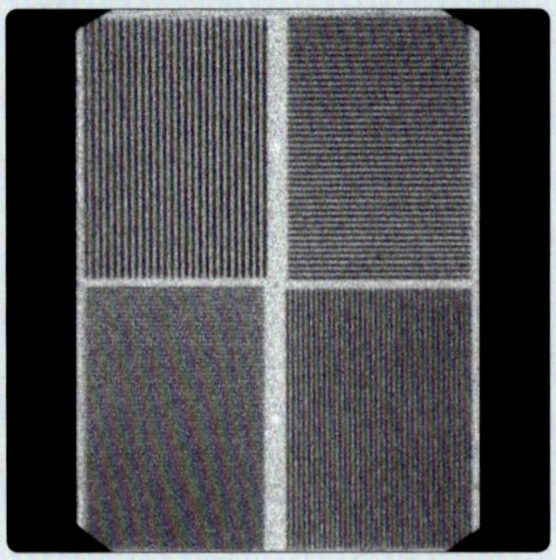

Planar imaging of ACR Jaszczak SPECT phantom is shown. Phantom base was placed directly onto an absorbent pad on the NM camera face (with collimators). This test is equivalent to the bars test of resolution.

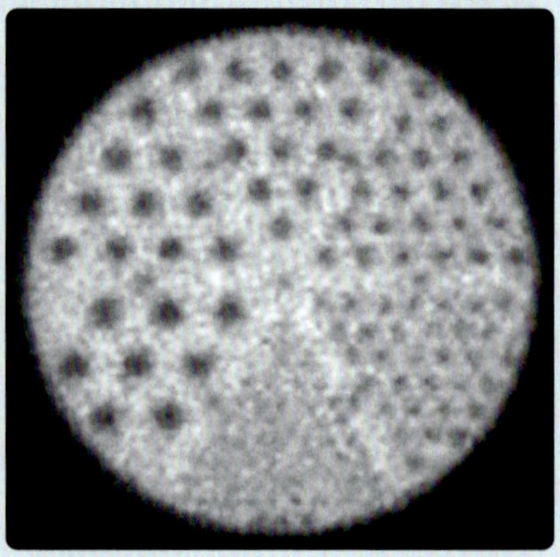

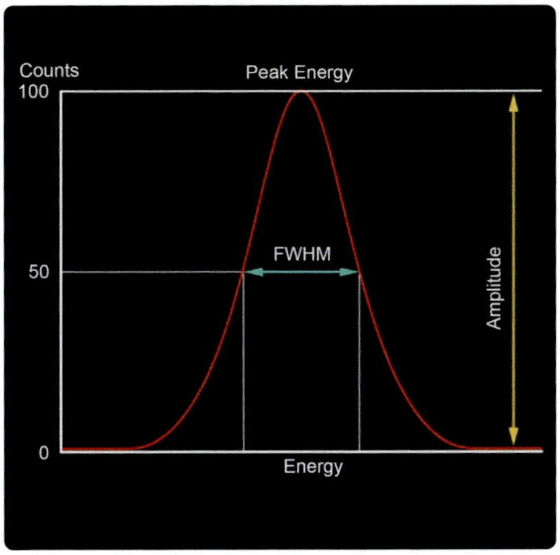

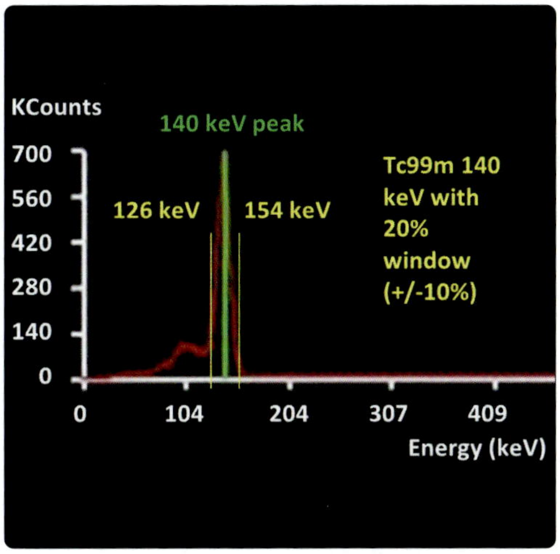

(Left) *Although the energy released by the radionuclide may be at just one energy (the peak energy), the camera system will detect a range of energies centered around the peak energy. The full width half maximum (FWHM) defines the width of this energy response.* **(Right)** *Tc-99m is typically acquired with a 20% window. Although the peak is at 140 keV, the 20% window (± 10%) sets the system up to acquire all counts between 126 keV (- 10%) and 154 keV (+ 10%).*

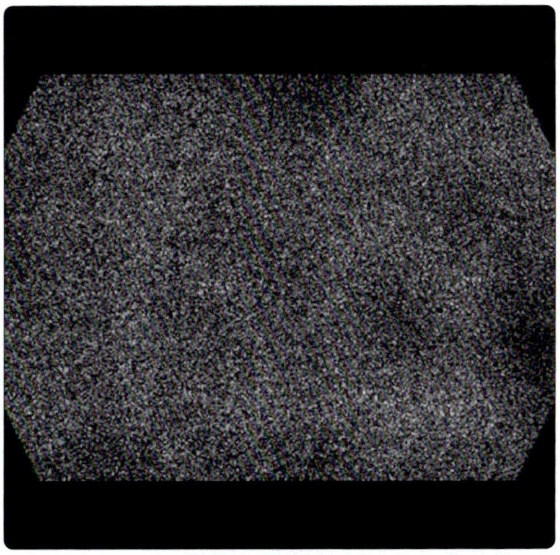

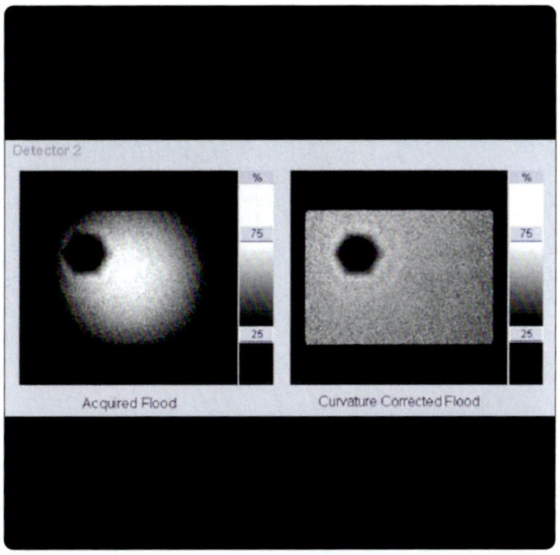

(Left) *Image uniformity test result with nonuniformity artifact caused by crystal hydration (sometimes called "measles") is shown. The sodium iodide scintillation crystal is sensitive to moisture and must be kept hermetically sealed.* **(Right)** *Intrinsic uniformity image test result of point source < 5 FOV is shown. Nonuniformity artifact is caused by a single photomultiplier failure.*

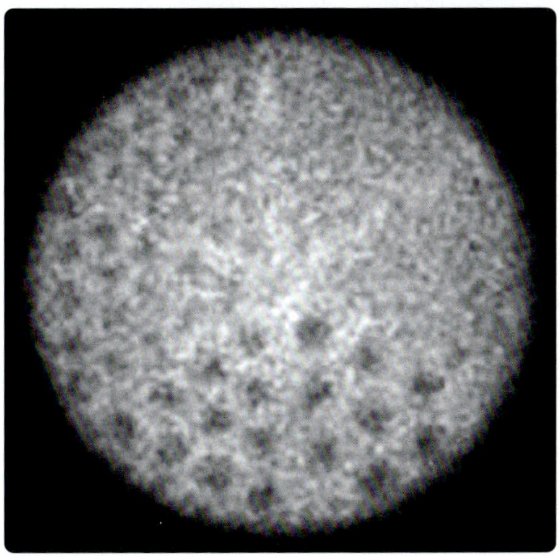

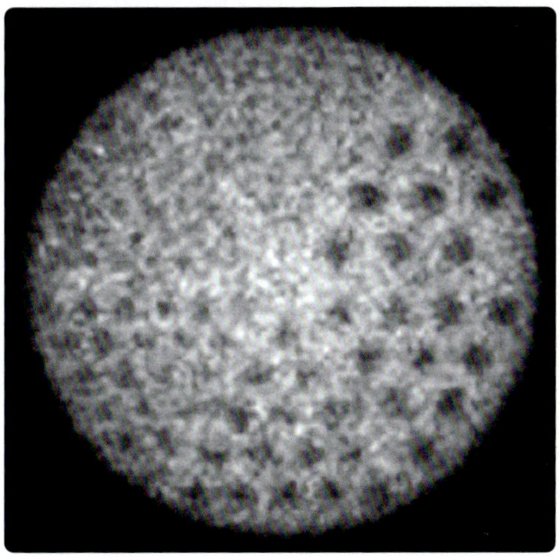

(Left) *Planar image of ACR Jaszczak SPECT phantom with Ga-67 is shown. Note that the resolution is less than what is seen for Tc-99m.* **(Right)** *Planar image of ACR Jaszczak SPECT phantom with Tl-201 is shown. Note that the resolution is less than what is seen for Tc-99m but more than what is seen for Ga-67.*

SPECT

KEY FACTS

SINGLE PHOTON EMISSION COMPUTED TOMOGRAPHY (SPECT)

- Acquisition
  - Number of views for step-wise acquisition: Typically 64-128
  - Arc of rotation of detector head(s): At least 180° required for reconstruction, but most often 360° is acquired for better image quality (resolution uniformity and correction)
  - Most systems are able to perform circular or oval/contoured orbit around patient
- Image reconstruction
  - Sinogram: Mapping of all of projected images as projection view vs. angle
    - Objects not centered in image will curve left and right through image as view changes
  - Additional filters: High pass, low pass, and band pass combination filters
  - 2D planar to 3D tomographic image reconstruction: Filtered backprojection or iterative methods
  - Attenuation correction
    - Attenuation of signal occurs for gamma photons coming from deeper depths, given erroneous view of radiopharmaceutical distribution
    - Attenuation correction, either by mathematically modeled method (such as Chang's method) or direct measurement (such as with CT on SPECT/CT system), corrects image so that signal reduction is not based on depth of source
- Bull's-eye artifact
  - Nonuniformity present in planar gamma camera image will appear in each projection view, creating round circle in reconstructed SPECT image

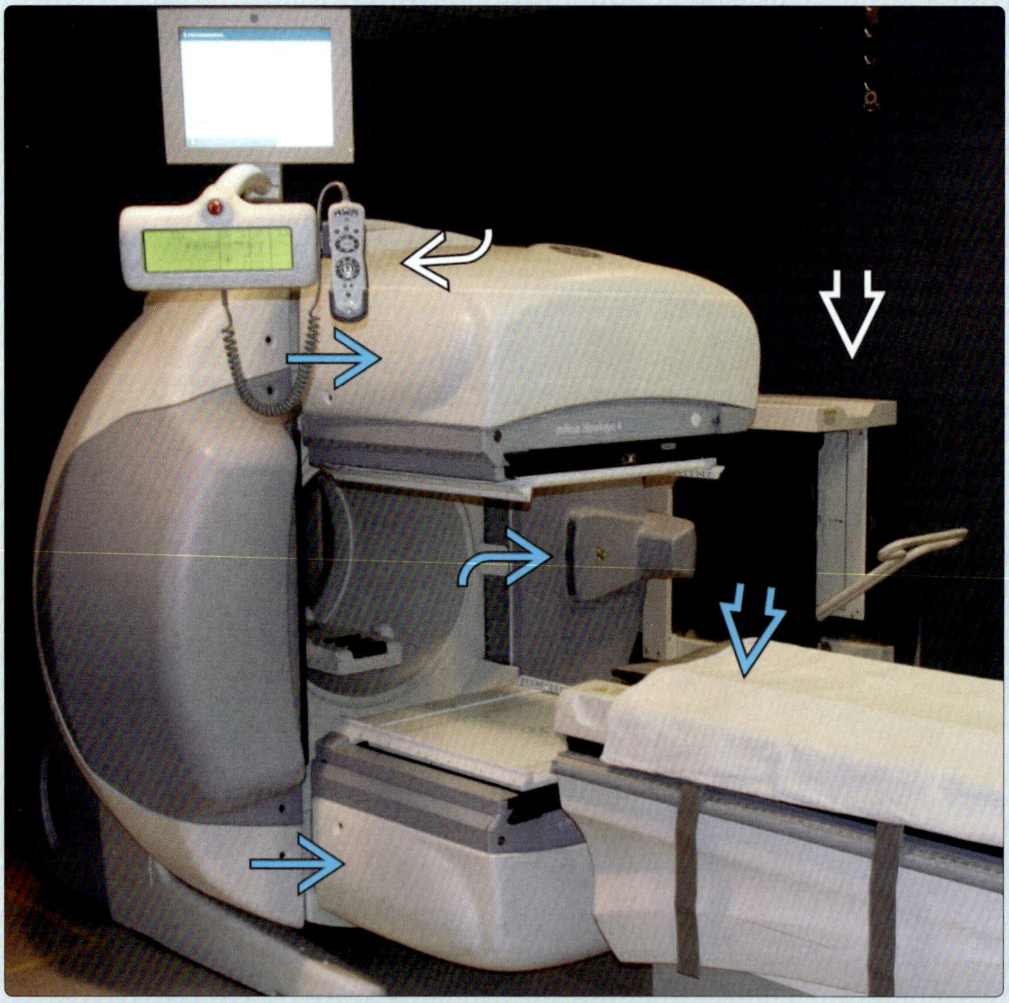

SPECT/CT gamma camera with 2 detector heads ➡ is shown. The 2 heads will travel around the patient as they detect the gamma photon image data during a SPECT acquisition. This unit also has CT capability ➡. The unit comes with a patient table ➡, a collimator cart to add and remove collimators ➡, and a control panel ➡.

SINGLE PHOTON EMISSION COMPUTED TOMOGRAPHY (SPECT)

SPECT Equipment

- 1, 2, or 3 head gamma detector systems rotate around patient, generating layers of 2D images that are reconstructed into 3D tomographic images
  - Use of more heads may result in greater system sensitivity
    - For same total acquisition time required for 1 head, 2-3x as much data can be acquired with 2 or 3 head systems
  - Use of more heads may result in reduced scan time
    - For same total acquisition counts required for 1 head, 2 or 3 heads can count simultaneously (multiple angular projections) in 1/2 to 1/3 total scan time
- Camera rotation: Step-wise or continuous
  - Step-wise: Camera heads typically stop for a number of seconds at each position around body to gather images that cover up to 360°
  - Continuous: Camera heads move continuously while rotating around patient to gather images that cover up to 360°
- Number of views for step-wise acquisition
  - Typically 64-128 views
  - Typically, for full 360° rotation, number of views should match square image matrix (e.g., 128 x 128 matrix should have 128 views)
- Arc of rotation of detector head(s): At least 180° required for reconstruction, but most often 360° is acquired for better image quality (resolution uniformity and correction)
  - If > 1 detector head (e.g., 2 or 3 head system) is used, each head only travels part of arc so that collectively they cover entire arc in less time
  - Most systems are able to perform circular or oval/contoured orbit around patient
    - Circular orbit
      - Detector head(s) maintain fixed distance from center of rotation, which typically results in head(s) farther from surface of patient being imaged in posterior or anterior views and closer for lateral views
    - Oval/contoured orbit
      - Detector head(s) adjust their movement to maintain fixed distance from surface of patient being imaged as they rotate around patient and table
      - Will appear to be oval pattern based on typically larger lateral diameter of human torso and table geometry
      - Objects closer to detector face will have greater image resolution, and thus contoured arc of rotation will typically provide better image resolution than circular orbit

Image Reconstruction

- Sinogram: Mapping of all of projected images as projection view vs. angle
  - Objects not centered in image will curve left and right through image as view changes
- 2D planar to 3D tomographic image reconstruction: Filtered backprojection or iterative methods
  - Backprojection reconstruction: In layering effect, each projected 2D planar view is added together
    - View of each projection is seen as detector sees it
    - Each view is added together via their projections to reconstruct image
    - Advantage: Simplicity of math results in fast image reconstruction
    - Disadvantage: Star artifact (if one object has high signal, it is more likely to be streaked across entire image with each projection)
  - Filtered backprojection reconstruction: Filter is used to reduce high intensity of edges of high signal data
    - Can reduce star artifact, but not eliminate it
  - Iterative reconstruction: Guess(es) of image are compared to projections of actual projection data
    - Guess of initial image is compared to actual acquired projection data
    - Error between guessed image and acquired projection data provides feedback to update guess of image
    - Process is repeated many times until error is reduced and guessed image nearly perfectly matches actual projection data
    - Advantage: Resulting image does not have star artifact
    - Disadvantage: Each iterative guess takes same time as single filtered backprojection reconstruction
      - More guesses = longer reconstruction time
- Additional filters: High pass, low pass, and band pass combination filters
  - High pass filters
    - Eliminate low-frequency data; edge enhancement but also noise enhancement (e.g., ramp filter)
  - Low pass filters
    - Eliminates high-frequency data; smoothing filter but also image detail reducer (e.g., Butterworth, Hamming, Hann & Parzen filters)
  - Band pass or combination filters: Combination low and high pass filters to optimize features
- Attenuation correction
  - Attenuation of signal occurs for gamma photons coming from deeper depths, given erroneous view of radiopharmaceutical distribution
  - Attenuation correction, either by mathematically modeled method (such as Chang's method) or direct measurement (such as with CT on SPECT/CT system), corrects image so that signal reduction is not based on depth of source

Bull's-Eye Artifact

- Nonuniformity present in planar gamma camera image will appear in each projection view, creating round circle in reconstructed SPECT image

SELECTED REFERENCES

1. Cherry S et al. Physics in Nuclear Medicine. 4th ed. Philadelphia: Saunders, 2012
2. Prekeges J. Nuclear Medicine Instrumentation. Burlington: Jones and Bartlett, 2011
3. Christian P et al. Nuclear Medicine and PET: Technology and Techniques. 5th ed. Maryland Heights: Mosby, 2004
4. Wagner RH et al. Questions & Answers in Nuclear Medicine. Maryland Heights: Mosby, 1999

Gamma Camera & SPECT Quality Control (QC) Tests

Test (Frequency)	Setup	Processing and Expected Results
Gamma Camera Planar QC (Failures Also Affect SPECT)		
Uniformity (daily for standard setup; quarterly recommended to check all collimators)	Intrinsic (collimator off) with point source of clinically used radionuclide (point source = small quantity of radionuclide in syringe or other small container) or extrinsic (collimater on) with flood source or fillable flood (per ACR 256 x 256, 10 million counts)	Uniform image without artifacts: In some cases requires curvature or dome correction if source close to camera face; high count may be performed (100-300 million counts) to recalibrate and fix some uniformity issues; nonuniformities can be caused by collimator damage, crystal damage, or PMT issues. Bull's-eye artifact caused by nonuniformity on planar image acquired at each angle around patient
Spatial resolution & linearity (weekly on most cameras)	4 quadrant bar phantom placed on camera face: Intrinsic (collimators off + point source) or extrinsic (collimators on + flood source) (per ACR: 512 x 512, 10 million counts); can also image base of Jaszczak SPECT phantom (per ACR 256 x 256, 0.6 million counts)	Bars (visualize line pairs in expected # of quadrants) or Jaszczak (visualize expected # of wedges of cold rods) based on camera and ACR criteria for Tc-99m: Bars: 2.5-2.9 mm quadrant is resolved; Jaszczak: 9.9 mm cold rod wedge is resolved
Energy spectrum (daily or automatic with each use)	Camera centers peak over current clinical radionuclide in use	Radionuclide peak is correctly positioned in center of acquisition window; windows improperly placed will cause image artifacts such as hot or cold PMT nonuniformity
Energy resolution & linearity (annually)	Acquire an energy spectrum (detected radionuclide energies vs. # of counts) of common clinical radionuclide(s)	Measure full width half maximum (FWHM) of resulting energy peak and compare it to manufacturer's specifications; linearity test done with multiple radionuclide photopeaks analyzed
Count rate response or maximum count rate (annually)	One method involves setting point source in lead pig under camera and then shielding top with layers of copper; as each copper sheet is removed, count rate increases until it maximizes and then drops	Peak drops after even more copper is removed due to dead time; maximum count rate obtained can be compared to manufacturer's specifications but will be slightly less due to differences in NEMA standard testing conditions at factory; compare year to year for significant changes
Count rate sensitivity (annually)	Known quantity (e.g., 1,000 uCi) of clinically used radionuclide is placed at set distance (e.g., 10 cm) from detector face and counted for set time (e.g., 1 minute)	Calculation is performed of uCi/minute with appropriate decay since source was checked by dose calibrator; compared year to year for significant changes
Multiple window spatial registration (annually; not required by ACR NM accreditation)	3 point sources of Ga-67 placed at 3 positions on face of gamma camera; all 3 are imaged 3x with windows around each of 3 energy peaks of Ga-67	3 resulting images are compared to ensure that point sources are placed at same physical location in image regardless of which of 3 energy peaks was acquired; if this test fails, service engineer will need to recalibrate uniformity with different radionuclide energies
SPECT QC		
Center of rotation (COR) (monthly)	Radionuclide point source is placed at set distance from camera face such that camera will rotate around source without changing distance from point source	Resulting location of point source is mapped vs. angle of rotation; any wobble in rotation is visible and measurable; too much wobble can cause image blur in resulting SPECT post-processed images
System image quality	Fill Jaszczak SPECT phantom with clinically used radionuclide (e.g., 10-20 mCi [370-740 MBq] Tc-99m) and acquire SPECT image (per ACR for Tc-99m, 32 million counts over 360° rotation or 180° for 2 detector heads, 120 x 120 or 128 x 128 matrix)	Per ACR, perform SPECT reconstruction using Butterworth or site filter and attenuation correction method (Chang or other); analysis of 3 sections of phantom: Uniformity, wedges of cold rods (spatial resolution) and cold spheres (contrast resolution); ACR minimum criteria for Tc-99m is uniformity (no artifacts or artifacts only on a few slices), rods (11.1 mm wedge resolved; less resolution than seen with planar imaging), and spheres (19.1 mm sphere resolved)

Mettler et al. Essentials of Nuclear Medicine Imaging, 6th Edition. Elsevier, 2012; American College of Radiology (ACR) Accreditation Standards

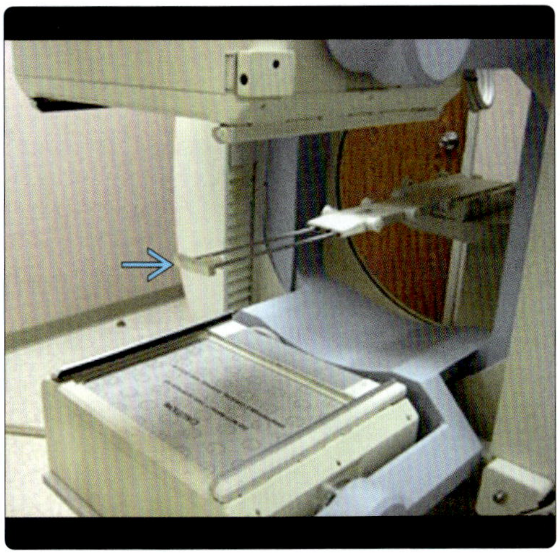

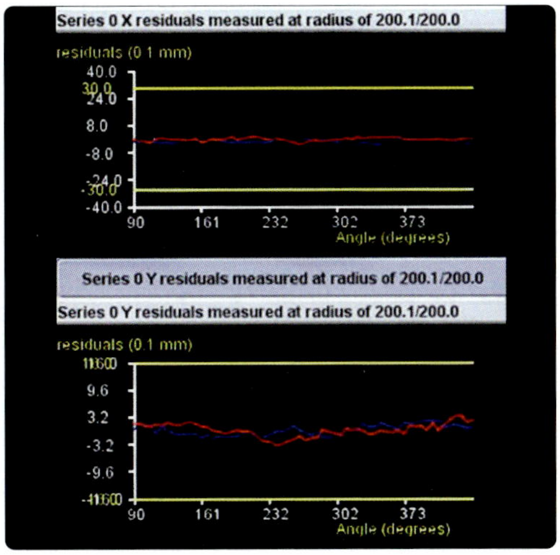

(Left) *Center of rotation (COR) test setup (± collimators) is shown. Point source (10 µCi Tc-99m)* → *is placed between 2 camera heads as cameras are rotated around it.* **(Right)** *COR test outcome is shown. The source is mapped for its position vs. the angle of the detector heads (red and blue represent detectors 1 and 2). Ideally, very little wobble is seen in the positioning. Each system will have its own acceptable criteria (here shown with the yellow lines). COR test failure can result in image blur.*

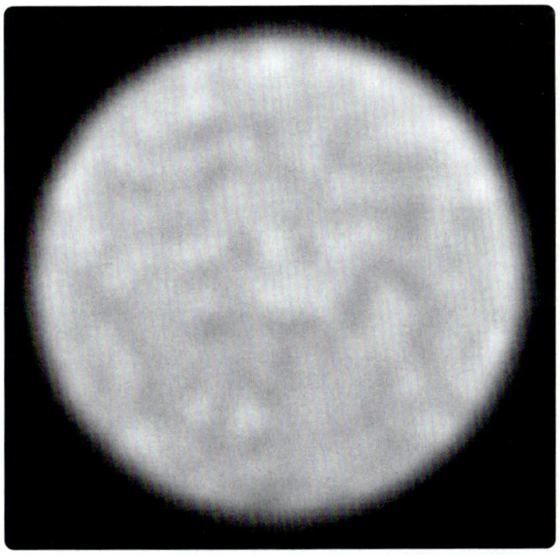

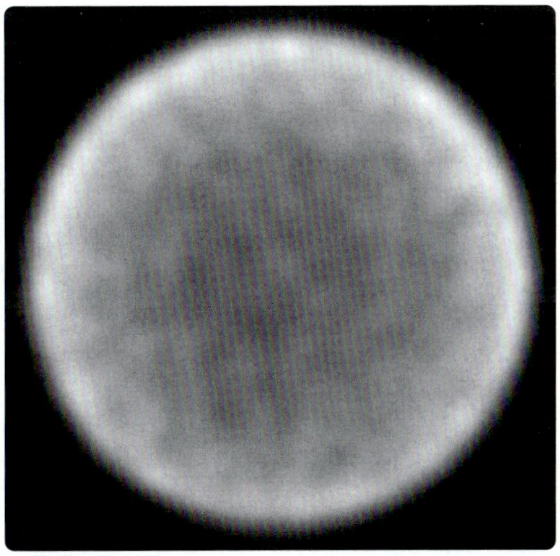

(Left) *Jaszczak SPECT phantom uniformity slice section after ACR specified acquisition (15 mCi Tc-99m, 30 million counts acquired over 180° rotation for 2 detector heads covering 360°) is shown, reconstructed with Chang attenuation correction and Butterworth filter.* **(Right)** *Jaszczak SPECT phantom uniformity slice section without attenuation correction is shown. Note that signal from deeper in phantom is darker than the edge due to attenuation; however, the radionuclide in the phantom is evenly distributed.*

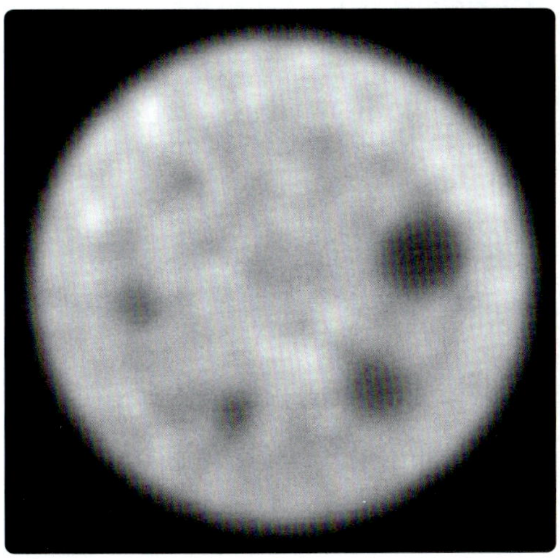

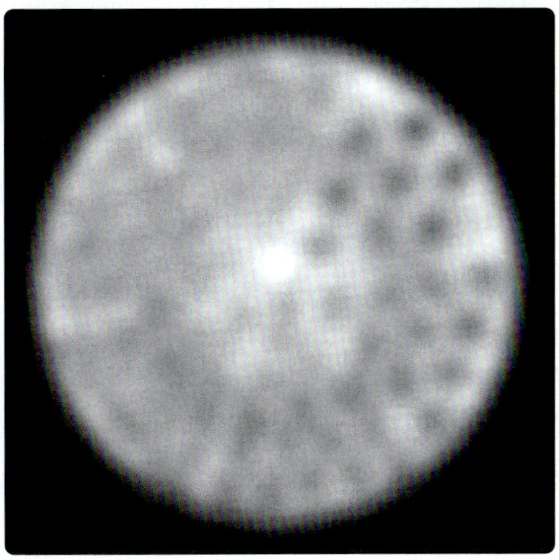

(Left) *Jaszczak SPECT phantom cold sphere slice section (same acquisition and processing as for uniformity image) is shown. This is a test of contrast resolution (larger objects seen against a background).* **(Right)** *Jaszczak SPECT phantom rod wedge slice section (same acquisition and processing as for uniformity image) is shown. This is a test of detail resolution. Note that the number of wedges visualized in the SPECT image is less than what was seen in the planar image from the gamma camera.*

KEY FACTS

POSITRON EMISSION TOMOGRAPHY (PET)

- Although called PET, image is actually created from 511 keV annihilation photons and not positrons emitted
- Positron (positively charged electron) only travels short distance before meeting electron and annihilating, creating two 511 keV photons
- Theoretically, these two 511 keV photons travel exactly 180° apart if positron and electron are at rest when they annihilate
- In reality, these two 511 keV photons are not 180° apart due to fact that positron and electron are not completely at rest when they annihilate (thus, minor error is produced in their projected location)

2D AND 3D ACQUISITION MODES

- 2D mode: PET is considered to have electronic collimation rather than actual collimation even with existence of septa
- 2D direct mode: Septa allow only photons emitted parallel to plane of detector ring to be detected and thus provide efficient rejection of annihilation photons that have been scattered in body
- 2D crossplain mode: With slight or no modification of lengths of septa, PET scanners also can acquire data from immediately adjacent rings, known as cross planes
- 2D high-sensitivity mode: In PET scanners with very small detector elements, number of cross planes can be increased even further to include crystal ring differences of ± 2, ± 3, and so forth
- 3D mode: Interplane septa are removed from PET scanner and data are obtained for all possible lines of response

ATTENUATION CORRECTION

- Most often performed with CT scanner on PET systems (PET/CT)

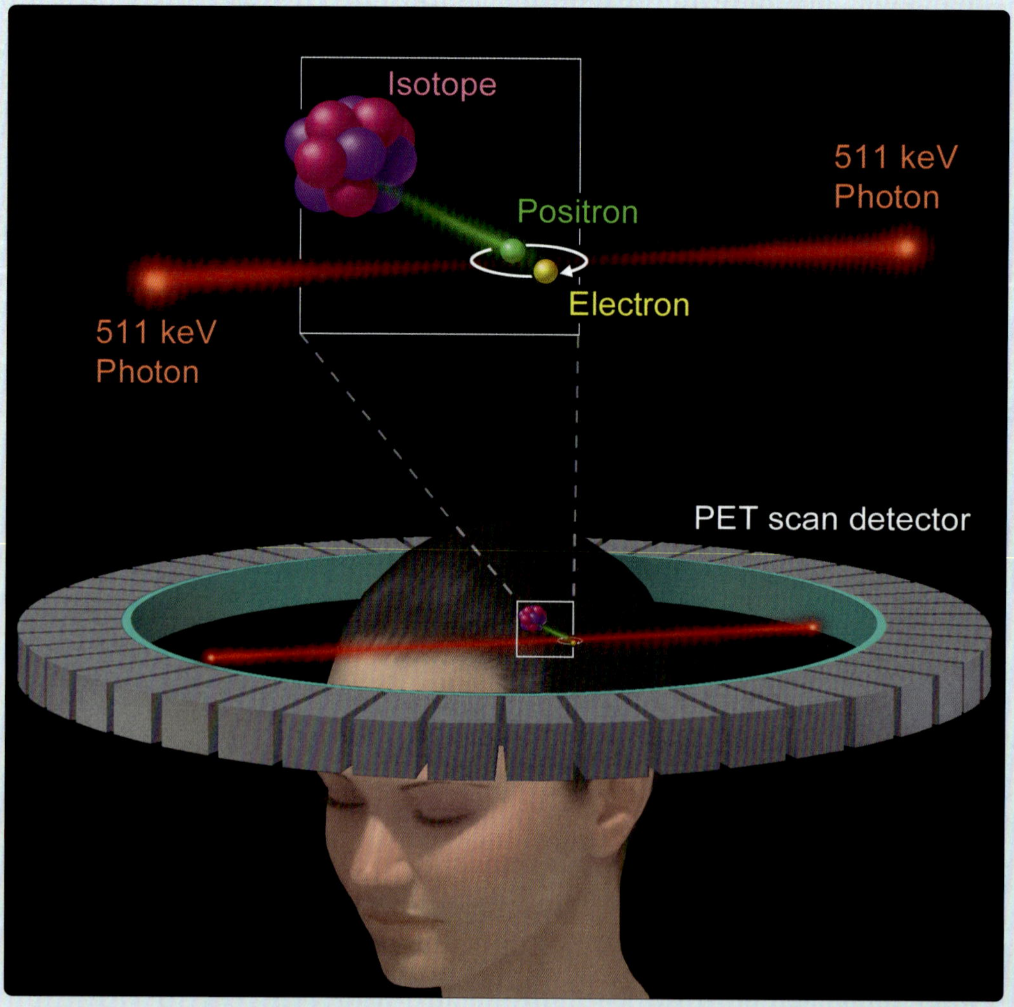

A patient is injected with a radioisotope that is a positron emitter. Fluorine-18 (F-18) is the most common positron emitter used, tagged to a sugar, fluorodeoxyglucose (FDG). Positron emission tomography (PET) scan involves detection of two 511 keV photons produced after positron annihilation (when the positron and an electron annihilate converting mass to energy in the form of two 511 keV photons).

TERMINOLOGY

Definitions

- Positron emission tomography (PET)
  - Utilizes radionuclides that emit positrons (beta +) as they decay
    - $\rho^+ \rightarrow \eta + \beta^+ + \nu$ (neutrino) + energy
    - Number of protons (atomic number) decreased by 1
    - Number of neutrons increased by 1
    - Mass number approximately same (= number of protons + number of neutrons)
    - ν (neutrino) is small and not important to imaging
  - Positron: Positively charged particle that travels ~ 1 mm before combining with electron, undergoing annihilation
  - Annihilation yields two 511 keV (0.511 MeV) gamma photons at 180° from one another
  - Ring of detectors surrounds patient and detects coincident gamma photons emitted, making 3D image

RADIONUCLIDE PRODUCTION

PET Detector Array Design

- PET cameras are designed to detect paired 511 keV photons generated from annihilation reaction of positron and electron
- By incorporating multiple opposing detectors in complete ring or other geometric array around patient, and operating each detector in array in coincidence with multiple detectors on other side of array, data for multiple projection angles can be acquired simultaneously
- With stationary ring or geometric array that completely surrounds patient, it is possible to acquire data for all projection angles simultaneously
  - Allows performance of relatively fast dynamic studies and reduction of artifacts caused by patient motion
- Series of small detectors in ring array detects each pair of gamma rays produced by annihilation event
  - Circular or hexagonal arrays of detectors for simultaneous collection of data from various directions in PET scanner
  - Each detector in array or ring is in coincidence with large number of detectors on its opposite side
- Via knowledge that they exited body 180° apart and by timing their appearance at each detector, exact location where annihilation occurred can be pinpointed
- Line of response
  - Line between 2 detectors that have detected true coincidence event
  - Assumes detection of annihilation event lies somewhere along line between detectors
- Coincidence detection
  - Uses opposing detectors operating in coincidence to detect simultaneous emission of two 511-keV photons created by annihilation
  - Depending on location of their origin, pair of 511 keV photons should strike opposing detectors at close to same time
  - Detector closest to positron-electron annihilation event picks up 511 keV photon first
  - Coincidence circuit checks simultaneity of photomultiplier (PMT) pulses to within ~ 15 nanoseconds
  - When coincident, single coincident event is recorded; otherwise, PMT pulses are rejected
- True coincidence (true events): When single annihilation event is recorded as hitting 2 opposing detectors at nearly same time (within nanoseconds), creating line of response
  - If event is true, only those annihilation photons produced in volume between detectors have chance of arriving at detectors simultaneously
  - Annihilation photons produced at locations outside of this volume will not reach detectors simultaneously (in true coincidence)
  - Thus such a pair of detectors measures radioactivity, without use of collimator per se, of small volume only (electronic collimation)
  - Note that PET does not use collimator per se, but septa will be used or not used to differentiate between 2D and 3D imaging
- Scatter events
  - 1 of 511 keV photons from annihilation event scatters in new direction before reaching detector and line of response is incorrectly positioned due to scattering event
- Random events
  - Two separate events (not same annihilation events) are incorrectly recorded as coming from single annihilation event because they are recorded as hitting 2 opposing detectors at nearly same time, creating line of response
  - Photons generated from separate sites in body may reach opposing detectors at same time
  - These separate events are incorrectly perceived as resulting from annihilation of single positron emitter occurring along line between detectors
  - Note that in some texts, random and scatter are grouped, although not always since they can be handled separately with post-processing
- Time of flight
  - Assumption that location of annihilation photon can be localized along line of flight of coincident photons by measuring time of arrival of each photon at opposing crystals
  - Only possible with very fast electronics; some scanners can utilize some time-of-flight data to improve positioning but not base it completely on time of flight
- Image reconstruction
  - Utilizes same back projection reconstruction or iterative techniques used for gamma camera SPECT reconstruction

Flow of Data and Processing

- Crystals convert gamma rays emitted from patient to photons of light, and photomultiplier tubes convert and amplify photons to electrical signals
  - Electrical signals are then processed by computer to generate images
- Table is then moved (typically 3-4x per head to thigh image acquisition) and process is repeated, resulting in series of tomographic images of body

Scintillators

- High-energy photons (mostly 511 keV) interact with scintillator material and are converted to visible light

- Common PET scintillators: Convert annihilation photons to light, which is then converted to electronic signal with PMT
  - Bismuth germanate (BGO)
  - Lutetium oxyorthosilicate (LSO)
  - Lutetium yttrium orthosilicate (LYSO)
  - Gadolinium orthosilicate (GSO)
  - Barium fluoride (BaF2)
- Scintillator + PMT combination
  - Light from scintillator is captured by PMT tube and light is converted to electrical energy and amplified

2D Direct Imaging

- PET is considered to have electronic collimation rather than actual collimation even with existence of septa for 2D imaging
- Septa allow only those photons emitted parallel to plane of detector ring to be detected and thus provide efficient rejection of annihilation photons that have been scattered in body
- Septa also reduce single-channel counting rate, thereby lowering random coincidence rate and minimizing dead time losses
- Each ring collects data from single slice
- Images can be reconstructed using filtered back projection or iterative approaches

2D Cross Plane Imaging

- With slight or no modification of lengths of septa, PET scanners also can acquire data from immediately adjacent rings, known as cross planes
- At center of scanner, cross planes fall exactly halfway between direct planes that are defined by individual crystal rings
- Because cross planes receive data from 2 different lines of response, they have roughly 2x sensitivity (and therefore twice the counting rates) as direct planes

2D High-Sensitivity Imaging

- In PET scanners with very small detector elements, the number of cross planes can be increased even further to include crystal ring differences of ± 2, ± 3, and so forth
- As larger ring differences are accepted, sensitivity increases
- However, there is loss of spatial resolution in axial direction, because of superposition of data that comes from axial disparate locations

3D Imaging

- In 3D acquisition mode, interplane septa are removed from PET scanner and data are obtained for all possible lines of response
- Typically, this leads to 4-8x improvement in sensitivity
- However, number of scattered photons and single-channel counting rates are also increased
- In 3D mode, important to place structures of interest as close as possible to center of axial FOV as possible
- Reconstruction of 3D PET data requires more complex reconstruction algorithms than 2D

3D PET Imaging

- Greater sensitivity (up to 8x or more)
- Increased scatter
- Higher random events and deadtime
- Loss in spatial resolution

Advantages of PET/CT

- Mechanically aligned functional and anatomical images
  - Fusion imaging: Images are not fused but overlaid via alpha blending
- CT provides attenuation correction information for PET images
- CT scan can be used for scatter correction

Attenuation Correction

- Most often performed with CT scanner on PET systems (PET/CT)
- Without attenuation correction
  - Lungs and skin may appear hot
  - Activity deep within body may have less signal due to tissue attenuation of photons
  - Focal uptake still apparent
- With attenuation correction
  - Appropriate distribution of radionuclides in imaging (reduces attenuation effect at greater depths in body)
  - Possibility of strong attenuates (metal objects or contrast) appearing spuriously hot; must compare to original unattenuated image to be sure hot spot is from localization of radionuclide

SELECTED REFERENCES

1. Saha GB. Basics of PET Imaging: Physics, Chemistry, and Regulations. Springer, 2004
2. Christian PE et al. Nuclear Medicine and PET: Technology and Techniques, 5th Edition. Mosby, 2004
3. Valk PE et al. Positron Emission Tomography: Basic Science and Clinical Practice. Springer, 2002

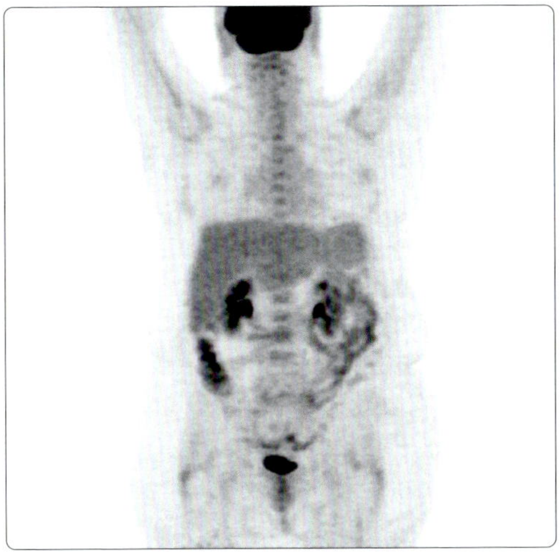

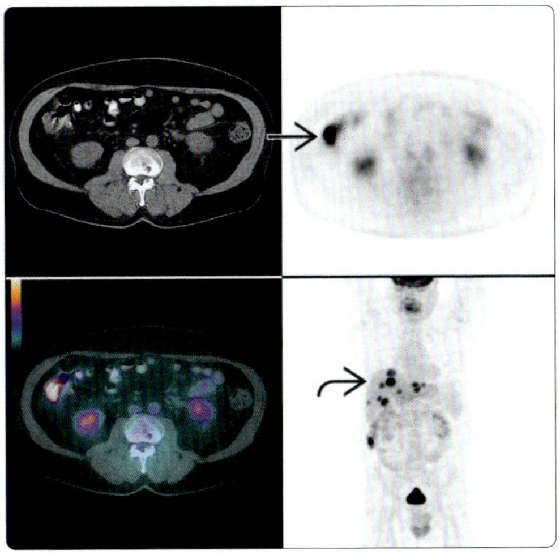

(Left) *Normal whole-body F-18 FDG PET is acquired on a time of flight scanner, which allows for better image resolution, especially in obese patients.* **(Right)** *F-18 FDG PET/CT shows primary colon carcinoma ⇨ and metastatic liver lesions ⇨. CT allows for attenuation correction and anatomic localization.*

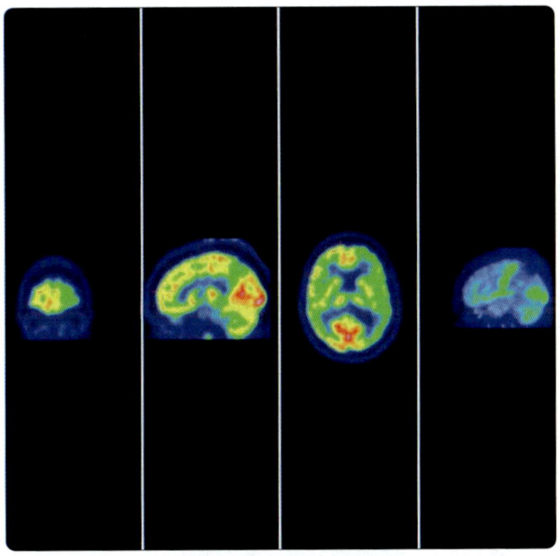

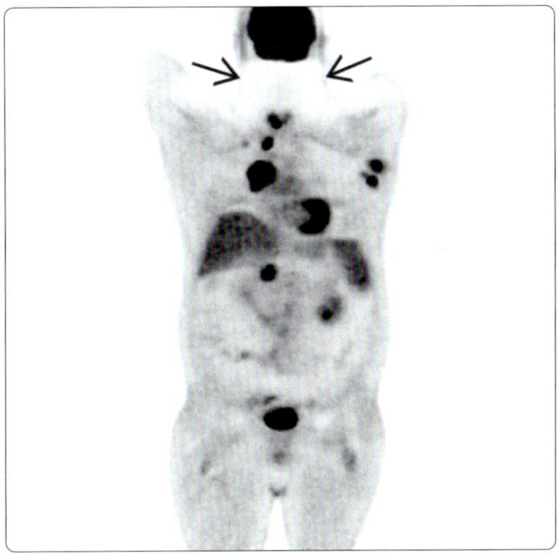

(Left) *F-18 FDG PET of the brain acquired in 3D mode shows increased sensitivity, but also increased scatter, during 3D acquisition compared to 2D. Proper positioning is paramount for image acquisition.* **(Right)** *Coronal F-18 FDG PET shows artifact in the head and neck region ⇨ from patient arm motion, creating a false attenuation map. The patient had their arms down for the CTAC and up for the PET, causing under correction of the emission data with the incorrect attenuation map.*

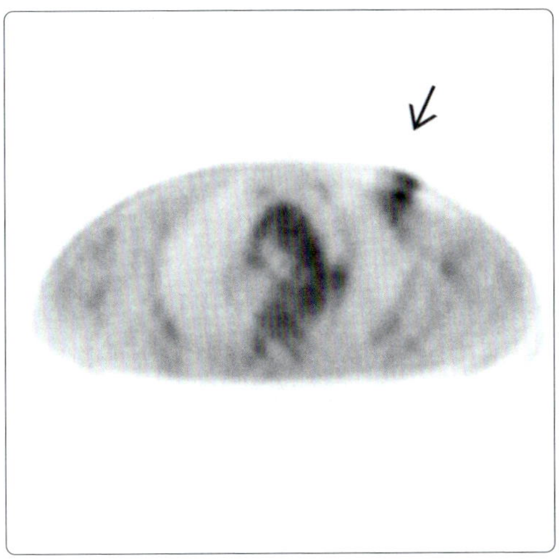

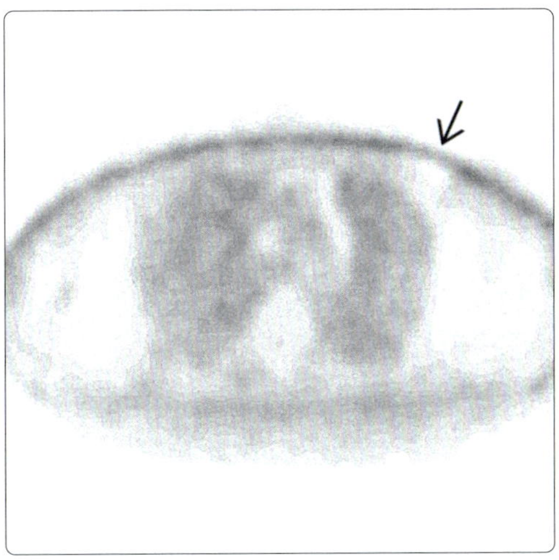

(Left) *PET attenuation corrected (AC) image from a patient with a left anterior chest wall pacemaker shows false increased uptake artifact on the left chest wall ⇨. The false uptake is due to the pacemaker attenuation during the CT scan.* **(Right)** *PET nonattenuated corrected (NAC) image in the same patient shows no abnormal activity in the left anterior chest wall ⇨.*

KEY FACTS

CLINICAL IMPLICATIONS

- Molecular effects of radiation
  - Photon of ionizing radiation delivers at least enough energy to eject electron from atom or molecule
  - Ionized particle and ejected electron can ultimately interact with other atoms or molecules
- Radiation interaction with cells
  - Short-term effects of ionizing radiation on cells and tissues
    - Changes in molecules, in proteins, DNA, RNA, and cellular structure, leading to cellular damage and apoptosis
  - Long-term effects of ionizing radiation on cells and tissues
    - Result from changes in mitochondrial and nuclear DNA
  - Irreparable damage can occur as well as mutations, which can be propagated within cell line
- Deterministic effects
  - Direct, generally acute, effects of excessive radiation (e.g., erythema, hair loss, nausea/vomiting, aplastic anemia)
  - Evident within minutes to weeks
  - Deterministic dose-response model typically follows linear or S-curve that starts at radiation dose > 0 (threshold)
- Stochastic effects
  - Probabilistic effects of radiation exposure (e.g., cancer and genetic mutations)
  - Latency period is required before stochastic effects become evident
  - No threshold amount; cannot be predicted on individual basis
  - Can be reduced in population by reducing cumulative radiation exposure to all individuals in population
  - Stochastic dose-response model typical follows linear or linear-quadratic curve that crosses through 0

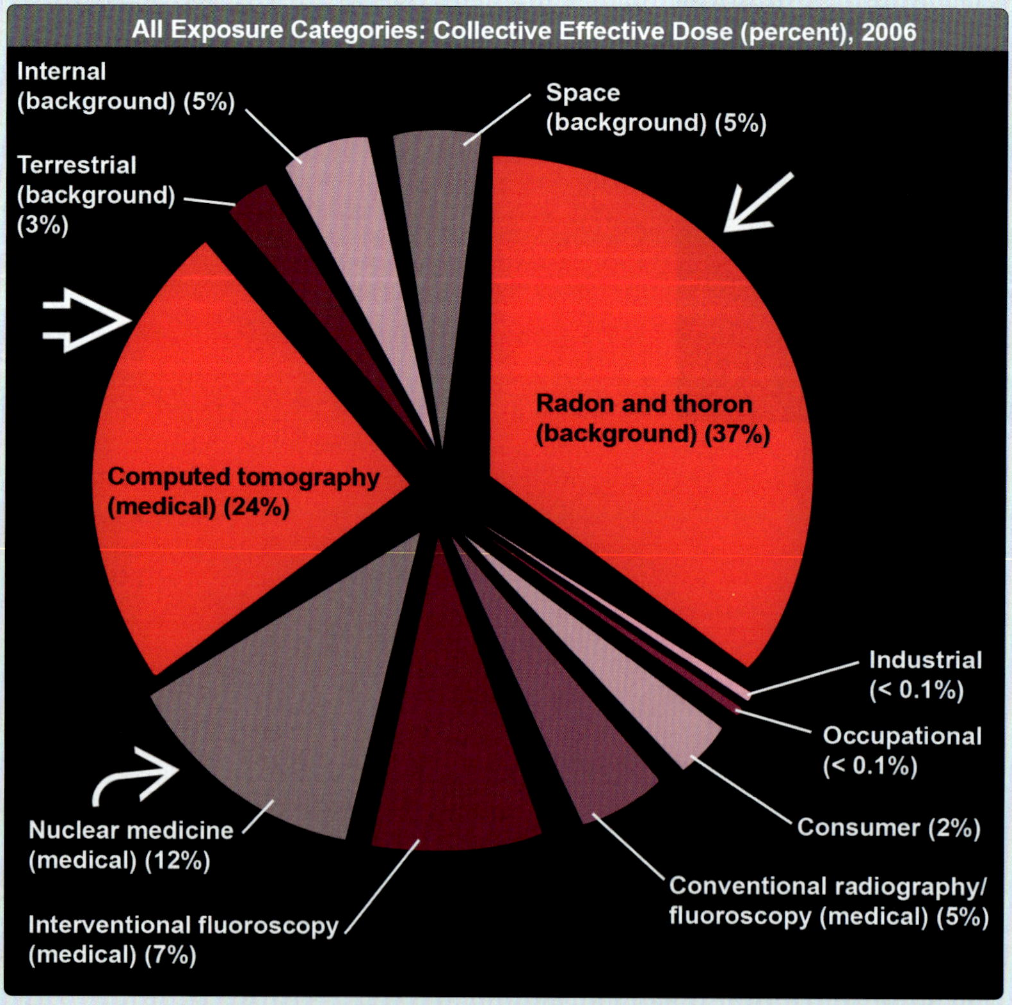

As of 2006, the largest source of collective effective dose to USA population was from radon and thoron background radiation at 37% ➡. CT scans rank 2nd at 24% ➡ and nuclear medicine ranks 3rd at 12% ➡. The largest contribution to medical radiation exposure is computed tomography.

TERMINOLOGY

Definitions

- **Radiation intensity**
  - Roentgen (R) (non-Standard International (SI) units); as measured with ionization chamber in milliRoentgen per hr (mR/hr)
- **Absorbed dose**
  - Total amount of energy deposited in material
    - Any type of radiation, any radiation intensity, any material
  - Expressed as radiation absorbed dose (rad) (non-SI units), or gray (Gy) (SI units)
    - 100 rads = 1 Gy; 1 rad = 10 mGy
  - 1 rad = absorption of 100 ergs per g of tissue
  - In nuclear medicine, this depends on many factors
    - t1/2 of radiopharmaceutical
    - Biological t1/2 of radiopharmaceutical
    - Percentage taken up by body and differential uptake in organs
    - Type of radiation emitted by radiopharmaceutical
  - Absorbed dose for different nuclear medicine studies is estimated based on biodistribution studies in animals
- **Equivalent dose**
  - Amount of radiation dose weighted based on damaging effects of type of radiation on tissue
    - Accounts for differences in types of radiation type and intensity
    - Based on relative biological effectiveness (RBE): Compares dose of standard radiation that yields biological response to dose of different radiation to produce similar biological response
    - For example, alpha particle with mass and charge (weighting factor Q of 20) will do more damage than gamma photon without mass or charge (weighting factor Q of 1)
  - Measured in roentgen equivalent man (rem) (non-SI units), or sievert (Sv) (SI units)
    - 100 rem = 1 Sv; 1 rem = 10 mSv
    - rem = rad x weighting factor (Q)
- **Effective dose**
  - Equivalent dose while accounting for tissue/organ sensitivity and specifc damage from radiation
  - Tissue-weighted sum of equivalent doses in all tissues/organs of body
  - For example, tissue weighting factor (Wt) is high for breast tissue at 0.12 (12%) but low for brain tissue at 0.01 (1%); tissue weighting factors summed for all organs in body should add up to 1 (100%)
  - Measured in rem (non-SI units) or Sv (SI units)
  - Useful in estimating long-term biological risks to population from radiation exposure
- **Direct effects**
  - Primarily from particulate & charged radiation (alpha, beta) where radiation directly damages cell
- **Indirect effects**
  - Primarily from gamma and x-ray photons (no mass or charge) that primarily cause chemical changes from interactions with water and other molecules that lead to secondary chemical changes and indirect cell damage

CLINICAL IMPLICATIONS

Molecular Effects of Radiation

- Ionizing radiation delivers at least enough energy to eject electron from atom or molecule
- Ionized particle and ejected electron can ultimately interact with other atoms or molecules

Deterministic Effects of Radiation

- Deterministic effects are direct, generally acute effects of excessive radiation above set threshold
- Evident within minutes to weeks, depending on type and amount of radiation and affected body parts
- Examples include skin burn, hair loss, nausea/vomiting, aplastic anemia
- Threshold amount of radiation has to be exceeded before deterministic effect occurs
  - Threshold varies by radiation type, energy distribution, person, and organ system
  - Lower frequency external radiation dose (e.g., UV rays from sunlight) will cause skin burn before aplastic anemia secondary to bone marrow destruction
  - Properly fractionated, modulated, high-frequency external dose (e.g., x-rays used in total body irradiation) will destroy bone marrow and induce aplastic anemia with minimal acute skin effects
- Acute radiation syndrome (radiation sickness) is deterministic effect of very high dose of radiation to whole body
- Deterministic effects can be reduced or eliminated by reducing time of exposure, increasing distance from radiation source, or increasing shielding

Stochastic Effects of Radiation

- Stochastic effects are probabilistic effects of radiation exposure
- Examples of stochastic effects include cancer and genetic mutations
- Latency period is required before stochastic effects become evident
  - Latency will vary with condition, but is typically on order of years to decades
  - Effects on leukemia rates can be seen after 2-7 years post acute exposure; other cancers can have latency periods of 20-50 years
- Stochastic effects do not have threshold amount and cannot be predicted on individual basis
  - Probability of effect generally increases with dose and type of radiation
  - Probability is determined when comparing outcomes between groups exposed to radiation vs. unexposed controls
- Stochastic effects can be reduced in population by reducing cumulative radiation exposure to all individuals in population

Dose-Response Models

- Radiation dose-response models represent amount of effect caused by dose of radiation
- These models are represented with linear or graphical curve, with x-axis tracking amount of radiation and y-axis indicating amount of effect

Comparison of Doses by Procedure

Exam/Procedure	Effective Dose in mSv (mrem)
Chest x-ray (PA and lateral)	0.1 (10)
20 mCi (740 MBq) Tc-99m MDP bone scan	4.4 (440)
CT from PET/CT	15 (1,500)
15 mCi (555 MBq) F-18 FDG PET	14 (1,400)

Stabin M et al. Radiation Dose Estimates for Radiopharmaceuticals. Radiation Internal Dose Information Center. IMPACTscan.org, 1996

Estimated Radiation Absorbed Doses in Adults for Common Radiopharmaceuticals

Radiopharmaceutical	Adult Total Body Effective Dose (rem/mCi)	Critical Organ and Dose (rad/mCi)
Tc-99m pertechnetate	0.014	Thyroid: 0.130
Tc-99m MDP	0.007	Bladder wall: 0.31
Tc-99m sulfur colloid	0.019	Liver: 0.338
Tc-99m MAG3	0.007	Bladder wall: 0.480
Tc-99m DTPA	0.006	Bladder wall: 0.27
Tc-99m MAA	0.015	Lung: 0.22
Tc-99m mebrofenin	0.02	Upper colon: 0.474
Tc-99m tetrofosmin resting	0.03	Gallbladder: 0.18
Tc-99m sestamibi resting	0.0167	Upper colon: 0.18
Tl-201 chloride	0.21	Thyroid: 2
Tc-99m HMPAO	0.013	Lacrimal gland: 0.258
Ga-67 citrate	0.26	Lower colon: 0.90
F-18 FDG	0.11	Bladder wall: 0.32
I-123 NaI (25% uptake)	0.043	Thyroid: 32.5
I-131 NaI (25% uptake)	0.71	Thyroid: 1,300

Adapted from Gopal B. Saha Fundamentals of Nuclear Pharmacy, 4th edition. Springer-Verlag, 1998; package insert data

- Linear, no-threshold model
  - Linear: Assumes that if high dose causes high degree of risk, then low dose will cause low degree of risk (but not zero risk)
  - No-threshold: Assumes no minimal amount of radiation dose is too small to cause effect
    - At low levels, no data to prove no effects vs. natural occurrence, but many regulations are conservatively based on assumption that low levels of radiation can cause effects
- Deterministic dose-response model
  - Typically follows linear or S-curve that starts at radiation dose > 0 (threshold)
- Stochastic dose-response model
  - Typically follows linear or linear-quadratic curve that crosses through 0
- Complex dose-response curves
  - Does not follow typical models, e.g., in populations whose genetic susceptibility makes them more sensitive to radiation effects

Radiation Epidemiology

- Sources of radiation exposure have shifted significantly over last 30 years
  - Medical radiation was ~ 15% of typical individual's total ionizing radiation exposure in 1980s
  - By 2006, medical radiation had increased to 48% of individual's total ionizing radiation exposure
- In 2006, collective sources of radiation exposure (collective effective dose)
  - Background radiation (primarily from radon): 37%
  - CT scans: 24%
  - Nuclear medicine: 12%

Internal Radiation Dosimetry

- Medical internal radiation dose (MIRD) method
  - Considers dose to each organ from radioactivity in that organ and radioactivity from surrounding organs
  - Considers amount of radioactivity and how long radioactivity remained at each location
  - Considers physical and biological t1/2 (effective t1/2)
- FDA-approved package inserts will include representative dose models for each radiopharmaceutical

SELECTED REFERENCES

1. Mahesh M: NCRP Report Number 160: its significance to medical imaging. J Am Coll Radiol. 6(12):890-2, 2009

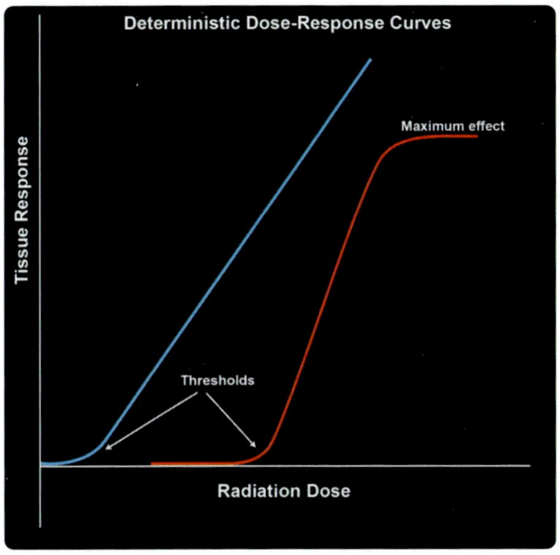

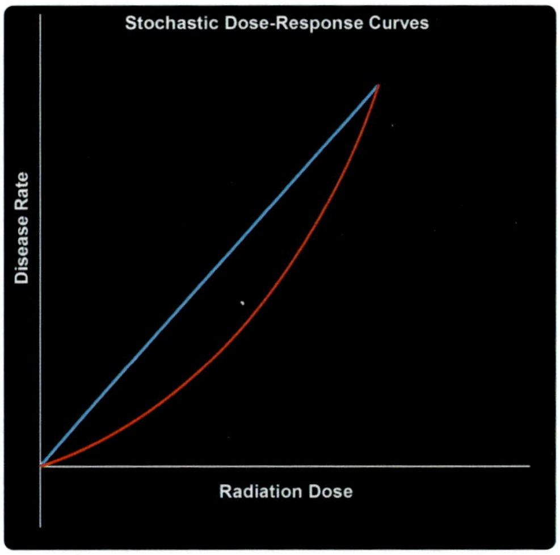

(Left) *A deterministic dose-response model typically follows a linear or S-curve that starts at a radiation dose > 0 (the threshold below which the effect will not occur). A plateau ("maximum effect" on the red S-curve) can occur if any increase in dose no longer increases the effect (e.g., complete hair loss).* **(Right)** *A stochastic dose-response curve follows a linear or linear-quadratic curve that crosses through 0. There is a probability of disease at any dose level and the probability increases with dose.*

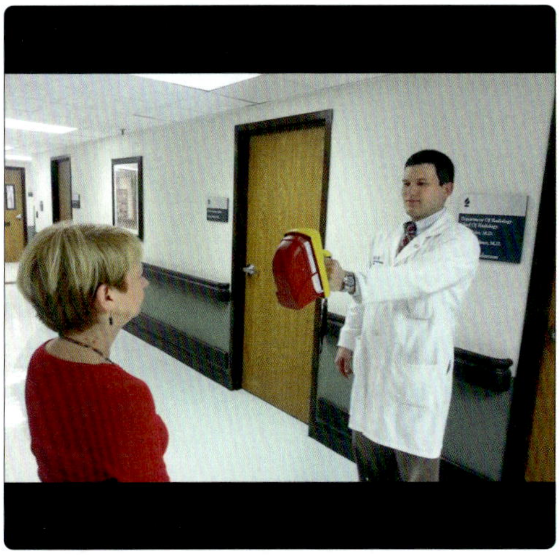

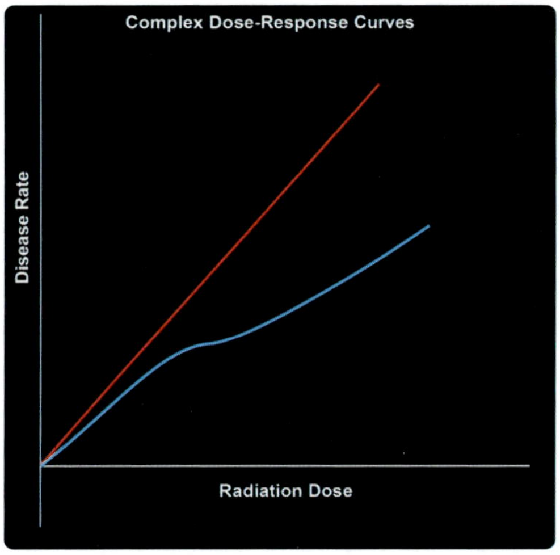

(Left) *An ionization chamber is being used to determine the radiation dose at 1 meter after I-131 NaI therapy. The NRC limit is 7 mrem/hr for patient release with detailed instructions to limit exposure to others.* **(Right)** *The nonlinear complex curve (in blue) shows a dose response for a population with a higher genetic susceptibility to the stochastic effect. This nonlinear complex curve could reveal the proportion of a susceptible subgroup (e.g., melanoma cases in fair-skinned vs. darker-skinned individuals).*

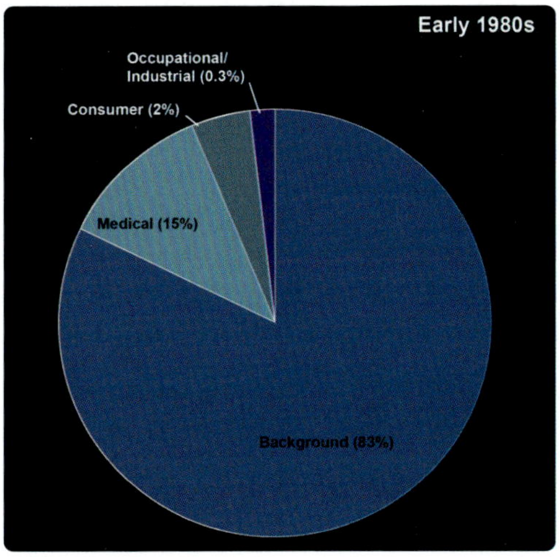

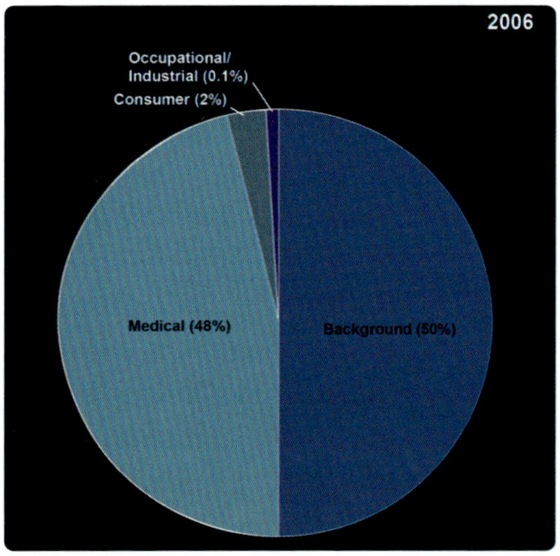

(Left) *In the 1980s, medical radiation composed 15% of a typical individual's total ionizing radiation exposure.* **(Right)** *By 2006, medical radiation had increased to 48% of an individual's total ionizing radiation exposure and the collective effective dose nearly doubled due to the increased medical use of radiation on USA population.*

SECTION 14
Safety

Medical Use of Byproduct Material

Standards for Protection Against Radiation

Transportation of Byproduct Materials

KEY FACTS

NRC REGULATIONS TITLE 10, CODE OF FEDERAL REGULATIONS PART 35: MEDICAL USE OF BYPRODUCT MATERIAL, SUBPART A

- Agreement states have entered into regulatory contracts with NRC giving them authority to license and inspect byproduct, source, or special nuclear material used or possessed within their borders
- Nuclear materials in federal agencies, such as VA hospitals, are regulated by NRC regardless of location
- Medical use: Intentional internal or external administration of byproduct material or radiation from byproduct material to patients or human research subjects under supervision of authorized user (AU)
- Preceptor: Individual who provides, directs, or verifies training and experience required for individual to become AU, authorized medical physicist, authorized nuclear pharmacist, or radiation safety officer
- Prescribed dosage: Specified activity or range of activity of unsealed byproduct material as documented in written directive or in accordance with directions of AU
- Sealed source: Any byproduct material encased in a capsule designed to prevent leakage or escape of byproduct material
- Therapeutic dosage: Dosage of unsealed byproduct material intended to deliver radiation dose to patient or human research subject for palliative or curative treatment
- Unit dosage: Dosage prepared for medical use for administration as single dosage to patient or human research subject without any further manipulation of dosage after it is initially prepared
- Written directive: Authorized user's written order for administration of byproduct material or radiation from byproduct material to specific patient or human research subject

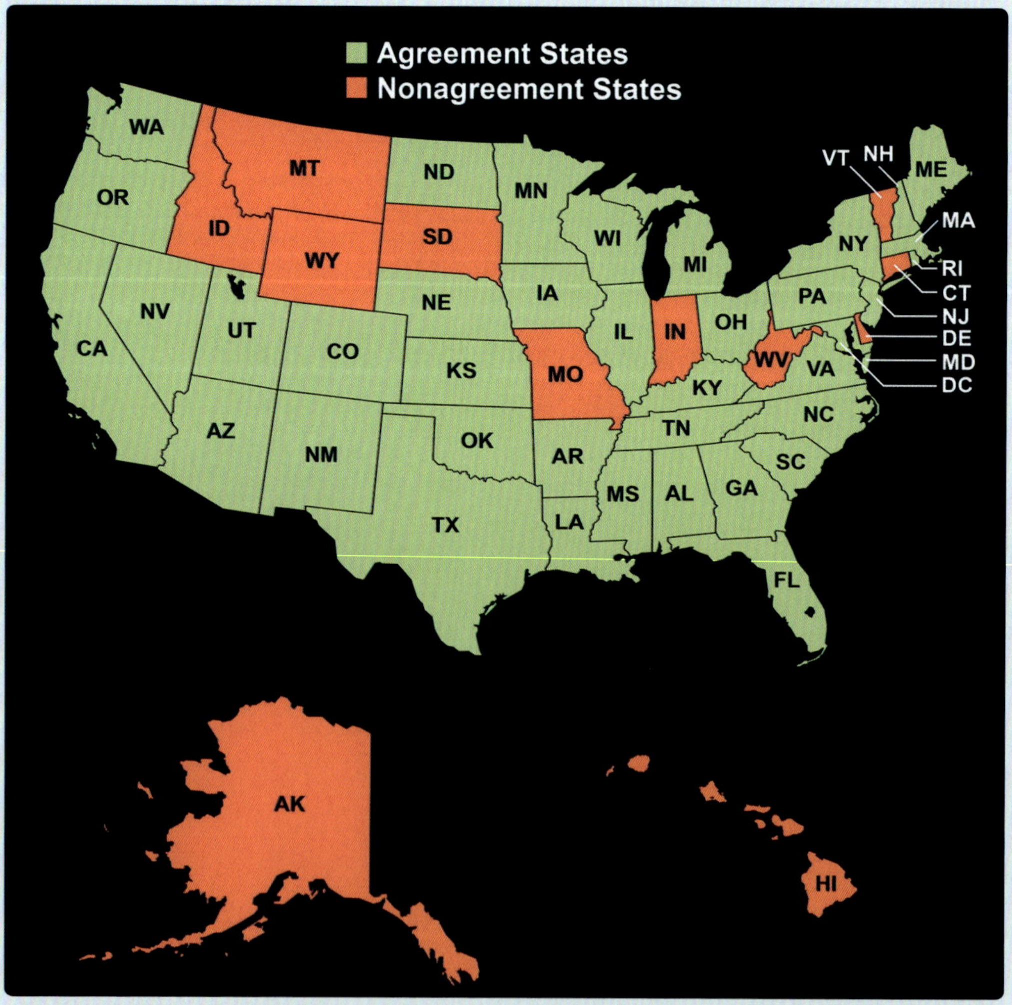

Agreement and nonagreement states are shown. Agreement states have signed an agreement with the NRC authorizing the state to regulate certain uses of radioactive materials within the state. As noted, the majority of the United States are agreement states.

NRC REGULATIONS TITLE 10, CODE OF FEDERAL REGULATIONS PART 35: MEDICAL USE OF BYPRODUCT MATERIAL, SUBPART A

35.1: Purpose and Scope

- This part contains requirements and provisions for medical use of byproduct material and for issuance of specific licenses authorizing medical use of this material
  - These requirements and provisions provide for radiation safety of
    - Workers
    - General public
    - Patients
    - Human research subjects

35.2: Definitions

- **Agreement State**
  - State with which (NRC or Atomic Energy Commission) has entered into effective agreement under Atomic Energy Act of 1954
    - 37 states have entered into agreements with NRC, and others are being evaluated
    - Agreement states have entered into regulatory contracts (agreements) with NRC giving them authority to license and inspect byproduct, source, or special nuclear material used or possessed within their borders
    - Nuclear materials in federal agencies, such as VA hospitals, are regulated by NRC regardless of location
- **Area of use**
  - Area set aside for purpose of receiving, preparing, using, or storing byproduct material
- **Authorized medical physicist**
  - Individual identified as authorized medical physicist or teletherapy physicist
- **Authorized nuclear pharmacist**
  - Pharmacist identified as authorized nuclear pharmacist
- **Authorized user**
  - Physician, dentist, or podiatrist identified as authorized user (AU)
- **Cyclotron**
  - Particle accelerator in which charged particles travel in outward spiral or circular path
    - Cyclotron accelerates charged particles at energies usually in excess of 10 MeV and is commonly used for production of short t1/2 radionuclides for medical use
- **Dedicated check source**
  - Radioactive source used to assure constant operation of radiation detection or measurement device over several months or years
- **Medical event**
  - Replaces previous term "misadministration"
    - Dose that differs from prescribed dose or dose that would have resulted from prescribed dosage by 5 rem (0.05 Sv) effective dose equivalent (EDE), 50 rem (0.5 Sv) to organ or tissue, or 50 rem (0.5 Sv) shallow-dose equivalent to skin
    - If medical event occurs, licensee must notify NRC, referring physician, and affected patient, unless (based on medical judgment) telling individual would be harmful
- **Medical institution**
  - Organization in which more than 1 medical discipline is practiced
- **Medical use**
  - Intentional internal or external administration of byproduct material or radiation from byproduct material to patients or human research subjects under supervision of authorized user
- **Positron emission tomography (PET) radionuclide production facility**
  - Facility operating cyclotron or accelerator for purpose of producing PET radionuclides
- **Preceptor**
  - Individual who provides, directs, or verifies training and experience required for individual to become an AU, authorized medical physicist, authorized nuclear pharmacist, or radiation safety officer
- **Prescribed dosage**
  - Specified activity or range of activity of unsealed byproduct material as documented in written directive or in accordance with directions of authorized user for procedures performed
- **Radiation safety officer (RSO)**
  - Individual identified as radiation safety officer on specific medical use license issued by NCR or Agreement State or medical use permit issued by Commission master material licensee
- **Sealed source**
  - Any byproduct material that is encased in a capsule designed to prevent leakage or escape of byproduct material
- **Therapeutic dosage**
  - Dosage of unsealed byproduct material intended to deliver radiation dose to patient or human research subject for palliative or curative treatment
- **Treatment site**
  - Anatomical description of tissue intended to receive radiation dose, as described in written directive
- **Unit dosage**
  - Dosage prepared for medical use for administration as single dosage to patient or human research subject without any further manipulation of dosage after it is initially prepared
- **Written directive**
  - AU's written order for administration of byproduct material or radiation from byproduct material to specific patient or human research subject

35.5: Maintenance of Records

- Each record required by this part must be legible throughout retention period specified by each Commission regulation
- Record may be original or reproduced copy or microform, provided that copy or microform is authenticated by authorized personnel and microform is capable of producing clear copy throughout required retention period
- Record may also be stored in electronic media with capability for producing legible, accurate, and complete records during required retention period
- Records such as letters, drawings, and specifications must include all pertinent information such as stamps, initials, and signatures

- Licensee shall maintain adequate safeguards against tampering with and loss of records

35.6: Provisions for Protection of Human Research Subjects

- Licensee may conduct research involving human research subjects only if using byproduct materials specified on license for uses authorized on license
- If research is conducted, funded, supported, or regulated by another federal agency that has implemented federal policy for Protection of Human Subjects (federal policy), licensee shall, before conducting research
  - Obtain review and approval of research from institutional review board, as defined and described in federal policy; and
  - Obtain informed consent, as defined and described in federal policy, from human research subject
- If research will not be conducted, funded, supported, or regulated by another federal agency that has implemented federal policy, licensee shall, before conducting research, apply for and receive specific amendment to its NRC medical use license
  - Amendment request must include written commitment that licensee will
    - Obtain review and approval of research from institutional review board, as defined and described in federal policy; and
    - Obtain informed consent, as defined and described in federal policy, from human research subject
- Nothing in this section relieves licensees from complying with other requirements in this part

35.7: FDA, Other Federal, and State Requirements

- Nothing relieves licensee from complying with applicable FDA, other federal, and state requirements governing radioactive drugs or devices

35.11: License Required

- Person may manufacture, produce, acquire, receive, possess, prepare, use, or transfer byproduct material for medical use only in accordance with specific license issued by Commission or Agreement State, or as allowed below
- Specific license is not needed for an individual who
  - Receives, possesses, uses, or transfers byproduct material in accordance with regulations in this chapter under supervision of authorized user, unless prohibited by license condition; or
  - Prepares unsealed byproduct material for medical use in accordance with regulations in this chapter under supervision of authorized nuclear pharmacist or authorized user, unless prohibited by license condition

35.12: Application for License, Amendment, or Renewal

- Application must be signed by applicant's or licensee's management
- Application for license for medical use of byproduct material must be made by
  - Filing original and 1 copy of NRC Form 313, "Application for Material License," that includes facility diagram, equipment, and training and experience qualifications of radiation safety officer, authorized user(s), authorized medical physicist(s), and authorized nuclear pharmacist(s); and
  - Submitting required procedures, as applicable
- Request for license amendment or renewal must be made by
  - Submitting original and 1 copy of either
    - NRC Form 313, "Application for Material License"; or
    - Letter requesting amendment or renewal; and
    - Submitting required procedures, as applicable
- In addition, application for license or amendment for medical use of byproduct material must also include information regarding any radiation safety aspects of medical use of material
  - Applicant shall also provide specific information on
    - Radiation safety precautions and instructions
    - Methodology for measurement of dosages or doses to be administered to patients or human research subjects; and
    - Calibration, maintenance, and repair of instruments and equipment necessary for radiation safety
  - Applicant or licensee shall also provide any other information requested by Commission
- Applicant that satisfies these requirements may apply for type A specific license of broad scope
- Facilities and equipment must be able to protect health and minimize danger to life or property
- License application must include diagram of facility and describe equipment necessary for radiation protection program
- For mobile diagnostic nuclear medicine services, applicant must submit a diagram of base facility or each base facility if multiple bases will be used
- Licensee has full responsibility in ensuring current license

35.13: License Amendments

- Licensee shall apply for and must receive license amendment before it
  - Receives, prepares, or uses byproduct material for type of use permitted under this part, but is not authorized on licensee's current license issued under this part
  - Permits anyone to work as authorized user, authorized nuclear pharmacist, or authorized medical physicist under license, except those who meet requirements
  - Changes RSOs (except when temporary RSOs)
  - Receives byproduct material in excess of amount or in different form, or receives different radionuclide than is authorized on license
  - Adds to or changes areas of use identified in application or on license
  - Changes address(es) of use identified in application or on license; and
  - Revises procedures, as applicable, where such revision reduces radiation safety
    - Including if change includes addition or relocation of either area where PET radionuclides are produced or PET radioactive drug delivery line from PET radionuclide/PET radioactive drug production area

35.14: Notifications

- Licensee shall provide Commission copy of board certification and written attestation(s) signed by
  - Preceptor, Commission, or Agreement State license
  - Permit issued by Commission master material licensee
  - Permit issued by Commission or Agreement State licensee of broad scope
  - Permit issued by Commission master material license broad scope permittee; or
  - Documentation that only accelerator-produced radioactive materials, discrete sources of radium-226, or both, were used for medical use or in practice of nuclear pharmacy
    - No later than 30 days after date licensee permits individual to work as authorized user, authorized nuclear pharmacist, or authorized medical physicist
- Licensee shall notify Commission no later than 30 days after
  - Authorized user, authorized nuclear pharmacist, radiation safety officer, or authorized medical physicist permanently discontinues performance of duties under license or has name change
  - Licensee permits authorized user or individual qualified to be RSO, function as temporary RSO, and perform functions of RSO
  - Licensee's mailing address changes or licensee's name changes, but name change does not constitute transfer of control of license
  - Licensee has added to or changed areas of use identified in application or on license where byproduct material is used
    - If change does not include addition or relocation of either area where PET radionuclides are produced or PET radioactive drug delivery line from PET radionuclide/PET radioactive drug production area
- Licensee shall send documents required in this section to appropriate address
- Bankruptcy proceedings must be reported to NRC within 24 hours after filing of bankruptcy petition
  - NRC must ensure there will be no public health or safety issues
  - However, licensee remains responsible for compliance with all regulatory requirements
- For diagnostic nuclear medicine licenses, NRC must be notified in writing within 60 days when license has expired or if decision made to permanently stop licensed activities at entire site
  - Licensees must certify disposition of licensed materials as well as ensure that facility is not contaminated to facilitate decommissioning

35.18 License Issuance

- Commission shall issue license for medical use of byproduct material if
  - Applicant has filed NRC Form 313 "Application for Material License"
  - Applicant has paid any applicable fee
  - Commission finds applicant equipped and committed to observe safety standards established by Commission in this chapter for protection of public health and safety; and
  - Applicant meets requirements of domestic licensing of byproduct material
- Commission shall issue license for mobile medical service if applicant
  - Meets requirements above and
  - Assures that individuals or human research subjects to whom unsealed byproduct material or radiation from implants containing byproduct material will be administered may be released following treatment

35.19: Specific Exemptions

- Commission may, upon application of any interested person or upon its own initiative, grant exemptions from regulations in this part that it determines are authorized by law and will not endanger life or property or common defense and security and are otherwise in public interest

SELECTED REFERENCES

1. United States Nuclear Regulatory Commission. NRC Regulations (10 CFR) Part 35: Medical Use of Byproduct Material. http://www.nrc.gov/reading-rm/doc-collections/cfr/part035. Published June 31, 2015. Accessed June 31, 2015

KEY FACTS

NRC REGULATIONS TITLE 10, CODE OF FEDERAL REGULATIONS PART 35: MEDICAL USE OF BYPRODUCT MATERIAL, SUBPART B

- In addition to radiation protection program requirements, licensee's management shall approve in writing
  - Requests for license application, renewal, or amendment before submittal to Commission
  - Any individual before allowing that individual to work as authorized user, authorized nuclear pharmacist, or authorized medical physicist
  - Radiation protection program changes that do not require license amendment
- Licensee's management shall appoint a radiation safety officer (RSO) who agrees in writing to be responsible for implementing radiation protection program
  - Licensee, through RSO, shall ensure that radiation safety activities are being performed in accordance with licensee-approved procedures and regulatory requirements
- Licensee shall establish authority, duties, and responsibilities of RSO in writing
- Licensees that are authorized for 2 or more different types of uses of byproduct material shall establish a radiation safety committee to oversee all uses of byproduct material permitted by license
  - Committee must include authorized user of each type of use permitted by license: RSO, representative of nursing service, and representative of management who is neither authorized user nor RSO
  - Committee may include other members licensee considers appropriate

TRC Form 12-1
08/04

Page 1 of 7

Department of State Health Services

RADIOACTIVE MATERIAL LICENSE

Pursuant to the Texas Radiation Control Act and Texas Department of State Health Services (Agency) regulations on radiation, and in reliance on statements and representations heretofore made by the licensee, a license is hereby issued authorizing the licensee to receive, acquire, possess and transfer radioactive material listed below, and to use such radioactive material for the purpose(s) and at the place(s) designated below This license is subject to all applicable rules, regulations and orders of the Agency now or hereafter in effect and to any conditions specified below

LICENSEE	
1 Name 2. Address	This license is issued in response to a letter Dated: February 9, 2015 Signed by:
	3. License Number
	Amendment Number 127
	PREVIOUS AMENDMENTS ARE VOID
	4. Expiration Date January 31, 2014

RADIOACTIVE MATERIAL AUTHORIZED

5. Radioisotope	6. Form of Material	7. Maximum Activity	8. Authorized Use
A. Any radio-active material with Atomic Number less than 84 and half life less than 120 days	A. Any except sealed sources	A. 50 millicuries of each isotope Total: 10 curies	A. Medical research, diagnosis and therapy.
B. Mo-99	B. Generators	B. 10 curies	B. Production of Tc-99m.
C. Tc-99m	C. Any	C. 10 curies	C. Medical research, diagnosis, and shielding evaluations.
D. Rb-81	D. Generators	D. 1 curie	D. Production of Kr-81m.
E. Kr-81m	E. Any	E. 1 curie	E. Medical diagnosis.
F. Xe-133	F. Any	F. 5 curies	F. Medical diagnosis.
G. H-3	G. Any	G. 0.1 curies	G. Medical research.
H. C-14	H. Any	H. 50 millicuries	H. Medical research.
I. P-32	I. Any	I. 200 millicuries	I. Medical research and therapy.
J. I-131; I-125	J. Any liquid or solid	J. 1 curie	J. Medical research, diagnosis and therapy.
K. Pd-103	K. Sealed source (Seeds)	K. 1 curie	K. Medical research and therapy.

* Texas Administrative Code (TAC) # U S Food and Drug Administration (FDA) * Investigational New Drug Application (IND)

This is an example of a radioactive material license issued by the state of Texas, which is an agreement state. Requests for a license application, renewal, or amendment fall under the responsibility of the radiation safety program management that is usually led by the radiation safety officer (RSO).

NRC REGULATIONS TITLE 10, CODE OF FEDERAL REGULATIONS PART 35: MEDICAL USE OF BYPRODUCT MATERIAL, SUBPART B

35.24: Authority and Responsibilities for Radiation Protection Program

- In addition to radiation protection program requirements, licensee's management shall approve in writing
  - Requests for license application, renewal, or amendment before submittal to Commission
  - Any individual before allowing that individual to work as authorized user, authorized nuclear pharmacist, or authorized medical physicist; and
  - Radiation protection program changes that do not require license amendment
- Licensee's management shall appoint radiation safety officer (RSO) who agrees in writing to be responsible for implementing radiation protection program
  - Licensee, through RSO, shall ensure that radiation safety activities are being performed in accordance with licensee-approved procedures and regulatory requirements
- For up to 60 days each year, licensee may permit authorized user or individual qualified to be RSO to function as temporary RSO and to perform functions of RSO
- Licensee may simultaneously appoint more than 1 temporary RSO if needed to ensure that licensee has temporary RSO that satisfies requirements to be RSO for each of different types of uses of byproduct material permitted by license
- Licensee shall establish authority, duties, and responsibilities of RSO in writing
- Licensees that are authorized for 2 or more different types of uses of byproduct material shall establish radiation safety committee to oversee all uses of byproduct material permitted by license
  - Committee must include authorized user of each type of use permitted by license: RSO, representative of nursing service, and representative of management who is neither authorized user nor RSO
  - Committee may include other members licensee considers appropriate
- Licensee shall provide RSO sufficient authority, organizational freedom, time, resources, and management prerogative, to
  - Identify radiation safety problems
  - Initiate, recommend, or provide corrective actions
  - Stop unsafe operations
  - Verify implementation of corrective actions
- Licensee shall retain record of actions taken

35.26: Radiation Protection Program Changes

- Licensee may revise its radiation protection program without Commission approval if
  - Revision does not require license amendment
  - Revision is in compliance with regulations and license
  - Revision has been reviewed and approved by RSO and licensee management
  - Affected individuals are instructed on revised program before changes are implemented
- Licensee shall retain record of each change

35.27: Supervision

- Licensee that permits receipt, possession, use, or transfer of byproduct material by individual under supervision of authorized user shall
  - Instruct supervised individual in licensee's written radiation protection procedures, written directive procedures, regulations of this chapter, and license conditions with respect to use of byproduct material
  - Require supervised individual to follow instructions of supervising authorized user for medical uses of byproduct material, written radiation protection procedures established by the licensee, written directive procedures, regulations of this chapter, and license conditions with respect to medical use of byproduct material
- Licensee that permits preparation of byproduct material for medical use by individual under supervision of authorized nuclear pharmacist or physician who is authorized user shall
  - Instruct supervised individual in preparation of byproduct material for medical use, as appropriate to that individual's involvement with byproduct material
  - Require supervised individual to follow instructions of supervising authorized user or authorized nuclear pharmacist regarding preparation of byproduct material for medical use, written radiation protection procedures established by the licensee, regulations of this chapter, and license conditions
- Licensee that permits supervised activities is responsible for acts and omissions of supervised individual

35.49: Suppliers for Sealed Sources or Devices for Medical Use

- For medical use, licensee may only use
  - Sealed sources or devices manufactured, labeled, packaged, and distributed in accordance with license issued under NRC requirements or equivalent requirements of Agreement State
  - Sealed sources or devices non-commercially transferred
  - Teletherapy sources manufactured and distributed in accordance with a license issued under NRC requirements or equivalent requirements of Agreement State

35.50: Training for Radiation Safety Officer

- Licensee shall require individual fulfilling responsibilities of RSO to be an individual who
  - Is certified by specialty board whose certification process has been recognized by Commission or Agreement State
    - Names of board certifications which have been recognized by Commission or Agreement State will be posted on NRC web page
  - To have its certification process recognized, specialty board shall require all candidates for certification to hold bachelor's or graduate degree from accredited college or university in physical science or engineering or biological science with minimum of 20 college credits in physical science
    - Have 5 or more years of professional experience in health physics (graduate training may be substituted for no more than 2 years of required experience) including at least 3 years in applied health physics; and

- Pass examination administered by diplomates of specialty board, which evaluates knowledge and competence in radiation physics and instrumentation, radiation protection, mathematics pertaining to use and measurement of radioactivity, radiation biology, and radiation dosimetry; or
- Hold master's or doctor's degree in physics, medical physics, other physical science, engineering, or applied mathematics from accredited college or university

- Have 2 years of full-time practical training &/or supervised experience in medical physics
  - Under supervision of medical physicist who is certified in medical physics by specialty board recognized by Commission or Agreement State; or
  - In clinical nuclear medicine facilities providing diagnostic &/or therapeutic services under direction of physicians who meet requirements for authorized users and
  - Pass examination, administered by diplomates of specialty board, that assesses knowledge and competence in clinical diagnostic radiological or nuclear medicine physics and in radiation safety; or
  - Has completed structured educational program consisting of both 200 hours of classroom and laboratory training in radiation physics and instrumentation and radiation protection; mathematics pertaining to use and measurement of radioactivity; radiation biology; and
  - Radiation dosimetry; and
  - 1 year of full-time radiation safety experience under supervision of individual identified as radiation safety officer on Commission or Agreement State license or permit issued by Commission master material licensee that authorizes similar type(s) of use(s) of byproduct material involving
    - Shipping, receiving, and performing related radiation surveys
    - Using and performing checks for proper operation of instruments used to determine activity of dosages, survey meters, and instruments used to measure radionuclides
    - Securing and controlling byproduct material
    - Using administrative controls to avoid mistakes in administration of byproduct material
    - Using procedures to prevent or minimize radioactive contamination and using proper decontamination procedures
    - Using emergency procedures to control byproduct material; and
    - Disposing of byproduct material; or
- Is a medical physicist who has been certified by specialty board whose certification process has been recognized by Commission or Agreement State and has experience in radiation safety for similar types of use of byproduct material for which licensee is seeking approval of individual as RSO, or
- Is an authorized user, authorized medical physicist, or authorized nuclear pharmacist identified on licensee's license and has experience with radiation safety aspects of similar types of use of byproduct material for which the individual has RSO responsibilities; and
  - Has obtained written attestation, signed by preceptor RSO, that individual has satisfactorily completed requirements, and has achieved level of radiation safety knowledge sufficient to function independently as RSO for medical use licensee; and
  - Has training in radiation safety, regulatory issues, and emergency procedures for types of use for which licensee seeks approval
    - This training requirement may be satisfied by completing training that is supervised by RSO, authorized medical physicist, authorized nuclear pharmacist, or authorized user, as appropriate, who is authorized for type(s) of use for which licensee is seeking approval

35.51: Training for Authorized Medical Physicist

- Licensee shall require authorized medical physicist to be an individual who
  - Is certified by specialty board whose certification process has been recognized by Commission or Agreement State (names of board certifications which have been recognized by Commission or Agreement State will be posted on NRC web page); to have its certification process recognized, specialty board shall require all candidates for certification to
    - Hold master's or doctor's degree in physics, medical physics, other physical science, engineering, or applied mathematics from accredited college or university
      - Have 2 years of full-time practical training &/or supervised experience in medical physics
      - Under supervision of medical physicist who is certified in medical physics by specialty board recognized by Commission or Agreement State; or
      - In clinical radiation facilities providing high-energy, external beam therapy (photons and electrons with energies ≥ 1 million electron volts) and brachytherapy services under direction of physicians; and
      - Pass examination, administered by diplomates of specialty board, that assesses knowledge and competence in clinical radiation therapy, radiation safety, calibration, quality assurance, and treatment planning for external beam therapy, brachytherapy, and stereotactic radiosurgery; or
    - Holds master's or doctor's degree in physics, medical physics, other physical science, engineering, or applied mathematics from accredited college or university; and has completed 1 year of full-time training in medical physics and additional year of full-time work experience under supervision of individual who meets requirements for authorized medical physicist for type(s) of use for which individual is seeking authorization
    - This training and work experience must be conducted in clinical radiation facilities that provide high-energy, external beam therapy (photons and electrons with energies ≥ 1 million electron volts) and brachytherapy services and must include
      - Performing sealed source leak tests and inventories
      - Performing decay corrections

- Performing full calibration and periodic spot checks of external beam treatment units, stereotactic radiosurgery units, and remote afterloading units as applicable; and
- Conducting radiation surveys around external beam treatment units, stereotactic radiosurgery units, and remote afterloading units as applicable; and
- Has obtained written attestation that individual has satisfactorily completed requirements, and has achieved level of competency sufficient to function independently as authorized medical physicist for each type of therapeutic medical unit for which individual is requesting authorized medical physicist status
- Written attestation must be signed by preceptor authorized medical physicist who meets NRC requirements, or equivalent Agreement State requirements for authorized medical physicist for each type of therapeutic medical unit for which individual is requesting authorized medical physicist status; and
- Has training for type(s) of use for which authorization is sought that includes hands-on device operation, safety procedures, clinical use, and operation of treatment planning system
- This training requirement may be satisfied by satisfactorily completing either training program provided by vendor or by training supervised by authorized medical physicist authorized for type(s) of use for which the individual is seeking authorization

35.55: Training for Authorized Nuclear Pharmacist

- Licensee shall require authorized nuclear pharmacist to be a pharmacist who
  - Is certified by specialty board whose certification process has been recognized by Commission or Agreement State (names of board certifications which have been recognized by Commission or Agreement State will be posted on NRC web page); to have its certification process recognized, specialty board shall require all candidates for certification to
    - Have graduated from a pharmacy program accredited by American Council on Pharmaceutical Education (ACPE) or have passed Foreign Pharmacy Graduate Examination Committee (FPGEC) examination
    - Hold current, active license to practice pharmacy
    - Provide evidence of having acquired at least 4,000 hours of training/experience in nuclear pharmacy practice; academic training may be substituted for no more than 2,000 hours of required training and experience; and
    - Pass examination in nuclear pharmacy administered by diplomates of specialty board, that assesses knowledge and competency in procurement, compounding, quality assurance, dispensing, distribution, health and safety, radiation safety, provision of information and consultation, monitoring patient outcomes, research and development; or
    - Has completed 700 hours in a structured educational program consisting of both 200 hours of classroom and laboratory training in radiation physics and instrumentation, radiation protection, mathematics pertaining to use and measurement of radioactivity, chemistry of byproduct material for medical use, and radiation biology; and
    - Supervised practical experience in nuclear pharmacy involving
      - Shipping, receiving, and performing related radiation surveys
      - Using and performing checks for proper operation of instruments used to determine the activity of dosages, survey meters, and, if appropriate, instruments used to measure alpha- or beta-emitting radionuclides
      - Calculating, assaying, and safely preparing dosages for patients or human research subjects
      - Using administrative controls to avoid medical events in administration of byproduct material; and
      - Using procedures to prevent or minimize radioactive contamination and using proper decontamination procedures; and
      - Has obtained written attestation, signed by a preceptor authorized nuclear pharmacist, that the individual has satisfactorily completed requirements and has achieved a level of competency sufficient to function independently as authorized nuclear pharmacist

35.59: Recentness of Training

- Training and experience specified must have been obtained within 7 years preceding date of application or individual must have had related continuing education and experience since required training and experience was completed

SELECTED REFERENCES

1. United States Nuclear Regulatory Commission. NRC Regulations (10 CFR) Part 35: Medical Use of Byproduct Material. http://www.nrc.gov/reading-rm/doc-collections/cfr/part035. Published June 31, 2015. Accessed June 31, 2015

KEY FACTS

NRC REGULATIONS TITLE 10, CODE OF FEDERAL REGULATIONS

- Each syringe/vial that contains unsealed byproduct material must be labeled to identify radioactive drug
- Licensee may authorize release from its control of any individual who has been administered unsealed byproduct material if total effective dose equivalent to any other individual from exposure to released individual is not likely to exceed 5 mSv (0.5 rem)
- Licensee may hold byproduct material with physical t1/2 of ≤ 120 days for decay-in-storage before disposal; before disposal, licensee must
    - Monitor byproduct material at surface and determine that its radioactivity cannot be distinguished from background radiation level with appropriate radiation detection survey meter set on its most sensitive scale
    - Remove or obliterate all radiation labels, except for radiation labels on materials that are within containers and that will be managed as biomedical waste after they have been released from licensee
- Unless otherwise directed by authorized user, licensee may not use dosage if dosage does not fall within prescribed dosage range or if dosage differs from prescribed dosage by > 20%
- Licensee shall determine and record activity of each dosage before medical use
- Licensee shall provide released individual or guardian with instructions, including written instructions, on actions to maintain doses to other individuals as low as reasonably achievable (ALARA) if total effective dose equivalent to any other individual is likely to exceed 1 mSv (0.1 rem)
- If total effective dose equivalent to nursing infant or child could exceed 1 mSv (0.1 rem), instructions must also include guidance on interruption or discontinuation of breastfeeding

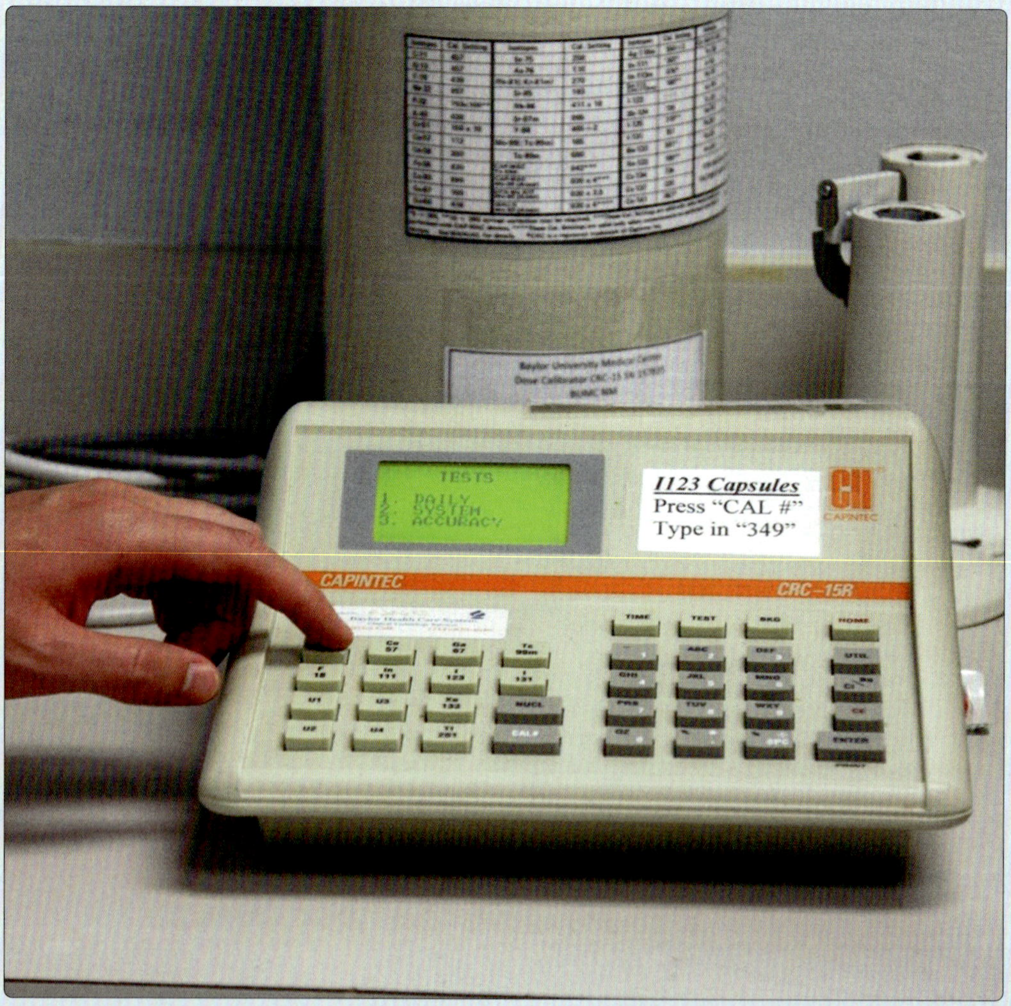

Before any activity is administered to a patient, the activity must be measured in a dose calibrator (shown) unless unit doses are being used. Unless otherwise directed by the authorized user, a licensee may not use a dosage if it does not fall within the prescribed dosage range or if it differs from the prescribed dosage by > 20%.

NRC REGULATIONS TITLE 10, CODE OF FEDERAL REGULATIONS

35.60: Possession, Use, and Calibration of Instruments Used to Measure Activity of Unsealed Byproduct Material

- For direct measurements, licensee shall possess and use instrumentation to measure activity of unsealed byproduct material before administered to each patient or human research subject
- Licensee shall calibrate instrumentation in accordance with nationally recognized standards or manufacturer's instructions
- Records must include
  - Model and serial number of instrument
  - Date of calibration
  - Results of calibration
  - Name of individual who performed calibration
- Licensee shall maintain record of instrument calibrations for 3 years

35.61: Calibration of Survey Instruments

- Licensee shall calibrate survey instruments used to show compliance with this part before 1st use, annually, and following repair that affects calibration
  - Calibrate all scales with readings up to 10 mSv (1,000 mrem) per hour with radiation source
  - Calibrate 2 separate readings on each scale to show compliance
  - Conspicuously note on instrument date of calibration
- Licensee may not use survey instruments if difference between indicated exposure rate and calculated exposure rate > 20%
- Record must include
  - Model and serial number of instrument
  - Date of calibration
  - Results of calibration
  - Name of individual who performed calibration
- Licensee shall maintain record of radiation survey instrument calibrations for 3 years

35.63: Determination of Dosages of Unsealed Byproduct Material for Medical Use

- Licensee shall determine and record activity of each dosage before medical use
- For unit dosage, this determination must be made by
  - Direct measurement of radioactivity
  - Decay correction, based on activity or activity concentration determined by
    - Manufacturer or preparer licensed NRC requirements or equivalent Agreement State requirements; or
    - NRC or Agreement State licensee for use in research in accordance with Radioactive Drug Research Committee-approved protocol or Investigational New Drug (IND) protocol accepted by FDA; or
    - PET radioactive drug producer licensed under NRC requirements or equivalent Agreement State requirements
- For other than unit dosages, this determination must be made by
  - Direct measurement of radioactivity
  - Combination of measurement of radioactivity and mathematical calculations
  - Combination of volumetric measurements and mathematical calculations, based on measurement made by
    - Manufacturer or preparer licensed NRC requirements or equivalent Agreement State requirements; or
    - PET radioactive drug producer licensed NRC requirements or equivalent Agreement State requirements
- Unless otherwise directed by authorized user, licensee may not use dosage if dosage does not fall within prescribed dosage range or if dosage differs from prescribed dosage by > 20%
- Licensee shall maintain record of dosage determinations for 3 years

35.65: Authorization for Calibration, Transmission, and Reference Sources

- Any person authorized for medical use of byproduct material may receive, possess, and use any of the following byproduct material for check, calibration, transmission, and reference use
  - Sealed sources, not exceeding 30 mCi (1.11 GBq) each, manufactured and distributed by person licensed under NRC requirements or equivalent Agreement State regulations
  - Sealed sources, not exceeding 30 mCi (1.11 GBq) each, redistributed by licensee authorized to redistribute sealed sources manufactured and distributed by person licensed under NRC requirements or equivalent Agreement State regulations
    - Providing redistributed sealed sources are in original packaging and shielding and are accompanied by manufacturer's approved instructions
  - Any byproduct material with t1/2 not longer than 120 days in individual amounts not to exceed 0.56 GBq (15 mCi)
  - Any byproduct material with t1/2 longer than 120 days in individual amounts not to exceed the smaller of 200 μCi (7.4 MBq) or 1,000x quantities in NRC (10 CFR) Appendix B of Part 30
  - Technetium-99m in amounts as needed

35.67: Requirements for Possession of Sealed Sources and Brachytherapy Sources

- Licensee in possession of any sealed source or brachytherapy source shall follow radiation safety and handling instructions supplied by manufacturer
- Licensee in possession of sealed source shall
  - Test source for leakage before first use unless licensee has certificate from supplier indicating that source was tested within 6 months before transfer to licensee; and
  - Test source for leakage at intervals not to exceed 6 months or at other intervals approved by Commission or Agreement State in Sealed Source and Device Registry
- To satisfy leak test requirements of this section, licensee shall measure sample so that leak test can detect presence of 0.005 μCi (185 Bq) of radioactive material in sample
- Licensee shall retain leak test records for 3 years
- If leak test reveals presence of 0.005 μCi (185 Bq) or more of removable contamination, licensee shall

  - Immediately withdraw sealed source from use and store, dispose, or cause it to be repaired; and
  - File report within 5 days of leak test
- Licensee need not perform leak test on following sources
  - Sources containing only byproduct material with t1/2 of < 30 days
  - Sources containing only byproduct material as gas
  - Sources containing 100 μCi (3.7 MBq) or less of beta or gamma-emitting material or 10 μCi (0.37 MBq) or less of alpha-emitting material
  - Sources stored and not being used; however, licensee shall test each such source for leakage before any use or transfer unless it has been leak tested within 6 months before date of use or transfer
- Licensee in possession of sealed sources shall conduct a semi-annual physical inventory of all such sources; licensee shall retain each inventory record for 3 years

35.69: Labeling of Vials and Syringes

- Each syringe and vial containing unsealed byproduct material must be labeled to identify radioactive drug
  - Each syringe shield and vial shield must also be labeled unless label on syringe or vial is visible when shielded
- Licensee shall ensure that each container of licensed material bears durable, clearly visible label bearing radiation symbol and "CAUTION, RADIOACTIVE MATERIAL"
  - Label must also provide sufficient information to permit individuals handling or using containers, or working in vicinity of containers, to take precautions to avoid or minimize exposures, such as
    - Radionuclide[s] present
    - Estimate of quantity of radioactivity
    - Date for which activity is estimated
    - Radiation levels
    - Kinds of materials
- Each licensee shall, prior to removal or disposal of empty uncontaminated containers to unrestricted areas, remove or deface radioactive material label or clearly indicate that container no longer contains radioactive materials

35.70: Surveys of Ambient Radiation Exposure Rate

- Licensee shall survey with radiation detection survey instrument at end of each day of use and all areas where unsealed byproduct material requiring written directive was prepared for use or administered
- Licensee does not need to perform surveys where patients are confined when they cannot be released
- Licensee shall retain record of each survey for 3 years

35.75: Release of Individuals Containing Unsealed Byproduct Material

- Licensee may authorize release from its control of any individual who has been administered unsealed byproduct material if total effective dose equivalent to any other individual from exposure to released individual is not likely to exceed 5 mSv (0.5 rem)
  - Current revision of NUREG–1556, Vol. 9, "Consolidated Guidance About Materials Licenses: Program-Specific Guidance About Medical Licenses" describes methods for calculating doses to other individuals and contains tables of activities not likely to cause doses exceeding 5 mSv (0.5 rem)
- Licensee shall provide released individual, or individual's parent or guardian, with instructions, including written instructions, on actions recommended to maintain doses to other individuals as low as is reasonably achievable (ALARA) if total effective dose equivalent to any other individual is likely to exceed 1 mSv (0.1 rem)
- If total effective dose equivalent to nursing infant or child could exceed 1 mSv (0.1 rem) assuming there was no interruption of breastfeeding, instructions must also include
  - Guidance on interruption or discontinuation of breastfeeding; and
  - Information on potential consequences, if any, of failure to follow guidance
- Licensee shall maintain record of basis for authorizing release of individual for 3 years after date of release
- Licensee shall maintain record of instructions provided to breast-feeding female for 3 years

35.80: Provision of Mobile Medical Service

- Licensee providing mobile medical service shall
  - Obtain letter signed by management of each client for which services are rendered that permits use of byproduct material at client's address and clearly delineates authority/responsibility of licensee & client
  - Check instruments used to measure activity of unsealed byproduct material for proper function before medical use at each client's address or on each day of use, whichever is more frequent
    - At minimum, check for proper function required by this paragraph must include constancy check
  - Check survey instruments for proper operation before use at each client's address; and
  - Before leaving client's address, survey all areas of use
- Mobile medical service may not have byproduct material delivered from manufacturer or distributor to client unless client has license allowing possession of byproduct material
  - Byproduct material delivered to client must be received and handled in conformance with client's license
- Licensee providing mobile medical services shall retain letter required and record of each survey for 3 years

35.92: Decay-in-Storage

- Licensee may hold byproduct material with physical t1/2 ≤ 120 days for decay-in-storage before disposal without regard to its radioactivity if it
  - Monitors byproduct material at surface before disposal and determines that its radioactivity cannot be distinguished from background radiation level with appropriate survey meter set to most sensitive scale and with no interposed shielding; and
  - Removes or obliterates all radiation labels, except for radiation labels on materials that are within containers and that will be managed as biomedical waste after they have been released from licensee
- Licensee shall retain record of each disposal for 3 years

SELECTED REFERENCES

1. United States Nuclear Regulatory Commission. NRC Regulations (10 CFR) Part 35: Medical Use of Byproduct Material. http://www.nrc.gov/reading-rm/doc-collections/cfr/part035. Published June 31, 2015. Accessed June 31, 2015

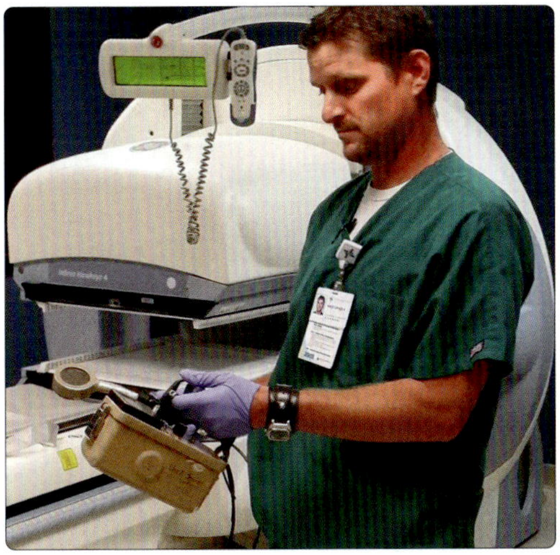

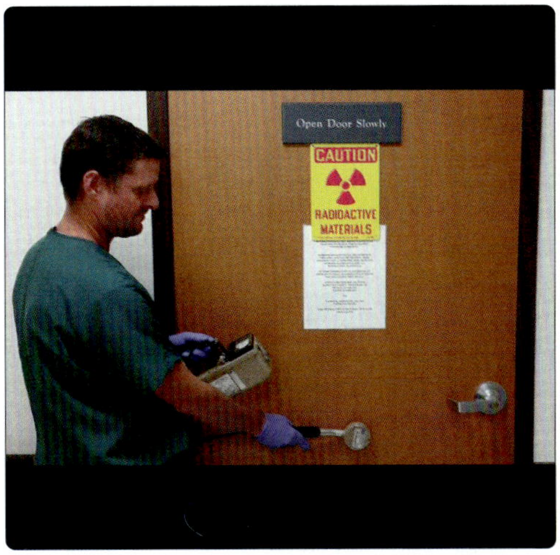

(Left) *A patient received a 100 mCi (3.7 GBq) dose of I-131 in this area. The NRC requires licensees to survey all areas where unsealed byproduct material requiring written directive was administered.* **(Right)** *Licensee may hold byproduct material with physical t1/2 of ≤ 120 days for decay-in-storage before disposal. A routine survey of the shielded door of the entrance to the decay-in-storage is shown.*

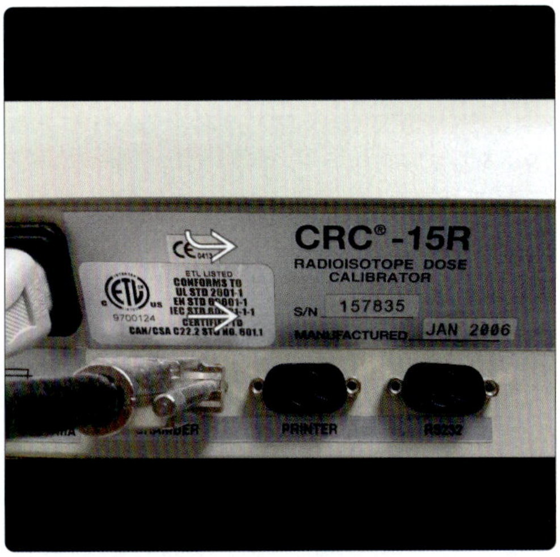

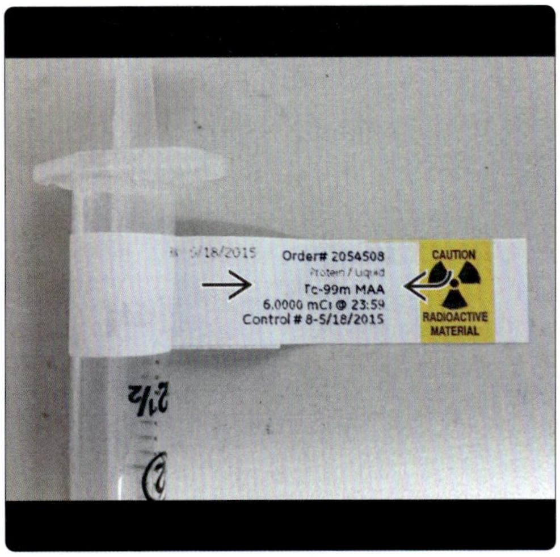

(Left) *Each licensee is required to calibrate instrumentation in accordance with nationally recognized standards or manufacturer's instructions recording the date, results, person performing the calibration, and model ➔ and serial number ➔ of the dose calibrator.* **(Right)** *Each syringe and vial containing unsealed byproduct material must be labeled to identify the radioactive drug ➔. It must also have a radioactive material label ➔.*

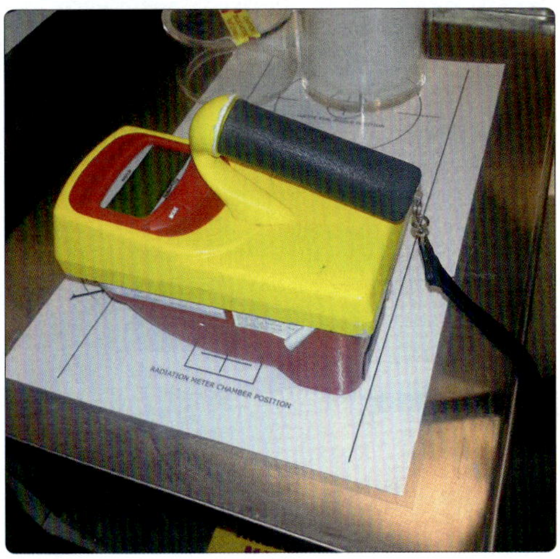

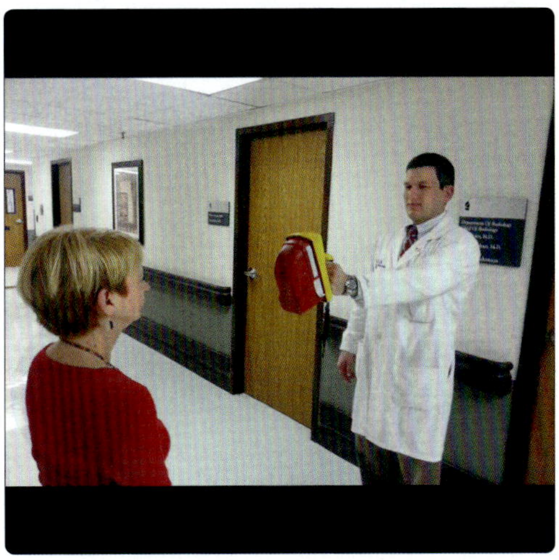

(Left) *Ionization detector is shown. This detector is a handheld, gas-filled detector that allows for accurate exposure measurements.* **(Right)** *Licensee may authorize release from its control of any individual who has been administered unsealed byproduct material if total effective dose equivalent to any other individual from exposure to released individual is not likely to exceed 5 mSv (0.5 rem).*

KEY FACTS

RADIOACTIVE SPILLS

- Goal is to minimize impact of radioactive contamination or unplanned exposure

MODEL SPILL PROCEDURE

- Medical needs attended first
- Spill procedure depends on many variables: Number of individuals affected, likelihood of contamination spread, types and surfaces contaminated, and radiation hazard of spilled material
- Notify all persons in area that spill has occurred
- Notify RSO immediately if major spill has occurred
- Prevent spread of contamination by isolating area and covering spill, if appropriate, with absorbent paper
- If minor spill, wear gloves, disposable lab coat, and booties; clean up spill with absorbent paper
- Survey area or contaminated individual with appropriate radiation survey instrument and check for removable contamination
- Check hands and clothing for self-contamination
- Decay any radioactive trash resulting from spill clean-up procedure for 10 half-lives or when activity reaches background

MINOR VS. MAJOR SPILL

- Threshold of 1, 10, or 100 mCi (37, 370 MBq, or 3.7 GBq) used to determine minor versus major spill
- 1 mCi (37 MBq) threshold: P-32, Sr-89, I-125, and I-131
- 10 mCi (370 MBq): Co-57, Ga-67, In-111, I-123, Sm-153
- 100 mCi (3.7 GBq): Tc-99m, Tl-201

GAS "SPILL"

- Evacuation time (T, in min) is calculated as: $T = V/Q \ln (A/CV)$
  - V = room air volume in mL
  - Q = total room air exhaust rate in mL/min
  - A = released activity of Xe-133 in μCi
  - C = restricted area DAC for Xe-133 (1×10^{-4} μCi/mL)

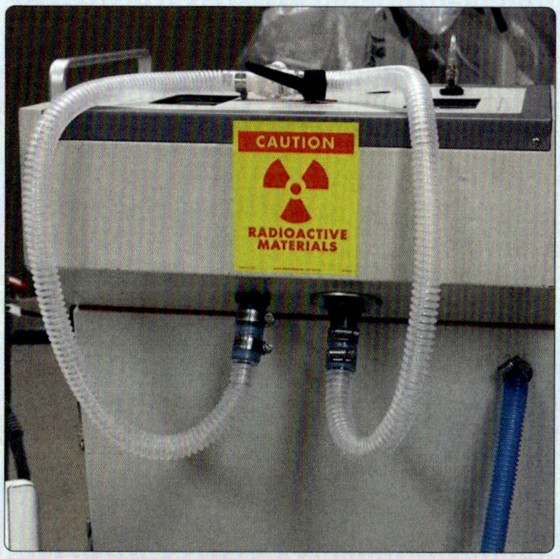

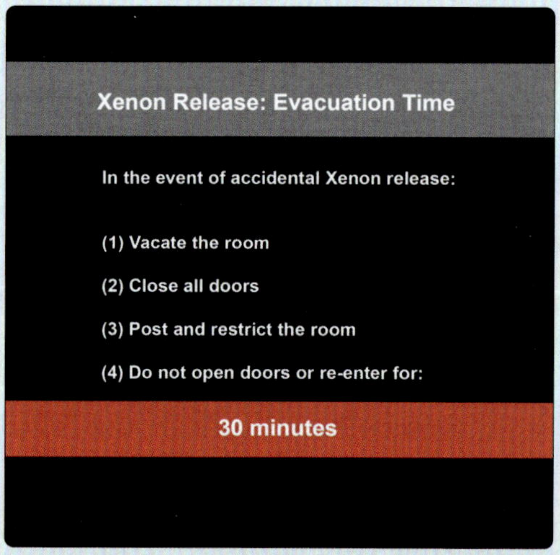

(Left) *Xe-133 trap is shown. These machines are used to trap the exhaled Xe-133 used for lung scintigraphy. For various reasons, the Xe-133 may leak out of this machine.* **(Right)** *An evacuation time is calculated for any room using radioactive gas. In this example, an evacuation time of 30 min is needed to clear this particular room of radioactive gas. The evacuation time is calculated from the room volume and total room air exhaust rate.*

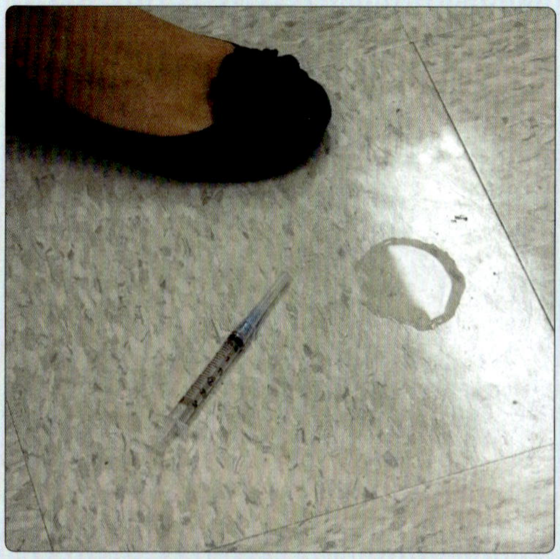

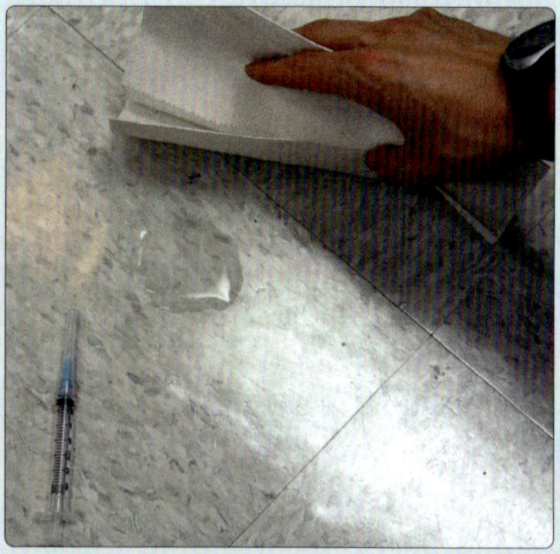

(Left) *A radioactive spill is shown. If this is a minor spill, once medical needs are met, the spill should be contained and then cleaned up.* **(Right)** *Radioactive spill clean up is shown. However, the technologist is not using proper protocol as he is not wearing gloves in this picture. During a minor spill, the technologist must wear gloves, a disposable lab coat, and booties, and clean up the spill with absorbent paper.*

10 CFR 20.1406 AND 20.1701

Preventing Contamination

- Applicants for licenses, other than renewals, must describe in application how facility design and procedures for operation will minimize, to extent practicable, contamination of facility and environment, facilitate eventual decommissioning, and minimize, to extent practicable, generation of radioactive waste
- Licensee shall use, to extent practical, process or other engineering controls (e.g., containment, decontamination, or ventilation) to control concentration of radioactive material in air

Radioactive Spills

- Goal is to minimize impact of radioactive contamination or unplanned exposure
- Spill procedure depends on many variables: Number of individuals affected, likelihood of contamination spread, types and surfaces contaminated, and radiation hazard of spilled material
- Always attend to medical needs first

Model Spill Procedure

- Notify all persons in area that spill has occurred
- Notify RSO immediately if major spill has occurred
- Prevent spread of contamination by isolating area and covering spill, if appropriate, with absorbent paper
- If clothing contaminated, remove article of clothing and place in plastic bag
- If individual is contaminated, rinse contaminated area with lukewarm water and wash with mild soap, using gloves
- Notify radiation safety officer or appropriate individual of any unusual circumstances immediately
- If minor spill, wear gloves, disposable lab coat, and booties; clean up spill with absorbent paper
- Place absorbent paper and all other contaminated disposable material in appropriately labeled radioactive waste containers
- Survey area or contaminated individual with appropriate radiation survey instrument, and check for removable contamination
  - If necessary, continue to decontaminate area or individual until decontamination activities no longer result in reductions in removable activity
  - If necessary, leave absorbent paper labeled "Caution: Radioactive Material" over area to prevent loosening of any fixed contamination
  - If necessary, shield spill area to reduce ambient exposure levels
- Check hands and clothing for self-contamination
- Report incident to radiation safety officer or appropriate supervisory personnel; if personnel contamination is found, skin dose will be evaluated
- Decay any radioactive trash resulting from spill clean-up procedure for 10 half-lives or when activity reaches background

Minor vs. Major Spill

- Threshold of 1, 10, or 100 mCi (37, 370 MBq, or 3.7 GBq) used to determine minor versus major spill; if the threshold for particular radionuclide is met, a major spill has occurred
  - Less than threshold is considered a minor spill for that radionuclide
- 1 mCi (37 MBq) threshold
  - P-32, Sr-89, I-125, and I-131
- 10 mCi (370 MBq) threshold
  - Co-57, Ga-67, In-111, I-123, Sm-153
- 100 mCi (3.7 GBq) threshold
  - Tc-99m, Tl-201

Spill Kit Contents

- Disposable gloves
- Housekeeping gloves
- Disposable lab coats
- Disposable head coverings
- Disposable shoe covers
- Roll of absorbent paper with plastic backing
- Masking tape
- Plastic trash bags with twist ties
- "Radioactive Material" labeling tape
- Marking pen
- Pre-strung "Radioactive Material" labeling tags
- Box of wipes
- Instructions for emergency procedures
- Clipboard with copy of Radioactive Spill Report Form for facility
- Pencil
- Appropriate survey instruments including batteries (for survey meters)
  - Survey instrument not necessarily in kit, but needed for spill procedure

Gas "Spill"

- In case of gas "spill" during ventilation exam during which Xe-133 is used, evacuation time must be implemented
- In event of evacuation, all individuals must leave room promptly while closing room door to minimize leakage
- Evacuation time can be based on conservative occupational limit specified for a restricted area (i.e., derived air concentration [DAC] of 1 × 10-4 μCi/mL for Xe-133)
  - Evacuation time (T, in min) is calculated as: $T = V/Q \ln (A/CV)$
    - V = room air volume in mL
    - Q = total room air exhaust rate in mL/min
    - A = released activity of Xe-133 in μCi
    - C = restricted area DAC for Xe-133 (1×10^{-4} μCi/mL)
  - Evacuation time varies, but can be in range of 15-45 min

SELECTED REFERENCES

1. United States Nuclear Regulatory Commission. NRC Regulations (10 CFR) Part 20: Standards for Protection Against Radiation. http://www.nrc.gov/reading-rm/doc-collections/cfr/part020. Published June 31, 2015. Accessed June 31, 2015

KEY FACTS

NRC REGULATIONS (10 CFR), PART 20, STANDARDS FOR PROTECTION AGAINST RADIATION, SUBPART M (REPORTS)

- Each licensee shall report by telephone, immediately after its occurrence becomes known to licensee, any lost, stolen, or missing licensed material in aggregate quantity ≥ 1,000x quantity specified in NRC Regulations (10 CFR) appendix C under such circumstances that it appears to licensee that exposure could result to persons in unrestricted areas
- Within 30 days after occurrence of any lost, stolen, or missing licensed material becomes known to licensee, report all licensed material in quantity > 10x quantity specified in NRC Regulations (10 CFR) appendix C to part 20 that is still missing at this time
- For reportable events each licensee shall submit a written report within 30 days after learning of any of the following occurrences
  - Doses in excess of occupational limits for adults or minors
  - Doses in excess of limits for embryo/fetus of declared pregnant woman
  - Doses in excess of limits for individual member of the public

NRC REGULATIONS (10 CFR), PART 20, STANDARDS FOR PROTECTION AGAINST RADIATION, SUBPART O (ENFORCEMENT)

- Commission may obtain injunction or other court order to prevent violation of provisions and payment of civil penalty
- Commission may impose criminal sanctions for willful violation of, attempted violation of, or conspiracy to violate any regulation issued

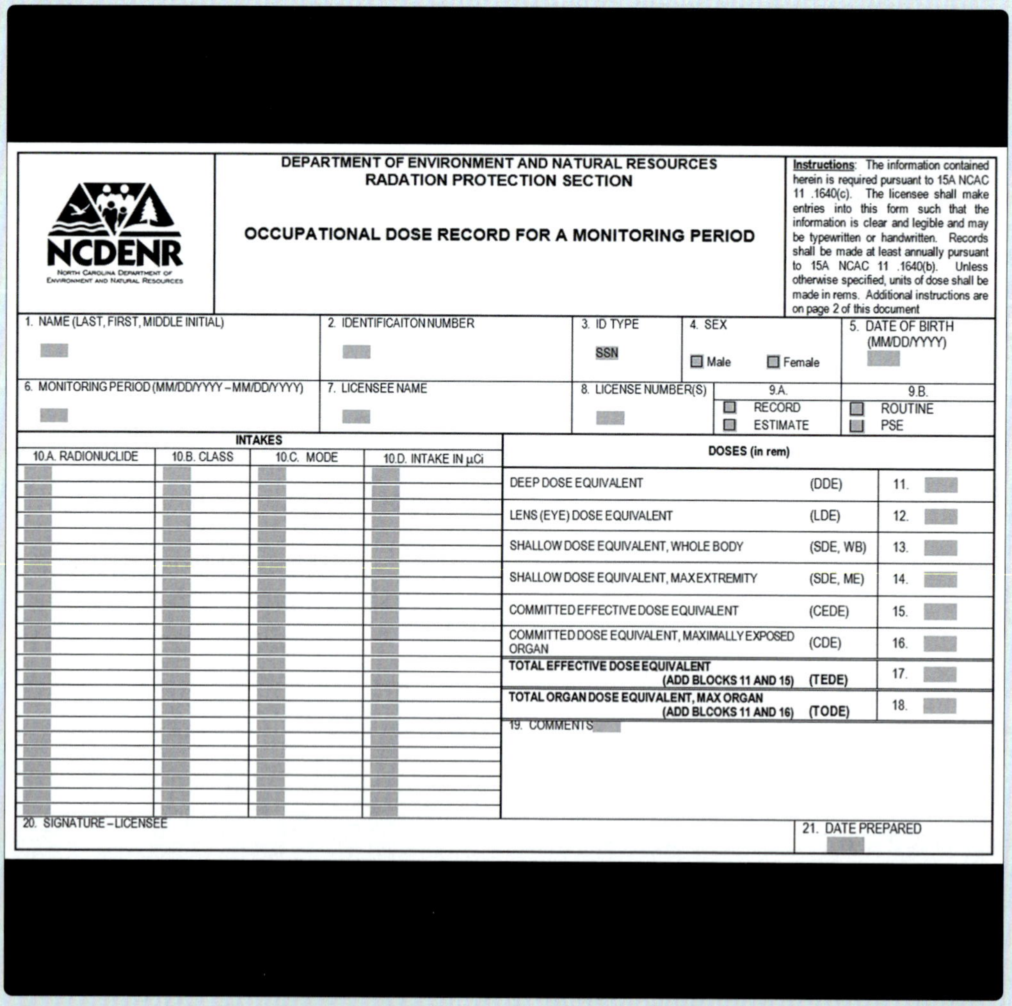

NCDENR
North Carolina Department of Environment and Natural Resources

DEPARTMENT OF ENVIRONMENT AND NATURAL RESOURCES
RADIATION PROTECTION SECTION

OCCUPATIONAL DOSE RECORD FOR A MONITORING PERIOD

Instructions: The information contained herein is required pursuant to 15A NCAC 11 .1640(c). The licensee shall make entries into this form such that the information is clear and legible and may be typewritten or handwritten. Records shall be made at least annually pursuant to 15A NCAC 11 .1640(b). Unless otherwise specified, units of dose shall be made in rems. Additional instructions are on page 2 of this document

1. NAME (LAST, FIRST, MIDDLE INITIAL)
2. IDENTIFICAITON NUMBER
3. ID TYPE — SSN
4. SEX — Male / Female
5. DATE OF BIRTH (MM/DD/YYYY)
6. MONITORING PERIOD (MM/DD/YYYY – MM/DD/YYYY)
7. LICENSEE NAME
8. LICENSE NUMBER(S)
9.A. RECORD / ESTIMATE
9.B. ROUTINE / PSE

INTAKES

10.A. RADIONUCLIDE	10.B. CLASS	10.C. MODE	10.D. INTAKE IN µCi

DOSES (in rem)

DEEP DOSE EQUIVALENT	(DDE)	11.
LENS (EYE) DOSE EQUIVALENT	(LDE)	12.
SHALLOW DOSE EQUIVALENT, WHOLE BODY	(SDE, WB)	13.
SHALLOW DOSE EQUIVALENT, MAX EXTREMITY	(SDE, ME)	14.
COMMITTED EFFECTIVE DOSE EQUIVALENT	(CEDE)	15.
COMMITTED DOSE EQUIVALENT, MAXIMALLY EXPOSED ORGAN	(CDE)	16.
TOTAL EFFECTIVE DOSE EQUIVALENT (ADD BLOCKS 11 AND 15)	(TEDE)	17.
TOTAL ORGAN DOSE EQUIVALENT, MAX ORGAN (ADD BLCOKS 11 AND 16)	(TODE)	18.

19. COMMENTS

20. SIGNATURE – LICENSEE

21. DATE PREPARED

A sample occupational dose record for an agreement state. If occupational dose limits are exceeded, this is considered a reportable event. Each licensee is required to submit a written report within 30 days after learning of such an occurrence.

NRC REGULATIONS (10 CFR), PART 20, STANDARDS FOR PROTECTION AGAINST RADIATION, SUBPART M (REPORTS)

20.2201: Reports of Theft or Loss of Licensed Material

- Telephone reports
  - Each licensee shall report by telephone as follows
    - Immediately after its occurrence becomes known to licensee, any lost, stolen, or missing licensed material in aggregate quantity ≥ 1,000x quantity specified in NRC Regulations (10 CFR) appendix C to part 20 under such circumstances that it appears to licensee that exposure could result to persons in unrestricted areas
    - Within 30 days after occurrence of any lost, stolen, or missing licensed material becomes known to licensee, all licensed material in quantity > 10x quantity specified in NRC Regulations (10 CFR) appendix C to part 20 that is still missing at this time
- Written reports
  - Each licensee is required to make written report within 30 days after making telephone report setting forth the following information
    - Description of licensed material involved, including kind, quantity, and chemical and physical form; and
    - Description of circumstances under which loss or theft occurred; and
    - Statement of disposition, or probable disposition, of licensed material involved; and
    - Exposures of individuals to radiation, circumstances under which exposures occurred, and possible total effective dose equivalent to persons in unrestricted areas; and
    - Actions that have been taken, or will be taken, to recover material; and
    - Procedures or measures that have been, or will be, adopted to ensure against a recurrence of loss or theft of licensed material
- Subsequent to filing written report, licensee shall also report any additional substantive information on loss or theft within 30 days after licensee learns of such information
- Licensee shall prepare any report filed with Commission pursuant to this section so that names of individuals who may have received exposure to radiation are stated in separate and detachable part of report
- Each licensee shall notify NRC as soon as possible but not later than 4 hours after discovery of event that prevents immediate protective actions necessary to avoid exposures to radiation or radioactive materials that could exceed regulatory limits or releases of licensed material that could exceed regulatory limits
  - Events may include fires, explosions, toxic gas releases, etc.

20.2202: Notification of Incidents

- Immediate notification: Notwithstanding any other requirements for notification, each licensee shall immediately report any event involving byproduct, source, or special nuclear material possessed by licensee that may have caused or threatens to cause any of the following conditions
  - Individual to receive
    - Total effective dose equivalent of 25 rems (0.25 Sv) or more
    - Lens dose equivalent of 75 rems (0.75 Sv) or more
    - Shallow-dose equivalent to skin or extremities of 250 rads (2.5 Gy) or more
  - Release of radioactive material, inside or outside restricted area, so that, had an individual been present for 24 hours, individual could have received intake 5x annual limit on intake
- 24 hour notification: Each licensee shall, within 24 hours of discovery of event, report any event involving loss of control of licensed material possessed by licensee that may have caused, or threatens to cause, any of the following conditions
  - Individual to receive, in period of 24 hours
    - Total effective dose equivalent exceeding 5 rems (0.05 Sv)
    - Lens dose equivalent exceeding 15 rems (0.15 Sv)
    - Shallow-dose equivalent to skin or extremities exceeding 50 rems (0.5 Sv)
  - Release of radioactive material, inside or outside of restricted area, so that, had an individual been present for 24 hours, individual could have received intake in excess of 1 occupational annual limit on intake
- Licensee shall prepare any report filed with Commission pursuant to this section so that names of individuals who have received exposure to radiation or radioactive material are stated in separate and detachable part of report
- Provisions of this section do not include doses that result from planned special exposures, that are within limits for planned special exposures

20.2203: Reports of Exposures, Radiation Levels, and Concentrations of Radioactive Material Exceeding Constraints or Limits

- Reportable events: Each licensee shall submit written report within 30 days after learning of any of the following occurrences
  - Doses in excess of any of the following
    - Occupational dose limits for adults
    - Occupational dose limits for minors
    - Limits for embryo/fetus of declared pregnant woman
    - Limits for individual member of public
    - Any applicable limit in license
  - Levels of radiation or concentrations of radioactive material in
    - Restricted area in excess of any applicable limit in license
    - Unrestricted area in excess of 10x any applicable limit set forth in this part or in license (whether or not involving exposure of any individual in excess of limits)
- Contents of reports
  - Each report must describe extent of exposure of individuals to radiation and radioactive material, including, as appropriate
    - Estimates of each individual's dose
    - Levels of radiation and concentrations of radioactive material involved
    - Cause of elevated exposures, dose rates, or concentrations

  - Corrective steps taken or planned to ensure against recurrence, including schedule for achieving conformance with applicable limits, ALARA constraints, generally applicable environmental standards, and associated license conditions
- Each report filed must include, for each occupationally overexposed individual
  - Name
  - Social Security number
  - Date of birth
  - Report must be prepared so that this information is stated in separate and detachable part of report and must be clearly labeled "Privacy Act Information: Not for Public Disclosure"

20.2204: Reports of Planned Special Exposures

- Licensee shall submit written report to administrator of appropriate NRC Regional Office within 30 days following any planned special exposure, informing Commission that planned special exposure was conducted and indicating date planned special exposure occurred and following information
  - Exceptional circumstances requiring use of planned special exposure
  - Name of management official who authorized planned special exposure and copy of signed authorization
  - What actions were necessary
  - Why actions were necessary
  - How doses were maintained ALARA
  - What individual and collective doses were expected to result, and doses actually received in planned special exposure
  - Licensee shall retain records until the Commission terminates each pertinent license requiring these records

20.2205: Reports to Individuals of Exceeding Dose Limits

- When licensee is required to report to Commission any exposure of identified occupationally exposed individual, or identified member of public, to radiation or radioactive material, licensee shall also provide individual a report on exposure data included in report to Commission
  - Report must be transmitted no later than transmittal to Commission

NRC REGULATIONS (10 CFR), PART 20, STANDARDS FOR PROTECTION AGAINST RADIATION, SUBPART O (ENFORCEMENT)

20.2401: Violations

- Commission may obtain injunction or other court order to prevent violation of provisions of
  - Atomic Energy Act of 1954, as amended
  - Title II of Energy Reorganization Act of 1974, as amended; or
  - Regulation or order issued pursuant to those Acts
- Commission may obtain court order for payment of civil penalty imposed under section 234 of Atomic Energy Act
  - For violations of
    - Any rule, regulation, or order issued
    - Any term, condition, or limitation of any license issued
  - For any violation for which license may be revoked

20.2402: Criminal Penalties

- Section 223 of Atomic Energy Act of 1954, as amended, provides for criminal sanctions for willful violation of, attempted violation of, or conspiracy to violate any regulation issued

SELECTED REFERENCES

1. United States Nuclear Regulatory Commission. NRC Regulations (10 CFR) Part 20: Standards for Protection Against Radiation. http://www.nrc.gov/reading-rm/doc-collections/cfr/part020. Published June 31, 2015. Accessed June 31, 2015

Quantities of Common Radionuclides To Be Reported to NRC if Lost or Stolen

Radionuclide	Quantity (mCi) 30 Day Reporting	Quantity (mCi) Immediate Reporting
I-131	0.1	10
I-123	1	100
In-111	1	100
F-18	10	1000
Ga-67	10	1000
Tc-99m	10	1000
Tl-201	10	1000
Xe-133	10	1000
**SI conversion factor: 1 mCi = 37 MBq.*		

Adapted from NRC Guide for Diagnostic Nuclear Medicine.

Written Directive Requirements

KEY FACTS

NRC REGULATIONS TITLE 10, CODE OF FEDERAL REGULATIONS

- Written directive must be dated and signed by an authorized user (AU) before administration of
  - I-131 sodium iodide > 30 μCi (1.11 MBq)
  - Any therapeutic dosage of unsealed byproduct material, or
  - Any therapeutic dose of radiation from byproduct material
- If, because of emergent nature of patient's condition, a delay in order to provide a written directive would jeopardize patient's health, oral directive is acceptable
  - Information contained in oral directive must be documented as soon as possible in writing in patient's record
  - Written directive must be prepared within 48 hours of oral directive
- Written directive must contain patient or human research subject's name and the following information
  - Dosage of any administration of quantities > 30 μCi (1.11 MBq) of sodium iodide I-131
  - For administration of therapeutic dosage of unsealed byproduct material other than sodium iodide I-131
    - Radioactive drug, dosage, and route of administration
- Written revision to existing written directive may be made if revision is dated and signed by an AU before administration of dosage of unsealed byproduct material
- If, because of patient's condition, a delay in order to provide a written revision to existing written directive would jeopardize patient's health, oral revision to existing written directive is acceptable
  - Oral revision must be documented as soon as possible in patient's record
  - Revised written directive must be signed by AU within 48 hours of oral revision
- Licensee shall retain copy of written directive for 3 years

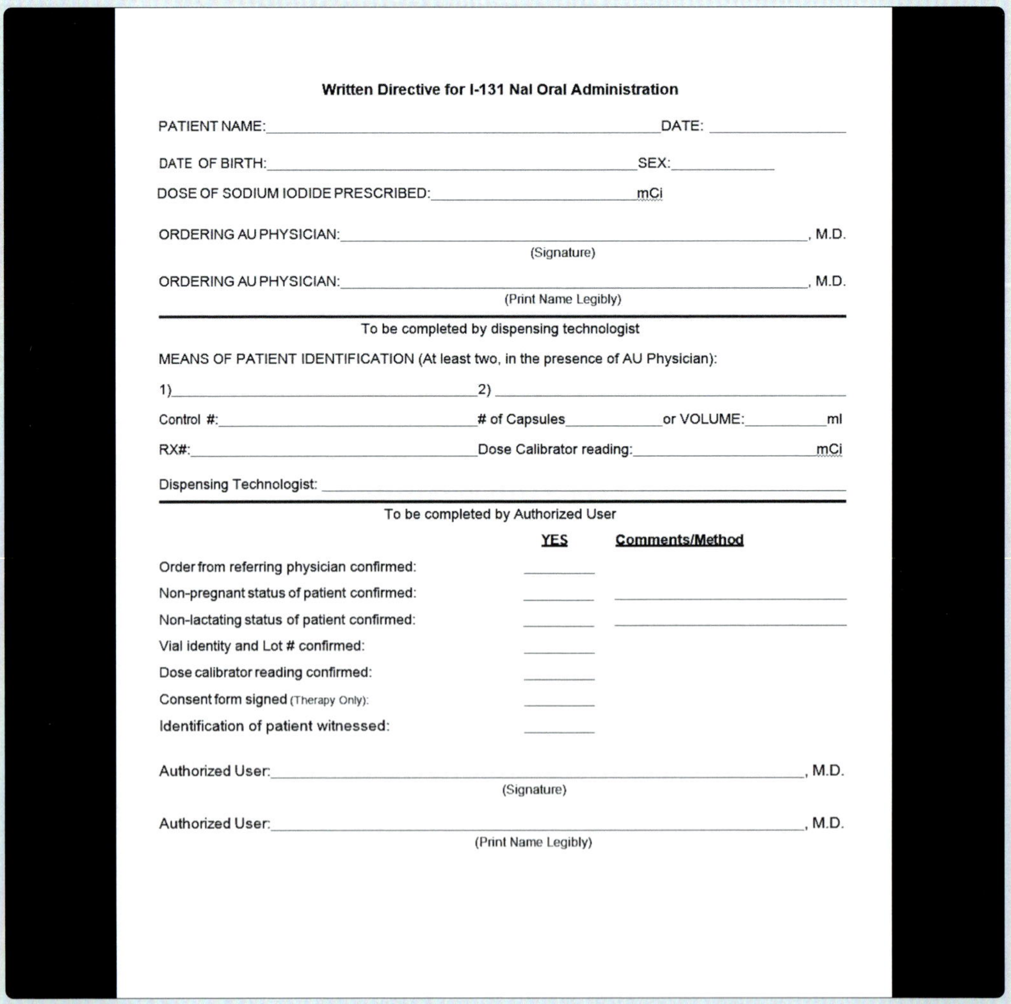

Written Directive for I-131 NaI Oral Administration

PATIENT NAME:________________________________ DATE: ____________

DATE OF BIRTH:________________________________ SEX:__________

DOSE OF SODIUM IODIDE PRESCRIBED:________________ mCi

ORDERING AU PHYSICIAN:________________________________, M.D.
(Signature)

ORDERING AU PHYSICIAN:________________________________, M.D.
(Print Name Legibly)

To be completed by dispensing technologist

MEANS OF PATIENT IDENTIFICATION (At least two, in the presence of AU Physician):

1)________________________ 2) ________________________

Control #:________________ # of Capsules__________ or VOLUME:__________ ml

RX#:________________ Dose Calibrator reading:________________ mCi

Dispensing Technologist: ________________________________

To be completed by Authorized User

	YES	Comments/Method
Order from referring physician confirmed:	______	
Non-pregnant status of patient confirmed:	______	____________
Non-lactating status of patient confirmed:	______	____________
Vial identity and Lot # confirmed:	______	
Dose calibrator reading confirmed:	______	
Consent form signed (Therapy Only):	______	
Identification of patient witnessed:	______	

Authorized User:________________________________, M.D.
(Signature)

Authorized User:________________________________, M.D.
(Print Name Legibly)

Sample written directive for administration of I-131 NaI is shown. Note that an authorized user must prescribe the dose and sign the form at the time of administration. This form must be kept for 3 years.

NRC REGULATIONS TITLE 10, CODE OF FEDERAL REGULATIONS

35.40: Written Directives

- Written directive
  - Written order dated and signed by an authorized user (AU) before administration of byproduct material to a specific patient or human research subject
    - Required before administration of I-131 NaI in amount > 30 μCi (1.11 MBq) or any therapeutic dosage of any other unsealed byproduct material
    - Written directives are generally not necessary in diagnostic nuclear medicine, as this activity typically not exceeded when performing thyroid uptake measurements
    - 30-μCi limit for I-131 applies only to I-131 NaI
      - Diagnostic studies with other I-131 labeled radiopharmaceuticals (e.g., I-131 metaiodobenzylguanidine, I-131 Hippuran, I-131 iodocholesterol) may be performed with activities > 30 μCi without need for written directive
- If, because of emergent nature of patient's condition, a delay to provide written directive would jeopardize patient's health, oral directive is acceptable
  - Information contained in oral directive must be documented as soon as possible in writing in patient's record
  - Written directive must be prepared within 48 hours of oral directive
- Written directive must contain patient or human research subject's name and the following information
  - For any administration of quantities > 30 μCi (1.11 MBq) of sodium iodide I-131
    - Dosage
  - For administration of therapeutic dosage of unsealed byproduct material other than sodium iodide I-131
    - Radioactive drug, dosage, and route of administration
- Written revision to existing written directive
  - May be made if revision is dated and signed by authorized user before administration of dosage of unsealed byproduct material
- If, because of patient's condition, a delay to provide a written revision to existing written directive would jeopardize patient's health, oral revision to existing written directive is acceptable
  - Oral revision must be documented as soon as possible in patient's record
  - Revised written directive must be signed by authorized user within 48 hours of oral revision
- Licensee shall retain copy of written directive for 3 years

35.41: Procedures for Administrations Requiring Written Directive

- For any administration requiring written directive
  - Licensee shall develop, implement, and maintain written procedures to provide high confidence that
    - Patient's or human research subject's identity is verified before each administration; and
    - Each administration is in accordance with written directive
- At minimum, procedures required in this section must address the following items applicable to licensee's use of byproduct material
  - Verifying identity of patient or human research subject
  - Verifying that administration is in accordance with treatment plan, if applicable, and written directive
  - Checking both manual and computer-generated dose calculations
  - Verifying that any computer-generated dose calculations are correctly transferred into consoles of therapeutic medical units
- Licensee shall retain copy of procedures for duration of license

SELECTED REFERENCES

1. United States Nuclear Regulatory Commission. NRC Regulations (10 CFR) Part 35: Medical Use of Byproduct Material. http://www.nrc.gov/reading-rm/doc-collections/cfr/part035. Published June 31, 2015. Accessed June 31, 2015

KEY FACTS

NRC REGULATIONS TITLE 10, CODE OF FEDERAL REGULATIONS: SUBPART A

- **Activity**: Rate of disintegration or decay of radioactive material; units are the curie (Ci) and the becquerel (Bq)
- **As low as reasonably achievable (ALARA)**: Making every reasonable effort to maintain exposures to radiation as far below dose limits as is practical consistent with purpose for which licensed activity is undertaken
- **Background radiation**: Radiation from cosmic sources; naturally occurring radioactive material, including radon (except as a decay product of source or special nuclear material); and global fallout and are not under control of licensee
- **Declared pregnant woman**: Voluntarily informed licensee, in writing, of her pregnancy and the estimated date of conception; declaration remains in effect until declared pregnant woman withdraws declaration in writing or is no longer pregnant
- **Distinguishable from background**: Detectable concentration of a radionuclide is statistically different from background concentration of that radionuclide in vicinity
- **Nonstochastic effect**: Health effects, severity of which varies with dose and for which a threshold is believed to exist; radiation-induced cataract formation is an example of nonstochastic effect (also called deterministic effect)
- **Occupational dose**: Dose received by an individual in course of employment in which individual's assigned duties involve exposure to radiation or to radioactive material from licensed and unlicensed sources of radiation
- **Stochastic effects**: Health effects that occur randomly and for which probability of effect occurring, rather than its severity, is assumed to be a linear function of dose without threshold; hereditary effects and cancer incidence are examples of stochastic effects

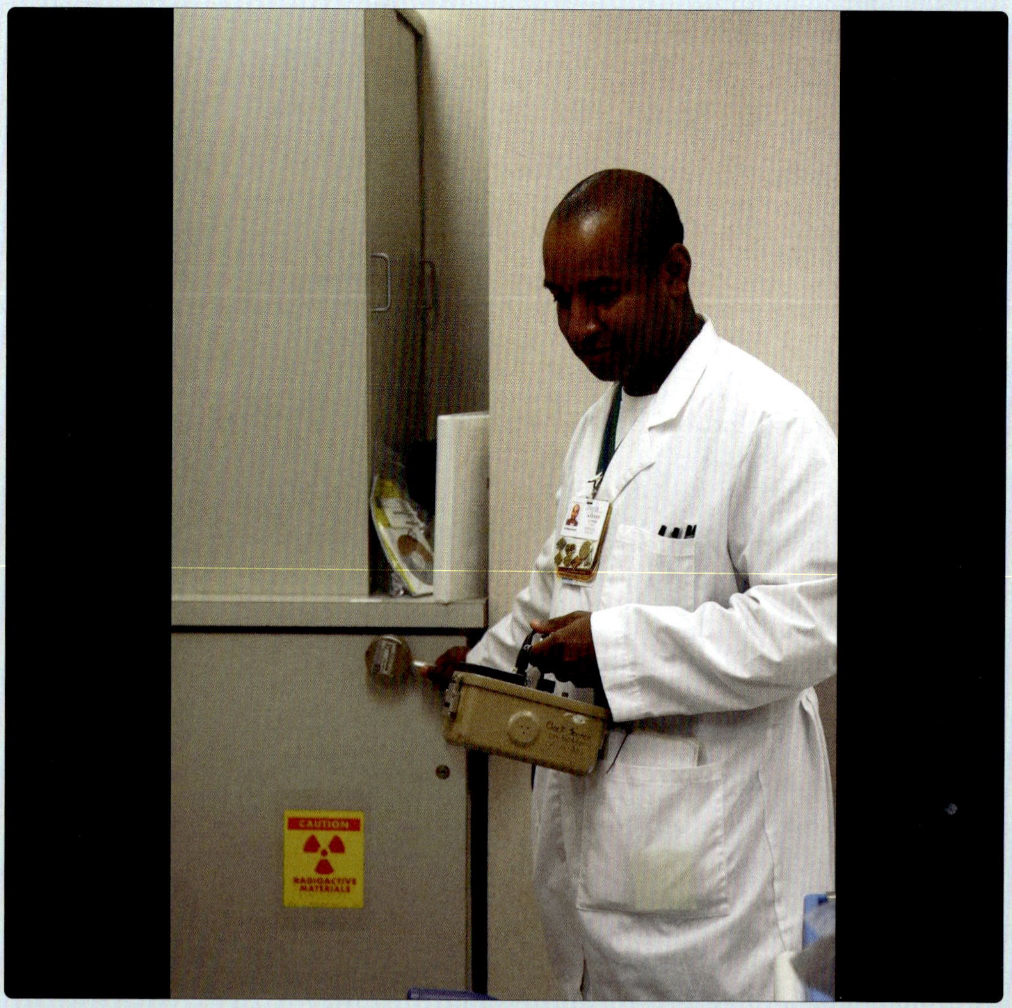

Technologist is shown performing a survey in a restricted area using a Geiger-Müller survey instrument. He is assessing the radiation level in the room and storage device as compared to background radiation levels. Occupational doses are affected by background radiation in the department.

NRC REGULATIONS TITLE 10, CODE OF FEDERAL REGULATIONS: SUBPART A

20.1001: Purpose

- Regulations in this part establish standards for protection against ionizing radiation resulting from activities conducted under licenses issued by Nuclear Regulatory Commission (NRC)
  - These regulations are issued under Atomic Energy Act of 1954 and Energy Reorganization Act of 1974
- It is the purpose of the regulations in this part to control receipt, possession, use, transfer, and disposal of licensed material by any licensee in such a manner that total dose to an individual (including doses resulting from licensed and unlicensed radioactive material and from radiation sources other than background radiation) does not exceed standards for protection against radiation prescribed in regulations in this part
  - However, nothing in this part shall be construed as limiting actions that may be necessary to protect health and safety

20.1002: Scope

- The regulations in this part apply to persons licensed by Commission to receive, possess, use, transfer, or dispose of byproduct, source, or special nuclear material or to operate production or utilization facility and to persons required to obtain certificate of compliance or approved compliance plan
- Limits in this part do not apply to doses due to background radiation, to exposure of patients to radiation for purpose of medical diagnosis or therapy, to exposure from individuals administered radioactive material, or to exposure from voluntary participation in medical research programs

20.1003: Definitions

- **Absorbed dose**: Energy imparted by ionizing radiation per unit mass of irradiated material
  - Units of absorbed dose are the rad (Rd) and the gray (Gy)
- **Accelerator-produced radioactive material**: Any material made radioactive by a particle accelerator
- **Activity:** Rate of disintegration (transformation) or decay of radioactive material
  - Units of activity are the curie (Ci) and the becquerel (Bq)
- **Airborne radioactive material**: Radioactive material dispersed in form of dusts, fumes, particulates, mists, vapors, or gases
- **Airborne radioactivity area**: Room, enclosure, or area in which airborne radioactive materials, composed wholly or partly of licensed material, exist in concentrations in excess of derived air concentrations (DACs) or to such a degree that an individual present in area without respiratory protective equipment could exceed, during hours an individual is present in a week, an intake of 0.6% of annual limit on intake (ALI) or 12 DAC-hours
- **As low as reasonably achievable (ALARA)**: Making every reasonable effort to maintain exposures to radiation as far below dose limits as is practical consistent with purpose for which licensed activity is undertaken, taking into account state of technology, economics of improvements in relation to state of technology, economics of improvements in relation to benefits to public health and safety, and other societal and socioeconomic considerations, and in relation to utilization of nuclear energy and licensed materials in public interest
- **Annual limit on intake (ALI)**: Derived limit for amount of radioactive material taken into body of adult worker by inhalation or ingestion in 1 year
  - ALI is smaller value of intake of given radionuclide in a year by reference man that would result in committed effective dose equivalent of 5 rems (0.05 Sv) or committed dose equivalent of 50 rems (0.5 Sv) to any individual organ or tissue
- **Background radiation**: Radiation from cosmic sources; naturally occurring radioactive material, including radon (except as a decay product of source or special nuclear material); and global fallout as it exists in the environment from the testing of nuclear explosive devices or from past nuclear accidents such as Chernobyl that contribute to background radiation and are not under the control of the licensee
  - Background radiation does not include radiation from source, byproduct, or special nuclear materials regulated by the Commission
- **Bioassay (radiobioassay)**: Determination of kinds, quantities or concentrations, and, in some cases, the locations of radioactive material in the human body, whether by direct measurement (in vivo counting) or by analysis and evaluation of materials excreted or removed from the human body
- **Byproduct material**
  - Any radioactive material (except special nuclear material) yielded in, or made radioactive by, exposure to the radiation incident to the process of producing or using special nuclear material
- **Collective dose**: Sum of the individual doses received in a given period of time by a specified population from exposure to a specified source of radiation
- **Commission**: NRC or its duly authorized representatives
- **Committed dose equivalent (HT,50)**: Dose equivalent to organs or tissues of reference (T) that will be received from an intake of radioactive material by an individual during the 50-year period following the intake
- **Committed effective dose equivalent**: Sum of the products of the weighting factors applicable to each of the body organs or tissues that are irradiated and the committed dose equivalent to these organs or tissues
- **Constraint (dose constraint)**: Value above which specified licensee actions are required
- **Controlled area**: Area, outside of a restricted area but inside the site boundary, access to which can be limited by the licensee for any reason
- **Critical group**: Group of individuals reasonably expected to receive the greatest exposure to residual radioactivity for any applicable set of circumstances

- **Declared pregnant woman**: Woman who has voluntarily informed the licensee, in writing, of her pregnancy and the estimated date of conception
  - The declaration remains in effect until the declared pregnant woman withdraws the declaration in writing or is no longer pregnant
- **Decommission**: To remove a facility or site safely from service and reduce residual radioactivity to a level that permits
  - Release of the property for unrestricted use and termination of the license; or
  - Release of the property under restricted conditions and termination of the license
- **Deep-dose equivalent**: Applies to external whole-body exposure; dose equivalent at tissue depth of 1 cm (1,000 mg/cm²)
- **Discrete source**: Radionuclide processed so that its concentration within material has been purposely increased for use for commercial, medical, or research activities
- **Distinguishable from background**: Detectable concentration of a radionuclide is statistically different from the background concentration of that radionuclide in the vicinity of the site or, in the case of structures, in similar materials using adequate measurement technology, survey, and statistical techniques
- **Dose or radiation dose**: Generic term that means absorbed dose, dose equivalent, effective dose equivalent, committed dose equivalent, committed effective dose equivalent, or total effective dose equivalent
- **Dose equivalent**: Product of the absorbed dose in tissue, quality factor, and all other necessary modifying factors at the location of interest
  - The units of dose equivalent are the rem and sievert (Sv)
- **Dosimetry processor**: Individual or organization that processes and evaluates individual monitoring equipment in order to determine the radiation dose delivered to the equipment
- **Effective dose equivalent**: Sum of the products of the dose equivalent to the organ or tissue and the weighting factors applicable to each of the body organs or tissues that are irradiated
- **Embryo/fetus**: Developing human organism from conception until the time of birth
- **Entrance or access point**: Any location through which an individual could gain access to radiation areas or to radioactive materials
  - This includes entry or exit portals of sufficient size to permit human entry, irrespective of their intended use
- **Exposure**: Being exposed to ionizing radiation or to radioactive material
- **External dose**: Portion of dose equivalent received from radiation sources outside body
- **Extremity**: Hand, elbow, arm below elbow, foot, knee, or leg below knee
- **Generally applicable environmental radiation standards**: Standards issued by Environmental Protection Agency (EPA) under authority of Atomic Energy Act of 1954, as amended, that impose limits on radiation exposures or levels, or concentrations or quantities of radioactive material, in general environment outside boundaries of locations under control of persons possessing or using radioactive material
- **Government agency**: Any executive department, commission, independent establishment, or corporation wholly or partly owned by United States of America, which is an instrumentality of the USA, or any board, bureau, division, service, office, officer, authority, administration, or other establishment in executive branch of government
- **High-radiation area**: Area, accessible to individuals, in which radiation levels from radiation sources external to body could result in an individual receiving a dose equivalent in excess of 0.1 rem (1 mSv) in 1 hour at 30 cm from radiation source or 30 cm from any surface that radiation penetrates
- **Hood**: Respiratory inlet covering that completely covers head and neck and may also cover portions of shoulders and torso
- **Individual monitoring means**
  - Assessment of dose equivalent by use of devices designed to be worn by an individual
  - Assessment of committed effective dose equivalent by bioassay or by determination of time-weighted air concentrations to which an individual has been exposed, i.e., DAC-hours; or
  - Assessment of dose equivalent by use of survey data
- **Individual monitoring devices (individual monitoring equipment)**: Devices designed to be worn by a single individual for assessment of dose equivalent such as film badges, thermoluminescence dosimeters (TLDs), pocket ionization chambers, and personal (lapel) air sampling devices
- **Internal dose**: Portion of dose equivalent received from radioactive material taken into body
- **Lens dose equivalent**: External exposure of lens of eye and is taken as dose equivalent at a tissue depth of 0.3 cm (300 mg/cm²)
- **Licensed material**: Source material, special nuclear material, or byproduct material received, possessed, used, transferred or disposed of under a general or specific license issued by Commission
- **Limits (dose limits)**: Permissible upper bounds of radiation doses
- **Lost or missing licensed material**: Licensed material for which location is unknown; includes material that has been shipped but has not reached its destination and whose location cannot be readily traced in transportation system
- **Member of the public**: Any individual except when that individual is receiving an occupational dose
- **Monitoring (radiation monitoring, radiation protection monitoring)**: Measurement of radiation levels, concentrations, surface area concentrations or quantities of radioactive material, and use of results of these measurements to evaluate potential exposures and doses
- **Nonstochastic effect**: Health effects, severity of which varies with dose and for which a threshold is believed to exist; radiation-induced cataract formation is an example of nonstochastic effect (also called deterministic effect)
- **NRC**: Nuclear Regulatory Commission or its duly authorized representatives
- **Occupational dose**: Dose received by an individual in course of employment in which individual's assigned duties involve exposure to radiation or to radioactive material from licensed and unlicensed sources of radiation, whether in possession of licensee or other person

- Occupational dose does not include doses received from background radiation, from any medical administration individual has received, from exposure to individuals administered radioactive material and released, from voluntary participation in medical research programs, or as a member of the public
- **Planned special exposure**: Infrequent exposure to radiation, separate from & in addition to annual dose limits
- **Public dose**: Dose received by a member of the public from exposure to radiation or to radioactive material released by a licensee, or to any other source of radiation under control of a licensee
  - Does not include occupational dose or doses received from background radiation, from any medical administration individual has received, from exposure to individuals administered radioactive material and released, or from voluntary participation in medical research programs
- **Quality factor (Q):** Modifying factor that is used to derive dose equivalent from absorbed dose
- **Quarter**: Period of time equal to 1/4 of the year observed by licensee (~ 13 consecutive weeks), providing that beginning of first quarter in a year coincides with starting date of year and that no day is omitted or duplicated in consecutive quarters
- **Radiation (ionizing radiation)**: Alpha particles, beta particles, gamma rays, x-rays, neutrons, high-speed electrons, high-speed protons, and other particles capable of producing ions
  - Radiation, as used in this part, does not include non-ionizing radiation, such as radio- or microwaves, or visible, infrared, or ultraviolet light
- **Radiation area**: Area, accessible to individuals, in which radiation levels could result in an individual receiving dose equivalent in excess of 0.005 rem (0.05 mSv) in 1 hour at 30 cm from radiation source or from any surface that radiation penetrates
- **Reference man**: Hypothetical aggregation of human physical and physiological characteristics arrived at by international consensus
  - These characteristics used by researchers and public health workers to standardize results of experiments and to relate biological insult to a common base
- **Residual radioactivity**: Radioactivity in structures, materials, soils, groundwater, and other media at site resulting from activities under licensee's control
  - Includes radioactivity from all licensed and unlicensed sources used by the licensee, but excludes background radiation
  - Also includes radioactive materials remaining at site as a result of routine or accidental releases of radioactive material at site and previous burials at site, even if those burials were made in accordance with NRC
- **Restricted area**: Area, access to which is limited by licensee for purpose of protecting individuals against undue risks from exposure to radiation and radioactive materials
  - Does not include areas used as residential quarters, but separate rooms in a residential building may be set apart as restricted area
- **Sanitary sewerage**: System of public sewers for carrying off waste water and refuse, but excluding sewage treatment facilities, septic tanks, and leach fields owned or operated by licensee
- **Shallow-dose equivalent**: Applies to external exposure of skin of whole body or skin of an extremity; taken as dose equivalent at tissue depth of 0.007 cm (7 mg/cm^2)
- **Stochastic effects**: Health effects that occur randomly and for which probability of effect occurring, rather than its severity, is assumed to be a linear function of dose without threshold; hereditary effects and cancer incidence are examples of stochastic effects
- **Survey**: Evaluation of radiological conditions and potential hazards incident to production, use, transfer, release, disposal, or presence of radioactive material or other sources of radiation
- **Total effective dose equivalent**: Sum of effective dose equivalent (for external exposures) and committed effective dose equivalent (for internal exposures)
- **Unrestricted area**: Area, access to which is neither limited nor controlled by licensee
- **Very high radiation area**: Area in which radiation levels from radiation sources external to body could result in an individual receiving an absorbed dose in excess of 500 rads (5 grays) in 1 hour at 1 m from radiation source or 1 m from any surface that radiation penetrates
  - At very high doses received at high dose rates, units of absorbed dose (e.g., rads and grays) are appropriate, rather than units of dose equivalent (rem and Sv)
- **Weighting factor (WT) for an organ or tissue**: Proportion of risk of stochastic effects resulting from irradiation of that organ or tissue to total risk of stochastic effects when whole body is irradiated uniformly; for calculating the effective dose equivalent
- **Whole body**: For purposes of external exposure, head, trunk, arms above elbow, legs above knee
- **Working level month (WLM)**: Exposure to 1 working level for 170 hours (2,000 working hours per year / 12 months per year = ~ 170 hours per month)

20.1004: Units of Radiation Dose

- **Gray (Gy)**: SI unit of absorbed dose; 1 gray is equal to an absorbed dose of 1 Joule/kilogram (100 rads)
- **Rad**: Special unit of absorbed dose; 1 rad is equal to an absorbed dose of 100 ergs/gram or 0.01 joule/kilogram (0.01 gray)
- **Rem**: Special unit of any of quantities expressed as dose equivalent; dose equivalent in rems is equal to absorbed dose in rads multiplied by quality factor (1 rem = 0.01 Sv)
- **Sievert**: SI unit of any of quantities expressed as dose equivalent; dose equivalent in sieverts is equal to absorbed dose in grays multiplied by quality factor (1 Sv = 100 rems)

20.1005: Units of Radioactivity

- 1 becquerel = 1 disintegration per second (s-1)
- 1 curie = 3.7 x 1,010 disintegrations per second = 3.7 x 1,010 becquerels = 2.22 x 1,012 disintegrations per minute

SELECTED REFERENCES

1. United States Nuclear Regulatory Commission. NRC Regulations (10 CFR) Part 20: Standards for Protection Against Radiation. http://www.nrc.gov/reading-rm/doc-collections/cfr/part020. Published June 31, 2015. Accessed June 31, 2015

KEY FACTS

NRC REGULATIONS (10 CFR) PART 20: STANDARDS FOR PROTECTION AGAINST RADIATION, SUBPART C (OCCUPATIONAL DOSE LIMITS)

- Licensee must develop policies/procedures to minimize radiation dose to workers from external exposure and internal contamination
- Radiation workers in nuclear medicine departments are exposed during 3 main activities: Dosage preparation and assay, injection, and patient imaging
- Licensee shall limit occupational dose to individual adults to the following dose limits
  - Total effective dose 5 rems (0.05 Sv)
  - Sum of deep-dose equivalent and committed dose equivalent to any individual organ other than lens of eye = 50 rems (0.5 Sv)
  - Lens dose equivalent of 15 rems (0.15 Sv)
  - Shallow-dose equivalent of 50 rem (0.5 Sv) to skin of whole body or to skin of any extremity
- Annual occupational dose limits for minors are 10% of annual dose limits for adult workers
- Licensee shall ensure that dose equivalent to embryo/fetus during entire pregnancy, due to occupational exposure of declared pregnant woman, does not exceed 0.5 rem (5 mSv)
  - Additional 0.05 rem (0.5 mSv) allowed during remainder of pregnancy if limit exceeded at time of pregnancy declaration
- Annual total effective dose equivalent to individual members of public from licensed operation does not exceed 0.1 rem (1 mSv)
- Dose in any unrestricted area from external sources, exclusive of dose contributions from patients administered radioactive material and released does not exceed 0.002 rem/hr (0.02 mSv/hr)

(Left) *Radiation workers in nuclear medicine departments are exposed during 3 main activities: Dosage preparation and assay, injection, and patient imaging. The annual effective dose equivalent limit for the whole body is 5 rems (50 mSv).* **(Right)** *An L-block is being used to shield the body and lens of the eyes from the radioactive source. The annual occupational dose limit to the lens of the eye is 15 rems (.15 Sv).*

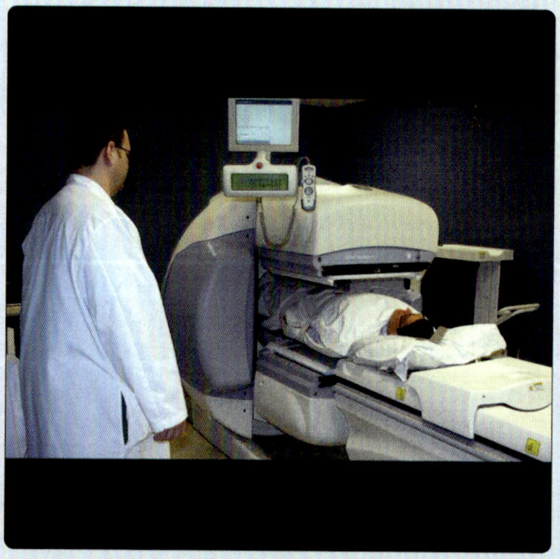

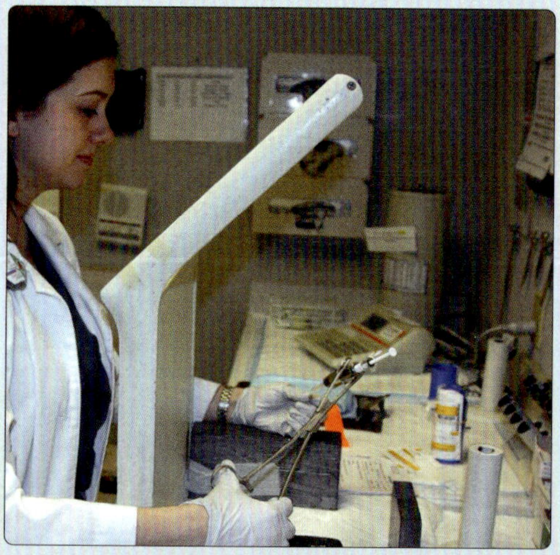

(Left) *The annual occupational dose limit to the hand is 50 rems (500 mSv).* **(Right)** *The dose equivalent to the embryo/fetus during the entire pregnancy, due to the occupational exposure of a declared pregnant woman, should not exceed 0.5 rem. An additional 0.05 rem (0.5 mSv) allowed during the remainder of the pregnancy if limit exceeded at the time of pregnancy declaration.*

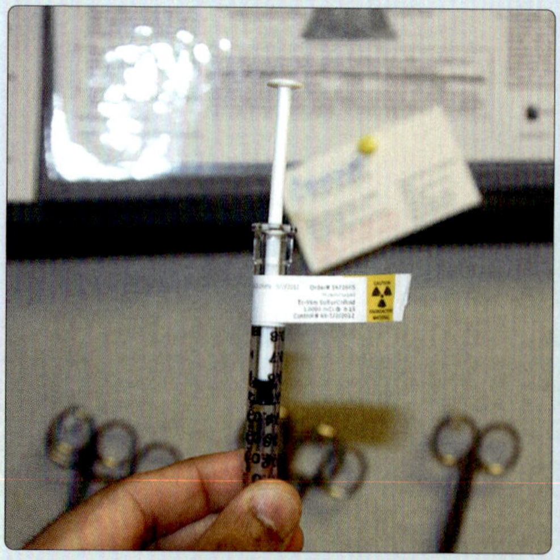

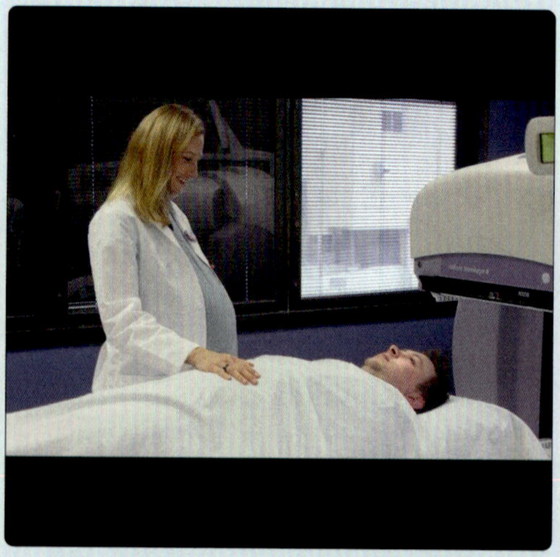

NRC REGULATIONS (10 CFR) PART 20: STANDARDS FOR PROTECTION AGAINST RADIATION, SUBPART C (OCCUPATIONAL DOSE LIMITS)

Introduction

- Based on principles of radiation protection, licensee must develop policies and procedures to minimize radiation dose to workers from both external exposure and internal contamination
- Radiation worker dose monitoring can demonstrate compliance with regulatory limits on radiation dose and principles of as low as reasonably achievable (ALARA)
- Radiation workers in nuclear medicine departments are exposed during 3 main activities: Dosage preparation and assay, injection, and patient imaging

20.1201: Occupational Dose Limits for Adults

- Licensee shall limit occupational dose to individual adults to the following dose limits
  - Annual limit, which is the more limiting of
    - Total effective dose equivalent = 5 rems (0.05 Sv); or
    - Sum of deep-dose equivalent and committed dose equivalent to any individual organ or tissue other than lens of eye = 50 rems (0.5 Sv)
  - Annual limits to lens of eye, skin of whole body, and skin of extremities, which are
    - Lens dose equivalent of 15 rems (0.15 Sv), and
    - Shallow-dose equivalent of 50 rem (0.5 Sv) to skin of whole body or to skin of any extremity
- Doses received in excess of annual limits, including doses received during accidents, emergencies, and planned special exposures, must be subtracted from limits for planned special exposures that individual may receive during current year and during individual's lifetime
- When external exposure is determined by measurement with external personal monitoring device, deep-dose equivalent must be used in place of effective dose equivalent, unless effective dose equivalent is determined by dosimetry method approved by NRC
  - Assigned deep-dose equivalent must be for part of body receiving highest exposure
  - Assigned shallow-dose equivalent must be dose averaged over contiguous 10 cm^2 of skin receiving highest exposure
  - Deep-dose equivalent, lens-dose equivalent, and shallow-dose equivalent may be assessed from surveys or other radiation measurements for purpose of demonstrating compliance with occupational dose limits, if individual monitoring device was not in region of highest potential exposure, or results of individual monitoring are unavailable
- Derived air concentration (DAC) and annual limit on intake (ALI) values may be used to determine individual's dose and demonstrate compliance with occupational dose limits
- Licensee shall reduce dose that individual may be allowed to receive in current year by amount of occupational dose received while employed by any other person
- Licensee is not required to monitor internal component of occupational radiation dose of workers with radioactive gases or aerosols (e.g., Xe-133 or Kr-81m gas and Tc-99m aerosols)
  - Licensee must use process or other engineering controls (e.g., containment, decontamination, or ventilation) to extent practical to control concentrations of radioactive material in air

20.1206: Planned Special Exposures

- Licensee may authorize adult worker to receive doses in addition to and accounted for separately from doses received under annual limits provided that each of the following conditions is satisfied
  - Licensee authorizes planned special exposure only in exceptional situation when alternatives that might avoid dose estimated to result from planned special exposure are unavailable or impractical
  - Licensee (and employer if employer is not licensee) specifically authorizes planned special exposure, in writing, before exposure occurs
  - Before planned special exposure, licensee ensures that individuals involved are
    - Informed of purpose of planned operation
    - Informed of estimated doses and associated potential risks and specific radiation levels or other conditions that might be involved in performing task; and
    - Instructed in measures to be taken to keep dose ALARA considering other risks that may be present
  - Prior to permitting individual to participate in planned special exposure, licensee ascertains prior doses during lifetime of individual for each individual involved
  - Licensee does not authorize planned special exposure that would cause individual to receive dose from all planned special exposures and all doses in excess of limits to exceed
    - Numerical values of any dose limits in any year; and
    - 5x annual dose limits during individual's lifetime
  - Licensee maintains records of conduct of planned special exposure and submits written report
  - Licensee records best estimate of dose resulting from planned special exposure in individual's record and informs individual, in writing, of dose within 30 days from date of planned special exposure
    - Dose from planned special exposures is not to be considered in controlling future occupational dose of individual, but is to be included in evaluations

20.1207: Occupational Dose Limits for Minors

- Annual occupational dose limits for minors are 10% of annual dose limits specified for adult workers

20.1208: Dose Equivalent to Embryo/Fetus

- Licensee shall ensure that dose equivalent to embryo/fetus during entire pregnancy, due to occupational exposure of declared pregnant woman, does not exceed 0.5 rem (5 mSv)
- Licensee shall make efforts to avoid substantial variation above uniform monthly exposure rate to declared pregnant woman so as to satisfy limit
- Dose equivalent to embryo/fetus is sum of
  - Deep-dose equivalent to declared pregnant woman; and
  - Dose equivalent to embryo/fetus resulting from radionuclides in embryo/fetus and radionuclides in declared pregnant woman

- If dose equivalent to embryo/fetus is found to have exceeded 0.5 rem (5 mSv), or is within 0.05 rem (0.5 mSv) of this dose, by the time woman declares pregnancy to licensee, licensee shall be deemed to be in compliance if additional dose equivalent to embryo/fetus does not exceed 0.05 rem (0.5 mSv) during remainder of pregnancy

NRC REGULATIONS (10 CFR) PART 20: STANDARDS FOR PROTECTION AGAINST RADIATION, SUBPART D (RADIATION DOSE LIMITS FOR INDIVIDUAL MEMBERS OF PUBLIC)

20.1301: Dose Limits for Individual Members of Public

- Each licensee shall conduct operations so that
  - Total effective dose equivalent to individual members of public from the licensed operation does not exceed 0.1 rem (1 mSv) in 1 year, exclusive of dose contributions from background radiation, from any administration the individual has received, from exposure to individuals administered radioactive material and released, from voluntary participation in medical research programs, and from licensee's disposal of radioactive material into sanitary sewerage
  - Dose in any unrestricted area from external sources, exclusive of dose contributions from patients administered radioactive material and released does not exceed 0.002 rem (0.02 mSv) in any 1 hour
- If licensee permits members of public to have access to controlled areas, limits for members of public continue to apply to those individuals
- Licensee may permit visitors to individual who cannot be released to receive radiation dose > 0.1 rem (1 mSv) if
  - Radiation dose received does not exceed 0.5 rem (5 mSv); and
  - Authorized user has determined before visit that it is appropriate
- Licensee or license applicant may apply for prior NRC authorization to operate up to an annual dose limit for individual member of public of 0.5 rem (5 mSv); licensee or license applicant shall include the following information in this application
  - Demonstration of need for and expected duration of operations in excess of limit
  - Licensee's program to assess and control dose within 0.5 rem (5 mSv) annual limit; and
  - Procedures to be followed to maintain dose ALARA

20.1302: Compliance With Dose Limits for Individual Members of Public

- Licensee shall make or cause to be made, as appropriate, surveys of radiation levels in unrestricted and controlled areas and radioactive materials in effluents released to unrestricted and controlled areas to demonstrate compliance with dose limits for individual members of public
- Licensee shall show compliance with annual dose limit by
  - Demonstrating by measurement or calculation that total effective dose equivalent to individual likely to receive highest dose from licensed operation does not exceed annual dose limit; or
  - Demonstrating that
    - Annual average concentrations of radioactive material released in gaseous and liquid effluents at boundary of unrestricted area do not exceed value limits set by NRC
    - If individual was continuously present in unrestricted area, dose from external sources would not exceed 0.002 rem (0.02 mSv) in 1 hour and 0.05 rem (0.5 mSv) in 1 year

SELECTED REFERENCES

1. United States Nuclear Regulatory Commission. NRC Regulations (10 CFR) Part 20: Standards for Protection Against Radiation. http://www.nrc.gov/reading-rm/doc-collections/cfr/part020. Published June 31, 2015. Accessed June 31, 2015

Annual Dose Limits

	Non-SI	SI
Total effective dose (whole body)	5 rem	50 mSv
Lens	15 rem	150 mSv
Skin/organ/extremity	50 rem	500 mSv
Total effective dose (fetus)	0.5 rem	5 mSv
Minor	10% above adult limits	10% above adult limits
Public	0.1 rem	1 mSv

Occupational dose limits are shown for all but the public limit. Total effective dose to the fetus assumes a declared pregnancy.

KEY FACTS

HOT LAB

- Access to hot lab should be restricted
- Do not eat, drink, smoke, apply cosmetics, or store food in hot lab

MO-99/TC-99M GENERATOR

- Parent: Mo-99; daughter: Tc-99m
- Given longer t1/2 of Mo-99 (67 hr) vs. shorter t1/2 of Tc-99m (6 hr), transient equilibrium achieved
  - Must be ≤ 0.15 µCi Mo-99/mCi Tc-99m (0.15 kBq Mo-99/MBq Tc-99m); if this activity ratio is exceeded, dosage cannot be administered
- Impurities
  - Radionuclidic: Mo-99 breakthrough
  - Radiochemical: Hydrolyzed reduced/free pertechnetate
  - Chemical: Aluminum in eluate

DOSE CALIBRATOR

- Typically found in hot lab
- Typically ± 20% dose range is allowable by NRC
- Dose calibrator quality control (QC) time intervals (all performed at installation initially)
  - Accuracy: Annually
  - Constancy: Daily
  - Linearity: Quarterly
  - Geometry: After repair or moving instrument
- Ionization chamber device that can measure radioactivity
- No sodium-iodide crystal
- Activity ionizes inert gas, producing measurable charge
- Cannot determine energy of item placed in calibrator
- Required to be used on all radiopharmaceutical dosages prepared in department or derived from Mo-99/Tc-99m generator
- Unit doses from outside commercial nuclear pharmacy do not require dose calibrator measurements

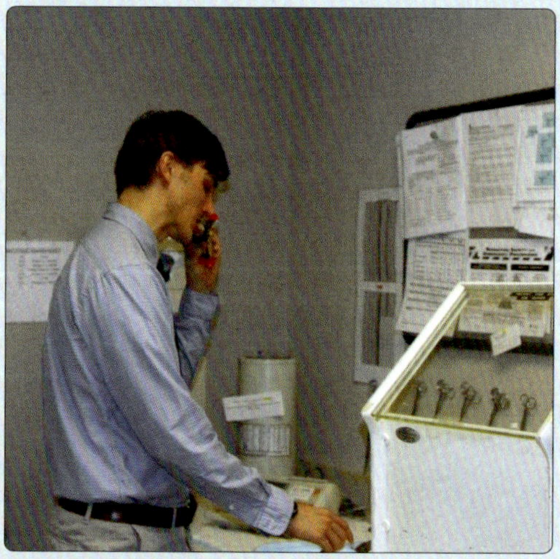

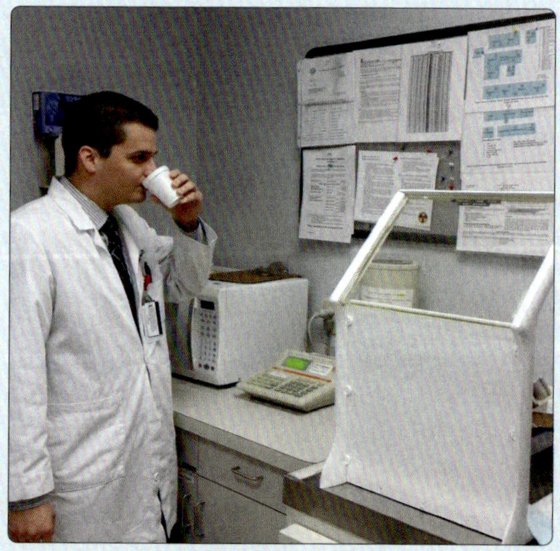

(Left) *No food is allowed in the hot lab for consumption by workers. This person is also not wearing a white coat to protect from contamination, and should be counseled by the radiation safety officer or the supervisor of the department.* **(Right)** *This individual should not be drinking in the hot lab, and should be counseled by the radiation safety officer or the supervisor of the department.*

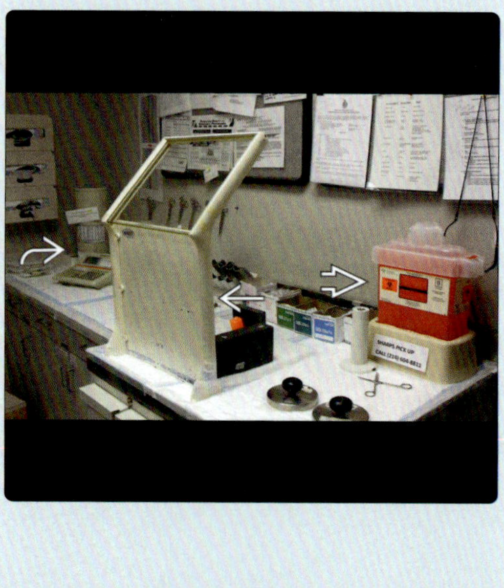

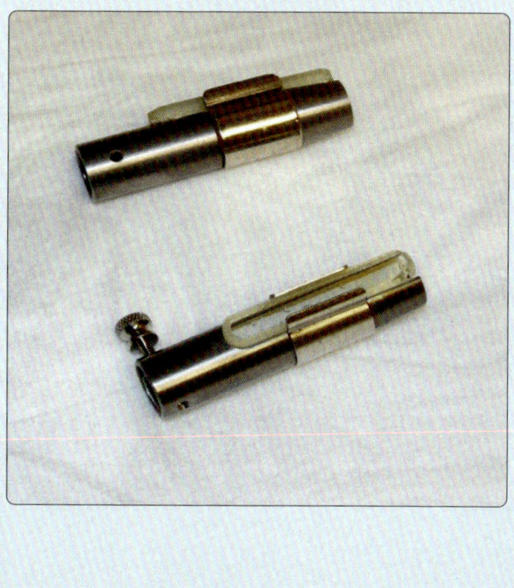

(Left) *A lead shield ➔ is in place to reduce radiation exposure to the technologist. Using principles of ALARA, radiopharmaceuticals should be handled behind this shield. A dose calibrator ➔ and a sharps container ➔ for radioactive needles are also present.* **(Right)** *Syringe shields are shown. Although these are not required, they can reduce the hand exposure to radiation workers when handling gamma emitters. Beta emitters should be shielded with glass or plastic to avoid bremsstrahlung x-ray exposure.*

CLINICAL IMPLICATIONS

Hot Lab

- Radiation exposure limited by time, distance, and shielding
- Receive, store, &/or prepare radiopharmaceuticals administered to patients for nuclear medicine studies
- Proper signage required on entrance indicating radioactive materials
- Radiation safety officer (RSO) numbers are listed
- Access to hot lab should be restricted
  - Propping door open would be violation of Nuclear Regulatory Commission (NRC) regulations
- Walls and doors are shielded
- Work areas are usually covered with absorbent material to allow ease of clean up and containment if spills occur
- Lead shield with leaded glass used to shield technologists as they prepare dosages
- Unit dosages typically delivered to & always stored in hot lab
- Survey meters, typically Geiger-Mueller or sodium iodide probes are kept here
- Workers should wear laboratory coats or other protective clothing and use disposable gloves
- Do not eat, drink, smoke, apply cosmetics, insert or remove contact lenses, or store food in hot lab
- Never pipette by mouth
- Workers should monitor hands and body for contamination when leaving

Mo-99/Tc-99m Generator

- Most common generator
- Parent: Mo-99; daughter: Tc-99m
  - Given longer t1/2 of Mo-99 (67 hr) vs. shorter t1/2 of Tc-99m (6 hr), transient equilibrium achieved
- Elution typically occurs in 24-hour intervals to maximize Tc-99m activity
- Saline is passed through system such that Tc-99m eluate is in form of sodium pertechnetate ($^{99}mTcO_4^-$)
- Aluminum columns in generator absorb nearly all Mo-99
- Mo-99 breakthrough
  - Mo-99 activity present in any Tc-99m preparation must be determined
    - Must be ≤ 0.15 μCi Mo-99/mCi Tc-99m (0.15 kBq Mo-99/MBq Tc-99m); if this activity ratio is exceeded, dosage cannot be administered
  - Mo-99 concentration of 1st eluate after receipt of Mo-99/Tc-99m generator must be measured and recorded
- Tc-99m impurities
  - Radionuclidic: Mo-99 breakthrough
    - Test with dose calibrator
    - Can cause poor image quality and will increase patient radiation dose
  - Radiochemical: Hydrolyzed reduced/free pertechnetate
    - Test with thin layer chromatography
    - Free pertechnetate: Salivary glands, thyroid, stomach, and urinary tract visualized
    - Hydrolyzed Tc-99m: Liver and spleen visualized
  - Chemical: Aluminum in eluate
    - Colorimetric test; aurintricarboxylic acid spot test
    - If eluate placed on test strip is more red than control, too much Al^{3+}

Dose Calibrator

- Typically found in hot lab
  - Ionization chamber device that can measure radioactivity
    - No sodium iodide crystal; activity ionizes inert gas, producing measurable charge; cannot determine energy of item placed in calibrator
  - Required to be used on all radiopharmaceutical dosages prepared in department or derived from Mo-99/Tc-99m generator
  - Unit doses from outside commercial nuclear pharmacy do not require dose calibrator measurements
  - Typically ± 20% range is allowable by NRC; authorized user may extend that range on any specific case or create more broad range for all prescribed dosages
  - Dose calibrator quality control (QC) time intervals (all performed at installation initially)
    - Accuracy: Annually
      - Reference sources of at least 2 radioisotopes are separately placed in dose calibrator and activity reading on each scale recorded
      - For each source, measured activity on each scale & its current actual activity should agree within 10%
    - Constancy: Daily
      - Reference source, such as Co-57, Ba-133, Ge-68, Cs-137, is placed in dose calibrator and the activity reading on each scale is recorded; day-to-day readings should agree within 10%
    - Linearity: Quarterly
      - Decay method
      - Start with high-activity (30-500 mCi [1.11-18.5 GBq]), independently calibrated Tc-99m source and assay its activity at constant intervals over 2-3 consecutive days
      - Measured activities vs. time plotted on semilogarithmic graph, & best-fit straight line is drawn
      - For each data point
      - Difference between measured activity & activity on best-fit straight line at that point should be < 10%
      - Shield method
      - Lead sleeves of increasing thickness placed in dose calibrator with Tc-99m source; by interposing increasing decay-equivalent thicknesses (as specified by manufacturer of set of lead sleeves) between source & sensitive volume of dose calibrator, decay-equivalent activity measured for each sleeve
      - By interposing increasing decay-equivalent thicknesses (as specified by manufacturer of set of lead sleeves) between source and sensitive volume of dose calibrator
      - Decay-equivalent activity measured for each sleeve
    - Geometry: After repair or moving instrument
      - To ensure sample size & geometry do not affect readings, know quantity & activity of Tc-99m is diluted & measured; as more dilution is achieved with same known activity, reading shouldn't change

SELECTED REFERENCES

1. Zanzonico P: Routine quality control of clinical nuclear medicine instrumentation: a brief review. J Nucl Med. 49(7):1114-31, 2008

KEY FACTS

NRC REGULATIONS TITLE 10, CODE OF FEDERAL REGULATIONS: SUBPART L (RECORDS) AND SUBPART M (REPORTS)

- Licensee shall retain record of each radiation protection program change made for 5 years
- Licensee shall retain copy of each written directive, record of instrument/radiation survey calibrations, disposal of licensed material, and Mo-99 concentration for 3 years
- Licensee shall report any event, except for event that results from patient intervention, in which administration of or radiation from byproduct material results in
  - Dose that differs from prescribed or would have resulted from prescribed dose by > 0.05 Sv (5 rem) effective dose equivalent, 0.5 Sv (50 rem) to organ or tissue, or 0.5 Sv (50 rem) shallow dose equivalent to skin
- Medical event: Dose that differs from prescribed dose or dose that would have resulted from prescribed dosage by > 0.05 Sv (5 rem) effective dose equivalent, 0.5 Sv (50 rem) to organ or tissue and total dose delivered differs from prescribed dose ≥ 20%, or wrong radiopharmaceutical, wrong route of administration, or administration to wrong individual occurs
- Licensee shall notify by telephone NRC Operations Center no later than next calendar day after discovery of medical event and submit written report to NRC within 15 days
- Licensee shall provide notification of medical event to referring physician and also notify individual subject of medical event no later than 24 hours after its discovery
- Licensee shall report any dose to embryo/fetus > 50 mSv (5 rem) dose equivalent as result of administration of byproduct material or radiation from byproduct material to pregnant individual unless dose to embryo/fetus was specifically approved, in advance, by authorized user

Written Directive for I-131 NaI Oral Administration

PATIENT NAME: ______________________ DATE: __________

DATE OF BIRTH: ______________________ SEX: ________

DOSE OF SODIUM IODIDE PRESCRIBED: ______________ mCi

ORDERING AU PHYSICIAN: ______________________ M.D.
(Signature)

ORDERING AU PHYSICIAN: ______________________ M.D.
(Print Name Legibly)

To be completed by dispensing technologist

MEANS OF PATIENT IDENTIFICATION (At least two, in the presence of AU Physician):

1) ______________ 2) ______________

Control #: ______________ # of Capsules ________ or VOLUME: ________ mL

RX#: ______________ Dose or Calibrator reading: ______________ mCi

Dispensing Technologist: ______________________

To be completed by Authorized User

	YES	Comments/Method
Order from referring physician confirmed:	______	
Non-pregnant status of patient confirmed:	______	______________
Non-lactating status of patient confirmed:	______	______________
Vial identity and Lot # confirmed:	______	
Dose calibrator reading confirmed:	______	
Consent form signed (Therapy only):	______	
Identification of patient witnessed:	______	

Authorized User: ______________________ M.D.
(Signature)

Authorized User: ______________________ M.D.
(Print Name Legibly)

A written directive must be signed by an authorized user before the administration of I-131 NaI greater than 30 µCi (1.11 MBq) or any therapeutic dosage of unsealed byproduct material.

NRC REGULATIONS TITLE 10, CODE OF FEDERAL REGULATIONS: SUBPART L (RECORDS) AND SUBPART M (REPORTS)

35.2024: Records of Authority and Responsibilities for Radiation Protection Programs

- Licensee shall retain record of actions taken by licensee's management for 5 years
  - Must include summary of actions taken and signature of licensee management
- Licensee shall retain copy of both authority, duties, and responsibilities of radiation safety officer (RSO), and signed copy of each RSO's agreement to be responsible for implementing radiation safety program for duration of license
  - Records must include signature of RSO and licensee management

35.2026: Records of Radiation Protection Program Changes

- Licensee shall retain record of each radiation protection program change made for 5 years
  - Must include copy of old and new procedures, effective date of change, and signature of licensee management that reviewed and approved change

35.2040 Records of Written Directives

- Licensee shall retain copy of each written directive for 3 years

35.2041 Records for Procedures for Administrations Requiring Written Directive

- Licensee shall retain copy of procedures for duration of license

35.2060: Records of Calibrations of Instruments Used to Measure Activity of Unsealed Byproduct Materials

- Licensee shall maintain record of instrument calibrations for 3 years
  - Must include
    - Model and serial number of instrument
    - Date of calibration
    - Results of calibration
    - Name of individual who performed calibration

35.2061: Records of Radiation Survey Instrument Calibrations

- Licensee shall maintain record of radiation survey instrument calibrations for 3 years
  - Must include
    - Model and serial number of instrument
    - Date of calibration
    - Results of calibration
    - Name of individual who performed calibration

35.2063: Records of Dosages of Unsealed Byproduct Material for Medical Use

- Licensee shall maintain a record of dosage determinations for 3 years
- Record must contain
  - Radiopharmaceutical
  - Patient's or human research subject's name, or identification number if one has been assigned
  - Prescribed dosage, determined dosage, or notation that total activity is < 1.1 MBq (30 μCi)
  - Date and time of dosage determination
  - Name of individual who determined dosage

35.2067: Records of Leaks Tests and Inventory of Sealed Sources and Brachytherapy Sources

- Licensee shall retain records of leak tests for 3 years
  - Must include
    - Model number and serial number, if one has been assigned, of each source tested
    - Identity of each source by radionuclide and its estimated activity
    - Results of test
    - Date of test
    - Name of individual who performed test
- Licensee shall retain records of semi-annual physical inventory of sealed sources and brachytherapy sources required for 3 years
  - Must include
    - Model number of each source, and serial number if one has been assigned
    - Identity of each source by radionuclide and its nominal activity
    - Location of each source
    - Name of individual who performed inventory

35.2070: Records of Surveys for Ambient Radiation Exposure Rate

- Licensee shall retain a record of each survey for 3 years
  - Must include
    - Date of survey
    - Results of survey
    - Instrument used to make survey
    - Name of individual who performed survey

35.2075: Records of Release of Individuals Containing Unsealed Byproduct Material or Implants Containing Byproduct Material

- Licensee shall retain record for 3 years of basis for authorizing release of individual if total effective dose equivalent is calculated by
  - Using retained activity rather than activity administered
  - Using occupancy factor < 0.25 at 1 m
  - Using biological or effective t1/2; or
  - Considering shielding by tissue
- Licensee shall retain record for 3 years that instructions were provided to breastfeeding female if radiation dose to infant or child from continued breastfeeding could result in total effective dose equivalent exceeding 5 mSv (0.5 rem)

35.2080: Records of Mobile Medical Services

- Licensee shall retain copy of each letter permitting use of byproduct material at client's address
  - Each letter must clearly delineate authority and responsibility of licensee and client and must be retained for 3 years after last provision of service
- Licensee shall retain record of each survey for 3 years
  - Must include
    - Date of survey

- Results survey
- Instrument used to make survey
- Name of individual who performed survey

35.2092: Records of Decay-in-Storage

- Licensee shall maintain records of disposal of licensed materials for 3 years
  - Must include
    - Date of disposal
    - Survey instrument used
    - Background radiation level
    - Radiation level measured at surface of each waste container
    - Name of the individual who performed survey

35.2204: Records of Molybdenum-99, Strontium-82, and Strontium-85 Concentrations

- Licensee shall maintain record of Mo-99 concentration or Sr-82 and Sr-85 concentration tests for 3 years
  - Must include
    - For each measured elution of Tc-99m: Ratio of measures expressed as kBq of Mo-99 per MBq of Tc-99m (or μCi of molybdenum per mCi of technetium), time and date of measurement, and name of individual who made measurement
    - For each measured elution of Rb-82: Ratio of measures expressed as kBq of Sr-82 per MBq of rubidium-82 (or μCi of Sr-82 per mCi of rubidium), kBq of Sr-85 per MBq of Rb-82 (or μCi of Sr-85 per mCi of rubidium), time and date of measurement, and name of individual who made measurement

35.2310: Records of Safety Instruction

- Licensee shall maintain record of safety instructions for 3 years
  - Must include
    - List of topics covered
    - Date of instruction
    - Name(s) of attendee(s)
    - Name(s) of individual(s) who provided instruction

35.3045: Report and Notification of Medical Event

- Licensee shall report any event, except for an event that results from patient intervention, in which administration of byproduct material or radiation from byproduct material results in
  - Dose that differs from prescribed dose or dose that would have resulted from prescribed dosage by > 0.05 Sv (5 rem) effective dose equivalent, 0.5 Sv (50 rem) to organ or tissue, or 0.5 Sv (50 rem) shallow dose equivalent to skin
    - Total dose delivered differs from prescribed dose ≥ 20%
    - Total dosage delivered differs from prescribed dosage ≥ 20% or falls outside prescribed dosage range
  - Dose that exceeds 0.05 Sv (5 rem) effective dose equivalent, 0.5 Sv (50 rem) to organ or tissue, or 0.5 Sv (50 rem) shallow dose equivalent to skin from any of the following
    - Administration of wrong radioactive drug containing byproduct material
    - Administration of radioactive drug containing byproduct material by wrong route of administration
    - Administration of dose or dosage to wrong individual or human research subject
- Licensee shall report any event resulting from intervention of patient or human research subject in which administration of byproduct material, or radiation from byproduct material results or will result in unintended permanent functional damage to organ or physiological system, as determined by physician
- Licensee shall notify by telephone Nuclear Regulatory Commission (NRC) Operations Center no later than next calendar day after discovery of medical event
- Licensee shall submit written report to appropriate NRC Regional Office within 15 days after discovery of medical event
  - Written report must include
    - Licensee's name
    - Name of prescribing physician
    - Brief description of event
    - Why event occurred
    - Effect, if any, on individual(s) who received administration
    - What actions, if any, have been taken or are planned to prevent recurrence
    - Certification that licensee notified individual (or individual's responsible relative or guardian), and if not, why not
  - Report may not contain individual's name or any other information that could lead to identification of individual
- Licensee shall provide notification of event to referring physician and also notify individual subject of medical event no later than 24 hours after its discovery, unless referring physician personally informs licensee either that he or she will inform individual or that, based on medical judgment, telling individual would be harmful
- Licensee is not required to notify individual without first consulting referring physician
  - If referring physician or affected individual cannot be reached within 24 hours, licensee shall notify individual as soon as possible thereafter
- Licensee may not delay any appropriate medical care for individual, including any necessary remedial care as result of medical event, because of any delay in notification
  - Notification of individual subject of medical event may be made instead to that individual's responsible relative or guardian
- If verbal notification is made, licensee shall inform individual, or appropriate responsible relative or guardian, that written description of event can be obtained from licensee upon request
  - Licensee shall provide such written description if requested
- Aside from notification requirement, nothing in this section affects any rights or duties of licensees and physicians in relation to each other, to individuals affected by medical event, or to that individual's responsible relatives or guardians
- Licensee shall
  - Annotate copy of report provided to NRC with
    - Name of individual subject of event; and
    - Social security number or other identification number, if one has been assigned, of individual subject of event; and

- Provide copy of annotated report to referring physician, if other than licensee, no later than 15 days after discovery of event

35.3047: Report and Notification of Dose to Embryo/Fetus or Nursing Child

- Licensee shall report any dose to embryo/fetus > 50 mSv (5 rem) dose equivalent as result of administration of byproduct material or radiation from byproduct material to pregnant individual unless dose to embryo/fetus was specifically approved, in advance, by authorized user
- Licensee shall report any dose to nursing child as result of administration of byproduct material to breastfeeding individual that
  - Is > 50 mSv (5 rem) total effective dose equivalent or has resulted in unintended permanent functional damage to organ or physiological system of child, as determined by physician
- Licensee shall notify by telephone NRC Operations Center no later than next calendar day after discovery of dose to embryo/fetus or nursing child
- Licensee shall submit written report to appropriate NRC Regional Office within 15 days after discovery of dose to embryo/fetus or nursing child
  - Written report must include
    - Licensee's name
    - Name of prescribing physician
    - Brief description of event
    - Why event occurred
    - Effect, if any, on embryo/fetus or nursing child
    - What actions, if any, have been taken or are planned to prevent recurrence
    - Certification that licensee notified pregnant individual or mother (or mother's or child's responsible relative or guardian), and if not, why not
  - Report must not contain individual's or child's name or any other information that could lead to identification of individual or child
- Licensee shall provide notification of event to referring physician and also notify pregnant individual or mother, both hereafter referred to as mother, no later than 24 hours after discovery of event, unless referring physician personally informs licensee either that he or she will inform mother or that, based on medical judgment, telling mother would be harmful
- Licensee is not required to notify mother without first consulting with referring physician
  - If referring physician or mother cannot be reached within 24 hours, licensee shall make appropriate notifications as soon as possible thereafter
- Licensee may not delay any appropriate medical care for embryo/fetus or for nursing child, including any necessary remedial care as result of event, because of any delay in notification
  - Notification may be made to the mother's or child's responsible relative or guardian instead of mother
- If verbal notification is made, licensee shall inform mother, or mother's or child's responsible relative or guardian, that written description of event can be obtained from licensee upon request
  - Licensee shall provide such written description if requested
- Licensee shall
  - Annotate copy of report provided to NRC with
    - Name of pregnant individual or nursing child subject of event
    - Social security number or other identification number, if one has been assigned, of pregnant individual or nursing child subject of event
  - Provide copy of annotated report to referring physician, if other than licensee, no later than 15 days after discovery of event

35.3067: Report of Leaking Source

- Licensee shall file report within 5 days if leak test reveals presence of 185 Bq (0.005 μCi) or more of removable contamination
- Report must be filed with appropriate NRC Regional Office with copy to Director, Office of Nuclear Material Safety and Safeguards
  - Report must include
    - Model number and serial number, if assigned, of leaking source
    - Radionuclide and its estimated activity
    - Results of test
    - Date of test
    - Action taken

35.4001 and 35.4002: Violations and Criminal Penalties

- Provisions allow licence to be revoked and civil and possibly criminal sanctions for willful violation of, attempted violation of, or conspiracy to violate any regulation

SELECTED REFERENCES

1. United States Nuclear Regulatory Commission. NRC Regulations (10 CFR) Part 35: Medical Use of Byproduct Material. http://www.nrc.gov/reading-rm/doc-collections/cfr/part035. Published June 31, 2015. Accessed June 31, 2015

KEY FACTS

NRC REGULATIONS (10 CFR) PART 20: STANDARDS FOR PROTECTION AGAINST RADIATION, SUBPART G

- Control of exposure from external sources in restricted areas
  - "CAUTION, RADIATION AREA" posted in all areas where it is possible for individual to receive dose > 5 mrem (0.05 mSv) in any 1 hour at 30 cm from radiation source
  - Licensee shall post each airborne radioactivity area with conspicuous sign or signs bearing radiation symbol and "CAUTION, AIRBORNE RADIOACTIVITY AREA" or "DANGER, AIRBORNE RADIOACTIVITY AREA"
  - Licensee shall post each area or room in which there is used or stored amount of licensed material with conspicuous sign or signs bearing radiation symbol and "CAUTION, RADIOACTIVE MATERIAL(S)" or "DANGER, RADIOACTIVE MATERIAL(S)"
  - Unrestricted area has dose rate of < 2 mrem (0.02 mSv) in any 1 hour and < 100 mrem (1 mSv) in 1 year
    - Reception area, waiting room, file room, bathrooms, and hallways
  - Restricted areas have dose rates exceeding those of unrestricted area limits and require control of access and not accessible to public
    - Byproduct material will be received, prepared, used, administered, and stored
  - Licensee shall use, to extent practical, process or other engineering controls (e.g., containment, decontamination, or ventilation) to control concentration of radioactive material in air

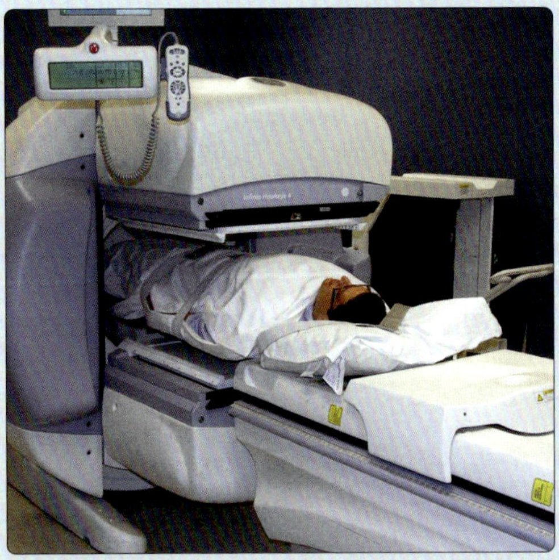

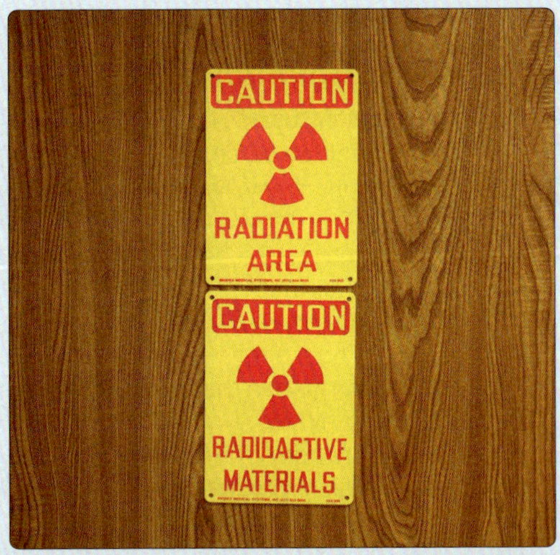

(Left) *The patient imaging area is a restricted area. A patient is shown being scanned on a SPECT/CT camera. Proper signage is required on the entrance door.* **(Right)** *Radiation area implies that an individual may receive a dose > 5 mrem (0.05 mSv) in any 1 hour at 30 cm from the radiation source. This is the door to a SPECT/CT room where radiopharmaceuticals are also administered so a radioactive materials sign was also placed.*

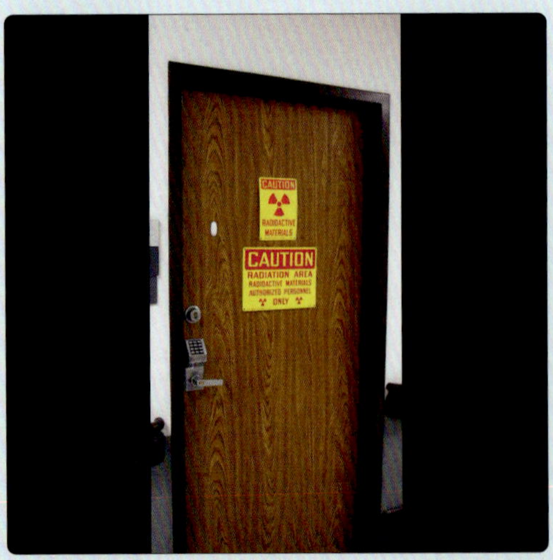

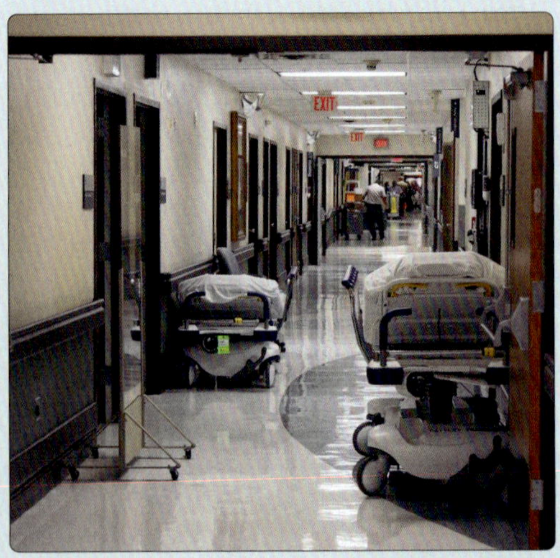

(Left) *The door to the nuclear medicine hot lab should have restricted access by lock and key, badge access, or keypad.* **(Right)** *Hallways of the nuclear medicine department are generally unrestricted areas. The dose rate must be < 2 mrem (0.02 mSv) in any 1 hour and <100 mrem (1 mSv) in 1 year.*

STANDARDS FOR PROTECTION AGAINST RADIATION, SUBPART G

20.1901: Caution Signs

- **Standard radiation symbol**: Unless otherwise authorized by Commission, the symbol prescribed by this part shall use magenta, purple, or black on yellow background in three-bladed design
  - Cross-hatched area is to be magenta, purple, or black, and background is to be yellow
- **Exception to color requirements for standard radiation symbol**: Licensees are authorized to label sources, source holders, or device components containing sources of licensed materials that are subjected to high temperatures, with conspicuously etched or stamped radiation caution symbols and without color requirement
- **Additional information on signs and labels**: In addition to contents of signs and labels, licensee may provide, on or near required signs and labels, additional information to make individuals aware of potential radiation exposures and to minimize exposures

20.1902: Posting Requirements

- **Posting of radiation areas**: Licensee shall post each radiation area with conspicuous sign or signs bearing radiation symbol and "CAUTION, RADIATION AREA"
  - Posted in all areas where possible for individual to receive dose > 5 mrem (0.05 mSv) in any 1 hour at 30 cm from radiation source
- **Posting of high radiation areas**: Licensee shall post each high radiation area with conspicuous sign or signs bearing radiation symbol and "CAUTION, HIGH RADIATION AREA" or "DANGER, HIGH RADIATION AREA"
  - Posted in all areas where individual might receive deep-dose equivalent of 0.1 rem (1 mSv) in 1 hour at 30 cm from radiation source
- **Posting of airborne radioactivity areas**: Licensee shall post each airborne radioactivity area with conspicuous sign or signs bearing radiation symbol and "CAUTION, AIRBORNE RADIOACTIVITY AREA" or "DANGER, AIRBORNE RADIOACTIVITY AREA"
- **Posting of areas or rooms in which licensed material is used or stored**: Licensee shall post each area or room in which there is used or stored amount of licensed material with conspicuous sign or signs bearing radiation symbol and "CAUTION, RADIOACTIVE MATERIAL(S)" or "DANGER, RADIOACTIVE MATERIAL(S)"

Unrestricted Areas

- Dose rate of < 2 mrem (0.02 mSv) in any 1 hour and < 100 mrem (1 mSv) in 1 year
  - Reception area, waiting room, file room, bathrooms, offices, and hallways

Restricted Areas

- If dose rate exceeds limits of unrestricted area, control of access must be put in place
  - Byproduct material will be received, prepared, used, administered, and stored, hot lab, patient imaging rooms, thyroid uptake room

20.1601: Control of Access to High Radiation Areas

- Licensee shall ensure that each entrance/access point to high radiation area has 1 or more of the following
  - Control device that, upon entry into area, causes level of radiation to be reduced below that level at which individual might receive deep-dose equivalent of 0.1 rem (1 mSv) in 1 hour at 30 cm from radiation source or from any surface that radiation penetrates
  - Control device that energizes conspicuous visible or audible alarm signal so that individual entering and supervisor of activity are made aware of entry; or
  - Entryways that are locked, except during periods when access to areas is required, with positive control over each individual entry
- In place of controls for high radiation area, licensee may substitute continuous direct or electronic surveillance capable of preventing unauthorized entry
- Licensee may apply to Commission for approval of alternative methods to control access
- Licensee shall establish controls in way that does not prevent individuals from leaving high radiation area
- Control is not required for each entrance or access point to room or other area that is high radiation area solely because of presence of radioactive materials prepared for transport and packaged and labeled in accordance with regulations of Department of Transportation provided that
  - Packages do not remain in area longer than 3 days; and
  - Dose rate at 1 m from external surface of any package does not exceed 0.01 rem (0.1 mSv) per hour
- Control of entrance or access to rooms or other areas in hospitals is not required solely because of presence of patients containing radioactive material, provided there are personnel in attendance who will take necessary precautions to prevent exposure of individuals to radiation or radioactive material in excess of limits established in this part and to operate within ALARA provisions of licensee's radiation protection program

STANDARDS FOR PROTECTION AGAINST RADIATION, SUBPART H

20.1701: Use of Process or Other Engineering Controls

- Licensee shall use, to extent practical, process or other engineering controls (e.g., containment, decontamination, or ventilation) to control concentration of radioactive material in air

20.1702: Use of Other Controls

- When not practical to apply process or other engineering controls to control concentrations of radioactive material in air to values below those that define airborne radioactivity area, licensee shall increase monitoring and limit intakes by one or more of the following means
  - Control of access, limitation of exposure times, use of respiratory equipment, or other controls

SELECTED REFERENCES

1. United States Nuclear Regulatory Commission. NRC Regulations (10 CFR) Part 20: Standards for Protection Against Radiation. http://www.nrc.gov/reading-rm/doc-collections/cfr/part020. Published June 31, 2015. Accessed June 31, 2015

Surveys and Monitoring

KEY FACTS

TERMINOLOGY

- Survey: Evaluation of radiological conditions and potential hazards
  - May be measurements (radiation levels measured with survey instruments or wipe tests), calculations, or a combination of measurements and calculations
  - Performed on facilities, equipment, personnel (during use, possession, transfer, or disposal of licensed material) restricted and unrestricted areas, sealed source leak testing, testing before waste disposal, testing after spills or other radiation incidents, checking incoming or outgoing packages, and products produced

CLINICAL IMPLICATIONS

- Xe-133 gas use requires trap and collecting system monthly checks
- Radiation safety officer or appropriate supervisory personnel must be notified if established radiation levels are exceeded in restricted or unrestricted areas
- Routine contamination surveys should initially be performed weekly in restricted areas, where workers may be exposed to radioactive contamination levels resulting in radiation doses > 10% of occupational dose limits
- Wipe tests analyzed by well counter
- No requirements describing level of removable contamination that trigger an action level for wipe surveys; value of 22,000 dpm/100 cm² is suggested as trigger level for wipe surveys
- Additional wipe surveys should be performed after spills or other radiation incidents
- Records from surveys describing location and amount of subsurface residual radioactivity identified at site must be kept for 3 years
- Licensee shall ensure that instruments and equipment used for quantitative radiation measurements (e.g., dose rate and effluent monitoring) are calibrated periodically for radiation measured

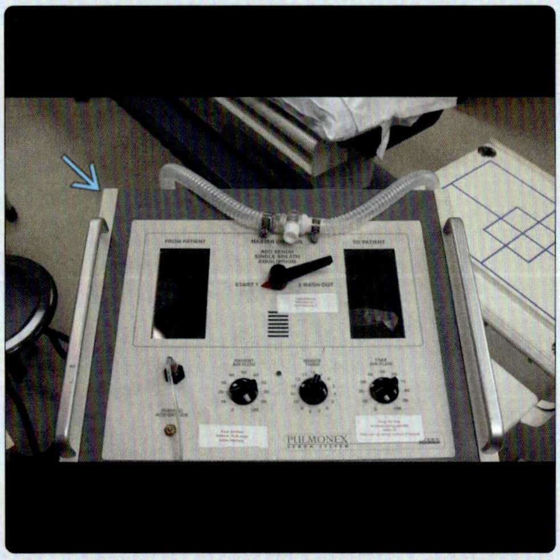

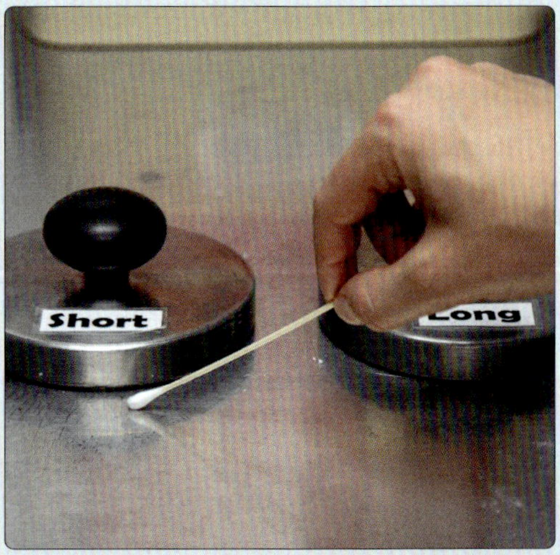

(Left) *Xe-133 gas use requires monthly checks of trap and collecting system* ➡. *In the case of a gas "spill," signage must be present that indicates evacuation time of the room. The door must be closed to minimize leakage to surrounding unrestricted areas.* **(Right)** *Routine contamination surveys should initially be performed weekly in restricted areas, where workers maybe exposed to radioactive contamination levels resulting in radiation doses > 10% of the occupational dose limits.*

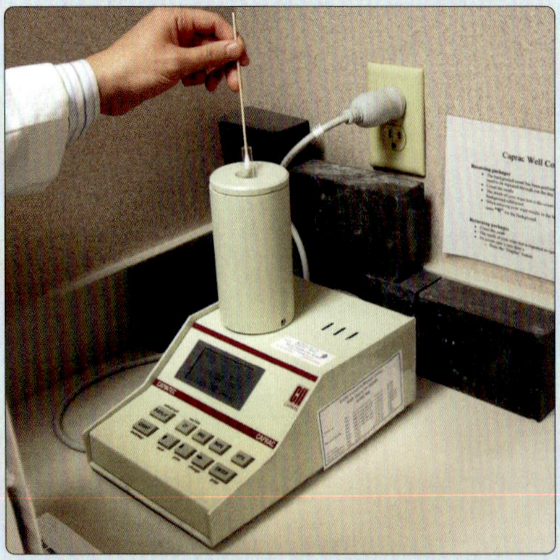

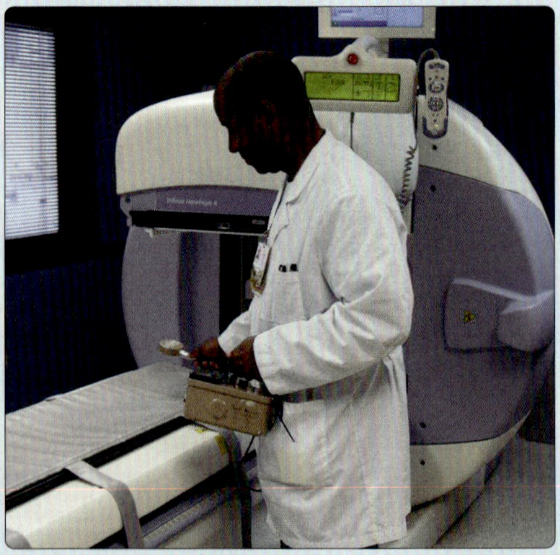

(Left) *A well counter should be used to analyze the wipe test. There are no requirements describing the level of removable contamination that may serve as an action level for wipe surveys. To be conservative, a value of 22,000 dpm/100 cm² is suggested as a trigger level for wipe surveys.* **(Right)** *A technologist is shown performing a routine weekly survey on equipment in a restricted area. If removable contamination is found, a spill-type procedure may be performed for decontamination.*

TERMINOLOGY

Definitions

- Survey: Evaluation of radiological conditions and potential hazards
  - May be measurements (radiation levels measured with survey instruments or wipe tests), calculations, or combination of measurements and calculations
  - Surveys performed for radioactive contamination present on surfaces of floors, walls, laboratory furniture, production line, packages, and equipment
  - Measurements of radioactive material concentrations in air for areas where radioactive materials are handled or processed in unsealed form, and areas that could expose workers or public to inhalation of radioactive material
  - Measurements of radioactive material concentrations in water that is released to environment or sanitary sewer
    - Radioactive excreta is not regulated by NRC and any amount can be introduced to sewer system
  - Bioassays to determine kinds, quantities, or concentration, and in some cases, location of radioactive material in human body; bioassay can be made by direct measurement (in vivo counting) or by analysis and evaluation of material excreted or removed from human body (in vitro counting)
  - Surveys of external radiation exposure levels in both restricted and unrestricted areas
- Surveys are performed on facilities, equipment, personnel, restricted and unrestricted areas, sealed source leak testing, testing before waste disposal, testing after spills or other radiation incidents, checking incoming/outgoing packages, and products produced
- Surveys should be performed on restricted areas, where workers may be exposed to radiation levels that might result in radiation doses > 10% of occupational dose limits, and unrestricted areas if radiation doses might exceed public dose limits

CLINICAL IMPLICATIONS

Surveys

- Institutions will typically survey areas including
  - Elution, preparation, assay, and administration of radiopharmaceuticals
  - Weekly surveys in all imaging areas and storage
  - End of day survey for radiopharmaceuticals requiring written directive
- Xe-133 gas use requires monthly checks of trap and collecting system
  - Ambient ventilation rates checked every 6 months
- Radiation surveys must be performed with sufficiently sensitive survey meter
- Radiation safety officer (RSO) or appropriate supervisory personnel must be notified if established radiation levels are exceeded in restricted or unrestricted areas
  - 5.0 mrem/hr (50 μSv) in restricted areas
  - 0.2 mrem/hr (2 μSv) in unrestricted areas
- Wipe tests
  - Routine surveys should initially be performed weekly in restricted areas, where workers may be exposed to radioactive contamination levels that might result in radiation doses > 10% of occupational dose limits
  - Unrestricted areas, where members of public may be exposed to radioactive contamination levels that might result in radiation doses that exceed public dose limits
  - Analyzed with appropriate detector system, such as sodium iodide well scintillation counter (shielded Geiger-Müller probe or uncollimated gamma camera also may be used for this purpose)
  - No requirements describing level of removable contamination that may serve as an action level for wipe surveys; to be conservative, a value of 22,000 dpm/100 cm² suggested as trigger level
  - Radiation safety officer (RSO) notified if limit exceeded
  - Additional wipe surveys should be performed after spills or other radiation incidents

NRC REGULATIONS (10 CFR): STANDARDS FOR PROTECTION AGAINST RADIATION, SUBPART F (SURVEYS AND MONITORING)

20.1501: General

- Each licensee shall survey areas, including subsurface, that are reasonable under circumstances to evaluate magnitude and extent of radiation levels, concentrations or quantities of residual radioactivity, and potential radiological hazards of radiation levels and residual radioactivity detected
- Records from surveys describing the location and amount of subsurface residual radioactivity must be kept for 3 years
- Licensee shall ensure that instruments and equipment used for quantitative radiation measurements are calibrated periodically for radiation measured
  - Records and serial number of instrument and person performing calibration kept for 3 years
- All personnel dosimeters (except for pocket ionization chambers and extremity dosimeters) that require processing to determine radiation dose must be processed and evaluated by dosimetry processor

20.1502: Conditions Requiring Individual Monitoring of External and Internal Occupational Dose

- Each licensee shall monitor occupational exposure from licensed and unlicensed radiation sources under control of licensee and shall supply and require use of individual monitoring devices & monitor effective dose equivalent of
  - Adults likely to receive, in 1 year, dose in excess of 10% of occupational dose limits
  - Minors likely to receive, in 1 year, from radiation sources external to body, deep dose equivalent in excess of 0.1 rem (1 mSv), lens dose equivalent in excess of 0.15 rem (1.5 mSv), or shallow dose equivalent to skin or extremities in excess of 0.5 rem (5 mSv)
  - Declared pregnant women likely to receive, during entire pregnancy, from radiation sources external to body, deep dose equivalent in excess of 0.1 rem (1 mSv); and
    - All occupational doses continue to be applicable to declared pregnant worker as long as embryo/fetus dose limit is not exceeded
  - Individuals entering high or very high radiation area

SELECTED REFERENCES

1. United States Nuclear Regulatory Commission. NRC Regulations (10 CFR) Part 20: Standards for Protection Against Radiation. http://www.nrc.gov/reading-rm/doc-collections/cfr/part020/ Published June 31, 2015. Accessed June 31, 2015

KEY FACTS

NRC REGULATIONS (10 CFR) PART 20, STANDARDS FOR PROTECTION AGAINST RADIATION, SUBPART K (WASTE DISPOSAL)

- Licensee shall dispose of licensed material
  - By transfer to authorized recipient such as waste disposal service company or original radiopharmacy for spent or unused doses or return of Mo-99/Tc-99m generators
  - By decay-in-storage locally in nuclear medicine department requiring restricted access and routine surveys
  - By release in effluents/sanitary sewerage
- Materials with t1/2 ≤ 120 days are appropriate for decay-in-storage
  - Containers should be shielded and restricted from public access
  - Seal container as needed and label with date sealed and longest t1/2 of radionuclide within
  - Once surface radiation reaches background levels, remove or deface any radioactive material labels
  - Discard as regular in-house waste, recycling, or infectious waste, as appropriate, only those containers that cannot be distinguished from background
  - Licensee shall maintain records of disposal of licensed materials for 3 years
    - Record must include
      - Date of disposal
      - Survey instrument used
      - Background radiation level
      - Radiation level measured at surface of each waste container
      - Name of individual who performed survey
- Excreta from individuals undergoing medical diagnosis or therapy with radioactive material are not subject to limitations

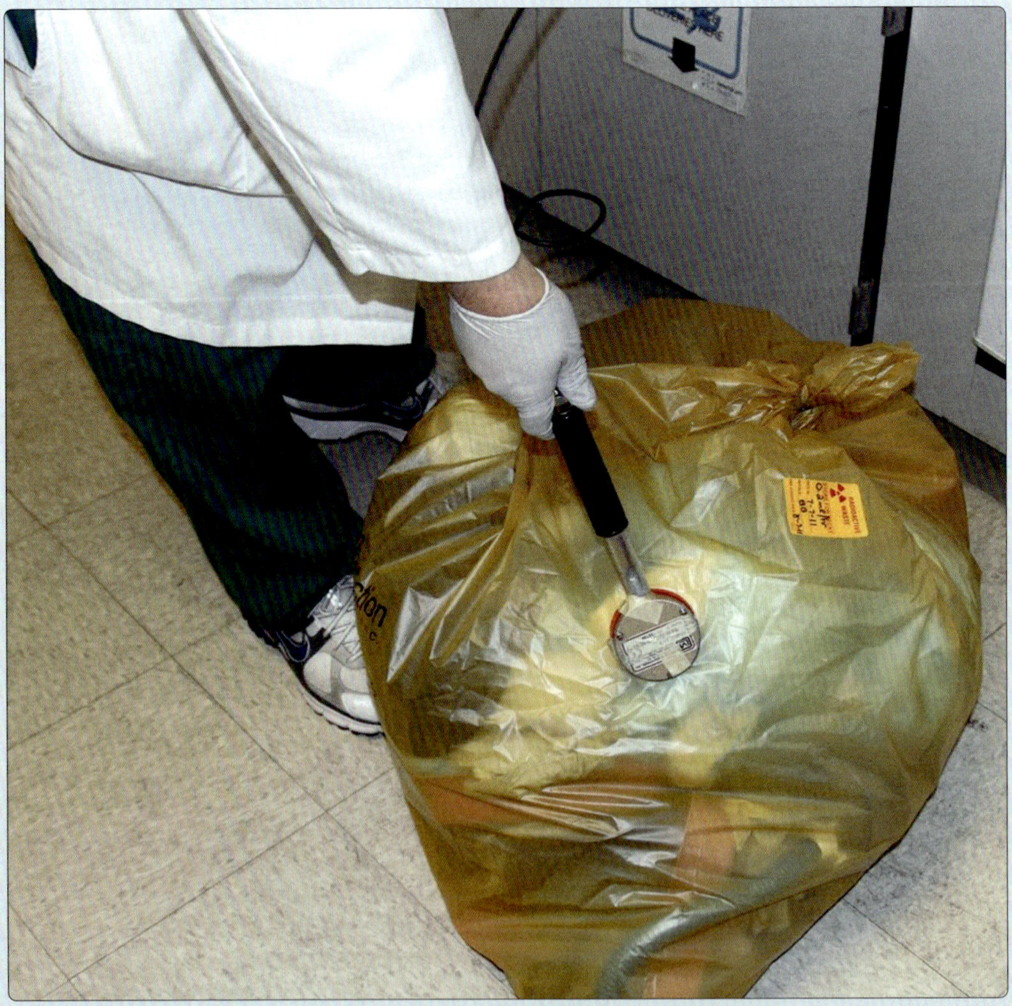

Technologist uses a Geiger-Müller detector to survey decay-in-storage material. Once the activity equals background levels, the radioactive labels are destroyed and the trash can be placed with regular trash.

NRC REGULATIONS (10 CFR) PART 20, STANDARDS FOR PROTECTION AGAINST RADIATION, SUBPART K (WASTE DISPOSAL)

20.2001: General Requirements

- Licensee shall dispose of licensed material only
  - By transfer to authorized recipient
    - Including waste disposal service company, **or**
    - Original radiopharmacy for spent or unused doses or return of Mo-99/Tc-99m generators
  - By decay-in-storage
    - Locally in nuclear medicine department requiring restricted access and routine surveys
  - By release in effluents/sanitary sewerage
- Person must be specifically licensed to receive waste containing licensed material from other persons for
  - Treatment prior to disposal
  - Treatment or disposal by incineration
  - Decay-in-storage
  - Disposal at land disposal facility
  - Disposal at geologic repository

20.2002: Method for Obtaining Approval of Proposed Disposal Procedures

- Licensee or applicant for license may apply to Commission for approval of proposed procedures to dispose of licensed material generated in licensee's activities
  - Each application shall include
    - Description of waste-containing licensed material to be disposed of, including
      - Physical and chemical properties important to risk evaluation
      - Proposed manner and conditions of waste disposal
    - Analysis and evaluation of pertinent information on nature of environment
    - Nature and location of other potentially affected licensed and unlicensed facilities
    - Analyses and procedures to ensure that doses are maintained as low as reasonably achievable (ALARA) and within dose limits in this part

Decay-in-Storage

- Materials with t1/2 ≤ 120 days are appropriate for decay-in-storage
- Storage could be designed to allow for differentiation of wastes with varying t1/2
- Containers should be shielded and restricted from public access
- Use separate containers, if possible, for different types of waste
  - e.g., needles vs. absorbent material vs. spent doses
- Seal container as needed and label with
  - Date sealed
  - Longest t1/2 of radionuclide within
- Recording surface radioactivity at time of storage may be performed
- Before disposal as regular waste, monitor and record results of monitoring for each container as follows
  - Remove any shielding from around container
  - Monitor (in low-level radiation area, if possible) all surfaces of each container
  - Remove or deface any radioactive material labels
    - Sharps boxes are not to be opened to check for &/or to remove any labels that may be affixed to syringes, vials, etc., already contained in box
    - Box should remain closed, and all radiation labels on box must be removed or defaced before disposal
  - Discard as regular in-house waste, recycling, or infectious waste as appropriate
    - Only those containers that cannot be distinguished from background
  - Return containers that can be distinguished from background radiation levels to storage area for further decay
- Licensee shall maintain records of the disposal of licensed materials for 3 years
  - Record must include
    - Date of disposal
    - Survey instrument used
    - Background radiation level
    - Radiation level measured at surface of each waste container, **and**
    - Name of individual who performed survey

20.2003: Disposal by Release Into Sanitary Sewerage

- Licensee may discharge licensed material into sanitary sewerage if each of the following conditions are satisfied
  - Material is readily soluble (or is readily dispersible biological material) in water
  - Quantity of licensed or other radioactive material that licensee releases into sewer in 1 month, divided by average monthly volume of water released into sewer by licensee, does not exceed concentration listed in NRC (10 CFR) table 3 of appendix B to part 20
  - If more than 1 radionuclide is released, the following conditions must also be satisfied
    - Licensee shall determine fraction of limit in NRC (10 CFR) table 3 of appendix B to Part 20 represented by discharges into sanitary sewerage by dividing actual monthly average concentration of each radionuclide released by licensee into sewer by concentration of that radionuclide listed in NRC (10 CFR) table 3 of appendix B to part 20
    - Sum of fractions for each radionuclide does not exceed unity
  - Total quantity of licensed and other radioactive material that licensee releases into sanitary sewerage system in 1 year does not exceed
    - 5 curies (185 GBq) of H-3
    - 1 curie (37 GBq) of C-14, **and**
    - 1 curie (37 GBq) of all other radioactive materials combined
- Excreta from individuals undergoing medical diagnosis or therapy with radioactive material is not subject to limitations

20.2004: Treatment or Disposal by Incineration

- Licensee may treat or dispose of licensed material by incineration
  - Only if they are authorized and specifically approved by Commission

20.2005: Disposal of Specific Wastes

- Licensee may dispose of the following licensed material as if it were not radioactive
  - 0.05 μCi (1.85 kBq) or less of H-3 or C-14 per gram of medium used for liquid scintillation counting
  - 0.05 μCi (1.85 kBq) or less of H-3 or C-14 per gram of animal tissue, averaged over weight of entire animal
    - Licensee may not dispose of tissue in manner that would permit its use either as food for humans or as animal feed
- Licensee shall maintain records

20.2006: Transfer for Disposal and Manifests

- Requirements of this section and appendix G to 10 CFR Part 20 are designed to
  - Control transfers of low-level radioactive waste by any waste generator, waste collector, or waste processor licensee, as defined in this part, that ships low-level waste
    - Either directly, or indirectly (through waste collector or waste processor), to licensed low-level waste land disposal facility
  - Establish manifest tracking system, **and**
  - Supplement existing requirements concerning transfers and recordkeeping for those wastes
- Any licensee shipping radioactive waste intended for ultimate disposal at licensed land disposal facility must
  - Document information required on NRC's uniform low-level radioactive waste manifest, and
  - Transfer this recorded manifest information to intended consignee
- Each shipment manifest must include certification by waste generator
- Each person involved in transfer for disposal and disposal of waste shall comply with requirements, including
  - Waste generator
  - Waste collector
  - Waste processor, **and**
  - Disposal facility operator
- Any licensee shipping byproduct material of definition of byproduct material intended for ultimate disposal at land disposal facility licensed must
  - Document information required on NRC's uniform low-level radioactive waste manifest, **and**
  - Transfer this recorded manifest information to intended consignee

20.2007: Compliance With Environmental and Health Protection Regulations

- Nothing in this subpart relieves licensee from complying with other applicable federal, state, and local regulations governing any other toxic or hazardous properties of materials that may be disposed of under this subpart

20.2008: Disposal of Certain Byproduct Material

- Licensed material as defined in definition of byproduct material may be disposed of, even though it is not defined as low-level radioactive waste
  - Therefore, any licensed byproduct material being disposed of at facility, or transferred for ultimate disposal at licensed facility, must meet requirements
- Licensee may dispose of byproduct material, as defined in definition of byproduct material, at disposal facility authorized to dispose of such material
  - In accordance with any federal or state solid or hazardous waste law
  - Including Solid Waste Disposal Act, as authorized under Energy Policy Act of 2005

SELECTED REFERENCES

1. United States Nuclear Regulatory Commission. NRC Regulations (10 CFR) Part 20: Standards for Protection Against Radiation. http://www.nrc.gov/reading-rm/doc-collections/cfr/part020. Published June 31, 2015. Accessed June 31, 2015

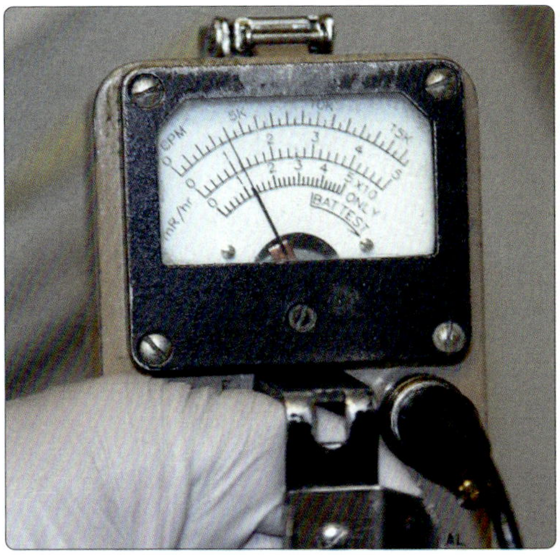
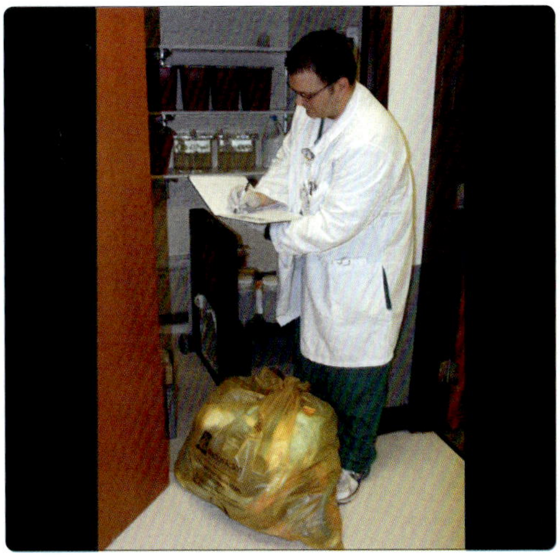

(Left) *A Geiger-Müller detector reads 1.2 mR/hr during a survey of decay-in-storage material. Background activity in this department is less than 1.2 mR/hr; therefore, continued storage is required.* **(Right)** *Records of all decay-in-storage must be made and kept for 3 years.*

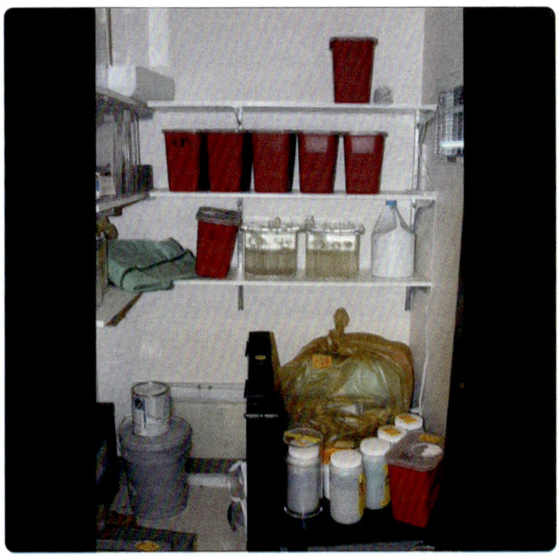
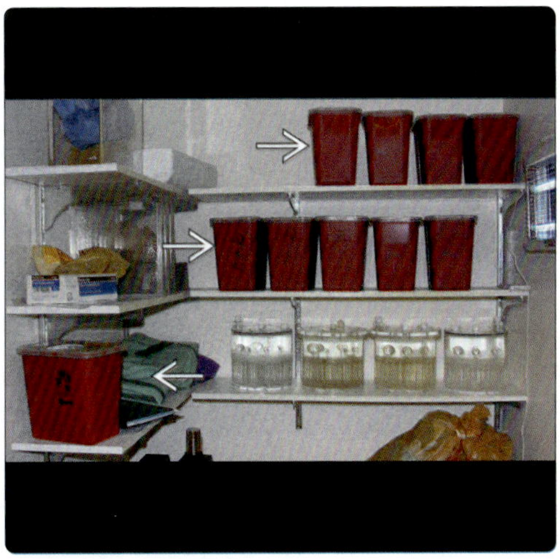

(Left) *Decay-in-storage closet is shown with sharps containers holding radioactive syringes/needles, radioactive trash, and supplies.* **(Right)** *Sharps containers ➡ should be kept in decay-in-storage separate from bags of other nonsharp material.*

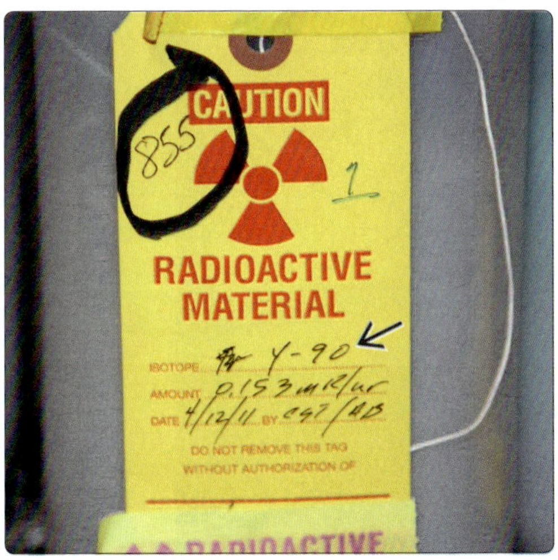

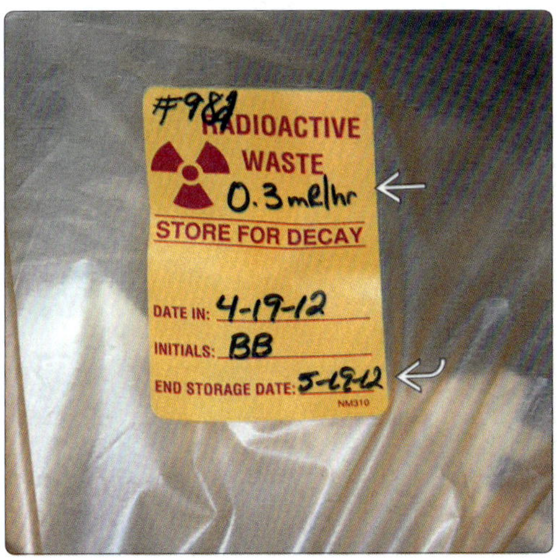

(Left) *Decay-in-storage for Y-90 ➡ is shown. With a t1/2 of 64 hours, the material should be kept until background levels are reached. Approximately 10 half-lives are typically needed.* **(Right)** *Radioactive trash with varying half-lives has a surface reading recorded ➡ and estimated end storage date ➡. In this case, 30 days should elapse between the date in and end storage date. Given the estimated 10 half-lives needed to decay to background, the longest t1/2 trash must be 3 days from either Ga-67, In-111, or Tl-201.*

KEY FACTS

NRC REGULATIONS (10 CFR): STANDARDS FOR PROTECTION AGAINST RADIATION, SUBPART J (PRECAUTIONARY PROCEDURES)

- Type A packages must demonstrate ability to withstand a series of tests without releasing contents; regulations require that package protects its contents and maintains sufficient shielding under conditions normally encountered during transportation
- White I: Almost no radiation; maximum allowable radioactivity is 0.5 mrem/hr (0.005 mSv/hr) on package surface
- Yellow II: Low radiation levels; maximum allowable radioactivity is 50 mrem/hr (0.5 mSv/hr) on package surface and 1 mrem/hr (0.010 mSv/hr) at 1 m from package
- Yellow III: Higher levels of radiation; maximum allowable radioactivity is 200 mrem/hr (2 mSv/hr) on package surface, and 10 mrem/hr (0.1 mSv/hr) at 1 m from package
- Number in transport index box indicates maximum radiation level measured (in mrem/hr) at 1 m from surface of package
- Must be done within 3 hours of receipt during normal working hours and no later than 3 hours from beginning of next working day if package was received after working hours
- If wipe sample indicates that removable radioactive contamination exceeds applicable limit (i.e., 6,600 dpm for wipe, based on wiped surface area of 300 cm^2 with removable contamination limit of 22 dpm/cm^2), notify appropriate individual and determine if package has contaminated any areas in facility
- Make a record for each package and retain for at least 3 years

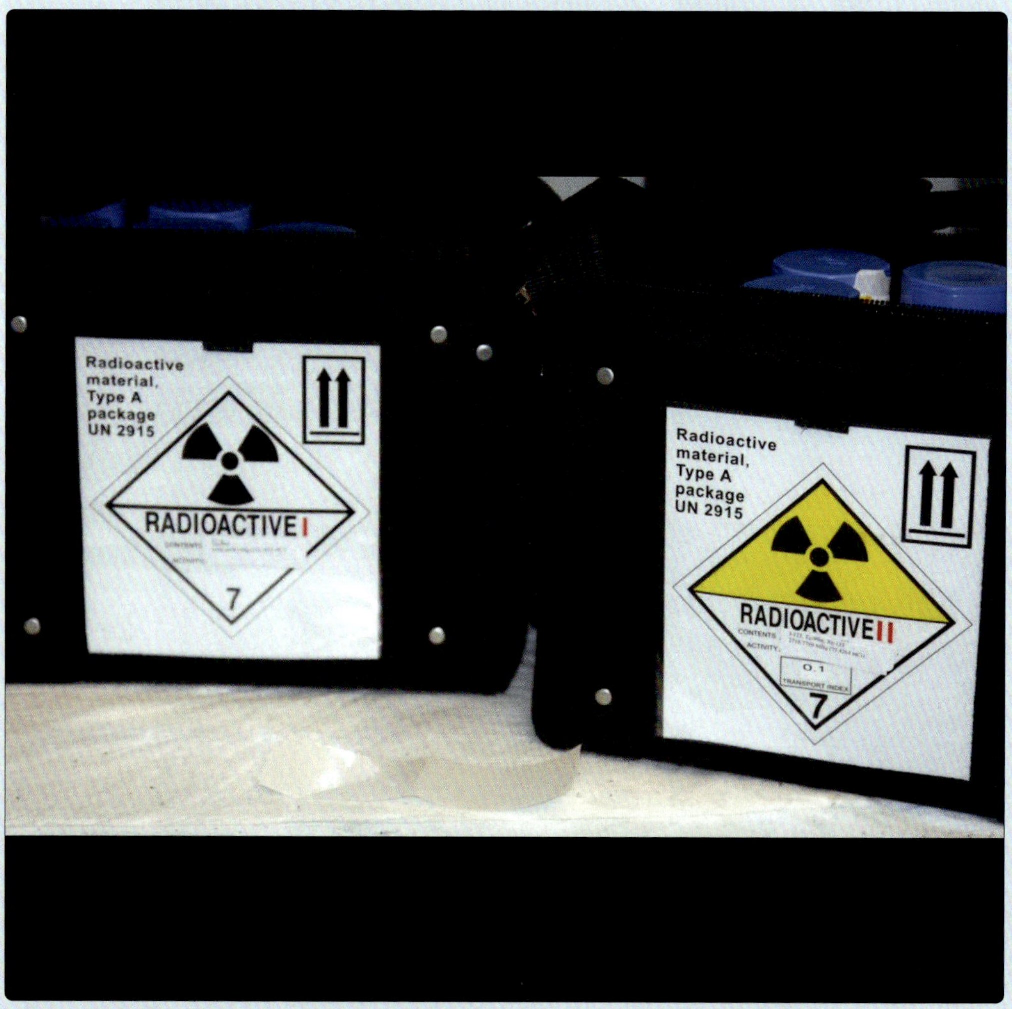

White I and yellow II packaging shown. The yellow II has a transportation index, which is the radiation exposure at 1 m. The shipping and receiving of packages is regulated by the Department of Transportation.

NRC REGULATIONS (10 CFR): STANDARDS FOR PROTECTION AGAINST RADIATION, SUBPART J (PRECAUTIONARY PROCEDURES)

20.1903: Exceptions to Posting Requirements

- Licensee is not required to post caution signs in areas or rooms containing radioactive materials for periods of < 8 hours, if each of the following conditions is met
  - Materials are constantly attended during these periods by an individual who takes precautions necessary to prevent exposure of individuals to radiation or radioactive materials in excess of limits established in this part and
  - Area or room is subject to licensee's control
- Rooms or other areas in hospitals that are occupied by patients are not required to be posted with caution signs provided that the patient could be released from licensee control

20.1904: Labeling Containers

- Licensee shall ensure that each container of licensed material bears a durable, clearly visible label bearing radiation symbol and "CAUTION, RADIOACTIVE MATERIAL" or "DANGER, RADIOACTIVE MATERIAL"
- Label must also provide sufficient information such as radionuclide present, estimate of quantity of radioactivity, date for which activity is estimated, radiation levels, kinds of materials, and mass enrichment to permit individuals handling or using containers, or working in vicinity of containers, to take precautions to avoid or minimize exposures
- Each licensee shall, prior to removal or disposal of empty uncontaminated containers to unrestricted areas, remove or deface radioactive material label or otherwise clearly indicate that container no longer contains radioactive materials

20.1905: Exemptions to Labeling Requirements

- Containers holding licensed material in limited quantities less than listed in Appendices B and C of NRC Regulations 10 CFR Part 20
- Containers attended by individual who takes precautions necessary to prevent exposure of individuals in excess of limits
- Containers in transport and packaged and labeled in accordance with regulations of Department of Transportation (DOT)
- Containers accessible only to individuals authorized to handle or use them, or to work in vicinity of, if contents are identified to these individuals by readily available written record (examples include containers in locations such as water-filled canals, storage vaults, or hot cells)
  - Record must be retained as long as containers are in use for purpose indicated on record
- Labeling of packages containing radioactive materials is required by DOT if amount and type of radioactive material exceeds limits for excepted quantity or article as defined and limited by DOT regulations

20.1906: Procedures for Receiving and Opening Packages

- Each licensee who expects to receive a package containing quantities of radioactive material in excess of type A quantity shall make arrangements to receive
  - Package when carrier offers it for delivery; or
  - Notification of arrival of package at carrier's terminal, taking possession of package expeditiously
- Each licensee shall
  - Monitor external surfaces of package with radioactive white I, yellow II, or yellow III label (as specified in DOT regulations for radioactive contamination, unless package contains only radioactive material in form of gas or in special form)
  - Monitor external surfaces of labeled package for radiation levels unless package contains quantities of radioactive material ≤ type A quantity
  - Monitor all packages known to contain radioactive material for radioactive contamination and radiation levels if evidence of degradation of package integrity, such as packages that are crushed, wet, or damaged
- Licensee shall perform monitoring as soon as practical after receipt of package, but not later than 3 hours after package is received at licensee's facility if it is received during licensee's normal working hours, or not later than 3 hours from beginning of next working day if it is received after working hours
- Licensee shall immediately notify final delivery carrier and NRC Operations Center, by telephone, when
  - Removable radioactive surface contamination exceeds limits or
  - External radiation levels exceed limits
- Each licensee shall
  - Establish, maintain, and retain written procedures for safely opening packages in which radioactive material is received
  - Ensure that procedures are followed and that due consideration is given to special instructions for type of package being opened

Transportation of Radioactive Materials

- Packaging
  - Type A packages must demonstrate ability to withstand a series of tests without releasing contents; regulations require that package protects its contents and maintains sufficient shielding under conditions normally encountered during transportation
  - Type B packages are used for radioactive materials that exceed limits of type A package requirements
    - Shippers use this type of package to transport materials that would present radiation hazard to public or environment
    - For this reason, type B package design must not only demonstrate its ability to withstand tests simulating normal shipping conditions, but it must also withstand severe accident conditions without releasing contents
- Labeling
  - White I: Almost no radiation; maximum allowable radioactivity is 0.5 mrem/hr (0.005 mSv/hr) on package surface

Radiation Level Limits by Package Label

Label Type	Package Surface Limit	Transportation Index
White I	0.5 mrem/hr	0 mrem/hr
Yellow II	50 mrem/hr	1 mrem/hr
Yellow III	200 mrem/hr	10 mrem/hr

Department of Transportation Limits. SI conversion: 1 mrem = 0.01 mSv.

- Yellow II: Low radiation levels; maximum allowable radioactivity is 50 mrem/hr (0.5 mSv/hr) on package surface and 1 mrem/hr (0.010 mSv/hr) at 1 m from package
- Yellow III: Higher levels of radiation; maximum allowable radioactivity is 200 mrem/hr (2 mSv/hr) on package surface and 10 mrem/hr (0.1 mSv/hr) at 1 m from package
- Package label is used when package is being shipped back with spent doses; radiation level at any point on external surface of package does not exceed 0.5 mrem/hr (0.005 mSv/hr)

- Transportation index (TI)
  - Yellow II and Yellow III labels have additional items called transport index box
    - Number in transport index box indicates maximum radiation level measured (in mrem/hr) at 1 m from surface of package
    - Transport index of 0.1 on radioactive III label indicates that radiation measured 1 m from surface of package should be < 0.1 mrem/hr
    - With exception of exclusive use shipments, maximum transport index for any shipment is 10 mrem/hr
  - Regulations limit exposure by restricting total of all transport indexes on any one vehicle, usually to < 50
  - If total shipment exceeds 200 mrem/hr, vehicle must be designated exclusively for purpose of transporting that shipment
  - Above transport index is contents line, which identifies material inside package
  - Reusable shipping containers that are empty, but possibly contaminated inside, are labeled "empty"

Model Procedure for Safely Opening Packages Containing Radioactive Material

- Cover all areas in hot lab at which packages will be received and opened, using disposable materials having plastic on one side and absorbent material on other
- Wear gloves to prevent hand contamination
- Check user ordering request to ensure that material received is material ordered, and inspect packages visually for any signs of damage
  - Must be done within 3 hours of receipt during normal working hours and no later than 3 hours from beginning of next working day if package was received after working hours
- If damage is noted, stop and measure external radiation levels at 1 m to determine whether radiation limit for package is exceeded (e.g., for white I-labeled package, limit is 0 mrem/hr)
  - If so, notify radiation safety officer or appropriate supervisory personnel
- If no damage, measure external radiation level at surface and again determine if it is above limit for package (e.g., for white I-labeled package, limit is 0.5 mrem/h [5 μSv/hr])
  - If so, notify appropriate individual
- Licensee will immediately notify final delivery carrier and NRC Operations Center if external radiation levels exceed 200 mrem/hr (2 mSv/hr) at any point on surface or 10 mrem/h (0.1 mSv/h) at 1 m
- Monitor external surfaces of package for radioactive contamination by performing wipe test
  - If wipe sample indicates that removable radioactive contamination exceeds applicable limit (i.e., 6,600 dpm for wipe, based on wiped surface area of 300 cm^2 with removable contamination limit of 22 dpm/cm^2), notify appropriate individual and determine if package has contaminated any areas in facility
  - Licensee will immediately notify final delivery carrier and NRC Operations Center
- If wipe test does not indicate contamination, remove packing slip
- Open outer package, following any instructions that may be provided by supplier
- Open inner package and verify that contents agree with packing slip
- Check integrity of final source container; if any reason to suspect contamination, wipe external surface to determine if any removable radioactivity
- Monitor packing material and empty package with radiation detection survey meter before discarding
  - If this material is contaminated, treat it as radioactive waste
  - If not, remove or obliterate radiation labels before discarding in normal trash or recycling
- Make a record for each package and retain for at least 3 years
  - Recording radionuclide, product name, chemical form/physical form, and lot number
  - Time, date, and activity at time of calibration
  - Time, date, and activity at time of receipt
  - Shipper's package identifying number, results of survey and wipe tests, and initials of person receiving package

SELECTED REFERENCES

1. United States Nuclear Regulatory Commission. NRC Regulations (10 CFR) Part 20: Standards for Protection Against Radiation. http://www.nrc.gov/reading-rm/doc-collections/cfr/part020/ Published June 31, 2015. Accessed June 31, 2015

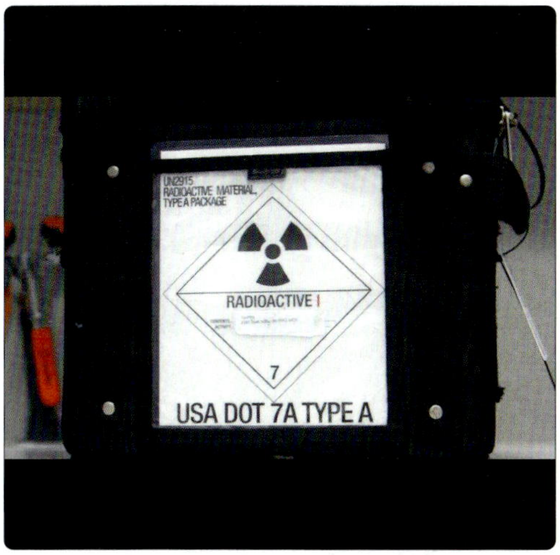

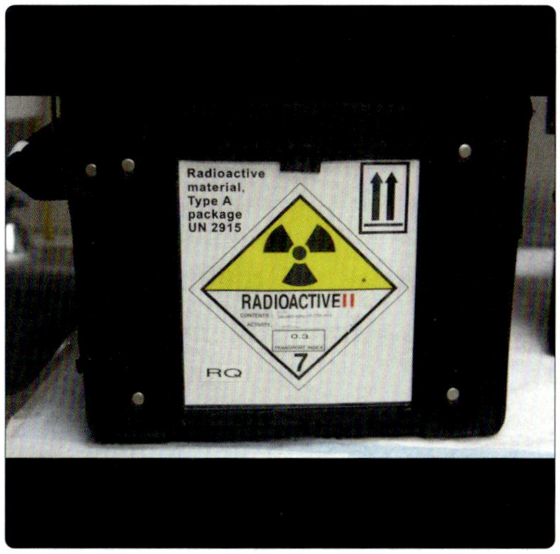

(Left) *A radioactive white I package is shown. The packages are inspected visually for any physical damage within 3 hours of receipt or no later than 3 hours from the beginning of the next working day if received after working hours.* **(Right)** *A radioactive yellow II package is shown. The maximum allowable radioactivity is 50 mrem/hr (0.5 mSv/hr) on the package surface, and 1 mrem/hr (0.010 mSv/hr) at 1 m from the package, which is the transportation index.*

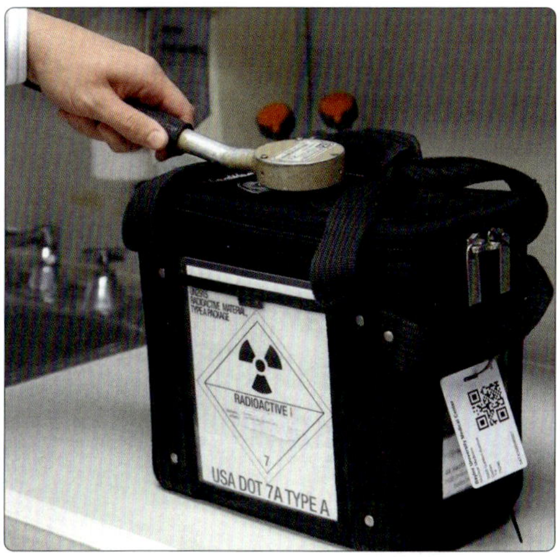

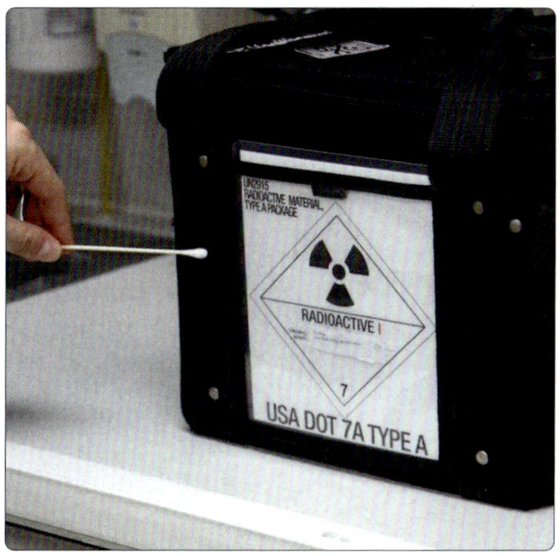

(Left) *A radioactive white I package is shown. These packages do not have a transportation index and should be surveyed at the surface, as shown.* **(Right)** *A wipe test is being performed on a radioactive white I package. If a wipe sample indicates that removable radioactive contamination exceeds the limit of 22 dpm/cm², the licensee will immediately notify the final delivery carrier and the NRC Operations Center.*

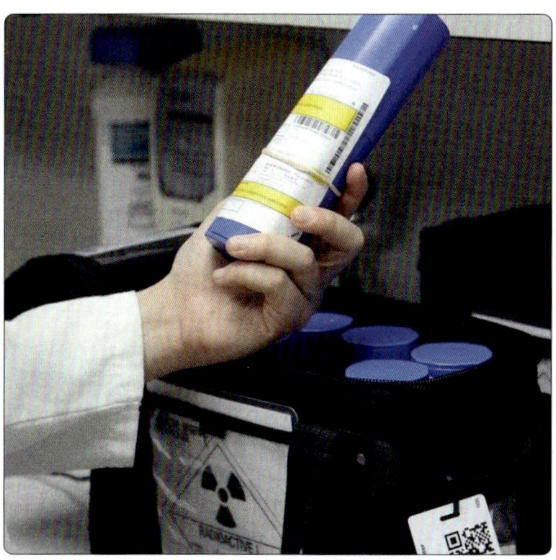

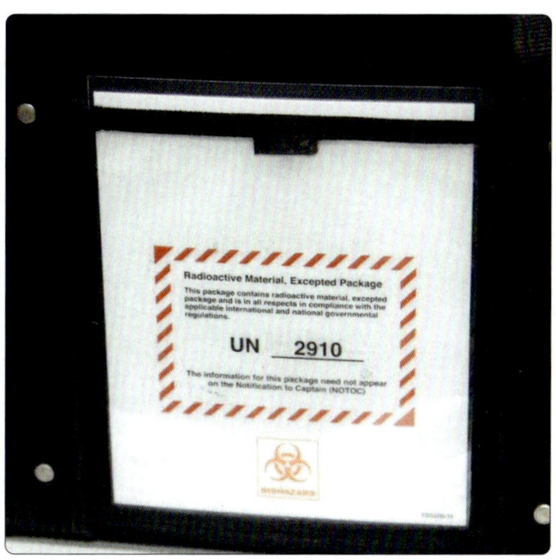

(Left) *The contents of a radioactive package should be checked to ensure the shipment received matches the packing slip.* **(Right)** *Radioactive labels can be turned around to the excepted package label once the contents are used and spent doses are ready to be shipped back to the nuclear pharmacy. The radiation level on the external surface of the package does not exceed 0.005 mSv/hr (0.5 mrem/hr).*

INDEX

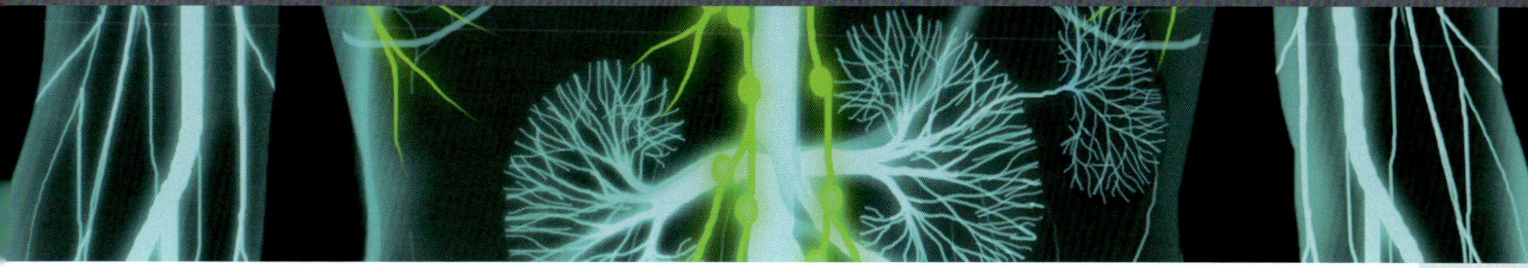

A

B

INDEX

INDEX

D

E

F

INDEX

INDEX

I

INDEX

J

K

L

INDEX

M

N

O

P

INDEX

Q

R

INDEX

S

T

INDEX

U

V

W

X

Y

Z